PEDIATRIC
PHYSICAL THERAPY

FIFTH EDITION

PEDIATRIC PHYSICAL THERAPY

FIFTH EDITION

Jan Stephen Tecklin, PT, MS

Professor
Department of Physical Therapy
Arcadia University
Glenside, Pennsylvania

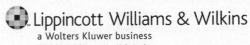
. Lippincott Williams & Wilkins
a Wolters Kluwer business
Philadelphia · Baltimore · New York · London
Buenos Aires · Hong Kong · Sydney · Tokyo

Sr. Acquisitions Editor: Emily Lupash
Product Development Editor: John Larkin
Production Project Manager: Marian A. Bellus
Marketing Manager: Leah Thomson
Manufacturing Manager: Margie Orzech
Designer: Stephen Druding
Compositor: S4Carlisle Publishing Services

Fifth Edition

351 West Camden Street
Baltimore, MD 21201

Two Commerce Square
2001 Market Street
Philadelphia, PA 19103

Printed in China

NOTICE TO READER: This publication contains information relating to general principles of medical care that should not be construed as specific instructions for individual patients. Manufacturers' product information and package inserts should be reviewed for current information, including contraindications, dosages, and precautions. It remains the responsibility of the practitioner to evaluate the appropriateness of a particular opinion or therapy in the context of the actual clinical situation and with due consideration of any new developments in the field and current drug information.

9 8 7 6 5 4 3 2

Library of Congress Cataloging-in-Publication Data

Pediatric physical therapy / [edited by] Jan S. Tecklin. — Fifth edition.
    p. ; cm.
Includes bibliographical references and index.
ISBN 978-1-4511-7345-1 (hardback)
I. Tecklin, Jan Stephen, editor of compilation.
[DNLM: 1. Physical Therapy Modalities.   2. Child.   3. Infant.   WB 460]
RJ53.P5
615.8'20832—dc23

                                                               2013041121

DISCLAIMER

Care has been taken to confirm the accuracy of the information present and to describe generally accepted practices. However, the authors, editors, and publisher are not responsible for errors or omissions or for any consequences from application of the information in this book and make no warranty, expressed or implied, with respect to the currency, completeness, or accuracy of the contents of the publication. Application of this information in a particular situation remains the professional responsibility of the practitioner; the clinical treatments described and recommended may not be considered absolute and universal recommendations.

The authors, editors, and publisher have exerted every effort to ensure that drug selection and dosage set forth in this text are in accordance with the current recommendations and practice at the time of publication. However, in view of ongoing research, changes in government regulations, and the constant flow of information relating to drug therapy and drug reactions, the reader is urged to check the package insert for each drug for any change in indications and dosage and for added warnings and precautions. This is particularly important when the recommended agent is a new or infrequently employed drug.

Some drugs and medical devices presented in this publication have Food and Drug Administration (FDA) clearance for limited use in restricted research settings. It is the responsibility of the health care provider to ascertain the FDA status of each drug or device planned for use in their clinical practice.

To purchase additional copies of this book, call our customer service department at **(800) 638-3030** or fax orders to **(301) 223-2320**. International customers should call **(301) 223-2300**.

Visit Lippincott Williams & Wilkins on the Internet: http://www.lww.com. Lippincott Williams & Wilkins customer service representatives are available from 8:30 am to 6:00 pm, EST.

With deep love, affection, respect and thanks to my
wife who has loved and supported me through almost fifty years of our lives
I love you Randee Lynn
and
in memory of my dear friend
Stephen Schecter

Heather Atkinson, PT, DPT, NCS
Clinical Specialist
Physical Therapy Department
Children's Hospital of Philadelphia
Philadelphia, Pennsylvania

Emilie J. Aubert, PT, DPT, MA
Associate Professor
Department of Physical Therapy
Marquette University
Milwaukee, Wisconsin

Jason Beaman, MPT, PCS
Staff Physical Therapist
Therapeutic and Rehabilitative Services
Nemours/duPont Hospital for Children
Wilmington, Delaware

Dolores B. Bertoti, PT, MS, PCS
Dean of Center for Academic Advancement
Associate Professor
Alvernia College
Reading, Pennsylvania

Anjana Bhat, PT, PhD
Assistant Professor in Kinesiology
Physical Therapy Program
University of Connecticut
Storrs, Connecticut

Amy Both, PT, MHS, ACCE
Assistant Professor and ACCE
Department of Physical Therapy
Health Science Campus
University of Toledo
Toledo, Ohio

Deborah Bubela, PT, PhD
Assistant Professor in Residence in Kinesiology
Physical Therapy Program
University of Connecticut
Storrs, Connecticut

Kathy Coultes, MSPT, PCS
Pediatric Clinical Specialist in Physical Therapy
Coordinator of Mercy Kids 4 Fitness Program
Mercy Fitzgerald Hospital
Darby, Pennsylvania

Michael Dilenno, PT, DPT, CSCS
Site Manager
The Children's Hospital of Philadelphia
Care Network, Primary Care
Nicholas and Athena Karabots Pediatric Care Center
Philadelphia, Pennsylvania

Jean M. Flickinger, MPT, PCS
Clinical Specialist
Physical Therapy Department
Children's Hospital of Philadelphia
Philadelphia, Pennsylvania

Rita F. Geddes, PT, MEd, DPT
Bucks County Intermediate Unit #22
Doylestown, Pennsylvania

Alan M. Glanzman, PT, DPT, PCS, ATP
Clinical Specialist
Physical Therapy Department
The Children's Hospital of Philadelphia
Philadelphia, Pennsylvania

Elliot M. Greenberg, PT, DPT, OCS, CSCS
Board Certified Specialist in Orthopaedic
    Physical Therapy
Sports Medicine & Performance Center
The Children's Hospital of Philadelphia
    Care Network
Pediatric & Adolescent Specialty Care, King
    of Prussia East
Philadelphia, Pennsylvania

Eric T. Greenberg, PT, DPT, SCS, CSCS
Board Certified Specialist in Sports Physical Therapy
Clinical Assistant Professor
Doctorate of Physical Therapy Program
Stony Brook University
Stony Brook, New York

Heather Hanson, PT, DPT, PCS
Physical Therapist III
The Children's Hospital of Philadelphia
Philadelphia, PA
Current position:
Physical Therapist
Step by Step Developmental Services
Rochester, New York

Faithe R. Kalisperis, MPT, DPT, C/NDT
Staff Therapist
Therapeutic and Rehabilitative Services
Nemours/duPont Hospital for Children
Wilmington, Delaware

Susan E. Klepper, PhD, PT
Assistant Professor of Clinical Rehabilitation &
  Regeneration Medicine
Columbia University, College of Physicians
  and Surgeons (CUMC)
Program in Physical Therapy
New York, New York

Rebecca Landa, CCC-SLP, PhD
Professor in Psychiatry
Johns Hopkins School of Medicine
Director, Hugo Moser Center for Autism and Related Disorders
Kennedy Krieger Institute
Baltimore, Maryland

Karen Yundt Lunnen, PT, EdD
Associate Professor and Head
Department of Physical Therapy
Western Carolina University
Cullowhee, North Carolina

Kirsten Hawkins Malerba, PT, DPT, PCS
Board Certified Specialist in Pediatric Physical Therapy
Department of Rehabilitation Services
Children's Healthcare of Atlanta
Atlanta, Georgia

Victoria Gocha Marchese, PT, PhD
Assistant Professor
Physical Therapy Department
Lebanon Valley College
Annville, Pennsylvania

Suzanne F. Migliore, PT, DPT, MS, PCS
Clinical Practice Coordinator
Physical Therapy Department
The Children's Hospital of Philadelphia
Philadelphia, Pennsylvania

Kathleen Miller-Skomorucha, OTR/L, C/NDT
Staff Occupational Therapist
Therapeutic and Rehabilitative Services
Nemours/duPont Hospital for Children
Wilmington, Delaware

Mary B. Schreiner, EdD
Chair of Education
Associate Professor
Alvernia University
Reading, Pennsylvania

Elena McKeogh Spearing, MA, DPT, PCS
Contract Physical Therapist
Dynamic Physical Therapy Solutions, Inc
Former Physical Therapy Manager
Children's Hospital of Philadelphia
Philadelphia, Pennsylvania

Elena Tappit-Emas, PT, MHS
Staff Therapist, School District of Philadelphia
Former Senior Therapist
Myelomeningocele Clinic
Children's Memorial Hospital, Chicago, Illinois
Private practice, Philadelphia, Pennsylvania

Jan Stephen Tecklin, PT, MS
Professor
Department of Physical Therapy
Arcadia University
Glenside, Pennsylvania

Diane Versaw-Barnes, PT, MS, PCS
Clinical Specialist-NICU
The Children's Hospital of Philadelphia
Philadelphia, Pennsylvania

Audrey Wood, PT, MS
OT/PT Clinical Specialist
Ken-Crest Services
Philadelphia, Pennsylvania

Bob Barnhart, PT, ScDPT, PCS
Director of Physical Therapy Program
Concordia University of Wisconsin
Mequon, Wisconsin

Martha Bloyer, PT, DPT, PCS
Director of Clinical Education and Clinical
  Assistant Professor
Department of Physical Therapy
Florida International University
Miami, Florida

Lisa Dannemiller, PT, DSc, PCS
Senior Instructor
Physical Therapy Program
University of Colorado
Aurora, Colorado

Leonard Elbaum, Ed.D, PT
Associate Professor
Department of Physical Therapy
Florida International University
Miami, Florida

Claudia B. Fenderson, PT, EdD, PCS
Professor
Physical Therapy Program
Mercy College
Dobbs Ferry, New York

Thomas Hudson, PT
Assistant Professor
Physical Therapy Deparment
Gannon University
Erie, Pennsylvania

Alison Kreger, PT, DPT, PCS, CKTP
Clinical Assistant Professor of Physical Therapy
Department of Physical Therapy
Wheeling Jesuit University
Wheeling, West Virginia

Alyssa LaForme Fiss, PT, PhD, PCS
Assistant Professor
Department of Physical Therapy
Mercer University
Atlanta, Georgia

Gary Lentell, DPT
Professor
Department of Physical Therapy
California State University, Fresno
Fresno, California

Janet Mutschler, PT, DPT
Assistant Professor, Director of Clinical Education
Department of Physical Therapy
University of Maryland Eastern Shore
Princess Anne, Maryland

Mary Elizabeth Parker, PT, PhD, NCS, PCS
Clinical Assistan Professor
Department of Physical Therapy
Texas State University-San Marcos
San Marcos, Texas

Claudia Senesac, PT, PhD, PCS
Clinical Associate Professor
Department of Physical Therapy
University of Florida
Gainesville, Florida

Elise Townsend, DPT, PhD, PCS
Associate Professor
Department of Physical Therapy
MGH Institute of Health Professions
Boston, Massachusetts

Jennifer Tucker, PT, DPT, PCS
Physical Therapy Instructor
Department of Health Professions
University of Central Florida
Orlando, Florida

The 5th edition of *Pediatric Physical Therapy*—"whooda thunk it" 27 years ago, in 1987, when the 1st edition was conceived. That this text is so well received and regularly adopted by many entry-level physical therapy programs in the United States and abroad is a testament primarily to the contributors. Two contributors, Dolores Bertoti and Elena Tappit-Emas, have been with the text through each of its five editions, and have always met deadlines and written and updated chapters in a very timely manner. The continuing goal that has guided the editor and many contributors through each edition is to provide a current description of major areas of practice in pediatric physical therapy for entry-level students and novice practitioners. Each edition has attempted to prepare entry-level students and new practitioners to begin pediatric care with a content that is supported by evidence, provides knowledge and insight within the diagnostic areas, and offers the tools by which to initiate and continue sound practice for the children with whom we work.

Organization

The book is organized into several sections based on the more common groups of disorders seen in infants and children. Chapter 1 stands alone and presents the issues of cultural sensitivity and family-centered care, to enhance understanding of these issues because the family is virtually always involved and we depend so often on a family's support and adherence with interventions. Chapter 2 focuses on the basics of chronologic motor development with a strong emphasis on the biomechanical aspects of that development. An entirely updated chapter on tests and measures of development, written by Kirsten Malerba, follows.

Neurologic and neuromuscular diseases and injuries are the focus for the next section of the text. The eight chapters in this section include one addition and one new group of authors. Jason Beaman and his associates have performed the daunting task of developing a completely new chapter about Cerebral Palsy with a strong section on gait. The new chapter, written by Anjana Bhat and colleagues, offers current information and discussion about autism spectrum disorders and is an important and current addition.

Chapters 13 through 15 discuss common musculoskeletal disorders and include two major revisions. Michael DiIenno

revised the chapter on major orthopedic disorders in children for Chapter 13. Elliot and Eric Greenberg (no relation) have updated and increased the evidence provided in Chapter 14 on sports injuries.

The final six chapters include several important and diverse groups of disorders. This section of the book includes one new chapter and a new author. Chapter 18 discusses a very contemporary topic—Obesity in Children—and was written by Kathy Coultes. Chapter 19, on Cardiac Disorders, was written by Heather Hansen, who is new to the book. The other chapters in this last section include updates to the previous edition.

Features

We have included extensive **Chapter Outlines** to help the student and the instructor focus on specific areas of information in the chapter. **Displays** have been included in an effort to provide greater depth of information, allowing information to be more inclusive without necessarily lengthening the text of the chapters. **Chapter Summaries** encapsulate and recapitulate the major points of information presented in each chapter. **Case Studies** help students hone their clinical decision-making skills with real-world situations.

Ancillaries

An interactive website is also included with this edition of *Pediatric Physical Therapy*. Instructors will have access to an Image Bank and PowerPoint lecture outlines. All of these resources are available at thePoint.lww.com/Tecklin5e.

The 5th edition of *Pediatric Physical Therapy* is much more than a timely update. It includes two chapters new to the book on autism and obesity, four entirely new chapters, and major updates for virtually all other chapters. In addition to the updates, the new authors in this edition have extensive experience in clinical care and regularly teach at the full-time faculty level or as an associated faculty member, and most have participated in clinical research. The authors represent the best in pediatric practice.

Jan Tecklin

ACKNOWLEDGMENTS

As in each previous edition, I would like to acknowledge the skill, creativity, knowledge, determination, and *generosity* of each of the authors who have contributed chapters to this 5th edition. Elena Spearing, a friend and former boss, updated Chapter 1, Providing Family-Centered Care in Pediatric Physical Therapy. Elena again, with her usual grace and agreeableness, coauthored Chapter 8, Traumatic and Atraumatic Spinal Cord Injury in Pediatrics, along with Heather Atkinson. Emilie Aubert authored two chapters despite, even more than most of us, dealing with a very stressful period of time. Her work under stress was, as in the past, outstanding and complete. Emilie updated her Motor Development chapter and again authored Chapter 12 on Adaptive Equipment and Environmental Aids for Children with Disabilities. Diane Versaw-Barnes and Audrey Wood completely rewrote Chapter 4 The Infant at High Risk for Developmental Delay. As I told them after the 4th edition, this extraordinarily comprehensive chapter could serve as a textbook on its own. Jason Beaman, a new author, along with his colleagues, dove in and completed the daunting Chapter 5 on Cerebral Palsy. We spoke regularly, and Jason was clearly up to the task and expanded the gait section of that chapter. Chapter 6, Spina Bifida, represents the fifth version of this comprehensive chapter by Elena Tappit-Emas who, along with Dolores Bertoti (coauthor of Chapter 10 with Mary Schreiner), has been with the text since the first edition in 1989, as noted in the Preface. Amy Both again updates her chapter, which discusses children with Traumatic Injury to the Central Nervous System: Brain Injury in Chapter 7, just as she did so successfully in the 3rd and 4th editions. Alan Glanzman, and Jean Flickinger coauthored and updated Chapter 9, Children with Myopathy and Related Disorders. I already mentioned Dolores Bertoti and the fifth version of Chapter 10 on Children with Mental Retardation written with Mary Schreiner. A new chapter to the 5th edition on Autism Spectrum Disorders by Anjana Bhat and colleagues Deborah Bubela and Rebecca Landa is an overdue and needed addition, and I appreciate the three coauthors' eagerness to participate. Emilie Aubert also updated Chapter 12, as noted above. Chapter 13, Orthopedic Management, has been completely written and revised by Michael DiIenno a new author to the 5th edition. Mike completed the chapter on time despite becoming a new dad and taking on a major increase in professional responsibilities, and I appreciate his ability to juggle several daunting projects. Chapter 14 about Sports Injuries in Children and Adolescents by Elliot Greenberg and Eric Greenberg is a great update that adds much evidence to support the interventions discussed about a multitude of injuries to young athletes. Susan Klepper has again presented the Juvenile Idiopathic Arthritis chapter (Chapter 15) which updates the 4th edition. Victoria (Tori) Marchese offers an update of her Pediatric Oncology in Chapter 16. Rehabilitation of the Child with Burns, by Suzanne Migliore revises and updates the discussion of the acute and long-term rehabilitation following serious burn injuries in Chapter 17. Heather Hanson, a new contributor, eagerly revised and updated Chapter 19 on Cardiac Disorders. I say "eagerly" because Heather's was the first completed chapter I received for review. I updated the Pulmonary Disorders chapter (Chapter 20) and attempted to focus on contemporary issues. Karen Lunnen, a friend since the early days of the Section on Pediatric Physical Therapy in the 1970s, and Rita Geddes have revised Physical Therapy in the Educational Environment, Chapter 21, with a focus on the clinical relevance of the topic.

I am deeply indebted to each author for the untold number of hours, moments of aggravation, and requests for the chapters to have been submitted "yesterday." I have incredible respect for each of these learned individuals, whom I think of as friends, who are also outstanding clinicians, mentors, scholars, and caregivers to children.

On a personal note:

I acknowledge the help over the past 27 years of the 41 colleagues across the United States who have been contributors to one or more editions of *Pediatric Physical Therapy*. Several of them I have not met face-to-face, but I have tried to mentor them using telephone, email, texts, and other modes in preparing chapters as best as I've been able. The most enjoyable parts of editing and compiling the 5th edition was to have the pleasure of including as authors five former students from Beaver College, which is now Arcadia University. These five include Diane Versaw-Barnes, Heather Baj Atkinson, Kathy Coultes, Elliot Greenberg, all graduates of the entry-level program, and Kirsten Hawkings Malerba, a graduate of our post-professional program.

I would be remiss if I did not acknowledge the support of the staff at Lippincott Williams & Wilkins. Notable among these folks has been Mr. John Larkin, our Managing Editor, who has nudged, pushed, cajoled, encouraged, but never nagged—and been largely responsible for the ultimate production of this book. To each and all of the folks above I offer my heartfelt appreciation and thanks.

CONTENTS

Contributors vii
Reviewers ix
Preface xi
Acknowledgments xiii

1 ▶ **Providing Family-Centered Care in Pediatric Physical Therapy** 1

Elena M. Spearing

PART I Development 15

2 ▶ **Motor Development in the Normal Child** 17

Emilie J. Aubert

3 ▶ **Assessment and Testing of Infant and Child Development** 69

Kirsten H. Malerba

PART II Neurological Disorders 101

4 ▶ **The Infant at High Risk for Developmental Delay** 103

Diane Versaw-Barnes and Audrey Wood

5 ▶ **The Infant and Child with Cerebral Palsy** 187

Jason Beaman, Faithe R. Kalisperis, and Kathleen Miller-Skomorucha

6 ▶ **Spina Bifida** 247

Elena Tappit-Emas

7 ▶ **Traumatic Injury to the Central Nervous System: Brain Injury** 301

Amy Both

8 ▶ **Traumatic and Atraumatic Spinal Cord Injuries in Pediatrics** 329

Heather Atkinson and Elena M. Spearing

9 ▶ **Neuromuscular Disorders in Childhood: Physical Therapy Intervention** 351

Alan M. Glanzman, Jean M. Flickinger, and Julaine M. Florence

10 ▶ **Intellectual Disabilities: Focus on Down Syndrome** 379

Dolores B. Bertoti and Mary B. Schreiner

11 ▶ **Autism Spectrum Disorders and Physical Therapy** 403

Anjana Bhat, Deborah Bubela, and Rebecca Landa

12 ▶ **Adaptive Equipment and Environmental Aids for Children with Disabilities** 423

Emilie J. Aubert

Part III Musculoskeletal Disorders 461

13 ▶ **Orthopedic Management** 463

Michael DiIenno

14 ▶ **Sports Injuries in Children and Adolescents** 501

Elliot M. Greenberg and Eric T. Greenberg

15 ▶ **Juvenile Idiopathic Arthritis** 541

Susan E. Klepper

PART IV Other Medical/Surgical Disorders 587

16 ▷ Pediatric Oncology 589
Victoria Gocha Marchese

17 ▷ Rehabilitation of the Child with Burns 611
Suzanne F. Migliore

18 ▷ Children with Obesity and the Role of the Physical Therapist 641
Kathy Coultes

19 ▷ Cardiac Disorders 657
Heather Hanson

20 ▷ Pulmonary and Respiratory Conditions in Infants and Children 679
Jan Stephen Tecklin

21 ▷ Physical Therapy in the Educational Environment 717
Karen Yundt Lunnen and Rita F. Geddes

Index 735

1

Providing Family-Centered Care in Pediatric Physical Therapy

Elena M. Spearing

Family-Centered Care
    Barriers to Providing Family-Centered Care
Families' Response to Medical Illness and Disability
Culture
    Diversity versus Sensitivity
    Influences on Cultural Identity
    Culture and Parental Expectations
    The Cultural Response to Illness
    The Cultural Response to Disability
    The Cultural Response to Death and Dying

Providing Family-Centered Intervention
    Cultural Desire
    Cultural Awareness
    Cultural Knowledge
    Cultural Skill
Benefits to Providing Family-Centered Care
Summary

▶ Family-centered care

The notion of family-centered care was first presented in the 1980s. It began in children's hospitals and pediatric units. This philosophy of care then spread to cancer units, maternity wards, mental health units, and various adult health care practices, where it is referred to as patient-centered care. Family-centered care is a philosophy recognizing that the family plays a vital role in ensuring the health and well-being of its members. Family-centered care also empowers the family to participate fully in the planning, delivery, and evaluation of health care services. It supports families in this role by building on the family members' individual strengths.[1,2]

Family-centered care is the foundation of pediatric physical therapy. Because a child is dependent on a caretaker, we must address both the child and the caretaker when we interact with a child receiving physical therapy.

The definition of family, in today's society, respects the notion that each family has unique characteristics and variables. Today, the family unit consists of "those significant others who profoundly influence the personal life and health of the individual over an extended period of time."[2] Families today come in all configurations and sizes and are not all traditional, married, two-biologic parent families. The 2010 U.S. Census reports that the number of husband–wife–own

children family households has decreased over the past 20 years despite increases in the total number of family households. The number of single-parent families, dual-income families, adoptive families, same-sex-parent families, and intergenerational families has steadily increased.[3]

Additionally, there is a "melting pot" of various cultural identities represented in the United States. The U.S. Census Bureau reported that the minority population continues to grow to an all-time high in 2012, with more people speaking languages other than English outside the home. The three fastest growing racial categories continue to be Asian and Pacific Islander, Hispanic, and "other."[3] This cultural factor presents additional challenges to health care providers who care for people with varying cultural and ethnic backgrounds.[4,5]

Historically, there has been a change in the developmental theory behind how pediatric physical therapy is provided (Display 1.1). This change has resulted in a shift from a reflex hierarchy model where a child develops on the basis of a set of primitive reflexes to one where a child develops as a result of the dynamic interaction of different systems that affect one another in the development of the child. In this dynamic system's model, all systems' components interact to produce meaningful, functional behavior.[6] The child's family is one of those systems. Similarly, pediatric care has shifted from being child focused, as in the 1980s, to currently being family focused.[1,7] Also, many center-based physical therapy service delivery models have been replaced by physical therapy service in the natural environment of the home and school. These initiatives help to promote family-centered care practice by the physical therapist.

Physical therapists who practice in the early intervention setting are mandated by law to provide care that respects a family's individualism. Those therapists have been charged with providing family-centered care since the initiation of Public Law 99-142 in 1975, Public Law 99-457 in 1986, and Public Law 102-119 in 1991.[1] Public Law 107-110 of 2001—No Child Left Behind (NCLB) and PL 108-446 of 2004, The Individuals with Disabilities Improvement Act—have similar mandates.[7,8] These laws placed the focus on revising and enhancing parents' involvement in the habilitation and education of the child.[1,9] Early studies showed that it was difficult to achieve this role on the basis of white middle-class families, and little attention was paid to social or ethnic differences. Additionally, enhancing parents' involvement is based on the assumption that the parents can participate in formal processes and, when necessary, draw on the availability of due process of the law. Family-centered care processes are also central to the development of the individualized family service plan (IFSP) and individualized education program (IEP), the required documentation for early intervention and educational services.

Physical therapists who practice in other pediatric settings, including the medically based inpatient and outpatient arenas, may be bound by health care accreditation standards, which recognize the importance of family-centered care. The Joint Commission on the Accreditation of Health Care Organizations has standards of care initiatives in place to address the needs of the family.[10] The Joint Commission has also developed publications to assist hospitals with meeting these standards.[11]

Collectively, the vision for family-centered care has included increasing support for the emotional and developmental needs of the child. Strategies for this include prehospitalization visits, presurgical education and preparation, 24-hour parental visitation and sibling visitation guidelines, and home care services. These initiatives have shifted from placing the family central not only to the child, but also to the child's plan of care.[12,13] Ultimately, this type of care results in a respect and a value for the parents as the ultimate experts in caring for their child.

Family-centered care involves the following themes[14,15]:

1. Respecting each child and his or her family
2. Honoring racial, ethnic, cultural, and socioeconomic diversity and its effect on the family's experience and perception of care
3. Recognizing and facilitating the choices for the child and family even in difficult and challenging situations
4. Facilitating and supporting the choices of the child and family about approaches to their care
5. Ensuring flexibility in organizational policies, procedures, and provider practices so services can be tailored to the needs, beliefs, and cultural values of each child and family
6. Sharing honest and unbiased information with families on an ongoing basis and in ways they find useful and affirming
7. Providing and ensuring formal and informal support for the child and parent and/or guardian during pregnancy, childbirth, infancy, childhood, adolescence, and young adulthood
8. Collaborating with families in the care of their individual child at all levels of health care, including professional education, policy making, and program development
9. Empowering each child and family to discover their own strengths, build confidence, and make choices and decisions about their health care

Barriers to Providing Family-Centered Care

Role conflict between families and health care professionals can impede the implementation of family-centered care. Often, this is very evident in the acute care setting. In the past, parents were expected to hand over the care of their children to the professionals and remain separate from them. Today, parents are expected to stay with their child and participate in their care. This example is also seen in the home care environment where parents are not afforded the respite care that they once were.

Role conflict contributes to role stress. Role stress is defined as "a subjective experience that is associated with lack of role clarity, role overload, role conflict, or temporary role pressures."[12] This stress can affect the communication process between health care provider and parent by causing one or the other to focus on the source of the stress as opposed to the underlying issues. Parents can be subjected to role stress owing to their child being ill, with exacerbation of that stress being associated with the child being hospitalized (Display 1.2).[12] The hospitalization of a child can be extremely stressful for even the most well-organized family. Many studies show that a professional can ease this stress by helping the parents understand the illness, help provide familiarity and comfort with the hospital setting, and encourage negotiating care of the child with health professionals.[12] Building a relationship with families and adapting styles to the individual learning styles, emotional stresses, and culture can lead to more effective intervention.[6] This has also been reported to improve developmental outcome and lead to enhanced cognitive and socioeconomic development in premature babies in the neonatal intensive care unit.[6]

The purpose of this chapter is to provide a framework for understanding the principles of family-centered care in order to enable the physical therapist to incorporate principles of family-centered care into their examination, assessment, and intervention techniques regardless of the pediatric practice setting. Themes of family-centered care cross not only practice settings, but also age and diagnosis. As these themes are threads across the pediatric spectrum of care, they are also threaded throughout the chapters of this textbook.

▶ Families' response to medical illness and disability

When parents are faced with the fact that their child has an illness or disability, their lives must change immediately. Some changes include readjusting the family's expectations and dealing with financial difficulties and health care systems and professionals. The most common initial responses include shock, disbelief, guilt, a sense of loss, and denial. After the period of denial, some parents may experience anger because of the stress of the medical issues as well as spousal disagreement or individual feelings of fault and guilt.[16]

As a result of these responses and concerns, there are many stresses for families with a child with a disability. Families raising a child with a disability will have different responses and means of adaptation. Factors that affect how a family responds include past life experiences, familial reactions to the child and the disability, and knowledge about health care and support systems. Supports can also vary. Sometimes there is a lack of understanding of the medical implications from those outside the family. There can also be feelings of embarrassment for the family. Professionals can use a cognitive approach to problem solving to help families examine their feelings and develop solutions for their own needs.

The effects of having a child with a disease or disability can not only affect the parents' relationship, but it can also have varied effects on siblings who also have individualized needs based on gender, birth order, and temperament. Siblings can also have mixed feelings toward their disabled sibling.[17] Some siblings may feel or be expected to have increased responsibility for the care of their siblings. Some siblings may have feelings of jealousy toward the sibling who has special needs.

A child with a disability may experience different effects as a result of his or her disability. By school age, most children are aware of their disability and may need help dealing with their feelings as they transition to school. The transition to school can be eased with education to the classmates prior to the disabled child entering school. Parents and professionals can assist with this planning. During adolescence, there may be particular new issues that emerge for a child with a disability. Feelings of comparing themselves and being part of a peer group are important for all adolescents and can present new challenges for those with chronic or new disabilities. Adolescents should also be acknowledged as having sexual interests. They should be educated on these feelings as well as trained in social skills. They should also be exposed to age-appropriate recreational skills, such as dancing, listening to music, and sports activities. Programs of inclusion help children to develop socialization skills and a good self-image.

Children with disability or illness may also have varying levels of understanding about their disease process or disability.[13] More recent data in the medical literature demonstrate that children with sickle cell disease provide their parents with information about their pain and assist with decision making. This should be kept in mind with children even as young as 5 years old.

The transition to adulthood is both important and difficult for patients and parents. Those individuals who remain dependent through adolescence tend to remain dependent through adulthood.[18] Adolescents who have the potential for independence but are having difficulties with separation may need assistance. Likewise, the family members may need assistance in supporting their child during this difficult time. Professionals should be partners with the family members and empower them to make decisions.

Disability as defined by the Americans with Disabilities Act is "physical or mental impairment that substantially limits one or more of the life activities of an individual, a record of such an impairment, or being regarded as having such an impairment."[19] Advances in medical technology, diagnosis, and treatment have resulted in decreased mortality rates for children with life-threatening conditions to survive well into adulthood.[18] The diagnosis of chronic illness or disability clearly impacts a family. How families respond to the diagnosis is a function of their adaptive capabilities.[16] What makes some families reorganize and become stronger, while others decline in function, become symptomatic, and sometimes disintegrate depends on family resilience according to Ferguson.[16] He describes eight aspects of resilient family processes as:

1. Balancing the illness with other family needs
2. Developing communication competence
3. Attributing positive meaning to the situations
4. Maintaining clear family boundaries
5. Maintaining family flexibility
6. Engaging in active coping efforts
7. Maintaining social integration
8. Developing collaborative relationships with professionals

A family's ability to be resilient or the extent of its resiliency is largely defined by society, time, place, and culture.[16]

Additionally, in studies dealing with disability, when looking at reaction to disability, there are three issues considered to be universal. They are as follows[20]:

1. The culturally perceived cause of a chronic illness or disability will play a significant role in determining family and community attitudes toward the individual. (This will be discussed later in this chapter.)
2. The expectations for physical survival for the infant or the child with a chronic disability will affect both the immediate care the child receives and the amount of effort expended in planning for future care and education.
3. The social role(s) deemed appropriate for disabled or chronically ill children and adults will help determine the amount of resources a family and community invests in an individual. This includes issues of education and training, participation in family and social life, and the long-range planning done by, or undertaken for, the individual over the course of a lifetime. In the history of literature on family reactions to having a child with a disability, there has been a shift in thinking. In the 19th century, with the flourish of specialization, the moral blame for disabilities was often placed on the parents. This set of beliefs most often placed the blame on poor mothers who made bad judgments. Reform schools, asylums, and residential schools all became apparent in the 19th century. This movement also led to special education schools after the turn of the century. The only way to deal with children that weren't "normal" was to turn the parenting over to professionals within the walls of these facilities.[12]

There was a major shift in thinking throughout the 20th century that included a reversal of the above assumptions. Professionals shifted to focusing on the damage that children with disabilities caused their families. The medical model began to analyze the family unit with terms such as *guilt, denial,* and *grief* and *role disruption, marital cohesiveness,* and *social withdrawal.*

Over the past few decades, a new approach has developed regarding the impact of a child's disability on the family. The recent approach includes models of stress and coping (adaptation) and models of family life course development. The adaptive family describes X—the potential family crisis—as an interaction of three factors: (1) an initial stressful event, combined with (2) a family's resource for dealing with the crisis and (3) the family's definition of the stressor.[16] This approach has allowed researchers to focus on the resiliency of the family and its ability to cope with a potentially stressful situation. There is a level of consensus today that identifies the varying ways that families with children with disabilities deal with stressful situations. There is great similarity to the way that families with children without disabilities deal with similar issues. There are also varying responses to how some deal with stressors. Sometimes, others can view stressors as benefits. Also, the response to stressors is cyclic and cumulative. Each stressor response affects others' responses.[16]

The evolving family concept also accepts that families evolve over time and tries to identify where they are in their developmental process. Similarly, families need to be considered across the continuum of care. This is especially true as their younger children age and approach adulthood. This line of thinking has allowed researchers to look at how and why some families are more resilient than others and also how extended coping with chronic disabilities affects families over time.

The supported family members look at internal and external resources that are available to them. How family members respond to difficulties depends on their supports. This also has root in societal and cultural assumptions. Recent research on family adaptation shows the following key themes[16]:

- There is a dominant body of literature that shows patterns of adjustment and well-being to be similar across groups of families of children with and without disabilities. This does show, however, that there are some developmental differences over the family life course.
- Additionally, there is an increasing recognition and growing research that a significant number of parents actually report numerous benefits and positive outcomes for their family associated with raising a child with a disability. These include coping skills (adaptability), family harmony (cohesiveness), spiritual growth or shared values, shared parenting roles, and communication.
- There are, obviously, stressors associated with having a child with a disability. The research continues to refine our understanding of why some families are more resilient than others in adapting to stress. Some research has suggested that the level of disability or family structure may not be as crucial as other factors (income, self-injurious behaviors, etc.). There are also differing patterns of adaptations along ethnic and cultural lines.[16]

▶ Culture

Culture affects how others view disability, how people with disabilities view themselves, and how people with disabilities are treated. The cultural context within which a disability is perceived is important to understanding the meaning of disability for a person or his or her family. It is also important to know the kinds of services to be provided to families and people with disabilities.

Culture can be defined in many ways. O'Connor defines culture as "the acquired knowledge people use to interpret experience and generate social behavior."[21] Other definitions include "the ever changing values, traditions, social and political relationships and a world view shared by a group of people bound together by a number of factors that can include a common history, geographic location, language, social class and/or religion."[22] An analysis of the various studies of culture yields the emergence of various similar themes[21]:

1. Culture is not innate or biologically inherited but, in fact, learned patterns of behavior.
2. Culture is transmitted from the older people to the young, from generation to generation.
3. Culture serves as a group identity and is shared by other members of the group.
4. Culture provides the individual or the members of a group with an effective mechanism for interacting with each other and their environment.

Diversity versus Sensitivity

There are many terms that are used today to refer to the impact of culture on health care. It is necessary to describe the two most common terms and their fundamental differences. *Cultural diversity* refers to having a range of cultures represented in an organization. This leads to a workforce that is more representative of the general population. In health care, diversity in the workplace leads to the increased potential of having similar cultures represented. By comparison, *cultural sensitivity* and effectiveness is a process of becoming "culturally competent" and striving toward the ability and availability to work effectively within the cultural context of a client, individual, family, or community regardless of the cultural background.[22]

Cultural sensitivity refers to the understanding that cultural differences exist. These differences are not necessarily better or worse, right or wrong, or more or less intelligent, but rather simply differences.[23] It is necessary to examine, in detail, attitude, behavior, and communication, which directly affect health care. It is important to realize that each person within a culture is an individual and should not be characterized or stereotyped on the basis of his or her cultural association. It is only through generalizations that one can gain a frame of reference and become more culturally aware.

Influences on Cultural Identity

There are various things that influence who we are and how we view illness and disability. These include our nationality, our race, and our ethnicity. Similarly, our socioeconomic status and education also play a role. Our society's view of illness and disability also influences our perception of the same. Other things like age, religion, and past experience shape our beliefs.

In addition to these, health care providers who were brought up in the U.S. culture are finding that their medical views are in conflict with the views of their patients from differing cultural backgrounds. Care provided in the past was monocultural and suited for the Euro-American culture. Traditionally, in medicine we have functioned under a "medical culture," one that values a "cure" and the expertise of those in the medical profession.[9]

This traditional model, however, is not as appropriate or relevant for those who are not of that "medical" cultural identity.[9] When this cultural disconnect occurs, the consequence is often disparities in the quality of care received by racial and ethnic minority populations. One example of this is the Tuskegee Syphilis Research Experiment, which occurred between 1932 and 1972. Three hundred and ninety-nine poor African American sharecroppers who were identified as having syphilis were told that they were being treated for the disease when they were unaware that they were control subjects.[24] This legacy has continued to affect the credibility and reputation of the medical industry for many African Americans who believe there are continuing racial and ethnic disparities in the health care system and mistrust the medical community.[24] Fortunately, these disparities are evolving with time but they still exist. Guerrero et al. found that black children have similar experiences as white children on overall family-centered care in models that adjust for socioeconomic factors. In contrast, there were still differences found on dimensions of overall family-centered care between white children and Latino children, irrespective of interview language and even with multivariate adjustment.[25]

Cultural and Parental Expectations

Many studies reveal that culture and acculturation are strong predictors of parental expectations of cognitive and social development. Most studies point to ethnic origin as the differentiating factor. More contemporary literature has determined that Western education and socioeconomic status were more predictive of differential beliefs than ethnic origin. This demonstrates that acculturation has a powerful effect on parenting styles and on parental beliefs about child development. What is even more profound is the difference between the description of mildly retarded, behaviorally disordered, and learning disabled between the parents and the professionals. Ethnographic studies have shown that there are sometimes differences related to culture, which emphasized that for some parents, a child's cognitive and social functioning has to be more limited for the concept of handicap or disabled to be applied. These statements are then interpreted by the professional as families being in "denial."[23] The following themes occur in a review of the literature on culturally appropriate services in the special education literature[9]:

1. There are cultural differences in definitions and interpretations of disability.
2. There are cultural differences in family coping styles and responses to disability-related stress.
3. There are cultural differences in parental interaction styles, as well as expectations of participation and advocacy.

4. There are differences in cultural groups' access to information and services.
5. There are negative professional attitudes to, and perceptions of, families' roles in the special education processes.
6. There is dissonance in the cultural fit of educational programs.

There are traditional cultural patterns associated with particular cultural groups. One example is that Asian groups attribute disability to spiritual retribution or reward. Similarly, there is an emphasis on the wholeness of the spirit within a disabled body. This is powerfully described in the novel *When the Spirit Catches You, and You Fall Down* by Anne Fatiman. It is demonstrated throughout the novel that this Hmong family attributed epilepsy to spiritual phenomena within the individual.[26]

The Cultural Response to Illness

How one views and responds to health, illness, and death is largely defined by his or her cultural values. Before detailing this, a distinction between disease and illness must be made.

Physicians diagnose and treat diseases, which can be defined as abnormalities in the structure and function of body organs and systems. Illnesses, on the other hand, are experiences of disvalued changes in states of being and cultural reactions to disease or discomfort.[27]

How a person understands and responds to illness is determined by what Kleinman calls "explanatory models." These are defined as "notions about an episode of sickness and its treatment that are employed by all those engaged in the clinical process."[27] Explanatory models address five major issues:

1. Etiology of the problem
2. Time and mode of onset
3. Pathophysiology of illness
4. Course of illness and degree and severity
5. Type of treatment that should be sought[28]

"Illness is culturally shaped in how we perceive, experience, and cope with disease based on our explanations of sickness, explanations specific to the social positions we occupy and systems of meanings we employ."[27] The role of traditional medicine and folk healing is based on cultural values. An estimated 70% to 90% of self-recognized episodes of sickness are managed outside of the formal health care system.[27] As Kleinman states, "folk healers deal with the human experience of illness." They seek to provide meaningful explanations for illness and respond to personal, family, and community issues surrounding illness.[27] Illness referred to as "folk illness" (i.e., illnesses that are recognized within a cultural group) may sometimes conflict with the biomedical paradigm.[29]

It is important to understand folk illness because people who experience "folk illness" may present to a medical practitioner and a "folk healer." Additionally, some "folk treatments" may be potentially hazardous. Finally, folk illness may be cultural interpretations of states of pathophysiology that may require medical attention. For many chronic problems, patients have reported greater improvement with marginal folk healers than with medical physicians. Kleinman attributes this improvement to folk healers' increased emphasis on "explanation" and a greater concordance of explanatory systems between healer and patient.[27]

For more serious illness, values and beliefs become even more crucial to understanding. Although the biologic manifestations of diseases are the same among cultural groups, individuals differ in the way they experience, interpret, and respond to illness. Explanatory models as well as coping styles have been shown to influence perceptions of illness.[27] Some have suggested that meanings are assigned using characteristic themes resulting from individual coping styles, knowledge, beliefs, and cultural background.[27] Viewing illness as a challenge regards the illness as something to be approached internally and mastered. The proper authorities are consulted, advice is followed, and life goes on. Illness as "God's will" is often perceived as beyond human control and may result in passive acceptance and resignation of what cannot be changed. This set of beliefs may result in less interest in aggressive procedures and may produce depression. Illness as a "strategy" describes using illness to secure attention or nurturing from parents, family, or health care professionals. Illness as a "value" may be the "highest form" of coping, where illness is viewed as an opportunity that can result in important insight into the meaning of life. Although meanings may be influenced by culture, they are not culture specific.[27]

Our expectations and perceptions of symptoms, as well as the labels we attach to sickness behaviors, are influenced by environment, family, and explanatory models. In addition, the way in which problems are communicated, how symptoms are presented, when and who is visited for care, how long one remains in care, and how care is evaluated are all affected by cultural beliefs.[30] Likewise, culture dramatically influences the reaction to and expression of pain, which has been learned throughout childhood.[30]

The Cultural Response to Disability

Research gives strong support to the argument that definitions of disability are socially constructed.[9,23] When disability is severe, studies show that although all groups recognize gross developmental, behavioral, or sensory impairments, their attributions differ widely as does the extent of stigma or value associated with that condition.[9,31] Responses to impairments vary through time, place, and culture. Over the course of history, societies have defined what did and did not constitute a disability or handicap. The past decade has seen changes in the conceptualization of the meaning of disability and the interplay between the possibility that an impairment becomes a physical handicap. Even more than physical limitations placed on the individual with a disability, attitudinal concepts and images affect treatment of an individual with a disability. The sources of concepts and images they produce are found in literature and art, television and movies, religious texts, and school books. Since these sources are all artifacts of culture, it is impossible to separate culture from attitudes toward disability.

For children with disabilities, the culturally perceived cause of a chronic illness or disability affects aspects of a family and community's attitudes toward that child.[20] In some cultures, disability is viewed as a form of punishment. Depending on the belief system, the individual with a disability, the family, or an ancestor has been targeted by God, or a god, for having sinned or violating a taboo. Witchcraft may also be strongly linked to disability as well as associated with that person who has been bewitched.[20]

Similarly, inherited disorders are frequently attributed to "running in the blood" or caused by a curse.[20,27] Closely related to this is the traditional belief that a disabled child may be the product of an incestuous relationship. In societies where there is a belief in reincarnation, disability may be seen as the result of a transgression in a previous life by parents of a child with a disability or the child itself. Some belief systems may emphasize the imbalance of humoral elements in the body as the cause of disability.[20]

All of these perceived causes identify the individual with the disability as responsible for that disability and suggests likely consequences on the person's place in the family. Additionally, where disability is seen as a punishment, the presence of a child with a disability may be a source of embarrassment to the family. Various types of neglect may be apparent, including isolation. In many cultures, the idea of early intervention is not in the mindset for medical and educational professionals.[20] There may also be strong social pressures placed on the family in these instances. Families may be reluctant to participate in therapeutic programs, fearing that these will call attention to their family member's physical and intellectual limitations.[20]

An understanding of traditional expectations for survival is also important. For some cultures, the belief that severely disabled children will simply not survive makes the allocation of medical and parental attention to healthy children more practical. Either neglecting a disabled child or overprotecting him or her because he or she is alive for only a short period of time can have serious implications for both health care services and psychological development. Moreover, how one is believed to be restored to health can have implications on long-term planning or arranging for special care, with members of some cultures feeling that "maybe God will make your baby all better on its own."[20]

Societies that limit occupational roles and social roles for individuals with disabilities can affect the time, energy, and expense invested in educating a child with a disability. Additionally, a gender bias, common in some cultures, may affect the degree to which a family is willing to spend money in order to obtain medical care. In these cultures, it may be perceived less justifiable to expend vast amounts of family resources on disabled female children than disabled male children.[20]

Failure to fully understand cultural beliefs and values toward disability may influence a family's care toward its disabled child. Consider the family members whose cultural beliefs lead them to feel that it is their responsibility to provide complete and total care for their disabled child. They may prefer to keep their child at home, unseen by even neighbors. They may hesitate to come forward for aid or advice, for various reasons, which may include poverty, fear, language barriers, or faith in traditional medical practices. When not viewed in a cultural context, this may be construed as neglect—the failure of parents to nurture and provide adequate ongoing education and emotional support.[23]

The Cultural Response to Death and Dying

The number of children with severe and complex neurodevelopmental disabilities and complex medical conditions who are surviving is increasing owing to advances in medical care and technology.[32] There can be conflict between palliative care at the end of life and cure-oriented treatment. Death and the customs surrounding it need to be addressed as they are highly influenced by cultural values. Expressions of grief and coping mechanisms vary from person to person but are related to cultural background.[33] The meaning of death, family patterns, including family roles during periods of grief, and the family's expectations for professional health care need to be understood. Professional attitudes regarding quality of life and appropriateness of care, the uncertainty of prognosis and the unique role of the child with a chronic disability, and the codependence between caregiver and child may all contribute to barriers to end-of-life care in this patient population.

The loss of a child with a chronic disability signifies not only loss of the child but loss of a lifestyle. Again, respecting the family's expertise when it comes to their child will assist with effective advanced care planning and implementation.[32]

▶ Providing family-centered intervention

The nursing literature has explored the process of cultural competence in the delivery of health care service, including a model for providing culturally competent interventions. This model for cultural competence includes cultural desire, cultural awareness, cultural knowledge, and cultural skill.[34]

Cultural Desire

The first requirement for cultural competence is "cultural desire." This is the motivation to "want to" engage in the process of becoming culturally aware, becoming culturally knowledgeable, becoming culturally skillful, and seeking cultural encounters.[34] Rather than doing it because it is required, cultural desire involves doing it because it is personally desired. It includes a genuine passion to be open and flexible with others, to accept differences and build on similarities, and to be willing to learn from others as cultural informants.

Cultural Awareness

Cultural awareness is the next step in achieving cultural competence and has been described as the self-examination and in-depth exploration of one's own cultural background.[34] This awareness involves recognizing one's biases, prejudices, and assumptions about individuals who are different. Without this self-awareness, there is a risk of imposing one's own beliefs, values, and patterns of behavior on one from another culture.

Cultural Knowledge

Cultural knowledge is the process of seeking and obtaining a sound educational foundation about diverse cultural and ethnic groups.[34] Obtaining this information does not refer to learning generalizations but to learning individual differences. Learning generalizations about specific cultural subgroups leads to the development of stereotypes. Understanding that there is as much intracultural difference and intercultural difference due to life experiences, acculturation to other cultures, and diversity within cultures will prevent us from imposing stereotypic patterns on our patients and families.

Cultural Skill

Cultural skill is the ability to collect cultural data regarding the patient's problem as well as performing a culturally based physical assessment.[34] There are many tools available to help collect this information via questions. One must also remember that it is a developmental skill to ask questions in a way that does not offend the patient or family. Listening and remaining nonjudgmental are effective and sensitive ways to obtain information. Additionally, having multiple cultural encounters is the way to refine or modify one's own belief about a cultural group and prevent stereotyping. Linguistic assessment is necessary to facilitate accurate communication. The use of specifically medically trained interpreters is important to the assessment process. Untrained interpreters, family members, and specifically children and siblings may pose a problem owing to lack of medical knowledge.

We must provide care that is not only culturally competent, but that also provides for low literacy skills. It is documented that people who have limited English proficiency experience obstacles when accessing health care.[35] They may experience delays in making appointments, and are also more likely to have misunderstandings regarding time, place, date, and location of appointment. People with low literacy skills may have difficulty communicating

with the health care professional and employees in the health care institution. These issues are more likely to exacerbate medical problems that require timely treatment or follow-up.[35]

In 1999, the U.S. Department of Health and Human Services (HHS) office of Minority Health developed standards of care within these areas. These standards were revised in 2007 (Display 1.3). In addition, the Office of Civil Rights and HHS enforce federal laws that prohibit discrimination by health care providers who receive funding from the HHS. Antidiscrimination laws are established by Section 504 of the Rehabilitation Act of 1973, title VI of the Civil Rights Act of 1964, title II of the Americans with Disabilities Act of 1990, Community Service Assurance provisions of the Hill–Burton Act, and the Age Discrimination Act of 1975. The laws mandate that providers who accept federal money must "ensure meaningful access to and benefits from health services for individuals who have limited English proficiency."[36] Using an interpreter and translating materials into languages and levels that can be read by those who have literacy deficiencies are important mandated tools.

Adults who have literacy deficiencies face many problems in understanding written and verbal materials that are provided to them. It is important to remember that while some readily admit their limitations regarding understanding verbal and written information, others may feel shameful and use strategies to hide their limitations. In these situations, one can use oral explanation and demonstration. Pictures, photographs, and visual cues also help to reinforce the information. Some people will also use family members to assist them with reading, and these family members may be important in the education process.

One can identify people with low literacy skills by looking for clues. An example is someone who gives excuses for not being able to read something or who cannot read back information that is provided. Some other strategies to providing information to those with low literacy skills include[37]:

- Remaining nonjudgmental
- Involving the patient/family
- Asking the patient simple questions
- Simplifying instructions
- Repeating the information many times
- Finding various ways to give the same message
- Organizing information so that the most important information is provided first
- Using audio-visual information
- Involving family and friends in the learning and reinforcing of information
- Asking the patient to recall the message in his or her own words or demonstrate the skill that is being taught
- Empowering individuals and families and fostering independence in their programs

Health care professionals and physical therapists should promote the sharing of information and collaboration

The CLAS standards are primarily directed at health care organizations[40]; however, individual providers are also encouraged to use the standards to make their practices more culturally and linguistically accessible. The principles and activities of CLAS should be integrated throughout an organization and undertaken in partnership with the communities being served.

Standard 1
Health care organizations should ensure that patients/consumers receive from all staff members effective, understandable, and respectful care that is provided in a manner compatible with their cultural health beliefs and practices and in preferred language.

Standard 2
Health care organizations should implement strategies to recruit, retain, and promote at all levels of the organization a diverse staff and leadership that are representative of the demographic characteristics of the service area.

Standard 3
Health care organizations should ensure that staff at all levels and across all disciplines receive ongoing education and training in CLAS delivery.

Standard 4
Health care organizations must offer and provide language assistance services, including bilingual staff and interpreter services, at no cost to each patient/consumer with limited English proficiency at all points of contact, in a timely manner during all hours of operation.

Standard 5
Health care organizations must provide to patients/consumers in their preferred language both verbal offers and written notices informing them of their right to receive language assistance services.

Standard 6
Health care organizations must assure the competence of language assistance provided to limited-English-proficient patients/consumers by interpreters and bilingual staff. Family and friends should not be used to provide interpretation services (except on request by the patient/consumer).

Standard 7
Health care organizations must make available easily understood patient-related materials and post signage in the languages of the commonly encountered groups and/or groups represented in the service area.

Standard 8
Health care organizations should develop, implement, and promote a written strategic plan that outlines clear goals, policies, operational plans, and management accountability/oversight mechanisms to provide CLAS.

Standard 9
Health care organizations should conduct initial and ongoing organizational self-assessments of CLAS-related activities and are encouraged to integrate cultural and linguistic competence-related measures into their internal audits, performance improvement programs, patient satisfaction assessments, and outcomes-based evaluations.

Standard 10
Health care organizations should ensure that data on the individual patient's/consumer's race, ethnicity, and spoken and written language are collected in health records, integrated into the organization's management information systems, and periodically updated.

Standard 11
Health care organizations should maintain a current demographic, cultural, and epidemiological profile of the community as well as a needs assessment to accurately plan for and implement services that respond to the cultural and linguistic characteristics of the service area.

Standard 12
Health care organizations should develop participatory, collaborative partnerships with communities and utilize a variety of formal and informal mechanisms to facilitate community and patient/consumer involvement in designing and implementing CLAS-related activities.

Standard 13
Health care organizations should ensure that conflict- and grievance-resolution processes are culturally and linguistically sensitive and capable of identifying, preventing, and resolving cross-cultural conflicts or complaints by patients/consumers.

Standard 14
Health care organizations are encouraged to regularly make available to the public information about their progress and successful innovations in implementing the CLAS standards and to provide public notice in their communities about the availability of this information.

---

among patients, families, and health care staff. Offering places such as a family resource center will give families opportunities to educate themselves around their child's needs. Also, developing programs that provide support to families in the community is an important related activity.

Some institutions have instituted family faculty.[38] These families have often been in similar situations and can act to encourage and facilitate parent-to-parent support. They also provide a network for families. Additionally, one must support family caregiving and decision making and help give them the tools to do so, even if one does not agree with the decision that is made. Institutions must involve patients and families in the planning, delivery, and evaluation of health care services. They should take feedback from families and incorporate that into program planning. They should also consider the family needs as well as the child's needs.

In summary, one provides culturally competent intervention by asking the right questions.[22]

▶ Benefits to providing family-centered care

Health care practitioners who practice family-centered care are aware that it can enhance parents' confidence in their roles and, over time, increase the competence of children and young adults to take responsibility for their own health care, particularly in the anticipation of the transition to adult services.[38] Family-centered care can improve patient and family outcomes, increase patient and family satisfaction, build on the child and family strengths, increase professional satisfaction, decrease health care costs, and lead to more effective use of health care resources, as shown in the following examples from the literature[38]:

- Family presence during health care procedures decreases anxiety for the child and the parents. Research indicates that when parents are prepared, they do not prolong the procedure or make the provider more anxious.
- Children whose mothers were involved in their posttonsillectomy care recovered faster and were discharged earlier than were children whose mothers did not participate in their care.
- A series of quality improvement studies found that children who had undergone surgery cried less, were less restless, and required less medication when their parents were present and assisted in pain assessment and management.
- Children and parents who received care from child life specialists did significantly better than did control children and parents on measures of emotional distress, coping during the procedure and adjustment during the hospitalization, the posthospital period, and recovery, including recovery from surgery.
- A multisite evaluation of the efficacy of parent-to-parent support found that one-on-one support increased parents' confidence and problem-solving abilities.
- Family-to-family support can have beneficial effects on the mental health status of mothers of children with chronic illness.
- Family-centered care has been a strategic priority at children's hospitals all over the country. Families participated in design planning for the new hospital, and they have been involved in program planning, staff education, and other key hospital committees and task forces.

Staff satisfaction also improves with family-centered care initiatives. The following points have been found:

- Staff report valuable learning experiences.
- A Vermont program has shown that a family faculty program, combined with home visits, produces positive changes in medical student perceptions of children and adolescents with cognitive disabilities.

- When family-centered care is the cornerstone of culture in a pediatric emergency department, staff members have more positive feelings about their work than do staff members in an emergency department that does not emphasize family-centered care.
- Coordination for prenatal care in a manner consistent with family-centered principles for pregnant women at risk of poor birth outcomes at a medical center in Wisconsin resulted in more prenatal visits, decreased rate of tobacco and alcohol use during pregnancy, higher infant birth rates and gestational ages, and fewer neonatal intensive care unit days. All these factors decrease health care costs and the need for additional services.
- After redesigning their transitional care center in a way that is supportive of families, creating 24-hour open visiting for families, and making a commitment to information sharing, a children's hospital in Ohio experienced a 30% to 50% decrease in their infants' length of stay.
- In Connecticut, a family support service for children with HIV hired family support workers whose backgrounds and life experiences were similar to those of the families served by the program. This approach resulted in decreases in HIV-related hospital stays, missed clinic appointments, and foster care placement.
- King County, Washington, has a children's managed care program based on a family participation service model. Families decide for themselves how dollars are spent for their children with special mental health needs as long as the services are developed by a collaborative team created by the family. In the 5 years since the program's inception, the proportion of children living in communication homes instead of institutions has increased from 24% to 91%. The number of children attending community schools has grown from 48% to 95%, and the average cost of care per child or family per month has decreased from approximately $6,000 to $4,100.

Benefits to the health care professional include[38]:

- A stronger alliance with the family in promoting each child's health and development
- Improved clinical decision making on the basis of better information and collaborative processes
- Improved follow-through when the plan of care is developed by a collaborative process
- Greater understanding of the family's strengths and caregiving capacities
- More efficient and effective use of professional time and health care resources
- Improved communication among members of the health care team
- A more competitive position in the health care marketplace
- An enhanced learning environment for future pediatricians and other professionals in training

- A practice environment that enhances professional satisfaction
- Greater child and family satisfaction with their health care
- Involving patients and families in change efforts in health care institutions helps deliver improvements in care processes, gains in health literacy, and more effective priority setting as well as more cost-effective use of health care and better outcomes.[39]

SUMMARY

It is important for us to examine our own belief systems to provide family-centered culturally competent care. First, we need to recognize the vital role families play in ensuring the health and well-being of its family members. It has been proposed that family members are equal members of the team.

Next, we need to acknowledge that emotional, social, and developmental supports are integral components of health care. Third, we need to respect the patient's and the family's choices and their values, beliefs, and cultural backgrounds. This can be accomplished by asking questions.

Finally, we can assume that families, even those living in difficult circumstances, bring important and unique strengths to their health care experiences.

"Family-centered care is a service delivery model that includes the manner in which the services match the needs identified by the family."[1] Although many people practice family-centered care, it is not widespread. Heath care professionals must adopt new practices and policies, and families and patients must learn new skills.

Today there are many government agencies that have been instituted around family-centered care initiatives. The Agency for Healthcare Research and Quality (AHRQ) (www.hhs.gov) and the Institute for Patient and Family Centered Care (www.ipfcc.org) are two examples. These organizations provide recommendations that include training programs to educate professionals both pre- and postprofessionally about their role in fostering family-centered care. Historically, these agencies began in an attempt to educate professionals around principles of family-centered care. In 1998, then Vice President Al Gore held a conference in Nashville regarding families and health. This conference set the stage for initiatives nationwide for recognizing the value of family-centered care in our health system. A Family Bill of Rights was originally developed by President Clinton. This Bill of Rights is posted in public areas in health care practices in multiple languages and made available to families as necessary.[14] At the family reunion conference, Vice President Gore also outlined a five-step action plan for bringing the powers of families into our health care system. This action plan can be used as a summary for this chapter. The plan is SMART. Its principles are as follows[14]:

Support families with information, education, understanding, and resources. Some examples of this are family resource centers, family advocacy groups, and family faculty.

Measure the effectiveness of programs. This can be done with outcome measures, qualitatively and quantitatively.

Ask the right questions. Determine the individual needs of the patient and family. This will decrease the tendency to make generalizations based on culture.

Respect that individual differences do occur and that they may be different from our own.

Train early on in the health care profession. Recognize that training is lifelong and ongoing.

Training programs should be in place to educate health care workers both pre- and postprofessionally about their role in fostering family-centered care. There is an urgent need for preservice training in multicultural practices.[14] Coursework for special educators and health professionals should be part of the preprofessional curriculum. There has been much published about specific cultural groups. This type of approach is promising for professionals who are being trained to work with specific groups of people. There is danger, however, in this method of training. It risks the development of stereotypes and assumptions that are not true. No individual training program can possibly address all the differences that are possible within groups. More effective methods of teaching cultural effectiveness include processes for a much broader conceptual approach. Many programs have developed their own methods. All have common themes: self-assessment, culturally effective knowledge of language, and the ability to apply the knowledge at both interpersonal and systems levels. Harry recommends an approach that is a habit of reflective practice that will lead to effective parent–professional collaboration without having a great deal of culturally specific information.[14] The approach includes developing culturally appropriate observation and interviewing skills, including asking questions that are open-ended. The federal government will continue to look at funding systems for programs and enact legislation to ensure that principles are being respected. If these principles are in place with our delivery of Physical Therapy Examination, Assessment and Intervention, it will serve to improve all aspects of the patient experience.

CASE STUDIES

CASE STUDY 1 **Roselyn** Roselyn is an 8-year-old girl with cerebral palsy. She lives with her mother, father, two brothers, one sister, grandmother, aunt, and four cousins in a small home in an urban environment. Roselyn's parents moved to the United States when they were teenagers. They have learned to speak English, but it is not their primary language spoken at home. Roselyn is unable to walk and does not attend school. Her family takes care of her every need. She rarely leaves the house except to go to church, where she is carried and doesn't have many friends her own age. She has a close family and enjoys many visits from friends and neighbors. Her family takes her regularly to the major medical center for all her medical care.

The professionals have recommended a special educational setting for Roselyn, where she would receive all her educational needs and therapies. The family has declined such a placement and prefers to homeschool her. She is not receiving any therapy at this time.

Many professionals who have seen Roselyn have tried to get the family to agree to outside help for Roselyn. They have stressed the importance of teaching her how to function independently. The family members insist that she does not need to do anything, because they will take care of her. They do not even want to get any type of special equipment to help them to take care of her. Roselyn has not had any acute medical issues; however, the team feels that Roselyn could do more for herself.

After many years of team recommendations not being followed by Roselyn's family, a new physical therapist offered to make a visit to the family's home to assess the situation. When she arrived, she found a very crowded living arrangement within a very small home. As she stayed to "visit," she observed a typical day in the life of Roselyn. She was amazed to see the whole family involved. One family member bathed and dressed her. Another family member fed her along with the rest of the family. When the other children went off to school, Roselyn's mother spent a few hours teaching her math and reading and doing "exercises" to make her strong. After lunch, Roselyn was carried outside and taken for a walk around the neighborhood and accompanied her father to the store for some groceries in a homemade wagon. After the children returned from school, Roselyn sat outside on the porch and watched the children as they played. They all included her in their games.

The physical therapist realized that Roselyn's family and neighbors had embraced her care as a team. They had developed strategies to care for her and included her in the family's activities. When speaking to Roselyn's mother, she sensed an enormous amount of sense of responsibility for Roselyn's disability, even referred to "punishment for sins that had been committed by her parents." It was obvious that Roselyn's family took great pride in her caretaking.

When the physical therapist returned from her visit, she shared the information that she received with the team. She took photos and video of the house and the equipment that the family used. All agreed that Roselyn was being cared for, but that perhaps they were going about helping her in the wrong way. They decided to have a social worker, who was of the same ethnic group, to work with the family on changing its understanding of the disability. Instead of focusing on changing what the family was doing, the team worked to support the family members in what they were doing. Very soon, the family accepted some help from the team. The team was able to give the family members suggestions to make it easier for them to care for Roselyn and

gave them suggestions for how she could play a more active role in the family and the community.

Clinic visits were not frustrating anymore as the team took a new approach to making recommendations to the family.

Points to Ponder

Was the team being family centered when they first worked with Roselyn and her family?

How did the therapist's visit change the perception of the team?

Why was the family so resistant to the recommendations that they made as a team?

How should the team proceed with their recommendations as Roselyn gets older?

CASE STUDY 2 **Daniel** Daniel is a 4-year-old boy who was admitted to the hospital for "a bad cough." His parents were not born in this country and spoke little English. There was no other family member with Daniel who spoke English, so the nurses and doctors attempted to get information to complete their assessment using gestures, pictures, and simple English. It appeared from the examination that Daniel had been ill for quite some time, without medical care. He was malnourished and had a severe productive cough with bloody sputum. He also had marks on his chest that appeared to be caused by a small object being rubbed on it. The professionals who examined Daniel felt that he had been neglected and discussed whether the authorities should be notified. The attending physicians decided to admit Daniel to the hospital for a workup. He called Social Services because of his concerns about the family and refused to allow the parents to accompany Daniel to his room. The family was left in the emergency room while Daniel was wheeled away, and security was called to restrain them there until Social Services arrived.

The social worker arrived to the situation and first went to speak to the doctor. The doctor said that he felt the parents neglected Daniel's needs and he was very concerned for Daniel's welfare. He added that Daniel had signs of abuse on his chest and was malnourished. It was his duty to call child protective services. In the meantime, Daniel was undergoing tests to determine what was wrong with him. The physician left to attend to Daniel as the social worker returned to the emergency room to speak with the parents.

The social worker met the parents and found out by simple cards with different languages what language they spoke. She was then able to get an interpreter through a language service. She collected basic facts about the boy and his current medical situation. She was also able to get a phone number to a neighbor of the family who was bilingual. She was able to convey to the parents that their son was going to have some medical tests to determine why he is sick and how to make him better.

The family's neighbor was able to come to the hospital to help to communicate with the family. It turned out that the boy had been sick for a few weeks and the family members were using traditional means to care for their son. "Coining," where a coin is rubbed on the ailing part of the body, was performed by the mother to "drive out the cough." The family also believed that a special diet of herbs and natural foods would cleanse his body and bring him back to health. It was very apparent to the social worker that they loved their son very much and were doing everything in their means to make him well.

She determined that they were not neglectful, but did not understand Western medicine and the importance that we as Americans place on our medical system. She spoke with the doctor and relayed, through the family interpreter, that the boy needed special treatment with medication. The family was scared as they did not trust the medical system. With the help of the interpreter, the nurses spent some time teaching the family some techniques, using pictures. The parents were allowed to be with their son. The nurses allowed the family to set up the child's room to allow "spiritual healing" to occur. They also took the time to explain everything that they were doing to the family.

A member of the family's church came to visit the boy and spoke with the nurses and doctor about some of the family's traditions, and they all decided on a few that the family would be able to carry out in the hospital room. For example, instead of prayer with the use of candles, the nurses obtained a battery-operated candle that used a light bulb for the flames. The family was also shown manual airway clearance techniques to perform in place of coining to assist Daniel with coughing.

The team held family meetings with Daniel's family frequently during his admission, with the use of medical interpreters. A mutual trust developed between the team and the family. Daniel began to get well and was discharged home with his family. He was followed as an outpatient and continued to enjoy a healthy and happy life.

Points to Ponder

How could the emergency room situation have been handled differently?

How did the social worker's behavior change the situation?

Do you think that the family of Daniel was negligent? Why or why not?

Did the doctor provide family-centered care? Why or why not?

What would you do if you were responsible for the care of this child?

REFERENCES

1. O'Neil ME, Palisano R. Attitudes toward family centered care and clinical decision making in early intervention among physical therapists. *Pediatr Phys Ther*. 2000;12:173–182.
2. McGrath JM. Family: essential partner in care. In Kenner C, Lott JW, eds. *Comprehensive Neonatal Care: An Interdisciplinary Approach*. 4th ed. St. Louis, MO: Saunders Elsevier; 2007:491–509.
3. *Census 2010 Profile*. Washington, DC:U.S. Department of Commerce, Economics, and Statistics Administration, U.S. Census Bureau; April 2012.
4. Reynolds D. Improving care and interactions with racial and ethnically diverse populations in healthcare organizations. *J Healthcare Manag*. 2004;49:4.
5. U.S. Department of Health and Human Services. *Health Communication in Health People 2010: Understanding and Improving Health*. 2nd ed. Washington, DC: U.S. Government Printing Office; 2010. Available at http://www.cdc.gov/nchs.
6. Sweeny J, Heriza CB, Blanchard Y, et al. Neonatal physical therapy. Part II: practice frameworks and evidence-based practice guidelines. *Pediatr Phys Ther*. 2010;22(1):2–16.
7. Iverson M, Shimmel J, Ciacera S, et al. Creating a family-centered approach in early intervention services—perceptions of parents and professionals. *Pediatr Phys Ther*. 2003;15:23–31.
8. ED.gov. U.S Department of Education. www.idea.ed.gov. Accessed November 16, 2013.
9. Harry B. Trends and issues in serving culturally diverse families of children with disabilities. *J Special Educ*. 2002;36:131–138.
10. The Joint Commission on the Accreditation of Healthcare Organizations. *Comprehensive Accreditation Manual for Hospitals*. Oak Brook, IL: Joint Commission Resources, Inc; 2006.
11. Wilson-Stronks A, Lee KK, Cordero CL, et al. *One Size Does Not Fit All: Meeting the Health Care Needs of Diverse Populations*. Oakbrook Terrace, IL: The Joint Commission; 2008. Available at: http://www.ipfcc.org/about/index.htm
12. Newton M. Family-centered care: current realities in parent participation. *Pediatr Nurs*. 2000;26:164–169.
13. Mitchell MJ, Lemanmek K, Palermo TM, et al. Parent perspectives on pain management, coping and family functioning in pediatric sickle cell disease. *Clin Pediatr (Phila)*. 2007;46(4):311–319.
14. Harvey J. Proceedings from the Family Re-Union 7 conference. Nashville, TN:Vanderbilt University; 1998. Available at: http://www.familycenteredcare.com. Accessed October 7, 2006.
15. The Institute for Family Centered Care. Patient and Family-Centered Care. Available at: http://www.familycenteredcare.com. Accessed October 7, 2006.
16. Ferguson P. A place in the family: an historical interpretation of research on parental reactions to having a child with a disability. *J Special Educ*. 2002;36:124–130.
17. Suris JC, Michaud PA, Viner R. The adolescent with a chronic condition. Part I: developmental issues. *Arch Disabled Child*. 2004;89:938–942.
18. Blum R. A consensus statement on health care transitions for young adults with special health care needs. *Pediatrics*. 2002;110:1304–1307.
19. Americans with Disabilities Act of 1990, Pub L 101-336.
20. Groce E, Irving Z. Multiculturalism, chronic illness and disability. *Pediatrics*. 1993;91(5):1048–1055.
21. McMillan A. Relevance of culture on pediatric physical therapy: a Saudi Arabian experience. *Pediatr Phys Ther*. 1995;7(3):138–139.
22. Camphina-Bacote J. Many faces: addressing diversity in health care. *Online J Issues Nurs*. 2003;8:1.
23. Anderson PP, Fenichel ES. *Serving Culturally Diverse Families of Infants and Toddlers with Disabilities*. Arlington, TX:National Center for Clinical Infant Programs; 1989.
24. Thomas SB, Quinn SC. The Tuskegee Syphilis Study, 1932–1972: implications for HIV education and AIDS risk programs in the Black community. *Am J Public Health*. 1991;81:1503.
25. Guerrero AD, Chen J, Inkelas M, et al. Racial and ethnic disparities in pediatric experiences of family-centered care. *Med Care*. 2012;48(4):388–393.
26. Taylor J. The story catches you and you fall down: tragedy, ethnography, and cultural competence. *Med Anthropol Q*. 2003;2:159–181.
27. Kleinman A. *Patients and Healers in the Context of Culture: An Exploration of the Borderline Between Anthropology, Medicine, and Psychiatry*. Berkeley, CA: University of California Press; 1980.
28. Parry K. Patient-therapist relations: culture and personal meanings. *Phys Ther*. 1994;2(10):88–345.
29. Pachtner LM. Culture and clinical care: folk illness beliefs and their implications for health care delivery. *JAMA*. 1994;271:690–694.
30. Munet-Vilaro F, Vessey JA. Children's explanation of leukemia: a Hispanic perspective. *Adv Nurs Sci*. 1990;15(2):76–79.
31. Spearing E, Devine J. A qualitative analysis of attitudes towards disability between Hispanic and Anglo-American families of children with chronic disabilities. *Pediatr Phys Ther*. 2004;16:65.
32. Graham RJ, Robinson WM. Intergrating palliative care into chronic care for children with severe neurodevelopmental disabilities. *J Dev Behav Pediatr*. 2005;26(5):361–365.

33. Lawson LV. Culturally sensitive support for grieving parents. *MCN Am J Matern Child Nurs.* 1990;15(2):76–79.

34. Gartner A, Lipisky D, Turnball A. *Supporting Families with a Child with a Disability.* Baltimore, MD:Paul H. Brooks Publishing Co; 1991.

35. Camphina-Bacote J. A model and instrument for addressing cultural competence in health care. *J Nurs Educ.* 1999;38:203–207.

36. Byrd W, Clayton LA. *An American Health Dilemma: A Medical History of African Americans and the Problem of Race.* New York, NY: Routledge; 2000.

37. National Standards for Culturally Linguistically Appropriate Services in Health Care. Washington, DC: U.S. Department of Health and Human Services; April 2007.

38. Bronheim S, Goode T, Jones W. *Policy Brief: Cultural and Linguistic Competence in Family Supports.* Washington, DC: National Center for Cultural Competence; 2006. Available at: http://gucchd.georgetown.edu. Accessed October 7, 2006.

39. Best A, Greenhalgh T, Lewis S, et al. Large-system transformation in health care: a realistic review. *Milibank Q.* 2012;90(3):421–456.

40. The Office of Minority Health. U.S Department of Health and Human Services. National Standards on Culturally and Linguistically Appropriate Services (CLAS). Available at: http://minorityhealth.hhs.gov/templates/browse.aspx?lvl=2&lvlID=15. Last updated April 2007. Accessed December 2012.

Development

I

Development

Motor Development in the Normal Child

Emilie J. Aubert
Photo credit to Ryan C. Aubert and Emilie J. Aubert

The Variability of Human Growth and Development

Developmental Theories
Maturational Theories
Behavioral Theories
Dynamic Systems Theories
Central Pattern Generators
Which Developmental Theory Is Correct?

Preterm Infants

Developmental Direction

The Neonate

Motor Development Goals

The Developmental Progressions
Prone Progression
Supine Progression
Rolling Progression
Sitting Progression
Erect Standing Progression
Stair Climbing

Balance

Fine Motor Development
Grasp
Release

The 2-to-7-Year-Old Child

Summary

Normal or typical development of abilities and skills in humans begins at the moment of conception. In normal conception and pregnancy, the **embryo** (conception through the 8th week of gestation) and the **fetus** (the 9th week of gestation until birth) develop according to a sequence and timing common to all humans.[1] Birth typically occurs at 40 weeks of gestation or 10 lunar months after conception, plus or minus 2 weeks.[2,3] Infants considered to be **term** or **full term** have a gestational age of 38 to 42 weeks.[2,3] Postpartum development of human behaviors is the continuation of that which began at conception. A person's development occurs over his or her life span as the body undergoes change. It has been said that human development is an ongoing process from the womb to the tomb.

After a child is born, change occurs at a relatively rapid rate compared with many changes in adulthood. Particularly notable during the first 24 months of life are the acquisition of and changes in gross and fine motor skills.

New gross and fine motor skills are definitely learned and refined after age 2, but many of these new and refined motor behaviors occur as the child or adult learns new skills needed for play, sports, and/or work. Also, new motor skills are acquired and refined as needed when the individual has particular age-appropriate functional requirements. Dr. Milani-Comparetti has referred to these as *appointments with function.*[4] Some of these appointments with function occur at relatively typical times in life, such as learning to independently don and doff one's jacket in time to begin kindergarten, learning to drive at age 16, or learning to tie one's own necktie when moving away from home to attend college. The chronologic ages of achievement of motor behaviors and skills are influenced by these appointments with function and numerous intrinsic and extrinsic factors, both prenatally and postnatally.[5]

Gestational and postgestational motor development usually occurs according to a typical sequence, pattern, and timing. However, after birth, extrinsic factors such as opportunity to learn and practice a skill, exposure to environmental pollutants, inadequate nurture and bonding, and parental and cultural childrearing practices may modify age of skill acquisition and possibly the sequence and pattern of the motor behaviors. As the child ages, more latitude must be allowed for the expression of differences in development as a result of the many and varied extrinsic factors (see Table 2.1).

Behaviors that develop in the human include gross motor, fine motor, cognitive, language, and personal–social behaviors. Although the emphasis of this chapter is on chronologic motor development, a thorough appreciation for and understanding of a child's development stems from knowledge regarding all developmental domains, as well as growth parameters such as strength and range of motion. Additionally, one must consider the development of and changes in the various systems of the body. All of

TABLE 2.1	Examples of Extrinsic Factors That Affect Motor Development	
Factor	**Example**
Opportunity	Stair climbing develops earlier in a child who must contend with stairs in the home, compared with children who are not permitted on stairs.
Environmental pollutants	Children raised in an environment of smoke from cigarette smoking may be delayed in developing motor skills and may have stunted growth.
Inadequate nurture and bonding	Infants who are not held to be fed may experience motor delay as well as failure to thrive.
Parental and cultural childrearing practices	Children placed supine to sleep may be slower to develop head control in prone and upright, prone-on-elbows posture, and rolling prone to supine.

these areas interact together as the child matures, grows, and develops.

The focus of this chapter is on normal or typical gross and fine motor development in the infant and toddler. The motor developmental sequence offers physical therapists a foundation for studying and understanding not only typical development, but also aberrant or atypical development of the child. This developmental sequence may be used as a basis for evaluating, assessing, and treating motor delays and deficiencies in both children and adults. The sequence, in particular, can play an important role in evaluating and treating people of all ages because identifiable components of motor behavior begin to evolve in specific aspects of the sequence. For example, in the prone-on-elbows or -forearms position typical of a 4-month-old infant, once able to assume the posture, the child begins to shift weight while maintaining the posture. This shifting of weight contributes the beginnings of movement components such as elongation of the trunk on the side bearing more weight (i.e., to the side the weight is shifted), unilateral weight bearing in the upper extremities to allow for visually directed reaching, and early accidental rolling from prone to supine. If the prone-on-elbows posture is not achieved or is delayed, the evolution of some of the mentioned movement components may be delayed, or the components may not develop.

Each stage of the motor developmental sequence has purpose and contributes to the overall development of the child. Therefore, various aspects of the sequence can be used in therapy, for adults and children, to facilitate the evolution of different movement components. In the evaluation and assessment of children, the typical timing of the acquisition of specific motor skills is linked to the determination of a **motor age**. Ideally, as an infant or toddler develops, the assessed motor age will be congruent with the child's chronologic age. A gap between the child's chronologic age and motor age, assessed according to established standards for age of skill or **milestone** development, is undesirable.[6-9] The greater the gap between chronologic age and motor

age, the more likely that the child is exhibiting a possible developmental problem.

In the **habilitation** of a developing child, established norms for the sequence, timing, and patterns of motor behaviors can be used not only to evaluate and assess the child, but also to set treatment goals and develop a treatment plan. This is not to say that the sequence must be followed in some strict manner when habilitating or rehabilitating a child or an adult. Rather, the sequence can be used as a guide, and it informs our understanding of the need for particular movement components in order to develop and refine particular functional motor skills.

Care must be taken when using the terms *normal* and *typical* when speaking about the motor development of a child, especially regarding age of milestone acquisition. Normal is defined as conformity with the established standards for humans.[10] Typical is defined as having the qualities of a particular group, in this case, human infants and children, so completely as to be representative of that group.[10] The reader should keep in mind that what is normal or typical motor behavior of humans at various ages is generally described in ranges. Such ranges exist because both motor development and individual motor skills are affected by numerous factors, in addition to the intrinsic biologic nature of the human. Even the intrinsic anatomy and physiology of a human are, in many ways, uniquely his or her own. For the purposes of this chapter, the terms normal and typical will be used synonymously.

Normative values for age of skill acquisition, based on a defined subject pool, are set forth in numerous norm-referenced developmental instruments.[6-9,11-14] Because the norms are based on a limited, albeit large, group of subjects and therefore established with certain cultural bias, extrinsic factors such as cultural customs, parental practices, and opportunity to learn skills may detract from or improve a child's score.[15-24] Therefore, this text emphasizes a rather broad range of achievement ages, based on several norm-referenced evaluation and assessment tools. Also, it is important to note that typical ages of achievement are usually based on full-term gestation in humans, which is 40 weeks.[2,3] Table 2.2 shows approximate expected ages of acquiring specific motor milestones for full-term infants.

▶ The variability of human growth and development

Although human birth, growth, and development have long histories, our understanding of these processes has increased and been refined over time. As we continue to study all aspects of human development, one characteristic of human development clearly stands the test of time. Human development is characterized by variability. In fact, lack of variability, either within one individual or when comparing an individual with textbook standards, is often a red flag. The less variable and more stereotypical a child's

TABLE 2.2 Ages of Motor Milestone Acquisition in Typical Full-term Infants		
Milestone	**Typical Age**	**Age Range**
Physiologic flexion	Birth	N/A
Turns head to side in prone	Birth	NA
Attempts to lift head in midline	1 mo	1–2 mo
Automatic stepping	Birth	N/A
Fencer's posture	2 mo	1–4 mo
Astasia	2 mo	N/A
Abasia	2 mo	N/A
Rolling supine to side-lying nonsegmentally	3 mo	2–4 mo
Beginning midline head control	3 mo	2–3 mo
Prone-on-elbows, head to 90 degrees, chin tuck	4 mo	3–5 mo
Hands to midline	4 mo	3–5 mo
Unilateral reaching prone-on-elbows	5 mo	4–6 mo
Prone-on-extended-arms	5 mo	4–6 mo
Pivot prone posture	5 mo	4–6 mo
Beginning intra-axial rotation	5 mo	4–5 mo
Rolling prone to supine, segmentally	5 mo	4–6 mo
Head lifting in supine	5 mo	4–6 mo
Supine, hands to knees and feet	5 mo	4–6 mo
Supine, hands to feet	5 mo	4–6 mo
Supine, feet to mouth	5 mo	4–6 mo
Propped sitting	5 mo	5–6 mo
Supine bridging	5 mo	5–7 mo
Rolling supine to prone, segmentally	6 mo	5–7 mo
Ring sitting, unsupported with full trunk extension and high guard	6 mo	5–7 mo
Transferring objects hand to hand	6 mo	5–7 mo
Independent sitting with secondary curves	8 mo	7–9 mo
Beginning quadruped	8 mo	7–9 mo
Beginning pull-to-standing	8 mo	7–9 mo
Creeping	10 mo	9–11 mo
Plantigrade posture	10 mo	10–12 mo
Plantigrade creeping	10 mo	10–12 mo
Pulls to standing and lowers self	10 mo	9–12 mo
Cruising	10 mo	9–11 mo
Pulls to standing through half-kneeling	12 mo	10–13 mo
Walking independently	12 mo	10–15 mo
Creeps up stairs*	15 mo	14–18 mo
Walks up stairs with help or handrail*	18 mo	16–20 mo

*Age of achievement of ascending and descending stairs depends greatly on motivation, opportunity, and experience.

movements are, the more likely that his or her development and movement are atypical.[25–27]

Motor development and motor behaviors vary because of the influence of numerous intrinsic (endogenous) and extrinsic (exogenous) factors, many of which we cannot influence or control. However, many intrinsic and extrinsic factors can be controlled and manipulated to optimize

fetal and infant development. For example, it is now known that fetal exposure to alcohol of unknown quantities can result in a child who has fetal alcohol syndrome (FAS), alcohol-related neurodevelopmental disorder (ARND), or alcohol-related birth defects (ARBD).[28–33] Children who have been exposed to alcohol or illicit drugs in utero have been found to exhibit delayed mental, motor, and/or behavioral development when compared with standardized norms at 1, 4, 12, and 18 months and 2, 3, and 5 years of age.[34–41] Furthermore, prenatal alcohol effects on fetal, infant, and child development are not totally known, and the effects can be compounded by other pre-, peri-, and postnatal risk factors.[35,40,42–45] Fetal alcohol exposure is something that can be controlled (i.e., eliminated) during pregnancy, thereby effectively eliminating the potential adverse effects of alcohol on growth and development. To the contrary, if a woman unexpectedly develops a disease process during pregnancy, the disease may impact the fetus and child negatively. However, this insult to the developing embryo or fetus may not have been preventable.

The variability of human motor development has been the subject of much study. Scientists and therapists have attempted to explain the differences in motor development between one person and another, and have tried to discover ways to optimize those factors that produce healthy motor behaviors and minimize those that have a negative impact.

A number of theories about how humans develop motor and other behaviors have been proposed. Brief descriptions of some of these theories follow. The reader should keep in mind that just as no two humans develop exactly alike, it is most likely that no single theory can explain developmental fact.

▶ Developmental theories

Developmental theories have been applied to all aspects of infant and child development, including physical, psychosocial, and cognitive. To effectively work with children, physical therapists need to have a broad understanding of all areas of infant and child development. However, physical therapists most definitely need a broad and deep understanding of the physical aspects of growth and development. Therefore, those developmental theories that adequately address a child's physical development are easiest to apply in physical therapy. Those theories will be emphasized in this brief discussion.

Maturational Theories

Maturational theories, also referred to as hierarchical theories, have been developed and advanced by people with familiar names such as Piaget, Gesell, Bayley, and McGraw, beginning in the early 1900s. The works of these developmental theorists continue to contribute heavily to our understanding of child development today.[6,29,46–50] Their legacies are seen in the clinics worldwide. For example,

Nancy Bayley's early work from the 1930s produced standardized scales for mental and motor development.[51-53] Her work continues to be a powerful clinical tool for assessing a child's mental and/or motor development, with a third edition of the *Bayley Scales of Infant Development* having been published.[6]

Maturational theories of development emphasize a *normal developmental sequence* that is common to all fetal, infant, and child mental and motor development. According to *maturationists*, the normal sequence of development evolves as the central nervous system (CNS) matures, and the CNS is the major driving force of development.[50,53-56] Hierarchical theory has been interpreted by some to suggest a strict, invariant sequence of development in all *normal* children.[50,51] However, others have interpreted hierarchical development in a less stringent manner, including many physical therapists that have practiced since the 1970s who understand the hierarchy of motor skills to be merely, but consistently, a roadmap. Nonetheless, many of these same therapists believe in the primacy of the CNS in dictating developmental sequence and timing.

Behavioral Theories

A behavioral theory of development is rooted in the works of Pavlov, Skinner, and Bandura, with emphasis on conditioning behavior through the use of a stimulus-response approach.[51,54] Behavior theory advocates modifying behavior through manipulating stimuli in the environment to create a response that positively or negatively reinforces a particular behavior.[51,57,58] This type of theory is used by physical therapists when they control the environment to elicit a predictable behavior. For example, a therapist may move a very distractible child from the physical therapy gym to a quiet room, in order to control or improve the child's ability to stay on task. Therapists also use a stimulus-response approach when they manipulate parameters such as intensity, rate, and frequency of application of a given treatment modality.[59] Regarding motor development, some of a child's motor behaviors (responses) are conditioned by positive or negative feedback to particular behaviors.[60,61] For example, one typically developing child evaluated by this author spent very little time creeping on hands and knees, showing a preference for plantigrade creeping on hands and feet. Engaging in the plantigrade creeping as a major form of locomotion seemed to be the result of conditioning. During this pre-walking stage of development, which happened to occur during the summer, the child spent considerable time playing outdoors on the family's concrete patio and sidewalk. It did not take him long to *learn* that the trio of rough surfaces, shorts, and creeping on hands and knees could cause great discomfort and even injury. The stimulus of the rough surface, with *givens* of hot weather and summertime apparel, conditioned a movement response that kept his bare knees off the rough surface, yet still allowed him to locomote and explore his environment.

Dynamic Systems Theories

The third and final developmental theory to be addressed here is the dynamic systems theory. This theory is based on the original work of Bernstein in 1967 and has been modified by numerous others more recently, including Thelen et al., Horak, Heriza, and Shumway-Cook and Wollacott.[5,50,51,53,54,62] Unlike the longitudinal and hierarchical maturation theories, which consider the CNS to be the predominate factor and manager, organizer, and regulator of development, dynamic systems theories see infant and child development as nonlinear and the result of many factors, both intrinsic and extrinsic, that impact the developing fetus and child. According to the dynamic systems theory, no one system (such as the CNS in the maturational theories) is the preeminent director of development. Instead, each fetus and child develops certain characteristics and skills based on the confluence of many factors.[5,50,51,53-55,62-64] While motor behaviors do seem to develop in the fetus, infant, and toddler according to a basic scheme, the sequence, timing, and quality of developmental milestones may be modified by numerous factors in any one fetus or child.

Factors that influence motor development in the human include genetic inheritance, errors and mutations in genetic transmission, maternal/fetal and child nutrition, fetal and infant exposure to toxins and other chemical substances, race, ethnicity, presence or absence of quality prenatal care, childrearing practices, socioeconomic level (which may have immense bearing on several of the other factors mentioned here), disease processes, and trauma. In addition, opportunity, cognitive abilities, level of stimulation, and motivation affect the learning of new motor skills in children and adults, as do the motor task at hand, the functional outcome desired, and the context for using a particular motor skill.[5,15,19-21,28,29,34,42,46,49-51,65-77]

In a dynamic systems view of growth and development, the CNS is merely one, albeit very important, influential system. Unlike a purely hierarchical or maturational viewpoint, a dynamic systems approach to development considers the profound influences of other body systems on the anatomic, physiologic, and behavioral qualities of the fetus and child (the organism). These other systems include the peripheral nervous, musculoskeletal, cardiopulmonary, and integumentary systems.

Central Pattern Generators

"Today the existence of networks of nerve cells producing specific, rhythmic movements, without conscious effort and without the aid of peripheral afferent feedback, is indisputable for a large number of vertebrates. These specialized neural circuits are referred to as 'neural oscillators' or 'central pattern generators' (CPGs)."[78] It is known that the brain stem has CPGs for rhythmic functions such as chewing, breathing, and swallowing.[50,78-80] The spinal cord has CPGs for functional locomotion.[78,81]

In the absence of afferent input, the CPGs can still produce stereotypic, rhythmic movements such as locomotion. This is not to say that sensory feedback is not an important factor in normal locomotion.[78] However, the idea that motor output can occur without first having sensory input is contrary to early thinking in this field of study.[59]

Which Developmental Theory Is Correct?

Motor development in humans and motor behaviors have been shown to be under the influence of supraspinal structures, spinal structures, peripheral sensory input, CPGs, dynamic environmental features, and neuromodulatory influences. Supraspinal centers that control human locomotion include the sensorimotor cortex, cerebellum, and basal ganglia.[78] Sensory afferents, from the periphery, are important regulators of movement, helping modify the patterns generated centrally so that movements can be constantly adapted to the environment, task, and task context.[78] Neuromodulators such as serotonin and dopamine are also thought to influence centrally generated locomotion in some vertebrates, but their role is not yet completely understood.[78]

Among the many theories of development, including those affecting motor development, probably no single theory can ever be considered the one and only correct theory. Rather, many different theories can be called upon to explain and predict fetal and child motor development. Principles from different theories can be combined to analyze, interpret, and even predict motor development. Many aspects of the dynamic systems approach probably come the closest to being the dominant theory of motor development used by physical therapists in the 21st century, because this approach, in itself, considers the impact of many variables on the creation, growth, and development of a human biologic system. Having said that, it is this author's opinion that many contemporary physical therapists, in an effort to de-emphasize the hierarchical aspect of development, risk under consideration of the basic motor development sequence that has characterized fetal and child development for thousands of years. Given the multitude of environments in which children have grown and developed over time, the similarities in the *normal developmental sequence* and motor milestone acquisition among infants and toddlers are simply too great to be ignored.

▶ Preterm infants

Because of the prematurity, **a preterm** or **premature** infant, defined as one with a gestational age of less than 38 weeks, may not exhibit motor skills consistent with his chronologic age.[3] The child born too early may demonstrate motor delays equivalent to the number of weeks premature.[82,83] In order to distinguish between delays that are the natural result of not having enough in utero time and delays caused by abnormal pathophysiology, the premature infant is evaluated and assessed according to an **adjusted age**. Adjusted

---

DISPLAY
2.1   Calculating Adjusted Age for Preterm Infants

Date of Birth (DOB):   April 21, 2006
Gestational age (GA):   31 weeks 6 days
Date of Assessment (Date):   December 28, 2006

Child's chronologic or postnatal age = 8 mo 1 wk = 33 wk
Gestational age in weeks = 32 wk
40-32 wk = 8 wk adjustment for prematurity
33 wk-8 wk = **25 wk gestation-adjusted age**
(6 mo 1 wk)*

Disagreement exists regarding the chronologic or postnatal age, from 12–18 months, a child should be before the clinician stops adjusting for prematurity, for the purpose of assessing motor development. A standard should probably be set in a particular clinic, with variations made on a case-by-case basis as necessary.

---

*For the purpose of clinical assessment of an infant's motor development, this child would have a corrected or adjusted age of 6 months. For research purposes, adjusted age should be calculated accurately to the months, weeks, and days. A computerized formula is often used. When administering a standardized test, adjusted age should be calculated accurately as well, using the formula given for a particular standardized instrument, as the formulas differ from one standardized test to another.

---

age is determined by subtracting the **gestational age** of the child, the number of weeks and days in utero, from 40 weeks. This remainder is then subtracted from the child's actual **chronologic age**, which is calculated from the date of the child's birth.[82,83] A sample adjusted age calculation is shown in Display 2.1.

▶ Developmental direction

Studying the typical sequence of motor development reveals a developmental direction that applies to most of development, although there are exceptions. Pertinent exceptions will be noted in the following discussion. Ten sequences of developmental direction are listed in Table 2.3, with examples of how these sequences are revealed in normal development. A few of these principles deserve additional attention to develop an understanding of the typical emergence of motor skills in humans.

Motor behavior in humans is at first reflexive in nature. As the organism matures, motor behaviors become more complex and eventually come under **cortical** or **volitional** control. This is an example of **reflex to cortical** developmental direction. Additionally, primitive reflex responses tend to be more generalized rather than localized responses. This **generalized or total movement before the development of localized movement** in a given area of the body is another example of developmental direction. A good example of a generalized response is the response seen in the **flexor withdrawal reflex**. This reflex is a **primitive reflex**

TABLE 2.3	Examples Reflecting Principles of Developmental Direction	
Principle	**Earliest Control/Response**	**Control/Response with Maturation**
Reflex control before cortical control	Asymmetrical tonic neck reflex causes limbs to move in response to the head position.	Child volitionally moves limbs independent of head position.
Total response before localized response	Neonate moves upper extremities in wide sweeps and at random.	Child gains control of individual joints to stabilize the shoulder for precise, visually directed reach and grasp.
Proximal control before distal control	Child develops shoulder and hip stability.	Elbow, then wrist, and knee, then ankle, stability develop.
Cephalic control before caudal control	Shoulders develop control and stability.	Hips develop control and stability.
Medial control before lateral control	Three ulnar fingers dominate first grasp.	Thumb and index finger dominate pincer grasp. Forefinger dominance develops.
Cervical control before rostral control	Child has motor control of mouth at birth.	Child develops ability to fix eyes and focus.
Gross motor control before fine motor control	Child stabilizes the shoulders and holds a baby bottle with both hands.	Child picks up tiny pellets and puts them in a small bottle.
Flexor muscle tone develops before extensor muscle tone	Neonate is dominated by physiologic flexion.	Flexor tone loses dominance, and extensor tone is more manifest to balance tone.
Extensor antigravity control develops before flexor antigravity control	Child lifts head in prone at 4 months of age.	Child lifts head in supine at 5 months of age.
Weight bearing occurs on flexed extremities before on extended extremities	Child bears weight on upper extremities flexed at elbows in prone-on-elbows.	Child bears weight on extended elbows in prone-on-extended-arms and quadruped.

that is present at birth and produces a total flexion response in the limb, either upper or lower, when the hand or foot, respectively, is exposed to a **noxious** or **nociceptive** stimulus (Fig. 2.1). The response to the stimulus in this reflex, because it is primitive and generalized, does not permit selective or isolated movements at the various joints of the limb when elicited. The flexor withdrawal reflex is present at birth and becomes partially integrated by 2 months of age.[46] However, vestiges of this reflex remain throughout

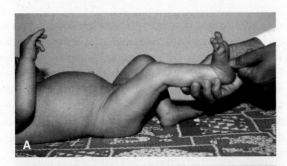
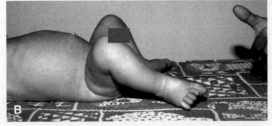

FIGURE 2.1 Flexor withdrawal reflex. A: Nociceptive stimulus to the sole of the foot. **B:** Flexor withdrawal response, total lower extremity flexion.

life as a protective mechanism for the hands and feet. The flexor withdrawal reflex is controlled at the level of the spinal cord in the CNS.[46] Most early or primitive reflexes are spinal cord reflexes, whereas the mature postural and balance responses are mediated in the midbrain and the cortex of the brain. The stimulus for a spinal cord reflex is an **exteroceptive** stimulus.[5] The receptors for exteroceptive stimuli are "peripheral end organs of the afferent nerves in the skin or mucous membrane, which respond to stimulation by external agents."[1,5,84,85] Another example of a **total response** developing before **localized response** is neonatal kicking. When the infant is first born, he or she moves in very random total patterns. In fact, full-term neonates, when compared with preterm neonates, exhibit a variety of neonatal kicking patterns, with differences in frequency, reciprocal movements, and intralimb *coupling*.[86–88] Coupling is defined by Heathcock et al. as similar timing of movement between joints within the same limb.[86] Heathcock et al. also found that full-term neonates were able to exhibit task-specific and purposeful lower extremity control compared with their preterm cohorts.[86] When some **neonates** kick, both lower limbs often move together, the infant being unable to consistently **dissociate** one lower extremity from the other. Also, when kicking, the pelvis frequently moves with the lower extremities, another example of lacking dissociation. In this case, the lack of dissociation is between the hips and pelvis. As the infant matures, he or she is consistently able to move the lower extremities while keeping the pelvis stable, and the right and left limbs can move independently of each other as well as reciprocally, all examples of dissociation. The ability to move the limbs independent of each other allows for **reciprocal kicking**, alternating kicks of the lower extremities. At this point, the infant is also able to move one lower extremity without moving the other and to move a joint within an extremity independent of the other joints in that extremity.

A third principle of developmental direction is **cephalocaudal** development. Generally, this principle is demonstrated in the development of motor control in that the head, upper trunk, and upper extremities develop motor control before the lower trunk and lower extremities. An example of cephalocaudal development of motor control is the development of stability of the scapulae and shoulders to maintain the prone-on-elbows posture, before the development of stability of the pelvis and hips as needed for the quadruped position (Fig. 2.2). An exception to cephalocaudal development is the development of muscle tone in the fetus. Studies of premature infants have shown that muscle tone develops in the lower extremities and lower body before tone in the upper extremities and upper body develops.[89]

Motor control also develops from **medial to lateral**; that is, control develops close to the median or midline of the body before developing more laterally. Midline stability of the neck and trunk develop before the more lateral shoulder and hip stability. During the first few weeks of life, the infant is relatively symmetric, with the exception of the head, which is turned to one side or the other in prone and supine. The second through fourth months of life are characterized in the term infant by asymmetry, as a result of the influence of reflex activity, most notably the **asymmetric tonic neck reflex (ATNR)**[90] (Fig. 2.3). The ATNR influence diminishes over those first months, thereby reducing reflex dominance and allowing the development of volitional control, as noted previously. Volitional control and developing stability begin medially in what is termed **midline activity**. As the ATNR wanes, the child is able to bring his head into midline and maintain it there, instead of being in the asymmetric cervical extension pattern of the ATNR, by 4 months of age. In addition, the child begins bringing his hands to midline, relying on the newly developed shoulder stability to use his hands together in midline (Fig. 2.4). Thus, by 6 months of age, the child demonstrates great symmetry.

Another example of this medial-to-lateral development is the development of grasp. To understand this, one must visualize the body in anatomic position. The ability to grasp and manipulate objects with the hands begins with

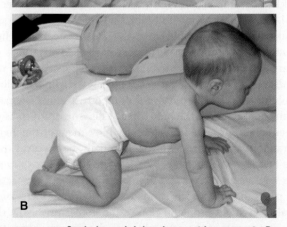

FIGURE 2.2 Cephalocaudal development in prone. A: Prone-on-elbows posture with prestance positioning of lower extremities; the more cephalic shoulder girdle exhibits stability. **B:** Quadruped posture; the more caudal hip exhibits stability as well.

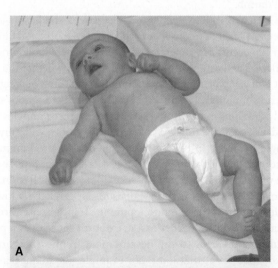

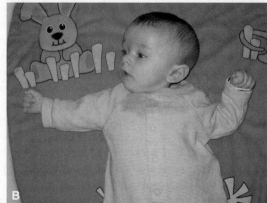

FIGURE 2.3 Asymmetric tonic neck reflex (fencer's posture) with head turned to right; note the extension of the face-side limbs and flexion of the skull or occiput-side limbs. **A:** Fencer's posture seen here in an infant 2 months of age. **B:** Fencer's posture waning.

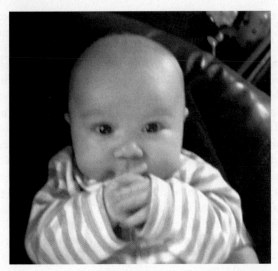

FIGURE 2.4 Notable symmetry of infant; head and hands are stable in midline.

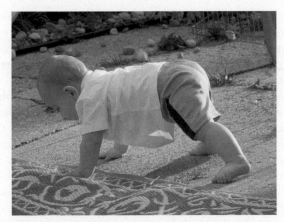

FIGURE 2.5 Plantigrade position with weight bearing on palms of hands and soles of feet; this is a transition posture between being on the floor and erect standing and may also be used as a locomotive form called plantigrade creeping.

predominant use of the ulnar fingers, which are more medial, before using the more lateral index finger (radial finger) and thumb.[91]

Control of the two major muscle groups, the flexors and extensors, also develops in a particular developmental direction and occurs in a general sequence. However, development of flexors and extensors differs depending on whether the infant is developing muscle tone, antigravity control, or weight-bearing function. Dominant **muscle tone** throughout the body develops in flexor muscles before extensor muscles, as readily seen in the full-term neonate who is born with **physiologic flexion**.[47,48,92] This physiologic flexion is a dominant flexor tone in all postures when at rest and with passive or active movement. Even in the absence of physiologic flexion, as seen in infants born preterm, extensor tone is relatively low.

In each posture, the development of antigravity movements and control occurs first in extensor muscles at a particular joint, prior to the development of the antagonist flexor muscles at that joint. For example, the infant learns to use his cervical extensors in the controlled antigravity movement of lifting his head in prone before he is able to lift his head against gravity in supine, which requires antigravity flexor control. However, to develop full and balanced control at a joint, both antigravity extensors and antigravity flexors are needed. Cephalocaudally developing trunk extensors for antigravity work develop before the flexors of the trunk. Therefore, the child is able to get into a prone-on-elbows posture by 4 months of age, using midline antigravity extensors, before he is able to bring his feet to his mouth in supine at 5 months of age. The foot-to-mouth activity requires antigravity flexor control of the trunk.

The weight-bearing function of the extremities occurs on flexed extremities before weight bearing occurs on extended limbs. In prone-on-elbows, the infant bears weight on flexed upper extremities, with relatively passive lower extremities. This developmental posture occurs before quadruped, wherein weight bearing is on extended upper extremities (the

elbows) and on flexed lower extremities (knees and hips) (see Fig. 2.2). The plantigrade creeping posture calls for weight bearing on the open hands and soles of the feet (Fig. 2.5). This posture is an example of weight bearing on extended upper extremities (elbows) and extended lower extremities (knees). In addition to exemplifying the rule of weight bearing, this progression from prone-on-elbows to the plantigrade creeping posture is also an example of cephalocaudal development.

Gross motor skills develop before fine motor skills, the infant being able to stabilize the shoulder with the large muscles of the shoulder before gaining control of the small muscles of the fingers and hand for fine motor skills. This exemplifies not only the **gross-to-fine** principle of developmental direction, but also the **proximal-to-distal** principle. Proximal refers to the part of an extremity, upper or lower, that is closest to the midline of the body. Distal means the part of the extremity farthest from the midline.

The neck and trunk muscles and all major joints of the extremities (i.e., shoulders, elbows, wrists, hips, knees, and ankles) develop according to certain stages of motor control. They develop mobility, stability, controlled mobility, and skill, as described by Sullivan et al.[85] This sequence was first described with different terminology, in the early 1960s by Margaret Rood.[59] In the upper extremity, the sequence unfolds in the following manner. The shoulder first develops mobility, the ability to move the upper extremity in space with the distal end, the hand, free. This is referred to as an **open-chain** movement.[93] The early movement of the infant is random and poorly controlled initially, but evolves over the first few weeks of life. Success with this ability to move the upper extremity at the shoulder in an open-chain activity paves the way for the shoulder to stabilize in the **closed-chain** activity of prone-on-elbows and -forearms.[93] Now, the distal segments of the extremity (i.e., the forearm, hand, and fingers) are not free in space. Rather, the extremity is performing a weight-bearing function, described by Rood as the stability aspect of motor behavior. Next, the infant demonstrates the ability to move the proximal joint, the shoulder in

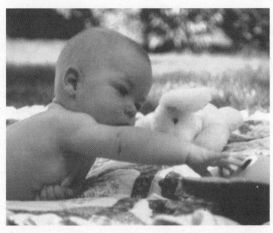

FIGURE 2.6 Unilateral weight bearing in prone-on-elbows posture with weight shift to the skull side and one upper extremity freed for reaching.

this example, over the distal extremity while the extremity is in a closed chain. This movement is seen as the development of weight shifting in the various weight-bearing postures of the upper extremities. Rood and others have described this phase as mobility superimposed on stability.[59,85] Eventually, the child is able to shift his weight entirely onto one or the other upper extremities for unilateral weight bearing. Then he begins to stabilize the non–weight-bearing shoulder with the hand free (open-chain activity), as the fingers move to grasp and manipulate an object, as seen in Figure 2.6. This represents the skill level denoted by Rood.[59,85]

The lower extremities follow the same sequence for developing mobility, stability, controlled mobility, and functional distal control. This sequence plays out again and again, for both the upper and lower extremities, in each of the developmental postures of prone-on-elbows,

prone-on-extended-arms, sitting, quadruped, and erect standing. In sitting without support and erect standing, the upper extremities play a vital role in providing stability of the upper body, even though they are not performing a weight-bearing function. This will be described later in this chapter when the sitting and erect standing sequences are explained.

▶ The neonate

The neonatal period in the infant is the first 28 days of post-partum life.[3] Full-term infants are born with **physiologic flexion** as described earlier, a prime example of muscle tone developing in flexor muscles before extensor muscles. This results in generalized moderate flexion in all positions of the neonate, prone, supine, held in sitting, vertical or horizontal suspension, and held in standing.[47,48,91,92] This flexor tone gradually diminishes over the first month of life in these full-term babies.

Babies who are preterm exhibit less physiologic flexion or the flexion is absent, depending on the child's gestational age.[94,95] The more weeks the child is preterm, the less likely he is to have the physiologic flexion. Instead, preterm infants are born with limbs and trunk relatively extended. This extension is not a dominance of extensor tone, but rather a lack of or diminished flexor tone. The reasons for this lack of flexor tone in the preterm infant are unknown. Several theories have been suggested, including intrauterine positioning and maternal hormonal influences.

In addition to lack of physiologic flexion in preterm neonates, other differences between full and preterm infants are noted at birth. These differences have been well described by Dubowicz and others, and a few of the major differences are shown in Table 2.4.[2]

TABLE 2.4	Differences Between Full-term and Preterm Neonates		
Tone and Movement Patterns	**Preterm Neonate (<32 wk)**	**Full-term Neonate (>36 wk)**	
Posture	Full extension	Physiologic flexion (full flexion)	
Scarf sign: arm passively moved across chest of child in supine with head midline	No resistance to passive movement	Resistance to passive movement before reaching midline	
Popliteal angle: passively move knee to chest; extend knee	Angle of extension between lower leg and thigh is 135 to 180 degrees	Angle of extension between lower leg and thigh is 60 to 90 degrees	
Ankle dorsiflexion: infant supine, passively flex foot against shin	Angle between lower leg and foot is 60 to 90 degrees	Angle between lower leg and foot <30 degrees	
Slip-through: infant in vertical suspension, holding under axillae	Completely slips through hands, does not set shoulders	Sets shoulders and does not slip through	
Pull-to-sit: child supine, pull-to-sitting by pulling gently on both upper extremities	Complete head lag	Head held in alignment with body	
Rooting reflex: child supine in midline, stroke corner of mouth	Absent	Head turns toward stimulus and mouth opens	
Sucking reflex: put nipple or clean finger in child's mouth	Weak or absent sucking response	Strong rhythmic sucking	
Grasp reflex: place finger horizontally in child's palm	Absent	Sustained flexion and traction	
ATNR: child supine with head in midline, passively turn head to one side	Absent	Upper and lower extremities on face side extend, extremities on skull-side flex	

Motor development goals

One goal of normal motor development is control of the body against gravity.[4] These antigravity movements generally develop first in the head, followed by development in the trunk (cervical to thoracic to lumbosacral), then in the lower extremities. Antigravity control in the lower extremities includes control at the three major joints of the hip, knee, and ankle. While the overall development of antigravity control is cephalocaudal, as revealed by the development of head control, then midline trunk control, and then lower extremity control, control at the various joints of the lower extremities may be occurring simultaneously, very close together in timing, or with the ankle being the lead joint.

Antigravity movements must develop in both extension movements and flexion movements. However, in mature, erect standing, the major body extensor groups are the antigravity muscles, as compared with their flexor antagonists. That is, the midline neck and trunk extensors, hip extensors, and knee extensors are the primary muscle groups that keep humans from surrendering to the force of gravity when upright.

A second goal of development is the ability to maintain the body's center of mass within the base of support.[4] The center of mass when standing is gradually and progressively rising as humans grow in height. Learning to maintain the body's center of mass within the base of support is accomplished as the infant and toddler develop righting, equilibrium, and tilting reactions. While these reactions develop and continue to be activated automatically, the typically developing individual can eventually control these automatic responses volitionally, as long as there are no intrinsic or extrinsic barriers to such control.

A third goal of motor development is the performance of intrasegmental and intersegmental isolated movements.[4] For example, even though various joints of the upper extremity move in a coordinated manner to produce an upper extremity functional skill, the individual joints, such as the elbow joint, must learn to move independently while the other upper extremity joints do not move. This is intrasegmental dissociation. Intersegmental dissociation, such as moving the head without moving the extremities or moving one lower extremity into flexion while moving the contralateral lower extremity into extension, must develop as well.

The developmental progressions

Rather than discussing motor development as a timeline of chronologically occurring events, this text will present the sequence of occurrences that leads to the development of various components of movement. This sequence includes various motor milestones and postures and movement within these postures. Because these events in the normal infant and toddler develop in an orderly sequence in each posture, these sequences will be referred to as **progressions**.

One of the earliest developmentalists, Myrtle McGraw, defined these progressions.[47] Prone, supine, rolling, sitting, and erect standing progressions will be presented, as well as various forms of locomotion in each progression.

Stabilizing in various postures is termed static posture and is in contrast to dynamic posture, the translation of those static postures into movement for locomotion, transitions between postures, and prehension.[48] These static and dynamic postures are often referred to as motor milestones. Particularly significant ages of performing certain milestones will be discussed. More detail of the age ranges for the achievement of these motor milestones can be found in Table 2.2. An important point to note is that the ages of acquisition of certain skills fall within ranges rather than at exact points in the developing child. Each developing child is unique, both in the intrinsic factors, biologic structure and function, and in the extrinsic factors that affect his or her development. This uniqueness must be remembered and considered, even though basic commonalities of anatomy, physiology, sequential development, and pathology exist.

Prone Progression

Prone Lying

At birth, the healthy, full-term neonate has physiologic flexion, which dominates the prone position.[96] In prone, the head is turned to one side (Fig. 2.7). This turning of the head to one side is the result of two primary influences. The first influence is a survival instinct, which allows the infant to turn his head to the side to clear his mouth and nose so he can breathe in prone, and the second is the influence of the ATNR.[46,97] Although the normal infant can be moved out of this pattern easily, the ATNR continues to influence head position in all postures, including prone, until the influence has completely subsided by approximately 4 months of age. Encountering considerable resistance to moving the child out of this ATNR-dominated fencer's posture may be an indication of atypical neuromotor development.[98,99]

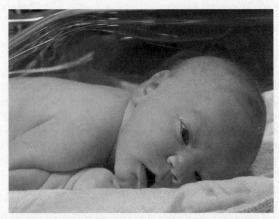

FIGURE 2.7 Neonate in prone; note the extreme shoulder adduction of the upper extremity with the elbow caudal to the shoulder in this infant only 2 hours after birth.

The hip flexion aspect of physiologic flexion is particularly strong in prone lying and is accompanied by a relative anterior tilt of the pelvis. The infant's knees are drawn underneath him with buttocks up in the air, and the exaggerated hip flexion and anterior tilt are preventing the pelvis from lying flat on the surface (Fig. 2.8). His weight is shifted forward onto his upper chest and face. When his head is turned to one side, the weight shifted onto the head is borne by the child's cheek on that side. The upper extremities are adducted into the side of the body with the elbows caudal to the shoulders. Hands are generally fisted, due to the strong influence of the hand grasp reflex. However, the hands frequently and spontaneously will open and can be opened passively in the normally developing infant. Persistently fisted hands that never open may indicate abnormal sensorimotor development.[98] Persistently fisted hands with the thumb flexed into the palm and held by the fingers is often a sign of pathology.[100–102]

As physiologic flexion diminishes over the first month, the infant begins falling more and more into gravity in both prone and supine. In prone, hip flexion decreases, allowing the buttocks to come down and the anterior pelvis to lie flat against the surface. Weight shifts away from the face, caudally toward the trunk and lower extremities. However, a relative anterior pelvic tilt is still present, albeit decreased (Fig. 2.9A-C). The diminished nature of the anterior pelvic tilt is not due to an active posterior tilt at this point but results simply from the loss of the physiologic flexion that kept the hips and knees flexed underneath the child's body.

As physiologic flexion disappears completely, the child lies flat on the surface in prone (Fig. 2.10). The hips are now passively extended and prepared for the beginning of active posterior pelvic tilt, which is an indication of the activation and development of the abdominal muscles (the trunk flexors) and the hip extensors. Without the buttocks in the air, the child's weight is no longer shifted forward onto the chest and cheek but instead is borne over all the body segments that are in contact with the surface. The infant at this point has no active antigravity control, with the exception of cervical extension, which is beginning to emerge.

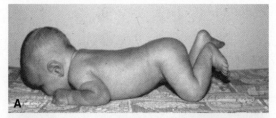
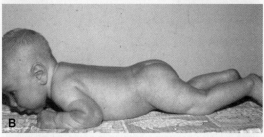
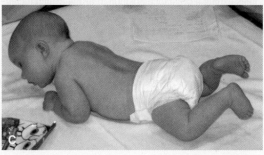

FIGURE 2.9 Neonate in prone. **A:** Note the anterior pelvic tilt and hip flexion, with buttocks up in the air; position prevents infant from lifting his head from the surface. **B:** As physiologic flexion diminishes, pelvis comes down toward the mat with decreasing hip flexion and anterior pelvic tilt; pelvis is flatter on the surface as caudal weight shifting evolves, making it easier for the child to begin to lift his head in prone. **C:** As anterior tilt continues to decrease, weight continues to shift caudally from head and upper chest to pelvis and lower extremities, improving attempts to lift head and attain prone-on-elbows, but pelvis is still in a relative anterior tilt, and upper extremities are held close to the sides with the elbows too caudal for weight bearing.

In the ensuing prone posture, the lower extremities are positioned in hip abduction, partial extension, and external rotation (Fig. 2.11). Knees are semiflexed and feet are dorsiflexed. This position of the lower extremities is the precursor to the position of the lower extremities in initial standing. Beginning at approximately 5 months of age, the

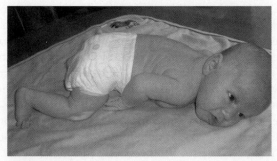

FIGURE 2.8 Physiologic flexion in a 3-week-old neonate; note that the shoulder adduction has decreased, and the hips and knees are still flexed with the buttocks up in the air.

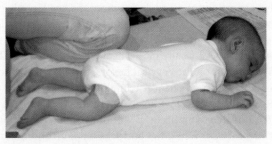

FIGURE 2.10 Physiologic flexion is gone; infant is flat in prone with elongated hip flexors and a relatively neutral pelvis.

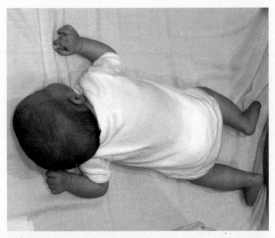

FIGURE 2.11 Once physiologic flexion has disappeared, lower extremities exhibit a prestance position in prone, which includes hip external rotation with slight flexion and abduction, slight flexion of the knee, and dorsiflexion of the ankle.

child will stand, with hands held or holding onto something such as the crib rails, with this same wide base of support, hips, knees, and feet mimicking the early lower extremity position seen in prone.

Prone-On-Elbows

To achieve the **prone-on-elbows** or prone-on-forearms posture, the next step in the prone progression, three things must happen: (1) stabilization of the pelvis, (2) head lifting with cephalocaudally progressing antigravity extensor control, and (3) movement of the upper extremities out of the neonatal position.

Head control in prone is the earliest antigravity control to develop. In order for the infant to begin experimenting with head control, he must move the head away from the support of the surface. To lift his head, he must actively contract his cervical extensors. At birth he was able to lift his head only briefly in prone to turn his head to the side for breathing. The first truly active attempts at lifting his head in prone are tenuous, at best (see Fig. 2.9). Body proportions of infants are different than those in older children and adults. In the infant, the head makes up approximately one-quarter of the body in length, causing the head to be proportionately large and heavy.[103] This compares with the body proportions of an adult, in whom the head is only one-eighth of height.[103] Maturation and practice of the skill of head lifting strengthen the cervical extensor muscles so that the infant can eventually lift his heavy head (Fig. 2.12). This ability depends on the cervical flexors, the anterior muscles, to lengthen through reciprocal inhibition.

Even with cervical extensors increasing in strength, the child is not able to lift his head without stabilizing in another part of his body. When the buttocks were up and the head was down, weight was shifted toward the head. If the head is to be up, the buttocks must be down, the weight must be

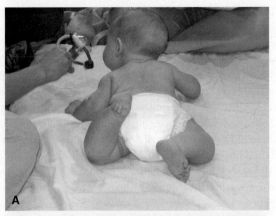

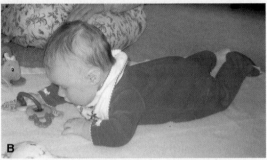

FIGURE 2.12 Infant has a relative posterior pelvic tilt, which promotes the use of the antigravity cervical extensors for head lifting in prone. **A:** Note the more abducted and forward position of the upper extremities and the prestance position of the lower extremities. **B:** Improved head lifting so that the face is at a 45-degree angle.

shifted caudally, and the pelvis must stabilize for head and midline upper trunk lifting. If one thinks of the child's head and upper trunk as being a lever arm, the fulcrum around which the lever arm turns for this movement is the pelvis, so the pelvis must be stabilized. This stabilization of the pelvis is achieved by recruiting abdominal muscles to tilt the pelvis posteriorly and hold it stable in a posterior tilt. With the help of the abdominal muscles to stabilize the pelvis in a relative posterior tilt, the infant begins actively lifting the head at approximately 2 months of age. By 3 months, cervical extension is adequate to lift the head such that the baby's face is at a 45-degree or greater angle with the surface, and head control is mostly due to antigravity extensor muscles (Fig. 2.12B and 2.13). As development of the spinal extensors progresses cephalocaudally, the upper thoracic extensors begin to strengthen and gain antigravity control. By 4 months, the baby is able to lift the head to 90 degrees. However, the chin of the infant who is able to lift his head to 90 degrees tends to jut forward slightly, with the neck hyperextended, during early successes in the prone-on-elbows and prone-on-extended-arms postures (Fig. 2.14). Although the infant has control of his cervical and upper thoracic antigravity extensors to lift the head to this face vertical position, one element of head control is still missing. Control at any joint in the body depends on a balance of muscles

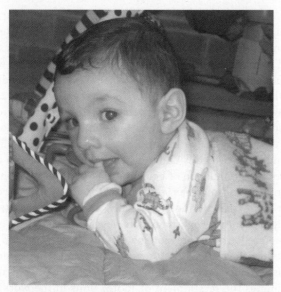

FIGURE 2.13 At 3 months of age, the child attains prone-on-elbows with the face at an angle greater than 45 degrees, not yet 90 degrees; note the forward position of elbows.

surrounding that joint. Therefore, head control is not complete until the antigravity cervical flexors have been activated and strengthened to balance the antigravity cervical extensors.

The child's ability to use his midline cervical extensors to lift his head is a sign of the diminishing ATNR and the development of active cervical flexors. Although the strength of the ATNR diminishes during the first 4 months, the waning influence continues to provide slight cervical asymmetric extension. Once the child begins to develop active cervical flexors to balance those extensors, the head is more easily brought to midline for lifting in prone. Continued strengthening of the cervical flexors, along with the activation of the serratus anterior muscles in the prone-on-elbows posture, contributes to what Bly refers to as a **chin tuck** when the head is lifted to 90 degrees so that the face is vertical (Fig. 2.2A).[104]

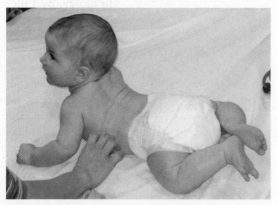

FIGURE 2.14 Infant in prone-on-extended-arms with face vertical (at 90 degrees) but with mild cervical hyperextension and without chin tuck.

The infant who is 4 months of age and has stable control of the head at 90 degrees, with the chin tucked, displays balanced cervical extensors and flexors. By comparison, head control of the 3-month-old child during head lifting is dominated by extensors that are not balanced by antigravity flexors, helping produce a chin that is not tucked.

Chin tuck appears, therefore, as a result of three developmental occurrences: (1) activation and strengthening of the cervical flexors, (2) reduction of the ATNR, and (3) activation and strengthening of the serratus anterior muscles. The infant uses the serratus anterior muscles to protract the shoulder girdle and work the elbows into the surface. Without the protraction provided by these muscles, the child may exhibit what Bly and others have termed *TV shoulders*.[104] In TV shoulders, the child's upper extremities are not worked into the surface. Rather, the shoulders elevate and the neck hyperextends, with the infant's occiput resting on his posterior cervical soft tissue, chin jutting forward. The face, in this position, is not at 90 degrees or vertical, and the child does not have active head control. With the shoulders elevated at the sides of the head, close to the ears, the head is passively supported. Consequently, persistence of the TV shoulders interferes with the development of active, antigravity head control and lateral head righting. TV shoulders also make it difficult to swallow, talk, and breathe, because of the cervical hyperextension.

If at 4 months of age the child exhibits cervical hyperextension with the occiput of the skull resting on the upper back, the cervical flexors and/or serratus anterior muscles are not activated or have insufficient strength. This is an example of how the developmental sequence and the movement components might be used to determine a plan of treatment. If a child exhibits TV shoulders while prone-on-elbows, the strength of the serratus anterior muscles as well as the strength of the cervical flexor and extensor muscles should be tested. Weakness of any of these muscles may account for the cervical hyperextension, at least in part. If the cervical extensors are weak, it is likely that they are too weak to maintain the head upright, and once the head is lifted, the child compensates for the inability to actively stabilize the neck. His head falls backward into hyperextension as a response to gravity. This is a pattern frequently seen in children who have delayed or abnormal sensorimotor development, such as children with cerebral palsy or other brain disorders. In such a case, one part of the physical therapy treatment plan would include strengthening the muscles that are weak and practicing control over those muscles.

The third element necessary for the child to achieve the prone-on-elbows milestone is a forward position of the elbows. The upper extremities, in the full-term neonate, are adducted closely into the body, or even slightly under the body, and extended at the shoulders, causing them to have a mechanical disadvantage in trying to lift the upper trunk and head (see Fig. 2.8). During the second month, at the time when the infant is first attempting to lift his head, upper extremity control at the shoulder begins to develop.

The infant gradually abducts and flexes the shoulders, bringing the elbows from underneath his body forward, more to a position underneath or just anterior to the shoulders. This enables the baby to bear weight on his elbows and forearms when he lifts his head. Figures 2.7 through 2.9, 2.12, and 2.13 show this progression. One important component of movement that begins to develop in this process is **scapulohumeral** elongation. Scapulohumeral elongation refers to the elongation of the axillary region as the humerus is flexed and/or abducted away from the body and therefore away from the scapulae. Without the ability to elongate this region, the child will not be able to get the elbows into position underneath the shoulders for the prone-on-elbows posture. Failure to elongate the axillary region will also interfere with reaching out in space, such as when an older child reaches out to grasp an object while sitting at his desk.

While the upper extremities are typically envisioned as limbs with important mobility functions, such as reach and grasp, and the lower extremities are visualized in terms of their weight-bearing functions, such as standing, all four extremities have both weight-bearing and mobility functions to perform. Prior to assuming the prone-on-elbows posture, the upper extremities have exhibited only mobility functions. The prone-on-elbows posture is the first call for the upper extremities to be weight bearing. This ability to weight-bear through the forearms, elbows, and shoulders foreshadows the weight bearing that will follow in the quadruped position.

Once the infant has achieved a stable prone-on-elbows position, in order to be functional he must be able to translate the position into movement while maintaining stability at the proximal joint, the shoulder. He begins to shift his weight from side to side, increasing the amount of weight bearing on each upper extremity as the weight is shifted to that side. Shifting weight side to side soon becomes shifting of weight in all directions, including forward, back, and diagonally. This weight shifting is a feature of all the milestone postures once the stability of each posture has been established. It is critical for the development of equilibrium and tilting responses for maintaining balance, as well as for functional use of the upper extremity. In the prone-on-elbows posture, if the baby does not learn to shift his weight, his upper extremities will not be able to develop controlled mobility functions. Essentially, he will be stuck. Without the appropriate development of weight shifting, the controlled mobility functions of reaching (open chain) and the closed-chain propulsion function of the upper extremities, needed for crawling and creeping, will not develop.

Weight shift is necessary for reasons other than just to free a limb for controlled mobility. Weight shift encourages elongation of muscles on one side of a joint or joints while the antagonist muscles shorten. In typical sensorimotor development, this elongation during weight shift occurs in the lateral trunk muscles on the side that is weight bearing or bearing most of the weight. For example, when

the child shifts his weight while in quadruped such that he unilaterally weight-bears on an upper extremity, the lateral trunk on the side bearing the weight is elongated (relaxed and stretched) while the lateral trunk on the side of the free upper extremity shortens (contracts), with lateral bending or flexion to that side (Fig. 2.15). Figures 2.16 through 2.21 show this elongation on the weight-bearing side in different postures and at different ages.

Weight shift also introduces the infant to vestibular stimulation, which is under his control, as opposed to the vestibular stimulation of being moved by another person or an object (rocking chair) or watching another person or object move (the crib mobile). Finally, when in full unilateral weight bearing, weight shift increases the weight borne, and therefore joint compression, on a particular side or limb up to twice the normal customary weight and compression. This increased weight on one limb or one side of the trunk facilitates the recruitment of motor units in the working muscles.[59,105]

Weight shifting in prone-on-elbows has another subtle, yet significant, effect on the baby's development. Babies are born with their forearms in relative pronation and are unable to supinate the forearms actively, even though the forearms can be moved passively into supination. As the baby shifts from side to side in prone-on-elbows, the weight shifting causes the forearm on the side to which he shifts

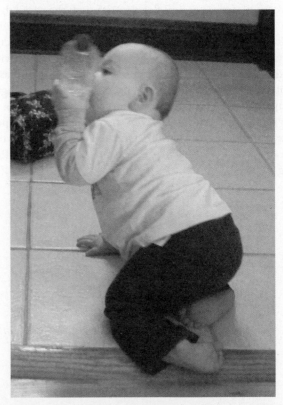

FIGURE 2.15 Unilateral weight bearing in the upper extremities from quadruped with elongation of the child's trunk on the side bearing the most weight, in this case his right side.

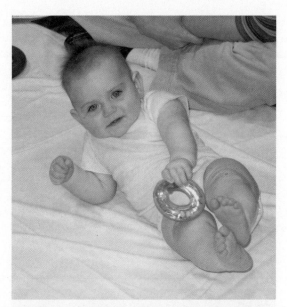

FIGURE 2.16 Weight shift to side-lying with elongation on the right (weight-bearing side).

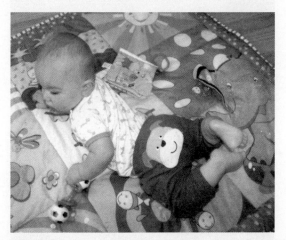

FIGURE 2.17 Prone-on-elbows with weight shift to skull side for unilateral weight bearing with elongation on the weight-bearing side.

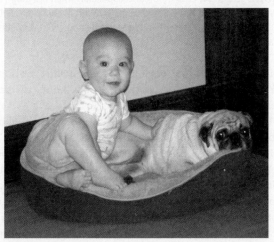

FIGURE 2.18 Sitting with weight shifted to child's left side with elongation of the weight-bearing side; note the crossing of midline with the lower extremity.

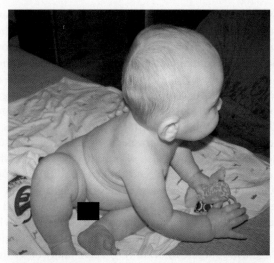

FIGURE 2.19 Sitting, shortening of the right side with weight shift to the left side; note the high degree of intra-axial rotation.

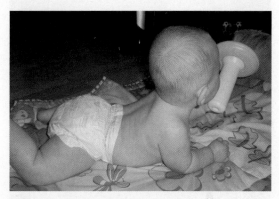

FIGURE 2.20 Prone-on-elbows, elongation on child's right side with reaching with the left hand.

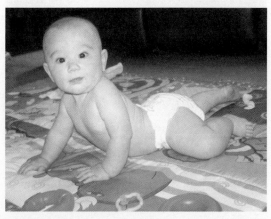

FIGURE 2.21 Prone-on-extended-arms with muscles of the weight-bearing anterior trunk, pelvis, and lower extremities elongated; also note the slight weight shift to child's right side with shortening of left lateral trunk musculature.

his weight to supinate, and the forearm on the side away from which he shifts pronates. The proprioceptive feedback from this reciprocal pronation and supination lays the foundation for emerging, active forearm supination. Without the ability to supinate the forearms, the infant would not develop the ability to reach for, grasp, and visually engage an object. With the forearm in pronation, the first two steps can be accomplished, but the dorsum of the hand blocks the child's view of the object grasped (Fig. 2.22). Lack of supination of the forearm is also responsible for spillage when children first attempt to feed themselves with a spoon. The child holds the spoon and captures the food with the forearm in pronation. As he brings the spoon toward his mouth, he needs to supinate in order to keep the bowl of the spoon level. Until he develops full active supination, spillage will continue to occur (Fig. 2.23). Many other functional activities across the life span depend on the ability to

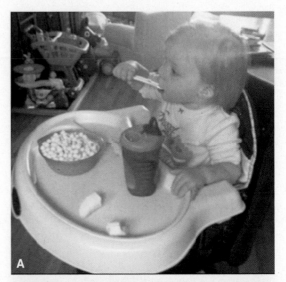

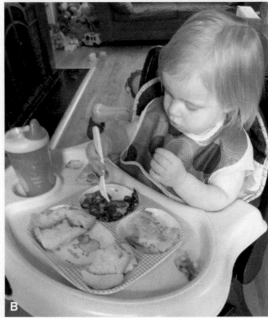

FIGURE 2.23 A: Lack of forearm supination when bringing the spoon to the mouth causes spillage. **B:** With the development of forearm supination, a child is able to use a spoon with very little spillage.

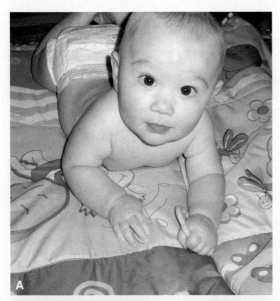

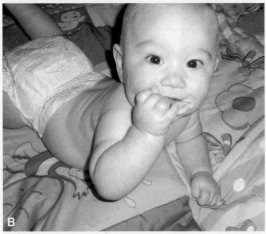

FIGURE 2.22 A: With forearm in pronation, visual examination of toy grasped in hand is blocked by the dorsum of the hand. **B:** The development of forearm supination allows visual examination of object and putting the object in the mouth with ease.

supinate the forearms, such as donning a shirt, buttoning and unbuttoning a shirt, turning a door knob, turning a steering wheel, and tying a bow.

As the child practices weight shift in prone-on-elbows, he begins to take an interest in reaching for toys from this position. First attempts at reaching while prone-on-elbows often fail because the child shifts his weight onto the side to which he is looking (Fig. 2.24). Eventually, the child learns from the error of his ways that his weight is shifted onto the very limb he needs to unweight in order to reach for the toy he sees. With practice of weight shifting in this posture and through trial and error, the child is eventually able to shift his weight to one elbow and forearm while looking in

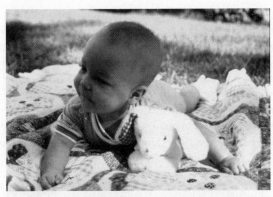

FIGURE 2.24 First attempts at visually directed reaching in prone-on-elbow or -extended-arms are often unsuccessful because the child shifts his weight in the direction that he is looking, and the arm nearest the object is not freed.

the opposite direction, thereby establishing visually directed reaching (Fig. 2.25).

Prone-On-Extended-Arms

Having secured the prone-on-elbows posture and having learned to shift his weight in different directions, the baby begins to lift himself farther from the surface. He pushes himself up into prone-on-extended-arms, working his open hands into the surface, using his triceps to extend his elbows, and actively using the serratus anterior muscles to protract and stabilize the shoulder girdle (Fig. 2.26A). The trunk extensors, continuing to activate and strengthen in a cephalocaudal direction, assist in this antigravity movement. The anterior thoracic muscles must elongate. The elbows, in the prone-on-extended-arms posture, illustrate the principle of weight bearing on extended limbs after first weight bearing on flexed limbs. In addition to the extended elbows, this posture is noted for increased antigravity extension using midline thoracic extensors, increased scapulohumeral

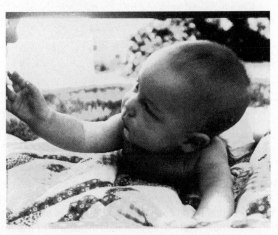

FIGURE 2.25 Eventually, the child learns to shift his weight to the skull-side limb, freeing the appropriate arm for reaching the object as he looks at it.

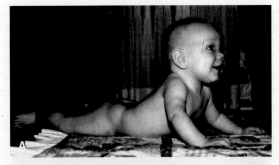

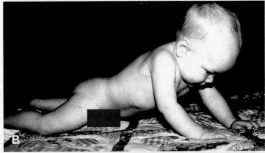

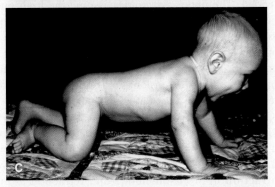

FIGURE 2.26 Transition from prone-on-extended-arms to quadruped. A: Prone-on-extended-arms. **B:** Push-up transition position. **C:** Quadruped.

elongation, a pelvis still in a relative posterior tilt in order to stabilize the lifted head and upper trunk, and comparatively passive lower extremities.

Although the lower extremities are decidedly passive in prone-on-elbows and prone-on-extended-arms, the position assumed by the lower extremities in these postures is predictive of later development and active use of the lower extremities. It is the same lower extremity position seen in the infant after the loss of physiologic flexion (Figs. 2.2A and 2.26A).

Once the child has begun to push into prone-on-arms with extended elbows, he begins to weight-shift in that posture, just as he did in the prone-on-elbows position. Weight shifting produces increased stability at the shoulder joints as more weight is accepted onto one or the other shoulder during weight shifting. Weight shifting to the side eventually produces unilateral weight bearing with the ability to reach and grasp, with the accompanying elongation of the trunk on the weight-bearing side. Posterior weight shift may actually cause him to move himself backward in this position, increasing scapulohumeral elongation. While pushing backward, the child may lift his buttocks from the surface, continuing to push his weight backward over the knees and into the quadruped posture, with weight on open hands. If he pushes with enough force, he may shift his weight backward onto his toes, rather than his flexed knees, in a "push-up" position (Fig. 2.26B). Eventually, the child succeeds in getting his weight shifted posteriorly onto his knees for hands-and-knees weight bearing (quadruped or four-point). He is definitely pleased with his accomplishment (Fig. 2.26C).

Pivot Prone

At approximately 5 months of age, the child develops an interesting skill that contributes to his pelvic and scapular mobility. The pivot prone posture or pattern, as seen in Figure 2.27, uses cephalocaudally progressing extension to extend the child's neck, midline trunk, and lower extremities. The pelvis is in an anterior tilt, with hips hyperextended. The upper extremities assume the **high guard** position with the scapulae adducted by the rhomboid muscles. The upper limbs are horizontally abducted at the shoulders and flexed at the elbows. This **retraction** of the shoulder girdle with the posturing of the upper extremities enhances the trunk extension. To assume the pivot prone pattern, the anterior musculature must elongate.

Once the child develops stability in the pivot prone position, he playfully moves alternately between pivot prone and prone-on-elbows. In this manner, he practices scapular and pelvic mobility. The shoulder girdle alternates between **protraction** in prone-on-elbows and retraction in pivot prone. The pelvic girdle moves between the posterior tilt of prone-on-elbows and the anterior tilt of pivot prone. Often, in his exuberance, the child actually pivots his body in a circle as he kicks his legs or quickly alternates between these two postures.

Quadruped

As in other postures, early attempts at the hands-and-knees posture are generally not refined, often because the lower extremities are not positioned optimally to accept weight

(Fig. 2.28). But with practice, the child soon masters another new skill. Refer again to Figure 2.2B. His open hands are aligned under flexed shoulders, and his knees are aligned under flexed hips. The active participation of the lower extremities in **quadruped**, also called **four-point**, requires stability around the hip joints caused by cocontraction of the hip musculature. The principles of developmental direction are illustrated well in quadruped. Weight bearing on flexed elbows has given way to weight bearing on extended elbows.

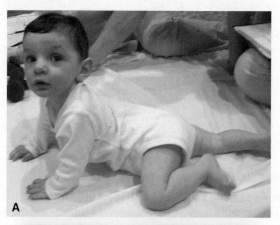

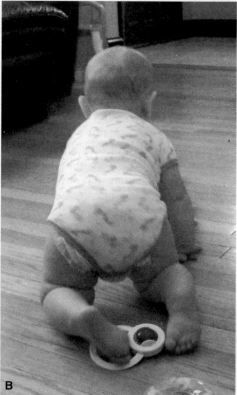

FIGURE 2.28 Immature quadruped position with hip abduction and external rotation, lower extremities in poor weight-bearing alignment; reciprocal and contralateral movement of extremities. **A:** Note the lumbar lordosis, an indication in quadruped that the abdominals are weak or not being activated. **B:** Improved quadruped position, but base of support is still wide, interfering with lateral weight shift for creeping.

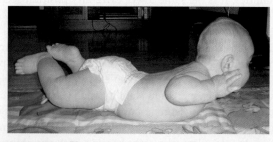

FIGURE 2.27 Pivot prone posture with elongation of anterior trunk and lower extremity musculature and retraction of shoulder girdle; only mid- and lower trunk are in contact with the supporting surface.

True to cephalocaudal development, the lower extremities now participate actively, unlike when in prone-on-elbows. Stability in quadruped increases, as it does in prone-on-elbows and prone-on-extended-arms, as the child moves into the weight-shifting phase of the quadruped posture. When weight is shifted posteriorly, with the upper extremities fixed in a closed-chain, scapulohumeral elongation is facilitated. The base of support in quadruped may be wide in initial attempts, particularly because of excessive abduction of the lower extremities (Fig. 2.28B). This wider base of support helps the child to be more stable. However, it interferes with adequate lateral weight shift, which is needed to achieve unilateral weight bearing. Unilateral weight bearing is necessary in both the upper and lower body to free one upper and one lower limb for the forward movement of creeping.

A stable quadruped position requires not only stable hips and shoulders, but also a stable trunk. Trunk flexors and extensors must balance each other to produce a flat back in the four-point position. When the child first achieves the quadruped posture, he generally displays the lumbar lordosis of the young infant whose abdominal musculature is not yet developed and strong. This is due to underdeveloped abdominal muscles as well as strong contraction of his hip flexors in order to stabilize. Overly active hip flexion is progravity fixing to increase muscle tone around the hip joints, and therefore stability. Increased hip flexion posturing leads to increased lumbar lordosis or anterior pelvic tilt. Development of the abdominals begins when the child first acquires the posterior tilt, which was essential for lifting of the head in prone. Concurrent with the achievement of a stable prone-on-elbows posture, with its posterior pelvic tilt resulting from activation of abdominal muscles, changes are taking place in the supine position to further recruit and strengthen abdominal muscles. Abdominal musculature continues to develop to balance the extensors of the trunk. With the balance of lumbar flexors and extensors, the quadruped position with a flat back is achieved (see Fig. 2.2B).

Locomotion in Prone

Locomotion is defined as movement from one place to another.[1] Six modes of locomotion develop in the prone position typically. In the order of development, they are scooting, crawling, pivoting in prone, rolling, creeping, and plantigrade creeping. Some locomotive forms may develop and be used nearly simultaneously, such as crawling and pivoting in prone, at approximately 5 months of age. Also, it is not unusual for one or more modes of locomotion not to develop in a given child. No long-term negative effects result from such failure. However, it is important for the child to develop, in other ways, any components of movement that typically develop or improve in the different forms of prone locomotion.

As early as a few days of age, the infant is able to move in the crib by wiggling and scooting. This is his first form of locomotion. Inevitably, an infant placed in the middle of a crib for a nap will find his way to a corner of the crib. It is thought that the closeness and security offered by a corner is comforting to the child, especially after 40 weeks in the close spaces of the womb. Because infants are able to wiggle and scoot, not even the youngest of babies should be left unattended on a raised surface such as a sofa, adult bed, changing table, or mat table, unless sufficient barriers of pillows and rolls have the infant contained.

During the first 2 months, when the infant is in prone or supine, he will wiggle and scoot as his chief form of locomotion. Once he attains and is stable in the prone-on-elbows position, he may locomote by crawling, moving his body forward by digging his elbows and forearms into the surface and extending his shoulders. **Crawling** is a locomotive form that infants may use from 3 months to 8 or 9 months of age. Crawling is defined as moving "slowly by dragging the body along the ground."[10,47,48,106] First attempts at crawling often produce a backward motion as the infant flexes his shoulders, instead of extending them. Once he achieves a forward progression, he may crawl by moving both forearms forward at the same time, or he may crawl by using reciprocal motions of the upper extremities (Fig. 2.29). This reciprocal motion is a precursor to reciprocal creeping, plantigrade creeping, and walking with reciprocal arm swing.

The defining component of crawling is that the child's belly is in contact with the floor. This compares with **creeping**, which means to move across the floor on hands and knees without the trunk being in direct contact with the surface.[10,46–49,106] While this distinguishing component may seem inconsequential, especially when the lay public often uses the terms synonymously, differentiating between crawling and creeping is important in the health care professions so that terminology is used consistently, leaving no room for misunderstanding.

In crawling, the lower extremities are basically passive while the upper extremities move either together or reciprocally. Crawling with nonreciprocal use of the upper extremities requires no trunk rotation, while reciprocal crawling does require rotation within the body axis. In **rotation** of the

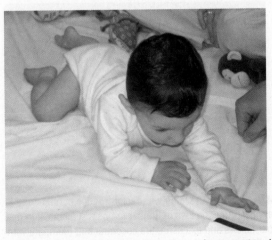

FIGURE 2.29 Crawling with reciprocal use of upper extremities.

trunk, either the upper or the lower trunk moves while the rest of the trunk remains stable. Rotation of the upper trunk means the upper trunk moves on a stable, nonmoving lower trunk. The converse is true as well. Reciprocal, contralateral creeping requires counterrotation, a progressively more complex movement. This contralateral movement requires counterrotation within the trunk. **Counterrotation** is defined as rotating the upper trunk to one side, while rotating the lower trunk in the opposite direction. Counterrotation of the trunk is a different movement from simple rotation of the trunk.

Pivoting in prone, as described previously, is a form of locomotion that some infants use in conjunction with crawling or rolling to move intentionally in a particular direction. For example, if the child wants to reach a toy that is out of his immediate space, he will often use a combination of these movements to direct himself appropriately to reach his goal.

Rolling from prone to supine and supine to prone, another means of locomotion, develops in the infant by 5 to 6 months of age. Still lacking an efficient locomotive form, once he achieves rolling from prone to supine and supine to prone, he may use a combination of rolling and crawling to move in a specific direction across the floor. The evolution of rolling will be discussed in a later section of this chapter.

At 6 to 7 months of age, while prone-on-extended-arms, he begins pushing his body backward, raising his buttocks into the air in attempts to get into quadruped (hands-and-knees posture). This position, also called four-point, is the position from which his next locomotive form, **creeping**, will develop. Both the upper and lower extremities participate equally in creeping (Fig. 2.30).

Once he is stable on hands and knees, the usual process of weight shifting in various directions occurs. With controlled weight shift he is able to lift one limb at a time, eventually lifting one upper extremity and the opposite lower extremity at once. This movement leads to creeping on hands and knees at approximately 9 to 11 months of age. Typical and refined creeping is both reciprocal and contralateral. In other words, the child advances one arm and the opposite leg at the same time (contralateral), reciprocating with the other arm and leg, which also move together. This contralateral movement requires not only rotation of the trunk, but also counterrotation. The reciprocal activity of creeping helps to refine intra-axial rotation and reciprocal use of the limbs, strengthening counterrotation for use in the higher levels of locomotion.

Plantigrade creeping, sometimes referred to as bear walking, is more of a transitional posture than a form of locomotion. However, some children do use the plantigrade position, open hands and plantar surfaces of the feet in closed-chain contact with the ground, to locomote. In many cases, this type of creeping may be the result of an environmental factor. For example, the child may choose plantigrade creeping over creeping in quadruped if he has bare knees and is on a concrete or other rough surface (see Fig. 2.31). This illustrates the dynamic nature of development. Many factors, in addition to maturation, influence the development of motor skills.

As a transitional posture, the plantigrade position is used by the child as one means of getting to standing from the prone position. In early attempts, the child may rely on being near furniture or a wall for assistance as he rises to standing, going through the plantigrade position to the upright standing posture.

Supine Progression

Supine Lying and Pull to Sitting

Like the prone progression, development in the supine position proceeds in a known sequence. The full-term neonate in supine has physiologic flexion, expressed in slight cervical flexion, with the head held toward midline, elbow flexion, posterior pelvic tilt, hip adduction, and hip and knee flexion. The feet are typically in the air and not touching the table surface. His hands are loosely fisted but are seen to open frequently, both at rest and with the infant's

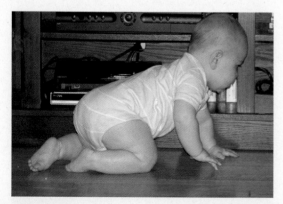

FIGURE 2.30 Creeping with reciprocal use of upper and lower extremities; note the loss of lumbar lordosis, an indication that lumbar flexors and extensors are cocontracting (compare with Fig. 2.28).

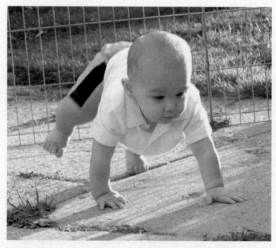

FIGURE 2.31 Plantigrade creeping, also called bear walking.

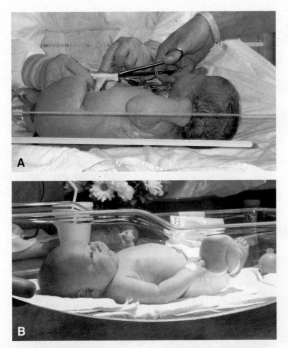

FIGURE 2.32 Physiologic flexion in supine in the full-term neonate; note that the feet are held above the supporting surface, and the hands and fingers are inconsistently in a fist. **A:** Physiologic flexion seen in infant only minutes old. **B:** Physiologic flexion in supine in infant 24 hours after birth. Note the inconsistently fisted hands of the neonate in both A and B.

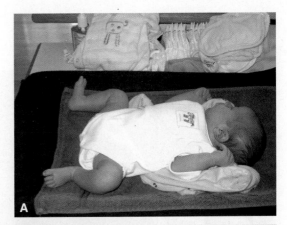
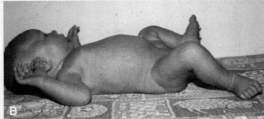

FIGURE 2.33 As physiologic flexion diminishes, **(A)** the hip and knee flexion gradually decrease, **(B)** allowing the feet to rest on the supporting surface.

random movements (Fig. 2.32). When the infant is **pulled to sitting**, the examiner gently pulling the infant's upper extremities at the wrists, the head is held in plane with the body and exhibits no **head lag**, mimicking active head control. Over the first month, as the physiologic flexion gradually disappears, the head falls away from midline to the side, elbows relax, and the hip and knee flexion dissipate, bringing the infant's feet down to the surface (Fig. 2.33). As the feet come down to the surface, the pelvis is pulled into a relative anterior tilt by gravity, now unopposed by physiologic flexion. Increasing hip abduction and external rotation begin to evolve. When pulled to sitting, head lag is present. This means that the infant's head, no longer being supported by the physiologic flexion, lags behind the rest of the body as the child is pulled toward the sitting posture. Antigravity flexors have yet to develop. Without active head control, the child's head falls backward into gravity when he is pulled toward the sitting posture. Over time, as the antigravity cervical flexors become stronger and active head control develops, the infant exhibits less and less head lag when pulled to sitting. After the initial period of head lag, which follows the loss of physiologic flexion, he will begin to hold his head in alignment with the body, in the same plane as the body. Then he learns to lead with his head as soon as the stimulus of being pulled to sitting occurs. Next in the sequence, the lower extremities begin to flex actively at the hips during the pull-to-sitting maneuver. Finally, the pull-to-sitting stimulus recruits cervical flexors, trunk flexors, and hip flexors. Figure 2.34 shows the pull-to-sitting sequence.

In supine, after the first month, the infant usually has his head turned to one side or the other, influenced by the ATNR. The ATNR is manifested in infants during wakefulness and sleep and diminishes over time, as seen in Figure 2.3. This reflex begins prenatally and is manifested by asymmetric extension of the neck, with accompanying predictable limb movements. Under the influence of the ATNR, when the head is turned to one side in slight hyperextension, cervical proprioceptors are stimulated. This causes the **face limbs**, the ipsilateral upper and lower extremities on the side to which the head is turned, to extend. The contralateral limbs, the **skull limbs** or **occiput limbs**, flex. The upper extremity manifestations of the ATNR are usually stronger than the lower extremity manifestations. The ATNR is seen in normal infants during the first 4 months of life, more as an attitude or assumed posture than a strong obligatory position. This posture is frequently termed the fencer's posture (see Fig. 2.3). Although this fencer's posture is evident in nearly all infants during this time period and is seen repeatedly in supine and supported sitting, the ATNR is not so strong in typical infants that it limits voluntary or passive movement of the extremities or head. If the ATNR presents stereotypically, is obligatory during those first months, or produces strong flexor or extensor tone in the extremities, this may be an indication of atypical neuromotor development. In the typical infant, the strength of the ATNR reflex is noted to diminish over time such that by 4 months it is evident inconsistently and finally disappears.[96,98,99,107]

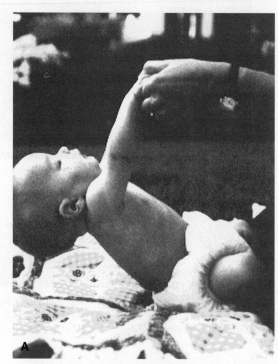

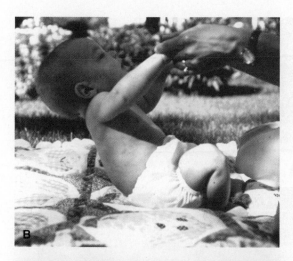

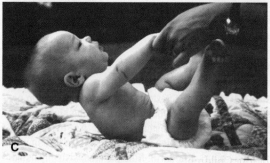

FIGURE 2.34 Pull-to-sitting sequence. A: Head lag when pulled to sitting, denoting lack of antigravity control of cervical flexor muscles. **B:** No head lag when pulled to sitting; as the child matures and control of antigravity cervical flexors develops, the child holds head in the same plane as his body. **C:** Cervical, trunk, and hip flexors exhibit active antigravity control when the child is pulled to sitting.

The ATNR is evidence of the infant's lack of dissociation. **Dissociation** is the ability of the human to move limbs independently from the head, move limbs independently from each other, move joints within the same limb independently, and move the body independently from the head. Head and limbs lack dissociation in a child manifesting an ATNR. The proprioceptors of the neck influence the position of the limbs, resulting in the posture as described. As the child matures and the ATNR loses its influence, the limbs no longer assume specific postures based on the position of the head, thereby demonstrating dissociation.

Another reflex that affects the supine and prone postures is the tonic labyrinthine reflex. The role of the tonic labyrinthine reflex in typical neuromotor development is not well understood, although it seems to provide an underlying predisposition for flexion tone in prone and extension tone in supine.[96,98,99,107] The receptors for this reflex are in the labyrinths of the ears and are responsive to the continuous forces of gravity. The basic functional skills of lifting the head in prone and supine and performing total body antigravity extension in prone (the pivot prone pattern) and antigravity flexion in supine (the feet-to-mouth pattern) are accommodated in the typical infant because resting tone and tone with initiation of movement are not excessive. However, the child with atypical development may

be influenced negatively by the tonic labyrinthine reflex, exhibiting extensor or flexor **hypertonus** that may prevent the development of antigravity contraction of the antagonist muscles in either or both postures. If tone is excessive in extensors in supine, for example, the flexor antagonists are not able to contract because the extensor muscles are not able to relax. This loss of **reciprocal inhibition**, the ability of antagonist muscles to relax or lengthen while agonist muscles contract or shorten, may be strong enough to cause sensorimotor impairment.

As the ATNR diminishes, the infant begins to appear more symmetric in supine (Fig. 2.35). The ability to bring his head to midline and hold it there is a significant milestone. Two processes interact to allow head-to-midline movement. Because the ATNR is an asymmetric influence on the posture of the head, as the ATNR diminishes the cervical extensors no longer contract as a reflex response. Rather, they relax, no longer keeping the head to one side. At the same time, this passive factor occurs in supine, the cervical flexors begin to work as antigravity muscles, helping to actively bring the head to midline. Eventually, the cervical flexors are strong enough to bring the head to midline and to lift the infant's head from the surface in supine (Fig. 2.36). These developmental achievements in supine are occurring during the second to fourth months, at the same time that

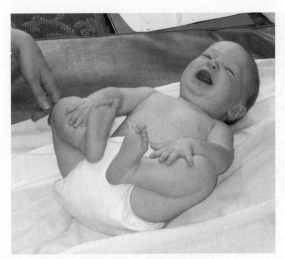

FIGURE 2.35 Postural symmetry exhibited by 6 to 7 months of age.

the cervical extensors are emerging as antigravity muscles in prone. Complete development of lifting of the head in prone (4 months) develops shortly before full lifting of the head in supine (5 months). When the cervical flexors contract to lift the head into flexion while in supine, the cervical extensors must elongate. This is another example of reciprocal inhibition. Children with neuromotor pathologies may lack the ability to lengthen or relax the cervical extensors.

As cephalocaudal development continues in supine, controlled movement of the upper extremities begins with volitional movement and subsequent stabilization of the shoulder joints. Whereas the achievement of prone-on-elbows develops the stability of the shoulder girdle in a weight-bearing function (closed chain), the supine position permits the development of shoulder stability for non–weight-bearing function (open chain).

During the first 3 months of life, the infant has little control over the placement and holding of the upper extremities in space. Attempts at grasping an object are made with the hands close to the body, because the child lacks the shoulder girdle stability and the strength to use his hands in space away from his body (see Fig. 2.4). With shoulder adduction, the upper extremities are held against the sides of the infant's body, providing stability in the only way the infant knows at this point. This process is referred to as **fixing**. Fixing is a normal process of development that occurs

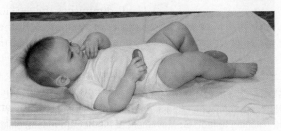

FIGURE 2.36 Lifting head in supine, an indication of well-developed antigravity cervical flexion.

with first attempts to stabilize the body, relative to gravity, in all postures. These first attempts, this fixing, are not true antigravity stability. Instead, they are a temporary means of stabilizing by fixing into gravity (**progravity**), until the appropriate muscles in a particular posture learn to stabilize or fix against gravity (**antigravity**).

Without the eventual emergence of muscle groups strong enough to work as antigravity muscles, development will be delayed. Fundamentally, antigravity muscle work is what keeps a person upright against gravity, whether in sitting, kneeling (tall kneeling or knee standing), quadruped, or standing erect. In normal mature bipedal movement, extensor muscles are the main antigravity muscles that keep humans upright. Consider the erector spinae, gluteus maximus, proximal hamstrings, and quadriceps muscles. In the supine position, however, the flexors act as antigravity muscles. Consider the cervical flexors, abdominal muscles, and hip flexors.

Once the infant develops shoulder stability using cocontraction of all of the muscles around the shoulder joint, he is able to reach out to grasp a toy (Fig. 2.37A), and thus begin the skills of grasp and manipulation. This process of fine motor development will take approximately 18 months to refine and will not be complete until approximately 30 months of age. Development of grasp and prehension will be discussed elsewhere in this chapter.

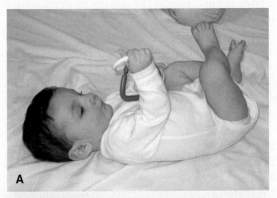
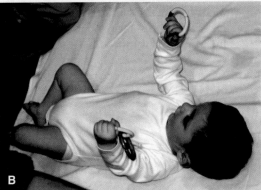

FIGURE 2.37 Reaching with upper extremities. A: Once stability is achieved in the shoulder girdle, the child can reach into space to grasp a toy; note the midline head and hands. **B:** Reaching well into space using antigravity control of the serratus anterior muscles; note the supine symmetry and concurrent but separate use of hands.

Hands to Knees and Feet, Feet to Mouth

Another developmental landmark occurs when the child reaches upward against gravity while in supine. As the pectoral muscles are being activated, so are the abdominals. The pectoral muscles are partially responsible for reaching the upper extremity toward the ceiling in supine (Fig. 2.37B). In order for this movement to occur, the serratus anterior muscles act in synergy, and the rhomboid muscles must elongate. These muscles, acting in concert, cause the shoulder girdle to protract. It is now that one sees the child's ability to reach for his mother or father's face while being diapered or dressed. Active use of the pectorals with reciprocal inhibition of the rhomboids, along with the recent inhibition of the ATNR, allows the child to reach upward and also to bring his hands to midline.

In supine at 5 months of age, as the child continues to gain ever-increasing control of his antigravity flexors, with reciprocal lengthening of antagonist extensor muscles, he begins to actively lift his lower extremities from the surface. Some foot-to-foot contact usually occurs (Fig. 2.38). Next he begins to reach for his knees and then his feet. At first he reaches his hand to the ipsilateral knee and foot, as seen in Figure 2.35. Eventually, he is able to cross midline with his upper extremities, placing a hand on the contralateral knee and/or foot (Fig. 2.39). This contact of the infant with his own body is important to the process of developing **body image** or **body scheme**.[97]

As the child flexes his hips to bring his feet toward his hands and head, his abdominals and hip flexors are gaining strength. Active contraction of the abdominal muscles causes the pelvis to tip posteriorly and the gluteus maximus and proximal hamstrings to elongate. The hips are in moderate flexion, abduction, and external rotation. His knees are flexed, and his feet are dorsiflexed and supinated (Fig. 2.40A).

The natural progression of hands to knees and hands to feet leads to the infant bringing his feet to his mouth. At 5 months of age, a child is very interested in oral stimulation. No longer under the influence of the rooting and sucking reflexes, he begins to use his mouth for more than eating. As he brings a foot toward his mouth, he exhibits

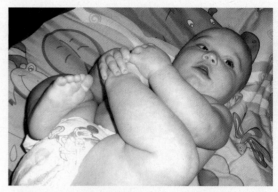

FIGURE 2.39 Supine, hand to contralateral foot.

feed-forward anticipation of putting his toes in his mouth (Fig. 2.40B). Putting his feet in his mouth, seen in Figure 2.40C, further develops body image. This activity also facilitates cognitive development. Infants learn about objects through touch, including the touch that accompanies

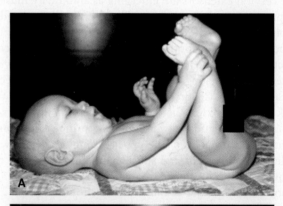

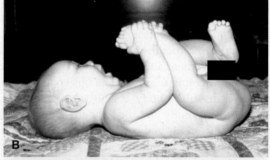

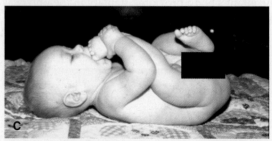

FIGURE 2.40 Foot-to-mouth sequence at 5 months of age. A: Note the elongation of posterior musculature and visually directed reaching to foot. **B:** Movement of foot toward mouth, child opening his mouth with feed-forward anticipation. **C:** Child puts foot into his mouth, one way of learning about his body.

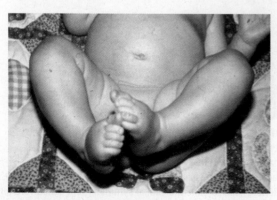

FIGURE 2.38 Supine at 5 months, foot-to-foot contact.

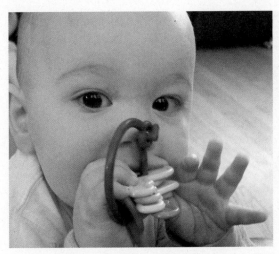

FIGURE 2.41 The activity of mouthing helps the infant develop form and shape perception as well as body image.

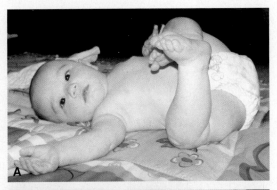

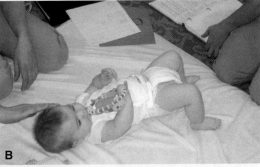

FIGURE 2.42 Development of pelvic mobility in supine. A: Feet toward head with posterior pelvic tilt. **B:** Bridging with anterior pelvic tilt.

placing objects in the mouth, a process referred to as **mouthing** (Fig. 2.41).

Pelvic stability, in a posterior pelvic tilt, is needed in prone for the infant to begin lifting his head in prone. In supine, at 5 months of age, the child puts his feet in his mouth, further enhancing the active posterior pelvic tilt. Once the posterior pelvic tilt is achieved and strengthened, the child begins to develop pelvic mobility. That is, he moves back and forth in supine between a posterior pelvic tilt and an anterior pelvic tilt. This is often observed during spontaneous play in supine, as the child brings his feet to his mouth with a posterior pelvic tilt. Then he lowers his feet to the surface, with a relative anterior tilt. Sometimes when he lowers his feet to the surface, he continues with active lumbar extension into the **bridging** posture, which requires more of the relative anterior tilt. In doing this, he works his feet into the surface (Fig. 2.42A and 2.42B). Developing pelvic mobility in supine allows the child to move back and forth between these two postures, in tandem with activities occurring in prone. At about the same time in development, approximately 5 months of age, the child practices pelvic mobility in prone. This requires alternating between the posterior tilt of prone on forearms and the anterior tilt of the pivot prone posture, as discussed previously.

Rolling Progression

Nonsegmental Rolling

Rolling develops in a two-stage progression. From birth to 6 months of age, the child performs **nonsegmental rolling**. **Segmental rolling** develops at approximately 6 months of age. Nonsegmental rolling, also referred to as **log rolling**, allows the child to roll from supine to side-lying. This movement is based on one of the infant reflexes, the **neck-righting reaction**. In the neck-righting reaction, the stimulation of proprioceptors in the neck as the child's head is turned actively or passively to one side causes the body to follow in one complete unit, without rotation within the vertebral column.[46,107] The neck-righting reaction gradually diminishes over time as another reaction, the **body-righting reaction acting on the body**, evolves.[46,107]

Segmental Rolling

The body-righting reaction acting on the body is a predominant factor in movement by 6 months of age. When the head is rotated to one side, the body reacts to the proprioceptive stimulus to the neck by following in the direction of the head turning, thus rolling toward that side. Now the movement within the vertebral column is segmental. That is, the different segments, the trunk, shoulder girdle, and pelvic girdle, as well as the upper and lower extremity on one side, are seen to respond sequentially, rather than moving as one unit (Fig. 2.43A). The sequence of movement of the various body segments is not identical in all people, nor is it always the same sequence in an individual. The baby may lead with the head, a lower extremity, an upper extremity, the pelvic girdle, or the shoulder girdle, and the other segments follow the lead segment (Fig. 2.43B, C, and D). Segmental rolling requires rotation within the body axis, the vertebral column. This rotation is referred to as **intra-axial rotation** and is facilitated by the body-righting reaction acting on the body, permitting the infant to roll from prone to supine and supine to prone.

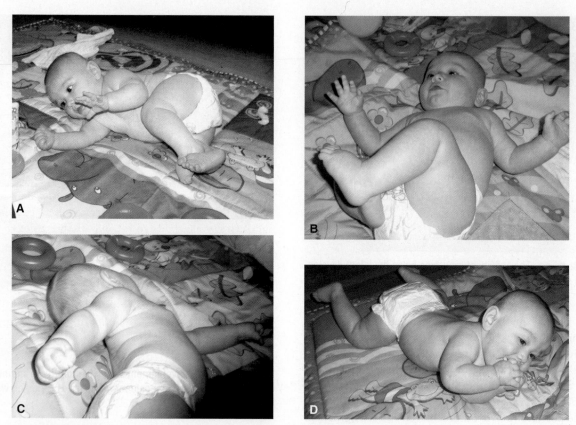

FIGURE 2.43 A: Intra-axial rotation develops, in part, as the result of the body righting acting on the body response. (B) Segmental rolling, supine to prone, leading with lower extrtemity; (C) prone to supine, leading with upper extremity; (D) prone to supine, leading with head.

Rolling Prone to Supine and Supine to Prone

Before the infant attempts to roll volitionally, rolling from prone to supine and supine to prone often occurs accidentally. Early on, the infant may roll accidentally from prone to supine because he pulls his knees underneath him and his buttocks are elevated. If the center of mass gets high enough, as a result of the elevated buttocks, the child may roll accidentally (Fig. 2.44). Accidental rolling, from prone to supine, may also occur as spinal extension progresses caudally, and the child achieves prone-on-elbows and prone-on-extended-arms. In this case, his center of mass becomes higher through the lifting of the head and upper trunk. Experimenting with the prone-on-elbows and prone-on-extended-arms postures, he becomes rather top-heavy and therefore may roll to supine accidentally. When this happens, the child may attempt to replicate the movement. Once able to replicate the movement, the child will practice this movement. Through trial and error and the increasingly strong body-righting reaction acting on the body, the child learns to roll segmentally from prone to supine, usually by 5 months of age (Fig. 2.45).

Rolling supine to prone also may occur as an involuntary movement initially. When the child is in supine around the age of 4 or 5 months, he may lift his pelvis from the surface

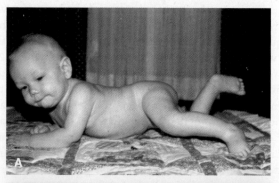

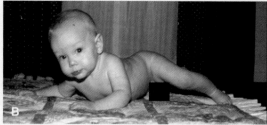

FIGURE 2.44 Accidental rolling prone to supine. A: In prone, the child lifts buttocks from the surface. **B:** As he lifts buttocks higher off the surface and pushes into the supporting surface with his foot, the child may accidentally roll prone to supine.

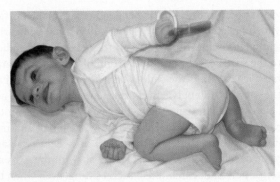

FIGURE 2.45 Segmental rolling prone to supine, leading with upper extremity.

on which he rests by plantar flexing his feet, working his feet into the surface. This bridging type of maneuver raises the center of mass, through the lower trunk, and may cause the infant to roll to one side or the other as he pushes a little harder into the surface with one foot, the foot contralateral to the direction to which he accidentally rolls. Trial-and-error practice, along with the strong body-righting reaction acting on the body, combines with other factors such as motivation, allowing the child to volitionally roll supine to prone by 6 months of age, using intra-axial rotation (Fig. 2.46). Although the age of acquisition of rolling skills may vary slightly, volitional rolling usually occurs from prone to supine before supine to prone, at 5 and 6 months, respectively.

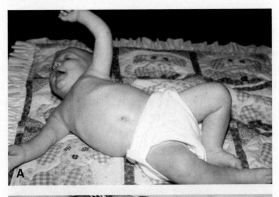

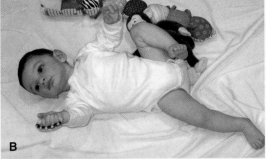

FIGURE 2.46 Segmental rolling supine to prone using intra-axial rotation. A: Rolling leading with upper extremity; note the scapulohumeral elongation. **B:** Segmental rolling leading with lower extremity; note the crossing of midline.

Once a child is able to roll volitionally, it is important that he learn to roll toward both left and right sides when in prone or supine. This will occur naturally in most cases, unless the infant encounters an obstacle to rolling to either left or right. Furniture, the side of the crib, or other environmental barriers may cause the child to always roll toward the same side. However, if such is the case, attentive parents and other caregivers can make sure the child is placed away from environmental obstacles and encouraged to roll toward both left and right sides during play. A child unable to roll toward one or the other side in the absence of environmental barriers or lack of opportunity may be exhibiting signs of neuromotor or musculoskeletal pathology. In such cases, the inability to roll in both directions should be viewed as a red flag, but is not in itself diagnostic.

The functional activity of rolling helps develop and secure several components of movement, as well as being a functional motor milestone in its own right. As the child learns to roll segmentally from prone to supine, the asymmetric cervical extension that he uses to initiate rolling during early attempts gives way to extension of the neck with lateral flexion and rotation. As the child gets to supine, he completes the roll using slight cervical flexion.

If the infant leads with the upper extremity when rolling supine to prone, he typically will bring one upper extremity across his chest, reaching toward the side to which he is rolling. This movement requires and encourages scapulohumeral elongation at the shoulder of the extremity with which he leads (Fig. 2.46A). Rolling supine to prone using intra-axial rotation also requires the lead upper or lower extremity, along with the other ipsilateral extremity, to cross midline (Fig. 2.46A and B). The ability to roll demonstrates dissociation of the right and left extremities as well as dissociation of the extremities and the head. If the upper or lower extremities are dependent on movements of the head in order to function, segmental rolling likely will not occur. In such a case, the ATNR may be influencing the limb movements. That is, turning of the head to one side in order to roll supine to prone causes the face-side extremities, upper more than lower, to extend in a pathologic pattern that blocks the ability to roll toward that side. Persistence of a primitive or obligatory ATNR may contribute to a child's inability to roll supine to prone. However, such reflex activity may actually be used by the child to roll prone to supine, using the abnormal asymmetric extensor tone of the ATNR and an elevated center of mass. This is also an atypical and pathologic pattern and is another red flag, particularly if the child does not have dissociation of the head and extremities and/or intra-axial rotation.

Sitting Progression

Supported Sitting

Preparation for sitting begins in the prone and supine positions as the child develops early components such as cephalocaudally progressing antigravity extension of the spine, pelvic mobility, intra-axial rotation, scapular mobility, and weight bearing on the upper extremities. During the neonatal period when the child is held in sitting, his posture is remarkable for extreme flexion of the spine, caused by the lack of antigravity extensor muscle control. In this posture, seen in Figure 2.47A, the infant's trunk exhibits what is termed a **complete C-curve**. The head is forward, with chin resting on the chest. Even though the child is at the mercy of gravity at this time and must be supported in sitting, the

pelvis of the typical child is perpendicular to the surface on which he sits (Fig. 2.47A). That is, he should be bearing weight on his ischial tuberosities. If the pelvis is perpendicular to the surface, the very top portion of the gluteal cleft is visible (Fig. 2.47B). If the child is bearing his weight, instead, on the sacrum, the pelvis is not perpendicular and the gluteal cleft is hidden from view. This weight bearing on the sacrum, referred to as **sacral sitting**, is a red flag and may be indicative of pathology. Regardless of a child's age and stage of development, it is atypical to sit with the extreme posterior pelvic tilt exhibited in sacral sitting, even when the spine is in the immature C-curve characteristic of the neonate. Note the position of the pelvis in all of the figures of children sitting in this chapter.

As the neonate develops, antigravity extension of the neck and trunk in sitting begins to appear. First, the cervical spine develops antigravity control, counteracting the infant's forward head position and lifting the head so that the face is vertical and the mouth is horizontal. As head control develops in supported sitting over the first 3 to 4 months, the child is also gaining increased antigravity extension in the prone position. At the same time, in the supine position, he is developing antigravity flexion control. Thus, head control, as provided by a balance of cervical flexors and extensors, evolves to keep the head upright against gravity when sitting. Additionally, the development of the chin tuck in the prone and supine positions secures the stable head in sitting by 4 months of age, even though the child still depends on external support to remain in a sitting position (Fig. 2.48).

Propped Sitting

At approximately 5 months of age, the child begins to exhibit his first abilities for sitting without the external support of either being held or sitting with a backrest. When put in the sitting position, the child attempts to prop with his upper extremities. With his weight shifted forward, the

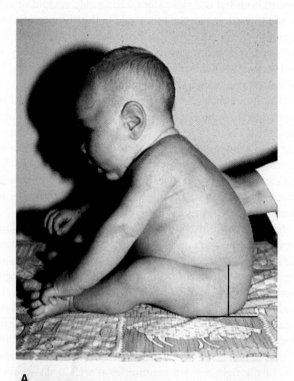

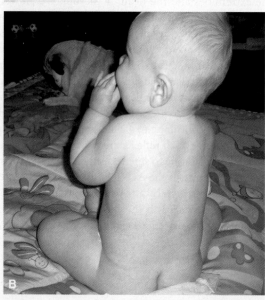

FIGURE 2.47 A: Supported sitting posture of neonate; note the lack of antigravity spinal extension and that the pelvis is perpendicular to the supporting surface. **B:** Sitting with full back extension, visible gluteal cleft indicates pelvis is perpendicular to surface.

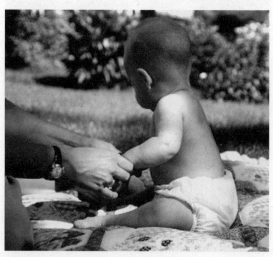

FIGURE 2.48 Supported sitting with full spinal extension; note the position of pelvis and stable head and neck.

child's hands are able to make contact with the surface. The **hand grasp reflex** has diminished and generally disappeared by 4 months of age, allowing the child's open hands to be placed on the floor in front of him. Thus, he begins the adventure of sitting, with his lower extremities out in front of him and his upper extremities once again performing in a major weight-bearing role. The two hands and the buttocks create a tripod base, which gives the infant a larger and more stable base of support than if he were to attempt to sit without the propping support of his upper extremities. This **propped sitting** posture is typical of an infant who is 5 months of age. As the infant feels increasingly secure in this posture, he will begin to rotate his neck to look around at his surroundings (Fig. 2.49). During propped sitting, the child fixes progravity, strongly contracting his hip flexors to increase his stability. He has not learned yet that his antigravity extensors will serve him better for remaining upright.

Mature stability against the forces of gravity in upright postures such as sitting and erect standing is attained through activation and strengthening of extensor muscles primarily. This antigravity extension of the trunk, hips, and knees develops over time in various postures. However, initial attempts at stability in upright postures are through the use of progravity contractions of trunk, hip, and knee flexors. Using progravity-stabilizing motor behaviors is referred to as **fixing into gravity** rather than **fixing against gravity**.

Ring Sitting

One major disadvantage of propping with the upper extremities while sitting is that the child cannot use his upper extremities for reaching and grasping objects. As his trunk

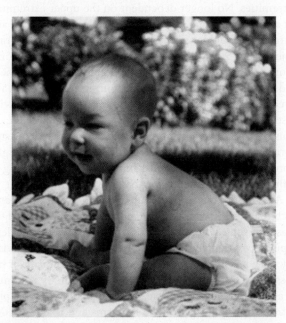

FIGURE 2.49 Propped sitting using the upper extremities to create a large base of support; note that pelvis is perpendicular to the supporting surface.

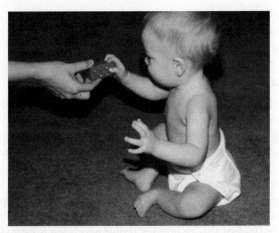

FIGURE 2.50 Independent ring sitting; note the high guard position of the upper extremities, used by the child to enhance trunk stability.

extension becomes stronger, the child is eventually able to rely less on the upper extremity support and the wide base, until he finally lifts his hands from the surface on which he sits. This new sitting posture is termed **ring sitting** because of the position of the lower extremities (Fig. 2.50).

Now the child is sitting more erect, pelvis still perpendicular to the surface, utilizing his ever-increasing trunk extension to remain upright against gravity. Although by this time, approximately 6 months of age, the child has adequate spinal extension to resist the pull of gravity while in sitting, he probably feels less stable in that posture than he is in actuality. In order to secure his trunk extension even more when sitting without propping or other external support, the child holds his upper extremities in the **high guard** position (see Fig. 2.50). The retraction of the shoulders in this position is analogous to the positioning of the upper extremities in the pivot prone posture and serves as an adjunct to the spinal extension. Contraction of the rhomboids increases the overall muscular activity in the child's posterior trunk, better securing him against gravity. This high guard position, using the rhomboid muscles to increase midline trunk stability against the pull of gravity, is seen again in the initial performance of tall kneeling and erect standing, as the child's center of mass moves higher in space relative to the supporting surface. However, the upper extremities, in the high guard position, are rendered virtually useless in terms of reaching for, grasping, and manipulating objects.

The lower extremities in ring sitting are flexed and externally rotated at the hips and flexed at the knees. The plantar surfaces of the feet are nearly touching or touching each other. The ankles may be pushed into moderate passive supination by contact with the surface. Ring sitting provides a relatively wide base of support as the externally rotated hips allow the lower extremities to rest on the floor. With the wider base of support and the high guard position, the child is able to sit independent of external support at this point, but he lacks the ability to independently achieve the sitting posture from the prone or supine positions. Rather, when placed in sitting, he is able to remain stable without falling as long as he does not attempt much movement while in this posture, lest he disturb his balance.

Other Independent Sitting Postures

As the child experiences increasing stability in independent sitting, he begins to move his lower extremities out of the ring position, into either a **half-ring** position or **long sitting** (Figs. 2.51 and 2.52). His ability to have one lower extremity in front of him with relatively neutral hip rotation and an extended knee, while the other hip is still in flexion and external rotation with a flexed knee, is a sign of developing dissociation between the two lower limbs. The child moves in and out of this position, varying which leg is extended, and is often seen to be in simple long sitting. In mature long sitting, the base of support is narrowed mediolaterally, allowing lateral weight shifting with ease.

The child develops a series of increasingly advanced sitting postures that do not require external support, including ring sitting, half–ring sitting, long sitting, and side sitting. He also develops short sitting (sitting with knees and hips flexed to approximately 90 degrees) on a child-size chair, climbing onto higher surfaces such as a child's high chair to sit, and getting into and sitting on an adult-size chair (Fig. 2.53). Depending on the environment and the individual child's motivation and opportunity, once the child achieves propped sitting followed by ring sitting, these various, more mature sitting postures may develop at different times for each child,

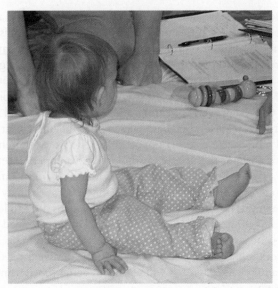

FIGURE 2.52 Long sitting with narrowed mediolateral base of support.

sometimes nearly concurrently. In each new sitting posture, the child repeats a series of motor behaviors that take him from a stable posture when placed, through being able to move in and out of the posture (the **transition**), to using his hands for prehension and object manipulation in each posture. These motor behaviors include antigravity performance, antigravity stabilization, weight shifting, intra-axial rotation, and transition between postures. Weight shifting in each posture is accompanied by elongation on the weight-bearing side.

As the child becomes more secure in ring sitting, he gradually relaxes the rhomboid muscles and lowers his upper extremities. No longer dependent on the upper extremities for stability in sitting, he is able to volitionally protract and retract the shoulder girdle in order to reach for and grasp objects (Fig. 2.54). At about the same time, he feels confident enough in his sitting that he is able to rotate his head and neck to look around and begin performing visually directed reaching. The stability that results from the wide base of support in ring sitting, however, is gained at the expense of lateral weight shifting. The wider the base of support in any posture, the more difficult it is to shift weight. Consequently, the child must move beyond ring-sitting to sitting postures with narrower bases of support.

At 6 months of age, the child's forearms are pronated such that, as he looks toward and reaches for an object, he grasps the object with his forearm pronated. Being unable to supinate volitionally, he is unable to inspect the object visually once it is in his hand (Fig. 2.50). It is also difficult or impossible to inspect the object with his mouth. By 8 months of age, he develops volitional supination and reciprocal pronation and supination of the forearms and is able to look at the object he has secured and put it in his mouth. The ability to reach, grasp, and supinate with either upper extremity makes it possible for him to take an object presented

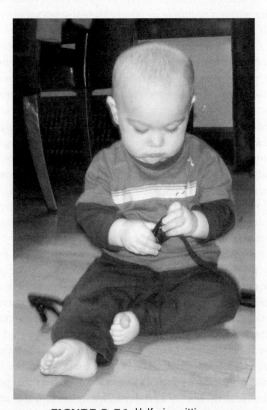

FIGURE 2.51 Half–ring sitting.

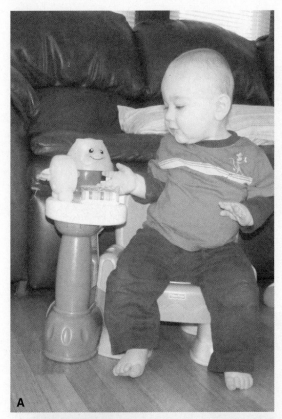

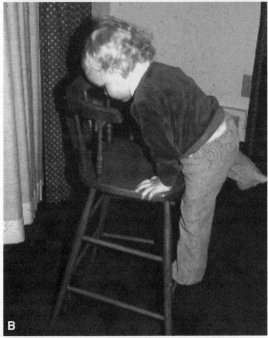

FIGURE 2.53 Sitting on surfaces of various heights. A: Short sitting on child-size chair. **B:** Climbing onto a high chair.

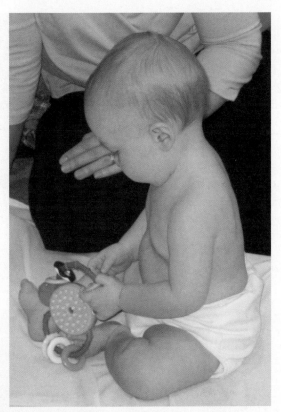

FIGURE 2.54 Ring sitting with no guard; note the bilateral use of hands in midline.

the ring-sitting posture, he is no longer influenced by the ATNR, so keeping his head in midline, using two hands in midline, and crossing midline with the head, eyes, and hands are easily achieved.

In propped sitting and ring sitting, the feet and ankles are notable for their passive positioning in supination (see Figs. 2.49 and 2.50). Therefore, at 5 and 6 months of age, these sitting positions reflect the supinated feet, hip flexion and external rotation, and knee flexion seen in the supine position when the child is bringing his feet to his mouth at 5 months of age. Also notable in the propped and ring-sitting postures is the child's tendency for progravity stabilization, using the hip flexors and abdominal muscles.

Once the child is stable in ring sitting and is able to move the head and limbs, he begins to use intra-axial rotation in sitting. This intra-axial rotation develops and strengthens by 5 to 7 months of age in prone and supine, allowing for segmental rolling. The intra-axial rotation also allows him to make transitions between postures, thus broadening his repertoire of sitting positions and increasing his independence as he learns to move from supine and prone to sitting and vice versa, using intra-axial rotation. See Figure 2.55 for one example of this transition from sitting to prone. Intra-axial rotation also serves to increase the accessibility of the space around the child, making more of his environment available for interaction as he uses the rotation to transition to quadruped and perhaps to creep (Fig. 2.56).

to him, inspect it, manipulate it by transferring the object from one hand to the other, and put it in his mouth. This bilateral hand activity also requires working in midline and crossing the midline of his body with his upper extremities, head, and eyes. By the time the typical child has achieved

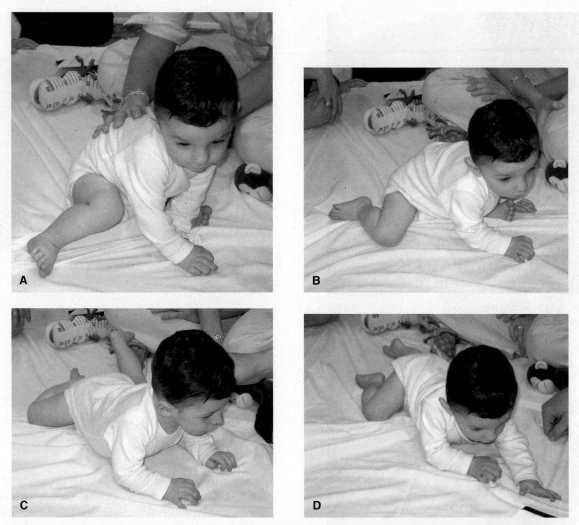

FIGURE 2.55 A–C: Sequence of transition from sitting to prone-on-elbows using intra-axial rotation. **D:** Reciprocal and contralateral crawling.

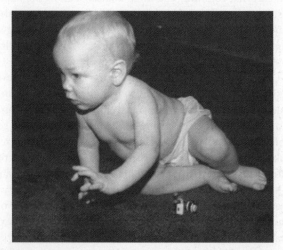

FIGURE 2.56 Intra-axial rotation is also used to increase the accessibility of the child's environment and for the transition between sitting and quadruped.

By 8 months of age, the child is able to sit independently. He has developed not only full antigravity extension of the back, but by the eighth month, sitting posture is characterized by the completion of the secondary curves of the spine (Fig. 2.57). These anterior–posterior curves, developing cephalocaudally, are the **cervical lordosis** and the **lumbar lordosis**. Now the child is able to move from prone or supine to sitting and return to prone or supine. He is also able to move in and out of the various sitting postures using the intra-axial rotation and can pull himself to standing.

Side sitting is a mature sitting posture that requires a number of motor components and abilities, including intra-axial rotation, dissociation, weight shifting, and elongation of the trunk on the weight-bearing side (Fig. 2.58). In side sitting, dissociation of the lower extremities is present, as evidenced by the hip external rotation and abduction of one lower extremity with internal rotation and adduction of the other hip. Sitting on a child-size chair

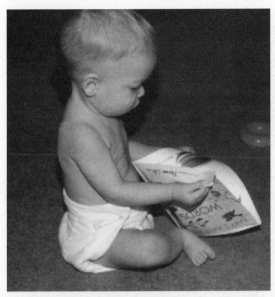

FIGURE 2.57 Sitting independently with secondary curves, the cervical and lumbar lordoses.

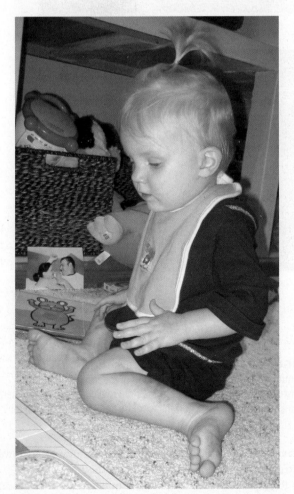

FIGURE 2.58 Side sitting; note the dissociation of the lower extremities.

requires the child to use another component of movement, eccentric contractions. Eccentric or lengthening contractions of the quadriceps, proximal hamstrings, and gluteus maximus muscles allow the child to lower himself slowly to the chair. As he lowers himself to sit, he shifts his weight posteriorly from the forefoot to the heel of the foot. Rising to standing from a small chair requires an anterior weight shift and concentric contractions of these same muscles.

Sitting on an adult-size chair, such as a sofa, is accomplished through a combination of several movements. This activity is often the first function that reveals a child's developing climbing skills. When a child begins to climb onto an adult-size chair, he usually uses considerable lateral trunk flexion to one side while he abducts and flexes the opposite hip. After months of practice, he begins to use more weight shifting to one side with accompanying elongation of the lateral trunk on that weight-bearing side, intra-axial counterrotation, and hip flexion of the opposite lower extremity. Figure 2.59 shows a series of movements used by a child to get into an adult-sized chair.

Locomotion in Sitting

Once children exhibit dissociation of the two lower extremities and are stable in half-ring sitting, some children actually develop a locomotive form in this posture called **hitching**. Hitching is when a child, while sitting on the floor, uses either foot to dig into the surface in order to scoot forward on his buttocks. Many children use hitching as a means of moving around in their environments before they learn to creep efficiently and can become quite adept at this form of locomotion.

Erect Standing Progression

Supported Standing

When held in standing during the neonatal period, the child bears partial weight on his lower extremities. His legs may be stiff with cocontraction, and the base of support is very narrow, with the feet supinated. Head control is absent, and his neck is flexed with the chin resting on the chest (Fig. 2.60). While in supported standing, tilting the child forward slightly will produce reflex stepping (automatic stepping) (Fig. 2.61).

By the end of 2 months of age, most infants lose the reflex stepping ability. Early developmentalists believed that the cessation of automatic stepping was simply a function of maturation of the child's CNS.[107] However, the groundbreaking studies of Esther Thelen in the early 1980s found that reflex stepping in infants whose lower extremities were weighted artificially was diminished. Babies who were held in standing in water increased their stepping rather than ceasing to step, presumably due to the effect of buoyancy on the lower extremities, and the stepping persisted beyond the

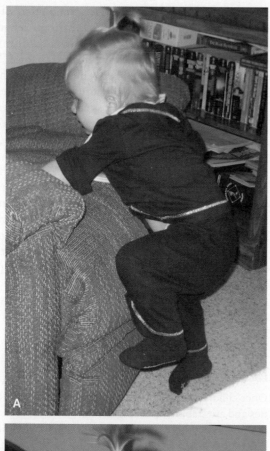

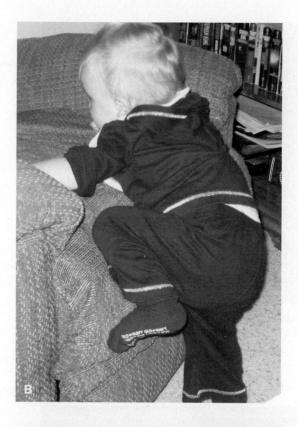

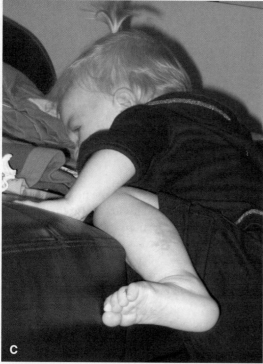

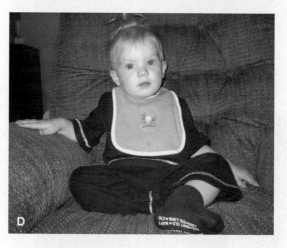

FIGURE 2.59 Climbing onto an adult-sized chair, early sequence A-D; note the lateral flexion of the trunk to the right (instead of shifting of weight to the right, which would cause lateral trunk flexion to the left) and the extreme abduction of the left hip.

usual age of dissolution of the stepping reflex. The conclusion drawn from these studies was that reflex stepping typically ceased at approximately 2 months of age, not because of programming and maturation of the CNS, but because the mass of the infant's lower extremities became such that it was too difficult for the infant to lift the heavy lower extremities.[108]

Regardless of the theory that one accepts for the cessation of automatic stepping, by the end of 2 months the typical child no longer produces this reflex stepping and

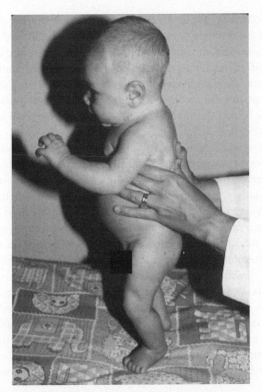

FIGURE 2.60 Supported standing in the neonate.

will often cease to take weight on the lower extremities when held in standing. This absence of automatic stepping is referred to as **abasia,** derived from the Greek words that mean *without step*.[1] The next stepping abilities will be

volitional. The lack of weight bearing through the lower extremities, which occurs typically during the third and fourth months, is the stage of **astasia**, literally meaning *without standing*.[1] This stage is temporary during normal development and may not be seen in all children.

During the first 4 months, head control has been developing in all postures, as control and balance of the antigravity cervical extensors and flexors progressed. By 5 months of age, his head secure in space, the infant volitionally begins to accept partial weight on the lower extremities during supported standing (Fig. 2.62). This milestone is characterized by moderate abduction, flexion, and external rotation of the hips, with knee flexion and pronation of the feet. This 5-month posture becomes even more exaggerated by 7 months of age, at which time the child is volitionally bearing full weight on his lower extremities (Fig. 2.63).

At 7 months, the child's poor anterior–posterior weight-bearing alignment and underdeveloped balance responses prevent him from standing alone without external support. He can stand and walk with his hands held (Fig. 2.63). His gait is characterized by hip external rotation and moderate abduction, giving him a wide base of support, and extremely pronated feet. The greater the abduction and external rotation of the hips, the more pronated the feet are. Typically, a fat pad masks the longitudinal arch of each foot, in babies and toddlers, increasing the pronated appearance of the feet. Hips and knees are flexed, creating continued poor anterior–posterior alignment for standing

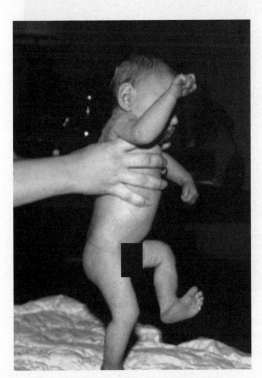

FIGURE 2.61 Automatic stepping of the neonate.

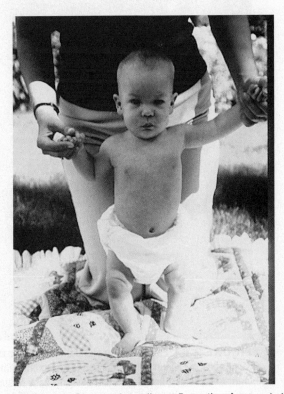

FIGURE 2.62 Supported standing at 5 months of age; note the flexed hips and knees.

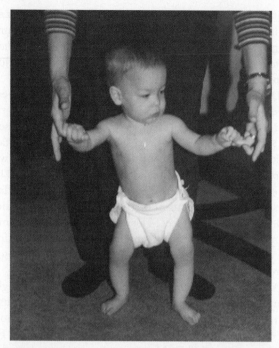

FIGURE 2.63 Supported standing at 7 months of age; note the wide base of support, hip and knee flexion, and pronation of feet.

without support. In correct mature weight-bearing alignment for standing, an imaginary straight line can be drawn in a parasagittal plane through the ear, shoulder, hip, knee, and lateral malleolus (Fig. 2.64A). In the immature standing posture, the imaginary line falls through the ear and shoulder but anterior to the hip joint and often slightly posterior to the knee joint, due to the flexion of the hips and knees (Fig. 2.64B and C).

The child begins pulling himself to standing in his crib at about this time (7 to 8 months). At first, this is accomplished by using the newly developed strength of the upper extremities, while the lower extremities remain essentially passive. Once standing, the child will frequently hold onto the crib rails for support while he bounces and experiments with this newly discovered standing ability. During his earliest attempts at supported standing in the crib, he finds that he is unable to get down. Lowering himself slowly to the mattress requires strong eccentric control of his hips and knees, something that he has not developed. Frustrated and tired of standing, he may simply let go of the crib rails and drop to sitting, thanks to gravity, or he may begin to cry, signaling to his parent his need for help. A parent will come and either take the child from the crib or put him down in

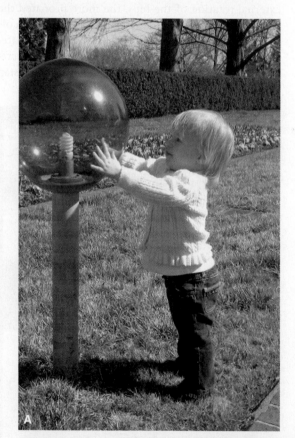

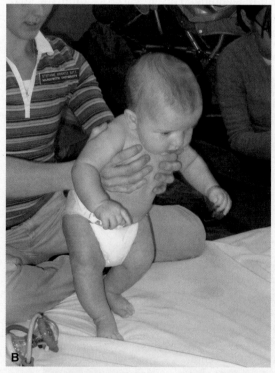

FIGURE 2.64 Ear-to-heel postural alignment for standing. A: Mature alignment; **(B)** inadequate and immature weight-bearing alignment for independent standing; note that the ear-to-heel weight line falls anterior to the hips and posterior to the knees, and also note the narrow base of support with supination of the feet. **C:** Improved postural alignment, but alignment is still inadequate for standing independently.

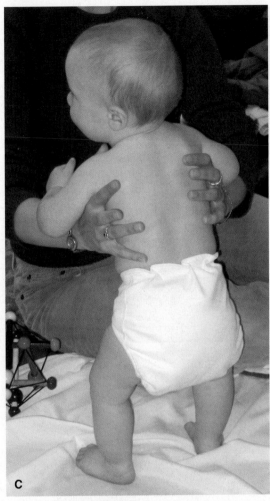

FIGURE 2.64 (continued)

prone or supine. Once this has happened, the child may realize that his actions were attention getting, so he will pull to standing once again, and the sequence of events repeats. This is great fun for the child to repeat these behaviors, as he discovers that his actions cause effects, oftentimes predictable effects.

Independent Standing

By 10 months of age, the child pulls himself to standing at furniture such as a sofa or low table. As seen in the sequence in Figure 2.65, now he gets to standing by going through the knee-standing (tall-kneeling) and half-kneeling postures and is adept at getting down with control. In the tall-kneeling posture, the base of support is kept relatively wide as the child's center of mass moves farther away from the floor. In order to achieve the half-kneeling posture, he must shift his weight to one side, elongating the trunk on that side, so that he is able to bring the unweighted limb forward and put his foot flat on the floor. This action, the

transition between the tall-kneeling and standing postures, requires intra-axial rotation, just as all transitional postures do. Once in half-kneeling, he uses his lower extremity muscles, particularly the hip extensors and knee extensors, to raise himself against gravity. He relies very little on the strength of the upper extremities as in past pull-to-standing attempts. Instead, the lower extremities do most of the work and the upper extremities help with balance. The same half-kneeling and tall-kneeling positions are used to get down to the floor from standing. With practice, these movements become very controlled and fast. Occasionally, he may simply let go of his support and drop quickly to the floor.

Cruising

Once standing at furniture, the child will play for long periods, going back and forth between the floor and the furniture, squatting and rising to stand repeatedly. He moves in and out of the various postures. Soon he begins stepping sideways while holding onto the furniture. This supported walking at 10 months of age is called **cruising** (Fig. 2.65C). He is able to work his way back and forth along the sofa or table and eventually begins to reach to other pieces of furniture to make his way around the room. Meanwhile, his anterior–posterior alignment is improving, with decreasing hip and knee flexion.[97] While standing at furniture, he can be seen to lift one or the other hand from the support, sometimes rotating his trunk to one side or the other while still maintaining his balance. Often, as he cruises around the furniture and reaches for the next piece of furniture, he briefly stands and maybe even takes one or two steps without support from either upper extremity. At times he stands briefly without touching the supporting surfaces. However, when walking forward without furniture for support, he still needs someone to hold his hand(s), but he is fast approaching the day when he will walk forward without holding the furniture or someone's hand. During the cruising phase of development, in addition to practicing his walking, the child's cruising movements contribute to the development and strengthening of hip abduction/adduction and eversion/inversion of the ankles as he sidesteps (Fig. 2.66). Even though the child walks, supported by holding onto furniture or someone's hand, the **plantar grasp reflex** may still be positive at 10 months of age, although considerably diminished and present inconsistently. The plantar grasp reflex is manifested by curling of the toes when the examiner places a finger horizontally at the base of the toes (Fig. 2.67). A positive plantar grasp causes the toes to flex or curl.[46,107] This reflex can also be observed spontaneously as curling of the toes when the child is in supported standing. Usually the complete dissolution of this reflex must occur before independent walking without support will develop. Gradually, over the next several weeks, he lets go of the adult's hand or the furniture, often standing independently for brief

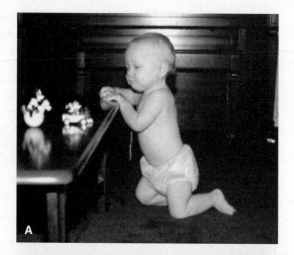

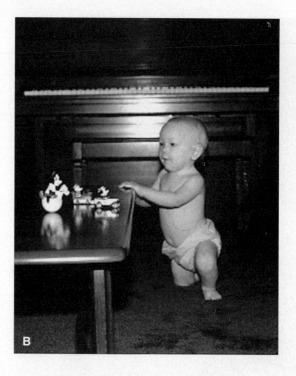

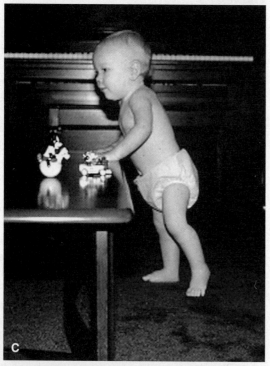

FIGURE 2.65 Pull-to-standing at furniture sequence. A: Tall kneeling. **B:** Half-kneeling; note the intra-axial rotation and the dissociation of the lower extremities. **C:** Erect standing at low table with cruising.

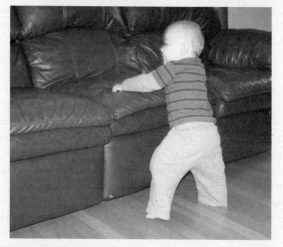

FIGURE 2.66 Cruising helps develop hip abduction for both mobility and stability (weight-bearing) functions.

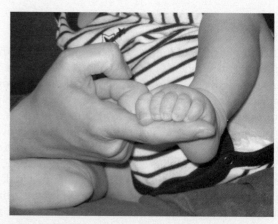

FIGURE 2.67 Plantar grasp, positive response.

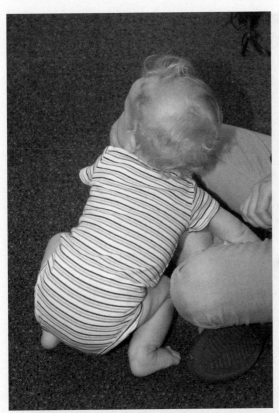

FIGURE 2.68 Squatting. The child frequently performs active squat to stand and back to squat and uses squat position as a play position.

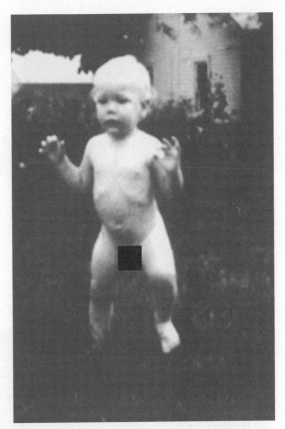

FIGURE 2.69 First independent walking with high guard positioning of upper extremities.

periods. When this happens, his upper extremities usually assume the high guard position for increased trunk stability.

During the development of standing, cruising, and walking, the child develops the ability to squat to play as well as squatting to pick up an object (Fig. 2.68). Often while standing at furniture, such as a sofa, the child can be seen to squat to pick up a toy, stand and place the toy on the sofa, and repeat this process many times. Also, he is able to spend great lengths of time in the squat position while playing. Squatting, therefore, is both a movement used to transition between postures and a posture in itself. Some have theorized that the active squat-to-stance-to-squat sequence facilitates cocontraction, and therefore stability, of the muscles surrounding the ankle joint. The theory is that the prolonged and maximal stretch to the muscle spindles of the ankle musculature fires both primary and secondary afferent endings.[59]

Independent Bipedal Locomotion

First independent forward walking generally occurs between 10 and 15 months of age, with the typical child walking at 12 months of age, plus or minus a month. At first, the child holds his upper extremities in the high guard position, the same position in which he held his arms during first independent sitting, in an attempt to increase stability against gravity by adducting the scapulae (Fig. 2.69). Posture

is characterized by improving but continuing poor, vertical alignment, with hips and knees flexed. Abduction and external rotation of the hips continue to provide a wide base of support. The child does not have heel strike initially, and the feet are still in considerable pronation.

As forward independent gait progresses over the next months, the shoulders lose much of the flexion of the high guard position, assuming a low guard position with elbows still flexed and hands just above the waist; fingers may be pointed upward or shoulders are adducted, and the hands are stabilized against the body, as shown in Figure 2.70. Then the upper extremities relax into full shoulder extension and hang at the child's sides. Over the next few weeks, reciprocal arm swing during gait is attained (Fig. 2.71).

With practice, the anterior–posterior postural alignment continues to improve with increasing hip and knee extension, decreasing hip abduction with narrowing of the base of support, and lessening of external rotation of the hips. Eventually, the child walks with good postural alignment, a narrow base of support, neutral pronation/supination of the feet, heel strike, push off, and reciprocal arm swing. The plantar fat pad does not completely disappear until approximately 2 years of age, at which time the longitudinal arches become visible.

Bipedal locomotion will continue to improve and progress over the next 2 to 4 years. Gait parameters for the

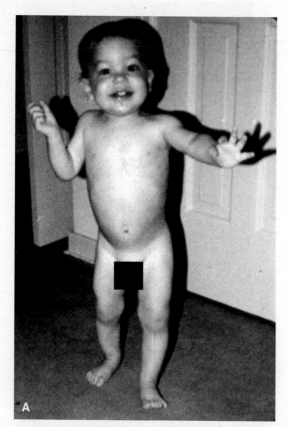
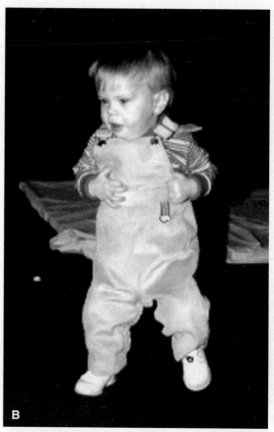

FIGURE 2.70 Independent walking. A: Note that the high guard position is decreasing, with the right upper extremity still in high guard, the left upper extremity being lowered with shoulder girdle protraction. **B:** Walking independently with low guard to enhance upright trunk stability.

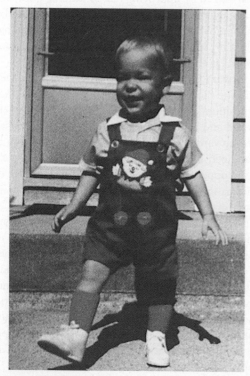

FIGURE 2.71 Mature independent walking with heel strike and reciprocal arm swing.

3-year-old child differ from early gait parameters at age 1 year.[109] These parameters include alignment of the lower extremities as well as various aspects of the gait cycle. As the child's gait matures, mediolateral alignment at the hip progresses from hip abduction to adduction, until the feet are approximately shoulders' width apart. At the knees, mediolateral alignment moves from genu varus at birth to approximately 12 degrees of genu valgus at 3 years of age. Then between 4 and 7 years of age, the valgus resolves to only 7 to 10 degrees. This change in alignment of the knees affects the mediolateral alignment of the hips, ankles, and feet as well.[109] Other gait parameters that change with growth and maturation are cadence, step and stride length, and velocity.[109] **Cadence**, the number of steps per minute, starts out very high in first independent walking. The 1-year-old child spends a decreased amount of time in single limb stance, compared with the 3-year-old and the adult. This is because the 1-year-old child has less strength and stability in his hips. Consequently, he takes more steps per minute, resulting in less time in single limb support.[109]

Gait **velocity**, the distance one covers in a specified amount of time, starts low and increases as the child ages.[109] Velocity is related to the length of one's step or stride. A **step** is measured from heel strike of one lower extremity to heel strike of the opposite lower extremity. **Stride**

length, measured from heel strike of one foot to heel strike of the same foot, is approximately twice the step length.[109] However, in a case where the step length of the two extremities differs considerably because of pathology affecting only one limb, in order to be accurate both step and stride length must be measured, instead of calculating stride length by multiplying the step length by two.

From 1 to 3 years of age, a child's step length and stride length increase, as do velocity and single limb stance time.[109] Single limb stance increases with increasing strength and balance abilities. Length of step and/or stride, and therefore gait velocity, increases as the child's lower extremities continue to grow in length, even well after age 3. Otherwise, gait at age 3 is considered to have parameters similar to those of an adult.[109] Various gait parameters at ages 1 year and 3 years are shown in Table 2.5.

Even though a toddler is able to walk fast, and his parents will often insist he is running, true running does not develop until 3 to 4 years of age. A **true run** is characterized by having both feet off the ground at the same time, unlike walking, where one foot does not leave the ground until the other foot makes initial contact.

Stair Climbing

Stairs present a considerable challenge to toddlers, as one might imagine. The typical **rise** of a step in a flight of stairs is 7 to 8 inches. For a 15-month-old child to negotiate stairs in erect standing would be the equivalent of an adult attempting to climb stairs with a knee-high rise (Fig. 2.72).

The ability to ascend and descend stairs is affected by a number of factors, most particularly, opportunity. Therefore, the age of achieving this milestone has considerable variability, although the sequence of achievement

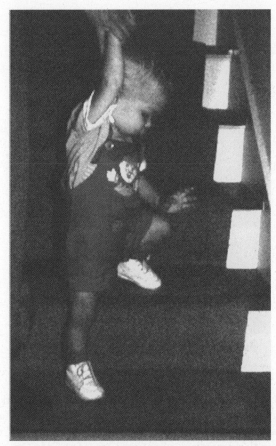

FIGURE 2.72 Descending stairs with hand held; note the rise of the step in relationship to the length of the child's lower extremity.

is much the same from one child to the next. A child who lives in a home without stairs, or at least without stairs that the child is permitted to climb, often develops stair-climbing skills at a later age than the child who has frequent daily encounters with stairs to get to and from his bedroom and/or toys.

The first ability to ascend and descend stairs is usually in the quadruped position (Fig. 2.73). The child learns to go up the stairs on his hands and knees, followed soon by coming down the stairs backward on his hands and knees. Sometimes children, in their first attempts at descending stairs, will try to do so in quadruped, but head first, with disastrous results if a caregiver is not nearby. With a bit of coaching, the child quickly learns through trial and error to descend the stairs backward on his hands and knees.

Ascending stairs generally develops to a more skillful level before descending stairs develops to the same level of skill. This sequence generally repeats itself in bipedal locomotion after the child has developed the ability to go up and down stairs using quadrupedal locomotion. Another feature of stair climbing that develops in a rather typical pattern is apparent once the child is climbing stairs while standing. Initially, bipedal stair climbing is performed by placing both feet on each step, in a manner that is called **marking time**.[48] Generally, the child will not begin doing steps one over one

TABLE 2.5	Gait Parameters in 1- and 3-Year-Old Children[a]		
Gait Parameter	1 Year of Age	3 Years of Age	Direction of Change
Base of support (pelvic span to ankle spread)	<1	≥1	↓
Step length	20 cm	33 cm	↑
Stride length (double the step length)	40 cm	66 cm	↑
Single limb stance	32% of gait cycle	35% of gait cycle	↑
Cadence (step frequency)	180 steps per minute	154 steps per minute	↓
Velocity (speed)	60 cm/sec	105 cm/sec	↑

[a]From Long TM, Toscano K. *Handbook of Pediatric Physical Therapy.* Philadelphia, PA: Lippincott Williams & Wilkins; 2001.

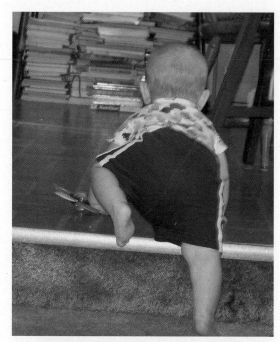

FIGURE 2.73 Ascending a step in quadruped.

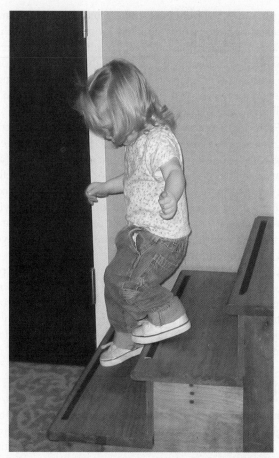

FIGURE 2.74 Descending stairs without upper extremity support.

(i.e., only one foot to each step) until he is close to 3 years of age, depending of course on how much trial and error and practice on stairs he has been afforded. This pattern of the feet is also dependent on the type of upper extremity support that is available. Stair climbing progresses as the upper extremity support decreases from using one handrail and/or an adult hand for support, to needing a handrail but no adult, and finally to needing no upper extremity support (Fig. 2.74). Of course, the speed with which the child develops increasingly more skillful stair-climbing abilities varies greatly, and like other skills, the ability to locomote on stairs may temporarily digress as unique and/or challenging circumstances, such as unusually steep stairs or the absence of a handrail, present themselves.

 Balance

Maintaining one's balance, that is, keeping one's center of mass within the base of support and effectively compensating when balance is disturbed, is a challenge to the developing child as he attempts and learns new motor skills. Following the achievement of a particular milestone or posture, a child must develop the ability to maintain his balance in that posture. Usually, as the child is bravely moving toward the next posture in the hierarchy, he continues to practice the newest learned posture, thereby developing new balancing skills in each successive posture. Balance skills make up the normal postural reflex mechanism. These balance skills are divided into four subgroups: righting reactions, tilting reactions, equilibrium reactions, and protective reactions. Each subgroup has a defined aspect of balance for which it is responsible. These subgroups operate on a continuum such that when one's balance is challenged, the reactions occur in a predictable order (see Display 2.2).

Righting reactions are responsible for securing the head in space and must develop in all planes.[46,107] When there is a disturbance in one's center of mass in any posture, **head-righting reactions**, also termed **labyrinthine righting reactions**, come into play first. If the disturbance is only slight and does not come close to moving the child's center of mass outside the base of support, the head-righting reactions suffice in bringing the body back into balance. When an individual's body is tilted in any direction, the head automatically rights itself; that is, no matter what the position of the body, the head moves to an upright position wherein the mouth is horizontal and the face is vertical, referenced to the floor or ground[46,107] (Fig. 2.75). If the disturbance is large enough to move the center of mass very near the edge of the child's base of support, then head righting occurs automatically, but it is not enough to maintain balance. Help is needed from the tilting or equilibrium reactions.

Tilting and equilibrium reactions, responsible for securing the position of the body in space when balance is challenged, are identical responses but are elicited by slightly different stimuli. A **tilting reaction** is the correct term to

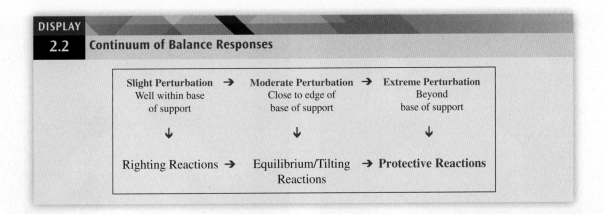

DISPLAY
2.2 **Continuum of Balance Responses**

Slight Perturbation	→	Moderate Perturbation	→	Extreme Perturbation
Well within base of support		Close to edge of base of support		Beyond base of support
↓		↓		↓
Righting Reactions	→	Equilibrium/Tilting Reactions	→	**Protective Reactions**

use when the surface on which the child is seated, standing, or otherwise positioned is moved, thus causing the child's center of mass to shift. When this happens, head righting occurs immediately. If the body senses that head righting is insufficient in itself, the tilting reactions are elicited.

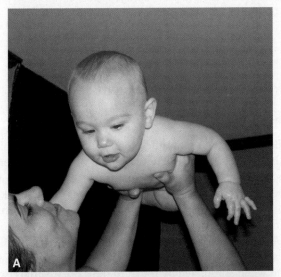

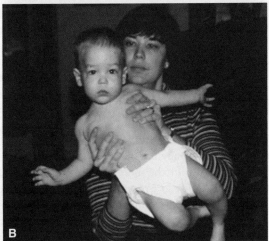

FIGURE 2.75 Positive labyrinthine righting reflex (head righting); face is maintained vertical with mouth horizontal in response to **(A)** ventral suspension and **(B)** a lateral tilt to the child's right.

The response looks like this. When on a balance board, ball, or other moveable surface, if the child is tilted to his left far enough to elicit the tilting reactions, lateral bending toward the right side occurs. If viewing the spine from a posterior vantage point, the vertebral column curves to the right, away from the direction toward which the child was tilted (Fig. 2.76). This returns the body's mass toward the center of the base of support. If the stimulus and the response are strong enough, the limbs enter into the response. In this case, the right shoulder and hip abduct, in an effort to help bring the body mass into the center of the base of support once again. An **equilibrium reaction** is identical to the tilting reaction, but the stimulus differs in that the individual is on a stationary surface instead of a mobile surface, and the force of the perturbation is directed at the child's body rather than the surface.[46,107] Tilting and equilibrium reactions develop in each successive posture shortly after the child develops stability in that posture and while he is beginning to experiment with and work on the next higher posture.

The final type of balance response is the protective response. In normal development, the protective response is responsible for regaining balance when the center of mass has been pushed beyond the borders of the base of support. When this happens, head-righting and tilting/equilibrium responses are elicited but are insufficient to regain control. Automatically, the child protects himself from the inevitable fall by sticking out his hand or foot (Fig. 2.77). This motion effectively moves the borders of the base of support outward, enlarging the base. In this manner, the body's mass is once again within the base of support, not because the body returned to being inside the base of support, as in the tilting/equilibrium reactions, but because the base of support has enlarged to once again capture the center of mass within its borders. The following example shows how protective responses are used in one of two ways to maintain balance and sometimes prevent injury. When one is standing in the aisle on a moving bus, and the driver suddenly slams on the brakes, if head-righting and tilting responses, both of which are elicited first, do not suffice in regaining balance, a person probably will do one of two things. Either he will take a step with one foot in order to increase the size of his

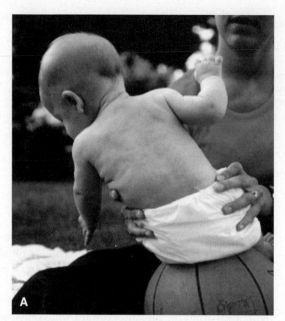 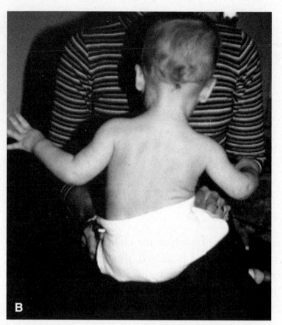

FIGURE 2.76 Test for tilting reaction in sitting. A: Response to a tilt to the left is negative but age appropriate because the child does not right his trunk. **B:** Response to same tilt is positive in older child, who laterally flexes his trunk away from the direction of the tilt.

base of support enough to regain balance within the base of support or he will fall forward. If he falls, as he nears the floor of the bus, one or both arms will reach out to help break the fall, creating a new and larger base of support and hopefully protecting the head and face from the potential impact. This second response is the reason people often fracture the distal end of the radius, the well-known Colles fracture, in a fall.[1]

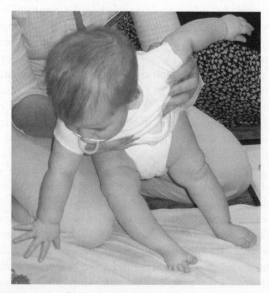

FIGURE 2.77 Protective extension of the upper extremity to the side.

▶ Fine motor development

Grasp

A discussion about motor development cannot be complete without attention to the development of grasp. Earlier in this chapter, the importance of proximal stability to the development of grasp and prehension was discussed. Like gross motor development, fine motor development occurs, in most typical cases, in a predictable order.

At birth, the full-term neonate has a hand grasp reflex. This reflex, which began in utero, is a reflex closing of the hand when stimulated by touch to the palmar surface with stretch of the intrinsic muscles of the hand. The response to this two-part stimulus is reflex grasping of the stimulating object. As long as the stimulus is in contact with the infant's hand, the fist remains closed. The grasp reflex is usually tested by the examiner placing his index finger into the infant's palm[46,107] (Fig. 2.78).

During the early months of life, the grasp reflex is intact, although it gradually weakens until disappearing at approximately 4 months of age. This means that until the reflex becomes naturally inhibited with time, anything that stimulates the palm of the infant's hand will elicit a reflex behavior. Such reflex grasp preempts voluntary grasping of objects. Therefore, attempts by the infant at voluntary grasp will not be successful until the hand grasp reflex has diminished and then disappeared. Even though this may mean that the child's early attempts at voluntary grasp are essentially thwarted, little is lost during those 4 months of active reflex behavior. This is because until approximately

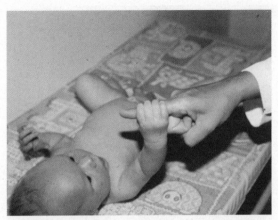

FIGURE 2.78 Hand grasp reflex is positive in response to tactile and proprioceptive stimuli from examiner's finger being placed in the infant's palm.

3 to 4 months of age, the child still lacks the stability in the shoulder joint needed for skillful reaching for and grasping of objects at will.

During the first 4 months, while the infant's grasp reflex diminishes, the child is gradually developing the ability to volitionally grasp an object, as seen in Figure 2.79 with the infant beginning to hold his bottle. He also develops the ability to stabilize his shoulders in order to reach for objects with some degree of accuracy and hold the upper extremity stable while grasping an object (Fig. 2.80A and B). The development of this shoulder stability is followed by the development of the child's ability to control the extremity enough to bring the object toward him for a closer look, to put it in his mouth, or to examine it with two hands (Fig. 2.81). Shoulder stability and the ability to perform a controlled reach arise from the infant's increasingly skillful weight bearing and weight shifting in the prone-on-elbows posture. It is complemented by such activities in supine as bringing the hands to midline (inhibition of the ATNR),

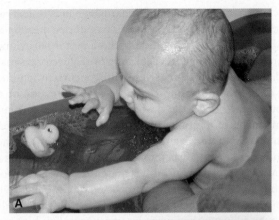
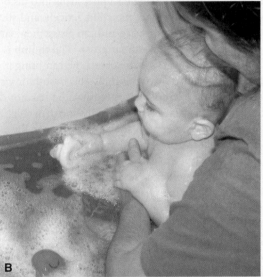

FIGURE 2.80 Sufficient shoulder stability to **(A)** reach away from body to grasp object; **(B)** note the pronated forearm with immature grasp.

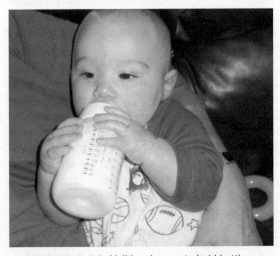

FIGURE 2.79 Volitional grasp to hold bottle.

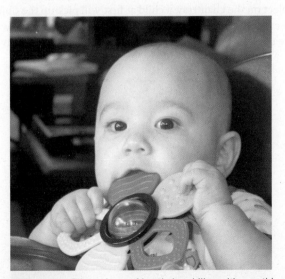

FIGURE 2.81 Bilateral use of hands in midline with mouthing; note beginning supination of forearms.

reaching hands to knees and eventually hands to feet, and reaching up to touch the caregiver's face during dressing and feeding activities. Accomplishing these motor behaviors in prone and supine requires activation of the pectoralis major and serratus anterior muscles, with concurrent lengthening of the rhomboid muscles, allowing protraction of the shoulders. Prior to the development of these particular components of motor behavior, the infant is unable to reach into space and stabilize the shoulder for grasp and prehension. Consequently, at 3 months of age, the child will take a toy such as a rattle only if it is presented close to his body, within 2 or 3 inches. This is because he cannot stabilize the shoulders when reaching into space, but he can stabilize them by adducting and fixing his upper arms into his body.

At 4 to 5 months of age, the child actively and successfully reaches for objects in space and can grasp them, at will, using the whole hand in a palmar grasp. The thumb is inactive initially. Once he grasps the object, he can bring it close to his face but is not able to put it into his mouth or visually inspect it with one hand. This is because he has not developed the ability to actively supinate his forearm (Fig. 2.82). Consequently, the dorsum of his hand is between his mouth and/or eyes and the object, and the object is essentially hidden from view. At 4 months of age, with a stable prone-on-elbows position, the child is beginning to shift weight. As mentioned earlier in this chapter, weight shifting in prone-on-elbows is the beginning of supination, as well as the ability to pronate and supinate the forearm reciprocally. As active, controlled supination develops and improves, the child begins to engage an object with his eyes, reach for the object, and grasp it. He then supinates his forearm as he brings the object close to his face. Now he can put it into his mouth, visually inspect it, touch it with both hands at once, and/or transfer the object from one hand to the other. Victory! (Fig. 2.83)

Although voluntary grasp at first is crude and palmar, the development of refined grasp progresses rather quickly in the large scheme of things. Sitting in a high chair with an object on the chair tray, a child at first will pick up the object by crudely raking it into his palm, using just his fingers, with the ulnar two fingers predominating.[48,110] This ulnar activity

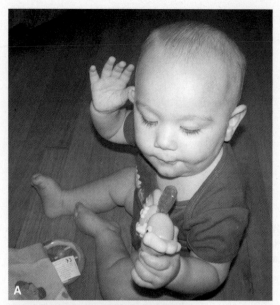

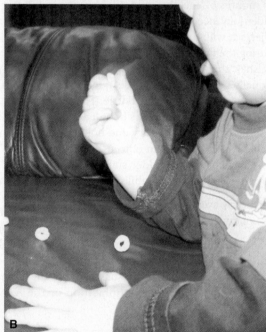

FIGURE 2.83 Forearm supination had developed, allowing **(A)** visual inspection of object and **(B)** putting objects in mouth with ease.

occurs long before the active participation of the thumb (radial activity), and it is a good example of the medial-to-lateral principle of developmental direction. In anatomic position, the ulnar fingers are medial and the thumb is lateral.

As grasp develops and becomes more refined, the child continues to use the fingers to palm the object, ulnar fingers still predominating, but radial fingers also participating. The thumb is still inactive. This type of grasp progresses to increasing dominance by the first two fingers. By 10 months of age, the child begins using a very active forefinger (index finger or first finger), and loves to poke and prod with that index finger.[17,51] This is the time when babies poke their

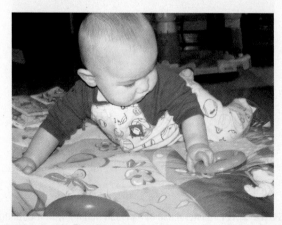

FIGURE 2.82 Reach and grasp with pronation of the forearm.

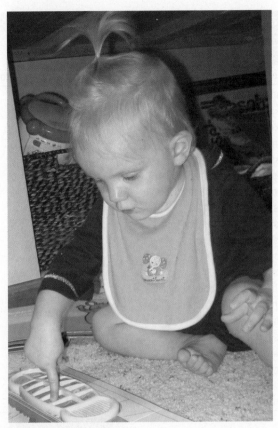

FIGURE 2.84 Forefinger (index finger) dominance, poking and prodding.

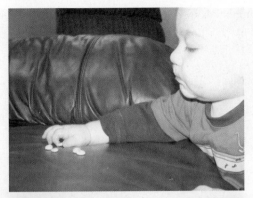

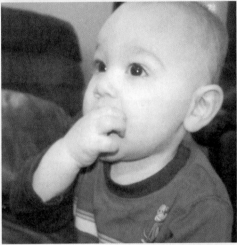

FIGURE 2.85 Pincer grasp to **(A)** pick up dry cereal and **(B)** put it in his mouth.

fingers in noses, eyes, and ears. They begin pointing at and poking nearly everything in sight. This poking with the forefinger continues to dominate fine motor activities for many months, as seen in this 15-month-old child in Figure 2.84. This obsession with the forefinger occurs at about the same time the thumb is becoming very active. At 10 months of age the child has a **pincer grasp**, using the thumb and first finger pad to pad.[48,110] Finger foods are very important to the child at this time as he develops the ability to pick up dry cereal pieces and put them in his mouth with considerable accuracy (Fig. 2.85). Also around 10 months of age, the child begins to use a *three-jaw chuck* type of grasp for larger objects, using the thumb, index, and second fingers[48,110] (Fig. 2.86).

Release

The development of release lags somewhat behind the development of grasp. Volitional release begins at approximately 11 months of age. Until that time, a child lets go of an object simply by relaxing the finger flexion. Not until 11 months of age does the child begin to intentionally release by actively extending his fingers.[48] The inability to actively and accurately release an object during those first 10 to 12 months of life is the root cause of the tendency to knock down the tower when trying to stack blocks. Until the child begins to gain some control over the release, he is able

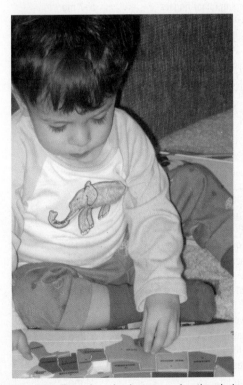

FIGURE 2.86 Three-jaw chuck grasp, using thumb, index finger, and second finger in a triangular pattern.

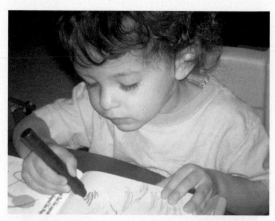

FIGURE 2.87 Using a crayon with opposite hand holding the paper.

TABLE 2.7	Advanced Motor Skills and Approximate Ages of Acquisition
Motor Skill	**Age of Acquisition**
Stands on low balance beam	2 yr
Walks straight line	3 yr
Walks circular line	4 yr
Balances on one foot for 3–5 sec	5 yr
Walks backward	18 mo
Jumps from bottom step	2 yr
Jumps off floor with both feet	28 mo
Hops 3 times	3 yr
Hops 8–10 times on same foot	5 yr
Hops distance of 50 feet	5 yr
Gallops	4 yr
Skips	6 yr
Catches ball using body and hands	3 yr
Catches ball using hands only	5 yr
Attempts to kick ball	18 mo
Kicks ball	2–3 yr
Hurls ball 3 feet	18 mo
Throws ball	2–3 yr
Fast walk	18 mo
True run with nonsupport phase	2–3 yr

TABLE 2.6	Development of Fine Motor Skills
Skill	**Age of Achievement**
Hand grasp reflex	Birth to 4–5 mo
Visual regard	Birth to 2 mo
Swipes with whole hand	2–3 mo
Visually directed reaching	3–5 mo
Midline clasping of hands	3–5 mo
Reaches out to grasp object	4–5 mo
Plays with feet; bangs objects together	5 mo
Crude palming, ulnar fingers predominating	5–7 mo
Transfers object from one hand to the other	6 mo
Lateral scissors grasp	8–9 mo
Pincer grasp, forefinger and thumb in opposition	10–11 mo
Forefinger dominance: poking and prodding with index finger	10–11 mo
Holds crayon	11 mo
Beginning voluntary release	11 mo
Uses graded pressure; varies pressure depending on object; uses finger tip with thumb opposition in fine pincer grasp	12 mo
Precision grasp with fine pincer and controlled release	15 mo
Scribbles on paper	15–18 mo
Holds paper with other hand when scribbling	18 mo
Puts object in container and dumps contents	18 mo
Builds tower of three cubes	18 mo
Turns pages of book, perhaps two or three at a time	21 mo
Turns pages of a book one at a time	24 mo
Unscrew jar lid	24 mo
Builds tower with eight cubes	30 mo

to place one block on top of another but causes the tower to fall when he tries to withdraw his hand.[48]

By 18 months of age, a child can grasp a pencil in the center using the pads of his fingers, put tiny pellets in a small bottle, stack a tower of three blocks, and mark with a crayon while holding the paper with the other hand[6,48,110] (Fig. 2.87). See Table 2.6 for approximate times of development of various fine motor skills.

▶ The 2-to-7-year-old child

During the first 2 years of life, the typical child develops the motor skills required for ordinary mobility and prehension. Further gross and fine motor development occur after the first 2 years, but these later-attained skills are more specific to an individual's play and work. These more advanced motor skills are developed and perfected more intentionally by each individual. Table 2.7 lists some of these more advanced skills and the approximate ages of acquisition.

SUMMARY

Normal motor development in humans usually occurs according to a particular sequence and timing. The sequence and timing are important to the clinician and can be used as guides in the physical therapy evaluation and treatment of children and adults. A thorough understanding of normal motor development is particularly germane to the study of abnormal neuromotor development in children. Although all humans share a common anatomy, physiology, and developmental sequence, one must keep in mind that many intrinsic and extrinsic factors, including pathology and culture, affect the sequence and timing of motor development in an individual.

REFERENCES

1. Dirckx JH. *Stedman's Concise Medical Dictionary for the Health Professions: Illustrated.* 4th ed. Baltimore, MD: Lippincott Williams & Wilkins; 2001.
2. Cowlin AF. *Women's Fitness Program Development.* Champaign, IL: Human Kinetics; 2002.
3. Bale JR, Stoll BJ, Lucas AO, eds. *Improving Birth Outcomes: Meeting the Challenge in the Developing World.* Washington, DC: The National Academies Press; 2003. Available at: http://www.iom.edu/CMS/3783/3915/16191.aspx. Accessed January 2, 2006.
4. VanSant AF. Should the normal motor developmental sequence be used as a theoretical model to progress adult patients? In: *Contemporary Management of Motor Control Problems: Proceedings of the II STEP Conference.* Fredricksburg, VA: Bookcrafters, Inc; 1991:95–97.
5. Shumway-Cook A, Woollacott MH. *Motor Control: Translating Research into Clinical Practice.* 4th ed. Baltimore, MD: Lippincott Williams & Wilkins; 2011.
6. Bayley N. *Bayley Scales of Infant and Toddler Development, Third edition (Bayley III).* San Antonio, TX: Pearson; 2005.
7. Stuberg WA, Dehne P, Miedaner J, et al. The Milani-Comparetti motor development screening test. 3rd ed. rev. Omaha, NE: University of Nebraska Medical Center; 1992.
8. Piper MC, Darrah J. *Alberta Infant Motor Scale.* Philadelphia, PA: WB Saunders; 1994.
9. Folio MR, Fewell RR. *Peabody Developmental Motor Scales, Second Edition, (PDMS-2).* San Antonio, TX: Pearson; 2000.
10. Friend JH, Guralnik DB, eds. *Webster's New World Dictionary of the American Language.* (College ed). Cleveland, OH: The World Publishing Company; 1960.
11. Provost B, Heimerl S, McClain C, et al. Concurrent validity of the Bayley Scales of Infant Development II Motor Scale and the Peabody Developmental Motor Scales-2 in children with developmental delays. *Pediatr Phys Ther.* 2004;16(3):149–156.
12. Connolly BH, McClune NO, Gatlin R. Concurrent validity of the Bayley-III and the Peabody Developmental Motor Scale-2. *Pediatr PhysTher.* 2012;24(4):345–352.
13. Campbell SK, Kolobe THA, Wright BD, et al. Validity of the Test of Infant Motor Performance for prediction of 6-, 9- and 12-month scores on the Alberta Infant Motor Scale. *Dev Med Child Neurol.* 2002;44(4):263–271.
14. Spittle AJ, Doyle LW, Boyd RN. A systematic review of the clinimetric properties of neuromotor assessments for preterm infants during the first year of life. *Dev Med Child Neurol.* 2008;50(4):254–266.
15. McClain C, Provost B, Crowe TK. Motor development of two-year-old typically developing Native American children on the Bayley scales of infant development II motor scale. *Pediatr Phys Ther.* 2000;12(3):108–113.
16. Valentini NC, Saccani R. Brazilian validation of the Alberta Infant Motor Scale. *Phys Ther.* 2012;92(3):440–447.
17. Jeng S, Yau K, Chen L, et al. Alberta infant motor scale: reliability and validity when used on preterm infants in Taiwan. *Phys Ther.* 2000;80(2):168–178.
18. Sanhueza AD. Psychomotor development, environmental stimulation, and socioeconomic level of preschoolers in Temuco, Chile. *Pediatr Phys Ther.* 2006;18:141–147.
19. Mayson TA, Harris SR, Bachman CL. Gross motor development of Asian and European children on four motor assessments: a literature review. *Pediatr Phys Ther.* 2007;19:148–153.
20. Tripathi R, Joshua AM, Kotian MS, et al. Normal motor development of Indian children on Peabody Developmental Motor Scales-2 (PDMS-2). *Pediatr Phys Ther.* 2008;20:167–172.
21. Santos DCC, Gabbard C, Goncalves, VMG. Motor development during the first year: a comparative study. *J Genet Psychol.* 2001;162(2):143–153.
22. Kelly Y, Sacker A, Schoon I, et al. Ethnic differences in achievement of developmental milestones by 9 months of age: the millennium cohort study. *Dev Med Child Neurol.* 2006;48(10):825–830.
23. Keller H, Yovsi RD, Voelker S. The role of motor stimulation in parental ethnotheories: the case of Cameroonian Nso and German women. *J Cross Cult Psychol.* 2002;3:398–414.
24. Kolobe THA. Childrearing practices and developmental expectations for Mexican-American mothers and the developmental status of their infants. *Phys Ther.* 2004;84(5):439–453.
25. Dusing SC, Harbourne RT. Variability in postural control during infancy: implications for development, assessment, and intervention. *Phys Ther.* 2010;90:1838–1849.
26. Vereijken B. The complexity of childhood development: variability in perspective. *Phys Ther.* 2010;90:1850–1859.
27. Hadders-Algra M. Variation and variability: key words in human motor development. *Phys Ther.* 2010;90(12):1823–1837.
28. Streissguth AP. *Fetal Alcohol Syndrome: A Guide for Families and Communities.* Baltimore, MD: Paul H. Brookes; 1997.
29. Edelman C, Mandle CL. *Health Promotion Throughout the Lifespan.* 5th ed. St. Louis, MO: Mosby, Inc; 2002.
30. Landgren M, Svensson L, Strömland K, et al. Prenatal alcohol exposure and neurodevelopmental disorders in children adopted from eastern Europe. *Pediatrics.* 2010;125(5): e1178–e1185. Available at: ww.pediatrics.org/cgi/doi/10.1542/peds.2009-0712. Accessed September 20, 2012.
31. Committee on Substance Abuse and Committee on Children With Disabilities. Fetal alcohol syndrome and alcohol-related neurodevelopmental disorders. *Pediatrics.* 2000;106(2):358–361.
32. Stratton K, Howe C, Battaglia F, eds. *Fetal Alcohol Syndrome: Diagnosis, Epidemiology, Prevention and Treatment.* Washington, DC: National Academy Press; 1996:4–21.
33. Astley SJ. Comparison of the 4-digit diagnostic code and the Hoyme diagnostic guidelines for fetal alcohol spectrum disorders. *Pediatrics.* 2006;118(4):1532–1545.
34. Kartin D, Grant TM, Streissguth AP, et al. Three-year developmental outcomes in children with prenatal alcohol and drug exposure. *Pediatr Phys Ther.* 2002;14:145–153.
35. U.S. Department of Health and Human Services. *Healthy people 2010.* Washington, DC: U.S. Department of Health and Human Services/Office of Public Health and Science; 1998.
36. Singer LT, Moore DG, Min MO, et al. One-year outcomes of prenatal exposure to MDMA and other recreational drugs. *Pediatrics.* 2012;130:407–413.
37. Lester BM, Tronick EZ, La Gasse L, et al. The maternal lifestyle study: effects of substance exposure during pregnancy on neurodevelopmental outcome in 1-month-old infants. *Pediatrics.* 2002;110(6):1182–1192.
38. Fetters L, Tronick EZ. Neuromotor development of cocaine-exposed and control infants from birth through 15 months: poor and poorer performance. *Pediatrics.* 1996;98(5):938–943.
39. LaGasse LL, Derauf C, Smith LM, et al. Prenatal methamphetamine exposure and childhood behavior problems at 3 and 5 years of age. *Pediatrics.* 2012;129(4):681–688.
40. Koseck K, Harris SR. Changes in performance over time on the Bayley scales of infant development II when administered to infants at high risk of developmental disabilities. *Pediatr PhysTher.* 2004;16(4):199–205.
41. Simmons RW, Thomas JD, Levy SS, et al. Motor response programming and movement time in children with heavy prenatal alcohol exposure. *Alcohol.* 2010;44(4):371–378.
42. LaGasse LL, Seifer R, Lester BM. Interpreting research on prenatal substance exposure in the context of multiple confounding factors. *Clin Perinatol.* 1999;26:39–54.

43. Messinger DS, Bauer CR, Das A, et al. The maternal lifestyle study: cognitive, motor, and behavioral outcomes of cocaine-exposed and opiate-exposed infants through three years of age. *Pediatrics.* 2004;113(6):1677–1685.

44. Arendt R, Angelopoulos J, Salvator A, et al. Motor development of cocaine-exposed children at age two years. *Pediatrics.* 1999;103(1):86–92.

45. Frank DA, Jacobs RR, Beeghly M, et al. Level of prenatal cocaine exposure and scores on the Bayley scales of infant development: modifying effects of caregiver, early intervention, and birth weight. *Pediatrics.* 2002;110(6):1143–1152.

46. Illingworth RS. *The Development of the Infant and Young Child: Normal and Abnormal.* New York, NY: Churchill Livingstone; 1980.

47. McGraw MB. *The Neuromuscular Maturation of the Human Infant.* New York, NY: Hafner Publishing; 1945.

48. Gesell A, Ilg FL. *Infant and Child in the Culture of Today.* New York, NY: Harper and Brothers Publishers; 1943.

49. Cech DJ, Martin ST. *Functional Movement Development Across the Life Span.* 2nd ed. Philadelphia, PA: W.B. Saunders; 2002.

50. Keshner EA. How theoretical framework biases evaluation and treatment. In: Lister MJ, ed. *Contemporary Management of Motor Control Problems: Proceedings of the II STEP Conference.* Fredricksburg, VA: Bookcrafters, Inc; 1991:37–47.

51. Effgen SK. *Meeting the Physical Therapy Needs of Children.* 2nd ed. Philadelphia, PA: F.A. Davis; 2013.

52. Bayley N. *The California Infant Scale of Motor Development.* Berkeley, CA: University of California; 1936.

53. Tecklin JS, ed. *Pediatric Physical Therapy.* 3rd ed. Philadelphia, PA: Lippincott Williams & Wilkins; 1998.

54. Horak FB. Assumptions underlying motor control for neurologic rehabilitation. In: Lister MJ, ed. *Contemporary Management of Motor Control Problems: Proceedings of the II STEP Conference.* Fredricksburg, VA: Bookcrafters, Inc; 1991:11–27.

55. Sugden D. Current approaches to intervention in children with developmental coordination disorder. *Dev Med Child Neurol.* 2007;49(6):467–471.

56. Salihagic-Kadic A, Medic M, Kurjak A. Neurophysiology of fetal behavior. *Ultrasound Rev Obstet Gynecol.* 2004;4(1):2–11.

57. Nader, K, Bechara A, van der Kooy D. Neurobiological constraints on behavioral models of motivation. *Annual Rev Psychol.* 1997;48:85–114.

58. Holland PC. Cognitive versus stimulus-response theories of learning. *Learn Behav.* 2008;36(3):227–241.

59. Stockmeyer SA. An interpretation of the approach of Rood to the treatment of neuromuscular dysfunction. *Am J Phys Med.* 1967;46:900–956.

60. Horne PJ, Erjavec M. Do infants show generalized imitation of gestures? *J Exp Anal Behav.* 2007;87(1):63–87.

61. Hauf P, Aschersleben G. Action-effect anticipation in infant action control. *Psychol Res.* 2008;72(2):203–210.

62. Spence JP, Clearfield M, Corbetta D, et al. Moving toward a grand theory of development: in memory of Esther Thelen. *Child Dev.* 2006;77(6):1521–1538.

63. Pin T, Eldridge B, Galea MP. A review of the effects of sleep position, play position, and equipment use on motor development in infants. *Dev Med Child Neurol.* 2007;49(11):858–867.

64. Bartlett DJ, Fanning JK, Miller L, et al. Development of the daily activities of infants scale: a measure supporting early motor development. *Dev Med Child Neurol.* 2008;50(8):613–617.

65. Rose-Jacobs R, Cabral H, Beeghly M, et al. The movement assessment of infants (MAI) as a predictor of two-year neurodevelopmental outcome for infants born at term who are at social risk. *Pediatr Phys Ther.* 2004;16:212–221.

66. Monson RM, Deitz J, Kartin D. The relationship between awake positioning and motor performance among infants who slept supine. *Pediatr Phys Ther.* 2003;15:196–203.

67. Dudek-Shriber L, Zelazny S. The effects of prone positioning on the quality and acquisition of developmental milestones in four-month-old infants. *Pediatr Phys Ther.* 2007;19:48–55.

68. Ravenscroft EF, Harris SR. Is maternal education related to infant motor development? *Pediatr Phys Ther.* 2007;19:56–61.

69. Abbott AL, Bartlett DJ, Fanning JE, et al. Infant motor development and aspects of the home environment. *Pediatr Phys Ther.* 2000;12(2):62–67.

70. Nervik D, Martin K, Rundquist P, et al. The relationship between body mass index and gross motor development in children aged 3 to 5 years. *Pediatr Phys Ther.* 2011;23(2):144–148.

71. Hanson H, Jawad AF, Ryan T, et al. Factors influencing gross motor development in young children in an urban welfare system. *Pediatr Phys Ther.* 2011;23(4):335–346.

72. Oriel KN, Frazier K, Lebron M, et al. The impact of the back to sleep campaign on gross motor development. *Pediatr Phys Ther.* 2006;18(1):102.

73. Smith MR, Danoff JV, Parks RA. Motor skill development of children with HIV infection measured with the Peabody developmental motor scales. *Pediatr Phys Ther.* 2002;14(2):74–84.

74. Majnemer A, Barr RG. Influence of supine sleep positioning on early motor milestone acquisition. *Dev Med Child Neurol.* 2005;47(6):370–376.

75. Marshall J. Infant neurosensory development: considerations for infant child care. *Early Childhood Edu J.* 2011;39(3):175.

76. Rodrigues LP, Saraiva L, Gabbard C. Development and construct validation of an inventory for assessing the home environment for motor development. *Res Q Exerc Sport.* 2005;76(2):140–148.

77. Bartlett DJ, Palisano RJ. Physical therapists' perceptions of factors influencing the acquisition of motor abilities of children with cerebral palsy: implications for clinical reasoning. *Phys Ther.* 2002;82(3):237–248.

78. MacKay-Lyons M. Central pattern generation of locomotion: a review of the evidence. *Phys Ther.* 2002;82:69–83.

79. Marder E, Calabrese RL. Principles of rhythmic motor pattern generation. *Physiol Rev.* 1996;76:687–717.

80. Jordan M, Brownstone RM, Noga BR. Control of functional systems in the brainstem and spinal cord. *Curr Opin Neurobiol.* 1992;2:794–801.

81. Grillner S. Locomotion in vertebrates: central mechanisms and reflex integration. *Physiol Rev.* 1975;55:247–304.

82. D'Agostino J. An evidentiary review regarding the use of chronological and adjusted age in the assessment of preterm infants. *J Spec Pediatric Nurs.* 2010;15(1):26–32.

83. Palisano RJ. Use of chronological and adjusted ages to compare motor development of healthy preterm and full-term infants. *Dev Med Child Neurol.* 1986;28(2):180–187.

84. Edwards S, ed. *Neurological Physiotherapy.* 2nd ed. New York, NY: Churchill Livingstone; 2002.

85. Sullivan PE, Markos PD, Minor MAD. *An Integrated Approach to Therapeutic Exercise: Theory & Clinical Application.* Reston, VA: Reston Publishing Company; 1982.

86. Heathcock JC, Bhat AN, Lobo MA, et al. The relative kicking frequency of infants born full-term and preterm during learning and short-term and long-term memory periods of the mobile paradigm. *Phys Ther.* 2005;85(1):8–18.

87. Piek JP, Carman R. Developmental profiles of spontaneous movements in infants. *Early Hum Dev.* 1994;39:109–126.

88. Thelen E, Ridley-Johnson R, Fisher D. Shifting patterns of bilateral coordination and lateral dominance in the leg movements of young infants. *Dev Psychobiol.* 1983;16:29–46.

89. Morgan A. Neuro-developmental approach to the high-risk neonate. (Notes from a seminar presented in Williamsburg, VA: November 3–4; 1984.) Cited in: Tecklin JS. *Pediatric Physical Therapy.* Philadelphia, PA: Lippincott Williams & Wilkins; 1999.

90. Clopton NA, Duvall T, Ellis B, et al. Investigation of trunk and extremity movement associated with passive head turning in newborns. *Phys Ther.* 2000;80(2):152–159.

91. Suzanne SD. *Neurological Development in the Full Term and Premature Neonate*. Amsterdam, Netherlands: Elsevier; 1977. Cited in: Bly L. *Motor Skills Acquisition in the First Year: An Illustrated Guide to Normal Development*. Tucson, AZ: Therapy Skill Builders; 1994.

92. Guzzetta A, Haataja L, Cowan F, et al. Neurological examination in healthy term infants aged 3–10 weeks. *Biol Neonate*. 2005;87:187–196.

93. Oatis CA. *Kinesiology: The Mechanics and Pathomechanics of Human Movement*. Philadelphia, PA: Lippincott Williams & Wilkins; 2004:106.

94. Piek JP. *Infant Motor Development*. Champaign, IL: Human Kinetics; 2006.

95. Dubowitz LMS, Dubowitz V, Mercuri E. *The Neurological Assessment of the Preterm and Full-Term Newborn Infant*. 2nd ed. London, UK: MacKeith Press, 1999.

96. Capute AJ. Early neuromotor reflexes in infancy. *Pediatr Ann*. 1986;15(3):217–222.

97. Bly L. *Motor Skills Acquisition in the First Year: An Illustrated Guide to Normal Development*. Tucson, AZ: Therapy Skill Builders; 1994.

98. Morgan AM, Aldag JC. Early identification of cerebral palsy using a profile of abnormal motor patterns. *Pediatrics*. 1996;98(4): 692–697.

99. Kornhaber L, Ridgway E, Kathirithamby R. Occupational and physical therapy approaches to sensory and motor issues. *Pediatri Ann*. 2007;36(8):484–493.

100. Koman LA, Smith BP, Shilt JS. Cerebral palsy. *Lancet*. 2004;363: 1619–1631.

101. Pooh RK, Ogura T. Normal and abnormal fetal hand positioning and movement in early pregnancy detected by three- and four-dimensional ultrasound. *Ultrasound Rev Obstet Gynecol*. 2004;4(1):46–51.

102. Jaffe M, Tal Y, Dabbah H, et al. Infants with a thumb-in-fist posture. *Pediatrics*. 2000;105:e41. Available at: http://www.pediatrics.org/cgi/content/full/105/3/e41. Accessed September 20, 2012.

103. Haywood KM, Getchell N. *Life Span Motor Development*. 3rd ed. Champaign, IL: Human Kinetics; 2001.

104. Bly L. *Normal and Abnormal Components of Movement*. Course notes presented in September 1984, Milwaukee, WI.

105. Umphred DA. *Neurological Rehabilitation*. 4th ed. St. Louis, MO: Mosby, Inc; 2001.

106. Norton ES. Developmental muscular torticollis and brachial plexus injury. In Campbell SK, Vander Linden DW, and Palisano RJ, eds. *Physical therapy for children*. 2nd ed. Philadelphia, PA: Saunders; 2000:p. 291.

107. Fiorentino M. *Reflex Testing Methods for Evaluating CNS development*. Springfield, IL: Charles C. Thomas; 1972.

108. Thelen E, Fisher DM. Newborn stepping: an explanation for a "disappearing" reflex. *Dev Psychol*. 1982;18:760–775.

109. Long TM, Toscano K. *Handbook of Pediatric Physical Therapy*. Philadelphia, PA: Lippincott Williams & Wilkins; 2001.

110. Erhardt RP. *Erhardt Developmental Prehension Assessment*. Laurel, MD: Ramsco Publishing; 1984. Cited in: Bly L. *Motor skills Acquisition in the First Year: An Illustrated Guide to Normal Development*. Tucson, AZ: Therapy Skill Builders; 1994.

Assessment and Testing of Infant and Child Development

Kirsten H. Malerba

Purposes of Developmental Testing
Basic Methods of Assessment
Tools for Assessment
  Guidelines for Selection of Tests
  Using Questions as Guidelines
Definitions
  Terms for Understanding Standardized
    Assessments

Overview of Tests
  Screening Tests
  Tests of Motor Function
  Comprehensive Developmental Scales
  Assessment of Functional Capabilities
  Outcome Measures
Integration of Information
Summary

Pediatric physical therapists are important members of the professional team involved in infant and child development. Pediatric physical therapists work to help children reach their maximum potential for functional independence through examination, evaluation, promotion of health and wellness, and implementation of a wide variety of interventions and supports.[1] Pediatric physical therapists collaborate with families and other medical, educational, developmental, and rehabilitation specialists to ensure a whole-child, comprehensive approach toward assessment of infant and child development.

Knowledge of motor development is central to the practice of pediatric physical therapy. Understanding the normal, orderly sequence of developmental achievement and patterns of integration is the basis upon which significant deviation in maturation is gauged.[2] From the knowledge of typical development, therapists can determine if a child is functioning at the expected norm for a given age through clinical observations and objective measurements, including developmental testing.

Purposes of developmental testing

The purposes of developmental testing include identifying risk of developmental delay, determining eligibility for services, intervention planning, documenting change over

time, determining efficacy of treatment over time, or for research purposes.

Developmental tests can be used as screening tools promoting early intervention for children at risk for delays in motor development.[3] The Committee on Children with Disabilities of the American Academy of Pediatrics recommends "all infants and children should be screened for developmental delays."[4] Developmental tests that are discriminative measures are used for determining eligibility for therapy services in early intervention or in school settings. Developmental tests also include evaluative measures, which are designed to measure change over time or response to an intervention.[3] Developmental tests can be used to plan interventions and measure progress over time as with curriculum-based assessments such as the Battelle Developmental Inventory 2 (BDI-2).[5] Finally, developmental tests are used as a clinical research tool when assessing reliability and validity of other developmental tests or for program evaluation.

Basic methods of assessment

The *Guide to Physical Therapist Practice*[6] offers a model of patient/client management, designed to maximize patient outcomes through a systematic, comprehensive approach to clinical decision making. The five elements of Examination, Evaluation, Diagnosis, Prognosis, and Intervention serve as a guide for therapists working with children who have been referred for physical therapy assessment.

Physical therapy examination is the first element in patient/client management consisting of obtaining patient/client history, performing a systems review, and selecting and administering tests and measures. The interview process for obtaining pertinent history includes identifying the family's concerns and needs related to the child's development, understanding the family's perception of the problem, and inquiring whether the developmental concerns impact daily family routines. The family's expectations, goals, and desired outcomes for physical therapy are important factors to identify during the interview process.

The review of the child's developmental and medical history provides valuable information and can be obtained through a questionnaire such as a case history form or through parent/client interview. The possible lack of reliability and bias of the parent should be considered in assessing the information gained in the history. When available, the medical records of a child may provide objective information regarding precautions, patient health status, previous medical history, suspected diagnosis, prognosis, medications, and other factors impacting the child's health. Other pertinent history, including information about the family and its genetic history, the pregnancy, labor, and delivery of the child, and the perinatal and neonatal events, should be obtained.

Therapists can gather a plethora of information about the child through clinical observations, often during the interview process. Is the child motivated to explore and move about in the environment, or is he or she more of an observer and active listener preferring to remain close to his or her family? If the child is mobile, what is the quality and symmetry of movement? How does the child's body respond to the effects of gravity? How does the child communicate with the parents and the therapist?

Developing a rapport with the family and child, assuring comfort in the environment, and being flexible and accommodating to the child's temperament, behavior, or special needs is a necessary skill for the pediatric physical therapist.

Selection of appropriate tests and measures for the examination depends on the purpose of the assessment. Kirshner and Guyatt describe three purposes of assessment: (1) Evaluative measures are used to determine change over time or change as the result of intervention, (2) Predictive measures are used to help identify children who will have delays in the future or to predict the outcome of the delay, and (3) Discriminative measures are used to distinguish between children who have a delay, impairment, functional limitation, or atypical development and those who do not.[7,8] Determining the most appropriate developmental test for the physical therapy examination is a key component of a valid developmental assessment.

▶ Tools for assessment

Guidelines for Selection of Tests

Careful and knowledgeable selection of tests is an important component of the physical therapy examination. If evaluators are unaware of the strengths, weaknesses, limitations, and restrictions of the tests being used, there is a high probability that an inappropriate test could be used, thus resulting in inaccurate or misinterpreted information.[9] Most published tests have some limitations or restrictions to their use, particularly regarding the ages and populations for whom they were developed and on whom they were standardized. These varied restrictions and limitations must be carefully examined and considered by the physical therapist in order to avoid choosing an inappropriate test, which could result in unintended misinterpretation of testing results.

In order to choose an appropriate test, some guidelines by which to evaluate a test are needed. Stangler and associates have proposed six criteria for evaluating a screening test that can be applied to any assessment test: (1) acceptability, (2) simplicity, (3) cost, (4) appropriateness, (5) reliability, and (6) validity. Every test may not fulfill each criterion; however, the test may be used knowledgeably if a therapist is aware of the limitations.[10]

Acceptability is defined as acceptance to all who will be affected by the test, including the children and families screened, the professionals who receive resulting referrals, and the community. *Simplicity* is the ease by which a test can be taught, learned, and administered. *Appropriateness* of screening tests is based on the prevalence of the problem to be screened and on the applicability of the test to the particular population. *Cost* includes the actual cost of equipment, preparation and payment of personnel, the cost of inaccurate results, personal costs to the person being screened, and the total cost of the test in relation to the benefits of early detection. In addition, tests must show both *reliability* and consistency between measurements, as well as *validity,* or the extent to which a test measures what it purports to measure.[10]

Using Questions as Guidelines

The choice of which developmental assessment is most appropriate for the examination depends on the response to the following questions[11]:

1. *For what purpose will the test be used?*
   - For identifying developmental delay
   - For determining eligibility for services
   - For research
   - For measuring the effect of therapy intervention
2. *What are the characteristics of the child?*
   - Age
   - Functional capability
   - Cognitive and language ability

3. *What content areas need to be assessed?*
   - Gross motor
   - Fine motor
   - Speech
   - Comprehensive assessment of functional capabilities
4. *What setting will the examination take place in?*
   - The child's natural environment (home, daycare, school)
   - Out-patient rehabilitation setting
   - In-patient hospital setting
   - Follow-up or specialty clinic
5. *What are the external constraints for the examiner?*
   - Time
   - Examiner experience and training
   - Space and equipment
   - Purchasing costs
   - Payor requirements or limitations

▶ Definitions

Terms for Understanding Standardized Assessments

An *age-equivalent score* is the mean chronologic age (CA) represented by a certain test score. For example, a raw score of 165 on the Locomotion subtest of the Peabody Developmental Motor Scales 2 (PDMS-2) represents an age equivalent to 53 months. Age-equivalent scores may be especially useful with developmentally delayed children for whom it may be impossible to derive a meaningful developmental index. Age-equivalent scores are easy for parents to understand, but they must be interpreted carefully because they can be misleading.

The *criterion-referenced test* is one in which scores are interpreted on the basis of absolute criteria (e.g., the number of items answered correctly) rather than on relative criteria, such as how the rest of the normal group performed. Such tests are usually developed by the teacher or researcher and can be used for research involving a comparison of groups, just as norm-referenced tests are used. Criterion-referenced tests are used to measure a person's mastery of a set of behavioral objectives. The tests represent an attempt to maximize the validity or appropriateness of the content based on that set of objectives. The *developmental quotient* is the ratio between the child's actual score (developmental age) on a test and the child's CA. An example is motor age / chronologic age equal to the motor quotient (MQ).

Norm-referenced or *standardized tests* use normative values as standards for interpreting individual test scores. The purpose of standardized tests is to make a comparison between a particular child and the "norm" or "average" of a group of children. Norms describe a person's test score relative to a large body of scores that have already been collected on a defined population. Examples of norm-referenced tests include the Bayley Scales of Infant and Toddler Development III (Bayley-III), the Peabody Developmental Motor Scales 2, and the Bruininks-Oserestsky Test of Motor Proficiency 2.

The *percentile score* indicates the number of children of the same age or grade level (or whatever is used for a source of comparison) who would be expected to score lower than the child tested. For example, a child who scores in the 75th percentile on a norm-referenced test has done better than 75% of the children in the norm group.

A *raw score* is the total of individual items that are passed or correct on a particular test. On many tests, this will require establishing a basal and ceiling level of performance. The number of items required to achieve a basal or ceiling level varies from one test to another.

Reliability refers to consistency or repeatability between measurements in a series. Types of reliability include interobserver and test–retest. Interobserver reliability describes the relationship between items passed and failed, or the percentage of agreement, between two independent observers. Simply stated, interobserver reliability is an index of whether two different testers obtain the same score on a test. Test–retest reliability is the relationship of a person's score on the first administration of the test to the score on the second administration. Simply stated, this type of reliability determines whether the same or similar scores are achieved when the test is repeated under identical conditions.

Standard error of measurement (SEM) is a measure of reliability that indicates the precision of an individual test score. The SEM gives an estimate of the margin of error associated with a particular test score and is related to the probability of observing a score at a given interval. The SEM can be used to develop confidence intervals for interpreting the accuracy of a test score.

Standard scores are expressed as deviations or variations from the mean score for a group. Standard scores are expressed in units of standard deviation (SD). When using standard scores, information is needed concerning the mean and SD of the standard score.

Validity is an indication of the extent to which a test measures what it purports to measure. *Construct validity* is an examination of the theory or hypothetical constructs underlying the test. *Content validity* assesses the appropriateness of the test or how well the content of the test samples the subject matter or behaviors about which conclusions must be drawn. The sample situations measured in the test must be representative of the set from which the sample is drawn. There are two types of *criterion-related validity*. *Concurrent validity* relates the performance on the test to performance on another well-known and accepted test that measures the same knowledge or behavior. *Predictive validity* means that the child's performance on the test predicts some actual behavior.

Sensitivity can be defined as the ability of a test to identify correctly those who actually have a disorder. High sensitivity results in few false-negative scores.

Specificity refers to the ability of the test to identify correctly those who do not have the disorder. High specificity results in few false-positive scores.

The *positive predictive value* of a test is defined as the proportion of true positives among all those who have positive results. The *negative predictive value* is the proportion of true negatives among all those who have negative screening results.

▶ Overview of tests

Developmental assessments may be considered in several broad categories. Screening tests are used to identify deficits in a child's performance that indicate the need for further services. Assessments of component functions address specific areas of functioning (e.g., gross motor ability or reflex status). Comprehensive developmental scales evaluate all areas of development. Functional assessments evaluate the essential skills that are required in the child's natural environments of home and school. Outcome and health-related quality-of-life (HRQOL) measures are used to assess patient functioning in multiple life domains.

The rest of the chapter reviews selected tests that are available for physical therapy evaluation. Some of the more widely known standardized evaluative procedures are presented, as are some tests that are not standardized but that have proven useful in clinical practice. The categories just mentioned are used for organization.

Screening Tests

Developmental screening is the process of proactively testing whole populations of children to identify those who are at high risk for clinically significant deviations or delay in development.[12] Screening tests are designed to be a brief assessment to identify children who would benefit from more intensive diagnosis or assessment. Screening tests may be parent-completed tools such as the Ages and Stages Questionnaire (ASQ) or the Parents' Evaluation of Developmental Status (PEDS) or directly administered tools by health care practitioners.[13]

Harris Infant Neuromotor Test

The Harris Infant Neuromotor Test (HINT) was developed to be used in clinical and research settings as an early screening for potential developmental disorders in both high- and low-risk infants.[14,15] Infants shown to be at a higher risk for developmental delay based on screening using the HINT would then be referred for more extensive assessment of motor delay.[14]

TEST MEASURES AND TARGET POPULATION The HINT measures infant motor behavior, behavioral state, head circumference, and parent/caregiver's concerns about the infant's development. The target population for the HINT is infants from 2.5 to 12.5 months of age and is intended for use by a wide variety of health care professionals, such as community health nurses, physical therapists, occupational therapists, physicians, and early childhood special educators.[16]

TEST CONSTRUCTION AND STANDARDIZATION The HINT was developed based on published research on early identification of neurodevelopmental difficulties, research involving the Movement Assessment of Infants (MAI), and the lead author's clinical experiences over 15 years.[17] The items assessing locomotion, posture, movement, stereotypical behaviors, behavioral state, and head circumference measurements were selected from previously published predictive validity studies. The parent/caregiver questionnaire was included in the HINT to ensure that parents' concerns are addressed. Normative data have been collected on 412 Canadian infants from 5 provinces and stratified by gender, maternal education, and ethnicity.[14]

TEST FORMAT

Type The test is a norm-referenced neuromotor, cognitive, behavioral screening tool.

Content The test comprises four sections: Section 1—infant's background information; Section 2—five questions assessing caregiver's perception of the infant's movement and play; Section 3—twenty-one items assessing the infant's motor skills in five positions (supine, prone, supine-to-prone transition, sitting, and standing), muscle tone, movement against gravity, cooperation, stereotypical behaviors, and head circumference; and Section 4—the tester's clinical impression of the infant's development[14] shows the HINT test items (Table 3.1).

Administration The test can be administered in approximately 15 to 30 minutes, depending on the infant's behavior and the skill of the administrator. Infant handling is minimal, and the test is meant to be primarily observational.

Scoring Throughout the testing session, the motor behaviors and movements observed are checked off in boxes on the score sheet to the right for each item. The corresponding score is to the right of the description of the behavior. Total scores are derived from a sum of all scores for each of the 21 motor behavior items.

Interpretation Lower HINT total scores indicate a more mature or more optimal infant development. For the HINT assessment, a total score falling within one SD of the mean for a particular age group is considered within normal limits. A score that is greater than one SD but less than two SD above the mean is considered suspect. Scores that are greater than two SD above the mean are considered atypical or abnormal.[14]

RELIABILITY AND VALIDITY Reliability and validity of the HINT was reported in a study of two high-risk infant follow-up programs in Vancouver, British Colombia.[16] The

TABLE 3.1	HINT Items		
Test Method	**Cognitive or Behavioral Development Items**		**Motor Development Items**
Observation (infant is observed in supine, prone, sitting, and standing positions)	• Behavior and cooperation • Presence of stereotypical behaviors		• Mobility, supine • Neck retraction, supine • Eye muscle control • Head position, prone • Upper extremity position, prone • Head position, sitting • Trunk position, sitting • Locomotion and transition skills • Posture of hands • Posture of feet • Frequency and variety of movements
Testing (infant is provided stimulation or is handled by the examiner to determine scores)	• Head circumference		• Visual following • Asymmetrical tonic neck reflex • Reaching from supine position • Passive range of motion in supine position • Head righting in transition from supine to prone to supine positions • Trunk mobility in transitions from supine to prone to supine positions • Passive range of motion in prone position

Items to be tested in Harris Infant Neuromotor Test. With permission from American Physical Therapy Association.

interrater, test–retest, and intrarater reliabilities of the total HINT score were all ≥0.98, well above the "benchmark" of 0.80. Concurrent validity with the Bayley Scales of Infant Development II (BSID-II) was assessed by comparing HINT total scores to raw scores for BSID-II Mental and Motor Scales. Moderately strong and significant relationships between scores on the HINT and BSID-II Mental Scales were identified, suggesting the HINT may be tapping early cognitive behaviors assessed in the first year of life. Using the Pearson product–moment correlation, the HINT and BSID-II Motor Scales correlated strongly at $r = -0.89$, $p < 0.01$.[16]

Concurrent validity between the HINT and the Alberta Infant Motor Scales (AIMS) was reported in a longitudinal study of 121 typical and at-risk infants.[18] Both the AIMS and the HINT were administered concurrently at two time points, 4 to 6.5 months and 10 to 12.5 months. The HINT total scores were strongly related to the AIMS total scores in at-risk infants at both time periods during the first year of life and in typical infants at ages 4 to 6.5 months. Correlation coefficients for the entire sample exceeded 0.80 at both assessment time points. Concurrent validity was also studied between the HINT and the Ages and Stages Questionnaire. Pearson product–moment correlations between the two test scores for 52 infants tested ranged from $r = -0.82$ to -0.84 ($p < 0.05$).[19]

ADVANTAGES/DISADVANTAGES The HINT was designed as a screening test that may appeal to community providers who are frequently involved in screening healthy infants.[18] The inclusion of caregiver comments regarding their level of concern for the infant's movement and play is a strength as it makes the HINT more family-centered. The HINT

differentiates itself from the AIMS or the Test of Infant Motor Performance (TIMP) screening items as it is aimed at not only identifying motor deficits, but also identifying early cognitive delays or behavioral difficulties.

The HINT normative sample is small (412 Canadian infants), relative to other infant motor assessments, and covers a narrow age range (2.5 to 12.5 months), which may limit its utility in pediatric settings with a broad age span of patients.

Bayley Infant Neurodevelopmental Screener

The Bayley Infant Neurodevelopmental Screener (BINS) is a screening tool designed to identify infants and young children who are at risk for developmental and neurodevelopmental delay.[20] It is mainly used in settings where high-risk infants are followed up, such as a developmental follow-up clinics or large-volume clinical and research programs.

TEST MEASURES AND TARGET POPULATION The BINS assesses four conceptual areas of ability: basic neurological function/intactness (posture, muscle tone, movement symmetry), expressive functions (gross, fine, and oral motor/verbal), receptive functions (visual, auditory, verbal), and cognitive processes (object permanence, goal-directedness, problem solving).[21] This screening test is appropriate for infants and young children from 3 to 24 months.

TEST CONSTRUCTION AND STANDARDIZATION The BINS was constructed from a subset of items from the BSID-II as well as items measuring neurological status. The BINS was standardized on more than 600 infants, stratified according to age, sex, ethnicity, region, and parent education.

TEST FORMAT

Type The test is a norm-referenced, standardized screening tool.

Content The BINS consists of six item sets assessing basic neurologic functions, receptive, expressive, and cognitive functions. Each set contains 11 to 13 items, depending on the child's age.

Administration/Scoring Each item in the BINS is scored "optimal" (1) or "nonoptimal" (0), and the total number of "optimal" items in each set is added yielding a summary score. The BINS can be administered in 15 to 20 minutes.

Interpretation For each of the item sets, three established summary cut scores identify an infant's level of risk for developmental delay, yielding three risk groupings: low risk, moderate risk, or high risk. The three-tiered framework is used to determine which infants need to be monitored (infants in the moderate risk status) and which infants should be enrolled in intervention programs (high risk).

RELIABILITY AND VALIDITY

Depending on the age of the child, test–retest reliability for the BINS ranges from 0.71 to 0.84. Interrater reliability was established and ranges from 0.79 to 0.96, with moderate to strong internal consistency.[20] During test standardization, the BINS demonstrated acceptable concurrent validity with the BSID-II.[20]

ADVANTAGES/DISADVANTAGES

The BINS is one of the few psychometrically sound screening tests for infants and young children at risk for developmental delay. It is brief and easily administered by a number of health care providers with a variety of backgrounds. The BINS has a high degree of sensitivity and specificity (75% to 86%), which is an important aspect of any screening test.[22] Limitations include difficulty clarifying the need for comprehensive developmental assessment for children whose BIN scores fall in the middle of the three-tiered classification system (those at moderate-risk group) and a need for clarification of criteria for many test items, including muscle tone.

Tests of Motor Function

Physical therapists use motor development assessment tools as part of the physical therapy examination to measure motor development and function. A large number of assessment tools are available that examine gross and fine motor function. The Test of Infant Motor Performance, the Alberta Infant Motor Scale, Gross Motor Function Measure and Gross Motor Function Classification System, Peabody Developmental Motor Scales 2, and Bruininks-Oseretsky Test of Motor Proficiency 2 (BOT-2) are described.

Test of Infant Motor Performance

Campbell and colleagues developed the Test of Infant Motor Performance (TIMP) for physical and occupational therapists to assess posture and movement of infants from 34 weeks postmenstrual age through 4 months corrected age.[23,24]

TEST MEASURES AND TARGET POPULATION

The TIMP quantitatively assesses motor development and is used to identify infants who might benefit from early intervention services. It assesses the postural control and alignment needed for age-appropriate functional activities involving movement in early infancy, including changing positions and moving against the force of gravity, adjusting to handling, self-comforting, and orienting the head and body for looking, listening, and interacting with caregivers. The TIMP is intended for use with infants in intensive care nurseries, developmental follow-up clinics, and early intervention programs.[25] The items in the test were designed to reflect the full range of motor maturity from 34 weeks' postconceptual age to 4 months postterm.

TEST CONSTRUCTION AND STANDARDIZATION

Version 1 of the TIMP was initially developed by Girolami for use in assessing the efficacy of neurodevelopmental treatment on posture and movement in prematurely born high-risk infants from 34 to 35 weeks' postconceptual age.[26] Several revisions to the original TIMP have occurred, including revision/elimination of test items and reduction in length of the assessment through Rasch analysis resulting in the 42-item TIMP.[27] Age standards developed from 990 U.S. infants reflecting distribution of race/ethnicity in the U.S. population are available.

TEST FORMAT

Type The test is norm-referenced with elicited and observed item components.

Content Version 5.1 of the TIMP contains an observed scale of 13 dichotomously scored items used to examine an infant's spontaneous movements such as head in midline and individual finger and ankle movements. An elicited scale of 29 items tests the infant's movement responses to various positions, sights, and sounds.

According to the test authors, the processes tested by the items include the following:

1. The ability to orient and stabilize the head in space and in response to auditory and visual stimulation in supine, prone, side-lying, and upright positions and during transitions from one position to another
2. Body alignment when the head is manipulated
3. Distal selective control of the fingers, wrists, hands, and ankles
4. Antigravity control of arm and leg movements

Administration/Scoring The test can be administered in 25 to 40 minutes, depending on the child's abilities, behavioral state, physiologic stability, and level of cooperation. Observations of spontaneous emitted behaviors/movements are rated present (1) or absent (0) throughout the course of the examination. Elicited items are administered according to standardized instructions and involve direct handling of the infant. Responses to these items are scored on a 3-, 4-, 5-, or 6-point rating scales that describe specific behaviors to be noted, ranging from less mature or minimal response to mature or full response, as defined individually for each test item. Total raw scores range from 0 to 142.

Interpretation Raw scores are transformed into standard scores and interpreted relative to the mean for the corresponding age group. Score sheets for plotting the infants' scores against percentile ranks provide age-equivalent scores. On the basis of previous research on predictive validity of the TIMP, the authors suggest a −0.5 SD below the mean for identifying infants who may require close monitoring and/or referral for intervention.[25]

RELIABILITY AND VALIDITY Test–retest reliability over a 3-day period is reported at $r = 0.89$ for infants from 34 weeks PCA to 4 months of age.[28] Intrarater reliability (ICC = 0.98 to 0.99) and interrater reliability (ICC = 0.95) are excellent.[29] Construct validity was assessed by determining the test's sensitivity for assessing age-related changes in motor skills and correlation with risk for developmental abnormality. The correlation between postconceptual age and TIMP performance measures was 0.83. Risk and age together explained 72% of the variance in TIMP performance ($r = 0.85$; $p < 0.00001$).[30] Concurrent validity between TIMP and AIMS raw scores at 3 months of age are reported at 0.64 ($p < 0.0001$) and 0.60 ($p < 0.0001$) between TIMP raw scores and AIMS percentiles.[31]

ADVANTAGES/DISADVANTAGES The TIMP has excellent test–retest and rater reliabilities and is designed specifically to assess infants born preterm and those at risk for poor motor outcome based on perinatal medical conditions. The predictive validity of TIMP scores at 3- to 12-month AIMS percentiles demonstrates a high sensitivity at 0.92 and a specificity of 0.76.[32] The TIMP scores at 3 months also demonstrate predictive validity for preschool motor performance using the Peabody Developmental Motor Scales, with a sensitivity of 0.72 and specificity of 0.91.[33] Due to the age specifications of this test, its clinical utility is limited to settings such as special care nurseries, developmental follow-up clinics, or early intervention services.

Alberta Infant Motor Scale

The Alberta Infant Motor Scale (AIMS) is an observational assessment scale constructed by Piper and Darrah to measure gross motor maturation in infants from birth through independent walking.[34] It was developed to incorporate components of motor development, which are deemed essential to the evaluation and treatment of at-risk infants. The AIMS is designed to (1) identify infants whose motor performance is delayed or aberrant relative to a normative group; (2) provide information to the clinician and parent(s) about the motor activities the infant has mastered, those

currently developing, and those not in the infant's repertoire; (3) measure motor performance over time or before and after intervention; (4) measure changes in motor performance that are quite small and thus not likely to be detected using more traditional motor measures; and (5) act as an appropriate research tool to assess the efficacy of rehabilitation programs for infants with motor disorders.

TEST MEASURES AND TARGET POPULATION The test is an assessment of gross motor performance designed for the identification and evaluation of motor development of infants from term (40 weeks after conception) through the age of independent walking (0 to 18 months of age). The AIMS not only focuses on achievement of motor milestones, but also assesses the motor aspects and mechanisms necessary to attain such milestones (e.g., weight-bearing, posture, and antigravity movement).[35] Sequential development of postural control relative to four postural positions: supine, prone, sitting, and standing is assessed through observation.

TEST CONSTRUCTION AND STANDARDIZATION The AIMS was constructed to fulfill three clinical purposes: the identification of different levels of motor performance, the evaluation of change in motor performance over time (through maturation or intervention), and the provision of useful information for the planning of motor-intervention strategies.[34] Test items were obtained through an exhaustive review of existing instruments and descriptive narratives of early motor development. Content validation of the instrument was accomplished through meetings with and a mail survey of Canadian pediatric physical therapists and consultation with an international panel of experts. A total of 58 items were included in the provisional test for reliability and validity testing. The establishment of norms for the AIMS involved data collection on 2,200 Albertan infants stratified by age and sex.[36]

TEST FORMAT

Type The test is norm-referenced, providing percentile ranks to determine an individual's motor performance relative to the reference group.

Content The test includes 58 items organized into four positions: prone, supine, sitting, and standing. The distribution of these items is as follows: 21 prone, 9 supine, 12 sitting, and 16 standing. For each item, certain key descriptors are identified that must be observed for the infant to pass the items. Each item describes three aspects of motor performance—weight-bearing, posture, and antigravity movements (Fig 3.1).

Administration/Scoring The administration of the test involves observational assessment, with minimal handling required. The surface of the body bearing weight, posture, and movement are assessed for each item. The scoring is recorded as "observed"/"not observed." For each of the four positions, the least mature and most mature item observed

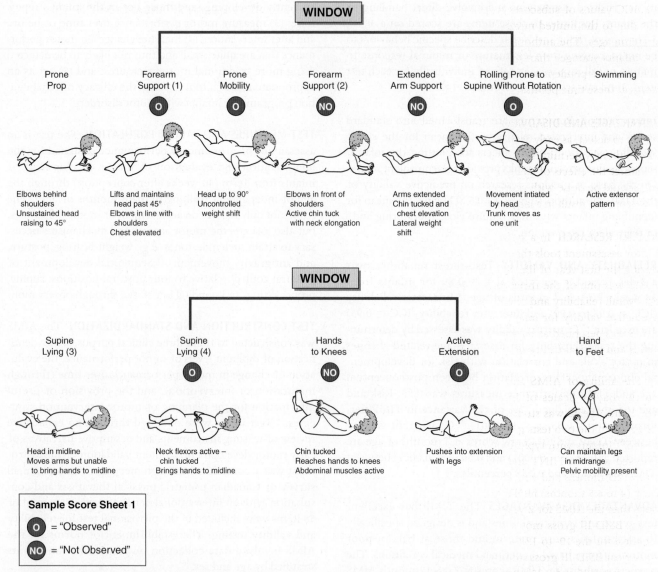

WINDOW

Prone Prop	Forearm Support (1)	Prone Mobility	Forearm Support (2)	Extended Arm Support	Rolling Prone to Supine Without Rotation	Swimming
	O	**O**	**NO**	**NO**	**O**	

Elbows behind shoulders
Unsustained head raising to 45°

Lifts and maintains head past 45°
Elbows in line with shoulders
Chest elevated

Head up to 90°
Uncontrolled weight shift

Elbows in front of shoulders
Active chin tuck with neck elongation

Arms extended
Chin tucked and chest elevation
Lateral weight shift

Movement intiated by head
Trunk moves as one unit

Active extensor pattern

WINDOW

Supine Lying (3)	Supine Lying (4)	Hands to Knees	Active Extension	Hand to Feet
O	**O**	**NO**	**O**	

Head in midline
Moves arms but unable to bring hands to midline

Neck flexors active – chin tucked
Brings hands to midline

Chin tucked
Reaches hands to knees
Abdominal muscles active

Pushes into extension with legs

Can maintain legs in midrange
Pelvic mobility present

Sample Score Sheet 1

O = "Observed"

NO = "Not Observed"

FIGURE 3.1 Sample score sheet for the AIMS. (Permission for use of this sample score sheet of the Alberta Infant Motor Scales [figure 4-1 in AIMS Manual] from Elsevier Publishers.)

in the assessment is recorded as "observed" and serves as the "window" of the infants' possible motor repertoire. Scores in each area (prone, supine, sitting, standing) are summed to yield a total score of items passed.

Interpretation The infant's total AIMS score is plotted on a graph to determine the percentile ranking of the infant's motor performance compared with the normative age-matched sample. The higher the percentile ranking, the less likely the infant is demonstrating a delay in motor development. As the AIMS is not a diagnostic test, implications of lower percentile rankings (10%) are not definitive, and the examiner's clinical judgment is required for decisions related to ongoing monitoring, referral for further diagnostic workup, and/or recommendations for intervention for motor delay.

RELIABILITY AND VALIDITY The original sample consisted of 506 (285 male, 221 female) normal infants, age stratified from birth through 18 months. One hundred twenty infants were scored on the AIMS, Peabody, and Bayley Scales for an assessment of concurrent validity, and 253 infants were each scored two or three times on the AIMS to assess the interrater and test–retest reliability of the AIMS.[36] The authors found an interrater reliability of 0.99 and a test–retest reliability of 0.99. Correlation coefficients reflecting concurrent validity with the Bayley and Peabody Scales were determined to be $r = 0.98$ and $r = 0.97$, respectively.[36] Pin et al. studied the intra- and interrater reliability in infants born at or before 29 weeks gestational age from 4 to 18 months chronologic age.[37] All of the ICC values were greater than 0.75 and the SEM less than 1.2. Although the AIMS is a reliable measurement tool to be used in this infant population, the ICC values of subscores were low at 4 and 18 months CA due to the limited number of test items at these two extreme ages. The authors caution about using the AIMS for infants younger than 4 months or after the infant has achieved independent walking, because of the limited test items at these time points.

ADVANTAGES AND DISADVANTAGES The AIMS provides the ability to detect, as early as possible, any deviations from the norm, thereby permitting early intervention to remediate or minimize the effects of dysfunction. Use of percentile ranking should be done with caution because a small change in raw score can result in a large change in percentile ranking.[38]

RECENT RESEARCH In a systematic review of nine neuromotor assessment tools that can be administered to infants during the first year of life, Spittle et al. concluded that the AIMS was one of the three tests demonstrating the highest overall reliability and one of the two with the strongest predictive validity for infants aged 8 to 12 months.[39] The AIMS was described as having the best psychometric properties and clinical utility of the five norm-referenced tests reviewed.

The ability of AIMS and the HINT to predict scores on the Bayley Scales of Infant Development (BSID) at age 2 and 3 years was studied to compare predictive validity between the two tests given during the infant's first year of life.[40] Infants with typical and at-risk development were assessed with the HINT and AIMS at 4 to 6.5 months and 10 to 12.5 months and with the BSID at 2 and 3 years. The early (4 to 6.5 months) HINT had higher predictive correlations than the AIMS for 2-year BSID-II motor outcomes and 3-year BSID-III gross motor outcomes. Correlations were identical for the 10- to 12.5-month HINT and AIMS scores and 3-year BSID-III gross motor ($r = 0.58$ and 0.58) and fine motor ($r = 0.35$ and 0.35) subscale.

Gross Motor Function Measure

The Gross Motor Function Measure (GMFM) is a clinical measure designed to evaluate change in gross motor function in children with cerebral palsy.[41]

TEST MEASURES AND TARGET POPULATION The test is designed to assess motor function or how much of an activity a child can accomplish. It is an evaluative index of gross motor function and changes in function over time, or after therapy, specifically for children with cerebral palsy. The original validation sample included children 5 months to 16 years old. The GMFM is appropriate for children whose motor skills are at or below those of a 5-year-old child without any motor disability. The Gross Motor Performance Measure (GMPM), an observational instrument assessing quality of gross motor movement, can be used in conjunction with the GMFM to evaluate change over time in specific qualitative features of motor behavior.[42]

TEST CONSTRUCTION AND STANDARDIZATION The GMFM was developed and tested according to contemporary principles of measurement design through a process of item selection, reliability testing, and validation procedures. The selection of items was based on a literature review and the judgment of pediatric clinicians. Items judged to be clinically important and measureable with the potential of showing change in the function of children were included. The original GMFM contains 88 items (GMFM-88). In an effort to improve the interpretability and clinical usefulness of the GMFM, Rasch analysis was applied to the GMFM-88, resulting in the GMFM-66.[43] The authors report that the GMFM-66 provides hierarchical structure and interval scoring that provides a better understanding of motor development in children with CP than the older GMFM-88.[44]

TEST FORMAT

Type The GMFM is a criterion-based observational measure.

Content The test includes 88 items that assess motor function in five dimensions: (1) lying and rolling; (2) sitting; (3) crawling and kneeling; (4) standing; and (5) walking, running, and jumping. With emphasis on maximizing a child's potential for independent function, the test measures whether a child can complete the task independently (with or without the use of aids), without any active assistance from another person.

Administration/Scoring For ease of administration, the items are grouped on the rating form by test position and arranged in a developmental sequence. For scoring purposes, items are aggregated to represent five separate areas of motor function. Each GMFM item is scored on a four-point ordinal scale. Values of 0, 1, 2, and 3 are assigned to each of the four categories; 0 = does not initiate; 1 = initiates (<10% of the task); 2 = partially completes (10 to <100% of the task); and 3 = task completion. A one-page score sheet is used to record results. Specific descriptions for how to score each item are found in the administration and scoring guidelines contained within the test manual. The 66 items that form the GMFM-66 are indicated on the scoresheet by shading and an asterisk. The time required to complete the GMFM-88 is approximately 45 to 60 minutes. As the GMFM-66 has 22 fewer items to be administered, it should require less time to administer the test.

Interpretation Each of the five dimensions contributes equal weight to the total score; therefore, a percent score is calculated for each dimension (child's score/maximum score × 100%). A total score is obtained by adding the percent scores for each dimension and dividing by five. A "goal total score" can also be calculated in order to increase the responsiveness of the measure by narrowing the focus to include selected GMFM dimensions most relevant to the child's goals. In order to interpret scores for the GMFM-66, a computer program, the Gross Motor Ability Estimator (GMAE) is required. The GMFM-66 score differs from the GMFM-88 score in that it has interval (as opposed to ordinal) properties.

RELIABILITY AND VALIDITY The test authors found intra-rater reliability for each dimension and the total score to range from 0.92 to 0.99 and interrater reliability to range from 0.87 to 0.99 (ICC).[3] The GMFM-66 is also highly reliable (ICCs = 0.97 to 0.99) and sensitive to change.[44, 45]

Construct validity of the GMFM-88 was demonstrated with significant linear relationships between gait speed and dimensions D (standing) ($r = 0.91$) and E (walking, running, and jumping) ($r = 0.93$).[46] More recently, the longitudinal construct validity of three scoring options (GMFM-88, GMFM-88 goal total, and GMFM-66) was evaluated in a 5-year follow-up study.[47] Forty-one children with cerebral palsy who were undergoing selective dorsal rhizotomy were monitored with the GMFM for 5 years. All three scoring options showed large longitudinal construct validity in the 5-year study. The GMFM-88 total and goal total scores revealed large changes in gross motor function earlier post-operatively than the GMFM-66 scores. Validity and reliability of two abbreviated versions of the GMFM-66 have also been reported.[48] Both the GMFM-66-IS (item set) and the GMFM-66-B&C (basal and ceiling approach) demonstrate high levels of validity (ICCs of 0.99) and reliability (ICCs greater than 0.98) and can be used in clinical practice or for research purposes.

During the course of validation of the original version of the GMFM, it became evident that a meaningful, valid, and reliable classification of children's functional mobility was needed to enhance communication among families and professionals and to provide a sound basis for stratification of children for research.[49] The Gross Motor Function Classification System for Cerebral Palsy (GMFCS), developed by Palisano and colleagues in 1997, was created to classify motor function in children with CP into one of five clinically meaningful levels (Table 3.2).[50]

From Level I (most able) to Level V (most limited), the GMFCS describes motor function within four age bands, from before a child's second birthday to between the 6th and 12th birthday. Motor function is described in "word pictures," focusing on function under ordinary circumstances, rather than on capacity as observed with formal tools such as the GMFM or PEDI. The GMFCS–E&R is the expanded and revised version of the GMFCS, with a revised 6- to 12-year age band, addition of a 12- to 18-year age band, with an expanded conceptual framework to coincide with the International Classification of Functioning, Disability, and Health.[50]

ADVANTAGES/DISADVANTAGES Debuse et al. completed a systematic review of outcome measures of activity for children with cerebral palsy.[51] The GMFM-88, GMFM-66, and the Pediatric Evaluation of Disability Inventory (PEDI) were the three outcome measures selected as most appropriate for testing function in children with cerebral palsy. Both the GMFM-88 and the PEDI exhibit high completion rates, confirming the relevance of these outcome measures to the functional ability of children with cerebral palsy. Long completion time and relative unidimensionality (testing only gross motor capacity in a controlled testing environment)

TABLE 3.2	General Headings for Each Level of GMFCS-E&R

General Heading for Each Level

LEVEL I—Walks without Limitations

LEVEL II—Walks with Limitations

LEVEL III—Walks Using a Hand-Held Mobility Device

LEVEL IV—Self-Mobility with Limitations; May Use Powered Mobility

LEVEL V—Transported in a Manual Wheelchair

Distinctions Between Levels I and II—Compared with children and youth in Level I, children and youth in Level II have limitations walking long distances and balancing; may need a hand-held mobility device when first learning to walk; may use wheeled mobility when traveling long distances outdoors and in the community; require the use of a railing to walk up and down stairs; and are not as capable of running and jumping.

Distinctions Between Levels II and III—Children and youth in Level II are capable of walking without a hand-held mobility device after age 4 (although they may choose to use one at times). Children and youth in Level III need a hand-held mobility device to walk indoors and use wheeled mobility outdoors and in the community.

Distinctions Between Levels III and IV—Children and youth in Level III sit on their own or require at most limited external support to sit, are more independent in standing transfers, and walk with a hand-held mobility device .Children and youth in Level IV function in sitting (usually supported) but self-mobility is limited. Children and youth in Level IV are more likely to be transported in a manual wheelchair or use powered mobility.

Distinctions Between Levels IV and V—Children and youth in Level V have severe limitations in head and trunk control and require extensive assisted technology and physical assistance. Self-mobility is achieved only if the child/youth can learn how to operate a powered wheelchair.

Permission from CanChild Website. http://Peds-QLTM.canchild.ca/en/measures/gmfcs_expanded_revised.asp

were reported as weaknesses or disadvantages of the test. While the GMFM-66 has 22 fewer items to test, allowing a faster completion time, it has floor effects in children with low motor ability and ceiling effects in children older than 5 years.[44] Careful consideration is required when determining whether to use the GMFM-88 or the GMFM-66 based on the child's motor abilities, ability to complete all test items required, and/or the clinician's knowledge and ability to use the Gross Motor Ability Estimator appropriately.

Peabody Developmental Motor Scales— Second Edition

The Peabody Developmental Motor Scales—Second Edition (PDMS-2) is the culmination of over a decade of research by the authors in response to reviewer's suggestions and feedback from examiners for improving the original Peabody Developmental Motor Scales (PDMS).[52,53]

TEST MEASURES AND TARGET POPULATION The PDMS-2 comprises six subtests that measure the interrelated gross and fine motor abilities that develop early in life. The PDMS-2 can be used by physical and occupational therapists, early intervention specialists, adapted physical education teachers, psychologists, diagnosticians, and others interested in examining the motor abilities of young children. It was designed to assess motor skills in children from birth through 6 years of age.

TEST CONSTRUCTION AND STANDARDIZATION The original PDMS was developed to improve on the existing instruments used for motor evaluation. Test items were obtained from validated motor scales, and new items were created based on studies of children's growth and development. Characteristics of the PDMS-2 include a larger normative sample of 2,003 children stratified by age residing in 46 states and one Canadian province, the addition of studies showing the absence of gender and racial bias, reliability coefficients for subgroups of the normative sample (e.g., individuals with motor disabilities, African Americans, Hispanic Americans, females, and males) as well as for the entire normative sample, and validity studies with special attention devoted to showing that the test is valid for a wide variety of subgroups as well as for the general population.[53]

TEST FORMAT

Type The PDMS-2 is a discriminative measure and is norm-referenced.

Content The PDMS-2 is divided into two components: the Gross Motor Scale and the Fine Motor Scale. The Gross Motor Scale contains 151 items divided into four subtests: Reflexes (birth to 11 months), Stationary (all ages), Locomotion (all ages), and Object Manipulation (12 months and older).

The Fine Motor Scale contains 98 items divided into two subtests: Grasping (all ages) and Visual-Motor Integration (all ages). Norms are provided for each skill category at each age level, as well as for total scores.

The results of the subtests may be used to generate three global indexes of motor performance called composites— the Gross Motor Quotient (GMQ), the Fine Motor Quotient (FMQ), and the Total Motor Quotient (TMQ).

Administration Both scales can be given to a child in approximately 45 to 60 minutes. To shorten testing time, entry points and basal and ceiling levels are used on all but one of the subtests (Reflexes). Examiners who give and interpret the PDMS-2 should have a thorough understanding of test statistics; general procedures governing scoring and interpretation; specific information about gross and fine motor ability testing; and development in children who are not progressing typically.[53] In order to achieve valid interpretation of a child's PDMS-2 performance, the scales must be administered exactly as specified in the Guide to Item Administration.

When the purpose of the test is eligibility or placement, instructional, or treatment programming for a child with disabilities, the examiner should administer an item as directed or adapt to fit the child's individual needs while retaining the intent of the item.

Scoring Each item on the PDMS-2 is scored as 0, 1, or 2. Specific criteria are given for each item, as are the general criteria for the numeric scores. Scores are assigned as follows:

0—The child cannot or will not attempt the item, or the attempt does not show that the skill is emerging.
1—The child's performance shows a clear resemblance to the item mastery criteria but does not fully meet the criteria. (This value allows for emerging skills.)
2—The child performs the item according to the criteria specified for mastery.

Scoring may be completed on a written summary sheet or by using the PDMS-2 Online Scoring and Report System.

Interpretation The PDMS-2 yields five types of scores: raw scores, age equivalents, percentiles, standard scores for the subtests, and quotients for the composites. From the raw scores calculated from each subtest, the age-equivalent and standard scores are obtained from the norms tables provided in the manual. The quotients for the fine motor, gross motor, and total motor composites are derived from summing the subtest standard scores and converting them to a quotient. After the standard scores and quotients have been determined, they may be plotted on the Motor Development Profile. This profile provides a means of visually comparing performance on the Gross Motor Scale and Fine Motor Scale and on the skill categories in each scale. Figure 3.2 presents an example of scoring the PDMS-2.

Item #	Ages in Months	Item name, Position, and Description	Score Criteria	Score
16	7	ROLLING *(Lying on back)* Shake Rattle at midline 12 in. above child. Lower rattle to surface on child's left, out of child's reach. Repeat procedure on opposite side	2　Rolls from back to stomach (both sides) 1　Rolls from back to stomach (on side only) 0　Remains on back	*2*
17	7	ROLLING *(Lying on back)* Attract child's attention to toy by shaking it to side of child. Repeat procedure on opposite side.	2　Rolls from back to stomach, leading with hips and thighs, folllowed by stomach and then shoulders (both sides) 1　Rolls from back to stomach (one side) 0　Remains on back	*2*
18	8	MOVING FORWARD *(Lying on stomach)* Place toy 5 ft. in front of child. Say, "Get the toy."	2　Moves forward using arms 1　Moves forward at least 2 ft. but less than 3 ftp. using arms 0　Moves less than 2 ft.	*1*
19	9	RAISING SHOULDERS & BUTTOCKS *(Lying on stomach)* Sit 3 ftp. in front of child. Hold your hands out to child and say, "Come here."	2　Raises and bears weight on hands and knees for 5 seconds and rocks back and forth for 2 cycles 1　Raises and bears weight on hands and knees for 1–5 seconds 0　Remains on stomach	*1*
20	9	CREEPING *(Hand and knees)* Place toy on floor 6 ft. in front of child. Say, "Get the toy." Move toy back as child approaches.	2　Creeps forward on hands and knees, using a cross-lateral pattern for 5 ft. 1　Creeps forward on hands and knees using cross-lateral pattern for 4 ft. or creeps without using cross-lateral pattern for 5 ft. 0　Remains stationary or moves on stomach	*0*
21	9	CREEPING *(Sitting)* Sit beside child on floor. Say, "Watch me." Demonstrate scooting by using your hands to propel your body forward on your buttocks to retrieve toy. Place toy 5 ft. in front of child. Say, "Scoot like I did and get the toy."	2　Maintains sitting posture and uses hands and legs to scoot forward 3 ft. 1　Maintains sitting posture and scoots forward 1–2 ft. 0　Moves less than 1 ft. forward	*0*

FIGURE 3.2 PDMS-2 item administration sample.

RELIABILITY AND VALIDITY The overall reliability of the PDMS-2 was studied by the test developers for three types of error variance-internal consistency, test–retest reliability, and interscorer reliability. The reliability coefficients for three composites and six subtests (Cronbach's $\alpha = 0.89$ to 0.97, test–retest $r = 0.82$ to 0.93, and interscorer $r = 0.96$ to 0.99) suggests a high degree of reliability. The magnitude of these coefficients strongly suggests that the PDMS-2 possesses little test error and that users can have confidence in its results.[53]

According to the authors, the content validity of PDMS-2 is based on established research on normal children's motor development and on other validated tests assessing motor development. The construct validity of the PDMS-2 was established by confirmatory factor analyses, with results demonstrating that the fine motor and the gross motor composites are two separate constructs within general movement. Connolly et al. explored the concurrent validity of BSID-II Motor Scales and the PDMS-2 in 15 typically developing 12-month-old infants.[54] A lack of concurrent validity between PDMS-2 and BSID-II Motor Scales standard scores was reported. Additionally, lack of agreement between age equivalents between the two tests was reported, except for locomotion. The investigators conclude that administration of the BSID-II and PDMS-2 may yield dissimilar findings in gross motor development for 12-month-old infants and may affect a child's eligibility for services. This information is valuable, however, to reinforce the importance of the physical therapists' overall assessment of the child (beyond reported objective assessment results) when determining the need for intervention.

ADVANTAGES/DISADVANTAGES The PDMS-2 is a standardized, reliable, and valid assessment tool with a broad age range for assessing infants and young children. Subtest composites can be scored separately, easing administration, and the 3-point scoring system enables examiners to identify emerging skills and to measure progress in children who are slow in acquiring new skills. Disadvantages of the PDMS-2 include absence of normative data on European children, long administration time for younger children, and the absence of a short form.[55]

Bruininks-Oseretsky Test of Motor Proficiency— Second Edition

The Bruininks-Oseretsky Test of Motor Proficiency— Second Edition (BOT-2) is the newest revision of the Bruininks-Oseretsky Test of Motor Proficiency (BOTMP) developed by Dr. Robert H. Bruininks.[56] The BOT-2 provides a comprehensive assessment of motor skills, including differentiated measures of fine and gross motor proficiency.[57]

TEST MEASURES AND TARGET POPULATION The BOT-2 is designed to assess gross and fine motor functioning in children and is used to support diagnosis of motor impairments, screen for motor deficits, assist in educational placement decisions, and can be used as a means for planning and evaluating various motor development curricula. The test is appropriate for children aged 4 through 21.[57]

TEST CONSTRUCTION AND STANDARDIZATION The revision of the Bruininks-Oseretsky Test of Motor Proficiency began in 2002 with a development team consisting of the authors, test directors, and researchers. The revision provided contemporary norms, improved test organization and content, and addressed current user needs. The BOT-2 has been standardized on a sample of 1,520 children from 38 states. Over 11% of the normative sample included children with disabilities. The sample selection was random and stratified across sex, race/ethnicity, socioeconomic status, and disability status within each of the 12 age groups.

TEST FORMAT

Type The BOT-2 is norm-referenced, and it involves individually administered tasks with direct observation and assessment of a child in a structured environment.

Content The BOT-2 assesses proficiency in four motor-area composites: Fine Manual Control, Manual Coordination, Body Coordination, and Strength and Agility. These four motor-area composites each comprise two of the eight BOT-2 subtests. The fifth composite, the Total Motor Composite, is devised from all eight subtests.

The relationship of the eight subtests to the composites is shown in Figure 3.3.

Administration The Complete Form can be administered in 40 to 60 minutes, with an extra 10 minutes needed to prepare the testing area. The Short Form (used for screening purposes) can be administered in 15 to 20 minutes, with an additional 5 minutes needed for area set up. The Short Form consists of 14 BOT-2 items carefully selected from all eight subtests and yields a single score of overall motor proficiency. Two short testing sessions are recommended for young children. Procedures for administration and scoring

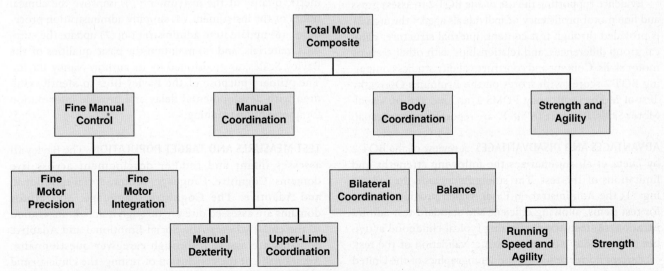

FIGURE 3.3 Relationship of the eight subtests of the Bruininks-Oseretsky Test of Motor Proficiency to the BOT-2 composites. (Adapted figures from the Bruininks-Oseretsky Test of Motor Proficiency, Second Edition [BOT-2]. Copyright 2005 NCS Pearson, Inc. Reproduced with permission. All rights reserved. "BOT" is a trademark, in the U.S. and/or other countries, of Pearson Education Inc. or its affiliates.)

of the test are well written and are shown in the manual. Materials needed to administer the BOT-2 are provided in the standardized test kit with the exception of stopwatch and tape measure.

Scoring Scoring may be completed using the BOT-2 ASSIST™ software or through hand scoring. The child's raw scores are recorded during the administration of the test and are converted first to point scores, then to standard scores, approximate age equivalents, and percentile rank (see Fig 3.4 for a sample record form for BOT-2). Five descriptive categories are also included on the scoring sheet to assist in communicating test results to examinees, parents, and teachers. The Total Motor Composite is derived from the sum of the four motor-area composite standard scores and is the most reliable and preferred measure of overall motor proficiency.

Interpretation Tables of norms are provided, and by comparing derived scores with the scores of subjects tested in the standardization program, users can interpret a child's performance in relation to a national reference group.

RELIABILITY AND VALIDITY Test–retest reliability coefficients for the subtests is in the upper 0.70s for examinees aged 4 through 7 and 8 through 12, and 0.69 for examinees aged 13 through 21. The mean of the composite correlation coefficients is in the low 0.80s for examinees aged 4 through 12, and is 0.77 for examinees aged 13 through 21.[57] Internal consistency reliability is high, with the mean subtest reliability in three age groups ranging from the high 0.70s to the low 0.80s.

Interrater reliability coefficients are extremely high at 0.98 and 0.99 for Manual Coordination, Body Coordination, and Strength and Agility composites. The Fine Motor Control composite coefficient is also high at 0.92.

Evidence supporting the use of the BOT-2 to assess gross and fine motor proficiency of individuals aged 4 through 21 is provided through test content, internal structure, clinical group differences, and relationships with other tests of motor skills. Content and construct validity studies comparing BOT-2 scores with scores on the Bruininks-Oseretsky Test of Motor Proficiency, PDMS-2, and the Test of Visual-Motor Skills, Revised (TVMS-R) are reported in the manual.

ADVANTAGES AND DISADVANTAGES A review of the BOT-2 by Dietz et al. summarizes the following strengths and limitations of the test. The strengths include the following: (1) the Administration Easel, which provides photos for test items, allowing efficient and standard test administration; (2) test items reflecting typical childhood activities (face validity); (3) the construct validation of the test; (4) current norms reflecting the demographics of the United States; and (5) moderate to strong interrater and test–retest reliabilities of the Complete Form Total Motor Composite and Short Form.[58] The reported limitations include (1) weak

test–retest reliability coefficients for some subtests and motor-area composites for some age groups; (2) the scoring process can be time intensive and tedious; and (3) the difficulty of the items for 4-year-old children who are developing typically or 5-year-old children with delays.

RECENT RESEARCH Motor proficiency in children with neurofibromatosis type 1 (NF1) was assessed using the BOT-2.[59] Twenty-six children with NF1, aged 4 to 15 years, participated in the study. Participant scores relative to age- and sex-matched test norms demonstrated significantly lower scores ($p < 0.05$) for the Total Motor Composite ($z = -1.62$) and 7 of the 8 subtests. The results indicate the BOT-2 is useful in identifying and characterizing delays in motor proficiency in children with NF1.

Comprehensive Developmental Scales

Comprehensive developmental scales assess all areas of infant and child development and are well suited for multidisciplinary and area assessment teams. Developmental areas assessed include physical, cognitive, communication, social-emotional, and adaptive language, complying with Part C of Individuals with Disabilities Education Act (IDEA) regulations for service eligibility for early intervention and special education services.[60]

Bayley Scales of Infant and Toddler Development— Third Edition

The Bayley Scales of Infant and Toddler Development— Third Edition (Bayley-III) is a revision of the BSID-II.[61,62] The revision was conducted to improve the quality and to enhance the utility of the Bayley Scales and had several major goals: (1) update the normative data, (2) develop 5 distinct scales, (3) strengthen the psychometric quality of the instrument, (4) improve the clinical utility of the instrument, (5) simplify administration procedures, (6) update item administration, (7) update the stimulus materials, and (8) maintain the basic qualities of the Bayley Scales, as envisioned by its author, Nancy Bayley. The primary purpose of the Bayley-III is to identify children with developmental delay and provide information for intervention planning.

TEST MEASURES AND TARGET POPULATION The Bayley-III assesses infant and toddler development across five domains: Cognitive, Language, Motor, Social-Emotional, and Adaptive. The Cognitive, Language, and Motor domains are assessed directly through item administration to the child, whereas the Social-Emotional and Adaptive domains are assessed through caregiver questionnaire. Additionally, at the conclusion of testing, the clinician and caregiver complete the Behavior Observation Inventory to assess whether the child's testing performance is typical of his or her ability. The Bayley-III is individually

BOT 2

Bruininks-Oseretsky Test
of Motor Proficiency, *Second Edition*
Robert H. Bruininks & Brett D. Bruininks

	Year	Month	Day
Test Date	2006	10	2
Birth Date	1998	7	1
Chronological Age	8	3	1

Preferred Drawing Hand: (Right) Left
Preferred Throwing Hand/Arm: (Right) Left
Preferred Foot/Leg: (Right) Left

Norms Used: ☒ Female ☐ Male ☐ Combined

Examinee Name KaLeah Nelson   Sex Female   Grade 2

Examiner Name Dan Kotter   School/Clinic Whittier Clinic

	Total Point Score	Scale Score Mean = 15, SD = 5 (Tables B.1–B.13)	Standard Score Mean = 50, SD = 10 (Tables B.4–B.7)	Confidence Interval (90%) or 95% (Tables C.1–C.4) Band	Interval	%ile Rank (Tables B.4–B.7)	Age Equiv. (Tables B.14–B.16)	Descriptive Category (Table C.13)
1 Fine Motor Precision	38	18		+ − 4	14 − 22		9:0–9:2	Average
2 Fine Motor Integration	38	18		+ − 4	14 − 22		10:0–10:2	Average
Fine Manual Control	Sum 36		57	+ − 7	50 − 64	76		Average
3 Manual Dexterity	28	17		+ − 4	13 − 21		8:9–8:11	Average / Well–Above
7 Upper-Limb Coordination	37	25		+ − 3	22 − 28		12:6–12:11	Average
Manual Coordination	Sum 42		65	+ − 6	59 − 71	93		Above Average
4 Bilateral Coordination	17	10		+ − 3	7 − 13		5:9–5:9	Below Average
5 Balance	27	8		+ − 3	5 − 11		5:2–5:3	Below Average
Body Coordination	Sum 18		35	+ − 6	29 − 41	7		Below Average
6 Running Speed and Agility	30	14		+ − 4	10 − 18		7:3–7:5	Average
8 Strength Push-up Knee (Full)	25	20		+ − 4	16 − 24		12:6–12:11	Above Average
Strength and Agility	Sum 34		56	+ − 7	49 − 63	73		Average

Sum 213

Total Motor Composite 54 + − 4   50 − 58   66   Average

	Total Point Score	Standard Score (Tables B.8–B.13)	Confidence Interval: 90% or 95% (Tables C.3, C.4) Band	Interval	%ile Rank (Tables B.8–B.13)	Descriptive Category (Table C.3)
SHORTForm Push-up Knee Full			+ − 4	50 − 58	66	

DIRECTIONS

Complete Form

During the testing session, record the examinee's performance on each item.

After the testing session, convert each item raw score to a point score using the conversion table provided. For items needing two trials, convert the better of the two raw scores. Then, record the point score in the appropriate oval in the Point Score column.

For each subtest, add the item point scores, and record the total in the oval labeled Total Point Score and on the appropriate line on the cover page.

Short Form

During the testing session, record the examinee's performance on each Short Form item, listed on page 8.

After the testing session, convert each item raw score to a point score using the conversion table provided. For items needing two trials, convert the better of the two raw scores. Then, record the point score in the appropriate oval in the Point Score column.

Finally, add the item point scores for all 14 Short Form items, and record the total in the oval labeled Total Point Score and on the appropriate line on the cover page.

FIGURE 3.4 Recording form for the eight subtests of the Bruininks-Oseretsky Test of Motor Proficiency. (Adapted figures from the Bruininks-Oseretsky Test of Motor Proficiency, Second Edition [BOT-2]. Copyright 2005 NCS Pearson, Inc. Reproduced with permission. All rights reserved. "BOT" is a trademark, in the U.S. and/or other countries, of Pearson Education Inc. or its affiliates.)

administered to infants and children between 1 month and 42 months of age.

TEST CONSTRUCTION AND STANDARDIZATION
The original BSID was derived from several infant and child developmental scales and a broad cross-section of infant and child research.[63] The creation of items for the Bayley-III was based on developmental research and theory that identifies behaviors typical for normal development in young children. Item administration for all three of the Bayley Scales (BSID, BSID-II, and Bayley-III) occurs in a modified power sequence; that is, items are typically ordered according to their degree of difficulty. The BSID-II contained three scales: Mental, Motor, and Behavior rating. The creation of a separate Language Scale for the Bayley-III reduced the number of items within the BSID-II Mental Scale, allowing expansion of cognitive concepts and constructs to be assessed in the Bayley-III Cognitive Scale. The normative information in the Bayley-III is based on a national standardization sample representative of the U.S. population for infants 1 month through 42 months of age. The sample included 1,700 children divided into 17 age groups composed of 100 participants. Stratification along parent education level, race / ethnicity, and geographic region was completed for the normative sample.

TEST FORMAT

Type The test is norm-referenced. Information is obtained by direct observation and interaction with the child.

Content The Bayley-III contains the following scales: (1) Cognitive-items assess sensorimotor development, exploration and manipulation, object relatedness, concept formation, memory, and other aspects of cognitive functioning; (2) Language-items assess receptive and expressive communication; (3) Motor-items assess fine motor and gross motor skills; (4) Social-Emotional-items assess social and emotional milestones in children based on the Greenspan Social-Emotional Growth Chart: A Screening Questionnaire for Infants and Young Children; and (5) Adaptive Behavior-items assess adaptive skill functioning in daily life based on Adaptive Behavior Assessment System, Second Edition (Display 3.1).[64,65]

Administration The time required for administration of the Bayley-III varies with test familiarity, specific strengths and limitations of the child, and test session behavior. For children aged 12 months and younger, administration time is approximately 50 minutes for the entire battery. For children 13 months and older, the total administration time is 90 minutes. Based on an age-specific start point, the child must receive a score of 1 on the first three consecutive items to move forward (basal level). If the child scores a 0 on the first age-specific item, the examiner goes to previous age-specific item and applies the same rule. The test is discontinued for the particular scale when the child receives scores of 0 for five consecutive items (ceiling level).

Scoring and Interpretation The Bayley-III Record Form is used to record the scores for each item in the Cognitive Scale and the Receptive and Expressive Communication, Fine Motor, and Gross Motor subtests. If the child meets the scoring criteria for the particular item, the examiner circles "1," and if the child does not meet the criteria, a "0" is circled. The raw scores for each subtest are summed (Total Raw Score) and then converted to Scaled Scores, Composite Scores, Percentile Rank, and Confidence Intervals using tables provided in the manual. Discrepancy comparisons may be completed to determine whether the differences between subtests are statistically significant (critical values) and how frequently the discrepancy occurred in the standardization sample (base rates). The Adaptive Behavior and Social-Emotional Scales are completed by the caregiver, and behavior frequencies are summed for a Total Raw Score. The Behavior Observation Inventory is completed after testing is concluded.

To facilitate interpretation, the Scaled Scores and Composite Scores can be plotted on the Scaled Score Profile or Composite Score Profile graphs. Scaled Scores range from 1 to 19, with a mean of 10 and an SD of 3. The Composite Scores range from 40 to 160, with a mean of 100 and an SD of 15.

RELIABILITY AND VALIDITY
The overall reliability coefficients of the Bayley-III subtests range include 0.86 (Fine Motor), 0.87 (Receptive Communication), and 0.91 (Cognitive, Expressive Communication, and Gross Motor).[61] According to the authors, the reliability coefficients for the Cognitive Scale are comparable to those of the Mental Developmental Index of the BSID-II. The reliability coefficients for the composite scales are higher at 0.93 (Language Composite) and 0.92 (Motor Composite).

Content validity of the Bayley-III was established by comprehensive literature and expert reviews resulting new items and subtests to improve content and relevance. The Bayley-III assesses a broad spectrum of tasks for the entire age range with relevance to the constructs being measured.[61] Correlation studies were conducted between the Bayley-III and the PDMS-2 on a sample of 81 children aged 2 to 42 months. The authors report very little difference between the means of the Bayley-III composites and the PDMS-2 quotients. The highest correlations were between the Fine Motor subtest and the Fine Motor Quotient ($r = 0.59$) and between the Gross Motor subtest and the Gross Motor Quotient ($r = 0.57$). More recently, Connolly et al. reported concurrent validity between the Bayley-III and the PDMS-2 with moderate to very high correlation for all groups between the Bayley-III Composite Scores and the PDMS-2 Total Motor Quotient Scores.[66] Evidence of validity through clinical utility studies among special group studies is also reported.

ADVANTAGES
The Bayley-III is the product of decades of research in infant and child development. The five distinct

3.1   BAYLEY-III Items to be Tested

Adaptive Behavior

- Communication
- Community use
- Functional preacademics
- Home living
- Health and safety
- Leisure
- Self-care
- Self-direction
- Social
- Motor

Cognitive

- Sensorimotor development
- Exploration and manipulation
- Object relatedness
- Concept formation
- Memory
- Habituation
- Visual acuity
- Visual preference
- Object permanence
- Plus other aspects of cognitive processing

Items measure age-appropriate skills including:

- Counting (with one-to-one correspondence and cardinality)
- Visual and tactile exploration
- Object assembly
- Puzzle board completion
- Matching colors
- Comparing masses
- Representational and pretend play
- Discriminating patterns

Language
Expressive communication

Assesses preverbal communications such as:

- Babbling
- Gesturing
- Joint referencing
- Turn taking
- Vocabulary development such as naming objects, pictures, and actions
- Morpho-syntactic development such as use of two-word utterances and use of plurals and verb tense

Receptive communication

Assesses preverbal behaviors and vocabulary development such as:

- The ability to identify objects and pictures that are referenced
- Vocabulary related to morphological development such as pronouns and prepositions
- Understanding of morphological markers such as plurals and tense markings

Motor
Fine motor

Fine motor skills associated with:

- Prehension
- Perceptual–motor integration
- Motor planning
- Motor speed

Items measure age-appropriate skills including:

- Visual tracking
- Reaching
- Object manipulation
- Grasping
- Children's quality of movement
- Functional hand skills
- Responses to tactile information (sensory integration)

Gross motor

Items assess:

- Static positioning (e.g., head control, sitting, standing)
- Dynamic movement including locomotion (crawling, walking, running, jumping, walking up and down stairs)
- Quality of movement (coordination when standing up, walking, kicking)
- Balance
- Motor planning
- Perceptual–motor integration (e.g., imitating postures)

Social-Emotional

- Determines the mastery of early capacities of social-emotional growth
- Monitors healthy social and emotional functioning
- Monitors progress in early intervention programs
- Detects deficits or problems with developmental social-emotional capacities

scales are designed to meet federal and state guidelines for early childhood assessment. The psychometric qualities and clinical utility have improved with the newest revision, while maintaining the basic qualities of the earlier Bayley Scales.

DISADVANTAGES The time to administer the assessment is lengthy, and can be difficult to complete in many health care settings. Concerns of underestimation of developmental delay by the Bayley-III was reported in a cohort study of 2-year-old children born extremely preterm/extremely low birth weight and those carried to term.[67] The authors urge caution in interpreting Bayley-III Scores for high-risk children in the absence of appropriate control groups.

Battelle Developmental Inventory—Second Edition

The Battelle Developmental Inventory—Second Edition (BDI-2) (published in 2005) is a comprehensive developmental assessment for children used to measure development in children with and without disabilities, to screen for children at risk for developmental delay, and to assist in development of individualized family service plans and individualized education plans.[5] It may be administered by a team of health care professionals or by an individual provider.

TEST MEASURES AND TARGET POPULATION The BDI-2 measures development in five domains: Adaptive, Personal-Social, Communication, Motor, and Cognitive. Each domain contains subdomains whose entry points in the test are determined by age or estimated ability of the child. The BDI-2 is appropriate for children from birth to 7 years, 11 months. The BDI-2 Screening Test is also available, consisting of a subset of items from the BDI-2 item pool.

TEST CONSTRUCTION AND STANDARDIZATION The original BDI, developed in 1984, has been used for determining children's eligibility for services as well as measuring change longitudinally in program-based studies, particularly for its assessment in the five domains of development listed in Part C of Individuals with Disabilities Education Act.[68] The BDI-2 is the result of a 5-year development process including updating of test items, refining the scoring criteria, revising the domain/subdomain structure, and new normative sampling. The new edition features colorful items and child-friendly manipulatives for all ages, new comprehensive norms, clear, scripted interview items with follow-up probes, computed or hand-scored processing, flexible administration, and an expanded range of items for all ages. The skills comprising the 450 test items were chosen based on their relationship to functional life skills and ability to be impacted by educational intervention. Normative data were collected on 2,500 children from birth to 7 years, 11 months, closely matching the 2000 U.S. Census.

TEST FORMAT

Type The BDI-2 is a norm-referenced and criterion-referenced comprehensive developmental assessment.

Content The five domains with subdomains include (1) Adaptive: Personal Responsibility and Self-care; (2) Personal-Social: Adult Interaction, Self-Concept and Social Growth, and Peer Interaction; (3) Motor: Fine Motor, Gross Motor, and Perceptual Motor; (4) Communication: Expressive and Receptive; and (5) Cognitive: Perceptual Discrimination/Conceptual Development, Reasoning and Academic Skills, and Attention and Memory.

Administration The BDI-2 contains three administration procedures: structured test, observation, and parent interview. Instructions are provided for determining which procedure is best for each item. This administration flexibility is useful when an item may be difficult to assess during the testing procedure or if a child refuses to participate. Additional descriptions of test-accommodation procedures for children with various impairments and disabilities are provided in the manual. The complete BDI-2 can be administered in 60 to 90 minutes, and 10 to 30 minutes for the Screening Test.

Scoring/Interpretation The BDI-2 can be hand scored or scored with optional scoring software, BDI-2 Data Manager™. The child's performance is scored based on standardized criteria using a simple three-point scoring system (2 = milestone achieved, 1 = milestone emerging, 0 = milestone not achieved). At the subdomain level, norm-referenced scores are provided (scaled scores with a mean of 10; SD = 3; score range, 1 to 19). The subdomain scores combine to form the five BDI-2 domain scores and the overall BDI-2 Developmental Quotient (standard scores with a mean of 100, SD = 15, score range from 40 to 160). Percentiles and Confidence Intervals are provided for the domain scores and Developmental Quotient. Additionally, age-equivalent tables are provided. The BDI-2 Data Manager Software provides consistency in determining raw score totals and norm-referenced scores. Narrative reports can be generated for parents and professionals, as well as score reports and aggregate reports for program evaluation purposes.

RELIABILITY AND VALIDITY Overall test score reliability is reported in the manual at 0.99.[69] Internal consistency using the split-half method is reported as reliabilities across ages. Reliabilities on domains averaged 0.90 to 0.96, and 0.85 to 0.95 on subdomains. Concurrent and criterion validity was obtained with the original BDI, BSID-II, WJIII, Denver II, PLS-4, Vineland SEEC, and WPPSI-III. The BDI-2 exceeds the recommended level of accuracy for testing (0.75) with a sensitivity of 0.83 and a specificity of 0.85. Spies et al. assessed the use of the BDI-2 as an early screener for autism spectrum disorders and reported high sensitivity (0.94) with a determined cut-off score of 96 (1.5 SD from the mean of the autism spectrum disorders group).[70]

ADVANTAGES/DISADVANTAGES The BDI-2 has a flexible framework for gathering information and can be used by multiple providers. Specific guidelines for providers working with children with developmental disabilities assists in assessment administration, and the inclusion of a screening test is beneficial in settings with time constraints. The three-point scoring system of 0, 1, and 2 accounts for emerging and developing skills. The time required to administer the complete battery of items is a limitation, and providers may have difficulty scoring the test when there is disagreement between observation and interview data.

Assessment of Functional Capabilities

Functional assessments examine what the child does in the context of daily life across multiple domains. What a child actually does in the community may be entirely different from their physical capability to perform the activity. It is important, therefore, to assess functional performance as well as functional capacity. Functional assessments are often grounded in a similar conceptual framework as the World Health Organization's International Classification of Functioning, Disability and Health (ICF).[71,72] The approach is to assess the child's participation in daily routines, the activities performed, and the environmental and personal factors that contribute to the child's daily function.

According to Haley, the concept of disability and functional assessment incorporates the following key concepts:

1. A child may have serious motor impairments that are not always reflected by the level of functional limitation or disability.
2. Functional deficits may or may not lead to a restriction in social activities and important childhood roles.
3. Environmental factors, family expectations, and contextual elements of functional task requirements play an important role in the eventual level of disability and handicap of the child.[73]

Comprehensive functional assessment instruments contain mobility, transfer, self-care, and social function items; they include measurement dimensions of assistance and adaptive equipment; and they incorporate developmental stages of functional skill attainment.[74] Functional assessments give pediatric physical therapists information on how a child's disability or movement disorder impacts task requirements of daily-life routines.

Pediatric Evaluation of Disability Inventory

The Pediatric Evaluation of Disability Inventory (PEDI) is a comprehensive clinical assessment of functional capabilities as well as performance in children between the ages of 6 months and 7.5 years.[75] The PEDI is intended to be used as an instrument to detect functional deficits or delays, as an evaluative instrument to monitor progress in pediatric rehabilitation programs, and/or as an outcome measure for program evaluation, either in pediatric rehabilitation setting or in an educational setting.

TEST MEASURES AND TARGET POPULATION The PEDI measures both the capability and performance of functional activities in three content domains: (1) self-care, (2) mobility, and (3) social function. Capability is measured by the identification of functional skills for which the child has demonstrated mastery and competence (Display 3.2).

Functional performance is measured by the level of caregiver assistance and environmental modifications needed to accomplish major functional activities.

The PEDI is designed to assess children ranging in age from 6 months to 7.5 years. Although the PEDI was created

---

DISPLAY 3.2 Functional Skills Content of the PEDI

Self-care Domain	Mobility Domain	Social Function Domain
Types of food textures	Toilet transfers	Comprehension of word meaning
Use of utensils	Chair/wheelchair transfers	Comprehension of sentence complexity
Use of drinking containers	Car transfers	Functional use of expressive communication
Toothbrushing	Bed mobility/transfers	Complexity of expressive communication
Hairbrushing	Tub transfers	Problem resolution
Nose care	Method of indoor locomotion	Social interactive play
Handwashing	Distance/speed indoors	Peer interactions
Washing body and face	Pulls/carries objects	Self-information
Pullover/front-opening garments	Method of outdoor locomotion	Time orientation
Fasteners	Distance/speed outdoors	Household chores
Pants	Outdoor surfaces	Self-protection
Shoes/socks	Upstairs	Community function
Toileting tasks	Downstairs	
Management of bladder		
Management of bowel		

Used with permission from Haley SM, Coster WJ, Ludlow LH, et al. *Pediatric Evaluation of Disability Inventory (PEDI): Development, Standardization and Administration Manual.* Boston, MA: New England Medical Center Hospital and PEDI Research Group; 1992:13.

and standardized for the evaluation of young children, it can be used to evaluate older children whose functional abilities fall below those expected of 7.5-year-old children with no disabilities.

TEST CONSTRUCTION AND STANDARDIZATION Content

and measurement scales for the PEDI underwent numerous revisions prior to the publication of the final version. Initial content was based on the available literature, previous functional and adaptive tests, and the clinical experience of the authors and consultant involved. A Development Edition was field-tested on more than 60 handicapped children and their families. The scales' comprehensiveness and representativeness of content was evaluated by external content experts. Revisions based on the field testing and the content validity study were then incorporated into the final PEDI items to establish the Standardization Version.

Normative data for the PEDI were gathered from May 1990 to June 1991 from 412 children and families distributed throughout Massachusetts, Connecticut, and New York. This sample from the Northeast region closely approximated most of the demographic characteristics of the U.S. population as defined by the 1980 U.S. Census data. Additionally, three groups of children, totalling 102, with disabilities, made up clinical samples for validation purposes.

TEST FORMAT

Type The PEDI can be used for both discriminative purposes such as determination of eligibility for intervention services (with norm-referenced standard scores) as well as evaluative purposes such as determining change following intervention (with criterion-referenced scores).[72]

Content The content areas of self-care, mobility, and social function are assessed through three sets of measurement scales: Functional Skills, Caregiver Assistance, and Modifications. The Functional Skills Scales were designed to reflect meaningful functional units within a given activity. The Caregiver Assistance Scales measure disability of children with respect to the amount of help they need to carry out functional activities. The Modifications section provides a frequency count of the type and extent of environmental modifications the child depends on to support functional performance.

Administration The PEDI can be administered by clinicians and educators who are familiar with the child or by structured interview of the parent. The PEDI's focus on typical performance requires the respondent to have had the opportunity to observe the child on several different occasions in order to gain an accurate picture of the child's typical performance. Administration through parent report will require 45 to 60 minutes. Administration guidelines, criteria for scoring each item, and examples are provided in the accompanying manual. Examiners should have knowledge about the item criteria used in the instrument and the methods employed in determining the child's level of assistance though specific training.

Scoring Items within the Functional Skills Scale are scored either a 1 (has capability) or a 0 (unable or has not demonstrated capability) for each of the content areas. Items within the Caregiver Assistance Scale are scored on a six-point rating scale from 0 (Total Assistance) to 5 (Independent), and the Modifications Scale is rated using a four-category scale from No Modifications to Extensive Modifications.

Scores are recorded in a booklet that also contains a summary score sheet that is used to construct a profile of the child's performance across the different domains and scales. A summary of rating criteria for the three sets of measurement scales is provided in Display 3.3.

Interpretation Raw scores are summed and transformed into two types of summary scores: normative standard scores and scaled scores. Separate summary scores are calculated for Functional Skills and for Caregiver Assistance in each of the three domains, thus yielding six normative standard scores and six-scaled scores. Normative standard scores provide a measure of the child's overall functional performance relative to age-related peers. Scores are interpreted relative to a mean of 50, with an SD of 10. Scaled scores, distributed along a scale from 0 to 100, describe where the child's performance falls relative to the maximum possible score on the PEDI. Scaled scores are not adjusted for age and, therefore, can be used to

---

DISPLAY

3.3 **Rating Criteria for the Three Types of Measurement Scales**

Part I: Functional Skills	Part II: Caregiver Assistance	Part III: Modification
(197 discrete items of functional skills)	(20 complex functional activities)	(20 complex functional activities)
Self-care, Mobility, Social function	Self-care, Mobility, Social function	Self-care, Mobility, Social function
0 = unable, or limited in capability to perform item in most situations	5 = Independent	N = No Modifications
	4 = Supervise/Prompt/Monitor	C = Child oriented (nonspecialized)
1 = capable of performing item in most situations, or item has been previously mastered and functional skills have progressed beyond this level	3 = Minimal Assistance	R = Rehabilitation Equipment
	2 = Moderate Assistance	E = Extensive Modifications
	1 = Maximal Assistance	
	0 = Total Assistance	

Used with permission from Haley SM, Coster WJ, Ludlow LH, et al. *Pediatric Evaluation of Disability Inventory (PEDI): Development, Standardization and Administration Manual.* Boston, MA: New England Medical Center Hospital and PEDI Research Group; 1992:16.

describe the functional status of children of all ages. In addition, frequency totals of the four levels of modifications can be calculated. These totals provide descriptive information on the frequency and the degree of modifications a child uses.

RELIABILITY AND VALIDITY The internal consistency reliability coefficients obtained from the normative sample range between 0.95 and 0.99. Interinterviewer reliability in the normative sample was very high (ICCs = 0.96 to 0.99) for the Caregiver Assistance Scales. Agreement on Modifications was also quite high, except for Social Function, where it was still adequate (ICC = 0.79).[75] Berg et al. investigated reliability of the Norwegian translation of the PEDI when administered to parents by an occupational therapist, physical therapists, or kindergarten teacher in typically developing children. Inter- and intrarater reliability was excellent with ICCs from 0.95 to 0.99.[76] Discrepancy between the different interviews was highest between parents and kindergarten teachers, with interrespondent reliability (ICC) from 0.64 to 0.74.

Content validity was examined using a panel of 31 experts to validate and confirm the functional content of the PEDI.[77] Data related to construct validity and concurrent validity indicate that the PEDI is a valid measure of pediatric function.[78] Preliminary data also support the discriminant and evaluative validity of the PEDI.[75] Concurrent validity between the WeeFim and the PEDI was investigated in children with developmental disabilities or acquired brain injuries.[79] The two tests were determined to measure similar constructs, with Spearman correlation coefficients greater than 0.88 for self-care, transportation/locomotion, and communication/social function.

ADVANTAGES AND DISADVANTAGES The PEDI represents a standardized clinical instrument for pediatric functional assessment. Rigorous methodology during its development has resulted in an instrument that is both valid and reliable. As the PEDI examines motor and self-care function, as well as participation (in the social function domain), it reflects the International Classification of Functioning, Disability, and Health domains of activity and participation.[51] In addition, the PEDI is an outcome measure that assesses the effect of a condition on a child in terms of his or her function across different domains, thus relating to how it affects his or her everyday life. Critiques from PEDI users include long administration time, small age range for normative values, translation issues, cultural differences in valued and important functional activities, and differing parental expectations for a child's developmental progression.[72] As the PEDI items are concentrated at the easier end of the functional continuum, it may not be ideal for older children or those with less severe disabilities.[80]

RECENT RESEARCH The Pediatric Evaluation of Disability Inventory—Computer Adaptive Test (PEDI-CAT) is a full revision of the PEDI based on years of experience, feedback, and formal research with the original PEDI.[81,82] The PEDI-CAT utilizes preinstalled software to estimate a child's abilities

from an item bank of 276 activities, measuring function in four domains: (1) Daily Activities, (2) Mobility, (3) Social/Cognitive, and (4) Responsibility. The revisions to the original PEDI include (1) new items extending the functional content assessed in self-care, mobility, and social functioning domains; (2) new 4-point difficulty scale replacing the dichotomous capable/unable scale; (3) addition of illustrations for self-care and mobility items; (4) replacement of Caregiver Assistance section with a new "Responsibility" section; and (5) creation of a CAT platform for content administration in each domain.[72] The CAT platform allows items to be administered based on previous responses, thus avoiding irrelevant items or items too easy or difficult for the child. Item administration begins in the middle range of difficulty or responsibility, and the response to that item dictates which item will appear next (easier or harder item). With the administration of subsequent items, the score is reestimated and either the assessment ends if a "stopping" rule has been satisfied or continues on with new items until the "stopping" rule has been met. The PEDI-CAT software then calculates and displays results, including an item map, age percentiles, and standard scores.[81]

Each of the PEDI-CAT domains is self-contained and can be administered individually or in a combination appropriate for assessment of the child. The level of difficulty for each domain is measured using a 4-point response scale: easy, a little hard, hard, and unable. The newest PEDI-CAT domain, Responsibility, measures the extent to which the individual or caregiver takes responsibility for performing complex, multistep tasks or life skills. The current PEDI – CAT website provides very helpful descriptions of the various domains, scoring, and recent publications regarding this computer-assisted test. www.pedicat.com/category/home - accessed 12/16/13.

Currently, two versions of the PEDI-CAT exist: the "Speedy-CAT," which requires only 15 or fewer items per domain to be administered, and the "Content-Balanced CAT," which includes approximately 30 items per domain with a balance of item content within each domain.[82] Concurrent validity and reliability of the PEDI-CAT mobility domain with the original PEDI Functional Skills Mobility Scale was investigated by Dumas et al.[82] Strong correlations between scaled scores ($r = 0.82$; $p < 0.001$) indicated strong agreement between the PEDI-CAT and the original PEDI, supporting concurrent validity. Intraclass correlation coefficients ranged from 0.3390 to 1.000, and agreement results ranged from 60% to 100% for eight items measured. Both assessment tools identified children with limitations with functional mobility, with the PEDI-CAT identifying a larger percentage of older children with functional limitations.

Functional Independence Measure for Children

The Functional Independence Measure for Children (WeeFIM) is the pediatric adaptation of the Functional Independence Measur (FIM) for adults of the Uniform Data System for Medical Rehabilitation (UDS).[83] The WeeFIM measures function in a developmental context and is intended to help monitor children with disabilities as they grow into adults who function at a maximum level of independence. The WeeFIM-II system includes the WeeFIM instrument, the WeeFIM instrument 0–3 Module, and an Internet-based software application with a report generator and quarterly aggregate reports.[84]

TEST MEASURES AND TARGET POPULATION The latest revision of the WeeFIM consists of 18 items within three domains—Self-care, Mobility, and Cognition—and is designed for use with children between the ages of 6 months and 7 years, but may be used with older children with developmental disabilities and mental ages less than 7 years.[82] The WeeFIM is a measure of disability, not impairment, and is intended to measure what a child with a disability actually does, not what they ought to be able to do or might be able to do if circumstances were different. The WeeFIM contains a minimum number of items and is designed to be useful across disciplines by trained clinicians.

TEST CONSTRUCTION AND STANDARDIZATION The WeeFIM was built on the organizational format of the FIM for adults and developed as a collaboration among an interdisciplinary team who reviewed gross motor, fine motor, receptive and expressive language, adaptive, cognitive, and educational instruments.[85] A normative sample of 417 children, aged 6 months to 8 years, without developmental delays was studied by Msall et al. A significant correlation was found between the age of the child in months and the total WeeFIM scores for children aged 2 to 5 years ($n = 222$, $r = 0.80$, $p < 0.01$).[85] Normative values for the WeeFIM are presented in the manual in 3-month intervals, with the first grouping from 5 to 7 months and the last grouping for children 83 months and older. Because the WeeFIM total ratings tend to flatten beyond 83 months at a total rating of 120, there is no additional breakdown provided beyond this age range.[84]

TEST FORMAT

Type The test is criterion based and is a descriptive measure of the caregiver and special resources that are required because of functional limitations.

Content The test consists of three domains: Self-care (eight items), Mobility (five items), and Cognition (five items) (Display 3.4).

Administration/Scoring Assessment using the WeeFIM should be based on direct observation of the child. If direct observation is not possible, assessments may be completed by interviewing parents or caregivers who are familiar with the child's everyday activities. Each of the 18 items to assess the child's function is rated on a seven-level ordinal scale, from (1) total dependence to (7) complete independence (Display 3.5).

The manual describes each of these levels as a general overview of the ratings and also provides specific guidelines for applying the levels scale for each of the 18 items.

DISPLAY 3.4 **WeeFIM Domains**

Self-care
1. Eating
2. Grooming
3. Bathing
4. Dressing—upper body
5. Dressing—lower body
6. Toileting
7. Bladder management
8. Bowel management

Mobility
9. Transfer chair, wheelchair
10. Transfer toilet
11. Transfer tub/shower
12. Crawl/walk/wheelchair
13. Stairs

Cognition
14. Comprehension
15. Expression
16. Social interaction
17. Problem solving
18. Memory

Interpretation The WeeFIM measures functional abilities and the "need for assistance" associated with varying levels of disability in children. The scores obtained are utilized as baseline descriptive clinical assessments of severity, assist in selection of treatment goals and evaluation of treatment, and aid in identifying the child and family's need for support. It is designed to track functional status and outcomes over time both in preschool years and in the early elementary school years.

DISPLAY 3.5 **Levels of Function for the WeeFIM**

No Helper
   7 = Complete independence (timely, safely)
   6 = Modified independence (device needed)

Helper

Modified Dependence
   5 = Supervision
   4 = Minimal assist (child = 75%–99%)
   3 = Moderate assist (child = 50%–74%)

Complete Dependence
   2 = Maximal assistance (child = 25%–49%)
   1 = Total assistance (child = 0%–24%)

RELIABILITY AND VALIDITY Test–retest and interrater reliability for the total WeeFIM are 0.99 and 0.95, respectively.[86,87] Data related to construct and discriminative validity indicate that the WeeFIM is a valid measure of disability related to functional independence.[88] Concurrent validity between WeeFIM and PEDI was reported by Ziviani et al., with Spearman correlation coefficients greater than 0.88 for self-care, transportation/locomotion, and communication/social function, indicating that the two tests measure similar constructs.[79]

ADVANTAGES AND DISADVANTAGES The WeeFIM has a short administration time from 10 to 15 minutes, and is useful for communicating a child's ability to cope with daily living tasks in a common language among health care providers. Use of the WeeFIM does require a subscription fee, and if institutions subscribe to a test database, accreditation of users is required. Information necessary for guiding clinical decision making may be difficult to extract from documentation of caregiver assistance alone.

School Function Assessment

The School Function Assessment (SFA) was developed by Coster, Deeney, Haltiwanger, and Haley in response to the need for an effective functional performance measure for children attending elementary school.[89] A reliable and valid assessment tool specific to the student's needs and abilities and performance within the school environment is necessary for effective evaluation and service planning.

TEST MEASURES AND TARGET POPULATION The SFA measures a student's performance of functional tasks which support participation in academic and social school-related activities for students in kindergarten through Grade 6. The SFA permits students with disabilities to use alternative methods to accomplish functional tasks, recognizing that function is defined primarily by what an individual is able to do.

TEST CONSTRUCTION AND STANDARDIZATION In 2002, Burtner et al. reported that the most frequently used assessment tools used in southwest states' school systems were assessments designed to measure only fine and gross motor skills.[90] In fact, many of the assessment tools utilized provide little information about the school-related abilities of the children being evaluated. Thus, the SFA was developed to fulfill the need for an effective functional assessment of student's performance in the context of the school environment. The SFA was standardized on a sample of 678 students comprising two groups: 363 students with special needs and 315 students in regular education programs at 112 sites in 40 states and Puerto Rico.[91]

TEST FORMAT

Type The SFA is a standardized, criterion-referenced assessment tool.

Content The SFA consists of three sections: Participation, Task Supports, and Activity Performance.[89,92] Participation is measured in six school activity settings: general or special education classrooms, playground, transportation to/from school, bathroom, transitions to/from class, and mealtimes. The Task Support section measures adaptations made and assistance given to the individual during school-related functions. The four scales in this section include Physical Task Support–Assistance, Physical Task Support–Adaptations, Cognitive/Behavioral Task Support–Assistance, and Cognitive/Behavioral Task Support–Adaptations. The Activity Performance section contains two major categories: Physical Tasks and Cognitive/Behavioral Tasks, measuring performance in school-related functional activities such as following school rules, using school materials, and communicating needs.

Administration/Scoring In the Participation section, a six-point rating system (1 = participation is extremely limited to 6 = full participation) is used for each of the six school activity settings to indicate whether the student's participation is similar to that of an age-related/grade peer. In the Task Supports section, a 4-point rating system (1 = extensive assistance/adaptation to 4 = no assistance/adaptation) is used to examine the extent of assistance and adaptations provided to the student. In the Activity Performance Section, the activities are rated on a four-point scale (1 = does not perform to 4 = consistent performance) with specific criteria defining performance. The raw scores for each section are converted to criterion scores on a 1 to 100 continuum using scoring tables provided in the SFA manual.[89] Criterion scores are then compared with criterion cut-off scores. Detailed guidelines for completion of the assessment are provided in the SFA *Rating Scale Guide* and the *Record Form* (Fig 3.5).

Interpretation Criterion scores are interpreted as a measure of the student's current functional performance relative to the overall participation, need for services, or functional performance represented in each particular scale. A score of 100 represents a criterion of full grade-appropriate functioning in a particular area. To identify when a student's performance is below what is expected of his or her same-grade peers, the criterion scores are compared with the criterion cut-off scores. The criterion cut-off scores were derived from the sample of students in regular education programs. Five percent or fewer from this population would be expected to have scores below these cut-off points.[91]

RELIABILITY AND VALIDITY Test–retest reliability estimates reported in the SFA manual ranges from $r = 0.90$ to $r = 0.98$ and internal consistency measure estimates (Cronbach's α) range from $\alpha = 0.95$ to 0.98.[89] Validity studies evaluating content were conducted during the development of the SFA. The SFA was determined to contain items that were both relevant and distinct among different levels of function and is both a comprehensive and relevant

PART II Task Supports

Directions: Read the description of each task provided below. Then refer to the rating criteria for Part II provided in the *Rating Scale Guide* to determine the rating that best describes the student's needs for additional help or for modifications to perform school-related functional tasks. Circle the appropriate rating next to each task. Sum the ratings within each scale to obtain the total raw score. Record the total raw score for each scale in the appropriate box.

Physical Tasks	ASSISTANCE	ADAPTATIONS
Travel: moving on all different types of indoor and outdoor surfaces; moving around obstacles, through congested or narrow spaces, or in a line; moving all distances required in school, including to and from transportation or playground; keeping pace with peers in all school situations, including evacuating the building as necessary.	1 ②3 4	①2 3 4
Maintaining and Changing Positions: moving self to and from positions, (including chair or wheelchair, standing, floor, and toilet); maintaining stable seated position on floor or toilet; maintaining functional position in seat for 1/2 hour of class instruction or seat work; boarding and disembarking from all vehicles.	1 ②3 4	①2 3 4
Recreational Movement: playing games involving physical activity, including throwing and catching during ball games; playing kickball; running, jumping, and climbing; and playing on both low and high playground equipment.	1 2 ③4	①2 3 4
Manipulation With Movement: transporting materials or belongings within and to and from classroom and in mealtime setting; carrying fragile objects or containers with spillable contents; picking up and setting down large and small objects; retrieving objects from table, storage space, or floor; opening and closing all types of doors.	①2 3 4	1 ②3 4
Using Materials: using all classroom tools effectively, including pencils, erasers, markers, scissors, stapler, tape, and glue; opening, closing, and turning pages in books; folding and securing papers; using art materials; and manipulating small game pieces.	①2 3 4	①2 3 4
Setup and Cleanup: retrieving, gathering, and putting away materials in classroom and lunchroom; opening food or classroom containers; setting up equipment or materials; disposing of waste; wiping up or tidying table top or desk.	①2 3 4	①2 3 4
Eating and Drinking: using all needed utensils; eating and drinking a typical meal, including drinking from a cup without spilling; using a napkin to wipe face and hands; completing mealtime/snack time tasks in the time allowed; drinking from student-accessible water fountain.	①2 3 4	1 ②3 4
Hygiene: toileting control; completing toileting tasks including wiping, flushing, or managing equipment; washing and drying hands; completing tasks within typical time limits; managing nose care; covering mouth when coughing or sneezing.	①2 3 4	①2 3 4
Clothing Management: putting on and taking off clothing as required for indoor and outdoor use, including fasteners (e.g., small buttons and zippers) and shoes; managing clothing for toileting purposes.	①2 3 4	①2 3 4

DW Respondent's Initials

	Physical Tasks	Assistance Raw Score	Adaptations Raw Score
		13	11

Complete any of the following three tasks that are applicable to this student in this school. Record raw scores in the optional tasks section of the Summary Score Form. Do not add these scores to the total raw scores on this page.

	ASSISTANCE	ADAPTATIONS
Up/Down Stairs: moving up and down a full flight of stairs (at least 12 steps); carrying objects up and down stairs; maintaining regular speed on stairs.	①2 3 4	①2 3 4
Written Work: producing written work (letters, words, and numbers) of acceptable quality; organizing items on lines, in columns, or on a page; copying from a textbook or blackboard; sustaining physical effort on written tasks; maintaining speed to keep up with peers.	1 2 3 4	1 2 3 4
Computer and Equipment Use: operating switches; using keyboard or mouse to carry out basic functions; inserting or removing tapes or diskettes; completing work on computer in a timely fashion.	1 2 ③4	①2 3 4

Reminder: Refer to the *Rating Scale Guide* for rating definitions and examples.

4

FIGURE 3.5 Case study form from the School Function Assessment (SFA). (Copyright 1998 NCS Pearson, Inc. Reproduced with permission. All rights reserved.)

assessment for students with disabilities in elementary school.[89] Hwang et al. examined the known-group validity of the SFA comparing scores of three different groups of children (general education students without disabilities, students with learning disabilities, and students with cerebral palsy).[93] Significant differences were found across all parts of the SFA among the three groups of students supporting validity of the SFA. Interrater reliability between occupational therapists and teachers administering the SFA was assessed on 16 students' ratings. Intraclass correlations demonstrated moderate relationships (ICCs from 0.68 to 0.73) between teachers and occupational therapists ratings.[92]

ADVANTAGES/DISADVANTAGES The SFA is based on current models of function and special education legislation, with content reflecting the functional requirements of elementary school environments utilizing transdisciplinary focus and language. The criterion-referenced scales measure meaningful functional change, and the separate scales delineate the students' function in specific performance areas. The SFA is useful for prioritizing needs in program planning, IEP development, and documenting progress and effects of intervention. To complete the entire SFA requires a lengthy time commitment up to 1.5 hours, although individual scales are reported to be completed in 5 to 10 minutes.

Outcome Measures

Pediatric outcome measures and HRQOL measures are used in clinical practice to improve patient–provider communication, improve patient/parent satisfaction, identify hidden morbidities, and assist in clinical decision making.[94] The development and utilization of HRQOL measures has increased over the last decade in an effort to improve patient health and determine the value of health care services.[95] The incorporation of HRQOL measures in clinical practice serves as a comprehensive evaluation of patient functioning across multiple life domains and can assist in targeting interventions based on patient-perceived needs.

Pediatric Quality-of-Life Inventory

The Pediatric Quality-of-Life Inventory™ (Peds-QL) is a modular instrument designed to measure health-related quality of life in healthy children and adolescents and those with acute and chronic illnesses.[96] The 23-item Peds-Q Generic Core Scales measure core dimensions of health as delineated by the World Health Organization, as well as school functioning. Peds-Q Condition-Specific and Disease-Specific Modules for asthma, arthritis, cancer, cardiac disease, cerebral palsy, rheumatology, and diabetes are also available for designated clinical populations. New disease-specific modules continue to be published through MAPI Research Trust.[97]

TEST MEASURES AND TARGET POPULATION The Peds-QL Generic Core Scales is a multidimensional questionnaire, measuring health-related quality of life pertaining to physical, emotional, social, and school functioning. Developmentally appropriate forms are available for children 2 to 4, 5 to 7, 8 to 12, and 13 to 18 years of age. The Peds-QL contains a pediatric self-report for children 5 to 18 years and a parent proxy report for children 2 to 18 years.

TEST CONSTRUCTION AND STANDARDIZATION The original Peds-QL 1.0 was designed from a pediatric cancer database as a generic quality-of-life inventory to be used across multiple pediatric populations. Further advancements in the measurement model, including additional constructs and items and a broader age range for child and parent proxy reports, led to additional revisions, with the most recent being Peds-QL 4.0. The initial field trial for the Peds-QL Generic Core scales was administered to 1,677 families (963 child self-report; 1,629 parent proxy report) recruited from pediatric health care settings.[98]

TEST FORMAT

Type The Peds-QL is a norm-referenced HRQOL outcome-measures questionnaire.

Content The Peds-QL contains four multidimensional scales: (1) Physical Functioning (8 items), (2) Emotional Functioning (5 items), (3) Social Functioning (5 items), and (4) School Functioning (5 items) and provides three summary scores: (1) Total Scale Score (23 items), (2) Physical Health Summary Score (8 items), and (3) Psychosocial Health Summary Score (15 items) (Fig 3.6).

Administration The Peds-QL Generic Core Scale is presented to the patient (self-report) or the caregiver (parent proxy) to complete, with approximate completion time of 5 minutes or less. The instructions for the Standard Version ask how much of a problem each item has been in the past 1 month. An Acute Version is available for the time interval of the past 7 days.

Scoring Response choices for the questions in each scale include (0) never a problem, (1) almost never a problem, (2) sometimes a problem, (3) often a problem, and (4) always a problem. Items are reverse scored and transformed to a 0- to 100-point scale (0 = 100, 1 = 75, 2 = 50, 3 = 75, 4 = 0), indicating a better health-related quality of life with higher scale scores. To create Scale Scores, the mean is computed as the sum of the items over the number of items answered. The Psychosocial Health Summary Score is the mean computed as the sum of the items over the number of items answered in the Emotional, Social, and School Scales. The Physical Health Summary Score is the same as the Physical Functioning Scale Score. The Total Scale Score is the mean

The **Child and Parent Reports** of the **PedsQL™** 4.0 Generic Core Scales for:

- Young Children (ages 5–7)
- Children (ages 8–12)
- And Teens (ages 13–18)

are composed of 23 items comprising 4 dimensions.

DESCRIPTION OF THE QUESTIONNAIRE:

Dimensions	Number of Items	Cluster of Items	Reversed scoring	Direction of Dimensions
Physical Functioning	8	1–8	1–8	
Emotional Functioning	5	1–5	1–5	
Social Functioning	5	1–5	1–5	Higher scores indicate better HRQOL.
School Functioning	5	1–5	1–5	

SCORING OF DIMENSIONS:

Item Scaling	5-point Likert scale from 0 (Never) to 4 (Almost always) 3-point scale: 0 (Not at all), 2 (Sometimes) and 4 (A lot) for the Young Child (ages 5–7) child report
Weighting of Items	No
Extension of the Scoring Scale	Scores are transformed on a scale from 0 to 100.
Scoring Procedure	**Step 1: Transform Score** Items are reserved scored and linearly transformed to a 0–100 scale as follows: 0=100, 1=75, 2=50, 3=25, 4=0 **Step 2: Calculate Scores** Score by Dimensions: • If more than 50% of the items in the scale are missing, the scale scores should not be computed, • Mean score = Sum of the items over the number of items answered. Psychosocial Health Summary Score = Sum of the items over the number of items answered in the Emotional, Social, and School Functioning Scales. Physical Health Summary Score = Physical Functioning Scale Score **Total Score:** Sum of the items over the numbers of items answered on all the Scales.
Interpretation and Analysis of Missing Data	If more than 50% of the items in the scale are missing, the Scales Scores should not be computed. if 50% or more items are completed: Impute the mean of the completed items in a scale.

FIGURE 3.6 PedsQL Version 4.0 example of Child Report (Ages 8-12). (http://PedsQLTM.pedsql.org/about_pedsql.html)

of the sum of all items over the number of items answered in all scales.

Interpretation In general, the higher the scores, the better the health-related quality of life. In published studies by the Peds-QL author, children in good health have scores around 83, whereas children in poor health have scores in the mid-60s to low 70s.[99]

RELIABILITY AND VALIDITY Internal consistency reliability for the Total Scale Score (α = 0.88 child, 0.90 parent report), Physical Health Summary (α = 0.80 child, 0.88 parent report), and the Psychosocial Health Summary Score (α = 0.83 child, 0.86 parent report) were reported as acceptable for group comparisons.[100] Construct validity was demonstrated using the known-group methods, between the Peds-QL 4.0 Generic Core Scales and the Peds-QL 3.0

Cancer Module.[99] The Peds-QL 4.0 Generic Core Scales are able to distinguish between healthy children and those with acute or chronic conditions and are related to indicators of morbidity and illness burden. Reliability, validity, and responsiveness to clinical change were also reported for the Peds-QL 4.0 Generic Scales and the Peds-QL Asthma Module Asthma Symptom Scale.[101]

ADVANTAGES/DISADVANTAGES The Peds-QL is a brief, easy-to-administer outcome measures tool that is used internationally across multiple health-related fields. It assessed multiple dimensions of health from both the parent's and the child's perspective and is applicable to several age groups. The Peds-QL measurement instruments (generic and disease-specific) may be utilized as an outcome measure in clinical trials, research, and in clinical practice as a measure of HRQOL. Disadvantages for generic quality-of-life measures such as Peds-QL include inability to assess relevant domains of functioning specific to disease processes and decreased sensitivity to measure small but meaningful changes that occur as a result of clinical intervention.[102]

Pediatric Outcomes Data-collection Instrument

The Pediatric Outcomes Data-Collection Instrument (PODCI), also known as the POSNA instrument, was created by the American Academy of Orthopedic Surgeons (AAOS) and the Pediatric Orthopedic Society of North America (POSNA) in 1997 as a comprehensive measure of musculo-skeletal outcomes associated with pediatric orthopedic problems.[103] It was created to measure outcomes that orthopedic treatment could affect: upper and lower extremity motor skills, relief of pain, and restoration of activity.

TEST MEASURES AND TARGET POPULATION The PODCI consists of an Adolescent Self-Report Outcomes Questionnaire, an Adolescent Parent-Report Outcomes Questionnaire, and a Pediatric Outcomes Questionnaire, which measure overall health, pain, and ability to participate in normal daily activities as well as vigorous physical activities. The Pediatric Outcomes Questionnaire is intended to be used for children 2 to 10 years through parent report; the Adolescent Parent-Report Questionnaire is intended for use in children between 11 and 18 years; and the Adolescent Self-Report Questionnaire is intended for youth and children 11 to 18 years who can complete the form independently. For the purposes of this chapter, the Pediatric Outcomes Questionnaire will be reviewed.

TEST CONSTRUCTION AND STANDARDIZATION The original POSNA instrument was constructed by the Pediatric Outcomes Instrument Development Group in 1994 as an outcomes questionnaire based on existing instruments, input from expert panellists, and pilot testing with patients/parents.[103] The instrument was revised after additional pilot testing determined important concepts and domains pertinent to pediatric functional health for the patient and parent study group. The Child Health Questionnaire (CHQ), a validated and reliable scale with national norms, was used as a benchmark for validity tests and comparisons for sensitivity to change. In 2000, the American Academy of Orthopedic Surgeons completed a normative data study for all of the outcome instruments to provide general, healthy population scale scores for comparison to patient scores.[104] A total of 20,631 valid responses were included in the study, providing an overall confidence interval of ±3% at a 95% confidence level.

TEST FORMAT

Type The PODCI is a norm-referenced functional HRQOL outcome-measures questionnaire.

Content The Pediatric Outcomes Questionnaire consists of 8 scales: (1) Upper Extremity and Physical Function Scale, (2) Transfer and Basic Mobility Scale, (3) Sports/Physical Functioning Scale, (4) Pain/Comfort Scale, (5) Treatment Expectations Scale, (6) Happiness Scale, (7) Satisfaction with Symptoms Scale, and (8) Global Functioning Scale. The questionnaire contains 86 questions.

Administration The Pediatric Outcomes Questionnaire is completed by a parent/guardian who has knowledge of the child's condition with approximate completion time of 10 to 20 minutes. Responses to questions are rated on various scales (ranging from 1 to 4, 5, or 6).

Scoring Standardized and normative scores can be calculated for each patient. The standard score is based on the mean of items in each scale. Although scales may have differing item values, for scoring purposes, all items are rescaled to range from 0 to 5 (i.e., 0 = lowest score possible and 5 = maximum score possible). Items comprising a given scale are then averaged over the total number of items answered and multiplied by 20 to have a range from 0 to 100. The final number is then subtracted from 100 to yield the patient's standardized score. Computation through Excel worksheets includes formulae for item recoding, computation of missing items, and known general population means and SDs. Using the actual mean and SD of the 0-to-100 scale from the general, healthy population, a formula is applied to derive the normative score.

Interpretation Standardized scores range from 0 to 100, with 0 representing the *most* disability, and 100 representing the *least* disability. The normative score as a measure based on the healthy populations mean provides a numeric measure of disability relative to this population.

RELIABILITY AND VALIDITY Internal reliability ranges from 0.82 to 0.95 in the adult scales and 0.75 to 0.92 in the adolescent scales, and test–retest reliability is 0.71 to 0.97.[103] The scales were correlated with physicians' assessments and the Child Health Questionnaire by patterns of results indicating construct validity. Construct validity between the Activity Scales for Kids (ASK) and the PODCI shows high correlation at $r \geq 0.78$.[105] Concurrent validity is reported between the Child Health Questionnaire (0.60 to 0.81), the GMFM (0.56 to 0.94), and the PEDI (0.50 to 0.81).[82]

ADVANTAGES/DISADVANTAGES As an outcome measure, the PODCI is highly correlated with parents and clinician's global physical function ratings and is able to distinguish between different diseases or different levels of disease severity. It addresses critical components of outcomes in disabled children: pain, physical function, and impact on the child's psyche. The PODCI is used extensively in orthopedic outcomes research in multiple diagnostic categories. Due to its length and complex scoring algorithms, it may not be feasible in some clinical settings.

▶ Integration of information

The administration of developmental assessments is just one component of a physical therapy assessment, as described by *The Guide to Physical Therapist Practice's*[6] model for patient/client management. *Examination* includes history, systems review, and selection of tests and measures. *Evaluation* is the dynamic process of the physical therapists' clinical judgment through analysis and synthesis of information obtained through the examination. *Diagnosis*, or physical therapy diagnosis, differs from a medical diagnosis. A physical therapy diagnosis is a term or label encompassing a cluster of signs related to impairments in one of the four systems of the body (musculoskeletal, neuromuscular, cardiopulmonary, or integumentary). For example, a child may have a medical diagnosis of cerebral palsy but a physical therapy diagnosis of muscle weakness. Formulating a physical therapy diagnosis helps determine the most appropriate intervention strategies. *Prognosis* pertains to the predicted optimal level of functional improvement and includes the frequency and duration of intervention, plan of care, and discharge criteria. Long-term and short-term goals are the objective measurements with time frames for achievement, whereas the expected outcomes included in prognosis are the changes anticipated as the result of implementing the physical therapy plan of care. Outcomes described by *Guide for Physical Therapist Practice* may include minimization of functional limitations and disability, optimization of health status, prevention of disability, and optimization of patient/client satisfaction.[6] The final component of the model includes Intervention, the purposeful and skilled interaction of the physical therapist with the patient/client. Coordination, communication, and documentation of care as well as patient/client instruction and procedural interventions (therapeutic exercise, functional training, etc.) are all components of Intervention.

DISPLAY
3.6   **Suggested Outline for a Narrative Report on the Results of Development Testing**

1. Identification information: child's name, date of birth, current age, date of evaluation
2. Reason for evaluation and source of referral
3. History
   a. Perinatal history
   b. Significant medical history
   c. Developmental history as presented by parents or other historian
4. Clinical observations
   d. Neurologic development: reflex development, muscle tone, equilibrium, and protective responses
   e. Musculoskeletal status: range of motion, manual muscle test, anthropometric measurements
   f. Sensory status: results of sensory testing, pain assessment, visual ability, and auditory ability
   g. Functional abilities: daily activities (e.g., feeding, toileting, dressing), assistive devices
5. Results of developmental assessments: include developmental age
6. Summary of findings
7. Recommendations

Re-examination, the process of using tests and measures to evaluate progress and to modify intervention,[6] may be performed periodically to review the appropriateness of the treatment program and to monitor the progress of the child.

Reports of physical therapy assessments are usually presented in narrative form. The purposes of a report are to clarify what has been heard and observed, to give the data on which recommendations for treatment are based, and to transmit this information in a clear and understandable way to others. Certain information is included for all patients, but each child's report should provide a specific description of the distinctive abilities and disabilities of that child.[106] An outline of a narrative report is given in Display 3.6.

SUMMARY

Several clinically useful and commonly used tools for assessment have been described, among which are screening tests, tests of motor function, comprehensive developmental assessments, functional assessments, and HRQOL outcome measures. The information gained from these assessments, when combined with the information obtained from an interview, medical and developmental history, and clinical observation, completes the comprehensive evaluation of a child. The guidelines presented for the selection of specific tests will aid the therapist in choosing the test most appropriate for the population to be assessed. The therapist should remember that a questioning attitude, based on and supported by knowledge of human growth and development, is necessary for a comprehensive evaluation.

REFERENCES

1. American Physical Therapy Association. *The ABC's of Pediatric Physical Therapy.* Alexandria, VA: Practice committee of the section of pediatrics, APTA; 2003.
2. Scherzer AL, Tscharnuter I. *Early Diagnosis and Therapy in Cerebral Palsy.* New York, NY: Marcel Dekker; 1982.
3. Russell DJ, Rosenbaum PL. Avery LM, et al. *Gross Motor Function Measure (GMFM-66 and GMFM-88) User's Manual.* London, UK: MacKeith Press; 2002.
4. American Academy of Pediatrics. Committee on Children with Disabilities. Developmental surveillance and screening of infants and young children. *Pediatrics.* 2001;108:192–196.
5. Newborg J. *Battelle Developmental Inventory.* 2nd ed. Itasca, IL: Riverside; 2005.
6. American Physical Therapy Association. Guide to physical therapist practice. Second edition. *Phys Ther.* 2001;81:9–746.
7. Kirshner B, Guyatt G. A methodologic framework for assessing health indices. *J Chronic Dis.* 1985;38:27–36.
8. Long T. Toscano K. *Handbook of Pediatric Physical Therapy.* 2nd ed. Philadelphia, PA: Lippincott Williams & Wilkins; 2002.
9. Lewko JH. Current practices in evaluating motor behavior of disabled children. *Am J Occup Ther.* 1976;30:413–419.
10. Stangler SR, Huber CJ, Routh DK. *Screening Growth and Development of Preschool Children: A Guide for Test Selection.* New York, NY: McGraw-Hill; 1980.
11. Tieman BL, Palisano R, Sutlive AC. Assessment of motor development and function in preschool children. *Ment Retard Dev Disabil Res Rev.* 2005;11:189–196.
12. Rydz D, Shevell MI, Majnemer A, et al. Developmental screening. *J Child Neurol.* 2005; 20(1):4–21.
13. Mackrides PS, Ryherd SJ. Screening for developmental delay. *Am Fam Physician.* 2011; 84(5):544–549.
14. Harris SR, Megens AM, Daniels LE. *Harris Infant Neuromotor Test (HINT) Test User's Manual Version 1.0 Clinical Edition (2009).* Chicago, IL: Infant Motor Performance Scales LLC; 2010.
15. Harris SR, Daniels LE. Content validity of the Harris Infant Neuromotor Test. *Phys Ther.* 1996;76:727–737.
16. Harris SR, Daniels LE. Reliability and validity of the Harris Infant Neuromotor Test. *J Pediatr.* 2001;139:249–253.
17. Harris SR, Megens AM, Backman CL, et al. Development and standardization of the Harris Infant Neuromotor Test. *Infants Young Child.* 2003; 16(2):143–151.
18. Tse L, Mayson TA, Leo S, et al. Concurrent validity of the Harris Infant Neuromotor Test and the Alberta Infant Motor Scale. *J Pediatr Nurs.* 2008;23:28–36.
19. McCoy SW, Bowman A, Smith-Blockley J, et al. Harris Infant Neuromotor Test: comparison of US and Canadian normative data and examination of concurrent validity with the ages and stages questionnaire. *Phys Ther.* 2009;89(2):173–180.
20. Aylward GP. *The Bayley Infant Neurodevelopmental Screener.* San Antonio, TX: The Psychological Corporation; 1995.
21. Aylward GP, Verhulst SJ. Predictive utility of the Bayley Infant Neurodevelopmental Screener (BINS) risk status classifications: clinical interpretation and application. *Dev Med Child Neurol.* 2000;42:25–31.
22. Council on Children with Disabilities, Section on Developmental Behavioral Pediatrics, Bright Futures Steering Committee, et al. Identifying infants and young children with developmental disorders in the medical home: an algorithm for developmental surveillance and screening. *Pediatrics.* 2006;118(4):1808–1809.
23. Campbell SK, Osten ET, Kolobe THA, et al. Development of the test of infant motor performance. *Phys Med Rehab Clin North Am.* 1993; 4(3):541–550.

24. Campbell SK. *The Test of Infant Motor Performance: Test User's Manual Version 2.0.* Chicago, IL: Infant Motor Performance Scales, LLC; 2005.
25. Campbell SK, Levy P, Zawacki L, et al. Population-based age standards for interpreting results on the test of infant motor performance. *Pediatr Phys Ther.* 2006;18:119–125.
26. Girolami GL, Campbell SK. Efficacy of a neuro-developmental treatment program to improve motor control in infants born prematurely. *Pediatr Phys Ther.* 1994; 6(4):175–184.
27. Campbell SK, Wright BD, Linacre JM. Development of a functional movement scale for infants. *J Appl Meas.* 2002;3(2):190–204.
28. Campbell SK. Test-retest reliability of the Test of Infant Motor Performance. *Pediatr Phys Ther.* 1999;11:60–66.
29. Lekskulchai R, Cole J. Effect of a developmental program on motor performance in infants born preterm. *Aust J Physiother.* 2001;47:169–176.
30. Campbell SK, Kolobe TH, Osten ET, et al. Construct validity of infant motor performance. *Phys Ther.* 1995; 75(7):585–596.
31. Campbell SK, Kolobe THA. Concurrent validity of the Test of Infant Motor Performance with the Alberta Infant Motor Scale. *Pediatr Phys Ther.* 2000;12:2–9.
32. Campbell SK, Kolobe THA, Wright B, et al. Validity of the Test of Infant Motor Performance for prediction of 6-, 9-, and 12- month scores on the Alberta Infant Motor Scale. *Dev Med Child Neurol.* 2002;44:263–272.
33. Kolobe THA, Bulanda M, Susman L. Predicting motor outcomes at preschool age for infants tested at 7, 30, 60, and 90 days after term age using the Test of Infant Motor Performance. *Phys Ther.* 2004;84:1144–1156.
34. Piper MC, Darrah J. *Motor Assessment of the Developing Infant.* Philadelphia, PA: WB Saunders; 1995.
35. Lee LLS, Harris SR. Psychometric properties and standardization of four screening tests for infants and young children: a review. *Pediatr Phys Ther.* 2005;17:140–147.
36. Piper MC, Pinnell LE, Darrah J, et al. Construction and validation of the Alberta Infant Motor Scale (AIMS). *Can J Public Health.* 1992;83(suppl 2):S46–S50.
37. Pin TW, de Valle K, Eldridge B, et al. Clinimetric Properties of the Alberta Infant Motor Scale in infants born preterm. *Pediatr Phys Ther.* 2010;22:278–286.
38. Fetters L, Tronick EZ. Neuromotor development of cocaine-exposed and control infants from birth through 15 months: poor and poorer performance. *Pediatrics.* 1996; 98(5):938–943.
39. Spittle AJ, Doyle L, Boyd RN. A systematic review of the clinimetric properties of neuromotor assessments for preterm infants during the first year of life. *Dev Med Child Neurol.* 2008;50:254–266.
40. Harris SR, Backman CL, Mayson TA. Comparative predictive validity of the Harris Infant Neuromotor Test and the Alberta Infant Motor Scale. *Dev Med Child Neurol.* 2010;52:462–467.
41. Russell DJ, Rosenbaum PL, Cadman DT, et al. The Gross Motor Function Measure: a means to evaluate the effects of physical therapy. *Dev Med Child Neurol.* 1989;31:341–352.
42. Can Child—Center for Childhood Disability Research. CanChild Website. http://www.canchild.ca/en/measures/gmpmqualityfm.asp. Accessed October 9, 2012.
43. Avery LM, Russell DJ, Raina PS, et al. Rasch analysis of the Gross Motor Function Measure: validating the assumptions of the Rasch model to create an interval-level measure. *Arch Phys Med Rehabil.* 2003; 84(5):697–705.
44. Russell DJ, Avery LM, Rosenbaum PL, et al. Improved scaling of the gross motor function measure for children with cerebral palsy: evidence of reliability and validity. *Phys Ther.* 2000; 80(9):873–885.
45. Shi W, Wang SJ, Liao YG, et al. Reliability and validity of the GMFM-66 in 0- to 3- year old children with cerebral palsy. *Am J Phys Med Rehabil.* 2006; 85(2):141–147.
46. Drouin LM, Malouin F, Richards CL, et al. Correlation between the Gross Motor Function Measure scores and gait spatiotemporal

measures in children with neurological impairments. *Dev Med Child Neurol.* 1996;38:1007–1019.

47. Josenby AL, Jarnlo G, Gummesson C, et al. Longitudinal construct validity of the GMFM-88 total score and goal total score and the GMFM-66 score in a 5-year follow up study. *Phys Ther.* 2009;89:342–350.

48. Brunton LK, Bartlett DJ. Validity and reliability of two abbreviated versions of the gross motor function measure. *Phys Ther.* 2011;91:577–588.

49. Rosenbaum PL, Palisano RJ, Bartlett DJ, et al. Development of the Gross Motor Function Classification System for cerebral palsy. *Dev Med Child Neurol.* 2008;50:249–253.

50. Palisano R, Rosenbaum P, Walter S, et al. Gross motor function classification system for cerebral palsy. *Dev Med Child Neurol.* 1997;39:214–223.

51. Debuse D, Brace H. Outcome measures of activity for children with cerebral palsy: a systematic review. *Pediatr Phys Ther.* 2011;23:221–231.

52. Folio MR, Fewell PR. *Peabody Developmental Motor Scales and Activity Cards Manual.* Allen, TX: DLM Teaching Resources; 1983.

53. Folio MR, Fewell RR. *Peabody Developmental Motor Scales.* 2nd ed. Austin, TX: Pro-Ed; 2000.

54. Connolly BH, Dalton L, Smith JB, et al. Concurrent validity of the Bayley Scales of Infant Development-II (BSID-II) and the Peabody Developmental Motor Scale II (PDMS-2) in 12- month old infants. *Pediatr Phys Ther.* 2006;18:190–196.

55. Cools W, De Martelaer K, Samaey C, et al. Movement skill assessment of typically developing preschool children: a review of seven movement skill assessment tools. *J Sports Sci Med.* 2009;8:154–168.

56. Bruininks RH. *Bruininks-Oseretsky Test of Motor Proficiency: Examiners' Manual.* Circle Pines, MI: American Guidance Services; 1978.

57. Bruininks R, Bruininks B. *Bruininks-Oseretsky Test of Motor Proficiency (BOT-2).* 2nd ed. Minneapolis, MN: NCS Pearson; 2005.

58. Deitz JC, Kartin D, Kopp K. Review of the Bruininks-Oseretsky test of motor proficiency, second edition (BOT-2). *Phys Occup Ther Pediatr.* 2007;27(4):87–102.

59. Johnson BA, MacWilliams BA, Carey JC, et al. Motor proficiency in children with Neurofibromatosis type 1. *Pediatr Phys Ther.* 2010;22:344–348.

60. Individuals with Disabilities Education Act Amendments of 1997, Pub L No 105–117, 20 USC, 1400 *et seq.*

61. Bayley N. *Bayley Scales of Infant and Toddler Development.* San Antonio,TX: The Psychological Corporation; 2006.

62. Bayley N. *The Bayley Scales of Infant Development-II.* San Antonio, TX: The Psychological Corporation; 1993.

63. Bayley N. *The Bayley Scales of Infant Development.* San Antonio, TX: The Psychological Corporation; 1969.

64. Greenspan S. *Greeenspan Social-Emotional Growth Chart.* San Antonio, TX: The Psychological Corporation; 2004.

65. Oakland T, Harrison P. *Adaptive Behavior Assessment System –II: Clinical Use and Interpretation.* San Diego, CA: Academic Press; 2008.

66. Connolly BH, McClune NO, Gatlin R. Concurrent validity of the Bayley-III and the Developmental Motor Scale-2. *Pediatr Phys Ther.* 2012;24:345–352.

67. Anderson PJ, DeLuca CR, Hutchinson E, et al. Underestimation of developmental delay by the new Bayley-III scale. *Arch Pediatr Adolesc Med.* 2010; 164(4):352–356.

68. Berls AT, McEwen IR. Battelle Developmental Inventory. *Phys Ther.* 1999; 79(8):776–783.

69. Newborg J, Stock JR, Wnek L, et al. *Battelle Developmental Inventory.* Allen, TX: DLM; 1988.

70. Spies M, Matson JL, Turygin N. The use of the Battelle Developmental Inventory-Second Edition (BDI-2) as an early screener for autism spectrum disorders. *Dev Neurorehabil.* 2011; 14(5):310–314.

71. World Health Organization. *International Classification of Functioning, Disability, and Health.* Geneva, Switzerland: World Health Organization; 2001.

72. Hayley SM, Coster W, Kao Y. Lessons from use of the Pediatric Evaluation of Disability Inventory: where do we go from here? *Pediatr Phys Ther.* 2010;22:69–75.

73. Haley SM. Motor assessment tools for infants and young children: a focus on disability assessment. In: Forssberg H, Hirschfeld H, eds. *Movement Disorders in Children.* Basel, Switzerland: S. Karger, AG; 1992:278–283.

74. Feldman AB, Haley SM, Coryell J. Concurrent and construct validity of the pediatric evaluation of disability inventory. *Phys Ther.* 1990;70:602–610.

75. Haley SM, Costern J, Ludlons LH, et al. *Pediatric Evaluation of Disability Inventory (PEDI): Development, Standardization and Administration Manual.* Boston, New England Medical Center Hospitals and PEDI Research Group; 1992.

76. Berg M, Jahnsen R, Froslie K, et al. Reliability of the Pediatric Evaluation of Disability Inventory (PEDI). *Phys Occup Ther Pediatr.* 2004;24:61–77.

77. Haley SM, Coster WJ, Faas RM. A content validity study of the Pediatric Evaluation of Disability Inventory. *Pediatr Phys Ther.* 1991;3:177–184.

78. Boyce WF, Gowland C, Hardy S, et al. Development of a quality-of-movement measure for children with cerebral palsy. *Phys Ther.* 1991; 71(11):820–828.

79. Ziviani J, Ottenbacher K, Shephard K, et al. Concurrent validity of the Functional Independence Measure for children (WeeFIM) and the Pediatric Evaluation of Disability Inventory (PEDI) in children with developmental disabilities and acquired brain injuries. *Phys Occup Ther Pediatr.* 2002;21:91–101.

80. McCarthy ML, Silberstein CE, Atkins EA, et al. Comparing reliability and validity of pediatric instruments for measuring health and wellbeing of children with spastic cerebral palsy. *Dev Med Child Neurol.* 2002;44:468–476.

81. Haley, SM, Coster WJ, Dumas HM, et al. *PEDI-CAT: Pediatric Evaluation of Disability Inventory-Computer Adaptive Test: Development, Standardization, and Administration Manual.* Boston, MA: CREcare, LLC; 2012. Available at http://pedicat.com.

82. Dumas HM, Fragala-Pinkman M. Concurrent validity and reliability of the pediatric evaluation of disability inventory-computer adaptive test mobility domain. *Pediatr Phys Ther.* 2012;24: 171–176.

83. Data Management Service of the Uniform Data System for Medical Rehabilitation and the Center for Functional Assessment Research: *Guide for Use of the Uniform Data System for Medical Rehabilitation, Including the Functional Independence Measure for Children (WeeFIM).* Version 1.5. Buffalo, NY: State University of New York at Buffalo; July 1991.

84. *The WeeFIM II Clinical Guide, Version 6.0.* Buffalo, NY: Uniform Data System for Medical Rehabilitation; 2006.

85. Msall ME, DiGaudio K, Duffy LC, et al. WeeFIM normative sample of an instrument for tracking functional independence in children. *Clin Pediatr (Phila).* 1994;33:431–438.

86. Msall ME, DiGaudio K, Duffy LC. Use of assessment in children with developmental disabilities. *Phys Med Rehab Clinics North Am.* 1993;4:517–527.

87. Ottenbacher KJ, Msall ME, Lyon NR, et al. Interrater agreement and stability of the Functional Independence Measure for children (WeeFIM): use in children with developmental disabilities. *Arch Phys Med Rehab.* 1997;78:1309–1315.

88. Thomas SS, Buckon CE, Phillips DS, et al. Interobserver reliability of the gross motor performance measure: preliminary results. *Dev Med Child Neurol.* 2001; 43(2):97–102.

89. Coster W, Deeney TA, Haltiwanger JT, et al. *School Function Assessment.* Boston, MA: Boston University; 1998.

90. Burtner PA, McMain MP, Crowe TK. Survey of occupational therapy practitioners in southwestern schools: assessments used and preparation of students for school-based practice. *Phys Occup Ther Pediatr.* 2002; 22(1):25–39.

91. School Function Assessment Technical Report. http://www.pearsonassessments.com/NR/rdonlyres/./SFA_TR_Web.pdf. Accessed October 11, 2012.

92. Davies PL, Soon PL, Young M, et al. Validity and reliability of the school function assessment in elementary school students with disabilities. *Phys Occup Ther Pediatr.* 2004;24(3):23–43.

93. Hwang J, Davies PL, Taylor MP, et al. Validation of school function assessment with elementary school children. *OTJR.* 2002; 22(2):1–11.

94. Varni JW, Burwinkle, TM, Lane MM. Health-related quality of life measurement in pediatric clinical practice: an appraisal and precept for future research and application. *Health Qual Life Outcomes.* 2005;3. Available at http://www.hqlo.com/content 3/1/34.

95. Fayers PM, Machin D. *Quality of Life: Assessment, Analysis and Interpretation.* New York, NY: Wiley; 2000.

96. PedsQL™ 4.0 Measurement Model. http://pedsql.org. Accessed October 11,2012.

97. MAPI Research Trust: PedsQL (Pediatric Quality of Life Inventory). http://www.mapi-trust.org/services/questionnairelicensing/catalog-questionnaires/84-pedsql. Accessed on October 11,2012.

98. Varni JW, Seid M, Rode CA. The PedsQL™: measurement model for the Pediatric Quality of Life Inventory. *Med Care.* 1999;37:126–139.

99. Varni JW, Burwinkle TM, Katz ER, et al. The PedssQL™ in pediatric cancer: reliability and validity of the pediatric quality of life inventory generic core scales, multidimensional fatigue scale, and cancer module. *Cancer.* 2002; 94:2090–2106.

100. Varni JW, Seid M, Kurtin PS. PedsQL™ 4.0: reliability and validity of the pediatric quality of life inventory version 4.0 generic core scales in healthy and patient populations. *Med Care.* 2001; 39:800–812.

101. Seid M, Limbers CA, Drscoll KA, et al. Reliability, validity, and responsiveness of the pediatric quality of life inventory™ (PedsQL™) generic core scales and asthma symptoms scales in vulnerable children with asthma. *J Asthma.* 2010;47:170–177.

102. Lim CMS. *Pain, Quality of Life, and Coping in Pediatric Sickle Cell Disease [dissertation].* Downtown Atlanta, Georgia: Georgia State University; 2009. Psychology Dissertations Paper 54.

103. Daltroy LH, Liang MH, Fossel AH, et al. The POSNA pediatric musculoskeletal functional health questionnaire: report of reliability, validity, and sensitivity to change. *J Pediatr Orthop.* 1998;18:561–571.

104. American Academy of Orthopedic Surgeons: Outcomes Instruments and Information. http://www.aaos.org/research/outcomes/outcomes_documentation.asp#pedsref. Accessed October 11,2012.

105. Pencharz J, Young NL, Owen JL, et al. Comparison of three outcomes instruments in children. *J Pediatr Orthop.* 2001;21: 425–432.

106. Knobloch H, Pasamanick B, eds. *Gesell and Armatruda's Developmental Diagnosis: The Evaluation and Management of Normal and Abnormal Neuropsychologic Development in Infancy and Early Childhood.* Hagerstown, MD: Harper & Row; 1974.

Neurological
Disorders

The Infant at High Risk for Developmental Delay

Diane Versaw-Barnes and Audrey Wood

**History and Evolution of the Philosophy
of Care in the Neonatal Intensive Care Unit**
  Introduction
**Levels of Newborn Intensive Care and
the Role of the Physical Therapist**
**Roles and Competencies of the Therapist
in the NICU**
**Theoretical Frameworks to Guide
Therapy**
  Dynamic Systems Theory
  Neuronal Group Selection Theory
  International Classification of Functioning,
    Disability, and Health
  Synactive Theory
  Developmental Care
  Family-Centered Care
**Developmental Foundations to Guide
Therapy**
  Embryogenesis and Neonatal Development
  Evolution of Tone, Reflexes, and Musculoskeletal
    Development
  Evolution of Sensory Responses
  Evolution of State Differentiation

Medical Foundations to Guide Therapy
  Language of the NICU
  Environmental Aspects of Intensive Care: Equipment
    and Technologic Supports
  Medical Issues of Prematurity
  Physical Therapy Assessment and Intervention:
    Issues of Prematurity
  Bronchopulmonary Dysplasia
  Physical Therapy Assessment and Intervention:
    Bronchopulmonary Dysplasia
  The Baby Who Requires Surgery
  Physical Therapy Assessment and Intervention
    for the Baby Who Requires Surgery
  The Baby with Neurologic Issues
  Physical Therapy Assessment and Intervention
    for the Baby with Neurologic Issues
  Medical Issues of the Late Preterm Infant
  Medical Issues of the Term Infant
  Physical Therapy Assessment and Intervention
    for the Late Preterm and Term Infants
Transition to Home
Neonatal Follow-up Services
Summary

History and evolution of the philosophy of care in the neonatal intensive care unit

Introduction

Mary Ellen Avery writes that all neonatologists, by definition, are pioneers, as they care for infants who would not have survived before.[1] The pioneering field of American neonatology has evolved over the past 150 years, its evolution affected by the changing cultural attitudes regarding babies, the technology explosion of the 20th century, and the erroneous assumptions of the first generation of health professionals caring for sick newborns.[2,3] Litanies of systemically implemented untested practices assumed to be beneficial for newborn infants later resulted in disastrous outcomes. The routine use of high amounts of supplemental oxygen resulting in blindness, or retrolental fibroplasia as it was known in the 1950s, is only one example.[4] Owing

to these humbling discoveries, evidence-based practice has moved to the forefront of current neonatology practice.[2]

American neonatology was born into a cultural ambivalence toward the newborn baby and the almost ubiquitous practice of home birthing. Newborn infant mortality was considered "expected reproductive loss," and there was a "silent understanding" that newborn infants had only "tentative claims to family membership."[4] Medical practices geared to saving sick newborns, or "weaklings" as they were termed, were considered futile, and were accompanied with the fear that surviving weaklings would go on to reproduce more weaklings, thus jeopardizing the entire community.[5] In addition, newborn babies were considered to be helpless, "mewling" and "puking" organisms who regarded the world as "blooming, buzzing, confusion" and were not considered capable of anything.[6]

Despite these misgivings, several American hospitals created units for the care of newborn infants. The concept of the newborn as a patient was novel, as the care of newborns was previously considered the territory of mothers.[7] The question of ownership of this newly identified patient led to a turf war between pediatricians and obstetricians.[5,7] In 1958, Virginia Apgar, the creator of the APGAR score for neonatal assessment, proposed that the newborn required his own medical caregiver, someone other than the delivering midwife or physician, who would be devoted to assessing and intervening for him.[7] The newborn became a patient in his own right, preparing the way for the emergence of the specialty practice of neonatology!

From the early 1900s till 1950, the prevailing philosophy of care in these first neonatal care units was a dogmatic "hands-off" policy to protect the babies from unnecessary handling and to provide them with favorable conditions for survival, such as warmth, cleanliness, and nutrition.[4] Even in this age of minimal treatment, untested standard practices like a thermal environment designed to reduce fluctuations in babies' body temperature, while maintaining a lower-than-typical body temperature, later proved inadequate for infant survival.[2,4] Mortality rates were very high for these fragile infants.[8,9]

As the knowledge and understanding of the unique needs of the newborn increased, and with the undeniable success of medical interventions like exchange transfusions and antibiotics in the late 1940s and 50s, the initial "hands-off" philosophy of neonatology gave way to an attitude of "therapeutic exuberance." Neonatology began to take on the challenge of supporting the survival of all infants through passionate interventions.[3,4,10] The technologic advances of the mid-20th century supplied these passionate interventions in the form of radiant warmers, ventilators, total parental nutrition, and central line access. The need for clinicians with expert skills and knowledge in order to provide the most appropriate care for newborns led to the regionalization and specialization of neonatal care.[3]

In 1970, the American Academy of Pediatrics (AAP) added neonatology as a subspecialty with board certification, and in 1975 the Committee on Perinatal Health published guidelines for regional perinatal centers. Brazelton's[11] *Neonatal Behavioral Assessment Scale*, published in 1973, authoritatively replaced the concept of the newborn as a mewling and puking organism with a new understanding of the newborn infant as a competent partner in social interaction.

Neonatal medicine was succeeding in that very low birth weight (VLBW) (i.e., less than or equal to 1500 g or 3 lb, 5 oz) infants were now surviving, however, with increased incidences of cerebral palsy (CP), respiratory disorders, blindness, cognitive delays, and hearing impairments.[8,9] Early intervention programs emerged in the mid-1970s to address the developmental needs of the survivors of neonatal intensive care. The womb was thought to provide a rich sensory environment of which the preterm infant (infant born at less than 37 weeks gestational age [GA]) was deprived. The initial philosophy of "minimal handling" for sick newborns was changing to embrace the belief that the varied tactile, vestibular, proprioceptive, and auditory conditions of the womb should be simulated in the neonatal intensive care unit (NICU) for these babies.[8,9]

Medical and technologic advances of the 1980s and 1990s brought more sophisticated respiratory monitors and therapies, such as nitric oxide, extracorporeal membrane oxygenation (ECMO), pulse oximetry, and surfactant replacement therapy, further reinforcing the need for specialization of NICU caregivers and regionalization of newborn intensive care. In the 1980s, as NICU graduates demonstrated developmental outcomes that were frequently atypical, infant follow-up programs were formalized and infant stimulation programs proliferated. The Education for All Handicapped Children Amendments passed in 1986 required states to provide early intervention services for families and infants with developmental delays or at risk for delays.

Research in the late 1970s demonstrating the aversive impact of the NICU environment on the infant's behavior, growth, and development led to the questioning and the reconceptualization of the sensory stimulation appropriate for a preterm and/or critically ill infant. Modifications of the constant harsh lighting, excessive noise, and intrusive procedures ("environmental neonatology") became important in the philosophy of caring for high-risk infants.[12,13] In addition, the cost of providing this highly specialized care for sick newborns continued to emphasize the need for regionalization of newborn intensive care.[8,9] The synactive theory of development, the creation of Heidelise Als published in the early 1980s, expanded the work of Brazelton and provided a framework for understanding and interpreting the infant's behaviors (physiologic, movement and muscle tone, waking/sleeping, and social interaction) as a window into the baby's overall regulation.[14] In addition, the importance of the family as a constant in the infant's life launched a new focus of family-centered care, which continues to this day. The philosophy of care for infants shifted to individualizing care to support each infant's unique capabilities while partnering with each family to care for the infant.[7,15]

A decade into the 21st century, optimal NICU care is defined as one that is developmentally supportive,[16] family-focused, culturally sensitive,[17] and evidence-based. Neonatology is characterized by a very guarded attitude toward new approaches and changing established protocols. There is a commitment to ensuring that new treatments are tested and proven to be efficacious. Systematic reviews have proliferated and are helpful in appraising and interpreting available research on a topic. Participation in institutional databases to promote benchmarking, the comparison of practices among different institutions, in order to identify the best clinical practice is now the standard in neonatology.[2]

Levels of newborn intensive care and the role of the physical therapist

In 2004, the AAP Committee on the Fetus and Newborn expressed the need for nationally applicable uniform definitions of the levels of newborn intensive care. Besides reinforcing the importance of an organized regional plan of neonatal care, these definitions assist in comprehensive benchmarking among NICUs (which facilitates the comparisons of health outcomes, cost, and utilization of resources), assist the public in seeking appropriate care, minimize the need for development of definitions by payers, and promote consistent standards of service for each level of intensive care. The three levels of newborn intensive care first proposed in 1976, as part of the efforts of the March of Dimes to improve maternal and neonatal outcomes, were refined and expanded on the basis of a survey of 880 NICUs by the committee in 2001. The Committee proposed three categories of care[18] (Table 4.1):

- Basic Neonatal Care (Level I)
- Specialty Neonatal Care (Level II)
- Subspecialty Neonatal Care (Level III)

A level I nursery is a well-baby nursery where healthy newborns are evaluated and cared for. This basic level of neonatal care is the minimum requirement for any hospital providing inpatient maternity care. Level I nurseries have the capacity to stabilize and care for stable late preterm infants (35 to 37 weeks GA), perform neonatal resuscitation at every delivery, and stabilize preterm and ill newborns for transfer to a facility providing specialty care.[18] Small community hospitals where babies are routinely delivered have this level of newborn nursery.

A level II nursery (specialty) is capable of providing the basic care that a level I nursery provides as well as caring for moderately ill infants who have medical problems that are anticipated to resolve rapidly, and infants recovering from serious illness treated in a level III nursery. A level II nursery is considered to be an intermediate or step-down from a level III nursery and provides continuing care, intravenous medications or alimentation, tube feedings, and oxygen support. Neonatologists and neonatal nurses staff these intermediate-level nurseries, which are usually contained in regional or community hospitals. Level II care is differentiated into two categories (IIA and II B) on the basis of the capacity to provide assisted ventilation for an interim period until a baby can be transferred or up to 24 hours. Level IIB nurseries must have the equipment and personnel continuously available to provide the latter as well as to address emergencies.[18]

A level III (subspecialty) nursery is a NICU that provides highly specialized services for the sickest and most fragile infants. Level III units must have personnel, for example, neonatologists, neonatal nurses, respiratory therapists, and equipment available 24 hours 7 days/week to provide life support for as long as needed.[18] Level III units are usually part of teaching hospitals and affiliated with a medical school. Neonatologists, neonatology fellows, clinical nurse specialists, neonatal nurse practitioners, and specially trained nurses staff level III nurseries and provide complex medical interventions, advanced diagnostic testing, surgery, and respiratory support for technologically dependent and medically fragile infants.[9] Level III nurseries are further subdivided into three categories on the basis of the means to provide minor versus major surgery, including cardiac surgery, and conventional versus a range of advanced respiratory supports such as high-frequency ventilation (HFV) and ECMO.[18]

Physical therapists are rarely consulted to see babies in level I nurseries, but may be consulted for a specific musculoskeletal issue. In level II nurseries, physical therapy intervention may involve handling for specific developmental needs. When working with fragile infants and their families in a level III nursery, the therapist needs to use skilled ongoing observation to discern the needs of the baby and provide recommendations regarding positioning, energy conservation, pain management, environmental design, caregiving, and medical management. These observational skills are essential so that the baby is not further stressed by unnecessary handling.

In order to implement care in this way, therapists working in the NICU must have a good knowledge base, a strong

TABLE 4.1	Levels of Neonatal Care
Level I	Basic Neonatal Care
Level I	• Neonatal resuscitation at delivery • Postnatal care and evaluation for healthy newborns • Stabilization and care for physiologically stable late preterm infants aged 35–37 wk gestational age • Stabilization for ill infants and infants <35 wk gestation prior to transfer
Level II	Specialty Neonatal Care
Level II A	• Level I capabilities • Resuscitate and stabilize ill or preterm infants prior to transfer • Care for infants ≥32 wk gestation and ≥1500 g • Provide care for infants convalescing after intensive care
Level II B	• Level II A capabilities • Provide mechanical ventilation or CPAP for <24 hr
Level III	Subspecialty Neonatal Care
Level III A	• Level II B capabilities • Comprehensive care for infants <1000 g and born <28 wk gestational age • Provide CMV • Provide minor surgery (central venous catheter placement or inguinal hernia repair)
Level III B	• Level III A capabilities • Provide advanced respiratory support • On-site and timely access to range of pediatric medical subspecialists • Provide urgent and routine imaging and interpretation of results • Provide major surgery (repair of abdominal wall defects, necrotizing enterocolitis, myelomeningocele)
Level III C	• Level III B capabilities • Provide extracorporeal membrane oxygenation (ECMO) • Provide surgery for complex cardiac malformations requiring cardiopulmonary bypass

understanding of the theoretical and developmental frameworks that guide therapy, and the medical framework that drives care (Table 4.2). These areas will be addressed in this chapter; however, developmental intervention in an NICU is a complex subject, and the reader is referred to the list of additional reading materials in the references section at the end of this chapter.

 ## Roles and competencies of the therapist in the NICU

The role of the therapist working in the NICU is very different from other areas of physical therapy practice. The neonatal therapist provides consultation, diagnosis, intervention, and family support to extremely fragile infants and families within a very stressful and fast-paced intensive care environment. In addition to understanding a wide range of neonatal conditions, medical interventions, and their potential to impact future development, the neonatal therapist must be a careful observer, good collaborator, and effective communicator.[2,9,19,20] Physical therapists have a special role to play as part of the NICU team owing to their expertise in movement, postural control, and neurodevelopment. However, the neonatal therapist must also have specialized knowledge and skills to work with very vulnerable infants and their families (see Table 4.2). The ability to make decisions quickly in terms of an infant's stability and need for external supports is necessary, as an infant's status can change rapidly.

TABLE 4.2	Areas of Knowledge for Neonatal Therapists

- Typical and atypical development
- Fetal and newborn development
- Development and interaction of sensory systems in preterm and full-term neonates
- Medical conditions of preterm and full-term neonates and interventions
- General function and safety regarding lines and medical equipment
- Neonatal preterm and full-term behaviors and social development
- Family dynamics, grief/loss process, attachment, parenting in the NICU
- Ecology and culture of the NICU
- The physical environment of the NICU and the effects on high-risk neonates
- Theoretical frameworks supporting care in the NICU
- Neonatal Practice guidelines
- Description, administration, psychometric properties, and interpretation of results of neonatal assessments
- Risk factors associated with developmental outcome
- Evidence-based practices for positioning and intervention with high-risk infants
- Teaching strategies for families and caregivers
- Safety regarding car seats and infant positioning equipment
- Early intervention, community resources, neonatal developmental follow-up programs

In this environment, interventions that might otherwise be considered benign may have serious immediate and far-reaching consequences.[9,19,20]

Therapy in the NICU is considered to be an advanced level of pediatric physical therapy practice[9,19–22] that needs to be achieved through education and mentored clinical practice. The American Association of Physical Therapy has established guidelines for therapists practicing in the NICU,[20,23] which include specific roles, competencies, knowledge areas, and precepted clinical training. The clinical practice guidelines were originally published in 1989[24] and updated in 1999[25] and again in 2009.[20] The most recent version of the guidelines is divided into two sections: Part I presents clinical training modules, clinical training competencies, and decision-making algorithms, whereas Part II discusses frameworks and evidence from the literature that support practice of therapists in the NICU. Physical therapy neonatal fellowship programs have been developed to provide the advanced knowledge and mentored practice required to develop highly skilled individuals who provide evidence-based family-centered developmental interventions and to foster research in the setting of the NICU.

An evidence-based clinical pathway developed for neonatal Physical therapists has also been recently published. The Infant Care Path for Physical Therapy in the NICU addresses observation and assessment, intervention, family support and education, and teamwork among the various disciplines that provide care to high-risk infants and their families in the NICU.[26–31] The written pathway provides a framework and knowledge that neonatal Physical therapists can use to further develop a research-based practice. While the pathway is a useful tool, neonatal therapists should individualize assessment and interventions specific to the infant, family, and NICU environment.

Theoretical frameworks to guide therapy

Dynamic Systems Theory

Dynamic systems theory describes a model of human development in which behaviors emerge because of the interaction of many subsystems.[32–36] There is no hierarchy; all subsystems are on an equal level, each complex, composed of many elements and unique to the individual. Both internal and external elements affect development; the environment is as equally important as the individual. In this model, the infant is not a passive recipient of information or change, but rather an active participant in which a developmental behavior assembles from the interaction of the many subsystems within the context of the environment and specific to the task. The progression of development is nonlinear; instead, there are series of states of stability, instability, and reorganization.[32–34,36–38] The individual is always trying to move toward homeostasis and reorganizes around the shift from stability to instability. These periods of instability or transition are important as the system has sufficient flexibility to explore and select new solutions or develop new behaviors. Therapeutic interventions are considered to be most effective at this time as the system can more easily be influenced or shifted.[32,34,36]

The dynamic systems framework can be used to evaluate and establish care for the high-risk infant in the NICU (Fig. 4.1).[25] The interaction of the multiple subsystems within the infant as well as the interaction of the infant and the environment influence the health and development of the individual infant. The infant subsystems include body structure, physiology, and behavior. The environment includes the physical environment of the nursery, multiple caregivers and support personnel, and family. Changes to

the intrinsic systems or the environment can have either positive or negative effects. These changes can produce stability to support function or interfere to cause disorganization and potentially maladaptive behaviors. A small change in one system component can have a large effect on another system and ultimately affect function.[25,32,37,38]

The therapist must understand the history, current status of the infant's system, and the environment, taking into consideration the effect caregiving/therapy will have on that particular infant.[25,34] The therapist must support the interactions that allow functional behaviors to develop, decrease infant stress, and understand the implications of the environment. At the same time, the therapist must assist the family and other caregivers in recognizing how they too can be supportive to the infant's health and development.

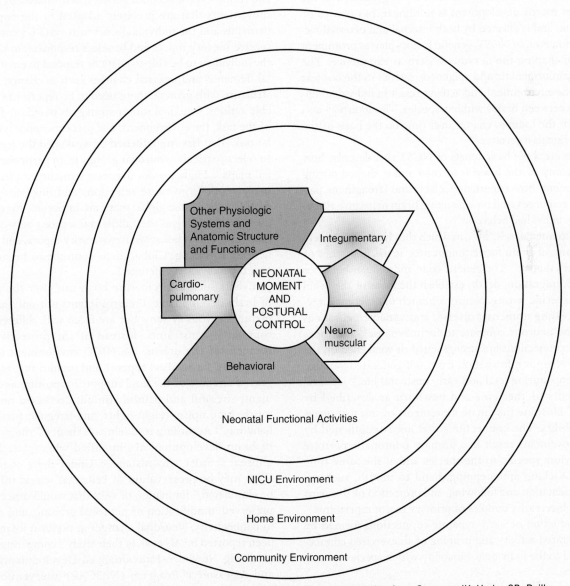

FIGURE 4.1 Dynamic systems theory in the NICU. (Reprinted with permission from Sweeney JK, Heriza CB, Reilly MA, et al. Practice guidelines for the physical therapist in the NICU. *Pediatr Phys Ther*. 1999;11(3):120.)

The therapist needs to be aware of transition periods when developmental interventions can be safely implemented and guide families to utilize these same strategies.

Neuronal Group Selection Theory

A theoretical concept of how the nervous system becomes organized, stores information, and creates new behavioral patterns was developed by Gerald Edelman.[39,40] According to this theory, called Neuronal Group Selection Theory (NGST), the brain is dynamically organized into populations of cells containing individually variable networks. The structures and the function of these networks are selected by evolution, the environment, and behavior. The units of selection are composed of hundreds to thousands of strongly interconnected neurons that work as functional units and are referred to as neuronal groups.[41]

NGST like dynamic systems theory is grounded in the idea that motor development is nonlinear, has phases of transition, and is affected by both internal and external factors.[42] However, in NGST, genetic factors play as prominent a role in shaping the nervous system as experience. The interaction of genetic and epigenetic factors in the context of specific environment and activity result in individual differences between brains within a species. This interplay also allows for the brain to change over time on the basis of the afferent signals it receives.[39]

There are three basic tenets of NGST that describe how the anatomy of the brain is formed and is shaped during development, how experience selects and strengthens patterns of responses, and how resulting brain maps give rise to uniquely individual behavior.[43]

Developmental selection, in which the characteristic neuroanatomy of brain formation occurs, is the first tenet of Edelman's theory.[43] The genetic code and cellular behavior (division, migration, death) establish the areas of the brain but not specific wiring. Neurons branch in different directions, creating immense, diverse, and variable neural circuits. The neurons compete to form synapses, and these synaptic connections are strengthened or weakened on the basis of afferent information from self-generated variable movements during fetal and early postnatal life.[44] General movements of the fetus and newborn as described by Pretchl[45] illustrate the innate movements of this first phase of variability. The connections that are strengthened by these movements result in a primary neuronal repertoire of behaviors specific to the species and at the same time unique. Kicking and stepping, hand to mouth, sucking, visual orientation and following, and projection of the arms toward objects are examples of primary motor repertoires.[45] Overproduction of early synaptic connections formed by self-generated activity and pruning of unexercised connections lead to the individual variability within species-specific behaviors.

Edelman's[43] second tenet involves the development of a secondary repertoire of functional circuits through experiential selection. As the infant interacts with new environmental situations after birth, connections are formed and strengthened. Secondary repertoires of functional connections that meet environmental constraints and support successful, goal-directed movements arise from the neuronal groups of the primary repertoires through experience, repetition, and exploration.[41] The secondary repertoires contain the motor synergies necessary for skilled functional movement as well as memory and other functions. During this phase of secondary variability, the individual explores a variety of movements, and sensory feedback from this exploration shapes the selection of effective strategies. This process continues throughout life, with changing environmental constraints and functional needs.[46-49]

The third tenet of NGST describes how the first two processes interact to form neural maps that connect neuronal groups throughout the nervous system. Massive parallel and reciprocal connections between neuronal maps produce movements that are precisely adapted to the contextual demands and the individual's nervous system's capacity to receive sensory inputs and to select responses. In order for the individual to be able to adapt or respond to environmental demands and internal changes such as change in body structure with growth, there need to be repertoires of variable actions. The final motor strategy is based on demands of the task, the environment, and past experience with similar tasks that has strengthened or weakened the tendencies to select particular neuronal groups from particular neuronal maps.[43] Higher-order dynamic structures called global maps result from these selections and link sensory and motor maps. These global maps are important for development and learning as they allow connections between local maps and motor behavior, new sensory inputs, and greater neural processing. Global maps continue to be modified over the individual's lifetime.[49]

Events such as premature birth can alter the process of brain development. Preterm infants not only have less mature nervous systems but are faced with different environmental constraints. Instead of the protective environment of the uterus, the NICU environment involves equipment for medical support and monitoring, effects of gravity and loss of the fluid support for posture and movement, stressful and painful stimuli, decreased nurturing touch, loud noise, bright lights, and irregular patterns of handling.[23] According to Edelman's theory,[39] the processes of brain development are modified when placed under unusual sensory circumstances. Under these conditions, there may be preservation of cells that would otherwise be eliminated, elimination of cells that would otherwise be preserved, modification of neuronal pruning, and changes in connectivity. Neuronal changes in preterm infants have been reported by Als et al. in their study[50] comparing infants receiving Newborn Individualized Developmental Care and Assessment Program (NIDCAP) intervention with infants receiving standard NICU care. The infant's health status, growth, neurobehavior, brain structure by magnetic resonance imaging (MRI), and neurophysiology by electroencephalography (EEG) were assessed at 2 weeks and 9 months. The authors reported that the infant receiving the NIDCAP care had better neurobehavioral function and more mature fiber structure in the cortex of the brain.[50]

Neonatal physical therapists need to consider the impact of the NICU environment and caregiving practices on the immature and developing brain. The formation of brain structure and function may be affected by these early and atypical sensory and motor experiences. Each infant has different genetic, maturational, and intra- and extrauterine environmental experiences, and the effect of the NICU environment and practices may have a different influence on brain development and function. Therefore, the effect of physical therapy assessment and intervention on brain architecture and maturation must be considered and adapted to meet the needs of the individual infant.

International Classification of Functioning, Disability, and Health

Models of enablement fit well with systems theories as they relate to human development and function. These models present interrelated frameworks for describing the many factors that influence not only an individual's health, but also how the environment influences health and function or participation. The model developed by the World Health Organization (WHO), the *International Classification of Functioning, Disability, and Health* (ICF), emphasizes health and functioning rather than disability and looks at development and function as a multilevel, multifactorial, dynamic process and emphasizes the need to consider the effects of the environment on the process.[51–53]

The components of the ICF framework include body function and structures, activities and tasks, and participation. Instead of starting with the pathophysiology, this model looks at what the individual wants or needs to do and then considers the individual factors that support or interfere with participation. The contextual factors of the individual and the environment are taken into consideration as well as the role of environment in supporting or limiting function/participation.

Although the NICU is a unique setting for physical therapy practice, the ICF model can be applied to guide assessment and intervention.[23] The physical therapist working with high-risk infants in this environment can use the framework to guide him or her in addressing functional and structural integrity of body parts and systems, promoting the development of postural and motor activities, and promoting appropriate interaction between the infant, the physical environment, and the family, NICU staff, and consultants. As with a child of any age, the contextual factors of the individual infant, family, and environment must be addressed in order to provide effective intervention. For example, the functional goal for an infant may be to socially interact with his or her family while being held. After a thorough assessment, the therapist needs to consider what components are required for this activity to be successful for the infant and family as well as those components that may interfere. The therapist may assist the family in positioning the infant in optimal alignment to support physiologic functions such as respiration and in swaddling to maintain the posture, and may assist the infant in bringing his or her hands to his or her face for calming and behavioral organization; the therapist may also dim the lights, reduce the sound in the area to decrease stress and promote arousal, and support the family in recognizing the infant's cues for interaction. In addition, the therapist, family, and NICU staff can work together to find the most optimal times for the infant to be successful in these interactions. Throughout an infant's NICU course, the physical therapist can address goals to promote activity and participation by supporting body structures and functions, family and caregiver education, and addressing environmental and other contextual factors. Atkinson and Nixon-Cave[54] have published a clinical reflection tool to assist in translating the ICF model into practice that can be applied to infants and families in the NICU.

Synactive Theory

The synactive theory of infant development, proposed by psychologist Heidelise Als,[14] is a model to understand and interpret the behavior of preterm infants and is similar to the dynamic systems approach in that multiple influences contribute and mutually influence the baby's functioning. The fetus from conception onward is thought to be organizing five distinct but interrelated subsystems: autonomic (governing basic physiologic functioning, e.g., heart rate, respiratory rate, visceral functions); motor (governing postures and movements); state (governing ranges of consciousness from sleep to wakefulness); attention/interaction (governing the ability to attend to and interact with caregivers); and self-regulatory (governing the ability to maintain balanced, relaxed, and integrated functioning of all four subsystems). These subsystems continually react and influence each other, thus the term *synactive*.[55–57] Babies born at term have completed the maturation of these subsystems to the degree that, in general, they are able to demonstrate brief periods of social interaction with a caregiver while maintaining stability in the physiologic, motoric, and state subsystems (Fig. 4.2). They can also utilize strategies to regulate the various subsystems when the environment poses a threat to their stability; for example, when eye contact with a parent becomes too intense, a term infant may yawn, look away briefly, stretch, tuck his or her head to his or her trunk, and bring the hands together (strategies represented by the attention/interaction and motor subsystems) before returning to gaze again at a parent's face.

In babies born before term, the maturation of the five subsystems is interrupted. In addition, babies born before term have lost the uterine supports for these subsystems (autonomic supports like temperature regulation, placental

MODEL OF THE SYNACTIVE
ORGANIZATION OF BEHAVIORAL DEVELOPMENT

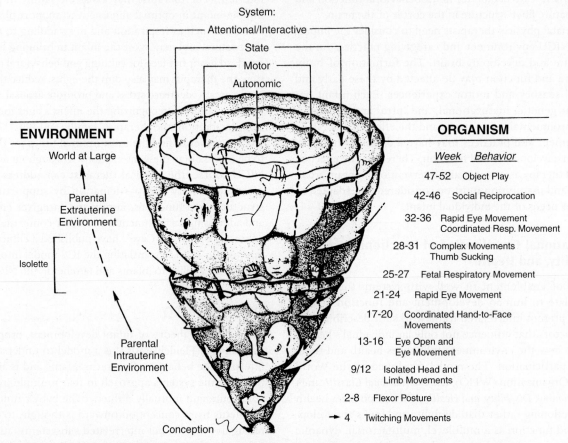

System:
Attentional/Interactive
State
Motor
Autonomic

ENVIRONMENT

World at Large

Parental
Extrauterine
Environment

Isolette

Parental
Intrauterine
Environment

Conception

ORGANISM

Week   Behavior

47-52   Object Play

42-46   Social Reciprocation

32-36   Rapid Eye Movement
Coordinated Resp. Movement

28-31   Complex Movements
Thumb Sucking

25-27   Fetal Respiratory Movement

21-24   Rapid Eye Movement

17-20   Coordinated Hand-to-Face
Movements

13-16   Eye Open and
Eye Movement

9/12   Isolated Head and
Limb Movements

2-8   Flexor Posture

4   Twitching Movements

FIGURE 4.2 Model of the synactive organization of behavioral development. (Reprinted with permission from Als H. Toward a synactive theory of development: promise for the assessment and support of infant individuality. *Infant Ment Health J.* 1982;3(4):234.)

nutrition delivery, waste removal, oxygen delivery, and carbon dioxide removal; motoric supports like the containment of the uterine wall and the buoyancy of the amniotic fluid; state supports like the diurnal cycles of the mother's sleep–wake cycle; and attention/interaction supports like diminished visual and auditory input). Babies born before term are required to complete the maturation of each subsystem while also negotiating more independent functioning, such as breathing, feeding, eliminating wastes, maintaining postures, and moving against gravity, and while also enduring bright lighting, harsh noises, frequent handling, and multimodal stimulation. The preterm baby is adapted for functioning in the womb, but is required to function outside the womb at a crucial time in development and, therefore, faces a very challenging existence.[14,55–58]

Developmental Care

Applying this synactive theory of infant development through systematic serial observations of the baby is

a very helpful way to identify the baby's areas of success at coping and areas of vulnerability. It is important to communicate these strengths and vulnerabilities to the parents and caregivers and to identify strategies to support the baby as he or she receives this necessary intensive care.[14,55,56,58–60] The process of systematic serial observations has led to a broad array of interventions to minimize the stress of the NICU for the infant and to individualize the caregiving to the infant's tolerance. These interventions include strategies to decrease noise and light levels, minimize handling of the infant, protect infant sleep states, promote understanding of infant behavioral cues, and promote relationship-based caregiving.[61] This approach to newborn intensive care is called the NIDCAP.[59] Ideally, NIDCAP observations are scheduled every 7 to 10 days and include viewing the baby at a baseline for 10 to 20 minutes before nursing care or procedure, throughout the care session or procedure, and after the session or procedure until the baby returns to baseline functioning[59,62] (Fig. 4.3). During this time, the

OBSERVATION SHEET   Name: _____   Date: _____   Sheet Number _____

Time:	0-2	3-4	5-6	7-8	9-10
Resp: Regular					
Irregular					
Slow					
Fast					
Pause					
Color: Jaundice					
Pink					
Pale					
Webb					
Red					
Dusky					
Blue					
Tremor					
Startle					
Twitch Face					
Twitch Body					
Twitch Extremities					
Visceral/ Resp: Spit up					
Gag					
Burp					
Hiccough					
BM Grunt					
Sounds					
Sigh					
Gasp					
Motor: Flaccid Arm(s)					
Flaccid leg(s)					
Flexed/Tucked Arms Act. Post.					
Flexed/Tucked Legs Act. Post.					
Extend Arms Act. Post.					
Extend Legs Act. Post.					
Smooth Mvmt. Arms					
Smooth Mvmt. Legs					
Smooth Mvmt. Trunk					
Stretch/Drown					
Diffuse Squirm					
Arch					
Tuck Trunk					
Leg Brace					
Face: Tongue Extension					
Hand on Face					
Gape Face					
Grimace					
Smile					

Time:	0-2	3-4	5-6	7-8	9-10
State: 1A					
1B					
2A					
2B					
3A					
3B					
4A					
4B					
5A					
5B					
6A					
6B					
AA					
Face (cont.): Mouthing					
Suck Search					
Sucking					
Extrem.: Finger Splay					
Airplane					
Salute					
Sitting On Air					
Hand Clasp					
Foot Clasp					
Hand to Mouth					
Grasping					
Holding On					
Fisting					
Attention: Fuss					
Yawn					
Sneeze					
Face Open					
Eye Floating					
Avert					
Frown					
Ooh Face					
Locking					
Cooing					
Speech Mvmt.					
Posture: (Prone, Supine, Side)					
Head: (Right, Left, Middle)					
Location: (Crib, Isolette, Held)					
Manipulation:					
Heart Rate					
Respiration Rate					
TcPO₂					

FIGURE 4.3 NIDCAP observation sheet. (Reprinted with permission from Als H. Reading the premature infant. In: Goldson E, ed. *Nurturing the Premature Infant: Developmental Intervention in the Neonatal Intensive Care nursery.* New York, NY: Oxford University Press; 1999:37.)

observer is watching for signs of stability and stress from each subsystem (Table 4.3) while recording environmental events and caretaking tasks. The infant's strategies for self-regulation, whether successful or unsuccessful, are then noted, and recommendations to support the infant in his or her attempts at organizing and self-soothing are made as well as recommendations for environmental modification, caregiving, and parental involvement.[14,55,57–60] Formal training through the NIDCAP regional training centers is required for reliability and certification in NIDCAP. However, using the principles and applying the synactive model to understand a baby's behavior is a helpful way to guide caregivers in developmentally supportive interventions through observations of nursing care.

The synactive model of preterm behavior identifies the autonomic subsystem and the motoric subsystem as the

TABLE 4.3 Signs of Stability and Stress in the Preterm Infant

System	Signs of Stability	Signs of Stress
Autonomic	Smooth, regular respirations	Respiratory pauses, tachypnea, gasping
	Pink, stable coloring	Paling, perioral duskiness, mottled, cyanotic, gray, flushed, ruddy
	Stable digestion	Hiccups, gagging, grunting, emesis, tremors, startles, twitches, cough, sneeze, yawn, sigh, gasp
Motor	Smooth, controlled posture and muscle tone	Fluctuating muscle tone
	Smooth movements of extremities and head	Flaccidity of trunk, extremities, and face
	Hand/foot clasp, leg brace, finger fold, hand to mouth, grasp, suck, tuck, hand hold	Hypertonicity of trunk and extremities
		Frantic diffuse activity
State	Clear, well-defined sleep states	Diffuse sleep with twitches, jerky movement, irregular breathing, whimpering sounds, grimacing, and fussing
	Focused alertness with animated facial expression	Diffuse wakeful periods with eye floating, glassy-eyed, strained appearance, staring, gaze aversion, panicked, dull look, weak cry

Adapted from Als H. Toward a synactive theory of development: promise for the assessment and support of infant individuality. *Infant Ment Health J.* 1982;3(4):237–238.

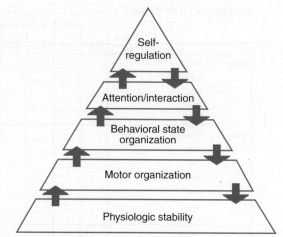

FIGURE 4.4 Pyramid of the synactive theory of infant behavioral organization with physiologic stability at the foundation. (Used with permission from Sweeney JK, Swanson MW. Low birth weight infants: neonatal care and follow-up. In: Umphred DA, ed. *Neurological Rehabilitation.* 4th ed. St. Louis, MO: Mosby; 2001:205.)

two core subsystems on which the rest of the infant's functioning is based (Fig. 4.4). Together, these two subsystems are the basis for the baby to achieve higher functioning like awaking (state subsystem) and gazing at a parent's face (attention/interaction subsystem). A therapist can recommend and intervene to support the motor system through positioning and containment, and in so doing can support the autonomic subsystem as well as the state and interactional subsystems as each system continually interacts and influences the others.[15,55,56,58] The systematic individualization of caring for an infant is the root of developmentally supportive care.[61,63] The knowledge and understanding of how one baby differs from another can only be gleaned by intense observation of the infant in interaction with his or her environment. Using this individualized knowledge of the baby's strengths and vulnerabilities to guide the provision of care has been shown to result in short-term benefits to the baby such as shorter hospitalization resulting in less costly care, decreased use of ventilator, earlier attainment of oral feeds, and improved growth. Long-term benefits include improved neurobehavioral functioning and enhanced brain structure in later infancy, advantages in expressive language and neurologic organization and function at 3 years, and improved attention and visual/spatial perception at 8 years.[50,57,58,60–62,64–68] Critics of the research on developmental care point out that studies have shown conflicting results, have utilized small sample sizes, and have demonstrated outcomes that may not be clinically significant. Some studies also have serious methodologic flaws in the designs, such as neglecting to blind the outcome assessors and allowing the control and experimental groups to receive the same interventions. The critics of developmental care have not found harmful effects to result from the application of the developmental care philosophy in the NICU, but question whether the benefits are real.[69,70] It is not prudent to implement a philosophy because it does no harm if there are no substantial benefits, as this may detract from other approaches that may prove truly beneficial. Given the abstract nature of the developmental care philosophy and relationship-based caregiving, it is no surprise that it is difficult to study, let alone to teach and implement. During NIDCAP observations, the authors have observed infants becoming progressively exhausted, limp, and passive during routine care, as their attempts to organize are continually thwarted by the noncontingent responses of the caregivers. In contrast, infants have been observed to maintain behavioral and physiologic stability when their caregivers are attentive and responsive to their cues. In addition, research on some specific techniques of supporting a baby during care (e.g., facilitated tucking and nonnutritive sucking [NNS]) have shown significant positive results.[71–79] It is not surprising that preterm infants would also need extra and special supports to cope with intensive care, given the emotional dependency that characterizes the infant and toddler periods.

Family-Centered Care

Family-centered care is a philosophy of patient care delivery for the maternal–child health division based on respect, collaboration, and support between health care professionals and patients' families. It is a philosophy that recognizes the family (defined as parents, children, and significant others) as the constant in the child's life and strives to include the family as partners in choosing and implementing the plan of care for the patient. Family-centered care also acknowledges that hospitalization is stressful for families and can potentially alter the integration of the child into the family and the development of the parental role.[80,81] In order to provide family-centered care in an NICU, a clinician must be knowledgeable about and sensitive to both the psychological tasks of pregnancy and the grief process.

Psychological Tasks of Pregnancy

In American culture, pregnancy is typically and naively regarded as a happy time of anticipation, and although that may be partially true, pregnancy is also a time of psychological turmoil. The 40 weeks of pregnancy provide a physical as well as a psychological preparatory period for the expectant parents. When this period is shortened, the baby and the parents may suffer from the incompletion of the pregnancy.[82–85] Bibring[86,87] has identified three psychological tasks of pregnancy, correlating with the three trimesters.[83,85] In the first trimester, parents accept the overwhelming news that their lives have begun a new phase of responsibility for a child (first task). Euphoria; inventorying one's childhood to evaluate his or her own parents' job at childrearing; maternal ambivalence, paternal ambivalence, and exclusion; feelings of helplessness and inadequacy; and fantasizing about the perfect baby and the perfect parent characterize this period.[83,88–90]

During the second trimester, the mother-to-be is confronted with the separateness of the baby as she begins to feel the fetal movements (second task). Although she feels a personal closeness to the baby, the mother's bodily changes and the baby's burgeoning movements make the individuality of the baby more real and apparent. She may enjoy the attention she receives from her changing shape. During this time, the mother continues to question herself about her adequacy as a parent. Concerns regarding the health and the potential to inflict harm on the fetus are prominent. Ambivalence toward the baby is still very much present for both parents, with fathers struggling with feelings of resentment and rivalry. Attachment to a baby requires time to develop.[83,85,88–90]

In the third trimester, the baby begins to be personified as names are chosen and rooms painted. In addition, the expectant mother recognizes patterns in fetal movement and is able to assign the baby a temperament and/or a gender on the basis of these patterns, further personifying the baby. The baby's individuality, revealed in his or her differing responses to the mother's music, food, or other environmental conditions, confirms his or her competence and capabilities, as well as demonstrates to the parents his or her ability to handle the rigors of labor and delivery.[83] Simultaneously, the mother-to-be is physically becoming increasingly uncomfortable and has difficulty sleeping, breathing, eating, and moving. She cannot get a break from being pregnant and this physical state leads to the third psychological task: being ready to give up the fetus.[84–86]

A full-term birth prepares the mother to cope with the shock of the separation of the baby from her body, and both parents to interact and bond with a particular baby. Parents who give birth prematurely are ill-prepared for these psychological tasks,[83] just as their babies are ill-prepared for independent living.[84] In addition, when a pregnancy or birth deviates from the expected, parents often feel guilty about failing to complete the pregnancy or about any complications the baby may experience.[84,91] The precariousness and unpredictability of an NICU have been shown to detract from completing the psychological tasks necessary for taking on the role of a parent. Instead, the psychological focus becomes the uncertainty and unpredictability of the situation, which distracts from the psychological task of preparing for a new family member and assuming the parental role.[90]

When babies are hospitalized at the critical time when parents should be establishing their relationships with their newborns and learning their parental roles, it is especially stressful.[92] The effects of this stress can continue for months after the NICU experience has ended and can pose severe threats to the parents individually and as a couple.[93] Indeed, the experience of having a baby who requires intensive care is a stressor significant enough to cause symptoms of post-traumatic stress disorder.[94–98] The development of post-traumatic stress disorder after life-threatening illnesses and medical procedures has been reported in the literature.[93] Research has shown that the families who endure the hospitalization and develop a positive outlook about the experience have children who develop better in the years after birth. Likewise, poor coping can have lasting detrimental effects on the child's development.[99,100] Therefore, it is important that clinicians working in the NICU recognize the stress families experience and establish supportive relationships with the families in an effort to support their individual coping styles. To do this, a clinician must understand the coping and grieving processes.

Coping and Grieving

Both coping and grieving have been described as a linear progression through distinct stages (e.g., shock, denial, anger, guilt, adjustment, and acceptance). However, this linear progression has not been validated empirically.[98,100] Instead, it is more helpful to understand grief and coping as ongoing processes involving circular progressions where previous issues and losses are resurrected and revisited.[99,101] The beneficial effects of plain old social support cannot be underestimated in the NICU setting. Approaching families with stereotyped expectations of a rigid time frame regarding their coping and grieving will result in the family feeling judged and will prevent the development of supportive relationships between families and staff, to the ultimate detriment of the baby.[99]

Providing Family-Centered Care in the NICU

The shock of a pregnancy, labor, and/or delivery gone awry, whether resulting in a fragile preterm baby or a full-term baby who requires intensive medical/surgical care, can linger with parents indeterminately. Parents of babies in an NICU are in crisis and should be cared for sensitively. It is important to understand the families' backgrounds (previous losses due to deaths, infertility, miscarriages, assistive reproductive technology, financial situation, current work and/or school responsibilities, current relational situations, and other life stressors). This can be accomplished by reading the social work consults and speaking directly with the social workers, nurses, psychologists, and families. The NICU therapist should not ignore this social history because it "does not change what I do with the baby." Rather, this background knowledge should guide how the therapist interacts with the family.

Every family in the NICU is grieving something, maybe the loss of the expected labor/delivery plan or perhaps the loss of the perfect child. This grief will resurrect past losses and can limit the parents' availability to establish an emotional bond with their infant. In addition, the interactional deprivation imposed by the intensive care the baby requires can prevent the families from knowing and connecting with their infant. The high-tech, crisis-prone NICU environment shocks and intimidates families. The families must ask permission to enter the unit as well as to touch or hold their infant, which creates a sense of lost ownership of their infant. Families may not want to risk emotional involvement with their fragile newborn who may later die.

Developmental care of an infant grows out of establishing a supportive and nurturing relationship with the infant. Likewise, family-centered care grows out of establishing a supportive and empowering relationship with the family. One of the goals of family-centered care is to facilitate the bonding process between the infant and the family and to assist the family in establishing emotional ties with their infant.[85,102] To be effective in this goal, therapists must be mindful of their own attitudes and nonverbal behaviors and must congruently communicate nonjudgmental acceptance of the family's emotions, coping methods, and pace. Therapists are responsible for crafting the relationship with the family and supporting and empathizing with their emotions while reflecting the strengths they observe in the family and the infant. Some suggestions to accomplish this include using the baby's name when talking about him or her; commenting on the baby's accomplishments; stating the baby's strengths; stating that the baby is attractive; commenting on the positive interactions between the baby and the family; emphasizing the parents' importance to the infant; pointing out the baby's preference for the parents; and emphasizing the parents' competence with tasks related to the infant's care.[54,102]

A family's human tendency to maintain hope for the future, that the professionals may be wrong, and that miracles can occur should be preserved. Hope is a motivating emotion, providing the energy to cope, work, strive, and stay involved with the infant. It sustains the impetus to maintain the emotional bond to the baby through visiting and interacting. Hope should not be destroyed, but neither should it be falsely fed with unrealistic expectations. Families in crisis with babies in an NICU deserve to hear congruent information from the medical team and the therapy team. This requires sensitivity, diplomacy, and good communication skills.[85]

▶ Developmental foundations to guide therapy

Embryogenesis and Neonatal Development

In this section, embryogenesis and the current understanding of muscle tone and sensory responses in the second half of gestation are discussed. The evolution of primitive reflexes is left out as it would not be prudent for a therapist today to try to elicit these reactions in a preterm infant for any reason, as it may cause unnecessary stress for the preterm infant. In addition, there is no benefit to a preterm infant to assess his or her muscle tone or sensory reactions solely to determine whether development is occurring appropriately. Rather, this information is included here to provide the neonatal therapist with an understanding of the preterm infant's development and struggle with the intrusiveness of the extrauterine environment at a critical time in his or her development.

Embryogenesis is a remarkable series of events. In 266 days, a 0.1-mm single large cell at fertilization increases in length by a factor of 5000, in surface area by a factor of 61 million, and in weight by a factor of 6 billion. During the pre-embryonic period, the first 2 weeks after fertilization of the oocyte by the sperm, cell division in the zygote forms three primary germ layers whose segmentation and axis formation are essential to the development of the human baby.[103] The ectoderm evolves into the skin, spinal cord, and teeth; the mesoderm into the blood vessels, muscles, and bone; and the endoderm into the digestive system, lungs, and urinary tract.[104] During the embryonic period (weeks 3 through 8), the mass of cells divides and differentiates into the more than 200 different cell types comprising the various organs of the body.[103] This is a result of amazing and complex processes that are precisely timed and interwoven. In the embryonic period, the cells initially are homogeneous, but increasing differentiation determines an exact biologic function for each cell. By the end of this period, the embryo has a heterogeneous structure. Any misstep in this process can result in demise or a major morphologic malformation in the embryo.[104] The nervous system, the first organ to initiate development and the last to complete development continuing well after birth, is very susceptible to insult. Other systems have shorter critical periods where an interruption or insult can cause a congenital anomaly[103] (see Fig. 4.5 for timing of major/minor anomalies).

In the first week after fertilization, the fertilized egg travels from the fallopian tube and reaches the uterus. In the second week, the fertilized egg, having undergone several mitotic cell divisions to reach the blastocyst stage, implants into the rich vascular wall of the uterus and by the end of the second week forms a primitive placenta. By the end of the third week, the embryo's blood is circulating in a U-shaped tube that later fuses to a single tube and undergoes partitioning into four chambers during weeks 4 to 7. In the fourth week, the embryo is now less than half a centimeter long. In 35 days, a single cell has grown and been transformed into more than 10,000 different cells. The changes are swift and the process so precise and predictable that the timing of a congenital defect can be pinpointed.[104] In addition, an ultrasound during the embryonic period can be used to date the pregnancy within 7 days.[105]

During the fetal period, weeks 9 through 36, the established organs and body parts of the embryo become refined and enlarged. The placenta serves as a barrier, removes wastes, and provides nutrition for the growing fetus, fulfilling the function of the fetal lungs, kidneys, intestines, and liver. In the third month, unbeknownst to the mother, the fetus is quite active, kicking and turning in its 8 oz of amniotic fluid.[104,106] All movement patterns present in a term newborn have been initiated by 15 weeks' gestation, including sucking, swallowing, breathing, and grasping the umbilical cord. Fetal responses to extrauterine stimuli (e.g., turning to auditory or visual stimulation, heart rate changes to environmental stimulation, and habituation to repeated stimuli) have been documented for decades.[107–109] Fetal activity also demonstrates cyclic fluctuations and circadian rhythms.[109]

The Competence of the Term Newborn

Before the 1900s, there were no formal structured examinations for the newborn; the newborn was perceived as disorganized, unstructured, and lacking in sensory and motor capacities. In the early 1900s, under the prevailing Sherrington reflex model, newborn reflexes were investigated and a standard neurologic test for newborns was

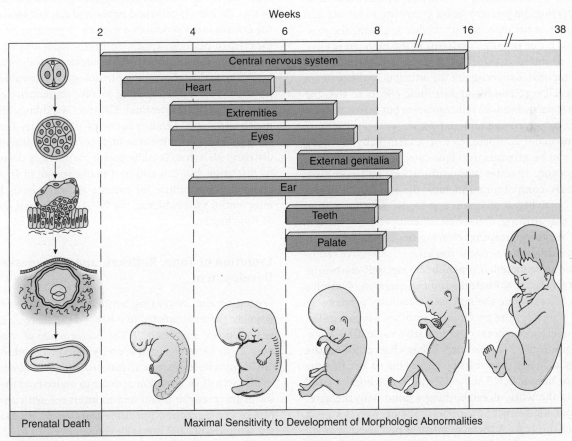

FIGURE 4.5 Embryogenesis and fetal development. (Modified from Rubin E, Gorstein F, Schwarting R, et al. *Pathology.* 4th ed. Baltimore, MD: Lippincott Williams & Wilkins; 2005.)

published. In the mid-1900s, the reflex model was expanded to include generalized motor functioning. Researchers looked at infants' active and passive muscle tone and considered infants able to modulate their behavior. Prechtl and Beintema[110] introduced the concept of infant state as distinct organizations of the brain and associated physiology, affecting how an infant responded to a stimulus. The infant was seen as actively generating responses and modulating performances. In the latter half of the 20th century, more complex infant functioning was appreciated. Infants demonstrated preferential gaze, sound discrimination, affective behaviors, coordination of movements and speech, and differing cries, and were considered "social beings."[111] With this newfound appreciation, the infant was perceived as "competent," no longer a passive recipient or blank slate on which the environment and the baby's caregivers could write.[6,111] Comparetti[107] wrote of fetal competencies for induction and participation in labor/delivery (automatic walking and positive support to locate and engage the baby's head in the birth canal and collaborate in the expulsion process from the womb) and for survival (rooting and sucking for feeding). Brazelton saw the baby as an active participant in the social tasks of eliciting caregiving and initiating the bonding process, organizing his or her own autonomic and state responses in order to modify the stimulation from the environment while maintaining his or her own stability.[11]

Likewise, Heidelise Als[55–59] has written numerous articles portraying the preterm infant as striving to initiate and maintain his or her own stability while completing the maturation of his or her organ systems in the high-stress environment of intensive care. Dr. Als has passionately worked to teach caregivers to recognize the attempts of the preterm infant to self-regulate, to support these efforts so that the baby not only succeeds at self-regulation but learns to trust his or her caregivers and him- or herself.

The neonatal competencies of a term baby allowing survival can be grouped into four categories: physiologic, sensorimotor, affective/communication, and complex. Physiologic competencies include the functional maturity and capability of all organ systems to allow breathing, feeding, and growing. Sensorimotor competencies include rooting, sucking, grasping, clearing the airway in prone, and horizontal and vertical tracking.[112] Affective/communication competencies include crying, self-consoling, eye contact, facial animation, and eye aversion. Complex competencies include the newborn's auditory preferences (mother's voice), taste preferences (mother's breast milk), visual preferences (faces), and imitative capacities (sticking tongue out).[113] Brazelton[11,83] has characterized the newborn as being on a mission to get his or her parents to care for him or her. The healthy term newborn is a full partner in the work of establishing a bond with the caregiver. Contrast this with the preterm infant, who is a weak partner in this task. A preterm infant is perceived as small and unattractive and is less responsive and more difficult to calm, and his cry elicits negative emotions in the caregiver.

Mothers of preterm infants experience less synchronous interactions, play fewer games, work harder to engage, and derive less gratification from their infants.[114] Thus, the bonding process is at risk between a preterm infant and his or her family.

A Competent Feeder

Feeding has been described as the infant's "primary work,"[9] and the coordination of sucking, swallowing, and breathing requires considerable skill as well as energy.[115] Nevertheless, every day, term newborn infants feed successfully. It is a typical and basic competency of a newborn term baby, who plays a very active role in the whole process, from waking and crying to communicate hunger, rooting to find the feeding source, pacing and coordinating sucking with swallowing and breathing, and digesting and eliminating a volume of food, to gaining weight and growing. In a preterm or sick full-term baby, failure with feeding can occur in any one or more of these areas. Sick or preterm babies may have learned an oral aversion as a result of their NICU care. A sick or preterm infant may lack the balance of flexion/extension to attain the appropriate alignment of neck extension and chin tuck to assist sucking and swallowing and breathing, or residual lung disease may cause the infant to breathe too fast to allow time for sucking and swallowing. A preterm baby may not self-regulate physiologic capacities so that the baby is calm and awake and can self-soothe when the environment produces a stressor. A preterm infant may experience periodic apnea, or bradycardia and be unable to manage the coordination of sucking, swallowing, and breathing without becoming physiologically unstable. Other potential obstacles to feeding involve immaturity or problems of the gastrointestinal (GI) tract including reflux and malabsorption.[115] Feeding is one of the primary functional tasks of a newborn infant and generally a requirement for discharge to home. Feeding problems not only delay hospital discharge, but can also be a major source of frustration and feelings of failure for parents and caregivers. Feeding interventions for babies in the NICU are beyond the scope of this chapter.

Evolution of Tone, Reflexes, and Musculoskeletal Development

Owing to the increasing sophistication of technology, younger preterm infants, just beyond the halfway mark of gestation, are surviving.[116] The preterm age of viability is now 23 to 24 weeks' gestation. A therapist working in an NICU must be intimately acquainted with fetal development in the last half of gestation in order to understand the behavior of the preterm infant and to intervene with and assess him or her. Suzanne Saint-Anne Dargassies[117] in 1955 studied 40 nonviable and previable fetuses from 20 to 27 weeks' gestation to determine the neurologic characteristics of fetal maturation. (At that time, the viability threshold was

27 weeks' gestation, and Dargassies studied these premature infants before they died.) She found that periods of 1 week were long enough to distinguish one stage from another, until 26 weeks, and then the rate of change slowed down. Dargassies observed spontaneous facial activity (excluding tongue and lips) very early; distal responses were manifest before proximal; gallant reflex (trunk incurvation) was completely present at 20 weeks; and active movements, elicited movements, and primary reflexes improved slowly in quality, duration, and completeness. She saw a complete lack of passive muscle tone in extremities and trunk, although this was hard to investigate because of "edema, sclerema, and death agony,"[117] and she observed babies from 21 weeks responding differently to tactile and painful stimuli.[117]

Dargassies[117] also studied 100 viable preterm infants from 28 weeks' to 41 weeks' gestation and observed maturational stages in 2-week segments during this time period. She created "maturative" criteria for infants at 28, 30, 32, 35, and 37 weeks and analyzed differences between term newborns and former preterms at 40 weeks' gestation. According to Dipietro,[108] the period between 28 and 32 weeks' gestation is a transitional one for a fetus. Heart rate, activity, state organization, responses to vibroacoustic stimulation, and the coupling between fetal activity and heart rate are variable with peaks and plateaus in presentation. By gestational weeks 31 to 32, the variability has stabilized and the rate of development has slowed so that a baby at 32 weeks' gestation will demonstrate less startle responses, increasing periods of quiescence, increasing state organization, mature levels of vibroacoustic responsiveness, and increasing abilities to habituate to stimuli. These patterns continue to mature through term age; however, a 32-week fetus behaves more like a term infant than a younger fetus. This transitional period parallels the period of rapid increases in neural development and myelination, including cortical vagal responses and sulcation.[108]

Allen and Capute[116] studied 42 preterm infants, none whom developed CP, from 24 to 32 weeks' gestation with weekly neurodevelopmental examinations, and found that flexor tone, recoil, and hyperreflexia appeared 2 to 3 weeks earlier in the lower extremities (33 to 35 weeks) than the upper extremities (35 to 37 weeks). Trunk tone (measured on ventral suspension) was manifest at 36 to 40 weeks. Neck tone was poor with greater than one-half the babies at term-corrected age continuing with a head lag in pull-to-sit. Primitive reflexes and deep tendon reflexes (DTRs) appeared in lower extremities before upper extremities. (Presence of asymmetric tonic neck reflex [ATNR] was detected in lower extremities first at 31 weeks and in upper extremities at 34 weeks.) They found that the evolution of tone, DTRs, and primitive and pathologic reflexes proceeded in an orderly sequential pattern (i.e., lower extremities to upper extremities and distal to proximal).[116]

Preterm infants, in addition to the previously described hypotonia, also have a decreased ratio of type I (slow twitch) muscle fibers to type II (fast twitch) compared with infants at term. This results in muscular fatigue (particularly respiratory muscles) in preterm infants. Preterm infants also demonstrate incomplete ossification of bones, ligamentous laxity, and connective tissue elasticity compared with term infants. The combination of these unique characteristics of preterm infants places them at the mercy of gravity and the surfaces on which they lie. Just as fetal movements or lack thereof are thought to contribute to the shaping of joints, skulls, and spinal curves of babies in utero, preterm infants can fall victim to positionally induced deformities in the NICU. These include skull-shaping abnormalities like dolichocephaly (increased anterior–posterior diameter of the head) and plagiocephaly (flattening of posterior–lateral skull due to preferred head and neck rotation to one side), as well as extremity misalignment.[118]

Research comparing former preterm infants at term age (37 to 42 gestational weeks) and term newborns has demonstrated differences in tone and reactivity in the two groups. Unlike infants born at term, preterm infants miss the experience of a crowded uterus to limit their range of active movement and to support the development of flexor tone. In contrast to term infants who are tucked and contained in utero, preterm infants experience gravity, as well as intravenous lines, support boards, and other restraints, during this period of maturational-related hypotonia. For these reasons, at term age, a former preterm infant and a term newborn will demonstrate differences in muscle tone. Former preterm infants at term age demonstrate less flexor tone of extremities and poorer flexor/extensor balance of head and neck, and in addition have greater range of motion in French angles, as well as greater active range of motion, than their term newborn counterparts.[119,120] Former preterm infants at term age are more reactive, demonstrating more startles, tremors, brisk reflexes, and a shorter attention span than their term counterparts.[117,120] Former preterms may also demonstrate toe walking during automatic walking, while their full-term counterparts demonstrate heel–toe walking.[117]

In addition, brain development of former preterm infants at term-corrected age differs from brain development of babies born at term. Newborn term infants show better behavioral functioning of autonomic, motoric, state, and attention/interactional subsystems, as well as higher amplitudes in EEG and photic-evoked responses and increased gray/white matter differentiation and myelination, than healthy former preterm infants at term age. Some of these differences may be explained by the cumulative complications of preterm birth; however, the developmentally inappropriate sensory stimulation of an NICU may also affect preterm brain development.[121–123]

Evolution of Sensory Responses

Research demonstrates neurosensory development in animals to follow a sequential pattern, first touch, then movement, smell and taste, hearing, and lastly sight. Stimulation of a particular system during development can be essential for the development of that system. However, if the stimulus is too intense or is atypically timed, it can interfere with the development of that and other sensory systems.[124] Preterm infants are forced to complete the development and maturation of their sensory systems while in an intensive care environment. The effects of this environment on the developing brain are not fully understood and are only beginning to be studied.

Tactile System

Four different sensory abilities comprise the tactile system: touch, temperature, pain, and proprioception. The first three sensory receptors are housed in the skin, and the last is composed of receptors from not only the skin, but also joints and muscles. The skin is the largest organ, and therefore touch is the largest sensory system as well as the first to develop.[125,126]

THE PROBLEM OF PAIN Pain comprises one of the sensory modalities of the tactile system. Pain assessment and management has been increasingly recognized as an integral component in the care of high-risk infants in the NICU. At one time, it was standard practice for infants to have no anesthesia or analgesia for painful procedures like circumcision, central line placement, or patent ductus arteriosus (PDA) ligation[75] as babies were believed to be incapable of feeling or remembering pain. However, over time, research has established that preterm infants not only experience and respond to painful stimuli, may be more sensitive to pain, and that there are both short-term and long-term consequences to pain that continue into infancy and childhood.[127] Neonates exposed to repeated painful and noxious stimuli show different behavioral and physiologic responses to pain, may be less reactive to painful stimuli, and demonstrate more somatization as toddlers than infants not exposed to painful stimuli. At 8 to 10 years, children who were exposed to painful and noxious stimuli as infants rated medical pain significantly higher than psychosocial pain.[128] Furthermore, research has found repeated skin-breaking procedures in very preterm infants to have a relationship with poorer cognitive and motor function.[129]

Pain receptors appear initially around the mouth at 7 weeks' gestation and spread to the entire body. Ascending pain pathways in the peripheral nervous system and spinal cord are functional by 20 to 22 weeks' gestation.[125,130,131] The neuroanatomic, neurophysiologic, and neuroendocrine systems are developed enough to allow the perception of pain in preterm and term infants, and their physiologic and hormonal pain responses are similar or exaggerated compared with adults or older children.[125,126,128] Increased sensitivity to pain in preterm infants less than 36 weeks GA has been attributed to decreased levels of expression of dopamine, serotonin, and norepinephrine in the preterm spinal cord, which are important for pain modulation. Also, inhibitory

fibers from the periaqueductal gray area do not release neurotransmitters until 46 to 48 weeks postconceptual age (PCA). Repeated invasive procedures can produce hyperalgesia and allodynia (pain caused by a stimulus not typically associated with pain), leading to long-term changes in pain processing, postnatal growth, brain structure, and neurodevelopment.[130,132-136]

Hospitalized neonates experience frequent routine medical touch and handling by staff members, as opposed to contacts with family. Routine touch for the care of hospitalized infants consists of repositioning, temperature taking, diaper changes, palpation to reinforce taping or to check the status of intravenous lines and organ systems, etc. Infants in an NICU experience an average of 40 to 70 contacts, with some infants experiencing 100 contacts per 24-hour period.[137-140] While not all interventions are painful, these activities may be very stressful for preterm infants.[141] Hellerud & Storm[142] observed that diaper changes produced increased physiologic and behavioral changes. Over time, tactile events may become more stressful as preterm infants exhibit not only hperalgesia but also allodynia as a result of central sensitization. Environmental factors such as lighting and sound can also contribute to stress in the preterm infant.

Infants in the NICU are also subjected to repeated painful procedures and noxious stimuli, such as heel sticks, intravenous line placement, and suctioning of endotracheal tubes, which are performed on a routine basis in addition to frequent handling.[74,75,143] Cignacco[144] reported that preterm infants experience 10 to 15 painful procedures per day, up to 22 procedures per day in the first 2 weeks of life. Cameron et al.[145] found increased pain scores continued long after the painful procedure in preterm infants. The greater survival of extremely low birth weight (ELBW) infants makes these high-risk infants more susceptible to the effects of pain and stress due to longer periods of exposure.[146] Although the frequency of and response to acute painful procedures is recognized, there is little understanding about the chronic pain experienced from medical conditions associated with prematurity or an NICU stay such as necrotizing enterocolitis, intraventricular hemorrhage, or prolonged mechanical ventilation.[147] While painful and stressful interventions are part of the life-sustaining care experiences of babies in an NICU, they can have long-term effects on growth and development.[133,148,149] Strategies to minimize or prevent pain and stress should be an essential part of the infant's care plan.

THE PROBLEM OF PAIN ASSESSMENT Pain is described as "an unpleasant sensory and emotional experience associated with actual or potential tissue damage, or described in terms of such damage."[131] The gold standard of pain assessment in older children and adults is patient report of pain. Since babies are unable to verbalize their pain, comprehensive, valid, and reliable pain assessment in an NICU is complex and requires the identification of multiple responses, both physiologic and behavioral.[128,135,147,150] Vulnerability to pain is expressed by preterm infants through specific pain behaviors, physiologic changes, changes in cerebral blood flow, and cellular and molecular changes in pain processing pathways.[131] Physiologic responses to pain include increase or decrease in heart rate, increase or decrease in respiratory rate, increased blood pressure, increased intracranial pressure, decreased oxygen saturation, decreased peripheral and cerebral blood flow, skin color pallor or flushing, diaphoresis, and palmar sweating.[135,151] Behavioral signs including facial responses (eye squeeze, brow buldge, nasolabial narrowing), extension of arms and legs, and finger splay have been associated with pain in preterm infants.[146,152] Term and preterm babies respond differently to pain, a fact that adds to the difficulty with pain assessment in babies in an NICU. Preterm babies are less robust than full-term infants in expressing pain through crying or moving; therefore, GA is an important consideration when assessing pain in an infant.[135,150,153] Equipment and lines may further impede their ability to demonstrate movements associated with pain. Critically ill infants may mimic preterm infants in their incapacity to display vigorous pain responses; therefore, a lack of behavioral pain responses should not be interpreted as a lack of pain.[128,134,150] The Joint Commission on Accreditation of Healthcare Organizations (JCAHO) has termed pain assessment the "fifth vital sign," and the standard of care now requires routine assessment of neonatal pain utilizing a standardized assessment scale of neonatal pain[154] and appropriate interventions to reduce and alleviate pain (see Table 4.4 for commonly used methods of pain assessment in newborns). There are a wide variety of tools to assess pain in neonates; for example, Duhn and Medves[155] identified over 40 assessments in their 2004 review. The authors recommend that infant population, setting, and type of pain experienced should be taken into consideration along with the psychometric strength of the instrument when choosing a pain scale.[155]

Despite recommendations for pain assessment and management in newborns from organizations such as the AAP and JCAHO,[154] the understanding of the infant's capability to feel pain and strategies to manage pain are underemployed

in NICUs.[128,147,151,156,157] Carbajal et al.[156] reported that 40% to 90% of infants do not receive preventive or effective treatment for pain. Obstacles to implementation of nonpharmacologic and pharmacologic pain supports include health practitioners' concerns regarding side effects, toxicity, and physiologic dependence for pharmacologic agents, and lack of understanding of effectiveness of nonpharmacologic supports in pain reduction.[128,147,158] Nonpharmacologic interventions are strategies to relieve pain while promoting the infant's self-regulatory capacities.[157] Physical therapists working in the NICU need to be familiar with physiologic and behavioral assessment of pain in young infants, as well as with a variety of environmental and behavioral strategies to reduce pain. They also need to be vigilant in anticipating the potential for pain for babies in the NICU and to advocate for early and aggressive intervention to minimize pain for these patients.[26,106,146]

ENVIRONMENTAL AND BEHAVIORAL STRATEGIES FOR PAIN REDUCTION Nonpharmacologic interventions are the bases for pain management and should ideally be implemented consistently for any painful procedure or noxious touch in the NICU.[128,156] However, they should not substitute for pharmacologic therapy, which should be utilized in addition to nonpharmacologic pain supports for prolonged or moderate to severe pain in the infant. However, studies have shown that opioids are ineffective for procedural pain such as heel sticks[134,156] and nonpharmocologic strategies are recommended for these interventions.

Environmental strategies reduce pain indirectly by reducing the level of noxious stimuli present to the infant. Environmental strategies include dimming the lights or shading the eyes of the infant and reducing the noise around the infant's bed space by keeping pagers on vibrate mode, silencing alarms, shutting drawers and porthole doors softly, and talking in soft voices away from the bedside. Other environmental strategies include reducing the frequency of handling and painful procedures.[71] However, clustering of care activities has been shown to produce pain-like responses in

TABLE 4.4	Common Neonatal Pain Assessment Scales			
	CRIES	**Premature Infant Pain Profile (PIPP)**	**Neonatal Facial Coding Scale (NFCS)**	**Neonatal Infant Pain Scale (NIPS)**
Characteristics assessed	*C*rying	Gestational age	Brow bulge	Facial expression
	*R*equires additional O₂	Behavioral state	Eye squeeze	Cry
	*I*ncreased vital signs	Heart rate	Nasolabial furrow	Breathing patterns
	*E*xpression	O₂ saturation	Open lips	Arms
	*S*leeplessness	Brow bulge	Stretched mouth	Legs
		Eye squeeze	Lip purse	State of arousal
		Nasolabial furrow	Taut tongue	
			Chin quiver	
			Tongue protrusion	

From Anand KJS, International Evidence-Based Group for Neonatal Pain. Consensus statement for the prevention and management of pain in the newborn. *Arch Pediatr Adolesc Med.* 2001;155:173–180.

high-risk infants.[159,160] Neonatal therapists can assess infants' response to care activities and advocate for spacing out caregiving activities if determined to be more beneficial for the individual infant.[146]

Nonpharmacologic interventions include positioning via swaddling or facilitated tucking, (nonnutritive sucking) NNS, skin-to-skin holding (kangaroo care), and sucrose.[128,143,161] Facilitated tucking is a manual technique where a support person holds the baby's flexed limbs close to the baby's body during a noxious or painful procedure. Facilitated tucking has been demonstrated to minimize physiologic indices of pain, shorten cry, maintain sleep state, and reduce scores on the premature infant pain profile (PIPP) during heel stick, endotracheal suctioning, and routine caregiving.[72–76,162,163] Swaddling an infant can also provide the bodily containment important for pain relief in infants undergoing painful procedures.[74]

NNS will help reduce hospital stay and decrease fussing/crying and physiologic arousal during heel stick.[77–79,147,135,164] The practice of giving sucrose with or without NNS has been shown to decrease physiologic and behavioral pain indices as well as pain scores for babies undergoing heel stick or venipuncture and is considered safe and effective in reducing procedural pain.[144,165,166,167] Oral sucrose has its greatest analgesic effect when given intraorally 2 minutes prior to a procedure.[166–168] Studies have also shown that breast-feeding and NNS with breast milk to be effective nonpharmocologic pain management interventions for neonates.[169,170] Kangaroo care, or skin-to-skin, chest-to-chest holding, provides comforting multisensory stimulation (continual and full-body touch, warmth of parent's body, sound of the heartbeat, chest and respiratory movements, body odor, and voice) and is thought to trigger endogenous mechanisms resulting in an analgesic effect on neonates.[164] Studies of kangaroo care demonstrate marked reductions in crying, grimacing, and heart rate during heel sticks in newborn infants.[171] Physical therapists and the nursing and medical teams in the NICU should carefully watch the expression of stress and pain in the infant, as well as for opportunities to implement environmental and behavioral strategies to reduce neonatal pain and stress from noxious stimuli.

Vestibular System

The sensory end organs of the vestibular system, the three semicircular canals, and the otolith are housed inside the skull cavity (vestibule), which also contains the hearing sense organ, the cochlea. Both the hearing and the vestibular systems convert stimuli into electrical signals via the cilia. In the vestibular system, these signals are carried by the vestibular nerve to the brainstem and relayed to a variety of areas so that information regarding the baby's position in space can be interpreted, integrated, and used to guide movement and function.[126]

The vestibular system is one of the first to develop in utero, and the vestibular nerve is the first fiber tract to begin myelination at the end of the first trimester. By 20 weeks' gestation, this nerve has reached its full-size shape, and the other vestibular tracts have begun to myelinate.[126] The vestibular system is thought to be responsible for the fetus orienting to the head-down position prior to birth. The vestibular system is mature in the full-term newborn,[137] but modifications and growth in the synapses and dendrites of the vestibular pathways continue until puberty as the child learns to move and adapts to his or her changing body size and shape.[126]

The womb provides almost constant vestibular stimulation to the developing fetus, some contingent (fetal movement) and some noncontingent (maternal movements).[126,172] The preterm baby in an NICU experiences primarily immobilization and therefore reduced vestibular stimulation. The consequences of the constant vestibular stimulation a term baby experiences in utero and the lack of such with a preterm baby are unclear and there is little information to guide interventions with the vestibular system. Research on vestibular stimulation on the preterm infant is often carried out with other modes of stimulation, making it difficult to understand the effects of pure vestibular stimulation. Vestibular stimulation is known to enhance behavioral states; for example, slow rhythmic rocking is soothing and promotes quiet sleep, and fast arrhythmic vestibular stimulation increases activity and agitation.[9] Vestibular stimulation has not been demonstrated to affect feeding, weight gain, length of stay, or neurodevelopmental outcomes in hospitalized infants.[69] More research is needed in this area; however, gentle vestibular stimulation within the infant's tolerance levels and for a developmentally appropriate reason may be implemented in the NICU.[172]

Olfactory and Gustatory Development

Taste and smell are both chemical senses, initiated in response to specific molecules in the immediate environment and transmitted into electrical signals by neurons. Olfactory development begins at 5 weeks' gestation with the appearance of the nasal pit. At 8 weeks, the neurons in the olfactory bulb begin to develop and are mature by 20 weeks. By 11 weeks, the nostrils are replete with olfactory epithelia. The ability to smell begins at 28 weeks when the biochemical development of olfactory epithelia and neurons is completed.

Taste buds begin to mature at approximately 13 weeks when the fetus begins to suck and swallow. At term age, approximately 7000 taste buds are present over the perimeter of the tongue, soft palate, and upper throat.[126] Sucking and swallowing amniotic fluid stimulates the taste buds and influences their synaptic connections. The amniotic fluid is constantly changing, reflecting the mix of the maternal diet with the fetus' urination. The fetus experiences a variety of tastes and smells while in utero. Likewise, breast milk is flavored by maternal diet and the newborn is able to recognize his or her mother's breast milk, as its smell and taste are familiar to the infant. From 24 weeks until term, a fetus swallows approximately 1 L of amniotic fluid per day. Contrast this with the experiences of the preterm baby, who frequently has an orogastric tube and/or endotracheal tube in his or her mouth, tape on his or her face, and the taste of a rubber glove, medications, or vitamins in his or her mouth. In addition, the preterm infant does not get this constant swallowing practice, making the necessary coordination of sucking, swallowing, and breathing a challenge.[126]

Auditory System

By 24 weeks' gestation, the development of the cochlea and peripheral sensory end organs is complete, and the first blink/startle responses to vibroacoustic stimulation can be elicited. By 28 weeks, these responses are consistent; the hearing threshold is approximately 40 dB and decreases to 13.5 dB (approximating the adult levels) by 42 weeks PCA, demonstrating the continuing maturation of the auditory pathways. A preterm infant in the NICU is subjected to the noise of an NICU during the normal development and maturation of hearing. Exposure to this NICU noise may cause cochlear damage as well as cause sleep disturbances and disrupt the growth and development of the baby.[123,173] The bubbling of water inside a ventilator tubing or tapping on the outside of the incubator can result in noise that is 70 to 80 dB inside an incubator, whereas closing the porthole doors or the drawers under the incubator or dropping the head of the mattress can result in 90 to 120 dB noise.[173] Incubator covers reduce only the noise of objects striking the incubator. However, most noise in an incubator comes from the motor, drawer and door closures, and the infant's own crying.[174] Other common NICU sounds include alarms, overhead pages, beepers, telephones, traffic, and conversations. In one study, peak noise was in the 65- to 75-dB range, and most noise was due to human activity.[175] Normal conversation is typically in the 60-dB range, and whispering is between 20 and 30 dB.[173]

Contrast this with the sounds of pregnancy inside the womb (i.e., muffled maternal speech, maternal heart rate, and GI sounds), which are structured or patterned but not continuous or fixed. These sounds may also be contingent on maternal or fetal behavior and typically affect more than one sensory organ.[112] Background noise in the human uterus allows low frequencies of maternal speech to be discriminated. In utero, the maternal tissues attenuate sound frequencies greater than 250 Hz and thus shield the developing fetus. The sound environment of an NICU has levels of low- and high-frequency sound, and this may diminish the babies' exposure to maternal speech. The NICU provides a very different auditory sensory experience for the developing baby than the womb.

The AAP[173] recommends that noise levels in an NICU should not exceed 45 dB; in order to accomplish this, staff must be cooperative and NICU design and construction must support this. In addition to strategies to reduce noise from human or mechanical sources, new alternatives to the crowded and noisy state of current NICU designs have been suggested by Evans, Philbin,[176–178] and White.[179]

Visual System

Vision is the most complex human sense and the least mature at term birth. By 23 to 24 weeks' gestation, the major eye structures and the visual pathways are in place; however, the eyelids are fused, the optic media is cloudy, and there are remnants of embryonic tissue in the eye globe. A few immature photoreceptor cells occupy the retina, and retinal blood vessels in the posterior retina have begun to develop. From 24 weeks to term, the retina and visual cortex undergo extensive maturation and differentiation. At 24 to 28 weeks, the eyelids separate. However, the pupillary reflex is absent; the lid will tighten to bright light, but this fatigues easily. By 34 weeks, the pupillary reflex is present, and bright light causes lid closure without fatigue. Brief eye opening and fixation on a high-contrast form under low illumination may occur. Morante et al.[180] found that most 32-week gestation premature infants could perceive 1/2-inch stripes at 12 inches, and by 35 to 36 weeks most could perceive 1/4-inch stripes. At term, most infants could distinguish 1/8-inch stripes. Also, pattern preference matured from 34 weeks on as well. Unlike Saint-Anne Dargassies,[117] Morante et al.[180] found that former premature infants at 40 weeks did less well with visual acuity and pattern preference than term newborns. By 36 weeks, the infant will orient toward a soft light and demonstrate saccadic visual following horizontally and vertically. At term, infants see with acuity estimates of 20/400. They are farsighted with poor focusing for objects up close.[112]

Typically, visual maturation occurs in a dark womb, and does not require light exposure. However, the infants born prematurely are subjected to the harsh bright lighting of the NICU, which produces phototoxic effects in animals and can potentially impact brain development. Bilirubin lights to treat hyperbilirubinemia can produce light equivalent to greater than 10,000 foot-candles. Because of their visual immaturity, preterm infants should be shielded from ambient and supplementary light sources. Five foot-candles is desirable to encourage spontaneous eye opening. Although preterm infants will attend to black-and-white patterns, this can be stressful for them. Prolonged attention to black-and-white patterns has been associated with lower IQ in childhood. Visual stimulation may also interfere with typical auditory dominance, resulting in decreased attending to speech, and may disrupt the emergence of hand regard and visually directed reaching.[9,112,126]

Evolution of State Differentiation

True behavioral states in terms of a set of characteristic variables linked together may not be present in infants less than 36 to 37 weeks GA,[114,181] and preterm infants younger than 36 weeks do not possess a full capacity for control over states of arousal.[9] Brazelton and Nugent[182] define six states in their newborn assessment and pay close attention to the range, variety, and duration of the states a baby exhibits during an assessment (Table 4.5). Als[183] modifies these states for preterm infants, describing them as less well organized and less clearly defined than states a healthy term baby demonstrates. In preterm infants, sleep states predominate, and wakeful periods emerge for brief periods around 28 weeks and become more numerous at 30 weeks.[117] Preterm infant sleep states are disorganized with more motoric responses during sleep. Wakeful periods in preterm infants are brief and sporadic. The proportions of sleep and wake periods change as babies mature. Quiet alert times appear in preterm infants who are close to term age and have a degree of physiologic and motoric stability. Because the state system is foundational for attending and interacting, it is important

---

TABLE

4.5   State-Related Behaviors*

Sleep State	Behaviors
State 1A	Infant in deep sleep with obligatory regular breathing or breathing in synchrony with only the respirator; eyes closed; no eye movements under closed lids; quiet facial expression; no spontaneous activity; typically pale color.
State 1B	Infant in deep sleep with predominately modulated regular breathing; eyes closed; no eye movement under closed lids; relaxed facial expression; no spontaneous activity except isolated startles.
State 2A	Light sleep with eyes closed; rapid eye movements can be seen under closed lids; low-amplitude activity level with diffuse and disorganized movements; respirations are irregular and there are many sucking and mouthing movements, whimpers; facial, body, and extremity twitchings, much grimacing; the impression of a "noisy" state is given. Color is typically poor.
State 2B	Light sleep with eyes closed; rapid eye movements can be seen under closed lids; low activity level with movements and dampened startles; movements are likely to be of lower amplitude and more monitored than in state 1; infant responds to various internal stimuli with dampened startle. Respirations are more regular; mild sucking and mouthing movements can occur off and on; one or two whimpers may be observed, as well as infrequent sighs or smiles.

Transitional (Drowsy) States

State 3A	Drowsy or semidozing; eyes may be open or closed; eyelids fluttering or exaggerated blinking; if eyes are open, glassy veiled look; activity level variable with or without interspersed startles from time to time; diffuse movement; fussing and/or much discharge of vocalization, whimpers; facial grimace.
State 3B	Drowsy, same as above but with less discharge of vocalization, whimpers, facial grimace, etc.

Awake States†

State 4AL	Awake and quiet, minimal noisy activity, eyes half open or open but with glazed or dull look, giving the impression of little involvement and distance, or focused yet seeming to look through rather than at object or examiner, or the infant is clearly awake and reactive but has eyes closed intermittently.
State 4AH	Awake and quiet; minimal motor activity; eyes wide open, "hyperalert" or giving the impression of panic or fear; may appear to be hooked by the stimulus; seems to have difficulty in modulating or breaking the intensity of the fixation to the object or moving away from it.
State 4B	Alert with bright shiny animated facial expression; seems to focus attention on source of stimulation and appears to process information actively and with modulation; motor activity is at a minimum.

Active States

State 5A	Eyes may or may not be open, but infant is clearly aroused as is dictated by motor arousal, tonus, and distressed facial expression, grimacing, or other signs of discomfort. Fussing, if present, is diffuse or strained.
State 5B	Eyes may or may not be open but infant is clearly awake and aroused, with considerable, yet well-defined, motor activity. Infant may also be clearly fussing but not crying robustly.

Crying States

State 6A	Intense crying, as indicated by intense grimace and cry face, yet cry sound may be very strained or weak or absent; intensity of upset is greater than fussing.
State 6B	Rhythmic, intense, lusty crying that is robust, vigorous, and strong in sound.

*These are subgrouped into the states themselves and specific, typically attention-related behaviors. Various configurations of behaviors encompassing eye movements, eye opening and facial expressions, gross body movements, respirations, and tonus aspects are used in specific temporal relationships to one another to determine at what level of consciousness an infant is at a particular time. It is possible to make meaningful, systematic distinctions between dynamic transformations of various behavioral configurations that appear to correspond to varying states of availability and conscious responsiveness. The following spectrum of observable states is suggested: states labeled as A are "noisy," unclean, and diffuse; states labeled as B are clean, well-defined states.REF7. REF2.

†For 4A, two types of diffuse alertness are distinguished, 4 AL and 4 AH. L or H is marked instead of a check mark.REF8. REF3.

AA: Should the infant move into prolonged respiratory pause (e.g., beyond 8 seconds), AA should be marked. The infant has removed him- or herself from the state continuum.

More than one box per 2-minute time block can be marked, depending on the fluctuation and behavior the infant shows. Operationally, typically a 2- to 3-second duration of a behavioral configuration is necessary to be registered as a distinct state; however, even briefer excursions, especially into states 4 and 6, can be recorded reliably. Reprinted with permission from Als H. Reading the premature infant. In: Goldson E, ed. *Nurturing the Premature Infant: Developmental Intervention in the Neonatal Intensive Care nursery*. New York, NY: Oxford University Press; 1999:82–84.

to be familiar with and to assess the range and robustness of states available to an infant, as well as the ease of transition between states.[183]

▶ Medical foundations to guide therapy

Language of the NICU

The language of the NICU also reflects the crisis-driven nature of the intensive care required by these critically ill infants. Many complex procedures and diagnoses are referred to by acronyms, and the language can be intimidating for those who do not know what the terms mean. There is a list of commonly used abbreviations in Addendum A at the end of this chapter. In addition, a few key terms will be defined below.

GA refers to the length of time the baby was in the womb and is counted in weeks from the mother's last menstrual period to the baby's birth.[184] Term gestation is 37 to 41 and 6/7 weeks, and a baby born before 37 weeks is considered preterm. A baby born at 42 weeks or more is considered postterm.[185]

Correcting a baby's age is an important skill to understand and to teach to parents. The 40 weeks of gestation are so critical to development that it is unfair to ignore the time lost in utero when a preterm birth occurs. It is important that both the therapist and the family develop expectations for a baby on the basis of *corrected age* and not chronologic age. Chronologic age (CA) is defined as the age the baby is based upon his or her birthday. Corrected or adjusted age (AA) is defined as the age the baby is from his or her due date; a baby born at 28 weeks whose CA is 8 weeks would have an adjusted age of 36 weeks PCA (PCA = GA + CA or 28 weeks + 8 weeks). That same baby 4 weeks later would be considered 40 weeks PCA, or term. Once the baby has reached his term age, the number of weeks the baby missed in utero is subtracted from his CA, so that at 5 months CA, the baby's adjusted age is 3 months (6 months − 3 months [12 weeks (missed in utero) is 3 months early]). This age adjustment is important for assessing a former preterm infant's growth and development until 2 to 3 years as most catching up is completed by then.[186]

AGA, SGA, and LGA are acronyms for *appropriate for gestational age*, *small for gestational age*, and *large for gestational age*, respectively. These terms refer to the weight of the baby at birth. AGA refers to an infant whose weight at birth falls within the 10th and 90th percentiles for his or her age. A baby born 12 weeks early can be AGA, or a baby born at term can be AGA if his or her weight is within two standard deviations of the mean (10th to 90th percentiles) for babies born at that GA. A baby who is SGA has a weight that is *below the 10th percentile* (or below two standard deviations from the mean) for his or her age, and a baby who is LGA *weighs above the 90th percentile* (or above two standard deviations from the mean) for his or her age at birth

(Fig. 4.6). SGA infants can also be called IUGR, or *intrauterine growth restricted*. The etiology for this may be a chromosomal abnormality in the baby, congenital malformation, or congenital infection.[106] LGA may be due to large parents, maternal diabetes, or postmaturity (greater than 42 weeks' gestation), or the baby may have other genetic syndromes. Babies born LGA are at risk for birth trauma, especially brachial plexus injury or perinatal depression. They may also be more likely to have hyperinsulinism or polycythemia.[185]

Research correlating birth weight with outcome is common, and has led to additional acronyms.[9,185]

Acronyms Regarding Birth Weight		
NBW	Normal birth weight	2500 to 3999 g (5 lb 8 oz to 8 lb 13 oz)
LBW	Low birth weight	less than 2500 g (5 lb 8 oz)
MLBW	Moderately low birth weight	1500 to 2500 g (3 lb 5 oz to 5 lb 8 oz)
VLBW	Very low birth weight	less than 1500 g (3 lb 5 oz)
ELBW	Extremely low birth weight	less than 1000 g (2 lb 3 oz)
Micropreemies		less than 750 g (1 lb 10 oz)
Macrosomia		more than 4000 g (8 lb 13 oz)

The medical chart may describe the mother as a 32-year-old G5 P1223. G stands for gravida and P for para. These terms describe the number of maternal pregnancies and pregnancy outcomes, respectively. The mnemonic "Florida Power And Light" can be used to remember what the numbers following P mean. The first number stands for number of full-term births, the second for number of *p*reterm births, the third for number of *a*bortions (whether spontaneous or therapeutic), and the fourth for number of *l*iving children. In the case of G5 P1223, the mother had five pregnancies; one full-term infant, two preterm babies, two abortions, and a total of three living children. When only a single number follows the P, it represents the number of living children.

A scoring system to evaluate the physical condition of newborn infants after delivery was developed by Virginia Apgar[187] in 1953, and the name APGAR has evolved into an acronym for this scale. A is for *appearance*, P is for *pulse*, G is for *grimace*, A is for *activity*, and R is for *respiration* (Table 4.6). These scores are generally assigned for the first and fifth minute of life if the baby does not require extensive resuscitation. Should the score reflect apnea or bradycardia with an Apgar score of less than 6, resuscitation is begun. A score in the range of 3 to 4 indicates the need for bag and mask ventilation; a score of 5 to 7 requires blow-by oxygen; and a score of 8 to 10 is considered typical for term newborns, and the infant does not require resuscitation.[188] An example of an Apgar score as recorded in the medical history is 8[1]9[5]. The Apgar score after 1 minute indicates the infant's changing condition and whether resuscitative efforts are adequate or need to be increased. For infants who require extensive resuscitation, Apgar scores may be

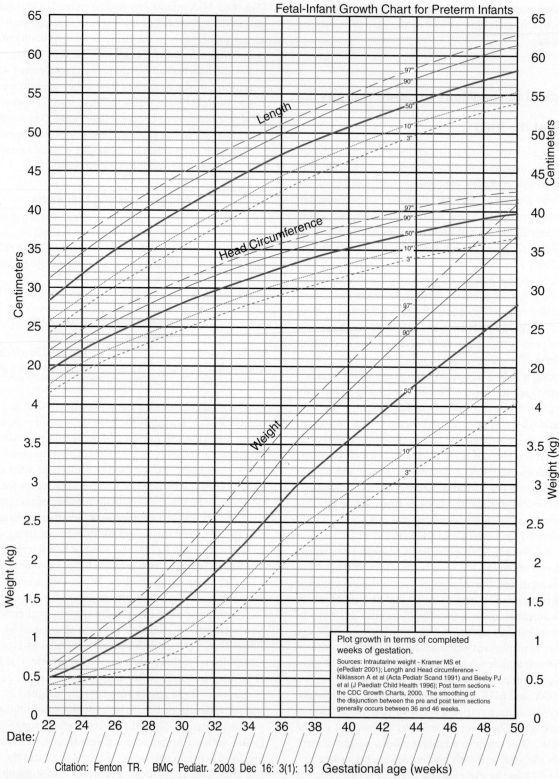

Fetal-Infant Growth Chart for Preterm Infants

Plot growth in terms of completed weeks of gestation.

Sources: Intrautarine weight - Kramer MS et (ePediatr 2001); Length and Head circumference - Niklasson A et al (Acta Pediatr Scand 1991) and Beeby PJ et al (J Paediatr Child Health 1996); Post term sections - the CDC Growth Charts, 2000. The smoothing of the disjunction between the pre and post term sections generally occurs between 36 and 46 weeks.

Date:

Citation: Fenton TR. BMC Pediatr. 2003 Dec 16: 3(1): 13   Gestational age (weeks)

FIGURE 4.6 Premature infant growth chart. (Adapted with permission from Babson SG, Benda GI. Growth graphs for the clinical assessment of varying gestational age. *J Pediatr.* 1976;89:814–820. Used with permission from Ross Products.)

TABLE
4.6 Apgar Score

Sign	Score		
	0	1	2
Heart rate	Absent	<100 bpm	100–140 bpm
Respiratory effort	Absent	Slow, shallow	Good, crying irregular
Reflex irritability	No response	Grimace	Cough or sneeze
Muscle tone	Flaccid	Some flexion	Active motion of extremities
Color	Blue	Pink body, blue extremities	All pink

From Apgar V. A proposal for a new method of evaluation of the newborn infant. *Anesth Analg.* 1953;32(4):260–267.

taken every 5 minutes until the score is greater than 6 (i.e., $0^1 0^5 2^{10} 5^{15} 6^{20}$).[188,189]

Environmental Aspects of Intensive Care: Equipment and Technologic Supports

The NICU is built around the highly technical supports that can sustain an infant's life. This technology has exploded in the latter half of the 20th century, allowing more babies to survive. This technology also influences the climate, culture, and workspace of the NICU, and can give the NICU a much cluttered, very cold, and metallic appearance. Equipment commonly found in the NICU to support a baby is listed in Table 4.7 (Figs. 4.7 and 4.8).

The primary objective of assisted ventilatory support in high-risk infants is to optimize the infant's cardiopulmonary status while minimizing trauma to the airways and lungs. This is done by working to improve gas exchange at the lowest amount of inspired oxygen concentration (FiO_2) and the lowest pressures and tidal volume. The individual infant's condition will dictate how ventilatory support is provided.[190]

TABLE
4.7 Common Medical Equipment in the NICU

Radiant warmer	Open bed with low, adjustable, Plexiglas side rails on a height-and-angle adjustable table with overhead heat source, temperature monitor, and procedure lights.
Isolette	Enclosed incubator. Clear plastic unit or box enclosing the mattress with heat and humidity control. Access to infant is through side port holes or side opening.
Open crib	Small bassinet-style bed or small metal crib without a heat source.
Bag and mask	Ventilating system consisting of self-inflating bag with reservoir, flow meter, pressure manometer connected to a mask that fits over the infant's nose and mouth.
Oxy hood	Plexiglas hood that fits over the infant's head and provides controlled oxygen and humidification.
Nasal cannula	Humidified gas delivered via flexible tubing with small prongs that fit into the nares.
HFNC	Humidified gas (may be highly humidified) delivered at high flow rates via a nasal cannula.
CPAP	Continuous or variable flow of warmed humidified gas at a set pressure generated by a CPAP unit or mechanical ventilator and delivered by mask.
Vapotherm	Highly humidified, high-flow system of delivering gas via nasal prongs.
Mechanical ventilation	
CMV	Conventional mechanical ventilation. Positive pressure ventilators are more commonly used in the NICU and are constant-flow, time-cycled, pressure-limited devices.
HFJV	High-frequency jet ventilation delivers short pulses of heated, pressurized gas directly into the upper airway through a jet injector.
HFOV	High-frequency oscillating ventilator has a piston pump or vibrating diaphragm that produces a sinusoidal pressure wave that is transmitted through the airways to the alveoli.
iNO	Nitric oxide is an inspired gas delivered in combination with mechanical ventilation that acts as a vasodilator and vascular smooth muscle relaxant.
ECMO	Extracorporeal membrane oxygenation is a heart-and-lung bypass procedure that involves draining venous blood, supplementing it with O_2, and removing CO_2 by means of a membrane oxygenator and returning the blood to either venous or arterial circulations.
Vital signs monitor	Unit that displays monitoring of HR, RR, BP, and SaO_2.
Pulse oximeter	Measures oxygen concentration in the peripheral circulation with a bandage-type light sensor attached to the infant's arm or leg, which provides a pulse-by-pulse readout of percent oxygen saturation on the screen of the monitor.

(continued)

TABLE 4.7	Common Medical Equipment in the NICU (Continued)
Transcutaneous oxygen and carbon dioxide monitor	Noninvasive method for monitoring concentrations of O_2 and CO_2 through the skin.
Infusion pumps	Electric infusion pump that controls the flow and rate of fluids, intralipids, and transpyloric feedings.
Phototherapy	Fiberoptic or overhead bank or spot lights or fiberoptic blanket used to reduce hyperbilirubinemia.
Gavage tube	Oral or nasogastric tube used for feeding directly into the stomach. Transpyloric tubes are used for infants who can not tolerate oral or nasal tubes, have severe GER, or are at risk for aspiration.
PIV	Peripheral intravenous line, which may be used for fluids, nutrition, or antibiotics.
CVL	Central venous line used for prolonged parental feeding or antibiotics, or to draw blood.
PICC	Percutaneous inserted central catheter. Long, flexible catheter inserted through a peripheral antecubital vein and threaded centrally to the superior vena cava. PICC lines are used for prolonged parental feeding or antibiotics or to draw blood.
UA	Umbilical arterial line inserted through the umbilical artery into the abdominal aorta and is used for the first 5–7 days of life for monitoring arterial blood gases, infusion of fluids, and continuous blood pressure monitoring.
UV	Umbilical venous line inserted into umbilical vein and is used for the first 7–14 days of life and as the initial venous access, to infuse vasopressors, and for exchange transfusions, monitoring of central venous pressure, and infusion of fluids.

Continuous positive airway pressure (CPAP) provides a continuous flow of warmed, humidified gas at a set pressure to maintain an elevated end-expiratory lung volume while the infant breathes spontaneously.[190–193] CPAP can be delivered by mask, nasal prongs, or less frequently through an endotracheal tube.

The gas mixture delivered via CPAP can be either continuous flow or variable flow. In continuous flow, the system provides a noninterrupted supply of gas to the infant.

Bubble or water-seal CPAP is a type of continuous flow. The blended gas is delivered to the infant after being heated and humidified. The distal end of the tubing is immersed in sterile water or acetic acid to a specific level to provide the desired amount of CPAP.[192] Bubble CPAP can generate vibrations in the infant's chest at frequencies similar to those used in HFV.[194] Variable flow nasal CPAP (NCPAP) uses injector jets to deliver gas at a constant pressure through nasal prongs into each naris. The flow is able to change so that the infant does not have to exhale against the CPAP.[192]

CPAP is used to prevent alveolar and airway collapse and to reduce the barotrauma caused by mechanical ventilation. Indications for CPAP include the early treatment of respiratory distress syndrome (RDS), moderately frequent apneic spells, recent extubation, weaning chronically ventilator-dependent infants, and early treatment to prevent atelectasis in premature infants with minimal respiratory distress and

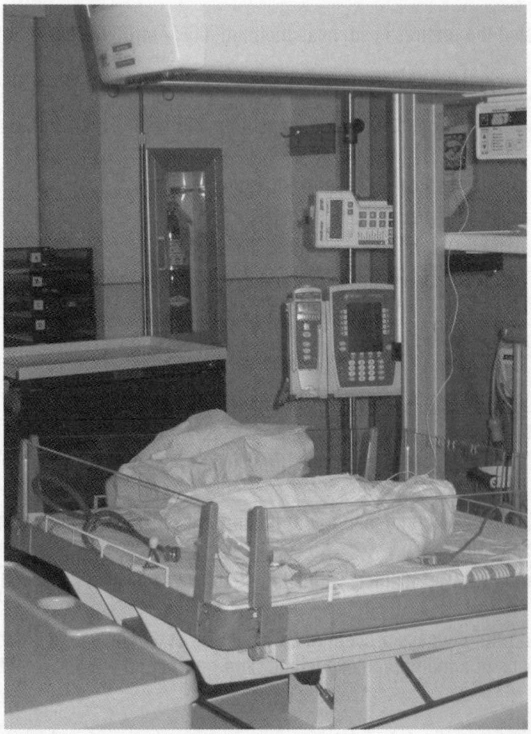

FIGURE 4.7 Radiant warmer bed set up for an admission to the NICU.

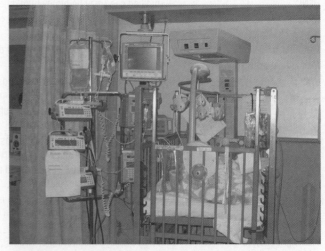

FIGURE 4.8 Crib with radiant warmer, infusion pumps, and monitor.

minimal need for supplemental oxygen. Negative aspects of NCPAP include gastric distension with high flows and excoriation or breakdown of the nasal septum when nasal prongs are used.[191–193]

The most common approach in the United States for treating respiratory failure in the NICU is with positive pressure ventilation.[195,196] The two types of positive-pressure mechanical ventilators are volume controlled or pressure limited. Volume-controlled ventilators deliver the same tidal volume of gas with each breath regardless of how much pressure is needed. While rarely used with newborn infants, volume ventilators designed specifically for neonates can be used in the presence of rapidly changing lung compliance.[190] Pressure-limited ventilators deliver gas until a preset limiting pressure is reached. The peak pressure delivered to the airway is constant, but the tidal volume with each breath is variable. Synchronized intermittent mandatory ventilation (SIMV), assist/control, and pressure support are adaptations of conventional pressure-limited ventilators and are also used in the NICU.

HFV utilizes extremely rapid ventilatory rates to deliver tidal volumes equal to or smaller than anatomic dead space. Continuous pressures are applied to maintain an elevated lung volume with superimposed tidal volumes provided at a rapid rate. The advantages of HFV over conventional ventilation are to provide adequate gas exchange at lower proximal airway pressures in lungs already damaged by barotrauma and volutrauma, and to preserve normal lung structure in the relatively uninjured lung.[197–200]

The three types of HFV used in the NICU are high-frequency positive pressure ventilation (HFPPV), high-frequency jet ventilation (HFJV), and high-frequency oscillating ventilation (HFOV).[197,200] HFPPV is produced by conventional ventilators or modified conventional ventilators set at a high rate.[199] HFJV delivers short pulses of heated, pressurized gas directly into the upper airway through a narrow cannula or jet injector.[199–201] The HFJV can maintain oxygenation and ventilation to wide ranges of lung compliance and patient size. HFOV has a piston pump or vibrating diaphragm that produces a sinusoidal pressure wave that is transmitted through the airways to the alveoli.[199,200] Small tidal volumes are superimposed over a constant airway pressure at a high respiratory rate.[202]

HFV is used primarily for infants who are failing conventional ventilation.[189,197] While outcome studies have been unable to demonstrate clear benefits of HFV over conventional mechanical ventilation (CMV), clinically HFV has been helpful in air leak syndromes, pulmonary interstitial emphysema (PIE), pre-/postcongenital diaphragmatic hernia (CDH) repair, meconium aspiration syndrome (MAS), and some forms of pulmonary hypoplasia.[199,200,202] HFV can also be used as a bridge to ECMO for infants with severe respiratory failure and may eliminate the need for ECMO in some infants.[199] Neonatal RDS is the most common lung disease treated with HFV in the NICU. HFJV has been shown to be most successful in the treatment of air leak syndromes,

while HFOV has shown better outcomes for infants with CDH, RDS, and persistent pulmonary hypertension of the newborn (PPHN).[199] The most serious side effect of HFV is an increase in long-term neurologic injury due to early periventricular leukomalacia (PVL) or severe intraventricular hemorrhage (IVH).[200] Some studies have found increased severe IVH in very premature infants treated with HFV versus CMV.[200,203] Other studies found no difference when other confounding variables were taken into consideration such as GA, type of delivery, early large PDA, and decreased superior vena cava blood flow (Fig. 4.9).[190,204]

Another form of ventilatory support that is beginning to be used with greater frequency in the NICU is high-flow nasal cannula. Studies have shown the high-flow nasal cannula to be as effective as NCPAP in providing positive end-distending pressure to the lungs of some infants with mild respiratory disease.

The advantage of nasal cannula over NCPAP is less irritation to the nasal spectrum.[205–207] The nasal cannula allows for greater comfort on the part of the infant and greater ease for the family or nurses to hold and care for the infant than mask or nasal prongs. Highly humidified high-flow nasal cannula is also used to provide higher flows of gas without the usual negative side effects of nasal cannula (i.e., drying, bleeding, or nasal septal breakdown due to the addition of high humidity).[208–212] Limited research is currently available regarding use of Vapotherm/highly humidified high-flow nasal cannula.

In December 1999, the U.S. Food and Drug Administration approved the use of inhaled nitric oxide (iNO) for the treatment of near-term and term infants with hypoxic respiratory failure. PPHN, RDS, aspiration syndromes, pneumonia, sepsis, and CDH are conditions that can cause hypoxic respiratory failure. The primary actions of nitric oxide are vasodilation and the relaxation of vascular smooth muscle, which increases blood flow to alveoli, improving oxygen and carbon dioxide exchange. Nitric oxide is a short-lived molecule, so that it affects the

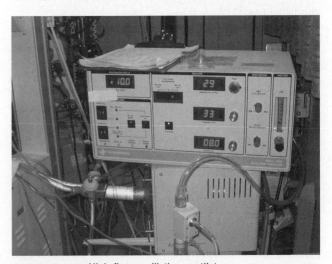

FIGURE 4.9 High-flow oscillating ventilator.

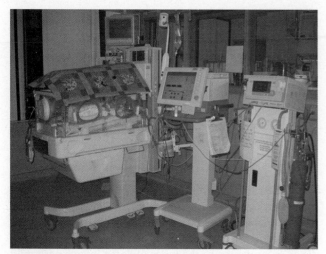

FIGURE 4.10 Conventional ventilator with nitric oxide tank.

pulmonary vascular smooth muscle without affecting systemic vasculature. Airway smooth muscle is also affected by nitric oxide, and the combined action of airway and vascular smooth muscle relaxation has been effective in the treatment of infants with ventilation–perfusion abnormalities (Fig. 4.10).[213,214]

Infants in the first week of life, who are 34 weeks' or greater GA with progressive hypoxic respiratory failure, meet the criteria for use of iNO as an adjunct to therapeutic interventions. The degree of illness and/or the modalities tried prior to the initiation of nitric oxide have not been clearly delineated. Nitric oxide is contraindicated for infants with congenital heart disease whose cardiopulmonary function depends on a right-to-left shunt or who have severe left heart failure.[215] While iNO has not been effective in treating infants with CDH, multicenter clinical trials have shown that iNO improves oxygenation and the outcome of near-term and term infants with hypoxic respiratory failure due to other conditions such as PPHN. Studies have also shown that iNO reduces the need for ECMO without increasing neurodevelopmental, behavioral, or medical abnormalities.[216–219]

The use of iNO in preterm infants is controversial, and there is no consensus on the timing for initiation, dosage, and length of time for iNO therapy with infants less than 34 weeks. In two studies of infants less than 32 weeks GA and body weight less than 1250 g requiring mechanical ventilation, those who received iNO demonstrated decreased incidence of bronchopulmonary dysplasia (BPD), less severe lung disease, decreased length of time requiring supplemental oxygen, decreased incidence of death, and no increased risk of brain injury. The benefits of iNO may be due to decreased airway resistance, which results in decreased need for supplemental oxygen, mechanical ventilation, and oxidative stress.[220,221]

ECMO is similar to a heart–lung bypass machine and provides rest and support for the baby's heart and lungs. ECMO is utilized with patients with cardiac and pulmonary

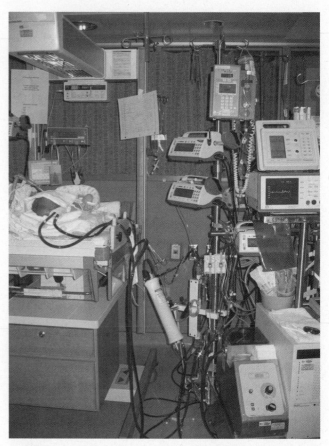

FIGURE 4.11 Infant on extracorporeal membrane oxygenation (ECMO).

dysfunction whose hypoxia is refractory to conventional therapies such as CMV and HFV. In the last decade, the use of surfactant, iNO, and HFV has replaced ECMO for patients with RDS, MAS, or pulmonary hypertension. ECMO continues to be implemented with patients with CDH, PPHN, and sepsis (Fig. 4.11).[222–226]

To initiate ECMO, catheters are inserted into the right side of the baby's neck and threaded to the heart in a process called "cannulation." The baby's unoxygenated blood drains via gravity (therefore, the baby's bed is elevated) through the catheters to the ECMO pump. The ECMO pump pushes the baby's blood through the ECMO circuit, where a membrane oxygenator acts as an artificial lung, removing carbon dioxide and providing oxygen to the blood. The oxygenated blood is then returned through the catheter into the baby. Babies receiving ECMO are sedated, paralyzed, and given pain medication. They are generally positioned in supine with their heads rotated to the left to allow access to the right neck vessels. These infants alsoare on large amounts of heparin, in order to prevent the blood from clotting when it contacts the catheters and the ECMO circuit.[227] The heparin, used to prevent clot formation, may cause the baby to bleed, the most significant complication of ECMO. Babies receive daily head ultrasounds to assess whether an intracranial hemorrhage (ICH) has occurred.

If present, ICH may be the reason to discontinue ECMO.[228] Babies who have received ECMO are at risk for developing atypical postures, tone, and movement patterns and require close developmental follow-up.[222-226] Babies post-ECMO, frequently demonstrate difficulties with oral feeding. Other neurodevelopmental morbidity includes seizures, hearing loss, hyperactivity, behavioral problems, CP, school failure, and developmental delay.[228] Although patients present with a variety of primary diagnoses requiring ECMO, after ECMO these patients demonstrate similar functional and neurodevelopmental outcomes, with the exception of babies with CDH. Patients with CDH have lower survival rates and higher morbidity, particularly in respiratory and digestive function, than other patients after ECMO.[224,229]

Medical Issues of Prematurity

Infants born prematurely are some of the most fragile in the NICU. They are at risk for multiple medical complications due to the immaturity of their body structures and organs, possible exposure to infections and teratogens, and the effects of the medical strategies and the technology required for minimizing illness and sustaining life. In this section, several of the more common medical conditions encountered in the NICU and the medical interventions used to treat them are discussed. The information provided is only a brief overview, and the reader is advised to consult neonatal medical texts, care manuals, and the original references cited at the end of this chapter for more in-depth detail.

Respiratory Distress Syndrome

RDS occurs as a result of pulmonary immaturity and inadequate pulmonary surfactant. Premature infants are predisposed to developing RDS owing to structural and physiologic immaturities, including poor alveolar capillary development, lack of type II alveolar cells, and insufficient production of surfactant. Surfactant is a substance produced by type II alveolar cells and lines the alveoli and small bronchioles. Decreased surfactant leads to respiratory failure due to increased alveolar surface tension, alveolar collapse, diffuse atelectasis, and decreased lung compliance. The preterm infant is further compromised by increased compliance of the chest wall due to the cartilaginous composition of the ribs, decreased type I fatigue-resistant muscle fibers in the diaphragm and intercostal muscles, and instability of neural control of breathing.[230-232]

Identification of RDS is made by prenatal risk factors, assessment of fetal lung immaturity, and postnatal clinical signs. Factors that affect lung maturity and increase predisposition for RDS include prematurity (GA less than 34 weeks), maternal diabetes (insulin appears to interfere with surfactant production), genetic factors (Caucasian race, siblings with history of RDS, and male gender), and thoracic malformations with lung hypoplasia.[233] Antenatal steroids are often used to accelerate lung maturity in the fetus and stimulate the production of surfactant. The National Institutes of Health (NIH)[234] in 2000 recommended that antenatal steroids be given to all pregnant women at 24 to 34 weeks' gestation who are at risk for preterm delivery within 7 days; however, there is a lack of consensus for the type of steroid used and the method of dosing. While a number of studies of antenatal steroid therapy have demonstrated increased surfactant production, decreased length of time on mechanical ventilation, and decreased incidence of IVH,[235] others have shown decreased fetal growth, increased mortality, and poor neurobehavioral outcomes.[236-240]

The diagnosis of RDS is based on history, clinical presentation, blood gas studies, and chest radiography. RDS can develop immediately after birth or within the first hours of life, depending on lung immaturity and perinatal events. Clinical signs of RDS include increased respiratory rate, expiratory grunting, sternal and intercostal retractions, nasal flaring, cyanosis, decreased air entry on auscultation, hypoxia, and hypercarbia. The lungs on chest radiography have a reticulogranular or "ground glass" appearance.[233]

Interventions for the premature infant with RDS depend on the severity of the disorder and include oxygen supplementation, assisted ventilation, and surfactant administration. Administration of prophylactic surfactant to intubated infants less than 30 weeks GA has been associated with initial improvement in respiratory status and a decrease in the incidence of RDS, pneumothorax, BPD, and IVH.[241] Current practice is moving away from prophylactic surfactant administration for infants who otherwise do not need to be intubated.[242-244] The Texas Neonatal Research Group[245] recommends that infants greater than or equal to 1250 g with mild to moderate RDS should not be electively intubated solely for the administration of surfactant.

Assisted mechanical ventilation has typically been the intervention of choice for infants with RDS. However, mechanical ventilation can cause airway damage in the form of barotrauma and volutrauma. HFV has been suggested as an alternative to conventional ventilation in order to decrease lung injury.[197-200] Positive pressure ventilation via nasal or nasal–pharyngeal prongs to address respiratory needs while limiting barotrauma from intubation has also been advocated.[194] Studies have shown the combination of early surfactant administration and NCPAP to improve the clinical course of RDS and decrease the need for mechanical ventilation.[246] According to Honrubia and Stark,[233] the use of CPAP with infants with RDS appears to prevent atelectasis, minimize lung injury, and preserve the functional properties of surfactant. The decision of which form of respiratory intervention to use is on the basis of the individual infant's clinical signs and chest radiography.

The prognosis of infants with RDS varies with the severity of the original lung involvement. Infants who do not require mechanical ventilation are more likely to have resolution of RDS with little or no long-term sequelae. However, the very immature ELBW infants may progress to chronic lung disease (CLD) or BPD owing to prolonged mechanical ventilation and the associated damage to the lungs. Infants with severe RDS are also at increased risk for ICH, retinopathy of prematurity (ROP), and necrotizing enterocolitis.[233]

In the acute stage of RDS, the infant is considered to be medically unstable and at risk for complications such as apnea, bradycardia, blood pressure variability, and IVH. Minimal environmental stimulation in the form of sound, light, and handling is often recommended to decrease infant stress. The physical therapist may perform observational evaluation of the infant using the NIDCAP to provide information to guide the delivery of care. Using this information, the therapist collaborates with the medical team and parents to develop a care plan to support overall growth and development. Suggestions for caregiving may include positioning, comfort, and protective measures.

Patent Ductus Arteriosus

The ductus arteriosus is a structure in the developing fetal heart that allows blood to bypass circulation to the lungs (Fig. 4.12). Since the fetus does not require the lungs to oxygenate blood, the flow from the right ventricle is shunted from the left pulmonary artery to the aorta. The ductus arteriosus typically closes within 10 to 15 hours after birth by constriction of medial smooth muscle. Anatomic closure is complete by 2 to 3 weeks of age, and factors that precipitate closure include oxygen, prostaglandin E_2 levels, and maturity.[247]

Oxygen appears to be the strongest stimulus for closure of the ductus.[248] The responsiveness of the smooth muscle to oxygen is related to GA. The premature infant has less of a response to oxygen in the environment due to decreased

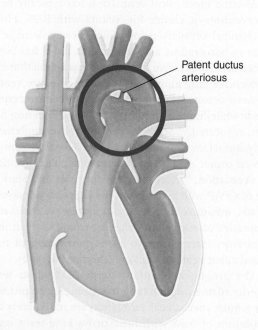

FIGURE 4.12 Illustration of PDA. (From the Anatomical Chart Company.)

sensitivity to oxygen-induced muscle contractions and high levels of prostaglandin E_2.[249] When the ductus fails to close, it is termed patent ductus arteriosus. In premature infants, the pulmonary vascular smooth muscle is not well developed, and there is a more rapid fall in pulmonary vascular resistance (PVR) than in full-term infants. The blood from the left side of the heart is shunted through the ductus to the right side, resulting in hypotension and poor perfusion, and can cause congestive heart failure from cardiovascular overload. Low mean blood pressure, metabolic acidosis, decreased urine output, and worsening jaundice due to poor organ perfusion are systemic consequences of left-to-right shunting.

The clinical signs of PDA include murmur, increased heart rate, and respiratory distress. Other symptoms associated with PDA are failure to gain weight, sepsis, congestive heart failure, and pulmonary edema. Diagnosis is made by chest radiography and echocardiography. Treatment is determined by the size of the PDA and clinical presentation. Initially, the PDA is treated with increased ventilatory support, fluid restriction, and diuretic therapy.[249] In symptomatic infants, indomethacin is used for nonsurgical PDA closure and is effective in approximately 80% of cases.[250,251] The use of indomethacin for prophylaxis in nonsymptomatic infants is controversial as side effects from the medication can occur. Symptomatic infants with a PDA that does not close after the second indomethacin treatment or infants for whom indomethacin is contraindicated undergo surgical ligation after echocardiographic documentation of the PDA.

Hyperbilirubinemia

Physiologic jaundice or hyperbilirubinemia is the accumulation of excessive amounts of bilirubin in the blood. Bilirubin is one of the breakdown products of hemoglobin from red blood cells. Hyperbilirubinemia commonly occurs in premature infants owing to immature hepatic function, increased hemolysis of red blood cells from birth injuries, and possible polycythemia (Fig. 4.13).

The primary concern in the treatment of hyperbilirubinemia is the prevention of kernicterus or the deposition of unconjugated bilirubin in the brain causing neuronal injury. The areas of the brain most commonly affected are the basal ganglia, cranial nerve nuclei, other brainstem nuclei, cerebellar nuclei, hippocampus, and anterior horn cells of the spinal cord.[252,253] Infants with chronic bilirubin encephalopathy can present with athetosis, partial or complete sensorineural hearing loss, limitation of upward gaze, dental dysplasia, and mild mental retardation. Kernicterus has become rare in preterm infants, but does still occur. Recent studies have shown an association between neurodevelopmental impairment and modest elevations in total serum bilirubin in ELBW infants.[254]

Premature infants are more susceptible to anoxia, hypercarbia, and sepsis, which open the blood–brain barrier, leading to deposition of bilirubin in neural tissue. Bilirubin

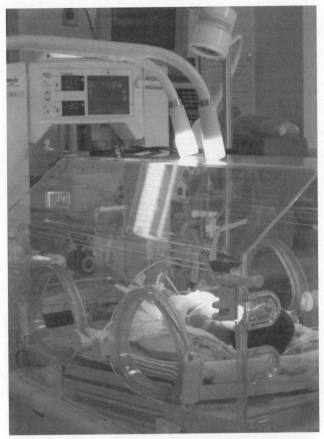

FIGURE 4.13 Phototherapy for hyperbilirubinemia. Note the motor stress signs demonstrated by the infant because of lack of boundaries.

toxicity in LBW infants may be more a reflection of their overall clinical status than a function of actual bilirubin levels.[252,255]

Hyperbilirubinemia is diagnosed by serum blood levels of bilirubin and treated with phototherapy or exchange transfusion. There are no consensus guidelines for treatment of infants less than 35 weeks GA with phototherapy or exchange transfusion. Generally, if phototherapy is not effective in reducing serum bilirubin levels or if there is a rapidly increasing bilirubin level, exchange transfusion is done.[256] Phototherapy is used to reduce serum bilirubin levels and is administered by fiberoptic blankets and bank or spot lights. Infants under phototherapy lights are naked except for a diaper and eye patches to protect their eyes in order to provide light exposure to the greatest surface area of skin. Exchange transfusion removes partially hemolyzed and antibody-coated red blood cells and replaces them with donor red blood cells lacking the sensitizing antigen. Bilirubin is removed from the plasma, and extravascular bilirubin binds to the albumin in the exchanged blood. The infant continues under phototherapy after the exchange transfusion.[252,257] Complications of exchange transfusion include hypocalcemia (which can cause cardiac arrhythmias), hypoglycemia, acid–base imbalance, hyperkalemia,

cardiovascular problems including perforation of vessels, embolization, vasospasm, thrombosis, infarction, volume overload and cardiac arrest, thrombocytopenia, infection, hemolysis, graft-versus-host disease, hypothermia, hyperthermia, and necrotizing enterocolitis.[252,253,257] There has been a dramatic decrease in the number of exchange transfusions performed on preterm infants due to more effective phototherapy and prevention of Rh hemolytic disease with Rh (D) immunoglobulin.[256]

Hyperbilirubinemia tends to decrease levels of arousal and activity. The infant may present with lethargy, hypotonia, and poor sucking ability.[256] Paludetto[257] and Mansi et al.[258] found that infants with moderate levels of hyperbilirubinemia demonstrate transient alterations in visual, auditory, social–interactive, and neuromotor capabilities. These findings are important considerations when performing a developmental assessment on an infant with increased levels of bilirubin.[9] Other issues to consider when assessing and planning treatment are the limitations imposed by phototherapy. When receiving phototherapy, the infant is generally positioned so that there is maximal exposure of body surfaces to the lights, limiting how some of the positioning devices and strategies are used for nesting and containment. The therapist will need to assist caregivers in creative ways to promote developmentally supportive postures and comfort without compromising the effectiveness of the phototherapy. Infants under the phototherapy lights need to have their eyes shielded to protect them from damage and to avoid any stress the bright lights may cause. Care must be taken to position eye shields so they are not too tight or too loose as either case can be extremely noxious to the sensitive, high-risk infant.

Gastroesophageal Reflux

Gastroesophageal Reflux (GER) has been defined as the involuntary movement of gastric contents in a retrograde fashion into the esophagus and above. The stomach contents that reflux can include acidic or alkaline gastric fluids, semisolids, feedings, enzymes, bile salts, or even air from crying or distended stomach that can move up to any portion of the esophagus, nasopharynx, oropharynx, or into the airway.[259–264]

All infants have some degree of reflux that is considered to be physiologic or asymptomatic if the infant is thriving well and the reflux resolves with maturation. Infants with asymptomatic GER may demonstrate small episodes of emesis; other infants may reswallow the refluxate without emesis. Infants with physiologic GER tend to grow and gain weight appropriately.[263] More frequent episodes of GER (pathologic GER) are referred to as GER disease or GERD and can burn the lining of the esophagus, resulting in inflammation, dysmotility, and pain.[265] These symptoms can lead to poor oral feeding patterns, oral aversion, and excessive crying due to pain. Blood loss in the emesis can lead to iron deficiency anemia. The result of severe reflux can be poor oral intake, poor weight gain, and malnutrition leading to failure to thrive.[266] Additional symptoms of GERD include apnea, aspiration, recurrent pneumonia, CLD, or larger airway inflammation.[267]

The most common mechanism of GER is relaxation of the lower esophageal sphincter (LES).[260] In addition, premature infants have shorter esophageal length and intraabdominal LES as well as smaller stomach capacity.[268,269] Risk factors that have been identified for neonatal GER include prematurity, birth asphyxia, perinatal stress, neonatal stress, delayed gastric emptying, congenital anomalies of the upper GI tract, acquired problems of the upper intestinal tract, diaphragmatic defects, respiratory disease, neurodevelopmental delays, ECMO, abdominal surgery, and medications. Acidic fluids can cause esophageal inflammation and further aggravate reflux. Higher risk for GER is associated with premature, stressed infants as well as those with CLD and congenital anomalies. Tone of the abdominal wall muscles, diaphragmatic activity, esophageal dysmotility, LES tone, and the physiologic immaturity of digestive function may be related to the increased incidence in these neonates.[264] Studies have demonstrated increased episodes of reflux with the presence of a nasogastric tube as it is an irritant and maintains the patency of the LES.[270–272]

The relationship between apnea, bradycardia and GER is controversial. Apnea and bradycardia occur frequently in preterm infants during and after feeding when GER is also frequently observed.[270] These apnea and bradycardia events may be related to GER owing to refluxate moving up into the esophagus, blocking the airway and causing obstructive apnea and subsequent bradycardia. Another proposed mechanism of apnea and bradycardia is due to the laryngeal reflex mechanism and laryngospasm.[273] However, research studies have not demonstrated a temporal relationship between GER events and apnea or bradycardia.[270,274,275] DiFiore[274] et al. suggested that apnea and GER may be observed to occur together owing to common risk factors.

Diagnosis of GER in neonates is by history, clinical evaluation, and studies including esophageal pH probe, esophogram, fluoroscopy or upper GI series, gastric scintography or milk scan, esophageal manometry, and endoscopy. History and clinical evaluation are important to rule out other conditions.[276] It is important to also identify whether the reflux is physiologic or pathologic, factors that make reflux worse, the mechanism of reflux, and the presence of complications caused by the reflux.

Nonpharmocologic management of GER in infancy often includes altering the type and delivery of feedings, positioning, and elevation of the head of the bed. Changes in the timing, volume, composition, and viscosity of feedings may assist in decreasing GER. The method of feeding, continuous versus bolus and feeding below the stomach, can also reduce the frequency of regurgitation. Continuous jejunal or duodenal feeding also reduces the risk of aspiration. However, there is also the risk of increased GER events due to use of chronic nasogastric or nasojejunal feeding tubes.[270]

Positioning the infant in supine, right side-lying, and infant seats has been associated with exacerbation of reflux. Prone, elevation of the head of the bed to 30 degrees, and left side-lying have been shown to decrease episodes of reflux.[276–279] Omari et al.[280] found that in healthy preterm infants, right side-lying is associated with increased transient LES relaxation and increased GER while at the same time increasing gastric emptying. Decreased gastric residuals have been reported in prone and right side-lying as compared with supine and left side-lying.[281,282] Chen[281] et al. suggested that preterm infants be positioned prone for the first 30 minutes postprandial and then change position to supine on the basis of behavioral cues. Van Wikk[283] et al. recommended repositioning from prone to left lateral position after first postprandial hour to decrease reflux. As both prone and lateral positioning have been associated with sudden infant death syndrome (SIDS), these positions are utilized with infants who receive cardiorespiratory monitoring.

Pharmacologic therapy is often initiated in the treatment of infants with GERD. The medications most often prescribed are antacids, histamine-2 receptor agonists, proton pump inhibitors, and prokinetics. These agents are used to neutralize or suppress acid and to promote gastric and/or esophageal motility.[284,285]

Surgery for pathologic GER may be considered for infants who have failed other management of GER and those with pulmonary symptoms from aspiration.[285] The most common antireflux surgical procedure is a fundoplication.[286] Partial or complete wrapping of the upper stomach or fundus around the esophagus is done to create a valve mechanism decreasing retrograde movement of stomach contents and promoting gastric emptying. Fundoplication is often performed in conjunction with feeding gastrostomy for infants requiring long-term tube feedings.[287]

Infants with GER and associated esophagitis may demonstrate pain behaviors that impact behavioral state organization and their ability to participate in activities with family and caregivers. Motor patterns observed may be of increased extension or arching of the head and trunk. Increased muscle tone may be noted in the extremities. Although the medical issues of GER need to be addressed primarily, the therapist in the NICU may be called upon to assist with positioning to minimize reflux and promote comfort. Ongoing neurodevelopmental assessments are required to determine the effect of reflux on behavior and how to adapt interventions to promote appropriate developmental competencies.

Necrotizing Enterocolitis

With an incidence of 1 to 3 per 1000 live births, necrotizing enterocolitis or NEC is one of the most common GI emergencies in the newborn infant.[288,289] Almost all NEC cases develop in preterm infants who have received enteral feedings,[290–292] and approximately 1% to 7.7% of NICU admissions are due to NEC.[288,289] NEC results from ischemic necrosis of the intestinal mucosa, resulting in intestinal infarction. While a portion of the terminal ilium and colon are affected in the majority of cases, NEC can affect the entire GI tract in severe cases.[288,290,293,294] Preterm infants are at the highest risk for NEC, and the incidence of NEC is inversely related to GA and birth weight.[288,295–297] Only 13% of NEC cases are reported in term infants and these babies typically have an underlying condition predisposing them to the disease, such as congenital heart disease, respiratory disease, sepsis, seizures, perinatal asphyxia, hypoglycemia, or intrauterine growth retardation.[288–301]

The etiology and pathogenesis of NEC remain unclear; it seems to be the result of multiple factors in a vulnerable baby. Prematurity and milk feeding are established risk factors in epidemiologic studies of NEC, although microbial bowel overgrowth, circulatory instability of the GI tract, and medications increasing intestinal mucosal injury or bacterial overgrowth are additional risk factors.[290,302–305]

NEC causes acute illness in the short term and is associated with long-term neurodevelopmental impairments in survivors, including CP, visual deficits, and intellectual challenges.[290,306] Male and female newborns are equally affected.[288,307] Although early detection and aggressive management has improved outcomes of survivors, overall mortality rates of 15% to 30% have been reported in the literature.[288,303,308] Mortality rates for babies with NEC are inversely related to birth weight and are higher for babies who require surgery.[288,308–313]

A baby developing NEC will present with both systemic signs and abdominal signs. Systemic signs include apnea, respiratory failure, lethargy, poor feeding, temperature instability, and hypotension. Abdominal signs include changes in feeding tolerance such as abdominal distension, tenderness, gastric residuals, vomiting of bile and/or blood, and/or bloody stools.[288,314–319] As NEC progresses, the infant may develop intestinal hemorrhage, gangrene, submucosal gas, and in some cases perforation of the intestines, sepsis, and shock.

The most important factor in determining outcome appears to be early diagnosis and treatment. Diagnosis is made by physical examination, and can be confirmed by abdominal X-ray with the presence of pneumotosis intestinalis (bubbles of gas observed in the intestinal wall); however, there is evidence to suggest that radiologic findings can vary by GA and may not be helpful in preterm infants.[288] Medical treatment is typically initiated in the absence of radiologic confirmation if clinical suspicion is high. The most commonly used uniform criteria for defining NEC is Bell's staging criteria originally published in 1978, and is based on systemic, intestinal, and radiographic findings; Bell's staging criteria has been modified to describe mildly and moderately ill babies in each of the three categories outlined below[309]:

- Stage I: Suspected NEC; infant demonstrates nonspecific systemic signs (temperature instability, apnea, and lethargy); abdominal signs such as abdominal distension, gastric residuals, emesis, and heme-positive stools; radiographic findings are normal or show mild bowel dilation.
- Stage II: Proven NEC; infant demonstrates symptoms of stage I plus absent bowel sounds and pneumotosis on abdominal radiography.
- Stage III: Advanced NEC; critically ill infant displaying, in addition to symptoms of stages I and II, hypotension, bradycardia, severe apnea, abdominal tenderness, acidosis, neutropenia, and disseminated intravascular coagulation. The infant may or may not show findings consistent with bowel perforation on abdominal radiography.[288,293,318,320–322]

Medical management is begun immediately when NEC is suspected and includes supportive care, such as bowel rest, discontinuation of enteral feeds, gastric suction to decompress the bowel, total parental nutrition, fluid replacement, antibiotics, close monitoring of laboratory values and GI tract (the latter by abdominal X-ray or ultrasound), and mechanical ventilation, if needed, to support the infant. Typically, abdominal radiographs are taken every 6 to 8 hours to detect progression of intestinal obstruction or possible perforation.

When NEC has been proven by changes on radiography, a pediatric surgeon is consulted to provide recommendations regarding the necessity for and timing of surgery. The goal of surgery is to conserve bowel length while not jeopardizing the baby. Surgical procedures include exploratory laparotomy and resection of necrotic bowel or primary peritoneal drainage (PPD). There is no hard evidence to recommend one procedure over the other, although PPD can be performed at the bedside under local anesthesia, will not require a reanastomosis surgery, and therefore may be preferred. Laparotomy typically entails resecting the involved portion of bowel, placing an ostomy and mucous fistula; less typically, if the affected bowel is short enough, the affected portion of the bowel can be resected and a primary anastomosis performed[304,320,290,323–329] (Fig. 4.14).

Complications of NEC include sepsis, meningitis, abscess, hypotension, shock, respiratory failure, and disseminated intravascular coagulation acutely and in the long term intestinal narrowing (stricture formation) and short bowel syndrome. Strictures requiring surgical resection are reported to occur in 9% to 36% of babies with NEC, while short bowel syndrome is reported to occur in 9% of infants who have received surgery for NEC. Short bowel syndrome results in chronic intestinal malabsorption and dependence on total parental nutrition. Babies with short bowel syndrome are at risk for sepsis, cholestasis, and liver failure, and may require eventual intestinal and hepatic organ transplantation.[304,321,330–332] Babies with NEC can endure long hospitalizations to manage these complications.

A spontaneous and isolated intestinal perforation in the newborn can also occur and needs to be differentiated from NEC. Spontaneous isolated intestinal perforations usually

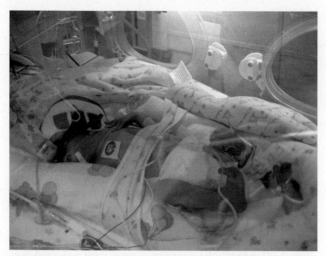

FIGURE 4.14 Infant with necrotizing enterocolitis with ostomy.

occur in preterm infants weighing less than 1500 g at birth. The perforation typically happens at the terminal ileum but can also occur in the jejunum or colon in the first 10 days of life. Risk factors for this include chorioamnionitis, maternal exposure to antibiotics before or at delivery,[333,334] and early administration of glucocorticoids.[333,334-337] Unlike NEC, a spontaneous intestinal perforation has an area of focal hemorrhagic necrosis with normal appearing bowel proximal and distal to the perforation and can be differentiated from NEC by presentation (hypotension and abdominal distension in the first 10 days of life with bluish discoloration of abdominal wall, radiographs showing pneumoperitoneum in the absence of pneumatosis intestinalis, and portal venous air). Initial management is similar to supportive care for NEC. Surgery is required, and like NEC can be either an exploratory laparotomy with bowel resection or PPD. There are no randomized controlled trials (RCTs) to recommend one procedure over another; however, babies receiving PPD are less likely to need an exploratory laparotomy. The drain is left in till drainage ceases; patency of the GI tract can be confirmed via a contrast study, or feeding can be started after bowel function has returned.[333,338-342]

The incidence of problems with growth and neurodevelopmental outcome of infants with NEC has been reported in comparison studies with other VLBW infants.[306,320,321,330,343] No growth or neurodevelopmental differences have been found in infants treated medically for NEC; however, in the population of infants treated surgically for NEC, significant differences in growth and neurodevelopmental functioning have been reported.[288,344,345] Infants with stages II and III NEC are reported to have lower head circumference and body length at 12 months and lower weight at 12 to 20 months than age-matched peers without NEC.[343] Neurodevelopmental outcome assessments performed on VLBW infants with stages II and III NEC and age-matched infants without NEC at 12 and 20 months corrected age demonstrate significantly lower general developmental quotients in infants with NEC at both 12 and 20 months. There is a higher incidence of

severe psychomotor retardation in infants with stage III NEC and multiple organ involvement.[343,309] Neurodevelopmental outcome may be better for babies with isolated perforation compared with NEC; however, the former babies appear to have a greater risk of developing ROP and PVL than infants without spontaneous perforation.[333,346-348]

Infants in the acute stages of NEC are critically ill and require constant monitoring by physicians and nurses. Therapists, more than any other professional on the NICU, are continually thinking how the present moment will affect the baby's current and future development. Therapists can advocate for the protection of the infant during the acute illness by minimizing environmental stimulation and handling, as well as careful attention to positioning with extra support for limbs with arterial or venous lines. The therapist should work in coordination with the medical team and family to assess the infant for signs of stress and comfort. Using this information, recommendations for individualized care can be made. As these infants are at risk for significant developmental delays, it is important that developmental intervention and developmental follow-up continue as their medical status improves and after discharge.

Germinal Matrix-Intraventricular Hemorrhage

GM-IVH is the most common type of brain lesion found in premature infants, occurring most frequently in infants less than 1500 g and at less than 32 weeks' gestation. The incidence of GM-IVH is inversely related to GA with the extremely premature being at greatest risk.[349-358] The hemorrhage typically originates in the subependymal layer of the germinal matrix and extends into the intraventricular space between the lateral ventricles (Fig. 4.15). During fetal development, this is the site of neuronal proliferation as neuroblasts divide and migrate to the cerebral parenchyma. The neuronal proliferation is complete by 20 weeks, while glial cell proliferation continues until approximately 32 weeks' gestation. The matrix decreases in size from 33 to 34 weeks and nearly complete involution occurs by 36 weeks' gestation.[349-351,358,359] These developmental changes in the brain influence the area and extent of the hemorrhage in the neonate.

A fragile and primitive capillary network supplies blood to this very metabolically active area. It is within this capillary network that periventricular hemorrhage–intraventricular hemorrhage (PVH-IVH) occurs. IVH is thought to be due to hypoxia and/or capillary bleeding resulting from the loss of cerebral autoregulation and an abrupt alteration in blood flow.[349,350,358,360,361] The alteration of cerebral circulation from autoregulation to pressure-passive circulation has been shown to be an important factor in the development of PVH-IVH. Hemorrhage can occur when the pressure-passive circulating pattern is compromised by fluctuations in cerebral blood flow and pressure. Factors associated with the loss of autoregulation are younger GA, ELBW, birth events, asynchrony of spontaneous and mechanical breaths, pneumothorax, rapid volume expansion, seizures, changes

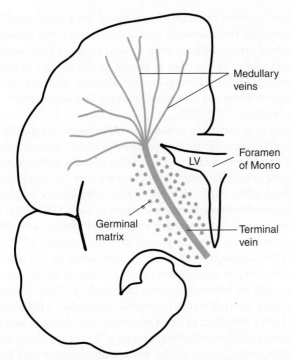

FIGURE 4.15 Diagram of the germinal matrix and the venous drainage of cerebral white matter. *LV,* lateral ventricular. (Reprinted with permission from Volpe JJ. *Neurology of the Newborn.* 4th ed. Philadelphia, PA: Saunders; 2001:432.)

in pH, $PaCO_2$, PaO_2, metabolic imbalances, tracheal suctioning, and noxious procedures of caregiving.[349,350,358,362–368]

IVHs are diagnosed by cranial ultrasound and classified according to severity.[351,358,369] A four-level grading system was developed by Papile et al.[357] and is still used by many neonatologists, neurologists, and radiologists. Volpe developed a different grading system in 1995 on the basis of neuropathologic and imaging studies. This scale uses three levels to grade IVHs. Grade I is a germinal matrix hemorrhage with no or minimal IVH. Grade II is an IVH occupying 10% to 15% of the intraventricular area without distension of the ventricles. Grade III is an IVH occupying greater than 50% of ventricular area and usually distends the lateral ventricle (Table 4.8).[349,350]

TABLE 4.8	Grading of Germinal Matrix–Intraventricular Hemorrhage (GM-IVH)
Grade	**Characteristic**
I	GMH with absent or minimal IVH
II	IVH occupying 10%–15% of the intraventricular area
III	IVH occupying >50% of ventricular area with ventricular distension
Periventricular hemorrhagic infarction	Intraparenchymal venous hemorrhage

Adapted with permission from Volpe JJ. *Neurology of the Newborn.* 4th ed. Philadelphia, PA: Saunders; 2001.

The neuropathologic complications of IVH include germinal matrix destruction, periventricular hemorrhagic infarction (PHI), and posthemorrhagic ventricular dilation (PVD).[349,350,355,361] PVL is frequently seen in infants with IVH, but is not caused by the hemorrhage itself.[349,355,358,370] Germinal matrix destruction and destruction of glial precursor cells is the result of germinal matrix hemorrhage. Destruction of glial precursor cells may negatively influence future development. Neurodevelopmental outcomes for infants with IVH are related to the severity of the hemorrhage. Vohr et al.[361] found that the LBW infants with IVH were more likely to develop CP. Spastic diplegic CP is most commonly associated with IVH due to the anatomic location of the corticospinal tracts.[350,359,361]

PHI was previously considered to be an extension of a large parenchymal hemorrhage or what Papile described as grade IV IVH. Neuropathologic and ultrasound studies have shown that the lesion represents a hemorrhagic venous infarction.[350,361,371] PHIs are generally large unilateral or asymmetric lesions dorsolateral to the lateral ventricle. This lesion is thought to be caused by obstruction of the terminal vein by a large IVH.[349,350,372] PHI generally occurs on the side of the larger IVH, and there is generally markedly decreased or absent flow in the terminal vein on that side. Studies have also described the lesion in the distribution of the medullary veins that drain into the terminal vein. Necrosis in this area can develop over time into a single large porencephalic cyst.[349] In the neonatal period, PHI is highly associated with an increased mortality rate as compared with IVH alone. Developmental outcomes associated with PHI are spastic hemiparesis, asymmetric quadriparesis, and cognitive deficits. The lower and upper extremities are equally affected in children with a history of PHI. Lesions due to extensive PHI cause more severe cognitive as well as motor deficits.[350,361]

PVD may occur days to weeks after the original IVH. The progressive ventricular dilation is due to a process that prevents the resorption of cerebrospinal fluid (CSF) and/or obstruction of CSF drainage due to a particulate clot. The injury to the brain from PVD is most likely due to hypoxia–ischemia and distension of the ventricle into the surrounding white matter, which may be more susceptible to additional injury after the effects of the initial hemorrhage.[350] The result of PVD is typically a bilateral cerebral white matter injury.[373] As there is a high incidence of arrest in the progression of ventriculomegaly without intervention, PVD is initially managed with close surveillance of ventricular size, head circumference, and clinical condition. Persistent slow ventricular dilation is treated with serial lumbar punctures to remove large volumes of CSF. Medications such as acetazolamide and furosemide can be used to decrease CSF production.[350,361] Rapidly progressive ventricular dilation with moderate to severe dilation, progressive head growth, and increasing intracranial pressure is managed initially with serial lumbar punctures followed by ventricular drainage of CSF with an external ventricular catheter or tunneled ventricular catheter that is connected to a subcutaneous reservoir.[350,361] Ventricular drainage is generally a temporary measure until a ventriculoperitoneal shunt can be placed. This type of shunt diverts CSF from the lateral ventricles into the peritoneal cavity.[350]

PVD occurs at a higher incidence in the extremely premature infant with ELBW as this is the population that is at greater risk for more severe IVH. With each additional week of gestation, the occurrence of PVD decreases. There is an increase in the incidence of PVD with each increase in the grade of IVH.[374] Murphy et al. found that the grade of IVH and need for inotropic support, such as dopamine or dobutamine, were significantly related to PVD requiring surgical intervention. PVD has been associated with neuromotor impairments and pronounced disability.[375–378] Krishnamoorthy et al.[369] demonstrated in their study that ventriculomegaly is an important antecedent of neuromotor sequelae and children with ventriculomegaly had a five times greater risk of developing CP independent of the grade of IVH.

While the incidence of IVH and PHI has decreased in recent years due to improvements in prenatal and postnatal preventative care, these lesions are still major factors for neurodevelopmental disability in ELBW infants.[350,355,374,379–382] The primary goal of prenatal management is to prevent or delay premature birth. Other strategies focus on providing support during labor and delivery, resuscitation, and plan for neonatal care. Since RDS is highly associated with IVH and PHI, treatments to decrease RDS such as the administration of prenatal steroids are utilized. Postnatal treatment focuses on preventing hypoxia or fluctuations in systemic and blood cerebral pressure. In addition to providing optimal respiratory and medical support, the principles of individualized developmentally supportive care are instituted to minimize stress during caregiving, decrease the potential for loss of physiologic stability, and decrease the risk of IVH.[56,360,383,384]

Periventricular Leukomalacia

PVL refers to specific areas of white matter necrosis adjacent to the external angles of the lateral ventricles. These areas involve the frontal horn and body, and optic and acoustic radiations. The incidence of PVL occurs most prominently in infants of less than 32 weeks' gestation who have survived more than a few days of postnatal life and have cardiorespiratory compromise.[349,350,385,386] Premature infants of younger GAs are at the greatest risk for white matter injury since these areas are poorly vascularized in the immature brain and contain precursors for oligodendrocytes, which are extremely sensitive to ischemia and infection.[349,350,359,385–387]

Focal periventricular necrosis and more diffuse white matter cerebral injury are the pathologic features of PVL. Focal necrosis is related to severe ischemia and occurs most often in infants at greater than 26 weeks' gestation.[349,350,372,386] The two main sites of focal injury are near the trigone of the lateral ventricles and the border

zones between the terminal arbors of the middle cerebral artery and the posterior cerebral artery or the anterior cerebral artery. Diffuse white matter injury is most apparent in infants at less than 26 weeks' gestation who develop atrophy, ventriculomegaly, and cortical underdevelopment with loss of oligodendrocytes and impairment in myelination.[349,350,372,386]

Areas of increased echodensity detected by cranial ultrasound are generally the first evidence of PVL. These echodensities represent areas of focal cellular necrosis due to axonal degeneration. Although echodensities may be transient or radiographic "flares" in some infants, other infants will demonstrate the characteristic evolution of focal PVL with the formation of cavitations that evolve into multiple cysts. This process occurs over the course of 1 to 3 weeks,[349,350,360,386] and the diagnosis of PVL will be dependent on the timing and number of cranial ultrasounds performed on the infant. More diffuse lesions less commonly undergo cystic changes and may go undetected by cranial ultrasound. MRI allows for better definition of brain structures and has been used to document diffuse white matter injury.[372]

The pathogenesis of the white matter destruction seen in PVL has been attributed to the interrelated factors associated with immature circulation and vascular structures of the preterm infant, impaired cerebral autoregulation, and the intrinsic vulnerability of the immature cerebral white matter neuroglia to ischemia–reperfusion.[349,350,370,372,386,388,389] Perinatal infection and the inflammatory response, including the release of proinflammatory cytokines, have also been shown to play an important role in the pathogenesis of PVL.[359,372,386,389–393] The effect of medications and other therapies used to treat complications of prematurity has been implicated in the pathogenesis of white matter injury.[394]

There is a strong association with mortality and long-term morbidity in infants with PVL. Death in infants with PVL in the neonatal period is usually attributed to the original insult, whether hypoxic, hemorrhagic, or infectious, rather than from PVL. Infants with PVL who survive the neonatal period are at high risk for neurodevelopment problems that affect motor, cognitive, and visual function.[268,378,382,386,391,392,395] Spastic diplegia, with or without hydrocephalus, is the most prominent long-term sequela of PVL. Han et al.[382] found that the presence of PVL was the "strongest and most independent risk factor" for the development of CP. The clinical presentation is one of motor disturbance in the lower extremities greater than the upper extremities owing to the anatomic location of the descending motor tracts (Fig. 4.16). In larger lesions extending further into the periventricular white matter, the upper extremities and cognitive functions will be more affected. Motor tracts associated with visual, auditory, and somesthetic functions can also be involved.[386,391,392] Extremely premature infants have been found to be at greatest risk for global motor and cognitive impairments.[352,353,370,396]

As with other injuries to the neonatal brain, the primary focus is prevention of prematurity, infection, hypotension,

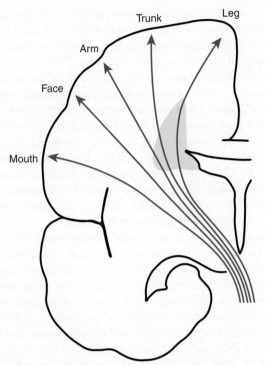

FIGURE 4.16 Illustrations of the periventricular area and motor tracts. (Reprinted with permission from Volpe JJ. *Neurology of the Newborn.* 4th ed. Philadelphia, PA: Saunders; 2001:432.)

and other associated factors. The initial management after the diagnosis of PVL is treating the primary cause and complications of the insult along with preventing further hypoxic–ischemic damage. Management strategies to prevent or minimize hypoxia, hypotension, acidosis, apnea, bradycardia, and infection are implemented. Developmental care strategies can be implemented to decrease stress and promote development. Serial cranial ultrasounds are done to monitor PVL, possible progression, and hydrocephalus.

Retinopathy of Prematurity

ROP is a vasoproliferative disorder of the developing retina of premature infants that can potentially result in visual impairment and blindness. The severity of ROP has been found to be predictive of poor neurodevelopmental outcome.[397] Premature infants are at higher risk for developing ROP due to the vasculogenesis and angiogenesis that typically occur in fetal life between 16 weeks and term. ROP is rarely diagnosed in full-term infants as vascularization of the retina is typically complete by 40 weeks.[398]

The incidence and severity of ROP is closely correlated with lower weight and GA at birth, twin gestation, and overall severity of illness.[399,400] Infants with extreme prematurity and VLBW have not only increased frequency of ROP but also more severe ROP.[401]

Other risk factors include poor postnatal weight gain, blood transfusions, and maternal factors such as hyperglycemia, smoking, and preeclampsia. The development of

ROP has been linked to exposure to large concentrations of oxygen since the 1940s[402]; however, the cause of ROP is presently thought of as multifactorial. Oxygen and non–oxygen-regulated growth factors have been associated with the development of ROP.[403] Genetic factors have also been implicated in the development of ROP.

The onset of ROP is marked by an alteration in the normal development of the blood vessels in the eye and has been described as a two-stage process. In the first phase, the premature infant is exposed to an environment that is more hyperoxic than the intrauterine environment. Hyperoxia suppresses growth factors, resulting in the cessation of normal vascular development, vasoconstriction of the immature retinal vessels, and capillary death.[404] The nonvascular area of the retina becomes hypoxic, which leads to the next phase of ROP. The second stage of ROP occurs around 32 to 34 weeks' postmenstrual age (PMA) and is characterized by a proliferation of new vessel growth at the junction between the avascular and vascularized retina due to the upregulation of growth and other factors in response to hypoxia.[404,405] If circulation and increased oxygenation to the avascular retina can be reestablished, ROP will regress and the excess vessels are resorbed. However, if there continues to be insufficient circulation and hypoxia, neovascularization into the vitreous occurs with uncontrolled vessel growth. These vessels are atypical in structure and prone to hemorrhage and edema. The pathologic growth of the vessels over time produces a fibrous scar, which places traction on the retina leading to detachment.[403]

The disease process usually peaks at 34 to 40 weeks and then regresses. In the majority of cases, the disease process regresses with resolution of the retinopathy. In severe cases, there may be visual impairment or blindness. Owing to the sequential progression of ROP and benefits of early diagnosis and treatment, ophthalmologists perform regularly timed retinal assessments on schedules on the basis of GA, comorbidities, and disease severity. The AAP[406] has developed guidelines for ROP screening examinations for preterm infants. According to these guidelines, infants with birth weight less than 1500 g or GA less than 30 weeks, as well as infants with birth weights between 1500 and 2000 g or GA greater than 30 weeks with complicated clinical course, including mechanical ventilation and supplemental oxygen, should be screened for ROP. The acute phase of screening is initiated on the basis of PMA as research has shown that there is better correlation of the onset of severe ROP with PMA. However, extremely preterm infants at less than 25 weeks' GA should be considered for earlier screening owing to the high risk factors. Ongoing examinations are performed according to a suggested schedule on the basis of retinal findings.[406] The acute phase of ROP screening ends when the risk of severe ROP is no longer present.[407]

ROP is classified by the location, stage, and extent of the pathophysiologic process using the International Classification of Retinopathy of Prematurity (ICROP).[406,407] The location indicates the distance that the atypically developing retinal blood vessels have traveled and is identified by how many clock hours of the eye's circumference are affected. The retina is divided into three concentric circles, which are known as zones (Fig. 4.17). The zones reflect the central to peripheral development of blood vessels.[398] Zone 1 is surrounding the optic nerve extending out to the macula. Zone 2 extends toward the nasal and temporal sides, and zone 3 extends further to the temporal side. The severity of the disease is classified in stages (Fig. 4.17). In stage 1, there is a thin line of demarcation separating the normal retina from underdeveloped, avascular areas. Stage 2 is when the demarcation becomes a thick, high ridge that protrudes into the vitreous humor. There is extraretinal fibrovascular proliferation along the edge of the ridge extending into the vitreous humor in stage 3. In stage 4, fibrosis and scarring develop, placing traction on the retina and leading to partial detachment. Stage 4 is further subdivided: in 4A, the partial detachment does not involve the macula, and in 4B the macula is involved. Stage 5 is complete detachment of the retina.[407]

Plus disease, occurring at any stage, is a severe form of ROP involving iris vascular engorgement, pupillary rigidity, and vitreous haze. In this form of ROP, the posterior retinal blood vessels become characteristically dilated and tortuous in appearance. Plus disease tends to progress very rapidly and requires intervention owing to increased risk of poor visual outcome.[398,407]

The category of pre-plus disease was added to the ICROP classification system in 2005 to describe the presence of vascular dilation and tortuosity but not severe enough to meet the criteria for plus disease. Pre-plus disease can progress to plus disease, and infants classified with pre-plus disease are followed very closely.[398,406,407] The severity for determination of surgery is described in terms of threshold and prethreshold. Threshold refers to conditions of five or more contiguous or eight cumulative clock hours of stage 3 with plus disease in zone 1 or 2. The risk of blindness is approximately 50% in threshold ROP, and surgical intervention is recommended.[398,407]

Prethreshold disease can be any of the following conditions: zone 1 ROP of any stage less than threshold, zone 2 ROP with stage 2 and plus disease, zone 2 ROP with stage 3 without plus disease, and zone 2 stage 3 with plus disease with four sections of stage less than threshold. Surgical intervention may be required for high-risk prethreshold ROP. The AAP[408] recommends treatment, if possible, within 72 hours of the detection of treatable threshold ROP. Follow-up is recommended 3 to 7 days after treatment to assess whether further treatment is required.

Ablative therapy is used in the treatment of ROP. Diode laser photocoagulation is now used over cryotherapy on the basis of the results of clinical studies demonstrating the superiority of laser treatment.[409,410] Timing of treatment has also moved to earlier stages of the disease on the basis of the Early Treatment for Retinopathy of Prematurity or ETROP study. In this study, laser decreased the progression and incidence of ROP; however, patients in the ETROP study still had poor visual outcomes.[411] This may be due to angiogenic factors that are not reduced by laser.

While retinal ablation is an effective management for the majority of cases of threshold ROP, there are cases that progress to retinal detachment. In these cases, surgical management with scleral buckling or vitrectomy is performed. Vitrectomy is a procedure that removes the scar tissue, pulling the retina forward. These procedures have had limited success in terms of functional visual outcomes.[412–415]

At this time, laser treatment is the only evidence-based therapy for ROP. Researchers are looking at pharmacologic

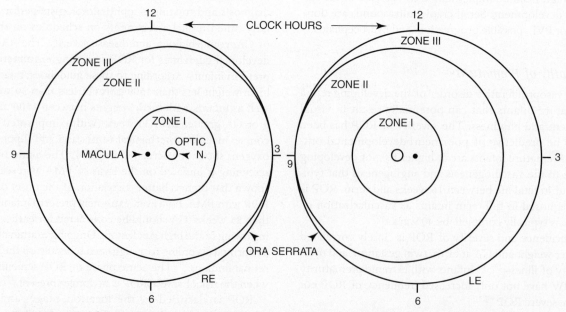

FIGURE 4.17 Schematic of the left and right eye showing the clock hours and the stages and zones of ROP. (Reprinted with permission from Committee for Classification of ROP. An International Classification of Retinopathy of Prematurity. *Arch Ophthalmol.* 1989;102(8):1131.)

treatments on the basis of ongoing studies of the pathogenesis of ROP. These interventions include anti-VEGF (vascular endothelial growth factor) agents, systemic beta-adrenergic receptor blockers, gene therapy, supplementation with omega-3 fatty acids, and IGF-1 (insulin-like growth factor-1).[410]

Presently there are no proven treatments to prevent ROP. Low oxygen saturation levels appear to reduce the incidence of ROP, but the optimum level of saturation has not been determined.[403,405] Methods that are used clinically for the prevention of ROP include preventing preterm birth, regulation of supplemental oxygen, nutrition to promote growth and weight gain, and minimizing other comorbidities of premature infants.

In order to prevent severe ROP and related visual impairment, screening examinations are necessary for preterm infants. However, pain and stress in infants undergoing ROP eye examinations have been documented in the literature.[416,417] Increased heart rate and blood pressure, and decreased oxygen saturation have been noted in infants undergoing eye exams. In addition, increased oxygen requirement, feeding intolerance, and apnea can occur for several hours after the eye exam.[418] The AAP[406] recommends that "all efforts be made to minimize discomfort and systemic effects of eye examinations."[419] Pretreatment with anesthetic eye drops has been studied with mixed results.[420,421] NNS on a pacifier, oral sucrose, and breast milk have been shown to decrease pain responses in preterm infants.[422–426] Other strategies used to comfort infants during eye exams include nesting, containment, and developmental care practices such as NIDCAP.[309,427,428] Physical therapists, as part of the developmental care team in the NICU, can play a role in educating family and caregivers to recognize an individual infant's cues of stress and comfort, identifying strategies to decrease pain and stress, and developing a plan for support during and following painful procedures such as ROP exams.

Chorioamnionitis

Cervicovaginal bacteria that invade the amniotic cavity and cause an inflammatory response in the membranes of the developing fetus cause chorioamnionitis. Chorioamnionitis is the most common cause of preterm labor. Most infants are not septic at birth as the placenta provides an efficient barrier. However, in cases where there is a fetal inflammatory response in addition to the maternal inflammatory response, babies may be more at risk for BPD, NEC, abnormalities on cranial ultrasound, and long-term neurologic impairment.[429] In addition, there has been evidence of an association between maternal intrauterine infection and the occurrence of fetal brain damage with subsequent neurologic deficits, with the strongest association between chorioamnionitis and PVL.[393,430]

Metabolic Bone Disease of Prematurity

The third trimester of fetal development is very important for bone formation. The essential nutrients for this process are provided most efficiently by the placenta when a baby is in utero. Approximately 80% of bone is produced between 24 and 40 weeks' gestation as the fetus accretes large amounts of calcium, phosphorus, and magnesium.[431–437] There is also mechanical stimulation to the bones as the fetus actively moves within the fluid-filled environment and pushes against the uterine wall. In addition, further mechanical loading of the skeletal system occurs during the third trimester as the infant is gaining muscle mass and being compressed by the cramped uterine space.[433–435] Prematurely born infants miss out on a portion or all of this period of bone formation and mineral accretion.

Metabolic bone disease of prematurity is defined as "postnatal bone mineralization that is less than intrauterine bone density at a comparable gestational age."[438] Preterm babies in the NICU are at risk for metabolic bone disease of prematurity, which has implications for their future growth[439] as well as putting them in danger of fractures in the present.[440] Risk factors that contribute to metabolic bone disease of prematurity include:

- Nutritional practices such as feeding restrictions, prolonged use of hyperalimentation, or the use of unfortified breast milk.
- Drugs such as corticosteroids and diuretics that cause increased mineral excretion.[433–437]
- Vitamin D deficiency, which is exacerbated by diseases that contribute to malabsorption such as cholestasis and NEC.
- A lack of mechanical stimulation, which can be intensified by sedatives, paralytics,[439] and supports for intravenous lines that immobilize tiny limbs.

Infants with metabolic bone disease of prematurity have fragile bones at high risk for fractures and positional deformities such as dolichocephaly and respiratory morbidities.[439]

Metabolic bone disease of prematurity can be challenging to diagnose as it may be asymptomatic until fractures occur or signs of rickets appear. Biochemical markers can be difficult to interpret, markers of bone formation lack sensitivity and specificity, and X-rays do not demonstrate osteopenia until significant demineralization has occurred.[439] Osteopenia can go unrecognized until a fracture occurs; there have been reports in the literature of fractures in preterm infants temporally associated with intravenous line placement.[441] Babies in the authors' NICU have also developed fractures that have been temporally associated with immunizations, intravenous line placement, heel sticks, and restraints used during a medical procedure. These developments have compelled the authors to advocate safe handling for all infants, especially replacing twisting and pulling limbs during line placement with repositioning the baby in order to allow the baby's limbs to maintain as neutral an alignment as possible. Other safe handling techniques include lifting an infant by placing one hand under the head and the other under the buttocks rather than picking up under the axilla or around the rib cage, and sliding your hand under the buttocks to lift for a diaper change, rather than grasping around the infant's ankles and lifting.[442]

The incidence of metabolic bone disease of prematurity is inversely related to GA and birth weight. ELBW infants (less than 1000 g) have an incidence of osteopenia of 50% to 60%; VLBW infants (less than 1500 g) have an incidence of osteopenia of 23%.[440] Fractures are reported in approximately 10% of VLBW infants at 36 to 40 weeks' PMA.[440] In the NICU, the prevention and treatment of bone disease in premature infants is aggressively managed through nutritional management. The medical staff carefully monitors the vitamins and minerals the infant receives through parenteral nutrition, human milk fortifiers, and/or preterm formula.[434–437] Even with carefully managed nutritional programs, cases of metabolic bone disease of prematurity still occur. Studies on the use of passive range of motion to promote bone formation in preterm infants have been reported in the literature[344,443–445]; however, these studies have small numbers of subjects and do not address the physiologic stress that handling can induce in this very fragile population. A Cochrane review[446] of eight trials to determine the effect of physical activity programs on bone mineralization, fractures, and growth in preterm infants. did not recommend it on the basis of the current evidence and cited the need for further studies with infants at high risk for metabolic bone disease of prematurity that address adverse events, long-term outcomes, as well as the contributions of nutrition.[446] Care must be taken when handling premature, VLBW infants in terms of their physiologic vulnerabilities as well as the increased risk of fracturing bone. In addition, attention should be paid to cranial molding with the use of positioning devices, varying postures, and including supine positions with head midline. The neonatal therapist should be advocating positioning and supports for infants that do not restrict movement and facilitate active movement. Intravenous lines for medications and endotracheal tubes providing respiratory support do need to be protected; however, babies should be allowed to initiate movement, which will allow opportunities for muscle strengthening and may contribute to bone strength.

Physical Therapy Assessment and Intervention: Issues of Prematurity

A complete history should include information from the medical chart, nursing and physician staff, and the family. Pertinent information from the medical chart includes prenatal history, birth history, history of the present illness, and family social history. Prenatal history consists of maternal age, circumstances regarding conception (the use of assistive reproductive technology), prenatal care and test results, complications during pregnancy, infections, illnesses, medications taken by the mother (licit and illicit,) interventions such as fetal/maternal surgery, maternal past medical history, and presence/treatment of preterm labor. Birth history includes GA at delivery, mode of delivery (spontaneous or induced vaginal delivery, with or without vacuum or forceps assist, or Cesarean section), weight, length, head circumference, Apgar scores (Table 4.6), infant's clinical presentation at delivery, necessary resuscitative efforts, and infant's need for ongoing interventions in the delivery room.

History of present illness includes an in-depth review of medical status by systems. A baby requires newborn intensive care because of the immaturity of his or her organs and the fragility of his or her physiologic function. In reviewing the chart, the therapist should attend to the baby's level of respiratory support, his or her requirements since birth, and his or her current needs, including modifications to sustain the baby through nursing care or feeding sessions. The therapist should note the frequency and severity of episodes of apnea, bradycardia, and oxygen desaturation, as well as interventions needed. Cardiovascular status is important to understand the health of the baby's other organ systems, in particular the central nervous system (CNS), respiratory system, and GI system. The baby's initial means of getting nutrition and how this has been tolerated, modified, regressed, and/or progressed should be understood as it provides a window into the baby's overall health, functioning, and ability to grow. Likewise, the baby's medications can impact his or her functioning and ability to stay alert and sustain a wakeful state. Infants who have required sedatives or narcotics for medical management may display signs and symptoms of withdrawal as the medications are being weaned.

Other medical problems that relate to the infant's current level of functioning and future risk include infections, metabolic issues, hyperbilirubinemia, genetic syndromes, congenital malformations, seizures, ICHs, and surgical issues. After a thorough review of the chart, the therapist should approach the nursing staff with questions to initiate a dialogue about the overall status of the infant. This should be followed by pertinent questions addressing the following: changes in status leading to changes in medical care, tolerance to nursing care, care procedures that lead to distress, and preferred comfort measures. If the family members are present, the therapist can seek to establish a relationship with them by initiating a dialogue about their baby. Through this process, the therapist can gain insight into the family's overall understanding of the infant's medical problems, their interpretation of the infant's behaviors, and their comfort in interacting with their baby. During this initial visit to the infant's bedside, the therapist is observing environmental information such as bed space location, levels of light and sound, and how the baby responds to the stresses in his or her immediate environment.

The therapist needs to observe the infant both at rest and during care activities with nursing or other health care professionals. During an observation of nursing or medical care, a baby may demonstrate sensitivity to environmental sounds. The therapist would then recommend strategies to minimize sounds such as encouraging staff to refrain from writing upon or placing objects on top of the isolette, quietly closing porthole and bedside cart drawers, keeping pagers on vibrate mode, and keeping voices low

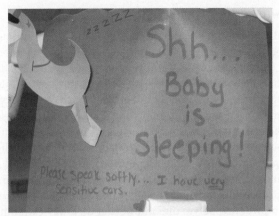

FIGURE 4.18 Signs such as this are used to alert staff and visitors that the infant is sensitive to sound.

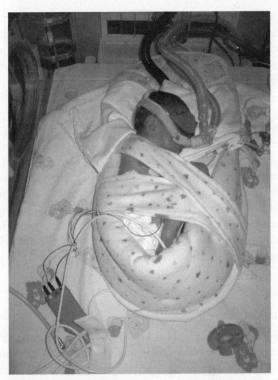

FIGURE 4.19 Infant positioned in a nest made from a Children's Medical Ventures Snuggle Up.

and conversations to a minimum. Large signs (Fig. 4.18) to keep noise down can be posted, indicating that the baby is stressed by sound so that all staff and visitors are aware of the need to keep noise to a minimum. If these measures are not sufficient, the baby's bed may need to be moved to a quieter space away from a sink, a trash can, or a heavily traveled corridor. Similarly, if a baby is sensitive to light, recommendations would be made to shield his or her eyes from bright light. Methods of modifying light include dimming the lights, covering the isolette, tenting the infant's face (by propping a blanket to shade the infant's eyes or draping a sheet over a crib), and cupping a hand over the infant's eyes during care. The physical environment of the NICU should be adapted with individual lighting for each bed space.[447]

A baby may also demonstrate frequent physiologic and motoric stress signs at rest as well as during intervention (Table 4.3). In order to assist the autonomic subsystem and the motor subsystem, the baby may benefit from firm containment through the use of positioning aides. Commercially made products or blanket rolls can be used to provide a nest that simulates the enclosed environment of the womb (Fig. 4.19).

During an observation, a baby may demonstrate unsuccessful attempts to self-calm. If the baby is unsuccessful at calming, he or she may become exhausted, limp, and physiologically compromised by the end of the caregiving episode. Suggestions for providing assistance for the baby's self-calming strategies include offering a pacifier, containing hands near face/mouth, and positioning legs in a tucked position near the baby's trunk. The caregiving may need to be paced to the infant's tolerance, and the infant allowed to rest after particularly disorganizing aspects of care (e.g., diaper change or suctioning). During the rest break, the baby should be contained from head to toe by spreading both hands to cover the infant and thus facilitating a tucked position. A blanket wrap can also be used to swaddle the infant and prevent the infant from exhausting him- or herself.[74,448–450]

Parent Education

Parent education should be a main focus of any neonatal physical therapy plan of care. Scale et al.[451] found that parents receiving early intervention services reported parent education on ways to support infant motor development to be more effective than direct physical therapy services. Dusing[452] found a combination of educational approaches to parent education to be most effective, including demonstrations, observations of assessment, written materials, and opportunities to ask questions. In order to be effective, parent education should be started early during the admission, ongoing throughout the hospitalization (not immediately before discharge), and have interdisciplinary collaboration.[453]

In order for parents to perform the challenging role of parenting, they need to understand the behaviors of a preterm baby, as well as the course of typical development and what to expect in the future. They need to be able to "read" their infants and respond supportively to them. When a therapist observes a baby interacting with his or her caregiver during nursing care, the therapist will discover the baby's areas of competence, strength, and vulnerability. Likewise, an NICU therapist, as a developmental specialist, will know the course of development and, therefore, is in a unique role to assist parents as they parent their infants. Parents have benefited in the short term and also in the long term from gaining awareness of their baby's interactive and developmental capabilities and responding appropriately to them.[454–457] The therapist can start the dialogue with the parents by asking, "How do you think your baby is doing?" and then listen to hear their concerns and their interpretations of the baby's behavior. This interaction will give the therapist a window into the parents' understanding of their baby. The therapist can invite the parents to watch the baby together, and the therapist can use that opportunity to point out the baby's unique capabilities, strategies of self-regulation, and sensitivities and vulnerabilities to the environment and medical care. The therapist can provide a synopsis of general components and patterns of infant development and guide the parent with recommendations to focus on the present. For an excellent review of parent teaching strategies, see the Lowman et al.[456] article on using developmental assessments in the NICU to empower families. Parenting is a challenging job at any stage of a child's development, but especially in infancy when children are not capable of articulating their needs and desires.

Kangaroo Care

Skin-to-skin holding, also known as kangaroo care, is an intervention that supports infant physiologic and behavioral stability and maturation as well as parent–infant interaction and attachment. This practice involves the parent holding the diaper-clad infant underneath his or her clothing, skin to skin, chest to chest,[458] and was initially used with preterm infants in Bogota, Columbia, during a time when there was limited availability of incubators.[459] Skin-to-skin holding has gained wider acceptance in the United States for use in the NICU over the past decade.

The benefits of skin-to-skin holding for the premature infant have been documented in several studies and include improved thermoregulation, improved respiratory patterns and oxygen saturations, decreased apnea and bradycardia, improved behavioral state organization, increased rates of weight gain, as an analgesic during painful procedures, and decreased length of hospitalization.[171,460-466] For parents, the benefits are increased maternal milk production, improved breast-feeding, opportunities for more positive interactions with their infant, and an overall more positive view of their infant.[466-468] Feldman and associates[468] found the parents of premature infants who used skin-to-skin holding to be more sensitive to their infant's cues, and to provide a better home environment after discharge. The infants in this study also had improved neurodevelopmental assessments at 6 months as compared with peers who received no skin-to-skin holding.

The initiation of skin-to-skin holding will vary between-institutions on the basis of GA, weight, and the acuity of the infant. Early in the infant's admission, the physical therapist can help to educate the family as to the benefits of skin-to-skin holding and then encourage the family to engage in the intervention as soon as the medical team approves the practice. The physical therapist can also assist the parents with positioning the infant for comfort and to ensure the most optimal position to promote physiologic stability and behavioral organization.

Positioning for Comfort

Preterm infants are more likely to experience muscular fatigue, particularly in the respiratory muscles.[118] Because of the combination of hypotonia, gravitational forces, and loss of uterine constraints, the infant develops postures of extension, leading to discomfort and an imbalance of flexion and extension. In order to support the respiratory and musculoskeletal systems and promote infant comfort, positioning should promote the following components of optimal alignment: neutral head and neck position and, if possible, slight chin tuck, scapular protraction to promote upper extremity flexion and hands midline (Fig. 4.20), flexion of the trunk with posterior pelvic tilt, and flexion of lower extremities with neutral abduction/adduction and rotation of the hips. Supports to assist the infant in maintaining optimal position can be fabricated using blanket rolls or commercially available devices. Children's Medical Ventures and Small Beginnings are two companies that manufacture and sell a variety of positioning products for use in the NICU.

The preterm infant needs to have regular positional changes in order to promote comfort, prevent skin breakdown, promote the development of the musculoskeletal system, promote gaseous exchange in all lung fields, and maintain head shape.[118,469-472] When medically tolerated, preterm infants benefit from prone positioning. Studies have shown that the prone position improves oxygenation and ventilation, improves cerebral venous return and lowers intracranial pressure, promotes self-calming and sleep states, and improves behavioral organization/self-regulation.[473-478] Grenier et al.[478] have found that infants placed in prone, whether nested or unnested, have the fewest stress behaviors compared with infants placed in either side-lying or supine. However, some nurseries have policies discouraging prone for babies who have umbilical lines or are intubated. It is best to know the nursery policy on prone positioning before recommending prone placement for an infant.

The unsupported prone position promotes shoulder retraction, neck hyperextension, truncal flattening, and hip

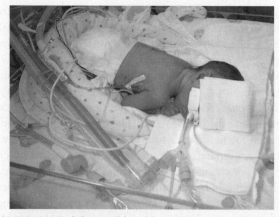

FIGURE 4.20 Infant positioned in prone position using anterior, midline roll under chest. The nest helps to promote flexion of the trunk, arms, and legs.

abduction/external rotation, which is uncomfortable and if left uncorrected can interfere with future motor development.[118,472] Infants placed in prone should have a thin roll under their chests to raise their chests from the surface and allow shoulder protraction and a more neutral neck alignment. A roll should be placed under the infant's hips to promote lower extremity flexion and a larger roll around the infant's sides and feet to promote boundaries.

Infants supported in side-lying also demonstrate decreased stress behaviors compared with supine. Other optimal effects of side-lying are symmetry and midline orientation of trunk and extremities, which promotes hands to mouth. In addition, in side-lying the respiratory diaphragm is placed in a gravity-eliminated plane, which lessens the work of breathing. GER is decreased in left side-lying, and gastric emptying is increased in right side-lying.[280,473,479] Blanket rolls are necessary to support infants placed in side-lying in order for side-lying to be beneficial to the infant. Unsupported side-lying has the potential to be stressful for the baby as it provides the least amount of postural support, making the preterm infant maintain body postures and self-organization on his or her own.[473,478,479] In his or her efforts to seek boundaries for postural control, a preterm baby is more likely to extend his or her neck and trunk to end ranges. These hyperextended postures are counterproductive, as tucking, flexion, and hands to face are the postures that promote comfort, calming, and self-regulation.[478]

Supine allows for maximal observation and access to the infant by caregivers. However, when compared with prone or side-lying, supine poses the most challenges for the infant biomechanically, organizationally, and physiologically. In supine, the forces of gravity pull the baby into neck extension, trunk extension, scapular retraction, anterior pelvic tilt, external hip rotation, and abduction. In addition, supine assists the baby as he or she actively extends. These postures do not promote calming and self-regulation. Studies of preterm infant positioning have found that infants move more and in a less-organized fashion in supine; have shorter and more interrupted sleep periods; have more labored, less-coordinated breathing; and have more episodes of GER.[480–482] Since supine is the most challenging position for the preterm infant, infants should be supported with rolls to promote midline symmetric flexion with head and trunk in midline, hands near mouth or face, and legs tucked close to the body with neutral hip position (Fig. 4.21). Benefits of supported supine include the unique potential for weight bearing on the posterior skull. For the older baby, supine allows increased visual exploration of the environment and face-to-face interaction. For the micropreemie during the first few days of life, supine prevents obstruction of cerebral venous drainage and increased cerebral blood flow.[483] In 1992, the AAP[484] initiated the "Back-to-Sleep" program, which advocates supine sleeping to prevent SIDS. Preterm infants are more at risk for SIDS and should be transitioned to supine sleeping prior to discharge from the hospital.[484]

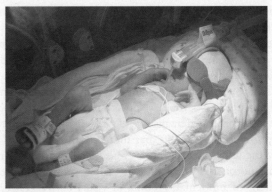

FIGURE 4.21 An infant positioned in the supine position using a nest made from a Children's Medical Ventures Snuggle Up around the legs and trunk, and a Frederick T. frog positioning aid around the head and neck to promote midline flexion.

The very medically fragile infant may be limited in positioning options owing to technologic supports (i.e., chest tubes, umbilical vein [UV]/umbilical artery [UA] lines, and ventilatory support) and medical conditions (i.e., gastroschisis [GS], omphalocele, prior abdominal surgery, and arthrogryposis). Under these circumstances, positioning supports to attain the most optimal alignment available are implemented. The goal is to promote physiologic stability and infant comfort rather than perfect biomechanical alignment. As the infant's condition improves, he or she is assessed for tolerance to positioning in better alignment and other positions.

The musculoskeletal consequences of poor alignment over time in a preterm baby include tightness of neck extensors, shoulder/scapular retractors, low back extensors, and hip abductors. Tight muscles predispose the infant to reinforce certain motor patterns while inhibiting others. The repetitive use of these motor patterns can cause the formation of dominant cerebral motor pathways and the regression of the less frequently used patterns. The effects of these muscle imbalances, malalignment, and dominant motor pathways can prevent the acquisition of developmental skills such as chin tuck and midline head postures, eye–hand regard and reaching, weight shifts, and rolling.[473,485,486] Delays in fine and gross motor development that interfere with play and exploration can delay cognitive development.[485] Research has demonstrated the persistence of an out-toeing gait in children as old as 4 to 6 years and the persistence of toe walking up to 18 months in former preterm infants.[118,487,488]

Positioning can also affect cranial molding and head shape. Preterm infants are more at risk for cranial deformations as their skulls are softer and thinner than full-term infants.[489–491] Head shaping can affect parental perceptions of infant attractiveness and can interfere with the attachment process.[492,493] Owing to the forces of gravity and the pressure of the mattress when lying with hi sor her head to the side, the preterm infant can develop an elongated anterior–posterior diameter of his or her skull. This is known as dolichocephaly and can interfere with the development of midline position of the head in supine. In addition, plagiocephaly or unilateral posterolateral head flattening can occur from prolonged supine positioning with a head preference and lack of head turning to the opposite side. Torticollis, unilateral shortening of the sternocleidomastoid muscle (SCM), can develop as a result of plagiocephaly and is characterized by ipsilateral head tilt and contralateral head rotation. Torticollis may influence the posture of not only the infant's head, but also his or her trunk, and may delay motor skill acquisition as well as prevent the development of binocular vision and visual convergence. To prevent cranial deformities and torticollis, commercially available gel pillows to disperse pressure across the skull can be used.[471,494-497] In addition, regular changes in the head position throughout the day and midline alignment of the head in supine can help to minimize cranial deformities and torticollis.

Neonatal Neurologic Assessment

As physical therapists, we strive to practice under the principle of beneficence—"above all, do no harm" to our patients. When working with the population of high-risk infants, the potential is always present to harm a baby when intervening with him or her. Using careful and skilled observations of the baby's physiologic status allows the therapist to decide on the competence of the infant to withstand an assessment and when to terminate or proceed with handling an infant. A skilled therapist will also collaborate with nursing staff to understand the baby's current medical status, tolerance to handling, and previous events of the day before undertaking any direct interaction with the baby. The infant should also be evaluated before, during, and after any assessment or intervention for signs of pain using the neonatal pain assessment approved by the medical facility.

If the results of this preliminary gathering of information show that the baby is easily stressed by the routines of the day, an observational assessment to identify the baby's attempts to regulate and difficulties tolerating care is warranted. The therapist would follow the steps for observational assessment and care as discussed previously in the "Developmental Care" section. As the infant demonstrates improving stability, the therapist should continue to weigh the inherent potential costs to the infant with an assessment that involves handling. When the baby can tolerate additional stimulation and is in a sleep state, serial responses to repeated light (flashlight across the eyes) and sound (a soft rattle) are used to assess the baby's ability to filter repetitive stimuli. This provides information regarding the stability of the sleep state and also gives the therapist a chance to determine the readiness for handling. If the baby becomes overly stressed and loses physiologic stability, the therapist should end the evaluation session and provide supports for regulation. However, if the baby is able to transition to an alert state and maintain physiologic stability, the therapist can proceed slowly with assessment that requires gentle handling. The authors do not recommend one standardized assessment tool. See Table 4.9 for a variety of standardized neonatal assessments. Throughout the assessment, the

TABLE 4.9	Standardized Neonatal Assessment Tools		
Name/Author	**Purpose**	**Description**	**Training**
Neurologic Assessment of Preterm and Full-Term Infants (NAPFI) Authors: Dubowitz V Dubowitz L[498,499]	To record the functional state of the nervous system and to document preterm infant neurologic maturation and recovery from perinatal insult Age: Preterm and full-term infants	Assessment of behavioral state, neurobehavior, posture, movement, muscle tone, and reflexes with passive manipulation. Emphasis on patterns of responses. Test cannot be quantified or compared with normative expectations for age over time. Time to administer: 15 min	Requires minimal training or experience. Items within the area of expertise of developmental therapists.
Neurobehavioral Assessment of the Preterm Infant (NAPI) Authors: Korner AF Thom VA[500]	To assess infant maturity, monitor progress, and detect lags in development and neurologically suspect performance. Age: 32–42 wk PCA	Assessment of state, behavior, reflexes, motor patterns, and tone. Most items overlap with other assessments and must be administered from rousing to soothing to alerting. Time to administer: 45 min	Training video available with manual.[501] To be used by any professional caring for or studying preterm infants in the intensive or intermediate care nursery.
Neonatal Behavioral Assessment Scale (NBAS) Author: Brazelton TB Nugent J[182]	To assess the infant's contributions to the interactional process. Age: 36–44 wk gestation	Consists of 28 behavioral items and 18 reflex items. Sequence of administration is flexible, and examiner seeks to elicit the infant's best performance. Time to administer: 30–45 min and scored in 15–20 min	Requires training for reliability in administration and scoring.[502] Trainees complete a four-phase process consisting of self-study, skill test, and practice (on 25 babies) before completing certification session.

Name/Author	Purpose	Description	Training
Assessment of Preterm Infant Behavior (APIB) Authors: Als H Lester BM Tronick EZ Brazelton TB[503,504]	To assess the individual behavioral organizational repertoire of the preterm infant. Age: Preterm infants	Based on the BNBAS but focusing on the preterm infant. Looks at the preterm infant's physiologic, motor, state, attentional–interactive, and regulatory systems. Time to administer: 30–45 min Scoring is labor-intensive.	Requires extensive training in the assessment as well as human development.
NICU Network Neurobehavioral Scale (NNNS) Authors: Lester BM Tronick EZ[111,505]	To assess neurologic integrity and behavioral functioning of infants at high risk. Stress scale to document signs of withdrawal. Age: 34–46 wk PCA Can be used in term, healthy infants, and high-risk infants (substance exposures and preterm infants). Infants <33 wk use just observational items.	Draws on NBAS, NAPI, APIB, Neurologic Examination of the Full-term Newborn Infant, and the Neurologic Examination of the Maturity of Newborn Infants. Items are grouped in packages, which are presented depending on infant state in a prescribed sequence. Can be modified for the very preterm, physiologically unstable infant. Time to administer: 30 min	Requires certification through 2- or 5-day training programs with certified trainers along with practice administering the test to infants in own facility. Amount of practice depends on experience, comfort handling infants, and clinical acumen.
Assessment of General Movements (GMA) Author: Einspieler C Pretchl HF Bos AF Ferrari F Cioni G[506,507]	To assess for early signs of brain dysfunction using qualitative measure. Age: 36 wk PCA to 4 mo Can be used with both preterm and full-term infants.	Infants are videotaped, and observational analysis of movements in terms of variety, fluidity, elegance, and complexity is performed. Video recording and analysis should be done longitudinally. Time: 1 hr initial videotape and 15-min follow-up tapes plus time for analysis	Two-day training required for basic principles. Practice of 100 recordings required to become a skilled observer. Training videotape available, which demonstrates qualitative aspects of movement.[508]
Test of Infant Motor Performance (TIMP) Authors: Campbell SK Girolami G Oston E Lenke M[509]	To identify motor delay in infants before 4 mo corrected age. Age: 34 wk gestation to 4 mo postterm	Consists of 13 observed items focusing on midline alignment, selective control, and quality of movement; 29 elicited items focusing on antigravity postural control elicited by handling typically experienced by an infant.	Workshops or self-study instructional CD.[510]
Alberta Infant Motor Scale (AIMS) Authors: Piper M Darrah J[511]	To identify motor delays, monitor individual development, and evaluate intervention. Age: 0–18 mo	Observational assessment of 58 transitional gross motor patterns and postures in supine, prone, sitting, and standing.	No training requirements specified. To be used by any professional with a background in infant motor development.

therapist needs to assess the baby's state control (i.e., the ability to maintain organized sleep states and demonstrate a range of states; see Table 4.5 for state-related behaviors).

Neuromotor examination, to be accurate, requires a baby to be in a calm, awake state as other states (sleep, crying) can affect muscle tone, range of motion, and active movement. It is generally safe to initiate a neuromotor examination on an infant who is medically stable, on room air, and in an open crib. However, this portion of the assessment can be most stressful to the infant; therefore, the therapist should proceed with caution while maintaining vigilance for signs of tolerance or fatigue. Components of a baseline assessment for a medically stable infant include observation of posture at rest, quality and quantity of active movements, palmar and plantar grasp reflexes, flexor recoil, traction responses, passive range of motion, and French angles (adductor, popliteal, heel to ear, dorsiflexion, and

scarf sign angles)[512,513](Figure 4.23) If the baby is tolerating these procedures, the therapist can move on to more intensive handling items, including pull-to-sit, slip through, ventral suspension, and prone, side-lying, and sitting placement. During this assessment, the therapist should be watching for an optimal time to elicit visual and auditory responses from the infant. This portion of the assessment should also be administered from least stressful to most stressful and unimodal to multimodal stimulation (i.e., inanimate object, blank face, animated face, face coupled with speech). During this time, the therapist needs to attend to the baby's responses to touch and movement through space and the baby's strategies to maintain organization in autonomic, state, and motor subsystems and calming strategies. The assessment allows the therapist a window into the baby's functioning at a single point in time; however, the baby's responses are based on his or her own level of maturity as well as contextual factors. Therefore, it is wise to serially examine an infant over time to gain an accurate picture of his or her function.

The therapist uses the information from the history, observation, and hands-on examination to determine the baby's strengths and needs and the family's strengths, needs, and expectations. The identified needs are prioritized and a plan of care is developed using interventions that challenge the baby within his or her range of tolerance. Recommendations are made so that the baby is appropriately challenged and supported by his or her family and caregivers throughout the week. For instance, a baby may have shown excessive extensor posturing and tight scapulohumeral and neck extensor musculature. The therapist would then recommend ways to incorporate flexion activities into daily routines and interactions with family and to avoid activities that promote excessive extension. As the baby develops and changes, these recommendations need to be updated.

Bronchopulmonary Dysplasia

BPD is the most common chronic lung disease of infancy (CLDI) associated with prematurity, and the incidence is closely and inversely related to birth weight and GA. The rates of BPD vary by definition applied, GA distribution, characteristics of the population, and medical center.[514] Despite advances in neonatal care, the incidence has not changed owing to the increased survival rate of extremely premature infants.[515–517]

Northway and colleagues[518] first described BPD in 1967 as a disease affecting both airway and lung parenchyma of preterm infants owing to injury caused by mechanical ventilation and oxygen therapy. The disease was characterized by airway injury and inflammatory response, lung parenchymal fibrosis and cellular hypoplasia, and areas of hyperinflation and atelectasis resulting in thickened and hyperreactive airways, decreased lung compliance due to fibrosis, increased airway resistance, impaired gas exchange with ventilation–perfusion mismatch, and air trapping.[519–521] Diagnosis was made on the basis of the need for supplemental oxygen at 36 weeks PMA, and radiographic changes.[522] Since that time, advances in management of preterm infants such as prenatal corticosteroids, postnatal surfactant, gentle ventilation techniques, and improved nutrition have changed the pathophysiologic characteristics of the disease.[516,523,524]

Infants with the "new" BPD are smaller and more immature than those originally studied by Northway. These infants present with less fibrosis and more uniform patterns of inflation; however, decreased alveolar formation and lung vascularization are still major factors in the disease process.[517,521,525,526] In the "new" BPD, there are fewer and larger simplified alveoli, fewer airway lesions, variable airway hypoplasia, variable interstitial fibroproliferation, dysmorphic vasculature, and atypical patterns of lung cell proliferation.[527,528] Owing to both changes in care practices

and presentation of BPD, the understanding of the pathogenesis and definition has continued to evolve.

In 2000, a consensus workgroup at the National Institutes of Child Health and Human Development (NICHD)/ National Heart, Lung, and Blood Institute (NHLBI) workshop proposed a severity-based definition of BPD.[528] According to this diagnosis, infants born at less than 32 weeks GA requiring supplemental oxygen at 28 days of life had a reassessment done at 36 weeks PMA. Those breathing room air were diagnosed with mild BPD. Those needing less than 30% FiO_2 were diagnosed with moderate BPD, and infants requiring greater than 30% FiO_2 and/or positive pressure ventilation were diagnosed with severe BPD. Walsh et al.[529] developed a physiologic definition for BPD on the basis of a physiologic test that uses objective criteria to establish the need for supplemental oxygen at 36 weeks PMA.[530] This physiologic definition compared with the NICHD/NHLBI definition resulted in a lower BPD rate and less variability in BPD rates in a multicenter study.[530] Recently, Massie et al.[531] published the Proxy-reported Pulmonary Outcome Score (PRPOS), which is scored by nurses before, during, and after care and feeding activities in order to discriminate between infants with no, mild, moderate, and severe pulmonary dysfunction.

Northway et al.[518] originally proposed four major factors in pathogenesis lung immaturity, respiratory failure, oxygen supplementation, and positive pressure ventilation. Research has supported these findings, and additional factors have been identified including inflammation, aberrations in lung growth and signaling pathways, derangements in transcription factors and growth factors, oxidative lung injury, and genetics.[514,532–534]

One of the greatest contributing factors to the development of BPD is the immaturity of the infant's lungs. Extremely premature birth occurs in the saccular stage of parenchymal development when the underdeveloped lung is very vulnerable to injury due to postnatal interventions such as mechanical ventilation and oxygen as well as the effects of inflammation due to infection.[535] Injury at this early stage of lung development can interfere with the development of alveoli and pulmonary microvasculature.[525,535–537]

Prenatal as well as postnatal factors may play a role in the development of BPD. Preeclampsia has been implicated as a risk factor for the development of BPD owing to the factors related to the development of the condition and the resultant effects on the infant such as oxidative stress, IUGR, and preterm birth.[538] Bose et al.[539] found fetal growth restriction to be highly predictive for BPD. In addition, intrauterine infection or colonization such as chorioamnionitis, one of the leading causes of preterm birth, may contribute to the development of BPD. The inflammatory process due to infection has been linked to the development of BPD.[537,540] Studies have shown that *Chlamydia trachomatis* and cytomegalovirus can cause slowly developing pneumonitis. Chorioamnionitis may increase the inflammatory response in premature lungs to injury caused by mechanical ventilation.[525,540,541] Other contributing factors for BPD include hyperoxia and hypoxia, early fluid overload and persistent left-to-right shunting through a PDA, undernutrition, familial airway hyperreactivity, genetic influences, and decreased surfactant synthesis.[517,521,524,525,535] Gender has also been found to be associated with susceptibility of preterm infants to BPD and severity of the disease.[517] Surfactant is synthesized later in gestation in the male fetal lung compared with the females, increasing the risk for acute respiratory distress.[522,542,543]

The most optimal method for prenatal prevention of BPD is the prevention of preterm birth. When premature delivery is inevitable, administration of prenatal steroids and gentle resuscitation with low levels of supplemental oxygen are medical interventions that improve lung maturity and protect lungs from damage respectively.[518,521,535] Postnatal medical treatment strategies are aimed at preventing or limiting the factors that set off the chain of pathogenic sequelae. Respiratory support is used only when necessary and at the lowest peak airway pressure needed to maintain adequate ventilation and decrease barotrauma.[516] NCPAP, iNO, and HFV have been utilized in an attempt to decrease trauma to the lungs.[535] Volume-targeted ventilation has been shown to decrease the incidence of BPD.[544] Target oxygen levels to prevent BPD and poor neurodevelopmental outcome in preterm infants continues to be investigated.[524] Careful fluid and nutrition management are used to provide hydration without overload and to promote growth.[517] Diuretic treatment is used to prevent cor pulmonale, congestive heart failure, and pulmonary edema.[535]Other treatments include infection control with careful monitoring and treatment of bacterial and fungal infections, and bronchodilator therapy is also used to decrease bronchospasm.[516] Corticosteroid treatment has been found to decrease bronchospasm and the inflammatory response; however, early use of inhaled corticosteroids has been associated with neurodevelopmental delay and CP.[524,545] The AAP recommends the use of postnatal corticosteroids on a case-by-case basis.[542] Strategies that may be used in the future to prevent the development of BPD in preterm infants include antioxidant and stem cell therapies.[516,517,524]

Complications associated with BPD are systemic hypertension, metabolic imbalance, hearing loss, ROP, nephrocalcinosis, osteoporosis, GER, and early growth failure.[387,394,396] Pulmonary artery hypertension (PAH) can develop owing to long-term morbidity and is associated with BPD due to pulmonary function abnormalities and reactive airways, neurodevelopmental delays, and growth failure.[546–565] Mortality risk is increased for infants with BPD and PAH.[546] The complications of BPD related to lung growth and function may continue into adolescence and early adulthood.[536,548] Balinotti et al.[536] reported impairment of alveolar development in infants and toddlers with BPD. Increased respiratory illness, respiratory symptoms (cough, wheeze, asthma), impaired pulmonary function tests, and compromised exercise capacity have been documented in preschool- and school-age children, adolescents, and young adults who had CLDI.[548]

Developmental outcomes vary in the literature; however, increased incidence of attention deficits, cognitive deficits, developmental coordination disorder, and poor visual-motor functioning have been found in infants with BPD.[350,352,353,551–559] Preterm infants diagnosed with BPD appear to be at greater risk for adverse neurodevelopmental outcome than preterm infants without BPD.[544,545] Singer et al.[554] found BPD to be a significant independent predictor of poor developmental outcome at 3 years of age. Severity of BPD, based on the NIH consensus definition, has been shown to have an independent adverse relationship with poorer cognitive, motor, behavioral, and language outcomes and CP.[551,558,559] Infants who require supplemental oxygen at 36 weeks PMA are at increased risk for global developmental impairment.[553,559] The incidence of CP has been shown to increase with severity of BPD.[551,552,553] Severity of CP, defined as higher Gross Motor Function Classification System (GMFCS) score and greater distribution of involvement (diplegia and quadriplegia), was found to occur at higher rates with increasing severity of BPD.[560] Van Marter et al.[561] reported that BPD with requirement for mechanical ventilation and supplemental oxygen at 36 weeks PMA was a strong predictor for diplegia and quadriplegia; however, BPD without mechanical ventilation requirement at 36 weeks PMA was not significantly associated with any form of CP. In addition, behavioral and social emotional problems associated with BPD have been reported in the literature.[561,562,563]

Physical Therapy Assessment and Intervention: Bronchopulmonary Dysplasia

The examination of the infant with BPD/CLD begins with a thorough review of medical history by systems as delineated in the "Medical Issues of Prematurity" section. The therapist needs to gather information as to past and current levels of functioning, with particular attention to respiratory status and level of respiratory support. It is important for the therapist to know the individual infant's baseline physiologic parameters and recognize that these may differ from age norms. It is imperative to interview the infant's nurse as to which activities the infant tolerates and which activities cause the baby to enter a cycle of respiratory instability. It is also important for the therapist to know the infant's scores on the pain assessment as recorded by nursing and to continue to assess for pain during the assessment. Babies with BPD are known for their ability to decompensate, have cyanotic episodes or "spells,"[564] and may require medical intervention to recover physiologic stability. When initiating the observation phase of the assessment, the therapist needs to assess heart rate, respiratory rate and pattern, and oxygen saturation at rest and during care activities. Any blood pressure concerns, edema of the trunk and extremities, and skin integrity issues should be noted. In terms of respiratory status, the infant with BPD/CLD may frequently demonstrate tachypnea, which is defined as a respiratory rate greater than

60 breaths per minute. These babies often exhibit paradoxic breathing and recruit accessory respiratory muscles rather than utilizing the typical pattern of abdominal breathing. The baby should be carefully assessed throughout the evaluation for signs of respiratory distress, including retractions of the chest wall, nasal flaring, grunting, and stridor.

A posture and musculoskeletal assessment of the baby provides information relevant to the baby's respiratory function as well as neuromotor development. When handling a baby with BPD, care should be taken owing to the high risk for fragile bones, as discussed in "Metabolic Bone Disease of Prematurity" section. The baby with BPD may develop compensatory motor patterns to assist respiration by opening up the airway and chest and to recruit accessory muscles. Typical posture that may be seen in babies with CLDI/BPD is hyperextension of the head and neck, shoulder elevation and retraction, trunk extension, and anterior pelvic tilt. These postures interfere not only with the development of efficient respiratory function, but possibly also with the infant's ability to develop self-calming, feeding, and fine and gross motor skills. Integumentary assessment should include the presence and integrity of scars on the trunk, specifically from PDA ligation, chest tubes, and abdominal surgery. These scars can cause limitations in trunk range of motion and lead to asymmetric trunk postures. Skin color and temperature should be assessed as indicators of perfusion to the trunk and extremities.

The therapist should attempt a neuromotor assessment as described in the "Physical Therapy Assessment and Intervention: Issues of Prematurity" section on the basis of the infant's physiologic stability and ability to tolerate handling during routine care activities. Prior to the initiation of a neuromotor examination, the therapist should consider which test items may be unduly stressful for the infant and modify the assessment accordingly. Modified hands-on assessment may include diaper change, repositioning, gentle facilitation of active movement, observation of general movements, recoil responses in the extremities, scarf sign, grasp reflex, and self-regulatory strategies.[27] The therapist should pay close attention to the physiologic responses and tolerance to handling. Throughout the assessment, work of breathing and oxygen saturation in the infant should be monitored. Infants with BPD have limited respiratory reserve, and a noxious test item may cause the infant to start a cycle of respiratory distress and compromise that requires medical intervention. Another concern is the energy cost and potential fatigue due to assessment even without severe respiratory decompensation.

A neurodevelopmental assessment needs to be completed as the infant's status allows. As with other areas of assessment, the infant with BPD may have decreased tolerance for developmental activities. Items and procedures of standardized assessment tools may need to be modified to accommodate the infant's level of tolerance. The therapist needs to respect the fact that breathing is always the baby's first priority and developmental activities need to be accomplished

secondarily. The therapist may need to start with modified hands-on assessment and then perform full hands-on assessment when the baby is able to tolerate the handling and length of time needed to complete a standardized test.[19,23,27]

Intervention for the infant with BPD is based on the information synthesized from the assessment. The first important consideration is the baby's reserve capacity and tolerance for activity. Timing of the intervention should be done with the knowledge of sleep patterns and other activities in the infant's schedule in order to avoid undue stress and fatigue. Infants with BPD may demonstrate episodes of irritability and restlessness owing to discomfort and/or hypoxemia. They may have difficulty sleeping because of these factors or disturbance from the environment and caregiving. The therapist can provide suggestions in terms of decreasing environmental stimulation, positioning to support the infant's respiratory status, and assisting the infant in transitioning to deeper sleep states. These activities are not only developmentally appropriate, but they also help to decrease stress and energy expenditure and promote lung healing and growth. As babies with BPD may spend many months in the NICU, it is important to continually assess the baby and progress intervention within his or her tolerance.

While posture and alignment should be assessed, the therapist must consider the baby's ability to tolerate a more optimal postural alignment while maintaining respiratory stability. Infants with BPD may use posture and postural muscles to assist respiration. Positioning to promote optimal alignment should be focused on ameliorating effects of atypical postures and promoting positions that allow for self-regulation, support respiration and future musculoskeletal and neuromotor development. One change should be made at a time followed by a period of observation to allow the infant to adjust to the change. It may be necessary to provide scar massage to improve the flexibility of scar tissue and thereby improve the flexibility and alignment of the trunk. Specific treatment strategies are discussed in detail in the care path developed by Byrne and Garber.[28]

The infant with BPD may have limited reserves for motor activities and social interaction owing to the high energy costs of the lung disease. It is extremely important that the therapist in the NICU learn to read the infant's cues of distress and availability for interaction. The therapist can assist parents in recognizing their infant's cues so they can provide comfort or social interactions appropriate to the infant's needs and availability. The parents can assist the infant in developing self-calming skills. This in turn helps to foster parental roles and enhances their abilities to care for their infant. The infant benefits from the parental interaction as well as the support to develop behavioral organization skills. Parents benefit from these opportunities to bond with their infant over the course of what can be a long hospitalization. The therapist must assess the best learning style for the parent and provide parent education to support independence with developmental interventions during hospitalization and after transition to home.[451,452]

Activities to promote motor skills and postural control can be built into routines of the day such as feeding, burping, diaper changes, and bathing.[28] Opportunities to practice developmental skills should be built into the infant's daily routines. Developmental activities should be appropriate to the infant's ability to interact and play. Suggestions for play positions and activities along with precautions based on the baby's cues should also be provided to the infant's family and care providers. Physical therapists should collaborate with other members of the care team to find creative ways to safely provide opportunities for supported upright and prone positions that can be integrated into daily routines and developmental play activities for infants who require long-term intubation. Shephard et al.[565] found improved neurodevelopmental outcomes and decreased readmission rates with a comprehensive interdisciplinary approach to the management of infants with BPD. Discharge planning should be addressed throughout admission and finalized as discharge approaches. It is important that parents feel comfortable with developmental interventions in order for continued participation in these activities at home.[451,453]

The Baby Who Requires Surgery

This section includes some of the more common fetal malformations that require surgical intervention in infancy, including CDH, omphalocele, GS, and tracheal esophageal fistula (TEF). Lastly, a brief review of fetal surgical interventions is included.

Congenital Diaphragmatic Hernia

CDH is a defect in the formation of the respiratory diaphragm during embryogenesis, and is estimated to occur in 1 per 2200 births.[566] During the 3rd to 16th week of gestation, when lung bronchi and pulmonary arteries are undergoing critical development,[566] the pleuroperitoneal cavity fails to close, allowing the developing abdominal viscera (bowel, stomach, liver) to protrude through the opening in the diaphragm into the hemithorax. The viscera compresses the developing lung on the ipsilateral side, resulting in decreased bronchial branching and lung mass (pulmonary hypoplasia)[568]; the contralateral lung may be affected as well if the herniated bowel causes a mediastinal shift, placing pressure on the contralateral lung.[569] Compression of the lung promotes overmuscularization of the pulmonary arterial tree, leading to pulmonary hypertension.[568] These changes then generate a dysfunctional surfactant system and a secondary surfactant deficiency.[570–572] The effects are most severe on the ipsilateral side of the diaphragmatic defect.[568]

Because the left hemidiaphragm is larger and closes later than the right, the defect occurs more frequently on the left (80% to 85%); right-sided CDHs occur in 10% to 15%, and bilateral herniation is rare.[571–573] Pulmonary hypoplasia and pulmonary hypertension caused by CDH can vary in severity and is responsible for the high neonatal mortality and long-term morbidity associated with CDH.[566]

The diagnosis of CDH is made by prenatal ultrasound, demonstrating the presence of abdominal contents in the pleuroperitoneal cavity and a mediastinal shift.[566,574] Prenatal diagnosis is improved by advancing GA, the presence of associated abnormalities, and when an experienced ultrasonographer performs the test. Mean age at prenatal diagnosis is 24 weeks.[575] Newborns with CDH, who are not diagnosed in utero, present with respiratory distress, barrel-shaped chest, scaphoid abdomen, absence of breath sounds on the ipsilateral side, presence of bowel sounds in the chest, displaced heart sounds, and chest X-ray showing abdominal contents in the hemithorax.[566]

Fifty to sixty percent of CDH cases are considered "isolated" or without associated anomalies. Pulmonary hypoplasia, intestinal malrotation, and cardiac dextroposition are considered part of the CDH sequence and are not associated anomalies. The other 40% to 50% of babies with CDH can have structural malformations (such as esophageal atresia [EA], omphalocele, and cleft palate), and chromosomal anomalies like trisomies 18, 13, and 21.[566] The majority of stillborn infants with CDH have associated anomalies like neural tube defects and cardiac anomalies.[575–577]

Prognosis for survival is worse for babies with an abnormal karyotype, severe associated anomalies, right-sided defect, liver herniation, and lower lung volumes. The severity of lung hypoplasia can be assessed by fetal MRI, or 3D sonography. Another useful prognostic measurement is the lung area–to–head circumference ratio. This is calculated by measuring the contralateral lung at the level of the atria and dividing it by the fetal head circumference.[574] The absence of liver herniation is the most reliable prenatal prognosticator of postnatal survival.[578]

Mothers with a prenatal diagnosis of CDH are counseled to deliver in a perinatal center with neonatal and pediatric surgical and ECMO capabilities.[579] The baby is monitored closely during pregnancy, labor, and delivery as the risk of fetal demise is 3% to 8%.[574] There is some evidence to suggest that delivery at slightly early-term gestation (37 to 38 weeks) helps to prevent the severity of pulmonary hypoplasia and pulmonary hypertension.[574]

Once the baby is born, the surgical repair is delayed until after the baby's pulmonary status and PAH have stabilized, which can take hours or days. Initial management involves intubation to prevent acidosis and hypoxia, which can increase the risk of pulmonary hypertension, gentle ventilation to prevent risk of barotrauma to hypoplastic lungs, and stomach decompression to avoid further lung compression. Umbilical arterial and venous lines are placed to provide medication and fluids. Medication to support blood pressure is administered to prevent right-to-left shunting. If the baby does not respond to the maximum conventional ventilatory therapy, he or she may be placed on ECMO. Children with CDH, whether they receive ECMO therapy or not, require close follow-up as there is a high incidence of sensorineural hearing loss, GER, failure to thrive, feeding problems, seizures, developmental delay, pectus excavatum, and scoliosis in these patients.[566,569]

Omphalocele

Defects in the anterior abdominal wall of the fetus are reported to occur in 1 per 2000 live births.[580] Less common defects include pentalogy of Cantrell, cloacal exstrophy, and body stalk defect; the two most common abdominal wall defects, omphalocele and gastroschisis, are described next.[580-582]

At the beginning of the sixth embryologic week, when the gut is developing faster than the embryonic body, a temporary physiologic herniation of the intestines into the base of the umbilical stalk occurs. Four weeks later, the intestines return into the embryologic abdominal cavity and the four ectomesodermal folds (caudal, cephalic, and two lateral) join to close the abdominal wall.[583] If the intestines fail to migrate back into the embryonic abdominal cavity, an omphalocele is formed, where the intestines are herniated into the base of the umbilicus.[584-586] If the abdominal wall fails to close, the liver may also herniate into the base of the umbilicus, resulting in a giant omphalocele.[587-589] Associated abdominal muscles, fascia, and skin are absent; however, the protruding sac containing fetal intestines, and liver, if present, is covered by the amnion and peritoneum membranes.

The incidence of omphalocele is approximately 1 per 5000 live births and is more common in women of young, less than 20 years, or advanced, greater than 40 years, maternal age.[590,591] Omphalocele occurs more frequently with fetal aneuploidy (35% to 60%) and structural anomalies (50% to 70%).[581,582,592,593] Reported associated syndromes include trisomy 13, 15, 16, 18, and 21, Beckwith–Wiedemann syndrome, pentalogy of Cantrell, and OEIS syndrome (omphalocele, exstrophy of the bladder, imperforate anus, spinal defects). Reported associated structural anomalies include congenital heart defects, diaphragmatic and upper midline defects, malrotation of the intestines, intestinal atresia, and genitourinary anomalies.[581,590,594] Babies with giant omphalocele (containing liver) are more likely to have a normal karyotype but a poorer neonatal outcome.[590,594-596] Amniotic fluid abnormalities (oligohydramnios or polyhydramnios) in the presence of omphalocele are associated with a poorer prognosis.[590]

Prenatal diagnosis is often made after positive maternal serum alpha-feto protein screen and/or by ultrasound before the 12th week if the omphalocele contains the liver or after the 12th week if not.[590] Because chromosomal abnormalities and structural anomalies are commonly present in babies with omphalocele, the obstetric workup typically includes a fetal karyotype, echocardiogram, and MRI. After prenatal diagnosis, the family is usually referred to pediatric surgeons, neonatologists, genetic counselors, and maternal–fetal medicine specialists, social work and other specialists on the basis of the presence of structural anomalies. Delivery at a tertiary care center is recommended; some physicians recommend Cesarean section[581,582]; however, the mode of delivery, surgical versus vaginal, has not been studied systematically. Most perinatologists recommend Cesarean deliveries for babies with omphalocele with liver herniation.[581,582,590,597] Fetal growth and well-being is monitored closely via serial ultrasounds and weekly fetal non-stress testing or biophysical profile monitoring. A quarter to more than a half of pregnancies deliver preterm,[590,597] and males are affected more than females.[595] The defect is associated with a small abdominal cavity.[585,586]

The postdelivery management of a newborn with an omphalocele includes the placement of an orogastric tube to decompress the stomach, intravenous access for antibiotics and fluids, airway stabilization, and ventilatory assistance. The omphalocele sac requires sterile dressings to minimize heat and fluid loss.[586,590,598] The amount of displaced intestine can vary from a small amount hardly distinguishable from an umbilical hernia to a massive amount with the entire midgut and liver present in the umbilical cord.[584] Depending on the size of the defect, surgical repair may be a primary or staged closure, or more recently, the topical application of an eschar-inducing agent to promote epithelization and a planned surgical closure later.[581,582] Babies with defects less than 2 cm have a primary direct closure. Babies with defects from 2 to 9 cm undergo a staged closure with a silo compression dressing. Babies with defects greater than 10 cm receive the topical dressing agent.[590]

In a staged closure, the baby is positioned in supine with the viscera suspended above the patient in a compression dressing called a silo.[581,582,585] The omphalocele is reduced gradually over several days to a week to return the viscera into the abdominal cavity.[585] While undergoing this process, the baby is paralyzed with a neuromuscular blockade while the fascial defect and abdominal wall are stretched with tissue expanders to accommodate the contents of the omphalocele sac. At closure, the surgeons usually perform an appendectomy to prevent an atypical presentation of appendicitis later in life and insert a gastrostomy tube for decompression. These babies often require aggressive ventilatory support postoperatively,[581,582,585,586,590,599] as the abdominal contents impede diaphragmatic movement and limit lung expansion. Owing to the large pressures required to expand the lungs against a large abdominal mass, BPD and CLD are frequent long-term consequences for these babies. Other long-term complications these babies can endure include feeding difficulties due to the prolonged period of decreased oral stimulation and tachypnea resulting from shallow breathing, and impaired growth.[581,582,586] Feeding intolerance can result in prolonged use of total parenteral nutrition and long hospitalizations.[585] In addition, the other anomalies associated with omphalocele have a major impact on the developmental outcome of the baby.[586]

Gastroschisis (GS)

Unlike omphalocele, a GS (Greek for "belly cleft") is a full-thickness abdominal wall defect, adjacent and usually to the right of the umbilicus. For reasons unclear, some evidence suggests a vascular compromise, in the tenth gestational week, when the four folds of the embryo should meet at the umbilicus and close the abdominal cavity, a defect in the abdominal wall occurs allowing the abdominal contents to leak out of the abdominal cavity.[580] Small bowel, stomach, colon, and ovaries can protrude and become thick, matted, and leathery as a result of contact with the amniotic fluid (chemical peritonitis).[583,584,600] GS is an isolated defect, often associated with prematurity and LBW but infrequently (10%) associated with congenital anomalies outside of the GI tract.[601,602] Other coexistent bowel abnormalities such as intestinal atresia and malrotation are present in 25% of the cases.[601,603] It has a higher incidence in younger (less than 20 years) primigravid mothers and mothers with a history of vasoconstrictive drug use and cigarette smoking.[583,600] The incidence of GS is reported to be 1 to 5 per 10,000, with prevalence increasing worldwide in a variety of geographic areas such as Hawaii, North Carolina, Georgia in the United States, and England, Ireland, and Canada.[583,601] Incidence is similar in males and females.[601,604–606] There is an increased familial risk of recurrence in families with a child with GS, which demonstrates that GS has a multifactorial etiology where environmental triggers as well as genetics contribute.[601,607–610]

GS is associated with elevated maternal serum alpha-fetoprotein screen; diagnosis is made by prenatal ultrasound showing a small abdominal wall defect to right of midline with visceral herniation of an intestinal mass floating freely in the amniotic fluid. A pregnancy with a diagnosis of GS is followed closely with serial ultrasounds every 2 to 4 weeks. Poor intrauterine growth is a poor prognostic feature.[594,601] Because there is an increased risk of third-trimester fetal demise, nonstress tests, biophysical profiles, and amniotic fluid indices are followed closely after 30 weeks.[601,611–615] As with omphalocele, best practice includes coordinating the delivery at a tertiary care center, although there are no evidence-based recommendations for timing or mode of delivery. Initial postnatal and surgical management is similar to babies born with omphalocele, where decompressing the stomach, stabilizing the airway, and wrapping the bowel in sterile dressings to preserve heat and minimize fluid loss are postnatal priorities.

Tracheal Esophageal Fistula (TEF)

Between the third and the sixth weeks of gestation, the primitive foregut is in the process of separating into the respiratory and alimentary tracts.[573] A defect in the lateral septation of the foregut into the esophagus and trachea causes a TEF.[616–618] TEF is the most common congenital anomaly of the respiratory tract with an incidence of 1 per 3500 live births.[616–621] Ninety-five percent of TEFs occur with EA; TEF is classified according to the anatomic configuration and is most commonly present (84%) as a proximal esophageal pouch and a distal TEF (type C).[584,616,619,621]

Many babies with TEF are not diagnosed prenatally. Babies with EA may present with polyhydramnios in utero[616,622] or present immediately after birth with an accumulation of oral secretions (due to ineffective swallowing), respiratory difficulties, and coughing, choking, and cyanosis with feeds. The medical staff is unable to pass a tube through the nose and into the stomach, and a radiograph may show the tube coiled in the upper esophageal pouch.

The rare TEF without EA (H type) is difficult to diagnose. Unlike babies with EA, babies with H type TEF may be asymptomatic at birth, or they may cough or choke with feeds. Diagnosis of an isolated TEF can be made on upper GI series where the contrast dye is pulled superiorly during the study or by use of 3D computed tomography (CT) scanning.[616,623–627] About half of babies with TEF also have other associated anomalies, often as part of the VACTERL association (vertebral anomalies, anal atresia, congenital heart defects, TEF, EA, renal abnormalities, limb deformities).[617,628]

Treatment of TEF/EA requires surgical ligation of the fistula and anastomosis of the esophagus; however, if the distance separating the two ends of the esophagus is great, a staged repair, including elongation of the esophagus, circular myotomies of the existing esophagus, or replacing the missing esophagus with a portion of the small or large intestine is required.[585,616,629–640] A gastrostomy tube is placed to allow feeding while the baby heals from surgery. Treatment of isolated TEF is less difficult; the fistula can be ligated and prognosis is good.[616,641–643]

Prognosis of TEF/EA is less assured and depends on the presence of other associated anomalies as well as the distance between the two esophageal pouches. Both short- and long-term complications of TEF/EA occur more commonly. Short-term complications include anastomotic leak, esophageal strictures, tracheomalacia, and disturbed peristalsis. Long-term complications include motility disorders, respiratory function abnormalities, and in some cases esophageal squamous cell cancer (Fig. 4.22).[420,585,616,644–650]

Fetal Surgery

The widespread use of prenatal imaging and diagnostic techniques beginning in the 1960s[651] has stimulated the development of a variety of methods to intervene during pregnancy to ameliorate the development of structural problems in the fetus. Fetal surgery has grown out of the understanding of the progression of an untreated condition and the belief that prenatal intervention could ameliorate damage to developing organs.[567,579,423,652] In 1982, the International Fetal Medicine and Surgery Society (IFMSS) formed and later established rigorous criteria for fetal surgery to protect both members of the maternal–fetal dyad. These guidelines include[653]:

1. Accurate diagnosis and prognosis must be possible.
2. No available postnatal effective therapy.
3. Experimental proof of safe effective prenatal intervention exists.
4. Interventions are done within a strict protocol by a trained multidisciplinary team.

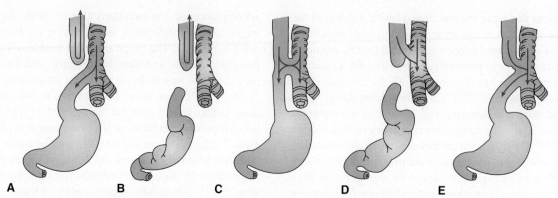

FIGURE 4.22 Esophageal atresia and tracheoesophageal fistula. (From Pillitteri A. *Maternal and Child Nursing.* 4th ed. Philadelphia, PA: Lippincott Williams & Wilkins; 2003.)

A commitment to evidence-based practice requires that all aspects of the practice of fetal surgery be tested for efficacy or harm for women and their babies; this includes the effects and timing of anesthesia, other pharmacologic agents, bed rest, and procedures on the mother and the fetus.[654]

In the 1990s, with the development of the laparoscope, minimally invasive fetal surgery was born and the possibility of vaginal delivery replaced the mandatory Cesarean section of open fetal surgery.[651,655] Minimally invasive fetal surgery includes needle techniques, where a sharp needle is introduced into the uterine cavity to sample blood or provide a transfusion, and endoscopic techniques, where a laser or other device is introduced to provide the intervention. Both techniques rely on ultrasound guidance.[655] These advances have improved outcomes over open fetal surgery techniques for both mother and baby such as decreased length of hospital stay and decreased incidence of placental abruption. However, there are two enduring complications of fetal surgery: amniotic fluid leakage and preterm (less than 37 weeks' gestation) prelabor rupture of membranes or PPROM.[651,655]

There are some diseases that require open fetal surgery using a maternal laparotomy, and hysterotomy and direct access to the fetus, such as resection of large congenital airway malformations, sacralcoccygeal teratomas, and repair of fetal myelomeningocele.[651]

The MOM's (Management of Myelomeningocele) trial, a multicenter RCT to examine the efficacy of prenatal versus postnatal repair of spina bifida ended in December 2010. Ninety-one subjects received fetal repair and 92 postnatal repair. The New England Journal of Medicine[656] reported results of 158 patients at 12 months of age. The prenatal surgery group had a 40% rate of shunt placement; the postnatal surgery had an 82% rate. At 30 months, the prenatal repair group demonstrated improved Bayley scores for mental development and motor function, decreased rates of hindbrain herniation at 12 months, and improved ambulation by 30 months. However, prenatal repair was associated with increased premature delivery as well as uterine dehiscence at

delivery.[656] On the basis of this RCT, fetal repair of MMC is now offered as standard of care in eight centers around the country.[657]

An additional fetal surgery success story involves babies with twin-to-twin transfusion syndrome (TTTS). A multicenter RCT showed a clear advantage in length of gestation, survival, and incidence of PVL associated with prenatal endoscopic laser ablation of communicating placental vessels over serial amnioreduction of polyhydramnios. Prenatal TTTS has become the most common indication for fetal surgery today.[651]

Currently, there are two RCTs being conducted in Europe for prenatal tracheal occlusion to treat CDH.[658] This is a different technique developed after a trial of open hysterotomy to perform a more typical postnatal repair prenatally.

Fetal surgery will continue to evolve in response to refinements in technique and technologic advances, progress in postnatal therapies, and as new insights into fetal pathophysiology are gained.

Physical Therapy Assessment and Intervention for the Baby Who Requires Surgery

Although a baby in an NICU who requires surgery may not have been born prematurely, he or she may demonstrate immaturity and instability in any of the subsystems described in the synactive theory. Babies who require surgery may experience more immobility and pain than other babies in the NICU. It is important that issues of pain be addressed before the therapist proceeds with any direct intervention.

As with any other examination, the therapist starts with a thorough review of the chart with particular attention to the indications for surgery, the surgical procedure, the outcome of the surgery, and any precautions or contraindications. The nurse should be interviewed to find out how the baby's pain is managed and whether the current pain management is adequate for the baby at rest and during nursing care. A baby who requires surgical intervention may also need technologic supports such as mechanical ventilation, chest tubes with or without suction, drains, or gastric suctioning devices. These supports can also add to the baby's discomfort as well as limit his or her ability to be positioned and moved. The therapist should assess the surgical incisions for how they are healing and for the presence of scar tissue. The healing process can be delayed by the presence of antibiotic-resistant bacteria and the risk of iatrogenic infections, which can prolong the baby's hospitalization. Prolonged illness, immobilization, and hospitalization can interfere with the baby's acquisition of developmental milestones as well as with his or her socialization and ability to bond, placing him or her at greater risk for delays. Living in a crisis-prone environment disadvantages children who "grow old in the NICU" as they experience multiple caregivers, limited interactions with family, and limited opportunities to move, practice developmental activities, and have typical sensory experiences. In addition, staff may feel challenged to provide the appropriate stimulation in the newborn intensive care setting.[659]

The assessment should also include the impact of the surgical intervention on the infant's respiratory function. The rate and the pattern of the baby's breathing should be examined as it may be influenced by the presence of scarring, thoracic and abdominal pressure changes, anatomic changes, pain, edema, and lack of musculoskeletal support. In addition, the above may also affect the baby's passive and active range of motion. For these patients, it is important to assess their developmental skills in an ongoing fashion.

Owing to the nature of the illness and intensive care these babies require, they often demonstrate developmental delays and the NICU therapist's role may change from primarily consultative to more traditional "hands-on" during the course of the infant's hospitalization.

Interventions for a baby who has had surgery can include positioning, mobilization of soft tissue, facilitation of sensory responses, postural control, and gross and fine motor activities. It is frequent for the initial portions of each therapy session to focus on mobilization techniques for alignment and flexibility prior to handling activities to promote developmental skills. It is not uncommon for babies who have required surgical intervention to their thoracic or abdominal areas to develop asymmetric postures. This may be due to the underlying anatomic lesion or result from postsurgical scarring and limitations to positioning. In addition, positioning programs can be developed and caregivers can be shown techniques to incorporate mobilization into daily routines. The therapist should provide developmentally appropriate activity suggestions to family and NICU staff. This can be in the form of direct teaching as well as posting play ideas at the infant's bedside.

The Baby with Neurologic Issues

The Baby with Asphyxia

Perinatal asphyxia is a result of a lack of oxygen (hypoxia) and/or a lack of perfusion (ischemia) to various organs.[660] The incidence of asphyxia is 2 to 6 per 1000 births.[378]

It is more frequent in preterm infants (60% in VLBW births), where it is usually associated with PVH/IVH,[430] and accounts for 20% of perinatal deaths. Asphyxia is more likely to occur in term infants of diabetic or toxemic mothers and is also associated with IUGR and breech presentation. Ninety percent of asphyxiated births are estimated to occur as a result of placental insufficiency during the antepartum or intrapartum periods.[660] However, cardiopulmonary anomalies of the fetus are also a risk factor for asphyxia.[430] All babies experience hypoxia during normal labor but not to a degree that is damaging. An umbilical cord or fetal scalp pH less than 7.0 may indicate substantial intrauterine asphyxia. Other supporting evidence includes the presence of meconium staining, abnormalities in fetal heart rate and rhythm, and an Apgar score of less than or equal to 3 for greater than 5 minutes. The organs most susceptible to damage during asphyxia are the kidneys, brain, heart, and lungs, with the most important consequence of perinatal asphyxia being hypoxic–ischemic encephalopathy (HIE).[660] There must be evidence of hypoxia and ischemia to make the diagnosis of HIE, and there may also be an underlying neurologic disturbance predisposing the baby to a hypoxic–ischemic event.[661]

HIE can range from mild to severe. Ten percent to 20% of term asphyxiated infants die, and the remainder who survive have a good chance of developing normally even in the presence of seizures in the neonatal period. However, there is a small group of severely asphyxiated infants who, having escaped death, will develop major neurologic sequelae, including CP, mental retardation, seizure disorder,[660] cortical blindness, hearing impairment, and microcephaly.[378] A baby who has been asphyxiated may develop any of the following five neurologic lesions:

1. Focal or multifocal cortical necrosis
2. Watershed infarcts (occurring in the boundary zones between cerebral and cerebellar arteries where blood flow is reduced with hypotension or hypoperfusion)
3. Selective neuronal necrosis (brainstem nuclei or Purkinje cells in the cerebellum)
4. Status marmoratus (necrosis of the thalamic nuclei and basal ganglia with myelination of astrocytic processes versus neurons)
5. PVL[378,430,660]

More extensive lesions occur with more severe asphyxia. Partial episodes of asphyxia result in diffuse cerebral necrosis, whereas total asphyxia spares the cortex and affects the brainstem, thalamus, and basal ganglia. The Sarnat clinical stages (Table 4.10) are used to estimate the severity of asphyxiation in infants greater than 36 weeks' gestation and are based on clinical presentation and duration of symptoms.[660] Asphyxiation in a preterm infant is more difficult to recognize owing to the brain immaturity, hypotonia, and immature reflexes. Premature infants may be protected from HIE by their immaturity, as the more mature the organism at the time of the asphyxia, the shorter the duration needed to cause brain damage.[430] The most effective intervention is prevention of asphyxia by establishing ventilation and perfusion and minimizing hypotension and hypoxia. Babies should be handled with care with the intention to minimize stress and to avoid fluctuations in blood pressure and sensory overload and to teach parents to do the same (Table 4.10).[378]

The Baby with Seizures

Seizures in the neonatal period are difficult to recognize and diagnose because the perinatal brain is functionally and morphologically immature. The electrical discharge underlying a seizure depends on synaptic connections, axonal/dendritic arborization, and myelination, making the well-organized motoric patterns of a seizure in an older infant unlikely in a newborn.[662] The expression of a seizure in a newborn generally manifests as chewing, lip smacking, sucking, apnea, and gaze abnormalities, probably due to the relative maturity of the limbic structures and their connections to the brainstem.[663] There are five types of seizure patterns:

1. Subtle seizures are the most common in term and preterm infants, comprising about 50% of all seizures in this population. They occur most commonly with other seizures. They may not demonstrate EEG correlation and may be refractory to anticonvulsant treatment. They include tonic horizontal deviation of the eyes, oral/buccal/lingual movements, swimming/bicycling movements, apnea, and other autonomic phenomena.[662,663]

2. Focal clonic seizures are characterized by localized clonic jerking with a fast contraction phase and a slower relaxation phase not associated with loss of consciousness. They are usually due to metabolic disturbances, an underlying structural lesion in the contralateral cerebral hemisphere, or focal traumatic injury, and have a good prognostic outcome.[662,663]

3. Multifocal clonic seizures consist of random clonic movement of a limb that migrates to other limbs. This

TABLE 4.10 Sarnat and Sarnat Stages* of Hypoxic–Ischemic Encephalopathy

Stage	Stage 1 (Mild)	Stage 2 (Moderate)	Stage 3 (Severe)
Level of consciousness	Hyperalert: irritable	Lethargic or obtunded	Stuporous, comatose
Neuromuscular control:	Uninhibited, overreactive	Diminished spontaneous movement	Diminished or absent spontaneous movement
Muscle tone	Normal	Mild hypotonia	Flaccid
Posture	Mild distal flexion	Strong distal flexion	Intermittent decerebration
Stretch reflexes	Overactive	Overactive, disinhibited	Decreased or absent
Segmental myoclonus	Present or absent	Present	Absent
Complex reflexes:	Normal	Suppressed	Absent
Suck	Weak	Weak or absent	Absent
Moro	Strong, low threshold	Weak, incomplete high threshold	Absent
Oculovestibular	Normal	Overactive	Weak or absent
Tonic neck	Slight	Strong	Absent
Autonomic function:	Generalized sympathetic	Generalized parasympathetic	Both systems depressed
Pupils	Mydriasis	Miosis	Midposition, often use poor light reflex
Respirations	Spontaneous	Spontaneous; occasional apnea	Periodic; apnea
Heart rate	Tachycardia	Bradycardia	Variable
Bronchial and salivary secretions	Sparse	Profuse	Variable
Gastrointestinal motility	Normal or decreased	Increased diarrhea	Variable
Seizures	None	Common focal or multifocal (6–24 hr of age)	Uncommon (excluding decerebration)
Electroencephalographic findings	Normal (awake)	Early: generalized low voltage, slowing (continuous delta and theta) Later: periodic pattern (awake): seizures focal or multifocal; 1.0–1.5 Hz spike and wave	Early: periodic pattern with isopotential pH Later: totally isopotential
Duration of symptoms	<24 hr	2–14 days	Hours to weeks
Outcome	About 100% normal	80% normal; abnormal if symptoms more than 5–7 days	About 50% die; remainder with severe sequelae

*The stages in this table are a continuum reflecting the spectrum of clinical states of infants over 36 weeks' gestational age.
From Sarnat HB, Sarnat MS. Neonatal encephalopathy following fetal distress: a clinical and electroencephalographic study. *Arch Neurol.* 1976;33:696.
Reprinted with permission from Aurora S, Snyder EY. Perinatal asphyxia. In: Cloherty JP, Eichenwald EC, Stark AR, eds. *Manual of Neonatal Care.* 5th ed. Philadelphia, PA: Lippincott Williams & Wilkins; 2004:542–543.

is rare in a newborn because of the immaturity of the newborn brain to propagate the discharge throughout the brain.[662,663]

4. Tonic seizures can be focal or generalized and resemble the decerebrate or decorticate posturing of older children involving tonic flexion or extension of the neck, trunk, and upper extremities with tonic lower extremity extension. Prognosis can vary, but in general is poor.[662,663]

5. Myoclonic seizures are characterized by twitching of one or several body parts and can include the head and trunk as well. They are distinguished from clonic seizures by their speed and irregular pattern. They are associated with diffuse CNS pathology and carry a poor prognosis.[662,663]

The underlying etiologies of a seizure in a newborn can include CNS trauma, metabolic abnormalities, infection, brain malformation, drugs, polycythemia, and focal infarct, and is unknown in 3% to 25% of cases. Recurrent or continuous seizures can cause biochemical effects leading to brain damage. The goal of medical intervention is to identify and treat the underlying cause of the seizure in addition to controlling the seizure through the administration of anticonvulsants. Prognosis depends on the precipitating condition as well as the duration of the seizures and the presence of tonic or myoclonic seizure patterns. Fifteen percent of babies die, 30% have long-term neurologic sequelae, and 55% have a normal outcome.[662,663]

Physical Therapy Assessment and Intervention for the Baby with Neurologic Issues

The therapist should begin the assessment with a thorough chart review as discussed previously. Particular attention should be paid to the neurology consultation, neuroradiographic studies (cranial ultrasound, MRI, CT scan), and EEGs in terms of the area of lesion(s), size of the lesion(s), and clinical findings. The therapist should be aware of the prognosis made by the physician and whether that information has been communicated to the family. The family members should also be interviewed to ascertain their level of understanding of their infant's condition and prognosis. Attention should also be paid to the medical/surgical intervention such as medications, CSF tapping, and shunting or ventriculostomy. During examination, the therapist should take into consideration the effects of medications such as anticonvulsants that can decrease arousal and muscle tone.

Prior to beginning a hands-on assessment, the therapist should speak to the infant's nurse and family about the events of the infant's day as this may affect the baby's energy level, sleep and awake schedule, and tolerance for the evaluation. The therapist needs to know whether the observed behaviors are typical for the infant. If the infant has seizures, the therapist should inquire as to the typical presentation of seizure activity and whether there are triggers for seizures. Other questions for the infant's nurse include timing of administration of seizure medication, presence and quality

of aroused states, observed active movement, and atypical posturing.

A crucial part of the assessment focuses on muscle tone; however, infant behavioral state impacts muscle tone and motor behaviors. Infants who have sustained a neurologic insult may present with atypical states that lack variety, lack smooth transitions, and limit interaction. For example, the infant may only display a sleep state or irritable wakeful state. Completing a neurologic assessment in either of these two states would limit the accuracy; however, the therapist can still obtain useful information by observing active movement of trunk and extremities. Active movement should be observed for symmetry, smoothness, variety, complexity, and isolation. The infant should be reassessed in a serial fashion for changes in behavioral state organization and neuromotor status. When appropriate, a neurologic assessment including reflexes, range of motion, and muscle tone should be completed. There are some babies who present with symmetric active movement but may demonstrate asymmetries in elicited responses. Examples include a brisk gallant response, stronger palmar/plantar grasp reflex on one side, and/or asymmetric French angles (Fig. 4.23). These may be subtle signs and should be monitored as they have been predictive of neuromotor outcomes.[664]

Intervention for infants with a neurologic insult should begin with adapting their environment to support their behavioral state. For the infant who is unable to achieve wakeful states, the therapist can suggest strategies to arouse the infant such as unswaddling, using a soothing voice, setting low illumination, tactile stimulation, diaper change, or a sponge bath. An infant who only displays irritability when awake may benefit from modifying the environment to decrease stimulation. These modifications include swaddling, NNS, containment, proprioceptive input, and facilitation of slow transitions to and from awake states. Once state issues have improved, the therapist will want to address neuromotor and musculoskeletal concerns. Owing to muscle tone and limited active movement, the infant may demonstrate tightness with range of motion and require interventions such as gentle stretching and splinting. A referral for occupational therapy services may be required to evaluate the need for hand splints. Strategies for positioning and handling to promote symmetric postures and movements should be provided to the family and caregiving staff.

Medical Issues of the Late Preterm Infant

The late preterm infant is born between 34 and 36 and 6/7 weeks GA and is formerly known as the "near-term" infant, a term that implies similar needs and care to the term infant. However, recently, it has been recognized that these infants are more vulnerable and have needs more similar to preterm infants. Late preterm births have risen in incidence over the past three decades in the United States, related both to an increase in medically indicated births and an increase in multiple deliveries as part of the use of assisted

Neurologic Development of the High-Risk Infant

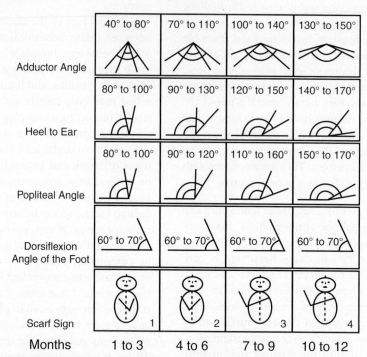

FIGURE 4.23 Symmetric active movement demonstrating asymmetries in elicited responses, as seen in these French angles. (Reprinted with permission from Ellison PH. Neurologic development of the high-risk infant. *Clin Perinatol.* 11(1):45 and adapted from Amiel-Tison C. A method for neurological evaluation within the first year of life. *Curr Probl Pediatr.* 1976;7(1):45.)

reproductive technology.[664–669] Late preterm births account for over 250,000 births per year.[664] The following section describes the medical issues of the late preterm infant.

The late preterm infant has higher morbidity, higher rates of hospital readmission through the first year, and may be at increased risk for long-term neurodevelopmental impairment compared with her term counterpart.[664,670–674] The multiple vulnerabilities are a result of the late preterm infant's overall immaturity. For example, terminal respiratory sacs and lung alveoli continue to mature through the 36th gestational week. The surfactant surge, typically occurring at 34 weeks, responsible for assisting this pulmonary maturation may be missed by the infant born in the late preterm period. The respiratory morbidities of the late preterm infant include transient tachypnea, persistent pulmonary hypertension, RDS, pneumonia, and respiratory failure requiring mechanical ventilation.[664,673,675–677] For each advancing week of gestation, an infant's need for respiratory intervention and vulnerability for respiratory morbidities decreases.[664,670,673,678] Another example of the late preterm infant's immaturity contributing to his vulnerability is the interplay of the underdeveloped hepatic bilirubin conjugation pathways, poor feeding and swallowing coordination, and not fully formed blood–brain barrier. These multiple immaturities increase the risk of prolonged jaundice and bilirubin-induced brain injury in the late preterm infant.[664,670,673,679,680] In addition, late preterm infants have less adipose tissue, larger surface area–to-weight ratio, and are less capable of generating heat, leading to hypothermia. Apnea and bradycardia are more common in the late preterm infant as well.[664,670,679–684] There is some evidence that long-term neurodevelopmental outcome can be affected in this population as well, with some researchers reporting increased incidences of both CP and intellectual disability,[664,684–689] although others have not reported this.[664,690]

Medical Issues of the Term Infant

While prematurity and its associated complications represent the concerns of a large number of infants in the NICU, there are a number of conditions that can cause full-term infants to require intensive care management. These infants are often very critically ill, have extended hospitalizations, and benefit from neonatal physical therapy services. A number of these more common conditions and related interventions are discussed in this section.

Meconium Aspiration Syndrome

In the presence of acute or chronic hypoxia, the fetus may pass meconium into the amniotic fluid prior to delivery. The act of gasping for the first breath may cause the infant to aspirate the meconium-stained amniotic fluid in the lungs where particles of meconium can obstruct airways, interfere with gas exchange, and result in respiratory distress with varying degrees of severity from mild respiratory distress to life-threatening respiratory failure requiring resuscitation.[691-694] Meconium staining is reported to occur in approximately 9% of births.[691-693]

MAS is presumed in newborn infants who, after being born through meconium-stained fluid, demonstrate respiratory distress that cannot be explained by another mechanism.[691,695] Approximately 2% to 10% of infants born through meconium-stained amniotic fluid demonstrate MAS.[691-693] The risk of meconium aspiration is largest in postmature infants as well as SGA infants.[691,696-699] Owing to changes in obstetric care in recent years in the United States, specifically a reduction in postmature births and monitoring of fetal well-being during labor, the incidence of MAS has declined.[691,698-701] Conditions of prolonged fetal compromise such as hypoxia, predating labor, and intrauterine infection have been associated with meconium aspiration and may lead to acute asphyxia during labor. Twenty to 33% of babies with MAS are depressed at birth and require resuscitation.[691,698,702-706] The meconium can have a direct toxic effect on the lung owing to chemical pneumonitis, infection, inflammation, and inactivation of surfactant, or it can occlude the airway trapping air distally in the lungs leading to lung distention, alveolar rupture, and pneumothorax.[691,707-709] Vasoconstriction of the pulmonary vessels in response to hypoxemia can contribute to the development of PPHN, a secondary effect of MAS.[694,703]

In the neonatal period, respiratory effects of meconium aspiration include marked tachypnea, cyanosis, use of accessory muscles for breathing, intercostal and subxyphoid retractions, barrel-chested appearance, and paradoxical breathing patterns with grunting and nasal flaring.[691] A subset of affected infants can be asymptomatic at birth and develop worsening respiratory distress as the meconium moves distally into smaller airways. Initial management of infants in the delivery room includes direct laryngoscopy to suction the hypopharynx and to intubate and suction the trachea before providing positive pressure ventilation. Infants with MAS may require supplemental oxygen or, if disease is severe, mechanical ventilation. In cases where the respiratory compromise progresses, management may require high-frequency ventilation, surfactant therapy, and nitric oxide.[691,698,710] Severely ill infants with meconium aspiration, PPHN, and respiratory failure that is not responsive to the above measures may require ECMO.[694] Infants with associated PPHN will have right-to-left shunting and a difference in pre- and postductal oxygenation saturations. Long-term pulmonary morbidity is common in babies with MAS and has been reported to include symptomatic coughing and wheezing consistent with reactive airway disease requiring bronchodilator therapy, and airway obstruction and persistent hyperinflation on pulmonary function tests

up to 11 years of age.[694,698,711] Neurodevelopmental outcome varies and depends on the injury to the CNS due to asphyxia.[694,711,712]

Persistent Pulmonary Hypertension of the Newborn

PPHN of the newborn is most commonly seen in term or postterm infants as the result of disruption in the typical transition from fetal to neonatal circulation. If PVR fails to drop after birth, the right-to-left shunting at the foramen ovale and ductus arteriosus that characterizes typical fetal circulation continues and results in severe hypoxemia. Hypoxia and alveolar atelectasis lead to pulmonary vasoconstriction and maintenance of pulmonary hypertension.[713,714]

The PVR can fail to drop owing to three types of abnormalities of the pulmonary vasculature. The pulmonary vasculature can be underdeveloped, with decreased cross-sectional area and result in a fixed elevation of PVR. This is the typical pathophysiology of PPHN in a diagnosis associated with lung hypoplasia, such as CDH. Secondly, pulmonary vasculature can develop with an abnormally thick and extensive muscle layer. Remodeling of the pulmonary vasculature typically occurs in 10 to 14 days after birth, at which time the PVR drops. This abnormality of pulmonary vasculature may have a genetic predisposition, be triggered by the use of nonsteroidal anti-inflammatory drugs during pregnancy, or associated with MAS. Lastly, a normally developed vascular bed may fail to dilate after birth because of adverse perinatal conditions such as a bacterial infection or perinatal depression.[714-718] PPHN has also been associated with maternal factors, including diabetes, or urinary tract infection. Perinatal asphyxia is the diagnosis most commonly associated with PPHN.[714,719]

PPHN is suspected in any infant with severe hypoxemia that is not responsive to the administration of 100% oxygen or positive pressure respiratory support such as CPAP or ventilation. PPHN is diagnosed by echocardiograph that shows normal heart structural anatomy with evidence of pulmonary hypertension, and right-to-left shunting through the ductus arteriosus and/or foramen ovale. PPHN is a medical emergency, and diagnosis and treatment need to be made promptly. Goals of treatment are to ensure adequate tissue oxygenation while promoting a decline in PVR. Interventions include supplemental oxygen, vasodilators, intubation and mechanical ventilation, iNO, ECMO, correction of metabolic acidosis, hemodynamic support, and correction of metabolic abnormalities and polycythemia.[713,714,719-721] Because agitation can cause a release of catecholamines that increases PVR, these babies may need to be sedated and pharmacologically paralyzed.[714]

The prognosis for infants with PPHN has improved significantly with improved delivery of mechanical ventilation, iNO, and ECMO. However, survivors are at risk for CLD, ICH, neurodevelopmental delays, and sensorineural hearing impairment.[719] Significant impairments have been found in survivors of moderately severe and severe PPHN in motor, cognitive, and hearing function.[714,721–728]

Therapists working with infants with PPHN need to be aware of potential cardiopulmonary compromise and support development without increasing infant stress and agitation. Family and other caregivers should be provided with suggestions to promote motor, social, and feeding skills while maintaining physiologic stability.[9] Therapists also need to be aware of associated sensory and neurodevelopmental risks and provide appropriate screening, family education, and follow-up services.

Fetal Alcohol Spectrum Disorder

Alcohol is a known teratogen throughout gestation, and since no safe threshold level has been established for alcohol ingestion during pregnancy, abstinence is recommended.[729] Current research has found that exposure of the fetus to alcohol can result in a variety of adverse outcomes, including growth abnormalities, CNS abnormalities, facial dysmorphisms, and congenital organ malformations.[350,730–732] The term *fetal alcohol spectrum disorder (FASD)* has been advocated for use as a result of the range of outcomes.[350,733–735] Reports of alcohol use (10.8%), including binge drinking (3.7%) and heavy drinking (1%), have been made by pregnant women from 15 to 44 years of age.[732,736] The prevalence of FASD is reported to be 0.3 to 1.5 cases per 1000 live births, with highest rates reported among blacks, American Indians, and Alaskan Natives.

The most severe form of FASD is fetal alcohol syndrome (FAS). The criteria for FAS include poor growth, CNS abnormalities, and distinct facial dysmorphisms, with or without confirmed alcohol ingestion[350,730–732,737–741] (Table 4.11). First described in detail by Jones and Smith in 1973,[737] FAS is one of the most common causes of intellectual disability worldwide. The effects of alcohol exposure are related to the amount, timing, and pattern of maternal alcohol consumption, as well as the individual rate of maternal metabolism of alcohol.[732,742–745]

Newborns exposed in utero to alcohol can demonstrate acute withdrawal symptoms, characteristics of FAS, or appear normal.[732] Heavy alcohol consumption around the time of conception and during the first trimester has been associated with alcohol-related birth defects, facial dysmorphology, and growth deficiencies,[729,732,746,747] whereas moderate consumption did not affect IQ at 8 years.[732,748] Exposure to alcohol during the second trimester has been associated with growth disturbances and learning deficits; exposure during the third trimester has been associated with deficits in longitudinal growth.[350,729,734] The hallmark of fetal alcohol exposure is severe growth retardation (length more affected than weight). Growth deficiencies continue postnatally, but weight is more affected than length.[350,738]

The most serious feature of FAS is disturbance of CNS development. Disorders of neuronal proliferation, migration, and midline prosencephalic formation occur as a

TABLE 4.11 Features of FAS	
Physical Features	**Neurodevelopmental Concerns**
Prenatal growth deficiencies/IUGR	Developmental delay
Postnatal growth deficiencies	Impaired cognitive function
Microcephaly	Speech impairments
Short palpebral fissures	Conductive hearing loss
Epicanthal folds	Sensorineural hearing loss
Midline facial hypoplasia	Behavioral issues
Short upturned nose	Mental retardation
Hypoplastic long or smooth philtrum	
Thin vermilion of upper lip	
Ear abnormalities	
Optic nerve hypoplasia	
Cardiac defects (ASD, VSD)	
Hydronephrosis	
External genitalia anomalies	
Abnormal palmar creases	
Joint abnormalities (hands, fingers, toes)	
Cutaneous hemangioma	

ASD, atrial septal defect; IUGR, intrauterine growth restriction; VSD, ventral septal defect.

result of the teratogenic effects of alcohol during the first two trimesters of pregnancy.[350] Microcephaly is present in almost all cases, with delayed neurologic development also present in a majority of cases of children with FAS. Kartin and associates[748] found lower-than-average developmental performance in preschool children exposed to alcohol and drugs prenatally. In addition to decreased intellectual functioning, hyperactivity, distractibility, decreased attention span, impaired speech and language development, and impaired visual memory affect functioning in school. Long-term effects on psychosocial function have also been reported.[350,732,733,735,749,741,748–752]

FAS may be difficult to recognize in the neonatal period and may be mistaken for other syndromes. Infants may have no signs of withdrawal if exposed to even moderate amounts of alcohol. Withdrawal signs of jitteriness, sleep disturbance, tremors, hypotonia, or GI symptoms may be seen in some infants exposed to very high levels of alcohol.[350,752,753] The infant may have been exposed to other substances in addition to alcohol and demonstrate more severe withdrawal symptoms because of these substances. Since facial and physical features of FAS may be subtle and the infant may not demonstrate signs of withdrawal, the diagnosis of FAS may not be made until later in the preschool or school-age years when inattention, hyperactivity, and learning problems are more apparent.[735,753,754] Children with late diagnosis may miss out on early intervention and other services that can address growth and developmental needs. Infants with known prenatal exposure to alcohol or suspected FAS should be referred for developmental follow-up services upon discharge from the hospital.[732,741]

Neonatal Abstinence Syndrome

Prenatal maternal narcotic use is typically accompanied by lifestyle choices that can affect the health of the fetus, including poor prenatal care, and high-risk behaviors that can lead to illnesses and infections. Prenatal maternal narcotic use results in fetal dependence on these substances. The drugs associated with dependence and withdrawal most commonly used during pregnancy are heroin, methadone, and prescription pain medicines.[755-758] Term infants demonstrate more severe withdrawal symptoms than preterm infants; there are several potential explanations for this including a lack of recognition of preterm withdrawal symptoms.[757,758] There is also greater storage of drugs in fat, leading to increased dependency on these substances with increasing GA. At birth, when the drugs are no longer being provided, the infant begins the process of withdrawal.[757,758]

The onset of symptoms for acute narcotic withdrawal can vary from the first hours of life to more than 5 days of age.[758-762] Symptoms are usually noted within 24 to 48 hours depending on type of drug, length of maternal use, GA of the infant, and last maternal dose.[350,755,759] It is not uncommon for infants to be exposed to multiple substances; withdrawal from multiple substances is more severe for infants than withdrawal from methadone or opiates alone.[756,757,759,763,764] Symptoms of withdrawal include irritability, tremors, seizures, apnea, increased muscle tone, inability to sleep, hyperactive DTRs, incoordination, hyperactive sucking, inefficient sucking and swallowing, and high-pitched, shrill cry.[755,757,759,764,765]

Treatment for symptomatic infants includes tight swaddling, holding, rocking, decreasing external stimulation of sound and light, and feeding with high-calorie formula as needed. Infants who are unable to respond to these supportive interventions require the addition of medication to their plan of care.[350,755-757,759,765,766] The decision to start pharmacologic intervention is based on objective measurement of symptoms recorded using a neonatal abstinence score as well as the presence of seizures, sleeplessness, and growth failure or weight loss. The most commonly used neonatal abstinence score is the system developed by Finnegan.[767,768] The NICU Network Neurobehavioral Scale (NNNS) incorporates features of the Finnegan scale but also assesses maturity, behavioral control, and self-regulation.[505] Decisions in terms of increasing or weaning of medications are also based on abstinence scores.[755-757,766] In several studies, opiates have been better at reducing withdrawal symptoms compared with phenobarbitol or supportive treatment alone, and the AAP recommends morphine or methodone.[757-760,755,756,769-771,772]

Infants with NAS may have lower birth weight, height, and head circumference. They often exhibit depressed or inconsistent interactive behaviors and have poor self-calming, which can impact development. In addition, treatment of NAS may require weeks to months of hospitalization, which can interfere with maternal bonding and overall development.[350,756,759,765,766] Developmental follow-up studies of infants with NAS have found a higher incidence of hyperactivity, learning and behavior disorders, and poor social adjustment.[766] The developmental performance of preschool children with prenatal alcohol and drug exposure has been reported as lower than expected for age.[773-775] It is unclear to what extent confounding variables such as environmental factors, maternal characteristics, tobacco use, polydrug use, poverty, and social factors associated with substance abuse are responsible for these outcomes versus prenatal substance exposure.[350,766] While it is difficult to make a direct link between neonatal substance exposure and developmental outcomes, these children and their families are clearly at risk for social, behavioral, and developmental problems. Therefore, close follow-up and maternal–child services including early intervention are warranted.[758,773,774]

Physical Therapy Assessment and Intervention for the Late Preterm and Term Infants

Full-term and late preterm infants in the NICU can be very fragile with complex medical conditions. When working with any preterm infant, the therapist should recall that at 35 weeks' gestation the preterm brain weighs 65% of a term infant's brain, and has fewer sulci.[665] This is a fact that highlights the rapid brain growth and development that an infant is experiencing during the late preterm period. Supporting the infant in growing and developing his or her brain as well as his or her other organs is a top priority for any neonatal therapist; all physical therapy interventions should be judiciously timed and administered so as not to interrupt an infant's sleep or cause additional stress to the burden of care a hospitalized infant already encounters. In addition, the cost of the intervention should be carefully weighed against proven benefits. Unfortunately, in neonatal physical therapy, there is little hard evidence for many interventions. It is also important that physical therapy interventions support the family in assuming parenting roles.

The physical therapist should start by completing a thorough chart review, including maternal/prenatal history, birth history, review of past and present problems by systems, medical test/study findings, medical/surgical interventions, medications, and the infant's response to interventions and medications, including neonatal pain assessments. If the infant is withdrawing from substance exposure, neonatal abstinence scores and any change in medical and/or pharmacologic intervention should be noted. Information regarding family psychosocial history and concerns should also be reviewed and discussed with the social worker if appropriate. The therapist should interview the infant's nurse for updated information regarding physiologic status, any changes in care, and the events of the day. A discussion with the family members as to their understanding of the infant's condition and their own concerns for their infant is a helpful starting point in developing a relationship with the family and planning therapy intervention, including family education.

The evaluation of the infant should begin with an observation of the type of respiratory support, presence of central or peripheral lines, and presence of feeding tubes, as these are not only indications of the fragility of the infant, but may also limit the infant's positioning and active movement. An observational assessment should include the vital signs, pattern of respiration, behavior, state, presence of edema, preferred postures, and active movement. The integumentary system should be assessed for the presence of skin breakdown or scars, which may interfere with alignment, mobility, and function.

Infants recovering from medical conditions such as MAS or PPHN of the newborn may not tolerate a hands-on assessment if they are still critically ill and requiring large amounts of medical support to promote physiologic function. Infants exposed to prenatal infections may also be very ill and unable to tolerate handling. While withdrawing from substance exposure, infants may not be able to tolerate the stimulation of handling. At this stage in the infant's hospital course, the therapist would be primarily consulting with the nursing staff and the family to make suggestions for positional and environmental modifications to promote comfort, physiologic function, and, if possible, positional alignment for future developmental tasks.

The assessment of the stable infant who is able to tolerate handling would include respiratory status and pattern/efficiency of breathing in different positions, integumentary status, behavioral state organization, posture and alignment, passive and active range of motion, muscle tone, presence and symmetry of reflexes, quantity and quality of active movement, postural control, response to sensory stimuli, pain assessment, visual tracking, auditory localization, and social/interaction skills. If appropriate, a standardized developmental assessment may be administered. Physical therapy intervention is then based on the individual infant's strengths and concerns. The concerns may be prioritized according to the infant's medical status and immediate needs in the NICU environment. It is important to be observant of the infant's cardiopulmonary status and behavioral cues when handling the infant and to help the family to understand that the infant may not be able to tolerate as much activity as other infants his or her age.

Infants withdrawing from prenatal substance exposure often require long hospital stays and present with unique needs. Generally older and more physiologically stable, it is not uncommon for these infants to demonstrate poor behavioral organization, extended deep sleep, agitated sleep, vacillation between sleep and crying states, and panicked awakening.[775] The assessment should include all the elements previously discussed and assessment of neonatal abstinence scores. Initially, recommendations for environmental modifications in order to decrease environmental

stress as well as caregiving recommendations to streamline and organize care to avoid overstimulation is essential. Assessing and promoting self-regulatory behaviors is also important. The infant may only tolerate comfort measures, particularly early in his or her withdrawal. Interventions should be graduated in order to allow the infant to become successful at self-soothing.[776] Interventions may include providing containment through bundling and deep pressure and facilitating flexion through positioning with tucked postures that promote hands-to-midline and -mouth. When providing stimulation to infants withdrawing from drug exposure, it is important to offer stimulation that involves only one or two sensory systems so as not to overload the infant. It is also important to be vigilant for early signs of distress (color changes, hiccups, frequent yawning, and/or decreasing eye contact) in order to prevent overstimulation.[777] Infant massage using firm strokes may be helpful to some infants and is a good bonding activity for parents. Gentle vestibular input in the form of gentle rocking or swinging can be effective for some infants. For infants who demonstrate hypertonia and extended postures, supine and standing positions should be minimized. For infants who demonstrate hypotonia, supportive positioning promoting symmetrical, flexed, and midline postures is important. When the baby is awake, gradual attempts at eye contact should be made to prevent overstimulation.[776,778] It is important to remember that these infants are older and to provide appropriate developmental intervention when the infant is awake and able to tolerate these activities. The therapist should work with the family members to understand the needs of the infant and help them learn calming and appropriate developmental interactions. An intervention priority is to promote attachment and bonding over the course of the hospitalization, which may be weeks to months.

Infants with prenatal alcohol exposure may not demonstrate signs of withdrawal or developmental concerns in the neonatal period. The therapist should perform a full assessment and address any needs or concerns. Whether or not there are specific findings on inpatient assessment, the infant should be referred for developmental follow-up at the time of discharge owing to the high risk of long-term developmental concerns.

▶ Transition to home

Normally, discharge planning begins on the first day of hospital admission; however, when caring for medically fragile high-risk infants whose survival is not certain, this may be premature. The exact date of discharge may not be predictable, but when an infant begins to demonstrate more consistent physiologic stability, steps can be initiated toward a discharge plan. Infants leaving the NICU often require unique long-term health care follow-up, and their families require time to learn their care. Current trends in health care for early discharge mean that families are required to care for younger, less stable infants, and therefore families should be included in the discharge process as soon as possible.

A good discharge plan is individually tailored to both the infant and his or her family with clearly identified goals. These goals should be communicated to the family and the medical team so as to eliminate duplication and fragmentation of family education and follow-up care, to prevent delays in access to health care, to establish links to resources for health and development in the community, and to promote success of the infant and family at home.[779–782] The medical team needs to assess the particular strengths and needs of the infant's family, including caretaking capabilities, resource requirements, social supports, and home physical facilities. The AAP[779] recommends that at least two family caregivers are able, available, and committed to learning and providing for the infant(s). Increased risk of attachment disturbances and abuse has been identified for children born prematurely and children with prenatal substance exposure. Family issues that put an infant at risk are lower education level, lack of social support, marital instability, fewer prenatal care visits, substance use, and fewer family visits during hospitalization. Active parent involvement and preparation for posthospital care demonstrate a family's readiness to care for the infant at home.[779,781]

Elements commonly identified as medical requirements for discharge from the NICU include sustained pattern of weight gain, maintenance of normal body temperature in an open environment, a successful mode of feeding (oral or tube feeding), and no episodes of apnea and bradycardia for 5 days.[779,781] Some level II and level III nurseries may have discharge requirements based on GA and weight. Feedings and medications need to be streamlined for home routines. Discharge teaching needs to be initiated early to allow the family time to process information and demonstrate proficiency. Families should be provided with blocks of time to provide care for their infant, and "rooming in" (where the parents spend the night in the hospital acting as sole caretakers for their infant) prior to discharge is recommended.[779,781]

The physical therapy regimen should also be modified for home implementation so that parents are able to carry out all of the infant's care without undue exhaustion. The therapist can assist the family in transition to the home environment in terms of positioning and providing appropriate sensory experiences and developmental activities. Positioning supports are common in the NICU; however, the AAP[374] has strongly recommended that the infants should be positioned on their backs for sleeping, and the sleep environment should be free of soft or loose bedding materials and stuffed toys or animals that could obstruct infant airways. The therapist can develop a plan to wean the infant of positioning supports and transition to back sleeping as necessary.[783] Positioning supports can be utilized and may be very important for some infants for play and activities while awake. Blanket rolls may be positioned behind the infant's shoulders and along the thighs while he or she is seated in an infant seat to promote symmetry and hands-to-midline.

It is important that the therapist educate the family in safe prone positioning for play when the infant is awake as this may be forgotten in light of the back-to-sleep recommendations. Supervised prone play while the infant is awake offers opportunities to strengthen shoulder, neck, and trunk musculature in preparation for future gross motor skills.

Infants who have required intensive care may continue to have sensitivities to light and sound after discharge to home. In order to help the infant transition successfully to the home environment, the therapist can help the parents to identify the infant's vulnerabilities and make home modifications and recommendations for appropriate settings. The parents may need to dim or shade bright lights and minimize sound around the infant in order to support regulation and to promote arousal and interaction. The therapist needs to role-model problem solving and ongoing adaptations to the infant's changing cues.

Developmental activities will also change over time as the infant matures. Parents will need to continue to correct the infant's age for prematurity in order to have an accurate framework of expectations, for instance, if the infant's Chronological age at discharge is 4 months, but the adjusted age is 1 month. Toys and play experiences should be targeted at the adjusted age. Activity recommendations should be specific to each infant; however, there are common elements for most babies in early infancy. Many babies who have had high-tech respiratory support, increased work of breathing, and GER, babies who have required supine positioning owing to medical status; and preterm infants who missed out on the cramping and crowding of the uterine experience may have difficulty initiating flexion of head, trunk, and limbs. Families should be educated in positioning and techniques to facilitate flexion within the infant's tolerance. For example, the parent places the infant on his or her lap, cradled by the thighs, to promote head midline, chin tuck, and shoulder protraction. The infant should be positioned so that his or her legs are flexed against the parent's abdomen. In this position, the infant can gaze at the parent's face to promote downward convergent gaze and chin tuck (Fig. 4.24). Other activities that fit into families'

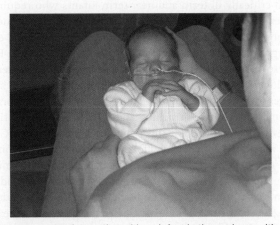

FIGURE 4.24 Interaction with an infant in the supine position on the parent's lap.

daily routines can also be provided. For infants whose age or adjusted age is at term or near term, activities should promote symmetry, flexion, and midline orientation.

In addition to providing families with home programs, referrals should be made to community resources such as early intervention. Early intervention services are programs throughout the United States and its territories funded by Federal and local governments that are mandated by the Individuals with Disabilities Education Act (IDEA). Early intervention services provide developmental services for children and their families. These programs can provide a variety of therapy and educational services for infants at risk for developmental delays or documented delays and their families. However, the period between referral to the program and initiation of services can be 45 days or longer.[784] Therefore, it may be necessary to set up interim services provided by outpatient or private home-based therapists until early intervention services can start. Interim services are particularly necessary when a child may need frequent monitoring of a splint or peripheral nerve injury such as brachial plexus injury.

▶ Neonatal follow-up services

Infants who have required neonatal intensive care are at high risk for both major and minor disabilities. Forty-eight percent of high-risk infants demonstrate transient neurologic abnormalities consisting of hypotonia or hypertonia, and 10% go on to demonstrate major neurologic sequelae such as CP, hydrocephalus, blindness, seizure disorder, and hearing impairment.[377,393,785–790] Minor neurodevelopmental and neurobehavioral impairments include IQ significantly lower than full-term siblings, "temperament problems, language delays, fine motor deficits, visual-motor deficits, sensory integration dysfunction, social incompetence, emotional immaturity, attention deficits, learning disorders, and ultimately diminished school performance."[791] These impairments are prevalent among survivors and become increasingly more apparent with age.[72,352,368,396,790–796] In addition, LBW infants and critically ill term and near-term infants who required intensive care have long-term health issues such as frequent rehospitalization, shunt complications, orthopedic and eye surgeries, CLD, and failure to thrive.[393,549,785,793,797,798] For these reasons, NICU graduates require specialized long-term follow-up services. The AAP recommends follow-up services for these developmental concerns as well as for organized postdischarge tracking and to provide information regarding outcomes for this population.[779,786] Most NICUs are associated with neonatal follow-up programs to monitor the outcomes for these high-risk neonates and to determine the effects of NICU interventions on outcomes. In addition, these programs maintain outcome databases, conduct single-center studies, and participate in larger multicentered studies. Tracking information includes growth parameters over time (head circumference, height, and weight), feeding

and nutrition, medication use, illnesses and hospitalizations, pain, home technology use (oxygen, apnea monitor, feeding tube/pump), sleep position and sleep patterns, car seat use, follow-up with other specialists, home environment, caretaking plan, parental concerns, and medical and neurologic examinations. Standardized developmental assessments are administered as part of the follow-up program. There are many from which to choose; the *Bayley Scales of Infant & Toddler Development* Edition III (BSID III) are the recognized standards for measuring infant development between 0 and 42 months. Many follow-up programs will administer the BSID III in conjunction with other domain-specific assessments for social and emotional development, gross and fine motor development, language and behavior development, and family function.[785,786] Babies should be seen in the follow-up program (not to be confused with the first pediatrician visit, which should occur the first week from discharge) at 4 months adjusted age unless the discharge team, physical therapist, community pediatrician, home-visiting nurse, or caregiver has concerns warranting earlier follow-up. Generally, babies who are discharged with technologic supports such as tracheostomy, supplemental oxygen, apnea monitor, and feeding tube are seen within the first month after discharge. The babies return for neonatal follow-up every 3 months for the first year, every 6 months in the second year, and yearly from 3 years adjusted age to school age. However, this schedule can change to more frequent follow-up if more specific concerns are being monitored. For infants who are followed as part of a study, the frequency may be determined as per the protocol for that particular study.

The follow-up team is usually composed of professionals from many disciplines and can include a developmental pediatrician, neonatologist, pediatric nurse practitioner, social worker, psychologist, nutritionist, and physical, occupational, and speech therapists. Administrative support staff includes a clinic coordinator, data manager, and secretary. Owing to the multidisciplinary nature of the follow-up clinic, the visits are highly coordinated for efficiency and to address the needs of the high-risk infants and their families. Families often perceive the clinic staff as "experts" in the care of their babies, and will utilize them as a resource and to confirm recommendations made by outside health care providers. Some members of the follow-up team may also have provided care for the infant and his or her family during hospitalization in the NICU, which may provide the family with a level of comfort and familiarity. In this way, the family's needs identified during the hospitalization can be more effectively followed, and the family may also feel more at ease to discuss new concerns. The social worker can identify and address financial issues and social risk factors such as poverty, housing, substance abuse, and lack of education, which can pose additional risks for the health and development of the infant. Studies have shown that environmental factors such as maternal years of education and socioeconomic status can mitigate or exacerbate the biologic risk factors typically associated with neonatal intensive care.[72,368,799,800,801]

Physical therapists bring a unique strength to the follow-up of high-risk infants as their background in kinesiology and development allows them to examine the qualitative aspects of infant movement. Understanding the fundamental components of a movement pattern allows the therapist to determine whether the infant is developing a balanced repertoire of movement patterns needed for the progression of development or is reusing the same maladaptive patterns that prevent this progression. It is helpful for physical therapists to take part in a neonatal follow-up clinic for their own understanding of development and long-term outcomes of high-risk infants. It is important that therapists observe the changes in infants over time as some of the "red flags" seen in the NICU may be transient and may be replaced by more typical movement patterns as the infant develops. It is also a good learning experience, albeit sad, to see babies who have seemingly left the NICU unscathed only to return to a follow-up clinic with atypical neurodevelopmental assessments. Although this is sobering, it can serve to challenge the therapist to seek out other assessment tools and look more closely for subtleties in infant performance. While participating in a follow-up clinic, therapists may also see the responsiveness or limitations of community resources and perhaps learn of new resources that may prove to be effective. In addition, therapists participating in neonatal follow-up programs have the opportunity to see family resilience and the challenges a family may face on the journey that began in the NICU. The experiences of neonatal follow-up care provide the therapist caring for infants in the NICU with a wealth of information, which should be used when intervening with infants in the NICU, providing discharge recommendations, and communicating with families regarding future outcomes.

SUMMARY

The last century has seen the evolution of the subspecialty of neonatology, and as this practice has changed over time, so too has the role of the physical therapist in the NICU. The increasing understanding of preterm infant development and the effects of the environment, neonatal care, and family involvement on the evolving infant systems has led to a unique and specialized opportunity for physical therapists to act as developmental specialists within the setting of the NICU. In order to effectively and appropriately fulfill this need, therapists require in-depth understanding and knowledge of medical conditions and interventions; fetal and infant behavior and development; family stresses related to pregnancy, childbirth, and transition to parenthood within the NICU; risk factors; and long-term outcomes. In addition, the therapist needs to have a mentored practice within the NICU setting and participate in a neonatal follow-up program. It is also important that the physical therapist be an integrated member of the team providing care for the high-risk baby and his or her

family. The physical therapist must take the initiative to keep abreast of the rapidly changing technology and management, and their effects on infant health and development. This requires keeping current with both physical therapy and neonatal literature.

The therapist practicing in the NICU requires the advanced knowledge and skills as outlined previously and the time, training, and mentoring to achieve the highest level of practice in order to provide the sensitive, knowledgeable, and supportive care the babies and their families deserve. To be a physical therapist in the NICU is a meaningful and rewarding role and is well worth the time and training.

CASE STUDIES

CASE STUDY 1 **Kayla** Kayla was born at 23 3/7 weeks' gestation with a birth weight of 570 g (1 lb 4 oz) (Fig. 4.25) to a married 30-year-old G2P2 mother who had good prenatal care. Maternal complications included Group B *Streptococcus*, bleeding at 22 weeks, and preterm labor at 23 3/7 weeks, at which time she was dilated and contracting. The infant was born via vaginal breech delivery with Apgar scores of 4 at 1 minute and 7 at 5 minutes. Resuscitative efforts in the delivery room included intubation, positive pressure ventilation, and surfactant. Kayla was transported to the NICU, where she was placed on conventional ventilator, and UA and UV lines were placed. Phototherapy was initiated because of bruising.

Because of worsening respiratory status, Kayla was placed on HFOV, which she received for 33 days before she was able to wean to CMV. She was able to be extubated and placed on CPAP after 2 months on the conventional ventilator. After 2 weeks on CPAP, Kayla was weaned to a nasal cannula, but had to be reintubated and placed on mechanical ventilation 2 weeks later because of sepsis. Kayla was extubated and placed on nasal cannula 2 weeks later. She was finally weaned off all respiratory support at 143 days of life.

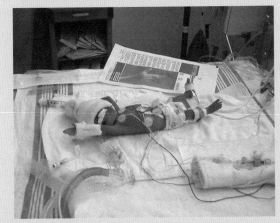

FIGURE 4.25 Kayla being stabilized after birth. Note the size of the infant versus the size of the glove wrapper.

Kayla's hospital course was complicated by severe BPD, pulmonary interstitial emphysema, large PDA requiring surgical ligation, hyperbilirubinemia, mild supravalvular pulmonic stenosis, and multiple bouts of sepsis, including meningitis, pseudomonas tracheitis, methicillin-resistant *Staphylococcus aureus* (MRSA), and pneumonia.

Pain Management

Pain management was initiated on Kayla's first day of life with the administration of morphine. She continued to receive morphine until day of life 34 when a tapered wean was completed. Morphine was restarted on day of life 120 when she required reintubation and mechanical ventilation. Kayla was weaned off morphine slowly beginning day of life 133 and ending on day of life 143. She tolerated this weaning process well, and neonatal abstinence scores were followed closely for any adverse response to withdrawal. Throughout her hospitalization, Kayla was assessed for pain by all staff. Pain assessments were also performed by the physical therapist and documented in the chart after each interaction with the therapist.

Physical Therapy Services

Kayla was referred for physical therapy services at 2 weeks of life (25 weeks' postconceptional age). The physical therapist reviewed Kayla's history by thoroughly reading her medical chart and discussing Kayla's status with her nurse. Kayla's nurse reported that she was very restless and became irritable with hands-on care. The physical therapist observed Kayla in her isolette before, during, and after caregiving activities. At this time Kayla was intubated, requiring HFOV, and was under phototherapy. She demonstrated increased extensor posturing of her head, trunk, and extremities and jerky restless movements prior to care. Sensitivity to sound and light were also noted. Kayla had very low tolerance to handling and position changes during care. Her stress signs included color changes, increased heart rate, oxygen desaturation, and motor stress signs of arching of head and trunk and extension of extremities. Kayla was unable to effectively utilize any self-calming behaviors and was difficult to calm with external supports. She did respond to facilitated tucking and firm touch when provided long enough for her to relax and settle into the position. After care she was pale and exhausted.

Physical Therapy Goals

Physical therapy goals at this time were as follows:

1. To decrease environmental stress
2. To promote calming behaviors
3. To promote flexed postures for calming and optimal body alignment for musculoskeletal development
4. To assist family and caregivers in identifying and responding to Kayla's cues
5. To provide education to the family regarding developmentally supportive care

Suggestions included:

1. Minimizing environmental stimulation by covering her isolette and shading her eyes from bright lights, alerting people to keep noise levels down around her bedside with a sign, and education
2. Pacing care activities, providing rest breaks with facilitated tucking, using slow movements and firm touch
3. Positioning in flexion in a deep nest and varying positions between prone, side-lying, and supine as tolerated
4. Allowing for hands to head and grasping, and offering the pacifier for self-calming

Kayla's mother visited every day and the physical therapist was able to meet with her to discuss Kayla's status and suggestions to support her development. Together, they looked at Kayla's cues and discussed strategies for calming and bonding. Kayla's father visited in the evening, and her mother shared the suggestions for developmentally supportive care with him.

For the next 2 months Kayla continued to be an extremely fragile, critically ill infant with high respiratory requirements, surgical ligation of her PDA, and episodes of sepsis. Physical therapists continued to observe Kayla and adjust her developmental care plan as appropriate. At 10 weeks of age (33 weeks' PCA), Kayla was able to wean from HFOV to the conventional ventilator. She continued to have low tolerance for handling, but was easier to console with the pacifier and firm touch/containment in flexion. She also demonstrated attempts at self-calming with hand-to-head, grasping, and foot-bracing behaviors. The physical therapist continued to work with the nursing staff and Kayla's family to develop care plans to promote self-calming, optimal positioning, and tolerance to caregiving activities. At this time Kayla's parents were practicing kangaroo care and holding Kayla daily (Fig. 4.26). The physical therapist was able to provide suggestions for positioning Kayla during kangaroo care.

Kayla made slow improvements medically, and at 36 weeks' PCA she still required mechanical ventilation. Her tolerance to handling and position changes was improving. She was able to

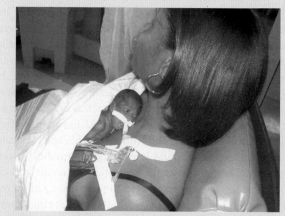

FIGURE 4.26 Kayla and her mother practicing kangaroo care, or skin-to-skin holding.

maintain a quiet, alert state using her pacifier and containment for support. Even with external supports she had limited tolerance for visual or social stimulation. Kayla was very sensitive to light and sound in the environment. Physical therapy examination revealed increased flexor posturing in her lower extremities, with full passive range of motion. She held her upper extremities in scapular retraction, shoulder abduction, and external rotation. Kayla had antigravity movement of her extremities through limited range of motion with jerky, tremulous quality of movement. She still frequently moved into extension rather than flexion. Despite the use of a gel pillow, the time spent on HFOV had left Kayla with flattening of the lateral sides of her head, or dolichocephaly. She held her head in extension with shortening of her capital and neck extensors. Tightness in her thoracic, lumbar, and sacral areas was also noted. Goals for Kayla included

1. Maintaining a quiet alert state for increasing duration of time
2. Improved ability to self-calm
3. Neutral head alignment with decreased tightness in cervical spine
4. Increased flexibility in lumbosacral spine
5. Decreased tightness in scapulae and shoulders
6. Increased antigravity flexion movement
7. An additional goal was for Kayla's family and caregivers to be independent in positioning and developmentally supportive activities.

The therapist continued to work with Kayla's family and nurses in reading her cues and progressing handling and social interactions to her tolerance. The therapist also provided positioning suggestions to promote midline alignment, flexion, and shoulder protraction. Gentle mobilization to her spine was provided, starting in the lumbosacral area and slowly moving proximally over the course of several weeks, based on Kayla's response.

Over the next month, Kayla was weaned off the ventilator to CPAP and then to nasal cannula. She had one setback in her respiratory stability because of sepsis, but was able to be weaned off all support by 43 weeks' PCA. The therapist continued to work on the previously stated goals until time of discharge to home. Concerns at the time of discharge included:

1. Sensitivity to light and sound
2. Limited tolerance to handling
3. Limited range of motion in cervical spine and shoulders
4. Delayed postural responses

Her strengths were robust and defined behavioral states, improved ability to self-calm, and greater availability for social interactions. She was able to visually fix on an object and track it to the left and right. Her parents were able to read Kayla's behavioral cues and respond appropriately. Suggestions for home were provided to her parents, who were able to demonstrate independence in performing these activities. Kayla was discharged to home at 45 weeks' PCA without any respiratory support and taking all feedings by bottle. Follow-up services included ophthalmology,

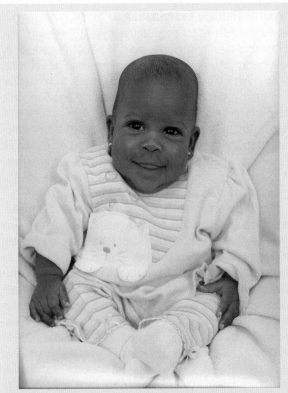

FIGURE 4.27 Kayla at 7.5 months chronologic age, or 3.25 months adjusted age.

special babies clinic (neonatal follow-up), cardiology, and early intervention services (Fig. 4.27).

CASE STUDY 2 Baby J

History

Baby boy J was born at 37 2/7 weeks' gestation via spontaneous vaginal delivery to a 24-year-old G4P3A1 AA mother with normal labs. He weighed 3.375 kg, had Apgar scores of $8^1 8^5$, and was taken to the well-baby nursery at the local hospital, where he developed respiratory distress without O_2 requirement on day of life 1. Chest radiography was negative. After being fed for 12 hours, he developed abdominal distention and was ill appearing. Abdominal radiography showed pneumatosis, and baby J was transferred to his local children's hospital for surgical evaluation. On day of life 3, he underwent laparoscopic surgery and had ileal cecectomy, with ileostomy and mucous fistula placement. Eleven centimeters of bowel was resected. Feeds were initiated on day of life 17, and baby J developed abdominal distention and emesis. On day of life 23, the upper gastrointestinal series showed possible stoma stenosis. He had a history of fungal line sepsis, treated with amphotericin. Baby J's parents were married and had two preschool-aged siblings; the eldest sibling received speech therapy through early intervention.

Physical Therapy Examination

Baby J was referred for physical therapy at 3.5 weeks of age. At that time his nutrition consisted of 5 mL of Pregestimil by mouth every 3 hours as well as hyperalimentation. His physical therapy examination was limited to the right side-lying position, in an effort to keep the stool from his stoma from draining into his abdominal wound, which had dehisced. He presented in a sleep state throughout the session with mildly distended abdomen, gauze pad over abdomen, colostomy with a small amount of yellow seedy stool, and a peripherally inserted central catheter (PICC) line in the left anterior calf. The CRIES pain score was 0 to 1 throughout examination.

Baby J did not habituate to light over 10 trials and habituated to rattle on sixth stimulus in sleep state. Muscle tone was mildly decreased in sleep state. Initial examination was limited on account of positioning precautions and sleep state. Baby J's physical therapy diagnosis was increased risk for developmental delays due to medical status and potential for prolonged hospitalization. He was to be followed by physical therapy two times per week for ongoing assessment, parent education, and developmental stimulation. Initial short-term goals (4 weeks) included alerting for 8 to 10 minutes per session, visually attending to face for 8 to 10 seconds, intact anterior and posterior head righting reactions in upright with support at upper chest, and parents to be independent with positioning baby for comfort. The long-term goal was age-appropriate developmental skills at 15 months. At baby J's second physical therapy session, he demonstrated slow state transitions with defined drowsy state and bright-eyed alert periods with visual regard for the therapist, cleared his airway in prone, and demonstrated intact anterior–posterior head righting reactions and symmetric flexor tone of his limbs. His active range of motion (AROM) was jittery with the presence of forearm rotation right to left. He did not demonstrate automatic walking.

Physical Therapy Course

Baby J's parents were frequently at his bedside with his older siblings. His family decorated his bed space with poems, photographs, and pictures from his siblings and extended family. His parents were receptive to suggested play ideas for baby J, which were explained, demonstrated, and posted at his bedside by his physical therapist. At next re-examination at 1.5 months of age, baby J had missed one session due to fever. He had developed a left head preference and was an animated baby who used yawning or sneezing to regulate intensity of social interactions. He had met all of his short-term goals, and new short-term goals (4 weeks) included the following: AROM of head/neck to right 45 to 60 degrees to follow visual cue two times per session, neutral head extension sustained in prone for 8 to 10 seconds, bat at toy in supine once per session, and sustain neutral head extension in upright for 10 to 18 seconds with support at upper trunk. Baby J continued to be seen twice weekly; however, on day of life 56 he underwent laparoscopic surgery for closure of his enterostomy and lysis of adhesions. Postoperatively, baby J developed a fever and was taken back to the operating room for exploratory laparoscopy on day of life 61, where an abscess was

discovered; the surgeons drained this abscess and reinforced his reanastomosis. After this latter surgery, physical therapy goals changed as baby J was intubated, irritable, stiff, and colonized with MRSA. The physical therapist provided baby J's parents with suggestions for comforting, handling, and positioning baby J as well as placement of visual stimulation in order to encourage neutral head alignment. New short-term goals (4 weeks) when baby J was 2.5 months old included tolerating prone placement without fussing for 90 to 180 seconds, extending head in prone for 3 to 5 seconds, approximating hands in midline in supine twice per session, and sustaining neutral head in upright for 8 to 10 seconds with support at axilla, and baby J's parents describing two developmentally appropriate activities for baby J. Baby J missed several physical therapy sessions after this latter surgery due to sleep state and critical medical status due to sepsis.

At the next re-examination at 3.5 months, baby J had transferred out of the NICU to an integrated care service to address his ongoing feeding issues. He demonstrated social smiles and could extend his head to 90 degrees in prone with elbows behind shoulders; he demonstrated head righting reaction in prone when the therapist imposed lateral weight shifts; he was able to sustain head in neutral in upright with bobbing. Occupational therapy became involved with him at this time and followed him twice weekly as well. New 4-week short-term goals included taking weight through lower extremities for 8 to 10 seconds in supported standing, sustaining lateral head RR in prone with imposed weight shift for 25 to 40 seconds bilaterally, maintaining 90-degree head extension in prone prop for 40 to 60 seconds with elbows in line with shoulders, and grasping rattle in hand with eye–hand regard two times per session. Baby J was seen twice a week for sensory and developmental stimulation. At 4.5 months of age, baby J completed the Test of Infant Motor Performance (TIMP) and performed within the normal limits for his age.

Baby J was discharged home shortly after that on oral feeds. His parents were trained in nasogastric tube placement and use in case baby J was unable to maintain oral feeds. He was to follow up with his pediatrician for developmental and medical monitoring. His parents were given suggestions for developmental activities for the present and upcoming 3 months.

REFERENCES

1. Avery ME. Neonatology. *Pediatrics*. 1998;2(1):270–271.
2. Robertson AF, Baker JP. Lessons from the past. *Semin Fetal Neonatal Med*. 2005;(10):23–30.
3. Nelson NM. A decimillennium in neonatology. *J Pediatr*. 2000;(137):731–735.
4. Silverman WA. Neonatal pediatrics at the century mark. *Pediatr Res*. 1990;27(6 suppl):S34–S37.
5. Baker JP. The incubator and the medical discovery of the premature infant. *J Perinatol*. 2000;(5):321–28.
6. Friedrich O. What do babies know? *Time*. August 15, 1983.
7. Philip AGS. The evolution of neonatology. *Pediatric Res*. 2005;58(4):799–815.
8. Pressler JL, Turnage-Carrier CS, Kenner C. Developmental care: an overview. In: Kenner C, McGrath JM, eds. *Developmental Care of Newborns and Infants: A Guide for Health Professionals*. Philadelphia, PA: Elsevier; 2004.

9. Vergara ER, Bigsby R. *Developmental and Therapeutic Interventions in the NICU*. Baltimore, MD: Paul H Brookes Publishing Co; 2004.

10. Robertson AF. Reflections on errors in neonatology: I. The "Hands-Off" years, 1920 to 1950. *J Perinatol*. 2003;(23):48–55.

11. Brazelton TB. *Neonatal Behavioral Assessment Scale*. 2nd ed. Philadelphia, PA: JB Lippincott Company; 1984.

12. Lucey JF. Is intensive care becoming too intensive? *Pediatrics*. 1977;(59 suppl):1064–1065.

13. Korones SB. Disturbance and infants' rest. In TD Moore, ed. *Iatrogenic problems in neonatal intensive care: Report of the 69th Ross Conference on Pediatric Research*. Columbus OH Ross Laboratories; 1976:94–97.

14. Als H. Toward a synactive theory of development: promise for the assessment and support of infant individuality. *Infant Ment Health J*. 1982;3(4):229–243.

15. Johnson B. Family centered care: four decades of progress. *Fam Syst Health*. 2000;18(2):137.

16. Gibbins S, Coughlin M, Hoath SB. Quality indicators: using the Universe of Developmental Care Model as an exemplar for change. In Kenner C, McGrath JC, eds. *Developmental Care of Newborns and Infants*. 2nd ed. Glenview, IL: National Association of Neonatal Nurses; 2010.

17. Stevens DC, Helseth CC, Kurtz JC. Achieving success in supporting parents and families in the neonatal intensive care unit. In Kenner C, McGrath JC, eds. *Developmental Care of Newborns and Infants*. 2nd ed. Glenview, IL: National Association of Neonatal Nurses; 2010.

18. Committee on Fetus and Newborn. Levels of neonatal care. *Pediatrics*. 2004;114(5):1341–1347.

19. Sweeney JK. Assessment of the special care nursery environment: effects on the high-risk infant. In: Wilhelm IJ, ed. *Physical Therapy Assessment in Early Infancy*. New York, NY: Church Livingstone; 1993.

20. Sweeney JK, Swanson MW. Low birth weight infants: neonatal care and follow-up. In: Umphred DA, ed. *Neurological Rehabilitation*. 4th ed. St. Louis, MO: Mosby; 2001.

21. Sweeney JK, Heriza CB, Blanchard Y. Neonatal physical therapy. Part I: clinical competencies and neonatal intensive care unit clinical training models. *Pediatr Phys Ther*. 2009;21:296–307.

22. Campbell SK. *Decision Making in Pediatric Neurologic Physical Therapy*. Philadelphia, PA: Churchill Livingstone; 1999.

23. Sweeney JK, Heriza CB, Blanchard Y, et al. Neonatal physical therapy. Part II: practice frameworks and evidence-based practice guidelines. *Pediatr Phys Ther*. 2010;22:2–16.

24. Scull S, Deitz J. Competencies for physical therapists in the neonatal intensive care unit (NICU). *Pediatr Phys Ther*. 1989;1:11–14.

25. Sweeney JK, Heriza CB, Reilly MA, et al. Practice guidelines for the physical therapist in the neonatal intensive care unit (NICU). *Pediatr Phys Ther*. 1999;11:119–132.

26. Campbell SK. Use of care paths to improve patient management. *Phys Occupat Ther Pediatr*. 2013;33(1):27–38.

27. Byrne E, Campbell SK. Physical therapy observation and assessment in the neonatal intensive care unit (NICU). *Phys Occupat Ther Pediatr*. 2013;33(1):39–74.

28. Byrne E, Garber J. Physical therapy intervention in the neonatal intensive care unit. *Phys Occupat Ther Pediatr*. 2013;33(1):75–110.

29. Garber J. Oral-motor function and feeding intervention. *Phy Occupat Ther Pediatr*. 2013;33(1):111–138.

30. Goldstein LA. Family support and education. *Phys Occupat Ther Pediatr*. 2013;33(1):139–161.

31. Barbosa VM. Teamwork in the neonatal intensive care unit. *Phys Occupat Ther Pediatr*. 2013;33(1):5–26.

32. Kamm K, Thelen E, Jenson JL. A dynamical systems approach to motor development. *Phys Ther*. 1990;70(12):763–775.

33. Heriza CB. Implications of dynamic systems approach to understanding infant kicking behavior. *Phys Ther*. 1991;71(3):222–234.

34. Heriza CB. Motor development: traditional and contemporary theories. Contemporary management of motor control problems. In: *Proceedings of the II Step Conference*. Alexandria, VA: Foundation of Physical Therapy; 1991.

35. Lockman JS, Thelen E. Developmental biodynamics: brain, body, behavior connections. *Child Dev*. 1993;64:953.

36. Thelen E. Motor development: a new synthesis. *Am Psychologist*. 1995;50(2):79–90.

37. Guiliani CA. Theories of motor control: new concepts for physical therapy. Contemporary management of motor control problems. In: *Proceedings of the II Step Conference*. Alexandria, VA: Foundation for Physical Therapy; 1991.

38. Horak FB. Assumptions underlying motor control for neurologic rehabilitation. Contemporary management of motor control problems. In: *Proceedings of the II Step Conference*. Alexandria, VA: Foundation for Physical Therapy; 1991.

39. Edelman GM. *Neural Darwinism: Theory of Neuronal Group Selection*. Oxford, UK: Oxford University Press; 1989.

40. Edelman GM. *Bright Air, Brilliant Fire: On the Matter of the Mind*. New York, NY: Basic Books Inc; 1992.

41. Sporns O, Edelman GM. Solving Bernstein's problem: a proposal for the development of coordinated movements by selection. *Child Dev*. 1993;64:960–981.

42. Hadders Algra M. The neuronal group selection theory: a framework to explain variation in normal development. *Dev Med Child Neurol*. 2000;42:566–572.

43. Edelman GM. Neural darwinism: selection and re-entrant signalling in higher brain function. *Neuron*. 1993;10:115–125.

44. Hadders Algra M. The neuronal group selection theory: promising principles for understanding and treating developmental motor disorders. *Dev Med Child Neurol*. 2000;42:707–715.

45. Prechtl HFM. Developmental neurology of the fetus. *Bailliere's Clin Obstetr Gynecol*. 1988;2(1):21–36.

46. Hadders Algra M. Variation and variability: key words in human motor development. *Phys Ther*. 2010;90:1823–1837.

47. Smith LB, Thelan E. Development as a dynamic system. *Trends Cogn Sci*. 2003;7(8):343–348.

48. Adolph KE. Learning in the development of locomotion. *Monogr Soc Res child Dev*. 1997;62(1–4):1–158.

49. Campbell SK. The child's development of functional movement. In: Campbell SK, Palisano RJ, Orlin MN, eds. *Physical therapy for Children*. 4th ed. St Louis, MO: Elsevier Saunders; 2012.

50. Als H, Duffy FH, McAnulty GB, et al. Early experience alters brain function and structure. *Pediatrics*. 2004;11(4):846–857.

51. World Health Organization. *International Classification of Functioning, Disability and Handicaps*. Geneva, Switzerland: World Health Organization; 2001.

52. Goldstein DN, Cohn E, Coster W. Enhancing participation for children with disabilities—application of the ICF enablement framework to pediatric physical therapist's practice. *Pediatr Phys Ther*. 2004;16(2):114–120.

53. Palisano RJ, Campbell SK, Harrris SR. Evidenced-based decision making in pediatric physical therapy. In Campbell SK, Palisano RJ, Orlin MN, eds. *Physical therapy for Children*. 4th ed. St Louis, MO: Elsevier Saunders; 2012.

54. Akinson HL, Nixon-Cave K. A tool for clinical reasoning for reflection using the International Classification of functioning, disability, and Health (ICF) framework and patient management model. *Phys Ther*. 2011;91(3):416–430.

55. Als H. Infant individuality: Assessing patterns of very early development. In: Call J, Galenson E, Tyson RL, eds. *Frontiers of Infant Psychiatry*. New York, NY: Basic Books; 1983.

56. Als H. A synactive model of neonatal behavioral organization: framework for the assessment of neurobehavioral development in the premature infant and for support of infants and parents in the neonatal intensive care environment. In: Sweeney JK ed. *The High Risk Neonate: Developmental Therapy Perspectives*. *Phys Occup Ther Pediatr*. 1986;6:3–55.

57. Als H, Lawhon G, Brown E, et al. Individualized behavioral and environmental care for the very low birth weight preterm infant at high risk for bronchopulmonary dysplasia: neonatal

intensive care unit and developmental outcome. *Pediatrics.* 1986;78(6): 1123–1132.

58. Als H, Lester BM, Brazelton TB. Dynamics of the behavioral organization of the premature infant: a theoretical perspective. In: Field TM, Sostek AM, Goldberg S, et al. , eds. *Infants Born at Risk.* New York, NY: Spectrum; 1979.

59. Als H. *Manual for the Naturalistic Observation of Newborn Behavior: Newborn Individualized Developmental Care and Assessment Program (NIDCAP).* Boston, MD: National NIDCAP Training Center; 1995.

60. Lawhon G, Melzar A. Developmental care of the very low birth weight infant. *J Perinatal Neonatal Nurs.* 1988;2(1):56–65.

61. Bowden VR, Greenberg CS, Donaldson NE. Developmental care of the newborn. *Online J Clin Innovations.* 2000;3(7):1–77.

62. Gilkerson L, Als H. Role of reflective process in the implementation of developmentally supportive care in the newborn intensive care nursery. *Infants Young Child.* 1995;7(4):20–28.

63. Chappel J. *Advancing Clinical Practice and Perspectives of Developmental Care in the NICU.* Morristown, NJ: 2004.

64. Als H, Lawhon G, Duffy FH, et al. Individualized developmental care for the very low-birth-weight preterm infant. *JAMA.* 1994;272(11): 853–858.

65. Becker PT, Grunwald PC, Moorman J, et al. Outcomes of developmentally supportive nursing care for very low birth weight infants. *Nurs Res.* 1991;40:150–155.

66. Becker PT, Grunwald PC, Moorman J, et al. Effects of developmental care on behavioral organization in very-low-birth-weight infants. *Nurs Res.* 1993;42(4):214–220.

67. Buehler DM, Als H, Duffy FH, et al. Effectiveness of individualized developmental care for low-risk preterm infants: behavioral and electrophysiologic evidence. *Pediatrics.* 1995;96(5):923–932.

68. Petryshen P, Stevens B, Hawkins J, et al. Comparing nursing costs for preterm infants receiving conventional vs. developmental care. *Nurs Econ.* 1997;15(3):138–150.

69. Symington A, Pinelli J. Distilling the evidence on developmental care: a systematic review. *Adv Neonatal Care.* 2002;2(4):198–221.

70. Symington A, Pinelli J. Developmental care for promoting development and preventing morbidity in preterm infants (Cochrane Review). *Cochrane Database Syst Rev.* 2002;4.

71. Franck LS, Lawhon G. Environmental and behavioral strategies to prevent and manage neonatal pain. *Semin Perinatol.* 1998;22(5): 434–443.

72. Hill S, Engle S, Jorgensen J, et al. Effects of facilitated tucking during routine care of infants born preterm. *Pediatr Phys Ther.* 2005;17: 158–163.

73. Ward-Larson C, Horn RA, Gosnell F. The efficacy of facilitated tucking for relieving procedural pain of endotracheal suctioning in very low birth weight infants. *Am J Matern Child Nurs.* 2004;29(3):151–156.

74. Taquino L, Blackburn S. The effects of containment during suctioning and heelstick on physiological and behavioral responses of preterm infants. *Neonatal Nurs.* 1994;13(7):55.

75. Corff KE, Seideman R, Venkataraman PS, et al. Facilitated tucking: a nonpharmacologic comfort measure for pain in preterm neonates. *J Gynecol Neonatal Nurs.* 1995;24(2):143–147.

76. Corff KE. An effective comfort measure for minor pain and stress in preterm infants: facilitated tucking. *Neonatal Netw.* 1993;12(8):74.

77. Corbo MG, Mansi G, Stagni A, et al. Nonnutritive sucking during heelstick procedures decreases behavioral distress in the newborn infant. *Biol Neonate.* 2000;77:162–167.

78. Field T, Goldson E. Pacifying effects of nonnutritive sucking on term and preterm neonates during heelstick procedures. *Pediatrics.* 1984;74(6):1012–1015.

79. Pinelli J, Symington A. How rewarding can a pacifier be? A systematic review of nonnutritive sucking in preterm infants. *Neonatal Netw.* 2000;19(8):41–48.

80. Kilbride HW, Thorstad K, Daily DK. Preschool outcome of less than 801 grams preterm infants compared with full term siblings. *Pediatrics.* 2004;113(4):742–747.

81. Galvin E, Boyers L, Schwartz PK, et al. Challenging the precepts of family-centered care: testing a philosophy. *Pediatr Nurs.* 2000;26(6):625–632.

82. Harrison H. The principles of family-centered neonatal care. *Pediatrics.* 1993;92(5):643–650.

83. Brazelton TB, Cramer BG. *The Earliest Relationship.* Reading, MA: Addison-Wesley Publishing Company Inc.; 1990.

84. Lawhon G. Management of stress in premature infants. In: Angelini DJ, Whelan Knapp CM, Gibes RM, eds. *Perinatal-Neonatal Nursing: A Clinical Handbook.* Boston, MD: Blackwell Scientific Publications; 1986.

85. Mercer RT. *Nursing Care for Parents at Risk.* Thorofare, NJ: Charles B Slack Inc; 1977.

86. Bibring GL. Some considerations of the psychological process in pregnancy. *Psychoanal Study Child.* 1959;14:113–121.

87. Bibring GL, Dwyer TF, Huntington DS, et al. A study of the psychological processes in pregnancy and of the earliest mother-child relationship. *Psychoanal Study Child.* 1961;16:9–24.

88. Cowan CP, Cowan PA. When Partners Become Parents: The Big Life Change for Couples. Mahwah, NJ: Lawrence Erlbaum Associates Publishers; 1999.

89. Cowan CP, Cowan PA. Interventions to ease the transition to parenthood. *Fam Relations.* 1995;44:412–423.

90. Cowan CP, Cowan PA, Heming G, et al. Transitions to parenthood his, hers, and theirs. *J Fam Issues.* 1985;6(4):451–481.

91. Stainton MC, McNeil D, Harvey S. Maternal tasks of uncertain motherhood. *Matern Child Nurs J.* 1992;20(3,4):113–1231.

92. Miles MS, Brunssen SH. Psychometric properties of the parental stressor scale: infant hospitalization. *Adv Neonatal Care.* 2003;3(4): 189–196.

93. Melnyk BM, Alpert-Gillis LJ, Hensel PB, et al. Helping mothers cope with a critically ill child: a pilot test of the COPE intervention. *Res Nurs Health.* 1997;20:3–14.

94. *Diagnostic and Statistical Manual of Mental Disorders.* 4th ed. Washington, DC: American Psychiatric Association; 1994.

95. Jotzo M, Poets CF. Helping parents cope with the trauma of premature birth: an evaluation of a trauma-preventive psychological intervention. *Pediatrics.* 2005;115(4):915–919.

96. Holditch-Davis D, Bartlett TR, Blickman AL, et al. Posttraumatic stress symptoms in mothers of premature infants. *J Obstet Gynecol Neonatal Nurs.* 2003;32(2):161–171.

97. Peebles-Kleiger MJ. Pediatric and neonatal intensive care hospitalization as traumatic stressor: implications for intervention. *Bull Menninger Clin.* 2000;64(2):257–280.

98. DeMier RL, Hynan MT, Harris HB, et al. Perinatal stressors as predictors of symptoms of posttraumatic stress in mothers of infants at high risk. *J Perinatol.* 1996;16(4):276–280.

99. Affleck G, Tennen H. The effect of newborn intensive care on parents' psychological well-being. *Child Health Care.* 1991;20(1):6–14.

100. Sydnor-Greenberg N, Dokken D, Ahmann E. Coping and caring in different ways: understanding and meaningful involvement. *Pediatr Nurs.* 2000;26(2):185–190.

101. Clubb RL. Chronic sorrow: adaptation patterns of parents with chronically ill children. *Pediatr Nurs.* 1991;17(5):461–466.

102. Pohlman S. Fathers role in the NICU care: evidence-based practice. In: Kenner C, McGrath JM, eds. *Developmental Care of Newborns and Infants: A Guide for Health Professionals.* St. Louis, MO: Mosby; 2004.

103. Kaplan S, Bolender DL. Embryology. In: Polin RA, Fox WW, Abman SH, eds. *Fetal and Neonatal Physiology.* 2nd ed. Philadelphia, PA: WB Saunders Co; 1998.

104. Graham EM, Morgan MA. Growth before term. In: Batshaw MA, ed. *Children with Disabilities.* 4th ed. Baltimore, MD: Paul Brooks Publishing Company; 1997.

105. MacKenzie AP, Stephenson CD, Funai AF. Prenatal assessment of gestational age. Available at: http://www.uptodate.com/contents/prenatal-assessment-of-gestational-age?detectedLanguage=en&source=search_result&search=prenatal+assessment+of+gestational+age&selectedTitle=1%7E150&provider=noProvider. Accessed April 2013.

106. Wilkens-Haug L, Heffner LJ. Fetal assessment and prenatal diagnosis. In: Cloherty JP, Eichenwald EC, Stark AR, eds. *Manual of Neonatal Care*. 5th ed. Philadelphia, PA: Lippincott Williams & Wilkins; 2004.

107. Comparetti AM. Pattern analysis of normal and abnormal development: the fetus, the newborn, the child. In: Slaton DS, ed. *Development of Movement in Infancy*. Chapel Hill, NC: UNC; 1980.

108. Dipietro JA. Fetal neurobehavioral assessment. In: Singer LT, Zeskind PS, eds. *Biobehavioral Assesment of the Infant*. NewYork, NY: The Guilford press; 2001.

109. Rivkees SA, Mirmiran M, Ariagno RL. Circadian rhythms in infants. *NeoReviews*. 2003;4(11):298–303.

110. Prechtl H, Beintema D. *The Neurological Examination of the Newborn Infant. Clinics in Developmental Medicine, 12*. London, UK: Heinemann Educational Books; 1964.

111. Lester BM, Tronick EZ. History and description of the neonatal intensive care unit network neuro-behavioral scale. *Pediatrics*. 2004; 113(3):634–640.

112. Glass P. Development of the visual system and implications for early intervention. *Infants Young Child*. 2002;15(1):1–10.

113. Morrissey K. Seminar in Pediatric Physical Therapy: Infant Development and Therapeutic Interventions. Fall Semester 1994. Hahnemann University Program in Pediatric Physical Therapy.

114. Yoos L. Applying research in practice: parenting the premature infant. *Appl Nurs Res*. 1989;2(1):30–34.

115. Hunter JG. Neonatal intensive care unit. In: Case-Smith J, ed. *Occupational Therapy for Children*. 4th ed. Philadelphia, PA: Mosby; 2001.

116. Allen MC, Capute AJ. Tone and reflex development before term. *Pediatrics*. 1990;85:393–399.

117. Dargassies SSA. *Neurological Development in the Full-Term and Premature Neonate*. Amsterdam, Netherlands: Exerpta Medica; 1977.

118. Sweeney JK, Gutierrez T. Musculoskeletal implications of preterm infant positioning in the NICU. *J Perinatal Neonatal Nurs*. 2002;16(1):58–70.

119. Palmer PG, Dubowitz LMS, Verghote M, et al. Neurological and neurobehavioral differences between preterm infants at term and full-term newborn infants. *Neuropediatrics*. 1982;13:183–189.

120. Mercuri E, Guzzetta A, Laroche S, et al. Neurologic examination of preterm infants at term age: comparison with term infants. *J Pediatr*. 2003;142:647–655.

121. Duffy FH, Als H, McNulty, GB. Behavioral and electrophysiological evidence for gestational age effects in healthy preterm and full-term infants studied two weeks after expected due date. *Child Dev*. 1990;61:1271–1286.

122. Huppi PS, Schuknecht B, Boesch C, et al. Structural and neurobehavioral delay in postnatal brain development of preterm infants. *Pediatr Res*. 1996;39(5):895–901.

123. Mouradian LE, Als H, Coster WJ. Neurobehavioral functioning of healthy preterm infants of varying gestational ages. *Dev Behav Pediatr*. 2000;21(6):408–416.

124. Graven SN. Sound and the developing infant in the NICU: conclusions and recommendations for care. *J Perinatol*. 2000;20: S88–S93.

125. McGrath JM. Neurologic development. In: Kenner C, McGrath JM, eds. *Developmental Care of Newborns and Infants: A Guide for Health Professionals*. St. Louis, MO: Mosby; 2004.

126. Lutes LM, Graves CD, Jorgensen KM. The NICU experience and its relationship to sensory integration. In: Kenner C, McGrath JM, eds. *Developmental Care of Newborns and Infants. A Guide for Health Professionals*. Philadelphia, PA: Elsevier; 2004.

127. Grunau RE, Whitfield MF, Petrie-Thomas J, et al. Neonatal pain, parenting stress, and interaction in relation to cognitive and motor development at 8 and 18 months in preterm infants. *Pain*. 2009;43(1-2):138–146.

128. American Academy of Pediatrics, Canadian Paediatric Society. Prevention and management of pain in the neonate: an update. *Pediatrics*. 2006;188(5):2231–2241.

129. Grunau RE. Early pain in preterm infants. A model of long-term effects. *Clin Perinatol*. 2002;29:373–394.

130. Bouza H. The impact of pain in the immature brain. *J Mat Fetal Neonatal MED*. 2009;22(9):722–732.

131. Hall RW, Anand JS. Physiology of pain and stress in the newborn. *NeoReviews*. 2005;6:e61–e68.

132. Taddio A. Opiod analgesic for infants in the neonatal intensive care unit. *Clin Perinatol*. 2007;27:S9–S11.

133. Gunau RE, Holsti L, Peters JWB. Long-term consequences of pain in human neonates. *Sem Fetal Neonatal Med*. 2000;11:268–275.

134. Anand KJ, Aranda JV, Berde CB, et al. Summary proceedings from the neonatal pain-control group. *Pediatrics*. 2006;117:39–52.

135. Johnston CC, Stevens BJ, Yang F, et al. Differential response to pain by very preterm neonates. *Pain*. 1995;61:471–479.

136. Brummeltre S, Grunau RE, Chau V, et al. Procedural pain and brain development in the premature newborn. *Ann Neurol*. 2012;71:385–396.

137. Harrison LH, Lotas MJ, Jorgensen KM. Environmental issues. In: Kenner C, McGrath JM, eds. *Developmental Care of Newborns and Infants: A Guide for Health Professionals*. Philadelphia, PA: Elsevier; 2004.

138. Syman A, Cunningham S. Handling premature neonates. *Nurs Times*. 1995;91(17):35–37.

139. Blackburn S, Barnard K. Analysis of caregiving events relating to preterm infants in the special care unit. In: Gottfried AW, Gaiter JL, eds. *Infants Under Stress: Environmental Neonatology*. Baltimore, MD: University Park; 1985.

140. Gottfried AW, Hodgman JE, Brown KW. How intensive is intensive care? An environmental analysis. *Pediatrics*. 1984;74:292–294.

141. Holsti L, Grunau RE, Oberlander TF. Is it painful or not? Discreet validity of the behavioural indicators of infant pain (BIIP) scale. *Clin J Pain*. 2008;24(1):83–88.

142. Hellerud BC, Storm H. Skin conduction and behavior during sensory stimulation of preterm and term infants. *Early Human Dev*. 2002;20:38–46.

143. Franck LS, Miaskowski C. Measurement of neonatal responses to painful stimuli: a research review. *J Pain Symptom Manag*. 1997;14(6): 343–378.

144. Cignacco EL, Sellam G, Stoffel L, et al. Oral sucrose and "facilitated tucking" for repeated pain relief on preterms: a randomized control trial. *Pediatrics*. 2011;129:299–308.

145. Cameron EC, Raingangar V, Khoori N. Effects of handling procedures on pain responses of very low birth weight infanst. *Pediatr Phys Ther*. 2007;19:40–47.

146. Holsti L, Grunau RE, Oberlander TF, et al. Body movements: an important additional factor in discriminating pain for stress in preterm infants. *Clin J Pain*. 2005;21:491–498.

147. Stevens B, Gibbins S, Franck LS. Treatment of pain in the neonatal intensive care unit. *Pediatr Clin North Am*. 2000;47(3):633–650.

148. Grunau RE, Whitfield MF, Holsti L, et al. Biobehavioral reactivity to pain in preterm infants: a marker of neuromotor development. *Dev Med Child Neurol*. 2006;48:471–476.

149. Vinall J, Miller SP, Chau V. Neonatal pain in relation to postnatal growth in infants born very preterm. *Pain*. 2012;153:1374–1381.

150. Johnston CC, Stevens BJ, Franck LS, et al. Factors explaining lack of response to heel stick in preterm infants. *J Obstet Gynecol Neonatal Nurs*. 2004;33(2):246–255.

151. Losocco V, Cuttini M, Greisen G, et al. Heel blood sampling in European neonatal intensive care units: compliance with pain management guidelines. *Arch Dis Child Fetal Neonatal Ed*. 2011;96(1): F65–F68.

152. Morison SJ, Grunau RE, Oberlander TF, et al. Are there developmentally distinct motor indicators of pain in preterm infants? *Early Human Dev*. 2003;72(2):131–146.

153. Craig KD, Whitfield MF, Grunau RV, et al. Pain in the preterm neonate: behavioral and physiological indices. *Pain*. 1993;52:287–299.

154. Joint Commission on Accreditation of Healthcare Organizations. Joint Commission Hospital Quality Report. Available at: www.jcaho.org.

155. Duhn LJ, Medves JM. A systematic integrative review of infant pain assessment tools. *Adv Neonatal Care.* 2004;4(3):126–140.

156. Carbajal R, Lenclen R, Jugie M, et al. Morphine does not provide adequate analgesia for acute procedural pain among preterm neonates. *Pediatrics.* 2005;115:1499–1500.

157. Stevens B, Johnston C, Franck L, et al. The efficacy of developmentally sensitive behavioral interventions and sucrose for relieving procedural pain in very low birth weight neonate. *Nurs Res.* 1999;48(1):35–43.

158. Hatch DJ. Analgesia in the neonate. *BMJ.* 1987;294:920.

159. Browne JV. Developmental care for high-risk newborns: emerging science, clinical application, continuity for newborn intensive care unit to community. *Clin Perinatol.* 2011;38:719–729.

160. Holsti L, Grunau RE, Shaney E. Assessing pain in preterm infants in the neonatal intensive care unit: moving to a "brain oriented" approach. *Pain Manag.* 2011;1(2):171–197.

161. Franck L. Some pain some gain reflections on the past two decades of neonatal pain research and treatment. *Neonatal Netw.* 2002;21(5):37–41.

162. Obeidat H, Kahalaf I, Callister LA. Use of facilitated tucking for nonpharmocologic pain management in preterm infants: a systematic review. *J Perinatol Neonat.* 2009;23(4):372.

163. Axelin A, Kirjavainen J, Salantera S, et al. Effects of pain management on sleep in preterm infants. *Eur J Pain.* 2010;14(7):752–758.

164. Cong X, Cusson RM, Walsh S, et al. Effects of skin to skin contact on autonomic pain responses in preterm infants. *J Pain.* 2012;13(7):636–645.

165. Stevens B, Yamada J, Beyene J, et al. Consistent management of repeated procedural pain with sucrose in preterm neonates: is it effective and safe for repeated use over time? *Clin J Pain.* 2005;21(6):543–548.

166. Stevens B, Yamada J, Lee GY, et al. Sucrose for analgesia in newborn infants undergoing painful procedures. *Cochrane Database Syst Rev.* 2013;DOI:10.1002/14651858.CD001069.pub4. Accessed April 2013.

167. Stevens B, Yamada J, Lee GY, et al. Sucrose for analgesia in newborn infants undergoing painful procedures. *Cochrane Database Syst Rev.* 2010;(1):CD001069:PMD:20091512. Accessed April 2013.

168. Gerall R, Cignacco E, Stoffel L, et al. Phsyiologic parameters after non pharmacologic analgesia in preterm infants: a randomized trial. *Act Paediatr.* 2013;DOI: 10.111/ apa.12288.

169. Shah PS, Herbozo C, Aliwalas LL, et al. Breast feeding or breast milk for procedural pain in neonates (review). *Cochrane Database Syst Review.* 2012;12.

170. Simonese E, Mulder PGH, van Beek RHT. Analgesic effect of breast milk versus sucrose for analgesia during heel lance in late preterm infants. *Pediatrics.* 2012;129:657–663.

171. Gray L, Watt L, Blass EM. Skin-to-skin contact is analgesic in healthy newborns. *Pediatrics.* 2000;105(1):4–19.

172. Turnage-Carrier CS. Caregiving and the environment. In: Kenner C, McGrath JM, eds. *Developmental Care of Newborns and Infants: A Guide for Health Professionals.* Philadelphia, PA: Elsevier; 2004.

173. American Academy of Pediatrics, Committee on Environmental Health. Noise: a hazard for the fetus and newborn. *Pediatrics.* 1997;100(4):724–727.

174. Philbin MK. Planning the acoustic environment of a neonatal intensive care unit. *Clin Perinatol.* 2004;31:331–352.

175. Chang YJ, Lin CH, Lin LH. Noise and related events in a neonatal intensive care unit. *Acta Paediatr.* 2001;42:212–217.

176. Evans JB, Philbin MK. The acoustic environment of hospital nurseries. *J Perinatol.* 2000;20(8):S105–S112.

177. Philbin MK. Some implications of early auditory development for the environment of hospitalized preterm infants. *Neonatal Netw.* 1996;15(7):71–73.

178. Philbin MK, Evans JB. Noise levels, spectra and operational function of an occupied newborn intensive care unit built to meet recommended permissible noise criteria. *J Acoustic Soc Ame.* 2003;114(4, part 2):2326 (#2aNS2).

179. White RD. Recommended standards for newborn ICU design. *J Perinatol.* 2003;23(1):5–21.

180. Morante A, Dubowitz LMS, Levene M, et al. The development of visual function in normal and abnormal preterm and full term infants. *Dev Med Child Neurol.* 1982;24:771–784.

181. Prechtl HFR, Fargel JW, Weinmann HM, et al. Postures and respiration of low-risk pre-term infants. *Dev Med Child Neurol.* 1979;21:3–27.

182. Brazelton TB, Nugent JK. The Neonatal Behavioral Assessment Scale. 3rd ed. London, UK: MacKeith Press; 1995.

183. Als H. Reading the premature infant. In: Goldson E, ed. *Nurturing the Premature Infant Developmental Intervention in the Neonatal Intensive Care Nursery.* New York, NY: Oxford University Press; 1999.

184. Pompa KM, Zaichkin J. The NICU baby. In: Zaichkin J, ed. *Newborn Intensive Care: What Every Parent Needs to Know.* Santa Rosa, CA: NICU Ink Book Publishers; 2002.

185. Lee, KG, Cloherty JP. Identifying the high risk newborn and evaluating gestational age, prematurity, post maturity, large for gestational age, and small for gestational age. In: Cloherty JP, Eichenwald EC, Stark AR, eds. *Manual of Neonatal Care.* 5th ed. Philadelphia, PA: Lippincott Williams & Wilkins; 2004.

186. Gregory S. Homeward bound. In: Zaichkin J, ed. *Newborn Intensive Care: What Every Parent Needs to Know.* 2nd ed. Santa Rosa, CA: NICU Ink Book Publishers; 2002.

187. Apgar V. A proposal for a new method of evaluation of the newborn infant. *Curr Res Anesth Analg.* 1953;32(4):260–267.

188. American Academy of Pediatrics, Committee on Fetus & Newborn, American College of Obstetricians & Gynecologists et al. The apgar score. *Pediatrics.* 2006;117(4):1444–1447.

189. American Academy of Pediatrics Committee on Fetus & Newborn, American College of Obstetricians & Gynecologists & Committee on Obstetric Practice. The apgar score. Pediatrics. 2006;117(4):1444–1447.

190. Eichenwald EC. Mechanical ventilation. In: Cloherty JP, Eichenwald EC, Stark AR, eds. *Manual of Neonatal Care.* 5th ed. Philadelphia, PA: Lippincott Williams & Wilkins; 2004.

191. Cameron J, Haines J. Management of respiratory disorders. In: Boxwell G. *Neonatal Intensive Care Nursing.* New York, NY: Routledge; 2000.

192. Wiswell TE, Pinchi S. Continuous positive airway pressure. In: Goldsmith JP, Karotin EH, eds. *Assisted Ventilation of the Neonate.* 4th ed. Philadelphia, PA: Saunders; 2003.

193. Czervinske MP. Continuous positive airway pressure. In: Czervinske MP, Barnhart SC, eds. *Perinatal and Pediatric Respiratory Care.* 2nd ed. Philadelphia, PA: Saunders; 2003.

194. Lee KS, Dunn MS, Fenwick M. A comparison of underwater bubble continuous positive airway pressure with ventilator derived continuous positive airway pressure in premature infants ready for extubation. *Biol Neonate.* 1998;73(2):69–75.

195. Spitzer AR, Greenspan JS, Fox WW. Positive-pressure ventilation-pressure-limited and time cycled ventilation. In: Goldsmith JP, Karotin EH, eds. *Assisted Ventilation of the Neonate.* 4th ed. Philadelphia, PA: Saunders; 2003.

196. Schwartz JE. New technologies applied to management of the respiratory system. In: Kenner C, Lott JW, eds. *Comprehensive Neonatal Nursing: A Physiologic Perspective.* 3rd ed. Philadelphia, PA: Saunders; 2003.

197. Meredith KS. High frequency ventilation. In: Czervinske MP, Barnhart SC, eds. *Perinatal and Pediatric Respiratory Care.* 2nd ed. Philadelphia, PA: Saunders; 2003.

198. Mammel MC. Mechanical ventilation of the newborn. *Arch Dis Child Fetal Neonatal Ed.* 2000;83(3):F224.

199. Mammel MC. High frequency ventilation. In: Goldsmith JP, Karotin EH, eds. *Assisted Ventilation of the Neonate.* 4th ed. Philadelphia, PA: Saunders; 2003.

200. Keszler M, Derand DJ. Neonatal high frequency ventilation: past, present, future. *Clin Perinatol.* 2001;28(3):579–607.

201. MacIntyre NR. High frequency jet ventilation. *Respir Care Clin N Am.* 2001;7(4):599–610.

202. Bouchet JC, Goddard J, Claris O. High frequency oscillatory ventilation. *Anesthesiology.* 2004;100:1007–1012.

203. Moriette G, Paris-Llado J, Walti H, et al. Prospective randomized multicenter comparison of high frequency oscillatory ventilation and conventional ventilation in preterm infants of less than 30 weeks with respiratory distress syndrome. *Pediatrics.* 2001;107(2):363–372.

204. Osborn DA, Evans N. Randomized trial of high frequency oscillatory ventilation versus conventional ventilation: effect on systemic blood flow in very premature infants. *J Pediatr.* 2003;143(2):192–202.

205. Sreenan C, Lemke RP, Hudson-Mason A, et al. High-flow nasal cannulae in the management of apnea of prematurity: a comparison with conventional nasal continuous positive airway pressure. *Pediatrics.* 2001;107(5):1081–1083.

206. Locke RG, Wolfson MR, Shaffer TH, et al. Inadvertent administration of positive-end-distending pressure during nasal cannula flow. *Pediatrics.* 1993;91(1):135–138.

207. Saslow JG, Aghar ZH, Nakhla TA, et al. Work of breathing using high flow nasal cannula in preterm infants. *J Perinatol.* 2006;26(8):476–480.

208. Walsh B. Comparison of Vapotherm 2000i with a bubble humidifier humidifying flow through a nasal cannula. *Respir Care.* 2003;48(18).

209. Kopelman AE, Holbert D. Use of oxygen cannulas in extremely low birthweight infants. *J Perinatol.* 2003;23:94–97.

210. Vapotherm. Available at: http://www.vtherm.com/forclinicians/lowflow.asp. Accessed June 2013.

211. Woodhead DD, Lambert DK, Clark JM, et al. Comparing two methods of delivering high-flow gas therapy by nasal cannula following endotracheal extubation: a prospective, randomized, masked, cross-over trial. *J Perinatol.* 2006;26(8):481–485.

212. Waugh JB, Granger WM. An evaluation of two new devices for nasal high flow gas therapy. *Respir Care.* 2004;49(8):902–906.

213. Panitch HB, Wolfson MR, Shaffer TH. Epithelial modulation of preterm airway smooth muscle contraction. *J Pediatr.* 1993;74(3):1437–1443.

214. Cullen AB, Wolfson MR, Shaffer TH. The maturation of airway structure and function. *NeoReviews.* 2002;3(7):e125–e130.

215. Williams LJ, Shaffer TH, Greenspan JS. Inhaled nitric oxide therapy in the nearly term or term infant with hypoxic respiratory failure. *Neonatal Netw.* 2004;23(1):5–13.

216. Neonatal Inhaled Nitric Oxide Study Group (NINOS). Inhaled nitric oxide in full-term and nearly term infants with hypoxic respiratory failure. *N Engl J Med.* 1997;336:597–604.

217. Neonatal Inhaled Nitric Oxide Study Group (NINOS). Inhaled nitric oxide in term and nearly term infants: neurodevelopmental follow-up of the neonatal inhaled nitric oxide study group (NINOS). *J Pediatr.* 2000;136(5):611–617.

218. Ellington M, O'Reilly D, Allred EN, et al. Child health status, neurodevelopmental outcome, and parent satisfaction in a randomized, controlled trial of nitric oxide for persistent pulmonary hypertension of the newborn. *Pediatrics.* 2001;107(6):1351–1356.

219. American Academy of Pediatrics, Committee on Fetus and Newborn. Use of inhaled nitric oxide. *Pediatrics.* 2000;106(2, part 1):344–345.

220. Ballard RH, Truog WE, Cnaan A, et al. Inhaled nitric oxide in preterm infants undergoing mechanical ventilation. *N Engl J Med.* 2006;355(4):343–353.

221. Kinsella JP, Cutter GR, Walsh WF, et al. Early inspired nitric oxide therapy in premature newborns with respiratory failure. *N Engl J Med.* 2006;355(4):354–364.

222. Ford JW. Neonatal ECMO: current controversies and trends. *Neonatal Netw.* 2006;25(4):229–238.

223. Rais-Bahrami K, Short BL. The current status of neonatal extracorporeal membrane oxygenation. *Semin Perinatol.* 2000;24(6):406–417.

224. Jaillard S, Pierrat V, Truffert P, et al. Two years follow-up of newborn infants after extracorporeal membrane oxygenation. *Eur J Cardiothorac Surg.* 2000;18(3):328–333.

225. Kim ES, Stolar CJ. ECMO in the newborn. *Am J Perinatol.* 2000;17(7):345–356.

226. Rais-Bahrami K, Wagner AE, Coffman C, et al. Neurodevelopmental outcome in ECMO vs near-miss ECMO patients at 5 years of age. *Clin Pediatr.* 2000;39(3):145–152.

227. Tappero EP. NICU technology. In: Zaichkin J, ed. *Newborn Intensive Care: What Every Parent Needs to Know.* 2nd ed. Santa Rosa, CA: NICU Ink Book Publishers; 2002.

228. Cooper M, Arnold J. Extracorporeal membrane oxygenation. In: Cloherty JP, Eichenwald EC, Stark AR, eds. *Manual of Neonatal Care.* 5th ed. Philadelphia, PA: Lippincott Williams & Wilkins; 2004.

229. Nield TA, Langenbacher D, Poulsen MK, et al. Neurodevelopmental outcome at 3.5 years of age in children treated with extra corporeal life support: relationship to primary diagnosis. *J Pediatr.* 2000;136(3):338–344.

230. Massery M. Chest development as a component of normal motor development: implications for treatment for pediatric physical therapists. *Pediatr Phys Ther.* 1991;3(1):3–8.

231. Make BJ, Hill NS, Goldberg AI, et al. Mechanical ventilation beyond the intensive care unit: report of a consensus conference of the American College of Chest Physicians. *Chest.* 1998;113(5):289S–344S.

232. Vohr BR, Cashore WJ, Bigsby R. Stresses & interventions in the neonatal intensive care unit. In: Levine MD, Carey WB, Crocker AC, eds. *Developmental-Behavioral Pediatrics.* 3rd ed. Philadelphia, PA: Saunders; 1999.

233. Honrubia D, Stark AR. Respiratory distress syndrome. In: Cloherty JP, Eichenwald EC, Stark AR, ed. *Manual of Neonatal Care.* 5th ed. Philadelphia, PA: Lippincott Williams & Wilkins; 2004.

234. National Institutes of Health. *Report of the Consensus Development Conference on Anti-natal Corticosteroids Revisited: Repeat Courses.* Bethesda, MD: National Institute of Child Health and Human Development; 2000.

235. Baud O. Antenatal glucocorticoid treatment and cystic periventricular leukomalacia in very preterm infants. *N Engl J Med.* 1999;341(16):1190–1196.

236. Banks BA, Cnaan A, Morgan MA, et al. Multiple courses of antenatal corticosteroids and outcome of premature neonates. *Am J Obstet Gynecol.* 1999;181:709–717.

237. Banks BA, Macones G, Cnaan A, et al. Multiple courses of antenatal corticosteroids are associated with early severe lung disease in preterm neonates. *J Perinatol.* 2002;22:101–107.

238. Jobe AH, Ikegami M. Biology of surfactant. *Clin Perinatol.* 2001;28:671–694.

239. Egerman RS, Mercer BM, Doss JL, et al. A randomized controlled trial of oral and intramuscular dexamethasone in the prevention of neonatal respiratory distress syndrome. *Am J Obstet Gynecol.* 1998;179(5):1120–1123.

240. Hack MF, Minisch N, Fanaroff A. Antenatal steroids have not improved the outcomes of surviving extremely low birth weight (ELBW) infants [<750 grams]. *Pediatr Res.* 1998;43(2):214A.

241. Soll RF. Surfactant treatment of the very premature infant. *Biol Neonate.* 1998;74(suppl 1):35–42.

242. Suresh GK. Current surfactant use in premature infants. *Clin Perinatol.* 2001;28:671–694.

243. Escobedo MB, Gunkel JH, Kennedy RA, et al. Texas Neonatal Research Group. Early surfactant for neonates with mild to moderate RDS: a multicenter randomized trial. *J Pediatr.* 2004;144(6):804–808.

244. Jobe AH. Surfactant for RDS: when and why? *J Pediatr.* 2004;144(6):A2.

245. Dani C, Bertini G, Pezzati M, et al. Early extubation and nasal continuous positive airway pressure after surfactant treatment for respiratory distress syndrome among preterm infants <30 weeks gestation. *Pediatrics.* 2004;113(6):e560–e563.

246. Park MK. *Pediatric Cardiology for Practitioners.* 4th ed. St Louis, MO: Mosby; 2002.

247. Heyman MA, Teitel DF, Liebman J. The heart. In: Klaus MH, Fanaroff AA, eds. *Care of the High-Risk Neonate.* 4th ed. Philadelphia, PA: Saunders; 1993.

248. Wechsler SB, Wernovsky G. Cardiac disorders. In: Cloherty JP, Eichenwald EC, Stark AR, eds. *Manual of Neonatal Care.* 5th ed. Philadelphia, PA: Lippincott Williams & Wilkins; 2004.

249. Gersony WM, Peckham GJ, Ellison RC, et al. Effects of indomethacine in premature infants with patent ductus arteriosus: results of a national collaborative study. *J Pediatr.* 1984;102(6):895–906.

250. Gersony WM. Patent ductus arteriosus. *Pediatr Clin North Am.* 1986;33(3):545–560.

251. Martin CR, Cloherty JP. Neonatal hyperbilirubinemia. In: Cloherty JR, Eichenwald EC, Stark AR, eds. *Manual of Neonatal Care.* 5th ed. Philadelphia, PA: Lippincott Williams & Wilkins; 2004.

252. Dennery PA, Seidman DS, Stevenson DK. Neonatal hyperbilirubinemia. *N Engl J Med.* 2001;334:581–590.

253. Poland RL, Ostrea EM. Neonatal hyperbilirubinemia. In: Klaus MH, Fanaroff AA, eds. *Care of the High Risk Neonate.* Philadelphia, PA: Saunders; 1993.

254. Maisels MJ, Watchko JF, Bhutani VK, et al. An approach to the management of hyperbilirubinemia in the preterm inants less than 35 weeks of gestation. *J Perinatol.* 2012;32:660–664.

255. AAP Subcommittee on Neonatal Hyperbilirubinemia. Neonatal jaundice and kernicterus. *Pediatrics.* 2001;108(3):763–765.

256. Patra K, Storfer-Isser A, Siner B, et al. Adverse events associated with neonatal exchange transfusion in the 1990's. *J Pediatr.* 2004;144:626–631.

257. Paludetto R, Mansi G, Raimondi F, et al. Moderate hyperbilirubinemia induces a transient alteration of neonatal behavior. *Pediatrics.* 2002;110(4):e50.

258. Mansi G, De Maio C, Araimo G, et al. "Safe" hyperbilirubinemia is associated with altered neonatal behavior. *Biol Neonate.* 2003; 83(1):19–21.

259. Jadcherla SR. Gastroesophageal reflux in the neonate. *Clin Perinatol.* 2002;29(1):135–158.

260. Omari TI. Lower esophageal sphincter function in the neonate. *NeoReviews.* 2006;7(1):e13–e17.

261. Jadcherla SK, Rudolph CD. Gastroesophageal reflux in the preterm neonate. *NeoReviews.* 2005;6:e87–e95.

262. Tipnis NA, Tipnis SM. Controversies in the treatment of gastroesophageal reflux in preterm infants. *Clin Perinatol.* 2009;36:153–164.

263. Noviski N, Yehuda YB, Yorum B, et al. Does the size of nasogastric tube affect gastroesophageal reflux in children. *J Pediatr Gastroenterol Nutr.* 1999;29:448–451.

264. Hammer D. Gastroesophageal reflux and prokinetic agents. *Neonatal Netw.* 2005;24(2):51–58.

265. Sherman PM, Hassell F, Fagundes-Nero U, et al. A global evidence-based consensus on the definition of gastroesophageal reflux in the pediatric patient. *Am J Gastroenterol.* 2009;104:278–298.

266. Menon AP, Schefft GL, Thach BT. Apnea associated with regurgitation in infants. *J Pediatr.* 1985;106(4):625–629.

267. Jadcherla SR. Upstream effect of esophageal distension: effect on airway. *Curr Gastroenterol Rep.* 2006;8(3):190–194.

268. Gupta A, Gulati P, Kim W, et al. Effect of postnatal maturation on the mechanics of esophageal propulsion in preterm human neonates: primary and secondary peristalsis. *Am J Gastroenterol.* 2009;104:411–419.

269. Jadcherla SR. Pathophysiology of aerodigestive pulmonary disorders in the neonate. *Clin Perinatol.* 2012;39:631–654.

270. Peter CS, Sprodowski N, Bohnhorst B, et al. Gastroesophageal reflux and apnea of prematurity. No temporal relationship. *Pediatrics.* 2002; 109(8):8–11.

271. Poets CF. Gastroesophageal reflux: a critical review of its role in preterm infants. *Pediatrics.* 2004;113(2):e128–e132.

272. Krishnamoorthy M, Muntz A, Liem T, et al. Diagnosis and treatment of respiratory symptoms of initially unsuspected gastroesophageal reflux in infants. *Am Surg.* 1994;60:783–785.

273. Davies AM, Koenig JS, Thatch BT. Upper airway chemoreflex responses to saline and water in preterm infants. *J Appl Phys.* 1988; 64(4):1412–1420.

274. DiFiore J, Arko M, Herynk B, et al. Characterization of cardiorespiratory events following gastroesophageal reflux in preterm infants. *J Perinatol.* 2010;30(10):683–687.

275. Poets CF. Gastroesophageal reflux and apnea of prematurity- coincidence not causation. *Neurology.* 2013;103:103–104.

276. Orenstein SR, Whittington PF. Positioning for prevention of infant gastroesophageal reflux. *J Pediatr.* 1983;103:534–537.

277. Tobin JM, McCloud P, Cameron DJS. Posture and gastroesophageal reflux: a case for left lateral positioning. *Arch Dis Child.* 1997;76: 254–258.

278. Ewer AK, James ME, Tobin JM. Prone and lateral position reduce gastroesophageal reflux in premature infants. *Arch Dis Child.* 1999;81:F201–F205.

279. Corvaglia, L Rotatori R, Ferlini M, et al. The effect of body positioning on gastroesophageal reflux in the premature infant: evaluation by combined impedence and pH monitoring. *J Pediatr.* 2007;151:591–596.

280. Omari T, Rommel N, Staunton E, et al. Paradoxical impact of body positioning on gastroesophageal reflux and gastric emptying in the premature infant. *J Pediatr.* 2004;145:194–200.

281. Chen SS, Tzeng YL, Gau BS, et al. Effects of prone and supine positioning on gastric residuals in preterm infants: a time series with cross-over study. *Int J Nurs Stud.* 2013; Available at: http://dx.doi.org/10.1016/j.ijnurstu.2013.02.009. Accessed May 2013.

282. Sangers H, de Jong PM, Mulder SE. Outcomes of gastric residuals whilst feeding preterm infants in various body positions. *J Neonatal Nurs.* 2012. Available at: http://dx.doi.org/10.1016/j.jnn. Accessed December 2012.

283. van Wijk MP, Bennigan MA, Dent J, et al. Effect of body position-changes on postprandial gastroesophageal reflux and gastric emptying in the healthy preterm neonate. *J Peds.* 2007;585–590.

284. Malcolm WF, Cotton M. Metoclopramide, H2 blockers, and proton inhibitors: pharmacology for gastroesophageal reflux in neonates. *Clin Perinatol.* 2012;39:99–109.

285. Czinn SJ, Blanchard S. Gastroesophageal disease in neonates and infants. When and how to treat. *Pediatr Drugs.* 2013;15:19–27.

286. Loots CM, Benniga MA, Omari M. Gastroesophageal reflux in pediatrics (patho) physiology and new insights in diagnosis and treatment. *Minerva Pediatir.* 2012;64(1):104–119.

287. Loots C, van Herwaarden MY, Benniga MA, et al. Gastroesophageal reflux, esophageal function, gastric emptying and the relationship to dysphagia before an after antireflux surgery in children. *J Pediatr.* 2013;162:526–573.

288. RJ Schanler. Clinical Features and Diagnosis of Necrotizing Enterocolitis in Newborns. *Up to Date*, April 17 2012. Available at: http://www.uptodate.com/contents/clinical-features-and-diagnosis-of-necrotizing-enterocolitis-in-newborns?source=search_result&search=NEC+totalis&selectedTitle=2%7E150. Accessed May 2013.

289. Kosloske AM. Epidemiology of necrotizing enterocolitis. *Acta Paediatr Suppl.* 1994;396:2.

290. RJ Schanler. Pathology and pathogenesis of necrotizing enterocolitis in newborns. *UptoDate*, March 18, 2013. Available at: http://www.uptodate.com/contents/pathology-and-pathogenesis-of-necrotizing-enterocolitis-in-newborns?source=search_result&search=necrotizing+enterocolitis&selectedTitle=4%7E150#references. Accessed May 2013.

291. Neu J, Weiss MD. Necrotizing enterocolitis: pathophysiology and prevention. *J Parenter Enteral Nutr.* 1999;23:S13.

292. Hunter CJ, Upperman JS, Ford HR, Camerini V. Understanding the susceptibility of the premature infant to necrotizing enterocolitis (NEC). *Pediatr Res.* 2008;63:117.

293. Neu J. Necrotizing enterocolitis: the search for a unifying pathogenic theory leading to prevention. *Pediatr Clin North Am.* 1996;43:409.

294. Ballance WA, Dahms BB, Shenker N, et al. Pathology of neonatal necrotizing enterocolitis: a ten-year experience. *J Pediatr.* 1990;117:S6.

295. Horbar JD, Badger GJ, Carpenter JH, et al. Trends in mortality and morbidity for very low birth weight infants, 1991-1999. *Pediatrics.* 2002;110:143.

296. Sankaran K, Puckett B, Lee DS, et al. Variations in incidence of necrotizing enterocolitis in Canadian neonatal intensive care units. *J Pediatr Gastroenterol Nutr.* 2004;39:366.

297. Lee SK, McMillan DD, Ohlsson A, et al. Variations in practice and outcomes in the Canadian NICU network: 1996-1997. *Pediatrics.* 2000;106:1070.

298. Wiswell TE, Robertson CF, Jones TA, et al. Necrotizing enterocolitis in full-term infants. A case-control study. *Am J Dis Child.* 1988;142:532.

299. Polin RA, Pollack PF, Barlow B, et al. Necrotizing enterocolitis in term infants. *J Pediatr.* 1976;89:460.

300. Ostlie DJ, Spilde TL, St. Peter SD, et al. Necrotizing enterocolitis in full-term infants. *J Pediatr Surg.* 2003;38:1039.

301. Lambert DK, Christensen RD, Henry E, et al. Necrotizing enterocolitis in term neonates: data from a multihospital health-care system. *J Perinatol.* 2007;27:437.

302. Kliegman RM, Walker WA, Yolken RH. Necrotizing enterocolitis: research agenda for a disease of unknown etiology and pathogenesis. *Pediatr Res.* 1993;34:701.

303. Holman RC, Stoll BJ, Clarke MJ, et al. The epidemiology of necrotizing enterocolitis infant mortality in the United States. *Am J Public Health.* 1997;87:2026.

304. McAlmon KR. Necrotizing enterocolitis. In: Cloherty JP, Eichenwald EC, Stark AR, eds. *Manual of Neonatal Care.* 5th ed. Philadelphia, PA: Lippincott Williams & Wilkins; 2004.

305. Reber KM, Nankervis CA. Necrotizing enterocolitis: preventative strategies. *Clin Perinatol.* 2004;31(1):157–167.

306. Rees CM, Pierro A, Eaton S. Neurodevelopmental outcomes on neonates with medically and surgically treated necrotizing enterocolitis. *Arch Dis Child Fetal Neonatal Ed.* 2007;92:F193–F198.

307. Rees CM, Eaton S, Pierro A. National prospective surveillance study of necrotizing enterocolitis in neonatal intensive care units. *J Pediatr Surg.* 2010;45:1391.

308. Snyder CL, Gittes GK, Murphy JP, et al. Survival after necrotizing enterocolitis in infants weighing less than 1,000 g: 25 years' experience at a single institution. *J Pediatr Surg.* 1997;32:434.

309. Schanler RJ. Management of Necrotizing Enterocolitis in Newborns. *UpToDate,* March 5, 2013. Available at: http://www.uptodate.com/contents/management-of-necrotizing-enterocolitis-in-newborns?source=search_result&search=NEC+totalis&selectedTitle=1%7E150#H20 Accessed May 2013.

310. Abdullah F, Zhang Y, Camp M, et al. Necrotizing enterocolitis in 20,822 infants: analysis of medical and surgical treatments. *Clin Pediatr (Phila).* 2010;49:166.

311. Fasoli L, Turi RA, Spitz L, et al. Necrotizing enterocolitis: extent of disease and surgical treatment. *J Pediatr Surg.* 1999;34:1096.

312. Fitzgibbons SC, Ching Y, Yu D, et al. Mortality of necrotizing enterocolitis expressed by birth weight categories. *J Pediatr Surg.* 2009;44:1072.

313. Horwitz JR, Lally KP, Cheu HW, et al. Complications after surgical intervention for necrotizing enterocolitis: a multicenter review. *J Pediatr Surg.* 1995;30:994.

314. Kliegman RM, Fanaroff AA. Necrotizing enterocolitis. *N Engl J Med.* 1984;310:1093.

315. Walsh MC, Kliegman RM, Fanaroff AA. Necrotizing enterocolitis: a practitioner's perspective. *Pediatr Rev.* 1988;9(7):219–226.

316. Yu VY, Tudehope DI, Gill GJ. Neonatal necrotizing enterocolitis: 1. Clinical aspects. *Med J Aust.* 1977;1:685.

317. Kliegman RM, Walsh MC. Neonatal necrotizing enterocolitis: pathogenesis, classification, and spectrum of illness. *Curr Probl Pediatr.* 1987;17:213–288.

318. Kanto WP, Hunter JE, Stoll BJ. Recognition and medical management of necrotizing enterocolitis. *Clin Perinatol.* 1994;21:335–346.

319. Stoll BJ, Kliegman RM. Necrotizing Enterocolitis. Clinics in Perinatology. Philadelphia, PA: Saunders; 1994.

320. Walsh MC, Kliegman RM. Necrotizing enterocolitis: treatment based on a staging criteria. Pediatr Clin North Am 1986;33:179–201.

321. Kleigman RM. Necrotizing enterocolitis: bridging the basic science with the clinical disease. *J Pediatr.* 1990;117(5):833–835.

322. Bell MJ, Ternberg JL, Feigin RD, et al. Neonatal necrotizing enterocolitis. Therapeutic decisions based upon clinical staging. *Ann Surg.* 1978;187:1.

323. Clark DA, Miller MJ. Intraluminal pathogenesis of necrotizing enterocolitis. *J Pediatr.* 1990;117:S64.

324. Morgan J, Young L, McGuire W. Slow advancement of enteral feed volumes to prevent necrotising enterocolitis in very low birth weight infants. *Cochrane Database Syst Rev.* 2011;CD001241.

325. Morgan J, Young L, McGuire W. Delayed introduction of progressive enteral feeds to prevent necrotising enterocolitis in very low birth weight infants. *Cochrane Database Syst Rev.* 2011;CD001970.

326. La Gamma EF, Browne LE. Feeding practices for infants weighing less than 1500 G at birth and the pathogenesis of necrotizing enterocolitis. *Clin Perinatol.* 1994;21:271.

327. Schanler RJ, Shulman RJ, Lau C, et al. Feeding strategies for premature infants: randomized trial of gastrointestinal priming and tube-feeding method. *Pediatrics.* 1999;103:434.

328. Bombell S, McGuire W. Early trophic feeding for very low birth weight infants. *Cochrane Database Syst Rev.* 2009;CD000504.

329. Caplan M. Is EGF the Holy Grail for NEC? *J Pediatr.* 2007;150:329.

330. Cikrit D, Mastandrea J, West KW, et al. Necrotizing enterocolitis: factors affecting mortality in 101 surgical cases. *Surgery.* 1984;96:648–665.

331. Salvia G, Guarino A, Terrin G, et al. Neonatal onset intestinal failure: an Italian Multicenter Study. *J Pediatr.* 2008;153:674.

332. Cole CR, Hansen NI, Higgins RD, et al. Bloodstream infections in very low birth weight infants with intestinal failure. *J Pediatr.* 2012;160:54.

333. Kim ES, Brandt ML. Spontaneous intestinal perforation of the newborn. Available at: http://www.uptodate.com/contents/spontaneous-intestinal-perforation-of-the-newborn?source=search_result&search=spontaneous+infant+performation&selectedTitle=3%7E150. Accessed May 2013.

334. Ragouilliaux CJ, Keeney SE, Hawkins HK, et al. Maternal factors in extremely low birth weight infants who develop spontaneous intestinal perforation. *Pediatrics.* 2007;120:e1458.

335. Gordon PV, Young ML, Marshall DD. Focal small bowel perforation: an adverse effect of early postnatal dexamethasone therapy in extremely low birth weight infants. *J Perinatol.* 2001;21:156.

336. Stark AR, Carlo WA, Tyson JE, et al. Adverse effects of early dexamethasone in extremely-low-birth-weight infants. National Institute of Child Health and Human Development Neonatal Research Network. *N Engl J Med.* 2001;344:95.

337. Gordon P, Rutledge J, Sawin R, et al. Early postnatal dexamethasone increases the risk of focal small bowel perforation in extremely low birth weight infants. *J Perinatol.* 1999;19:573.

338. Baird R, Puligandla PS, St. Vil D, et al. The role of laparotomy for intestinal perforation in very low birth weight infants. *J Pediatr Surg.* 2006;41:1522.

339. Blakely ML, Gupta H, Lally KP. Surgical management of necrotizing enterocolitis and isolated intestinal perforation in premature neonates. *Semin Perinatol.* 2008;32:122.

340. Cass DL, Brandt ML, Patel DL, et al. Peritoneal drainage as definitive treatment for neonates with isolated intestinal perforation. *J Pediatr Surg.* 2000;35:1531.

341. Chiu B, Pillai SB, Almond PS, et al. To drain or not to drain: a single institution experience with neonatal intestinal perforation. *J Perinat Med.* 2006;34:338.

342. Rao SC, Basani L, Simmer K, et al. Peritoneal drainage versus laparotomy as initial surgical treatment for perforated necrotizing enterocolitis or spontaneous intestinal perforation in preterm low birth weight infants. *Cochrane Database Syst Rev.* 2011;CD006182.

343. Sonntag J, Grimner I, Scholtz T, et al. Growth and neurodevelopmental outcome of very low birth weight infants with necrotizing enterocolitis. *Acta Paediatr.* 2004;89:528–532.

344. Hintz SR, Kendrick DE, Stoll BJ, et al. Neurodevelopmental and growth outcomes of extremely low birth weight infants after necrotizing enterocolitis. *Pediatrics.* 2005;115:696.

345. Martin CR, Dammann O, Allred EN, et al. Neurodevelopment of extremely preterm infants who had necrotizing enterocolitis with or without late bacteremia. *J Pediatr.* 2010;157:751.

346. Attridge JT, Herman AC, Gurka MJ, et al. Discharge outcomes of extremely low birth weight infants with spontaneous intestinal perforations. *J Perinatol.* 2006;26:49.

347. Adesanya OA, O'Shea TM, Turner CS, et al. Intestinal perforation in very low birth weight infants: growth and neurodevelopment at 1 year of age. *J Perinatol.* 2005;25:583.

348. Roze E, Ta BD, van der Ree MH, et al. Functional impairments at school age of children with necrotizing enterocolitis or spontaneous intestinal perforation. *Pediatr Res.* 2011;70:619.

349. Volpe JJ. Brain injury in the preterm infant. *Clin Perinatol.* 1997;24(3):567–583.

350. Volpe JJ. *Neurology of the Newborn.* 4th ed. Philadelphia, PA: Saunders; 2001.

351. Vohr B, Allen WC, Scott DT, et al. Early onset intraventricular hemorrhage in preterm neonates: incidence of neurodevelopmental handicap. *Semin Perinatol.* 1999;23(3):212–217.

352. Vohr B, Wright LL, Dusick AM, et al. Neurodevelopmental and functional outcomes for extremely low birth weight infants in the National Institutes of Child Health and Human Development Neonatal Research Network, 1993–1994. *Pediatrics.* 2000;105(6):1216–1226.

353. Vohr B, Allan WC, Westerveld M, et al. School-age outcomes of very low birth weight infants in the indomethacin intraventricular hemorrhage prevention trial. *Pediatrics.* 2003;111(4):e340–e346.

354. Larroque B, Morret S, Ancel PY, et al. White matter damage and intraventricular hemorrhage in very preterm infants: the EPIPAGE study. *J Pediatr.* 2003;(143):477–483.

355. Vohr B, Ment LR. Intraventricular hemorrhage in the preterm infant. *Early Human Dev.* 1996;44(1):1–16.

356. Lucey JF, Rowan CA, Shiono P, et al. Fetal infants: the fate of 4172 infants with birth weights of 410 to 500 grams-The Vermont Oxford Network experience (1996–2000). *Pediatrics.* 2004;113(4):1559–1566.

357. Papile LA, Burstein J, Burston R. Incidence and evolution of subependymal and intraventricular hemorrhage: a study of infants with birthweights less than 1500 grams. *J Perinatol.* 1978;92:529–534.

358. Papile LA. Periventricular-Intraventricular hemorrhage. In: Fanaroff AA, Martin RJ, eds. *Neonatal-Perinatal Medicine: Diseases of the Fetus and Infant.* 5th ed. Philadelphia, PA: Mosby; 1992.

359. Shalik L, Perlman JM. Hemorrhagic-ischemic cerebral injury in the preterm infant: clinical concepts. *Clin Perinatol.* 2002;29:745–763.

360. Cullens V. Brain injury in the premature infant. In: L Boxwell G, ed. *Neonatal Intensive Care Nursing.* New York, NY: Routledge; 2000.

361. Vohr BR, Garcia-Coll C, Mayfield S, Brann B, Shaul P. Oh W. Neurologic and developmental status related to the evolution of visual-motor abnormalities from birth to 2 years of age in preterm infants with intraventricular hemorrhage. *J Pediatr.* 1989 Aug.;115(2):296–302.

362. Bada HS, Korones SB, Perry EH, et al. Frequent handling in the neonatal intensive care unit and intraventricular hemorrhage. *J Pediatr.* 1990;117(1, part 1):126–131.

363. Bada HS, Korones SB, Perry EH, et al. Mean arterial blood pressure changes in premature infants and those at risk for intraventricular hemorrhage. *J Pediatr.* 1990;117(4):607–614.

364. Perlman JM, Thach B. Respiratory origins of fluctuations in arterial blood pressure in premature infants with respiratory distress syndrome. *Pediatrics.* 1988;81(3):399–403.

365. Perlman JM, McMenamin JB, Volpe JJ. Fluctuating cerebral blood velocity in respiratory distress syndrome: relationship to subsequent development of intraventricular hemorrhage. *N Engl J Med.* 1983;309(4):204–209.

366. Fanconi S, Duc G. Intratracheal suctioning in sick preterm infants: prevention of intracranial hemorrhage and cerebral hypofusion by muscle paralysis. *Pediatrics.* 1987;79:583–543.

367. Bregman J, Kimberlin LVS. Developmental outcomes in extremely premature infants. *Pediatr Clin North Am.* 1993;40(5):937–950.

368. Perlman JM. Cognitive and behavioral deficits in premature graduates of intensive care. *Clin Perinatol.* 2002;29(4):779–797.

369. Krishnamoorthy KS, Kuban KC, Leviton A, et al. Periventricular-intraventricular hemorrhage, sonographic localization, phenobarbital, and motor abnormalities in low birth weight infants. *Pediatrics.* 1990;85(6):1027–1033.

370. Zach T, Brown JC. Periventricular leukomalacia. *Emedicine J.* 2003. Accessed April 2003.

371. Shankaran S. Hemorrhagic lesions of the central nervous system. In: Stevenson DK, Benitz WE, Sunshine P, eds. *Fetal and Neonatal Brain Injury.* 3rd ed. New York, NY: Cambridge University Press; 1997.

372. Inder TE, Weels SJ, Mogride NB, et al. Defining the nature of cerebral abnormalities in the premature infant: a qualitative magnetic resonance imaging study. *J Pediatr.* 2003;143(2):171–179.

373. Scher MS. Fetal and neonatal neurologic consultations and identifying brain disorders in the context of fetal-maternal-perinatal disease. *Semin Pediatr Neurol.* 2001;8(2):55–75.

374. Murphy BP, Inder TE, Rooks V, et al. Posthemorrhagic ventricular dilation in the premature infant: natural history and predictors of outcome. *Arch Dis Child.* 2002;87:F37–F41.

375. Anonymous. Randomised trial of early tapping neonatal post hemorrhagic ventricular dilatation results at 30 months. *Arch Dis Child Fetal Neonatal Ed.* 1994;70(2):F129–136.

376. Allan WC, Sobel DB. Neonatal intensive care neurology. *Semin Pediatr Neurol.* 2004;11(2):119–128.

377. Peterson BS, Vohr B, Staib LH, et al. Regional brain volume abnormalities and longterm cognitive outcome in preterm infants. *JAMA.* 2000;284(15):1939–1947.

378. Blackburn ST. Assessment and management of the neurologic system. In: *Comprehensive Neonatal Nursing: A Physiologic Perspective.* 3rd ed. Philadelphia, PA: Saunders; 2003.

379. Jones MW, Bass WT. Perinatal brain injury in the premature infant. *Neonatal Netw.* 2003;22(1):61–67.

380. Schmidt B, Davis P, Moddemann D, et al. Long-term effects of indomethacin prophylaxis in extremely-low-birth-weight infants. *N Engl J Med.* 2001;344(26):1966–1972.

381. Ment LK, Vohr B, Allen W, et al. Change in cognitive function over time in very low-birth-weight infants. *JAMA.* 2003;289(6):705–711.

382. Han TR, Bang MS, Yoon BH, et al. Risk factors for cerebral palsy in preterm infants. *Am J Phys Med Rehabil.* 2002;81:297–303.

383. Westrup B, Bohm B, Lagercrantz H, et al. Preschool outcomes in children born very prematurely. *Acta Paediatr.* 2004;93:498–507.

384. Sizan, J, Ratynski N, Boussard C. Humane neonatal care initiative: NIDCAP and family centered neonatal care. Neonatal individualized developmental care and assessment program. *Acta Paediatr.* 1999;88(10):1172.

385. Zupan V, Gonzalez P, Laaze-Masmonteil T, et al. Periventricular leukomalacia: risk factors revisited. *Dev Med Child Neurol.* 1996;38(12):1061–1067.

386. Volpe JJ. Neurobiology of periventricular leukomalacia in the preterm infant. *Pediatr Res.* 2001;50(5):553–562.

387. Larroque B, Marret S, Ancel P-Y, et al. White matter damage and intraventricular hemorrhage in very preterm infants. The EPIPAGE study. *J Pediatr.* 2003;143:477–503.

388. Blumenthal I. Periventricular leukomalacia: a review. *Eur J Pediatr.* 2004;163:435–442.

389. Batten D, Kirtley X, Swails T. Unexpected versus anticipated cystic periventricular leukomalacia. *Am J Perinatol.* 2003;20(1):33–40.

390. Kadhim H, Tabarki B, Verellen G, et al. Inflammatory cytokines in the pathogenesis of periventricular leukomalacia. *Neurology.* 2001;56:1278–1284.

391. Dammann O, Kuban KC, Leviton A. Perinatal infection, fetal inflammatory response, white matter damage and cognitive limitations in children born preterm. *Ment Retard Dev Disabil Res Rev.* 2002;8(1):46–50.

392. Dammann O, Leviton A. Infection remote from the brain, neonatal white matter damage and cerebral palsy in the preterm infant. *Semin Pediatr Neurol.* 1998;5:190–201.

393. Wilson-Costello D, Borawski E, Freidman H, et al. Perinatal correlates of cerebral palsy and other neurologic impairment among very low birth weight children. *Pediatrics.* 1998;102(2):315–322.

394. Gressens P, Rogido M, Paindaveine S, et al. The impact of neonatal intensive care practices on the developing brain. *J Pediatr.* 2002;140:646–653.

395. Perrott S, Dodds L, Vincer M. A population-based study of prognostic factors in very preterm survivors. *J Perinatol.* 2003;23(2):111–116.

396. Lemons JA, Bauer CR, Oh W, et al. Very low birth weight outcomes of the national institute of child health and human development neonatal research network, January 1995 through December 1996. *Pediatrics.* 2001;107(1):E1–E8.

397. Msall ME, Phelps DC, DiGaudio KM, et al. Severity of neonatal retinopathy of prematurity is predictive of neurodevelopmental functional outcome at age 5.5 years. Behalf of the Cryotherapy for Retinopathy of Prematurity Cooperative Group. *Pediatrics.* 2000;106(5):998–1005.

398. Askin DF, Diehl-Jones W. Retinopathy of prematurity. *Crit Care Nurs Clin N Am.* 2009;21:213–233.

399. Filho JBF, Eckert GU, Valiatti B. The influence of gestational age on the dynamic behavior of other risk factors associated with retinopathy of prematurity. *Arch Clin Exp Ophthalmol.* 2010;248:893–900.

400. DiFiore JM, Bloom JN, Orge F, et al. A higher incidence of intermittent hypoxemic episodes is associated with sever retinopathy of prematurity. *J Peds.* 2010;157:64–73.

401. Koo KY, Kim JE, Lee SM, et al. Effect of severe neonatal morbidities on long term outcome of extremely low birthweight infants. *Korean J Pediatr.* 2010;53(6):694–700.

402. Terry TL. Extreme prematurity and fibroblastic overgrowth of persistent vascular sheath behind each crystalline lens. *Am J Ophthalmol.* 1942;25(2):203–204.

403. Chen J, Smith LEH. Retinopathy of prematurity. Angiogenesis. 2007;10:133–140.

404. Smith LEH. IGF-1 and retinopathy of prematurity in the preterm infant. *Bio Neonate.* 2005;88:232–244.

405. Cavalluro G, Filippi L, Bagnoli P, et al. The pathophysiology of retinopathy of prematurity: an update of previous and recent knowledge. *Arch Ophthalmol.* 2013;1–19.

406. AAP Section on Ophthalmology, American academy of Ophthalmology, American Academy for Pediatric Ophthalmology, et al. Policy Statement. Screening exam of premature infants for retinopathy of prematurity. *Peds.* 2013;131(1):189–195.

407. ICROP: An International Committee for the Classification of Retinopathy of Prematurity. The ICROP Revisited. *Arch Ophthalmol.* 2005;123:991–999.

408. Screening Examination of Premature Infants for Retinopathy of Prematurity. Policy Statement American Academy of Pediatrics. *Pediatrics.* 2001;108(3):809–811.

409. Ng EY, Connelly BP, McNamara JA, et al. A comparison of laser photocoagulation with cryotherapy for threshold retinopathy of prematurity at 10 years: part 1. Visual function and structural outcome. *Ophthalmology.* 2002;109(5):928–934.

410. Mutlu FM, Sanci SU. Treatment of retinopathy of prematurity: a review of conventional and promising new therapeutic options. *Int J Ophthalmol.* 2013;692:228–236.

411. Early Treatment for Retinopathy of Prematurity cooperative Group. Revised indications for the treatment of retinopathy of prematurity: results of the early treatment for retinopathy of prematurity randomized control trial. *Arch Ophthamol.* 2003;121:1684–1694.

412. Zuparncic JAF, Stewart JE. Retinopathy of prematurity. In: Cloherty JP, Eichenwald EC, Stark AR, eds. *Manual of Neonatal Care.* 5th ed. Philadelphia, PA: Lippincott Williams & Wilkins; 2004.

413. Stout AU, Stout JT. Retinopathy of prematurity. *Pediatr Clin North Am.* 2003;50(1):77–87.

414. Ertzbischoff LM. A systematic review of anatomical and visual outcomes in preterm infants after scleral buckle and vitrectomy for retinal detachment. *Adv Neonatal Care.* 2004;4(1):10–19.

415. Quinn GE, Dobson V, Barr CC. Visual acuity in infants after vitrectomy for severe retinopathy of prematurity. *Ophthalmology.* 1991;98(1):5–13.

416. Laws DE, Morten C, Weindly M, et al. Systemic effects of screening for retinopathy of prematurity. *Br J Ophthalmol.* 1996;80:425–428.

417. Rush R, Rush S, Micolau J, et al. Systemic manisfestations in response to mydrasis and physician examination during screening for retinopathy of prematurity. *Retina.* 2004;24:242–245.

418. Sun X, Lemyre B, Barrowman N, et al. Pain management during eye exams for retinopathy of prematurity in preterm infants: a systematic review. *Acta Paediatr.* 2010;99:329–334.

419. Kandesay Y, Smith R, Wright IMK, et al. Pain relief for premature infants during ophthalmology assessment. *J AA Pos.* 2011;15:276–280.

420. Marsh V, Young W, Dunaway K, et al. Efficacy of topical anesthetics to reduce pain in premature infants during eye examinations for retinopathy of prematurity. *Am Pharmacother.* 2005;29:829–833.

421. Mehta M, Mansfield T, Vander Veen DK. Effect of topical anesthesia and age on pain score during retinopathy of prematurity screening. *J Perinatol.* 2010;30:731–735.

422. Stevens B, Yamada J, Ohlsson A. Sucrose for analgesia in newborn infants undergoing painful procedures. *Cochrane Neonatal Rev.* Avaiable at: www.chochraneneonatal. Accessed May 2013.

423. da Costa MC, Eckert GU, Fortes BGB, et al. Oral glucose for pain relief during examination for retinopathy of prematurity: a masked randomized clinical trial. *Clinics.* 2013;68(2):199–203.

424. Boyle EM, Freer T, Khna-Orakai Z, et al. Sucrose and non-nutritive sucking for the relief of pain in screening for retinopathy:a randomized controlled trial. *Arch Dis Child Fetal Neonatal Ed.* 2006;91(3):F1 6–F168.

425. Rush R, Rush S, Ighani F, et al. The effects of comfort care on pain response in preterm infants undergoing screening for retinopathy of prematurity. *Retina.* 2005;25:59–62.

426. Mitchell A, Stevens B, Mungen N, et al. Analgesic effects of oral sucrose and pacifier during eye examinations for retinopathy of prematurity. *Pain Manag Nurs.* 2004;5:160–168.

427. Slevin M, Murphy JFA, Daly L, et al. Retinopathy of prematurity screening, stress related responses, the role of nesting. *Br J Ophthalmol.* 1997;81:762–764.

428. O'Sullivan A, O'Connor M, BrosnahanD, et al. Sweeter, soother, and swaddle for retinopathy screening: a randomized placebo controlled trial. *Arch Dis Child Fetal Neonatal Ed.* 2010;95(6):F419–F422.

429. Redline RW. Placental pathology. In: Fanaroff AA, Martin RJ, eds. *Neonatal-Perinatal Medicine Diseases of the Fetus and Infant.* 7th ed. St. Louis, MO: Mosby; 2002.

430. Vannucci RC, Palmer C. Hypoxia-ischemia: neuropathology, pathogenesis, and management. In: Fanaroff AA, Martin RJ, eds. *Neonatal-Perinatal Medicine Diseases of the Fetus and Infant.* 7th ed. St. Louis, MO: Mosby; 2002.

431. Demari S. Calcium and phophorus nutrition in preterm infants. *Acta Paediatr Supp.* 2005;94(449):87–92.

432. Huttner KM. Metabolic bone disease of prematurity. In: Cloherty JP, Eichenwald EC, Stark AR, eds. *Manual of Neonatal Care.* 5th ed. Philadelphia, PA: Lippincott Williams & Wilkins; 2004.

433. Miller M. The bone disease of preterm birth: a biomechanical perspective. *Pediatr Res.* 2003;53(1):10–15.

434. Krug SK. Osteopenia of prematurity. In: Groh-Wargo S, Thompson M, Cox J, eds. *Nutritional Care for High-Risk Newborns Rev.* 3rd ed. Chicago, IL: Precept Press Inc; 2000.

435. Rauch F, Schoenau E. Skeletal development in premature infants: a review of bone physiology beyond nutritional aspects. *Arch Dis Child Fetal Neonatal Ed.* 2002;86:F82–F85.

436. Rigo J, DeCurtis M, Pieltain C, et al. Bone mineral metabolism in the micropremie. *Clin Perinatol.* 2000;27:147–170.

437. Rigo J, Senterre J. Nutritional needs of premature infants: current issues. *J Pediatr.* 2006;149(3 supp):S80–S88.

438. Abrams SA. Calcium and Phosphorus Requirements of Newborn Infants. *Up to Date.* Available at: http://www.uptodate.com/contents/calcium-and-phosphorus-requirements-of-newborn-infants?source=search_result&search=metabolic+bone+disease+of+prematurity&selectedTitle=1%7E150#H12Feb 12,2013 Accessed June 2013.

439. Fewtrell MS, Cole TJ, Bishop NJ, et al. Nenonatal factors predicting childhood height in preterm infants: evidence for a persisting effect of early metabolic bone disease? *J Pediatr.* 2000;137:668–673.

440. Vachharajani AV, Mathur AM, Rao, R. Metabolic bone disease of prematurity. *NeoReviews.* 2009;10:e402–e411.

441. Jones S, Bell MJ. Distal radius fracture in a premature infant with osteopenia caused by handling during intravenous cannulation. *Injury.* 2002;33:265–266.

442. Osteogenesis Imperfecta Foundation. Available at: http://www.oif.org/site/DocServer/Infant_Care_Suggestions_for_Parents.pdf?docID=7213.

443. Eliakim A, Nemet D. Osteopenia of prematurity-the role of exercise in the prevention and treatment. *Pediatr Endocrinol Rev.* 2005;2(4):675–682.

444. Moyer-Mileur LJ, Brunstetter V, McNaught TP, et al. Daily physical activity program increases bone mineralization and growth in preterm very low birth weight infants. *Pediatrics.* 2000;106(5):1088–1092.

445. Litmanovitz I, Dolfin T, Friedland O, et al. Early physical activity intervention prevents decrease of bone strength in very low birth weight infants. *Pediatrics.* 2003;112(1):15–19.

446. Schulzke SM, Trachsel D, Patole SK. Physical activity programs for promoting bone mineralization and growth in preterm infants. *Cochrane Database Syst Rev.* 2007;(2):CD005387.

447. Browne J, Cicco R, Erikson D, et al. Recommended Standards for Newborn ICU Design. Available at: http://www.nd.edu/~kkolberg/frmain.htm. Accessed January 13, 2005.

448. Vanden Berg KA. Basic principles of developmental caregiving. *Neonatal Netw.* 1997;16(7):69–71.

449. Lawhon G. Providing developmentally supportive care in the neonatal intensive care unit: an evolving challenge. *J Perinatal Neonatal Nurs.* 1997;10(4):48–61.

450. Ohgi S, Akiyama T, Arisawa K, et al. Randomized controlled trial of swaddling versus massage in the management of excessive crying in infants with cerebral injuries. *Arch Dis Child.* 2004;89(3):212–216.

451. Scales LH, McEwen IR, Murray C. Parent's perceived benefits of physical therapists' direct intervention compared with parental instruction in early intervention. *Pediatr Phys Ther.* 2007;19:196–202.

452. Dusing SC, Van Drew C, Brown SE. Instituting parent education practices in the neonatal intensive care unit: an administrative case report of practice evaluation and statewide action. *Phys Ther.* 2012;92(7):967–975.

453. Dusing SC, Muraay T, Stern M. Parent preferences for motor development education in the neonatal intensive care unit. *Pediatr Phys Ther.* 2008;20:363–368.

454. Eiden RD, Reifman A. Effects of Brazelton demonstrations on later parenting: a meta-analysis. *J Pediatr Psychol.* 1996;21(6):857–868.

455. Culp RE, Culp AM, Harmon RJ. A tool for educating parents about their premature infants. *Birth.* 1989;16(1):23–26.

456. Lowman LB, Stone LL, Cole JG. Using developmental assessments in the NICU to empower families. *Neonatal Netw.* 2006;25(3):177–186.

457. Loo KK, Espinosa M, Tyler R, et al. Using knowledge to cope with stress in the NICU: how parents integrate learning to read the physiologic and behavioral cues of the infant. *Neonatal Netw.* 2003;22(1):31–37.

458. Gale G, VandenBerg KA. Kangaroo care. *Neonatal Netw.* 1998;17(5):69–71.

459. Sloan N, Camacho LWI, Rojas EP. Kangaroo mother method: randomized controlled trial of an alternative method of care for stabilized low-birth-weight infants. *Lancet.* 1994;344:782–785.

460. Acolet D, Sleath K, Whitelaw A. Oxygenation, heart rate and temperature in very low birthweight infants during skin-to-skin contact with their mothers. *Acta Paediatr.* 1989;78:189–193.

461. Fohe K, Kropf S, Avenarius S. Skin-to-skin contact improved gas exchange in premature infants. *J Perinatol.* 2000;20:311–315.

462. Feldman R, Eidelman AI. Skin-to-skin contact (kangaroo care) accelerates autonomic and neurobehavioral maturation in preterm infants. *Dev Med Child Neurol.* 2003;45:274–281.

463. Lundington-Hoe SM, Anderson GC, Swine JY, et al. A randomized control of kangaroo care and cardiorespiratory and thermal effects on healthy preterm infants. *Neonatal Netw.* 2004;23(3):39–48.

464. Johnston CC, Stevens B, Pinelli J, et al. Kangaroo care is effective in diminishing pain response in preterm neonates. *Arch Pediatr Adolesc Med.* 2003;157(11):1084–1088.

465. Bier JA, Ferguson AE, Morales Y, et al. Comparison of skin-to-skin contact with standard contact in low birth weight infants who are breast fed. *Arch Pediatr Adolesc Med.* 1996;150(12):1265–1269.

466. Anderson G. Kangaroo care and breastfeeding for preterm infants. *Breastfeeding Abstracts.* 1989;9(2):7.

467. Feldman R, Weller A, Sirota L, et al. Testing a family intervention hypothesis: the contribution of mother-infant skin-to-skin contact (kangaroo care) to family interaction, proximity, and touch. *J Fam Psychol.* 2003;17(11):94–107.

468. Feldman R, Eidelman AI, Sirota L, et al. Comparison of skin-to-skin (kangaroo) and traditional care: parenting outcomes and preterm infant development. *Pediatrics.* 2002;110(1):16–26.

469. Hemingway M, Oliver S. Water bed therapy and cranial molding of the sick preterm infant. *Neonatal Netw.* 1991;10(3):53–56.

470. Hemingway M, Oliver S. Bilateral head flattening in hospitalized premature infants. *Neonatal Intens Care.* 2000;13(6):18–22.

471. Hemingway M. Preterm infant positioning. *Neonatal Intens Care.* 2000;13(6):18–22.

472. Vaivre-Douret L, Ennouri K, Jrad I, et al. Effect of positioning on the incidence of abnormalities of muscle tone in low-risk, preterm infants. *Eur J Pediatr Neurol.* 2004;8:21–34.

473. Hallsworth M. Positioning the pre-term infant. *Clin Neonatal Nurs.* 1995;7(1):18–20.

474. Chang YJ, Anderson GC, Lin CH. Effects of prone and supine positions on sleep state and stress responses in mechanically ventilated preterm infants during the first postnatal week. *J Adv Nurs.* 2002;40(2):161–169.

475. Wolfson MR, Greenspan JS, Deoras KS, et al. Effect of positioning on the mechanical interaction between the rib cage and abdomen in preterm infants. *J Appl Physiol.* 1992;72(3):1032–1038.

476. Bjornson K, Deitz J, Blackburn S, et al. The effect of body position on the oxygen saturation of ventilated preterm infants. *Pediatr Phys Ther.* 1992;4(3):109–115.

477. Goldberg RN, Joshi A, Moscoso P, et al. The effect of head position on intracranial pressure in the neonate. *Crit Care Med.* 1983;11:428–430.

478. Grenier IR, Bigsby R, Vergara ER, et al. Comparison of motor self-regulatory and stress behaviors of preterm infants across body positions. *Am J Occupat Ther.* 2003;57(3):289–297.

479. Vohr BR, Cashore WJ, Bigsby R. Stresses and interventions in the neonatal intensive care unit. In: Levine MD, Carey WB, Crocker AC, eds. *Developmental-Behavioral Pediatrics.* Philadelphia, PA: Saunders; 1999.

480. Hashimoto T, Hiurs K, Endo S, et al. Postural effects on behavioral states of newborn infants: a sleep polygraphic study. *Brain Dev.* 1983;5:286–291.

481. Hadders-Algra M, Prechtl HFR. Developmental course of general movements in early infancy. I. Descriptive analysis of change in form. *Early Human Dev.* 1992;201–213.

482. Adams JA, Zabaleta IA, Sackner MA. Comparison of supine and prone noninvasive measurements of breathing patterns in fullterm newborns. *Pediatr Pulmonol.* 1994;18:8–12.

483. Pellicier A, Gaya F, Madero R, et al. Noninvasive continuous monitoring of the effects of head position on brain hemodynamics in ventilated infants. *Pediatrics.* 2002;109(3):434–440.

484. American Academy of Pediatrics. Task Force on Infant Sleep Position and Sudden Infant Death Syndrome. Changing concepts of sudden death syndrome: implications for infant sleeping environment and sleep position. *Pediatrics.* 2000;105(3):650–656.

485. van Heijst JJ, Touwen BCL, Vos JE. Implications of a neural network model of sensori-motor development for the field of developmental neurology. *Early Human Dev.* 1999;55(1):77–95.

486. de Groot L. Posture and motility in preterm infants. *Dev Med Child Neurol.* 2000;42:65–68.

487. Fay MJ. The positive effects of positioning. *Neonatal Netw.* 1988; 23–28.

488. Monterososso L, Kristjanson L, Cole J. Neuromotor development and the physiologic effects of positioning in very low birthweight infants. *J Obstet Gynecol Neonatal Nurs.* 2002;31(2):138–146.

489. Shaw JC. Growth and nutrition of the preterm infant. *Br Med Bull.* 1988;44(4):984–1009.

490. Clarren SK, Smith DW, Hanson JW. Helmet treatment for plagiocephaly and congenital muscular torticollis. *J Pediatr.* 1979;94(1): 43–46.

491. Kriewell TJ. Structural, mechanical, and material properties of fetal cranial bone. *Am J Obstet Gynecol.* 1982;143(6):707–714.

492. Budreau GK. The perceived attractiveness of preterm infants with caranial molding. *J Obstet Gynecol Neonatal Nurs.* 1989;18(1):38–44.

493. Budreau GK. Postnatal cranial molding and infant attractiveness: implications for nursing. *Neonatal Netw.* 1987;5(5):13–19.

494. Schwirian PM, Eesley T, Cuellar L. Use of water pillows in reducing head shape distortion in preterm infants. *Res Nurs Health.* 1986;9(3):203–207.

495. Geerdink JJ, Hopkins B, Hoeksma JB. The development of head positioning preference in preterm infants beyond term age. *Dev Psychobiol.* 1994;27(3):253–268.

496. Cartlidge PH, Rutter N. Reduction of head flattening in preterm infants. *Arch Dis Child.* 1988;63(7):755–757.

497. Chan JS, Kelley MC, Khan J. The effects of a pressure relief mattress on postnatal head molding in very low birth weight infants. *Neonatal Netw.* 1993;12(5):19–22.

498. Dubowitz L, Dubowitz V. *The Neurological Assessment of the Preterm and Full-Term Newborn Infant. Clinics in Developmental Medicine. No. 12.* Philadelphia, PA: Lippincott; 1981.

499. Dubowitz L, Dubowitz V, Mercuri E. *The Neurological Assessment of the Preterm and Full-Term Newborn Infant.* 2nd ed. London, UK: MacKeith; 1999.

500. Korner AF, Brown JV, Thom VA, et al. *Neurobehavioral Assessment of the Preterm Infant.* Rev 2nd ed. Van Nuys, CA: Child Development Media, Inc. 2000.

501. http://med.stanford.edu/NAPI. Last accessed November 2013.

502. www.Brazelton-Institute.com. Last accessed November 2013.

503. Als H, Lester BM, Tronick EZ, Brazelton. Manual for the assessment of preterm infant's behavior (APIB). In Fitzgerald HE, Lester BM, Yogman MW (Eds.). Theory and research in behavioural pediatrics (pp. 35-63). New York: Plenum Press, 1982b.

504. Als H, Butler S, Kosta S, McAnulty G. the assessment of preterm infant's behavior (APIB): furthering understanding and measurement of neurodevelopmental competence in preterm and full-term infants. *Ment Retard Devel Disabil Res Rev.* 2005; 11:94–102.

505. Lester BM, Tronick EZ. The neonatal intensive care unit network neurobehavioral scale procedures. *Pediatrics.* 2004;113(3): 641–667.

506. Einspieler C, Prechtl HFR, Bos, et al. *The qualitative assessment of general movements in preterm, term, and young infants.* London, UK: Mac Keith, 2004.

507. Einspieler C, Prechtl HFR, Ferrari F, et al. The qualitative assessment of general movements in preterm, term, and young infants-review of the methodology. *Early Human Dev.* 1997;50:47–60.

508. General Movements./www.general-movements-trust.info.Last Accessed June 2012.

509. Campbell Sk. The Test of Infant Motor Performance. Test user's manual version 2.0. Chicago: Infant Motor Performance Scales, LLC, 2005.

510. Available at: www.TheTIMP.com. Last accessed November 2013.

511. Piper MC, Darrah J. Motor assessment of the developing infant. Philadelphia: WB Saunders, 1994.

512. Ellison PH. Neurologic Development of the high-risk infant. *Clin Perinatol.* 11(1):45.

513. Amiel-Tison C. A method for neurological evaluation within the first year of life. *Curr Probl Pediatr.* 1976;7(1):45.

514. Van Marter LJ. Epidemiology of bronchopulmonary dysplasia. *Semin Fetal Neonatal Med.* 2009;14:358–366

515. Deakins KM. Bronchopulmonary dysplasia. *Respir Care.* 2009;54(9):1252–1262.

516. Kair LR, Leonard DT, Anderson JDM. Bronchopulmonary dysplasia. *Pediatr Review.* 2012;33(5):255–263.

517. Ali Z, Schmidt P, Dodd J, et al. Bronchopulmonary dysplasia: a review. *Arch Gynecol Obstet.* 2012;DOI 10.1007.

518. Northway WH, Rosan RC, Porter DY. Pulmonary disease following respirator therapy of hyaline-membrane disease. Bronchopulmonary dysplasia. *N Engl J Med.* 1967;16(276):357–368.

519. Goetzman BW. Understanding bronchopulmonary dysplasia. *Am J Dis Child.* 1986;40:332–334.

520. Abman S, Groothius J. Pathophysiology and treatment of bronchopulmonary dysplasia. *Respir Med.* 1994;41:277–307.

521. Philip AGS. Bronchopulmonary dysplasia: then and now. *Neonatology.* 2012;102:1–8.

522. Bancalari E, Abdenocir GE, Feller R, et al. Bronchopulmonary dysplasia: clinical presentation. *J Pediatr.* 1979;95(5 part 2):819–823.

523. Jobe AH. The new bronchopulmonary dysplasia. *Curr Opin Pediatr.* 2011;23:167–172.

524. Sosenko IRS, Bancalari E. New developments in the pathogenesis and prevention of bronchopulmonary dysplasia. In: Bancalari E & Polin RA, eds. *The Newborn Lung: Neonatology Questions and Controversies.* 2nd ed. Philadelphia, PA: Elsevier Saunders; 2012: 217–233.

525. Jobe AH, Bancalari E. Bronchopulmonary dysplasia. *Am J Respir Crit Care Med.* 2001;63(7):1723–1729.

526. Jobe AH. The new BPD. *NeoReviews.* 2006;7:e531–e545.

527. Husain AN, Siddiqui NH, Stocker JT. Pathology of arrested acinar development in post surfactant bronchopulmonary dysplasia. *Human Pathol.* 1998;29(7):710–717.

528. NICHD consensus: Jobe AH, Bancalari E. NICD/NHLBI/ORD Workshop Summary: Bronchopulmonary dysplasia. 2001;163: 1723–1729.

529. Walsh MC, Wilson-Costello D, Zadell A, et al. Safety, reliability, validity of a physiologic definition of bronchopulmonary dysplasia. *J Perinatol.* 2003;23:45145–45146.

530. Walsh Mc, Yao Q, Gettner PP, et al. National Institute of Child Health and Human Development Neonatal Research Network: Imapct of a physiologic definition of bronchopulmonary dysplasia rates. *Pediatrics.* 2004;114:1305–1311.

531. Massie SE, Tolleson-Rinehart S, DeWalt DA, et al. Development of a proxy-reported pulmonary outcomes scale for preterm infants with bronchopulmonary dysplasia. *Health Qual Life Outcomes.* 2011;9:55.

532. Thebaud B, Abman SH. Bronchopulmonary dysplasia: where have all the vessels gone? Roles of angiogenic growth factors in chronic lung disease. *Am J Respir Crit Care Med.* 2007;175:978–985.

533. Parker RA, Lindstrom Dp, Cotton RB. Evidence from twin study implies possible genetic susceptibility to bronchopulmonary dysplasia. *Sem Perinatol.* 1996;20:206–209.

534. Bhandari V, Bizzaro MS, Shetty, et al. Famial and genetic susceptibility to major neonatal morbidities in preterm twins. *Pediatrics.* 2006;117:1901–1906.

535. Askin DF, Diehl–Jones W. Pathogenesis and prevention of chronic lung disease in the neonate. *Crit care Nurs Clin N Am.* 2009;21:11–25.

536. Balinotti JE, Chakr VC, Tiller C. Growth of lung parenchyma in infants and toddlers with chronic lung disease of infancy. *Am J Respr Crit Care Med.* 2010;181:1093–1097.

537. Trembath A, Laughton MM. Predictors of bronchopulmonary dysplasia. *Clin Perinatol.* 2012;39:585–601.

538. Rugolo LMSS, Bentin MK, Petean CE. Preeclampsia: effect on the fetus and newborn. *NeoReviews.* 2011;12:e1298–e206.

539. Bose CL, Van Marter LJ, Laughan M, et al. Fetal growth restriction and chronic lung disease among infants born before the 28th week of gestation. *Pediatrics.* 2009;124:e450–e458.

540. Lahra M. Intrauterine inflammation, neonatal sepsis, and chronic lung disease: a 13–year hospital cohort study. *Pediatrics.* 2009;123(5): 1314–1319.

541. Speer CP. Inflammation and bronchopulmonary dysplasia. *Semin Neonatol.* 2003;8(1):29–38.

542. Fleisher B, Kulovich M, Hallman M, et al. Lung profile: sex differences in normal pregnancy. *Obstet gynecol.* 1985;66(3):327–330.

543. Henderson-Smart DJ, Hutchinson DA, Donoghue DA, et al. Prenatal predictors of chronic lung disease in very preterm infants. *Arch Dis Child Fetal Neoonatal Ed.* 2006;91:F40–F45.

544. Morely CJ. Volume limited and volume targeted ventilation. *Clin Perinatol.* 39(3):513–523.

545. Halliday M, Ehrenkranz RA, Doyle LW. Early (<8 days) postnatal corticosteroids for preventing chronic lung disease in ventilated very low birthweight preterm infants. *Cochrane Database Syst Rev.* CD002057.

546. Khemani E, McElhinney DB, Rhein L, et al. Pulmonary artery hypertension in formally premature infants with bronchopulmonary dysplasia: clinical features and outcomes in the surfactant era. *Pediatrics.* 2007;120:1260–1269.

547. Hintz SR, Kendrick DE, Wilson-Costello DE, et al. Early childhood neurodevelopmental outcomes are not improving for infants born <25 weeks gestational age. *Pediatrics.* 2011;127:62–70.

548. O'Reilly M, Sozo F, Harding R. The impact of preterm birth and bronchopulmonary dysplasia in the developing lung: long-term consequences for respiratory health. Doi:10.1111/1440-1681.12068.

549. Korhonen P, Laitmen J, Hyodymaa E, et al. Respiratory outcome in school aged, very-low-birth-weight children in the surfactant era. *Acta Paediatr.* 2004;93:316–321.

550. Lewis BA, Singer LT, Fulton S, et al. Speech and language outcomes of children with bronchopulmonary dysplasia. *J Commun Disord.* 2002;35(5):393–406.

551. Jeng SF, Hsu CH, Tsai PN, et al. Bronchopulmonary dysplasia predicts adverse developmental and clinical outcomes in very-low-birthweight infants. *Devel Med Child Neurol.* 2008;50:51–57.

552. Short E, Kirchner L, Asaad GR, et al. Developmental sequelae in preterm infants having a diagnosis of bronchopulmonary dysplasia: analysis using a severity-based classification system. *Arch Pediatr Adolesc Med.* 2007;161(11):1082–1087.

553. Ehrenkrantz RA, Walsh MC, Vohr BR, et al. National Institutes of Child Health and Human Development Neonatal Research Network. Validation of the National Institutes of Health consensus definition of bronchopulmonary dysplasia. *Pediatrics.* 2005;116(6):1353–1360.

554. Singer L, Yamashita TS, Lilien L, et al. A longitudinal study of developmental outcome of infants with bronchopulmonary dysplasia and very low birthweight. *Pediatrics.* 1997;100:987–993.

555. Karogianni P, Tsakaidis C, Kyriakidou M, et al. Nueromotor outcomes in infants with bronchopulmonary dysplasia. *Pediatr Neurol.* 2011;44(1):40–46.

556. Majnemer A, Riley P, Shevell M, et al. Severe bronchopulmonsry dysplasia increase risk for later neurological and motor sequelae in preterm survivors. *Dev Med Child Neurol.* 2000;42:53–60.

557. Skidmore MD, Rivers A, Hack M. Increased risk of cerebral palsy among very low birthweight infants with chronic lung disease. *Dev Med Child Neurol.* 1990;82:325–332.

558. Kobaly K, Schluchter M, Minich N, et al. Outcomes of extremely low birthweight (<1 kg) and extremely low gestational age (<28 weeks) infants with bronchopulmonary dysplasia: effects of practice changes in 2000 to 2003. *Peditraics.* 2008;121(1):73–81.

559. Natarajan G, Pappas A, Shankaran S, et al. Outcomes of extremely low birth weight infants with bronchopulmonary dysplasia: impact of the physiologic definition. *Early Hum Dev.* 2012;88:509–515.

560. Palisano RJ, Hanna SE, Rosenbaum PL, et al. Validation of a model of gross motor function for children with cerebral palsy. *Phys Ther.* 2000;80(10):974–985.

561. Van Marter LJ, Kuban KC, Allred E, et al. Does bronchopulmonary dysplasia contribute to the occurrence of cerebral palsy among infants born before 28 weeks gestation? *Arch Dis Child fetal Neonatal Ed.* 2011;96:F20–F29.

562. Spittle A, Treyvaud K, Doyle Lw, et al. Early emergence of behavioural and social–emotional problems in very preterm infants. *J Am Acad Child Adolesc Psychiatry.* 2009;28(9):909–918.

563. Anderson PJ, Doyle LW. Neurodevelopmental outcome of bronchopulmonary dysplasia. *Semin Perinatol.* 2006;30:227–232.

564. Abman S, Nelin LD. Management of the infant with severe bronchopulmonary dysplasia. In: Bancalari E & Polin RA, eds. *The Newborn Lung: Neonatology Questions and Controversies.* 2nd ed. Philadelphia, PA: Elsevier Saunders; 2012:407–425.

565. Shephard EG, Knupp AM, Welty SE. An interdisciplinary bronchopulmonary dysplasia program is associated with improved neurodevelopmental outcomes and fewer rehospitalizations. *J Perinatol.* 2012;32:33–38.

566. Hedrick HL, Adzick NS. Congenital Diapharagmatic Hernia in the Neonate. *UpToDate.* Available at: http://www.uptodate.com/ contents/congenital-diaphragmatic-hernia-in-the-neonate?source= search_result&search=congenital+diaphragmatic+hernia&selected Title=2%7E31; Jan 22, 2013. Accessed March 2013.

567. DiFiore JW, Fauza DO, Slavin R, et al. Experimental fetal tracheal ligation and congenital diaphragmatic hernia: a pulmonary vascular morphometric analysis. *J Pediatr Surg.* 1995;30(7):917.

568. Bloss RS, Aranda JV, Beardmore HE. Congenital diaphragmatic hernia: pathophysiology and pharmacologic support. *Surgery.* 1981; 89:518.

569. Bianchi DW, Crumbleholme TM, D'Alton ME. Diaphragmatic hernia. In: *Fetology Diagnosis and Management of the Fetal Patient.* New York, NY: McGraw-Hill; 2000.

570. Lotze A, Knight GR, Anderson KD, et al. Surfactant (beractant) therapy for infants with congenital diaphragmatic hernia on ECMO: evidence of persistent surfactant deficiency. *J Pediatr Surg.* 1994;29:407.

571. Wilcox DT, Glick PL, Karamanoukian HL, et al. Pathophysiology of congenital diaphragmatic hernia. IX: Correlation of surfactant maturation with fetal cortisol and triiodothyronine concentration. *J Pediatr Surg.* 1994;29:825.

572. Wilcox DT, Glick PL, Karamanoukian HL, et al. Pathophysiology of congenital diaphragmatic hernia. XII: Amniotic fluid lecithin/ sphingomyelin ratio and phosphatidylglycerol concentrations do not predict surfactant status in congenital diaphragmatic hernia. *J Pediatr Surg.* 1995;30:410.

573. West SE. Normal and abnormal structural development of the lung. In: Polin RA, Fox WW, Abman SH, eds. *Fetal and Neonatal Physiology.* 2nd ed. Philadelphia, PA: WB Saunders Co; 1998.

574. Hedrick HL, Adzick NS. Congenital Diapharagmatic Hernia: Prenatal Diagnosis and Management. *UpToDate.* Available at: http:// www.uptodate.com/contents/congenital-diaphragmatic-hernia-prenatal-diagnosis-andmanagement?source=search_result&search =cdh&selectedTitle=2%7E11 Jan, 11, 2013. Accessed March 2013.

575. Crane JP. Familial congenital diaphragmatic hernia: prenatal diagnostic approach and analysis of twelve families. *Clin Genet.* 1979; 16:244.

576. Puri P, Gorman F. Lethal nonpulmonary anomalies associated with congenital diaphragmatic hernia: implications for early intrauterine surgery. *J Pediatr Surg.* 1984;19:29.

577. Witters I, Legius E, Moerman P, et al. Associated malformations and chromosomal anomalies in 42 cases of prenatally diagnosed diaphragmatic hernia. *Am J Med Genet.* 2001;103:278.

578. Mullassery D, Ba'ath ME, Jesudason EC, et al. Value of liver herniation in prediction of outcome in fetal congenital diaphragmatic hernia: a systematic review and meta-analysis. *Ultrasound Obstet Gynecol.* 2010;35:609.

579. Bianchi DW, Crumbleholme TM, D'Alton ME. Invasive fetal therapy and fetal surgery. In: *Fetology Diagnosis and Management of the Fetal Patient.* New York, NY: McGraw-Hill; 2000.

580. Monteagudo, A. Prenatal sonographic diagnosis of fetal abdominal wall defects. *UpToDate.* Available at: http://www.uptodate.com/contents/prenatal-sonographic-diagnosis-of-fetal-abdominal-walldefects?source=search_result&search=omphalocele+gastroschisis&selectedTitle=3%7E60 Oct 31, 2012. Accessed March 2013.

581. Davis AS, Blumenfeld Y, Rubesova E, et al. Challenges of giant omphalocele: from fetal diagnosis to follow-up. *NeoReviews.* 2008: 9(8)e338–e346.

582. Emanuel PG, Garcia GI, Angtuaco TL. Prenatal detection of anterior abdominal wall defects with US. *Radiographics.* 1995;15:517–530.

583. Chabra S, Gleason CA. Gastroschisis: embryology, pathogenesis, epidemiology. *NeoReviews.* 2005:6(11):e493–e498.

584. Ross AJ. Organogenesis, innervation and histologic development of the gastrointestinal tract. In: Polin RA, Fox WW, Abman SH, eds. *Fetal and Neonatal Physiology.* 2nd ed. Philadelphia, PA: WB Saunders Co; 1998.

585. Thigpen TL, Kenner C. Assessment and management of the gastrointestinal system. In: Kenner C, Lott JW, eds. *Comprehensive Neonatal Nursing: A Physiologic Perspective.* 3rd ed. Philadelphia, PA: Saunders; 2003.

586. Bianchi DW, Crumbleholme, TM, D'Alton ME. Omphalocele. In: *Fetology Diagnosis and Management of the Fetal Patient.* New York, NY: McGraw-Hill; 2000.

587. Duhamel B. Embryology of exomphalos and allied malformations. *Arch Dis Child.* 1963;38:142.

588. Hutchin P. Somatic anomalies of the umbilicus and anterior abdominal wall. *Surg Gynecol Obstet.* 1965;120:1075.

589. Cyr DR, Mack LA, Schoenecker SA, et al. Bowel migration in the normal fetus: US detection. *Radiology.* 1986;161:119.

590. Stephenson, CD, Lockwood CJ, MacKenzie AP. Obstetrical Management of Omphalocele. *UpToDate.* Available at: http://www.uptodate.com/contents/obstetrical-management-of-omphalocele?source=search_result&search=omphalocele+gastroschisis&selectedTitle=1%7E60. May 24, 2012. Accessed March 2013.

591. Byron-Scott R, Haan E, Chan A, et al. A population-based study of abdominal wall defects in South Australia and Western Australia. *Paediatr Perinat Epidemiol.* 1998;12:136.

592. Chen CP. Chromosomal abnormalities associated with omphalocele. *Taiwan J Obstet Gynecol.* 2007;46:1–8.

593. Ledbetter DJ. Gastroschissis amd omphalocele. *Surg Clin North Am.* 2006;86(2):249–260.

594. Nicholas SS, Stamilio DM, Dicke JM, et al. Predicting adverse neonatal outcomes in fetuses with abdominal wall defects using prenatal risk factors. *Am J Obstet Gynecol.* 2009;201:383.e1–e6.

595. Nyberg DA, Fitzsimmons J, Mack LA, et al. Chromosomal abnormalities in fetuses with omphalocele. Significance of omphalocele contents. *J Ultrasound Med.* 1989;8:299.

596. Benacerraf BR, Saltzman DH, Estroff JA, et al. Abnormal karyotype of fetuses with omphalocele: prediction based on omphalocele contents. *Obstet Gynecol.* 1990;75:317.

597. Carpenter MW, Curci MR, Dibbins AW, et al. Perinatal management of ventral wall defects. *Obstet Gynecol.* 1984;64:646.

598. Townsend. Abdomen. In: *Sabiston Textbook of Surgery.* 16th ed. Philadelphia, PA: WB Saunders Co; 2001:1478.

599. Biard JM, Wilson RD, Johnson MP, et al. Prenatally diagnosed giant omphaloceles: short- and long-term outcomes. *Prenat Diagn.* 2004;24:434.

600. Bianchi DW, Crumbleholme TM, D'Alton ME. Gastroschisis. In: *Fetology Diagnosis and Management of the Fetal Patient.* New York, NY: McGraw-Hill; 2000.

601. Stephenson, CD, Lockwood CJ, MacKenzie AP. Obstetrical Management of Gastroschisis. *UpToDate.* Available at: http://www.uptodate.com/contents/obstetrical-management-of-gastroschisis?source=search_result&search=omphalocele+gastroschisis&selectedTitle=2%7E60 2/27/13. Accessed March 2013.

602. Moore TC. Gastroschisis and omphalocele: clinical differences. *Surgery.* 1977;82:561.

603. Abdullah F, Arnold MA, Nabaweesi R, et al. Gastroschisis in the United States 1988-2003: analysis and risk categorization of 4344 patients. *J Perinatol.* 2007;27:50.

604. Mastroiacovo P, Lisi A, Castilla EE. The incidence of gastroschisis: research urgently needs resources. *BMJ.* 2006;332:423.

605. Loane M, Dolk H, Bradbury I, et al. Increasing prevalence of gastroschisis in Europe 1980-2002: a phenomenon restricted to younger mothers? *Paediatr Perinat Epidemiol.* 2007;21:363.

606. Overton TG, Pierce MR, Gao H, et al. Antenatal management and outcomes of gastroschisis in the U. K. *Prenat Diagn.* 2012;32:1256.

607. Mac Bird T, Robbins JM, Druschel C, et al. Demographic and environmental risk factors for gastroschisis and omphalocele in the National Birth Defects Prevention Study. *J Pediatr Surg.* 2009;44:1546.

608. Chambers CD, Chen BH, Kalla K, et al. Novel risk factor in gastroschisis: change of paternity. *Am J Med Genet A.* 2007;143:653.

609. Mattix KD, Winchester PD, Scherer LR. Incidence of abdominal wall defects is related to surface water atrazine and nitrate levels. *J Pediatr Surg.* 2007;42:947.

610. Kohl M, Wiesel A, Schier F. Familial recurrence of gastroschisis: literature review and data from the population-based birth registry "Mainz Model". *J Pediatr Surg.* 2010;45:1907.

611. Crawford RA, Ryan G, Wright VM, et al. The importance of serial biophysical assessment of fetal wellbeing in gastroschisis. *Br J Obstet Gynaecol.* 1992;99:899.

612. Brantberg A, Blaas HG, Salvesen KA, et al. Surveillance and outcome of fetuses with gastroschisis. *Ultrasound Obstet Gynecol.* 2004;23:4.

613. Adair CD, Rosnes J, Frye AH, et al. The role of antepartum surveillance in the management of gastroschisis. *Int J Gynaecol Obstet.* 1996;52:141.

614. Towers CV, Carr MH. Antenatal fetal surveillance in pregnancies complicated by fetal gastroschisis. *Am J Obstet Gynecol.* 2008;198:686.e1.

615. Kuleva M, Salomon LJ, Benoist G, et al. The value of daily fetal heart rate home monitoring in addition to serial ultrasound examinations in pregnancies complicated by fetal gastroschisis. *Prenat Diagn.* 2012;32:789.

616. Oermann CM. Congenital anomalies of the intrathoracic airways and tracheoesophageal fistula. *UpToDate,* Jan 23, 2013. Available at: http://www.uptodate.com/contents/congenital-anomalies-of-the-intrathoracic-airways-and-tracheoesophageal-fistula?source=search_result&search=tef&selectedTitle=1%7E62. Accessed April 2013.

617. Crisera CA, Grau JB, Maldonado TS, et al. Defective epithelial-mesenchymal interactions dictate the organogenesis of tracheoesophageal fistula. *Pediatr Surg Int.* 2000;16:256.

618. Goyal A, Jones MO, Couriel JM, et al. Oesophageal atresia and tracheo-oesophageal fistula. *Arch Dis Child Fetal Neonatal Ed.* 2006;91:F381.

619. Depaepe A, Dolk H, Lechat MF. The epidemiology of tracheo-oesophageal fistula and oesophageal atresia in Europe. EUROCAT Working Group. *Arch Dis Child.* 1993;68:743.

620. Robb A, Lander A. Oesophageal atresia and tracheo-oesophageal fistula. Available at: linkinghub.elsevier.com/retrieve/pii/S0263931907001135. [Accessed on November 16, 2007]). Surgery (Oxford) 2007; 25:283.

621. Keckler SJ, St. Peter SD, Valusek PA, et al. VACTERL anomalies in patients with esophageal atresia: an updated delineation of the spectrum and review of the literature. *Pediatr Surg Int.* 2007; 23:309.

622. Pretorius DH, Drose JA, Dennis MA, et al. Tracheoesophageal fistula in utero. Twenty-two cases. *J Ultrasound Med.* 1987;6:509.

623. Karnak I, Senocak ME, Hiçsönmez A, et al. The diagnosis and treatment of H-type tracheoesophageal fistula. *J Pediatr Surg.* 1997;32:1670.

624. Laffan EE, Daneman A, Ein SH, et al. Tracheoesophageal fistula without esophageal atresia: are pull-back tube esophagograms needed for diagnosis? *Pediatr Radiol.* 2006;36:1141.

625. Nagata K, Kamio Y, Ichikawa T, et al. Congenital tracheoesophageal fistula successfully diagnosed by CT esophagography. *World J Gastroenterol.* 2006;12:1476.

626. Islam S, Cavanaugh E, Honeke R, et al. Diagnosis of a proximal tracheoesophageal fistula using three-dimensional CT scan: a case report. *J Pediatr Surg.* 2004;39:100.

627. Dogan BE, Fitoz S, Atasoy C, et al. Tracheoesophageal fistula: demonstration of recurrence by three-dimensional computed tomography. *Curr Probl Diagn Radiol.* 2005;34:167.

628. Shaw-Smith C. Oesophageal atresia, tracheo-oesophageal fistula, and the VACTERL association: review of genetics and epidemiology. *J Med Genet.* 2006;43:545.

629. Little DC, Rescorla FJ, Grosfeld JL, et al. Long-term analysis of children with esophageal atresia and tracheoesophageal fistula. *J Pediatr Surg.* 2003;38:852.

630. Orford J, Cass DT, Glasson MJ. Advances in the treatment of oesophageal atresia over three decades: the 1970s and the 1990s. *Pediatr Surg Int.* 2004;20:402.

631. Tsao K, Lee H. Extrapleural thoracoscopic repair of esophageal atresia with tracheoesophageal fistula. *Pediatr Surg Int.* 2005;21:308.

632. Krosnar S, Baxter A. Thoracoscopic repair of esophageal atresia with tracheoesophageal fistula: anesthetic and intensive care management of a series of eight neonates. *Paediatr Anaesth.* 2005;15:541.

633. Rothenberg SS. Thoracoscopic repair of esophageal atresia and tracheo-esophageal fistula. *Semin Pediatr Surg.* 2005;14:2.

634. Meier JD, Sulman CG, Almond PS, et al. Endoscopic management of recurrent congenital tracheoesophageal fistula: a review of techniques and results. *Int J Pediatr Otorhinolaryngol.* 2007;71:691.

635. Holcomb GW 3rd, Rothenberg SS, Bax KM, et al. Thoracoscopic repair of esophageal atresia and tracheoesophageal fistula: a multi-institutional analysis. *Ann Surg.* 2005;242:422.

636. Freire JP, Feijó SM, Miranda L, et al. Tracheo-esophageal fistula: combined surgical and endoscopic approach. *Dis Esophagus.* 2006;19:36.

637. Patkowsk D, Rysiakiewicz K, Jaworski W, et al. Thoracoscopic repair of tracheoesophageal fistula and esophageal atresia. *J Laparoendosc Adv Surg Tech A.* 2009;19(suppl 1):S19.

638. Varjavandi V, Shi E. Early primary repair of long gap esophageal atresia: the VATER operation. *J Pediatr Surg.* 2000;35:1830.

639. Spitz L. Oesophageal atresia treatment: a 21st-century perspective. *J Pediatr Gastroenterol Nutr.* 2011;52(suppl 1):S12.

640. van der Zee DC. Thoracoscopic elongation of the esophagus in long-gap esophageal atresia. *J Pediatr Gastroenterol Nutr.* 2011;52 (suppl 1):S13.

641. LaSalle AJ, Andrassy RJ, Ver Steeg K, et al. Congenital tracheoesophageal fistula without esophageal atresia. *J Thorac Cardiovasc Surg.* 1979;78:583.

642. Ko BA, Frederic R, DiTirro PA, et al. Simplified access for division of the low cervical/high thoracic H-type tracheoesophageal fistula. *J Pediatr Surg.* 2000;35:1621.

643. Teich S, Barton DP, Ginn-Pease ME, et al. Prognostic classification for esophageal atresia and tracheoesophageal fistula: Waterston versus Montreal. *J Pediatr Surg.* 1997;32:1075.

644. Choudhury SR, Ashcraft KW, Sharp RJ, et al. Survival of patients with esophageal atresia: influence of birth weight, cardiac anomaly, and late respiratory complications. *J Pediatr Surg.* 1999;34:70.

645. Konkin DE, O'hali WA, Webber EM, et al. Outcomes in esophageal atresia and tracheoesophageal fistula. *J Pediatr Surg.* 2003;38:1726.

646. Upadhyaya VD, Gangopadhyaya AN, Gupta DK, et al. Prognosis of congenital tracheoesophageal fistula with esophageal atresia on the basis of gap length. *Pediatr Surg Int.* 2007;23:767.

647. Engum SA, Grosfeld JL, West KW, et al. Analysis of morbidity and mortality in 227 cases of esophageal atresia and/or tracheoesophageal fistula over two decades. *Arch Surg.* 1995;130:502.

648. Antoniou D, Soutis M, Christopoulos-Geroulanos G. Anastomotic strictures following esophageal atresia repair: a 20-year experience with endoscopic balloon dilatation. *J Pediatr Gastroenterol Nutr.* 2010;51:464.

649. Michaud L, Gottrand F. Anastomotic strictures: conservative treatment. *J Pediatr Gastroenterol Nutr.* 2011;52(suppl 1):S18.

650. de Lagausie P. GER in oesophageal atresia: surgical options. *J Pediatr Gastroenterol Nutr.* 2011;52(suppl 1):S27.

651. Luks FI. New and/or Improved Aspects of Fetal Surgery. *Prenat Diagn.* 2011;31:252–258.

652. Deprest JA, Done E, Van Mieghem T, et al. Fetal surgery for anesthesiologists. *Curr Opin Anaesthesiol.* 2008;21:298–307.

653. International Fetal Medicine and Surgery Society. 1st annual meeting in 1982: consensus statement and registry developed. Available at: http://www.ifmss.org/AboutIFMSS/History/tabid/67/Default.aspx. Accessed April 2013.

654. Wu D, Ball RH. The Maternal Side of Maternal-Fetal Surgery. *Clin Perinatol.* 2009;36:247–253.

655. Beck V, Lewi P, Gucciardo L, et al. Preterm prelabor rupture of membranes and fetal survival after minimally invasive fetal surgery: a systematic review of the literature. *Fetal Diagn Ther.* 2012; 31:1–9.

656. Adzick NS, Thom EA, Spong CY, et al. For the MOMS investigators. A randomized trial of prenatal versus postnatal repair of myelomeningocele. *N Engl J Med.* 2011;364:993–1004.

657. MOMS trail. http://en.wikipedia.org/wiki/MOMS_Trial. Last Accessed April 2013.

658. Total Trial website. http://www.totaltrial.eu/?id=9. Accessed April 2013.

659. Jones MW, McMurray JL, Englestad D. The "geriatric" NICU patient. *Neonatal Netw.* 2002;21(6):49–58.

660. Aurora S, Snyder EY. Perinatal asphyxia. In: Cloherty JP, Eichenwald EC, Stark AR, eds. *Manual of Neonatal Care.* 5th ed. Philadelphia, PA: Lippincott-Raven; 2004.

661. Kuban KCK, Philiano J. Neonatal seizures. In: Fanaroff AA, Martin RJ, eds. *Neonatal-Perinatal Medicine Diseases of the Fetus and Infant.* 4th ed. St. Louis, MO: Mosby; 1998.

662. Yager JY, Vannucci RC. Seizures in neonates. In: Fanaroff AA, Martin RJ, eds. *Neonatal-Perinatal Medicine Diseases of the Fetus and Infant.* 7th ed. St. Louis, MO: Mosby; 2002.

663. du Plessis AJ. Neonatal seizures. In: Cloherty JP, Eichenwald EC, Stark AR, eds. *Manual of Neonatal Care.* 5th ed. Philadelphia, PA: Lippincott-Raven; 2004.

664. Lekskulchai R, Cole J. The relationship between the scarf ratio and subsequent motor performance in infants born preterm. *Pediatr Phys Ther.* 2000;12:150–157.

665. Barfield WD, Lee KG, Late Preterm Infants. *Up to date.* http://www.uptodate.com/contents/late-preterm-infants?source=search_result&search=late+preterm+infant&selectedTitle=1%7E42. April 2nd 2013. Accessed May 2013.

666. Spong CY, Mercer BM, D'Alton M, et al. Timing of indicated late-preterm and early-term birth. *Obstet Gynecol.* 2011;118:323.

667. Hamilton BE, Martin JA, Ventura SJ, et al. Births: Final data for 2007. *Natl Vital Stat Rep.* 2010;58:24. Available at: http://www.cdc.gov/nchs/data/nvsr/nvsr58/nvsr58_24.pdf. Accessed May 2013

668. Goldenberg RL, Culhane JF, Iams JD, et al. Epidemiology and causes of preterm birth. *Lancet.* 2008;371:75.

669. Schieve LA, Ferre C, Peterson HB, et al. Perinatal outcome among singleton infants conceived through assisted reproductive technology in the United States. *Obstet Gynecol.* 2004;103:1144.

670. Reddy UM, Wapner RJ, Rebar RW, et al. Infertility, assisted reproductive technology, and adverse pregnancy outcomes: executive summary of a National Institute of Child Health and Human Development workshop. *Obstet Gynecol.* 2007;109:967.

671. Wang ML, Dorer DJ, Fleming MP, et al. Clinical outcomes of near-term infants. *Pediatrics.* 2004;114:372.

672. Shapiro-Mendoza CK, Tomashek KM, Kotelchuck M, et al. Effect of late-preterm birth and maternal medical conditions on newborn morbidity risk. *Pediatrics.* 2008;121:e223.

673. Bird TM, Bronstein JM, Hall RW, et al. Late preterm infants: birth outcomes and health care utilization in the first year. *Pediatrics.* 2010;126:e311.

674. Engle WA, Tomashek KM, Wallman C, et al. "Late-preterm" infants: a population at risk. *Pediatrics.* 2007;120:1390.

675. Leone A, Ersfeld P, Adams M, et al. Neonatal morbidity in singleton late preterm infants compared with full-term infants. *Acta Paediatr.* 2012;101:e6.

676. Engle WA, Kominiarek MA. Late preterm infants, early term infants, and timing of elective deliveries. *Clin Perinatol.* 2008; 35:325.

677. Consortium on Safe Labor, Hibbard JU, Wilkins I, et al. Respiratory morbidity in late preterm births. *JAMA.* 2010;304:419.

678. Engle WA, American Academy of Pediatrics Committee on Fetus and Newborn. Surfactant-replacement therapy for respiratory distress in the preterm and term neonate. *Pediatrics.* 2008; 121:419.

679. Rubaltelli FF, Bonafe L, Tangucci M, et al. Epidemiology of neonatal acute respiratory disorders. A multicenter study on incidence and fatality rates of neonatal acute respiratory disorders according to gestational age, maternal age, pregnancy complications and type of delivery. Italian Group of Neonatal Pneumology. *Biol Neonate.* 1998;74:7.

680. Escobar GJ, McCormick MC, Zupancic JA, et al. Unstudied infants: outcomes of moderately premature infants in the neonatal intensive care unit. *Arch Dis Child Fetal Neonatal Ed.* 2006;91:F238.

681. Sarici SU, Serdar MA, Korkmaz A, et al. Incidence, course, and prediction of hyperbilirubinemia in near-term and term newborns. *Pediatrics.* 2004;113:775.

682. Hunt CE. Ontogeny of autonomic regulation in late preterm infants born at 34–37 weeks postmenstrual age. *Semin Perinatol.* 2006;30:73.

683. Ramanathan R, Corwin MJ, Hunt CE, et al. Cardiorespiratory events recorded on home monitors: comparison of healthy infants with those at increased risk for SIDS. *JAMA.* 2001;285:2199.

684. Henderson-Smart DJ, Pettigrew AG, Campbell DJ. Clinical apnea and brain-stem neural function in preterm infants. *N Engl J Med.* 1983;308:353.

685. Morse SB, Zheng H, Tang Y, et al. Early school-age outcomes of late preterm infants. *Pediatrics.* 2009;123:e622.

686. Petrini JR, Dias T, McCormick MC, et al. Increased risk of adverse neurological development for late preterm infants. *J Pediatr.* 2009;154:169.

687. Chyi LJ, Lee HC, Hintz SR, et al. School outcomes of late preterm infants: special needs and challenges for infants born at 32 to 36 weeks gestation. *J Pediatr.* 2008;153:25.

688. Talge NM, Holzman C, Wang J, et al. Late-preterm birth and its association with cognitive and socioemotional outcomes at 6 years of age. *Pediatrics.* 2010;126:1124.

689. Moster D, Lie RT, Markestad T. Long-term medical and social consequences of preterm birth. *N Engl J Med.* 2008;359:262.

690. McGowan JE, Alderdice FA, Holmes VA, et al. Early childhood development of late-preterm infants: a systematic review. *Pediatrics.* 2011;127:1111.

691. Gurka MJ, LoCasale-Crouch J, Blackman JA. Long-term cognition, achievement, socioemotional, and behavioral development of healthy late-preterm infants. *Arch Pediatr Adolesc Med.* 2010;164:525.

692. Garcia-Prats JA, Abrams SA. Clinical Features and Diagnosis of Meconium Aspiration Syndrome. *Up to date.* May 22, 2012. Available at: http://www.uptodate.com/contents/clinical-features-and-diagnosis-of-meconium-aspiration-syndrome?source=search_result& search=meconium+aspiration&selectedTitle=1%7E36#references. Accessed June 2013.

693. Singh BS, Clark RH, Powers RJ, et al. Meconium aspiration syndrome remains a significant problem in the NICU: outcomes and

694. Whitfield JM, Charsha DS, Chiruvolu A. Prevention of meconium aspiration syndrome: an update and the Baylor experience. Proc (Bayl Univ Med Cent). 2009; 22:128.

695. Garcia-Prats JA, Abrams SA. Prevention and management of meconium aspiration syndrome. *Up to date,* May 11, 2012. Available at: http://www.uptodate.com/contents/prevention-and-management-of-meconium-aspiration-syndrome?source=search_result&s earch=meconium+aspiration&selectedTitle=2%7E36. Accessed May 2013.

696. Fanaroff AA. Meconium aspiration syndrome: historical aspects. *J Perinatol.* 2008;28(suppl 3):S3.

697. Balchin I, Whittaker JC, Lamont RF, et al. Maternal and fetal characteristics associated with meconium-stained amniotic fluid. *Obstet Gynecol.* 2011;117:828.

698. Clausson B, Cnattingius S, Axelsson O. Outcomes of post-term births: the role of fetal growth restriction and malformations. *Obstet Gynecol.* 1999;94:758.

699. Lee JS, Stark AR. Meconium aspiration. In: Cloherty JP, Eichenwald EC, Stark AR, eds. *Manual of Neonatal Care.* 5th ed. Philadelphia, PA: Lippincott Williams & Wilkins; 2004.

700. Martin RJ, Fanaroff AA, Klaus MH. Respiratory problems. In: Klaus MH, Fanaroff AA, eds. *Care of the High-Risk Neonate.* 4th ed. Philadelphia, PA: Saunders; 1993.

701. Yoder BA, Kirsch EA, Barth WH, Gordon MC. Changing obstetric practices associated with decreasing incidence of meconium aspiration syndrome. *Obstet Gynecol.* 2002;99:731.

702. Shankaran S. The postnatal management of the asphyxiated term infant. *Clin Perinatol.* 2002;29(4):675–692.

703. Gelfand SL, Fanroff JM, Walsh MC. Controversies in the treatment of meconium aspiration syndrome. *Clin Perinatol.* 2004;31:445–452.

704. Dargaville PA, Copnell B, Australian and New Zealand Neonatal Network. The epidemiology of meconium aspiration syndrome: incidence, risk factors, therapies, and outcome. *Pediatrics.* 2006;117:1712.

705. Cleary GM, Wiswell TE. Meconium-stained amniotic fluid and the meconium aspiration syndrome. An update. *Pediatr Clin North Am.* 1998;45:511.

706. Wiswell TE, Tuggle JM, Turner BS. Meconium aspiration syndrome: have we made a difference? *Pediatrics.* 1990;85:715.

707. Wiswell TE, Bent RC. Meconium staining and the meconium aspiration syndrome. Unresolved issues. *Pediatr Clin North Am.* 1993;40:955.

708. Ghidini A, Spong CY. Severe meconium aspiration syndrome is not caused by aspiration of meconium. *Am J Obstet Gynecol.* 2001;185:931.

709. Tran N, Lowe C, Sivieri EM, et al. Sequential effects of acute meconium obstruction on pulmonary function. *Pediatr Res.* 1980;14:34.

710. Tyler DC, Murphy J, Cheney FW. Mechanical and chemical damage to lung tissue caused by meconium aspiration. *Pediatrics.* 1978;62:454.

711. Stoll BJ, Kliegman RM. Respiratory tract disorders. In: Berhman RE, Kliegman RM, Jenson HB, eds. *Nelson's Textbook of Pediatrics.* 17th ed. Philadelphia, PA: Saunders; 2004.

712. Beligere N, Rao R. Neurodevelopmental outcome of infants with meconium aspiration syndrome: report of a study and literature review. *J Perinatol.* 2008;28(S3):93.

713. Konduri GG. New approaches for persistent pulmonary hypertension of the newborn. *Clin Perinatol.* 2004;31:591–611.

714. Adams JM, Stark AR. Persistent Pulmonary Hypertension of the Newborn. *UpToDate,* November 20 2012. Available at: http://www.uptodate.com/contents/persistent-pulmonary-hypertension-of-the-newborn?source=search_result&search=pphn+of+newborn& selectedTitle=1%7E46#references. Accessed May 2013.

715. Levin DL. Morphologic analysis of the pulmonary vascular bed in congenital left-sided diaphragmatic hernia. *J Pediatr.* 1978;92:805

716. Geggel RL, Murphy JD, Langleben D, et al. Congenital diaphragmatic hernia: arterial structural changes and persistent pulmonary hypertension after surgical repair. *J Pediatr.* 1985;107:457.

717. Murphy JD, Rabinovitch M, Goldstein JD, Reid LM. The structural basis of persistent pulmonary hypertension of the newborn infant. *J Pediatr.* 1981;98:962.

718. Dhillon R. The management of neonatal pulmonary hypertension. *Arch Dis Child Fetal Neonatal Ed.* 2012;97:F223.

719. VanMarter LJ. Persistent pulmonary hypertension of the newborn. In: Cloherty JP, Eichenwald EC, Stark AR, eds. *Manual of Neonatal Care.* 5th ed. Philadelphia, PA: Lippincott Williams & Wilkins; 2004.

720. Lipkin PH, Davidson D, Spivak L, et al. Neurodevelopmental and medical outcomes of persistent pulmonary hypertension of the newborn in term neonates treated with nitric oxide. *J Pediatr.* 2002;140(3):306–310.

721. Walsh MC, Stark ER. Persistent pulmonary hypertension of the newborn. Rational therapy based on pathophysiology. *Clin Perinatol.* 2001;28(3):609–627.

722. Inhaled nitric oxide in term and near-term infants: neurodevelopmental follow-up of the neonatal inhaled nitric oxide study group (NINOS). *J Pediatr.* 2000;136:611.

723. Ellington M Jr, O'Reilly D, Allred EN, et al. Child health status, neurodevelopmental outcome, and parental satisfaction in a randomized, controlled trial of nitric oxide for persistent pulmonary hypertension of the newborn. *Pediatrics.* 2001;107:1351.

724. Rosenberg AA, Kennaugh JM, Moreland SG, et al. Longitudinal follow-up of a cohort of newborn infants treated with inhaled nitric oxide for persistent pulmonary hypertension. *J Pediatr.* 1997;131:70.

725. Robertson CM, Finer NN, Sauve RS, et al. Neurodevelopmental outcome after neonatal extracorporeal membrane oxygenation. *CMAJ.* 1995;152:1981.

726. Cohen DA, Nsuami M, Etame RB, et al. A school-based Chlamydia control program using DNA amplification technology. *Pediatrics.* 1998;101:E1.

727. Fligor BJ, Neault MW, Mullen CH, et al. Factors associated with sensorineural hearing loss among survivors of extracorporeal membrane oxygenation therapy. *Pediatrics.* 2005;115:1519.

728. Eriksen V, Nielsen LH, Klokker M, et al. Follow-up of 5- to 11-year-old children treated for persistent pulmonary hypertension of the newborn. *Acta Paediatr.* 2009;98:304.

729. Chang G. Alcohol Intake and Pregnancy. *UptoDate,* November 29 2012. http://www.uptodate.com/contents/alcohol-intake-and-pregnancy?source=search_result&search=alcohol+in+pregnancy&selectedTitle=1%7E150 Accessed May 2013.

730. Jones KL. *Smith's Recognizable Patterns of Human Malformation.* 5th ed. Philadelphia, PA: Saunders; 1997.

731. AAP Committee on Substance Abuse 1999–2000. Fetal alcohol syndrome & alcohol related neurodevelopmental disorders. *Pediatrics.* 2000;106(2):358–361.

732. LA Siellski Infant of mothers with substance abuse. *UptoDate,* July 1 2013. Available at: http://www.uptodate.com/contents/infants-of-mothers-with-substance-abuse?source=search_result&search=nas&selectedTitle=2%7E15. Accessed May 2013.

733. Jones MW, Bass WT. Fetal alcohol syndrome. *Neonatal Netw.* 2003;22(3):63–70.

734. Day NL, Jasperse D, Richardson G, et al. Prenatal exposure to alcohol: effect of growth & morphologic characteristics. *Pediatrics.* 1989;84(3):536–541.

735. Sokol RJ, Delaney-Black V, Norstrom B. Fetal alcohol spectrum disorder. *JAMA.* 2003;290(22):2996–2999.

736. US Department of Health and Human Services. Results from the 2010 National Survey on Drug Use and Health: Summary of National Findings. Substance Abuse and Mental Health Services Administration; Center for Behavioral Health Statistics and Quality, 2010. Available at: http://oas.samhsa.gov/NSDUH/2k10NSDUH/2k10Results.htm. Accessed October 2012.

737. Jones KL, Smith DW. Recognition of the fetal alcohol syndrome in early infancy. *Lancet.* 1973;2:9.

738. Jobe AR. Alcohol as a fetal neurotoxin. *J Pediatr.* 2004;194(3):338.

739. Mukherjee RAS, Hollins S, Turk J. Fetal alcohol spectrum disorder: an overview. *J Roy Soc Med.* 2006;99:298–302.

740. Hoyme HE, May PA, Kalberg WO, et al. A practical clinical approach to diagnosis of fetal alcohol spectrum disorders: clarification of the 1996 institute of medicine criteria. *Pediatrics.* 2005;115:39.

741. American Academy of Pediatrics. Committee on Substance Abuse and Committee on Children With Disabilities. Fetal alcohol syndrome and alcohol-related neurodevelopmental disorders. *Pediatrics.* 2000;106:358.

742. Warren KR, Li TK. Genetic polymorphisms: impact on the risk of fetal alcohol spectrum disorders. *Birth Defects Res A Clin Mol Teratol.* 2005;73:195.

743. Jacobson SW, Carr LG, Croxford J, et al. Protective effects of the alcohol dehydrogenase-ADH1B allele in children exposed to alcohol during pregnancy. *J Pediatr.* 2006;148:30.

744. McCarver DG, Thomasson HR, Martier SS, et al. Alcohol dehydrogenase-2*3 allele protects against alcohol-related birth defects among African Americans. *J Pharmacol Exp Ther.* 1997;283:1095.

745. Stoler JM, Ryan LM, Holmes LB. Alcohol dehydrogenase 2 genotypes, maternal alcohol use, and infant outcome. *J Pediatr.* 2002;141:780

746. Feldman HS, Jones KL, Lindsay S, et al. Prenatal alcohol exposure patterns and alcohol-related birth defects and growth deficiencies: a prospective study. *Alcohol Clin Exp Res.* 2012;36:670.

747. Alati R, Macleod J, Hickman M, et al. Intrauterine exposure to alcohol and tobacco use and childhood IQ: findings from a parental-offspring comparison within the Avon Longitudinal Study of Parents and Children. *Pediatr Res.* 2008;64:659.

748. Kartin D, Grant TM, Streissguth AP, et al. Three-year developmental outcomes in children with prenatal alcohol and drug exposure. *Pediatr Phys Ther.* 2002;14(3):145–153.

749. Streissguth AP, Aase JM, Clarren SK, et al. Fetal alcohol syndrome in adolescents and adults. *JAMA.* 1991;265:1961.

750. Spohr HL, Willms J, Steinhausen HC. Prenatal alcohol exposure and long-term developmental consequences. *Lancet.* 1993;341:907.

751. Spohr HL, Willms J, Steinhausen HC. Fetal alcohol spectrum disorders in young adulthood. *J Pediatr.* 2007;150:175.

752. Roussotte F, Soderberg L, Sowell E. Structural, metabolic, and functional brain abnormalities as a result of prenatal exposure to drugs of abuse: evidence from neuroimaging. *Neuropsychol Rev.* 2010;20:376.

753. Gardner J. Fetal alcohol syndrome: recognition and intervention. *J Matern Child Nurs.* 1997;22(6):318–322.

754. Koren G, Nulman I, Chudley AE, et al. Fetal alcohol spectrum disorder. *Can Med Assoc J.* 2003;169(11):1181–1185.

755. Schechner S. Drug abuse and withdrawal. In: Cloherty JP, Eichenwald EC, Stark AR, eds. *Manual of Neonatal Care.* 5th ed. Philadelphia, PA: Lippincott Williams & Wilkins; 2004.

756. Johnson K, Gerada C, Greenough A. Treatment of neonatal abstinence syndrome. *Arch Dis Child.* 2002;F2–F5.

757. AAP Committee on Drugs. Neonatal drug withdrawal. *Pediatrics.* 1998;10:1079–1088.

758. LA Sielslki. Neonatal Opiod Withdrawal (Neonatal Abstinence Syndrome. *UptoDate,* September 13 2012. Available at: http://www.uptodate.com/contents/neonatal-opioid-withdrawal-neonatal-abstinence-syndrome?source=search_result&search=nas&selectedTitle=1%7E15. Accessed May 2013.

759. Akera C, Ro S. Medical concerns in the neonatal period. *Clin Fam Pract.* 5(2):265.

760. Hudak ML, Tan RC, Committee on drugs, et al. Neonatal drug withdrawal. *Pediatrics.* 2012;129:e540.

761. Zelson C, Rubio E, Wasserman E. Neonatal narcotic addiction: 10 year observation. *Pediatrics.* 1971;48:178.

762. Kandall SR, Gartner LM. Late presentation of drug withdrawal symptoms in newborns. *Am J Dis Child.* 1974;127:58.

763. Wright ML, Robinson MJ. Neonatal abstinence syndrome. *Arch Dis Child Fetal Neonatal Ed.* 1995;73:F122.

764. Bada HS, Bauer CR, Shankaran S, et al. Central and autonomic systems signs with in utero drug exposure. *Arch Dis Child Fetal Neonatal Ed.* 2002;F106–F112.

765. Fike DL. Assessment and management of the substance-exposed infant. In: Kenner C, Lott JW, eds. *Comprehensive Neonatal Nursing: A Physiologic Perspective.* 3rd ed. Philadelphia, PA: Saunders; 2003.

766. D'Apolito K. Substance abuse: infant and childhood outcomes. *J Pediatr Nurs.* 1998;13(5):307–316.

767. Finnegan LP, Connaughton JF, Kron RE, et al. Neonatal abstinence syndrome: assessment and management. *Addict Dis.* 1975;2(1–2):141–158.

768. Finnegan LP. Neonatal abstinence syndrome: assessment and pharmacotherapy. In: Rubatelli FF, Granati B, eds. *Neonatal Therapy: An Update.* New York, NY: Exerpta Medica; 1986.

769. Osborn DA, Jeffery HE, Cole MJ. Opiate treatment for opiate withdrawal in newborn infants. *Cochrane Database Syst Rev.* 2010;DOI:CD002059.

770. Jackson L, Ting A, McKay S, et al. A randomised controlled trial of morphine versus phenobarbitone for neonatal abstinence syndrome. *Arch Dis Child Fetal Neonatal Ed.* 2004;89:F300.

771. Kandall SR, Doberczak TM, Mauer KR, et al. Opiate v CNS depressant therapy in neonatal drug abstinence syndrome. *Am J Dis Child.* 1983;137:378.

772. Finnegan LP, Michael H, Leifer B, et al. An evaluation of neonatal abstinence treatment modalities. *NIDA Res Monogr.* 1984;49:282.

773. Kaltenbach K, Finnegan LP. Perinatal and developmental outcome of infants exposed to methadone in-utero. *Neurotoxicol Teratol.* 1987;9:311.

774. Doberczak TM, Shanzer S, Cutler R, et al. One-year follow-up of infants with abstinence-associated seizures. *Arch Neurol.* 1988;45:649.

775. Bauer CR. Perinatal effects of prenatal drug exposure. Neonatal aspects. *Clin Perinatol.* 1999;26:87.

776. Huffman DL, Price BK, Langel L. Therapeutic handling techniques for the infant affected by cocaine. *Neonatal Netw.* 1994;13(5):9–13.

777. Marcellus L. Care of substance-exposed infants: the Current state of practice in Canadian hospitals. *J Perinat Neonatal Nurs.* 2002;16(3):51–68.

778. Forrest DC. The cocaine-exposed infant, Part II: intervention and teaching. *J Pediatr Health Care.* 1994;(8):7–11.

779. American Academy of Pediatrics. Committee on Fetus and Newborn. Hospital discharge of the high risk neonate—proposed guidelines. *Pediatrics.* 1998;102(2):411–417.

780. Kenner C, Bagwell GA, Torok LS. Transition to home. In: Kenner C, Lott JW, ed. *Comprehensive Neonatal Nursing: A Physiologic Perspective.* 3rd ed. Philadelphia: Saunders, 2003.

781. Zaccagnini L. Discharge planning. In: Cloherty JP, Eichenwald EC, Stark AR, eds. *Manual of Neonatal Care.* 5th ed. Philadelphia, PA: Lippincott Williams & Wilkins; 2004.

782. Hack M. The outcomes of neonatal intensive care. In: Klaus MH, Fanaroff AA, eds. *Care of the High-Risk Neonate.* 5th ed. Philadelphia, PA: Saunders; 2001.

783. Lockridge T, Taquino LT, Knight A. Back to sleep: is there room in that crib for both AAP recommendations and developmentally supportive care? *Neonatal Netw.* 1999;18(5):29–33.

784. Bailey DB, Hebbeler K, Scarborough A, et al. First experiences with early intervention: a national perspective. *Pediatrics.* 2004;113(4):887–896.

785. Hack MB, Wilson-Costello D, Friedman H, et al. Neurodevelopmental predictors of outcomes of children with birth weight of less than 1000 grams: 1992–1995. *Arch Pediatr Adolesc Med.* 2000;154(7):725–751.

786. Vohr BR, O'Shea M, Wright LL. Longitudinal multicenter follow-up of high-risk infants: why, who, when, and what to assess. *Semin Perinatol.* 2003;27(4):333–342.

787. Vohr B. Overview of infants and children with hearing loss. Part 1. *Ment Retard Dev Disabil Res Rev.* 2003;9(2):62–64.

788. Vohr B. Infants and children with hearing loss—part 2: overview. *Ment Retard Dev Disabil Res Rev.* 2003;9(4):218–219.

789. Bear LM. Early identification of infants at risk for developmental disabilities. *Pediatr Clin North Am.* 2004;51:685–701.

790. Wood NS, Marlow N, Costloe K, et al. Neurologic and developmental disability after extremely premature birth. *N Engl J Med.* 2000;343(6):378–384.

791. Bennett FC. Perspective: low birth weight infants: accomplishments, risks, and interventions. *Infants Young Child.* 2002; 15(1):vi–ix.

792. Wolf MJ, Koldewijn K, Beelen A, et al. Neurobehavioral and developmental profile of very low birthweight preterm infants in early infancy. *Acta Paediatr.* 2002;91:930–938.

793. Stewart JE. Follow-up of very-low-birth-weight infants. In: Cloherty JP, Eichenwald EC, Stark AR. *Manual Neonatal Care.* 5th ed. Philadelphia, PA: Lippincott Williams & Wilkins; 2004.

794. Davis DW. Cognitive outcomes in school-age children born prematurely. *Neonatal Netw.* 2003;22(3):27–38.

795. Foulder-Hughes LA, Cooke RW. Motor, cognitive, and behavioral disorders in children born very preterm. *Dev Med Child Neurol.* 2003;45(2):97–103.

796. Pinto-Martin J, Whitaker A, Feldman J, et al. Special education services and school performance in a regional cohort of low-birthweight infants at age nine. *Pediatr Perinatal Epidemiol.* 2004;18:120–129.

797. Latal-Hajnal B, von Siebenthal K, Kovari H, et al. Postnatal growth in VLBW infants: significant association with neurodevelopmental outcome. *J Pediatr.* 2003;143(2):163–170.

798. Smith VC, Zupancic JA, McCormick MC, et al. Rehospitalization in the first year of life among infants with bronchopulmonary dysplasia. *J Pediatr.* 2004;144(6):799–803.

799. McCormick MC. The outcomes of very low birth weight infants: are we asking the right questions? *Pediatrics.* 1997;99(6):869–875.

800. Weisglas-Kuperus N, Baerts W, Smrkovsky M, et al. Effects of biological and social development of very low birth weight children. *Pediatrics.* 1993;92(5):658–665.

801. Bayley N. Bayley Scales of Infant and Toddler Development, 3rd ed. San Antonio, Texas: The Psychological Corporation; 2006.

RECOMMENDED READINGS

Brazelton TB, Nugent JK. *Neonatal Behavioral Assessment Scale.* 3rd ed. London, England: Mac Keith Press; 1995.

Cloherty JP, Eichenwald EC, Stark AR, eds. *Manual of Neonatal Care.* 5th ed. Philadelphia, PA: Lippincott Williams & Wilkins; 2004.

Goldson E. *Nurturing the Premature Infant.* London, England: Oxford University Press; 1999.

Hunter JG. Neonatal intensive care unit. In: Case-Smith J, ed. *Occupational Therapy for Children.* 4th ed. St. Louis, MO: Mosby; 2001.

Kenner C, Lott JW, eds. *Comprehensive Neonatal Nursing: A Physiologic Perspective.* 3rd ed. Philadelphia, PA: Saunders; 2003.

Kenner C, McGrath JM, eds. *Developmental Care of Newborns and Infants: A Guide for Health Professionals.* Philadelphia, PA: Elsevier; 2004.

Mercer RT. *Nursing Care for Parents at Risk.* Thorofare, NJ: Charles B. Slack Inc; 1977.

Sweeney JK, Heriza CB, Blanchard Y. Neonatal physical therapy. Part I: clinical competencies and neonatal intensive care unit clinical training models. *Pediatr Phys Ther.* 2009;21:296–307.

Sweeney JK, Heriza CB, Blanchard Y, et al. Neonatal physical therapy. Part II: practice frameworks and evidence-based practice guidelines. *Pediatr Phys Ther.* 2010;22:2–16.

Sweeney JK, Swanson MW. Low birth weight infants: neonatal care and follow-up. In: Umphred DA, ed. *Neurological Rehabilitation.* 4th ed. St. Louis, MO: Mosby; 2001.

Vergara ER, Bigsby R. *Developmental and Therapeutic Interventions in the NICU.* Baltimore, MD: Paul H. Brookes Publishing Co; 2004.

Volpe JJ. *Neurology of the Newborn.* 4th ed. Philadelphia, PA: Saunders; 2001.

Zaichkin J. *Newborn Intensive Care: What Every Parent Needs to Know.* 2nd ed. Santa Rosa, CA: NICU Ink Book Publishers; 2002.

▶ Common Abbreviations

A	Apnea
ABG	Arterial blood gas
AGA	Appropriate for gestational age
AOP	Apnea of prematurity
APIB	Assessment of Preterm Infant Behavior
AROM	Artificial rupture of membranes
B	Bradycardia
BAER	Brainstem auditory-evoked potentials
BPD	Bronchopulmonary dysplasia
BPI	Brachial plexus injury
BW	Birth weight
CDH	Congenital diaphragmatic hernia
CHD	Congenital heart disease
CHD	Congenital hip dysplasia
CLD	Chronic lung disease
CMV	Conventional mechanical ventilation
CMV	Cytomegalovirus
CPAP	Continuous positive airway pressure
CS	Cesarean section
D	Desaturation
DOL	Day of life
ECMO	Extracorporeal membrane oxygenation
EGA	Estimated gestational age
ELBW	Extremely low birth weight
FAS	Fetal alcohol syndrome
Fio$_2$	Fraction of inspired oxygen
FT	Full term
G	Gravida
GA	Gestational age
GBS	Group B streptococcus
GER	Gastroesophageal reflux
GM	Germinal matrix
GMA	General Movement Assessment
HAL	Hyperalimentation
HC	Head circumference
HFFI	High-frequency flow interruption
HFJV	High-frequency jet ventilation
HFOV	High-frequency oscillatory ventilation
HFV	High-frequency ventilation

HIE	Hypoxic–ischemic encephalopathy
HMD	Hyaline membrane disease
HR	Heart rate
ICH	Intracranial hemorrhage
ICN	Intensive care nursery
IDVA	Intravenous drug abuse
IMD	Infant of diabetic mother
IMV	Intermittent mandatory ventilation
iNO	Inspired nitric oxide
IVH	Intraventricular hemorrhage
IUGR	Intrauterine growth retardation
LBW	Low birth weight
LGA	Large for gestational age
MAS	Meconium aspiration syndrome
MCA	Multiple congenital anomalies
MV	Mechanical ventilation
NAPI	Neurobehavioral Assessment of the Preterm Infant
NAS	Neonatal abstinence syndrome / neonatal abstinence scale
NBAS	Neonatal Neurobehavioral Assessment Scale
NC	Nasal cannula
NEC	Necrotizing enterocolitis
NICU	Neonatal intensive care unit
NIDCAP	Newborn Individualized Developmental Care and Assessment Program
NNNS	Neonatal Intensive Care Network Neurobehavioral Scale
NJ	Naso jejunal
NG	Nasal gastric
NO	Nitric oxide
NP	Nasal prongs
OC	Open crib
OD	Right eye
OG	Oral gastric
OS	Left eye
P	Para
PCA	Postconceptual age
PDA	Patent ductus arteriosus
PEEP	Positive end-expiratory pressure
PHI	Periventricular hemorrhage infarction

PIE	Pulmonary interstitial emphysema
PO	By mouth
PPHN	Persistent pulmonary hypertension of the newborn
PPV	Positive pressure ventilation
PROM	Premature rupture of membranes
PT	Preterm
PTL	Preterm labor
PVD	Posthemorrhagic ventricular dilation
PVL	Periventricular leukomalacia
RDS	Respiratory distress syndrome
ROM	Rupture of membranes
ROP	Retinopathy of prematurity
RR	Respiratory rate

Sao_2	Oxygen saturation
SGA	Small for gestational age
SIMV	Synchronized intermittent mechanical ventilation
TORCH	Congenital viral infections (toxoplasmosis, other infections, rubella, cytomegalovirus, herpes)
TPF	Toxoplasmosis fetalis
TPN	Total parenteral nutrition
TTN	Transient tachypnea of the newborn
UAC	Umbilical arterial catheter
US	Ultrasound
UVC	Umbilical venous catheter
VLBW	Very low birth weight

Equipment Resources

Children's Medical Ventures
275 Longwater Drive
Norwell, MA 02061
888-766-8443 (Parents)
800-345-6443 (Hospitals)
866-866-6750 (Education)

www.childmed.com
Small Beginnings Inc.
17525 Alder Street
Suite #28
Hesperia, CA 92345
800-676-0462
www.small-beginnings.com

The Infant and Child with Cerebral Palsy

Jason Beaman, Faithe R. Kalisperis, and Kathleen Miller-Skomorucha

(adapted from the chapter "The Infant and Child with Cerebral Palsy" by Jane Styer-Acevedo in 4th edition)

Definition
Incidence
Etiology
Diagnosis and Prognosis
Classification
   Spastic
   Dyskinetic
   Ataxic
   Hypotonic
Assessment of the Infant and Child with CP
   Assessment of Movement
   Assessment of Postural Control
   Assessment of Postural Tone
   Musculoskeletal Assessment
Gait
   Observational Gait Analysis
   Common Gait Deviations
   Hemiplegic Gait
   Diplegic Gait
   Quadriplegic Gait
   Athetotic Gait
   Ataxic Gait
Fine Motor, Adaptive, and Self-care Skills
Speech and Language Considerations
Establishing Functional Outcomes
Therapeutic Interventions
   Therapeutic Exercise, Strengthening, and Stretching
   Neurodevelopmental Treatment

   Therapeutic Handling
   Sensory Integration and Sensory Processing Disorder
   Modified Constraint-induced Movement Therapy
   Treadmill Training/Robotic Gait Training
   Electrical Stimulation
   Aquatics
   Hippotherapy
   Community Programs
Adaptive Equipment
   Seating and Positioning Equipment
   Standers
   Ambulation Aids
Neurologic Interventions to Treat Spasticity
   Neuromedical Interventions
   Neurosurgical Interventions
Orthopedic Interventions
   Spine/Neuromuscular Scoliosis
   Hip
   Knee and Lower Leg
   Ankle and Foot
Lower Extremity Orthoses
   Ankle–Foot Orthoses
   Supramalleolar Orthoses
   Foot Orthoses
   Combining Orthoses
Home Management
School-based Therapy
Summary
Case Studies

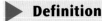

Definition

The International Workshop on Definition and Classification of Cerebral Palsy met in 2007 to refine the existing definition and classification of cerebral palsy (CP). They agreed upon the following definition of CP: "Cerebral palsy describes a group of permanent disorders of the development of movement and posture, causing activity limitations that are attributed to nonprogressive disturbances that occurred in the developing fetal or infant brain. The motor disorders of CP are often accompanied by disturbances of sensation, perception, cognition, communication and behavior as well as seizures and secondary musculoskeletal problems."[1,2] Beckung and Hagberg[3] found a variety of comorbidities in children with CP from ages 5 through 8. Forty percent of the children had mental retardation, which, when combined with the slow learners and persons with learning disabilities, increased to 75%; epilepsy occurred in 35% of the population; visual impairment in 20%; and hydrocephalus in 9%. Thirteen percent of the children had a combination of two impairments, and 15% had a combination of three impairments.[3] Additional associated problems include difficulty with speech in 25% and hearing impairments in 25%.[4] Stiller et al.[4] also found an increased frequency of visual impairments, as high as 40% to 50% in children with CP. Historically, children were diagnosed with CP if the insult occurred prenatally, perinatally, and postnatally. On the basis of the current definition, no upper age limit has been determined for postnatal onset.[1] For this reason, children are being diagnosed with CP throughout infancy and early childhood.

 ## Incidence

The US Collaborative Perinatal Project conducted by the National Institute of Neurological and Communicative Disorders and Stroke (NINCDS) is known as a landmark study for CP incidence and is still referred to in studies done today.[5] It was a study of 54,000 pregnant women from 12 urban teaching hospitals in the United States between 1959 and 1966. Of the women in the study, 46% were white, 46% were black, and most of the rest were Puerto Rican. The socioeconomic status of the sample was lower than that of the general population. The children born to these women had a regular schedule of examinations, including a general physical examination and a neurologic examination at both 1 and 7 years of age. Among the 38,533 children whose outcome was known at 7 years of age, 202 met the criteria for CP. Of the 202 children, 24 (12%) children had an acquired motor deficit secondary to a variety of factors in the early developing years, rather than congenital motor deficits occurring as a result of in utero factors or events at the time of labor and delivery. Infectious meningitis and trauma were the most common causes of acquired CP. In addition to the 202 children with CP who were alive at 7 years of age, 24 children with CP, most commonly with spastic quadriplegia, had died before 7 years of age. The following figures indicate the prevalence of CP based on the National Collaborative Perinatal Project:

5.2:1000—diagnosed as having CP

4.6:1000—when acquired cases of CP are excluded

2.6:1000—excluding mildly afflicted children (This figure more closely represents the prevalence of handicapping congenital CP.)

Further study of the population in the US Collaborative Perinatal Project indicated that there are "relatively low risks for cerebral palsy (1.3 to 2.9 per 1000) among children who had no abnormal signs, whether or not they had seizures in the nursery period."[6]

More recent studies of the incidence of CP prove it to be 2 to 3 per 1000 live births in the United States, the United Kingdom, Western Australia, Sweden, and Europe.[4,7–9] The survival of infants has improved over time but the prevalence of CP has remained the same with little change over the past 40 years. This may be due to the increase in CP within the population of preterm and very preterm infants.[7,8,10] The reported prevalence rate in twins is said to be 15 per 1000 live births, 80 per 1000 live births in triplets, and 43 per 1000 live births in quadruplets.[10] The rate increases to 40 to 100 per 1000 live births among babies born "very early or with very low birth weight."[9] In a British survey, it was shown that 100% of children noted to have CP in 1970 were still alive 10 years later, an increase in the numbers from the first survey done in 1958.[8]

 ## Etiology

There is no single specific cause of the constellation of symptoms known as CP. Rather, the potential causes of CP are known to occur in the prenatal stage of development and are also grouped with congenital problems in the perinatal or neonatal time period, and in the postnatal or postneonatal time period.[7,10] For a more complete list of the prenatal causes of CP, refer to Display 5.1; for the perinatal causes, refer to Display 5.2; and for the postneonatally acquired causes, refer to Display 5.3.

Prenatal events are thought to be responsible for about 75% of all CP. Perinatal asphyxia is thought to cause 6% to 8% of CP, with the underlying causes being unpreventable, and 10% to 18% of CP is thought to be caused postnatally.[7] The cause of CP in the majority of infants born at term in developing countries is due to prenatal influences and is not associated with significant neonatal encephalopathy.[11] Typically, one may see risk factors present in the infant or fetus (via medical testing) that may indicate a potential problem. Risk factors can be present before or during pregnancy, during labor and birthing, and in the period shortly after the birth of the infant.[7] Refer to Displays 5.4 through 5.8 for comprehensive lists of these risk factors.

Miller lists several possible congenital problems that can result in the infant and child with CP. These include schizencephaly, a segmental defect that causes a cleft in the brain; lissencephaly, a defect in the neuronal migration that normally goes toward the periphery of the brain but that then

DISPLAY 5.1	Prenatal Causes of CP

Vascular events such as a middle cerebral artery infarct

Maternal infections during the first and second trimesters such as rubella, cytomegalovirus, and toxoplasmosis

Less common: metabolic disorders, maternal ingestion of toxins, and rare genetic syndromes

DISPLAY
5.2   Perinatal Causes of CP

Problems During Labor and Delivery
Obstructed labor
Antepartum hemorrhage
Cord prolapse

Other Neonatal Causes
Hypoxic–ischemic encephalopathy
Neonatal stroke, usually of the middle cerebral artery
Severe hypoglycemia
Untreated jaundice
Severe neonatal infection

DISPLAY
5.4   Risk Factors Present Before Pregnancy

Maternal Factors
Delayed onset of menstruation
Irregular menstruation
Long intermenstrual intervals
Unusually short or long interval between pregnancies
Low social class in children with normal birth weight
Parity of three or more in preterm infants
Relationship with previous fetal deaths

Medical Conditions
Intellectual disability
Seizures
Thyroid disease

Paternal and Sibling Factors
Advanced paternal age (seen more frequently in those with athetoid dystonic cerebral palsy)
Motor deficit in sibling

---

results in a smooth brain, also known as decreased cerebral gyri; microcephaly and megalocephaly; cortical dysgenesis, a disorder of brain cortex formation; and defects in the normal formation and remodeling of synapses.[10] According to Hadders-Algra, approximately half of the created neurons die off (apoptosis), in particular during midgestation. Axons and synapses are also eliminated during the first decade or more of normal development. This shaping of the nervous system is guided by neurochemical processes and neural activity. The neural elements that best persist are those that fit the environment.[12] Therefore, changes in the formation of the developing nervous system can result in an infant with CP. However, the immature brain has much more plasticity or equipotentiality, terms used to define the

greater ability of the uninjured part to assume the function of the injured part of the brain.[10] Therefore, the response to injury is much different and makes diagnosis and prognosis difficult.

▶ Diagnosis and prognosis

The signs and symptoms of CP may be apparent in early infancy. Infants presenting with abnormal muscle tone, atypical posture, and movement with persistence of primitive reflexes may be diagnosed earlier than 2 years of age.[10] Milder cases of CP may not be diagnosed until 4 to 5 years of age.[13] Evaluation of the child's motor skills, neuroimaging, and evidence that symptoms are not progressing are key elements of this diagnosis. A correlation between clinical findings and neuroanatomy is possible to a limited degree. Neuroimaging of the brain, such as cranial ultrasound, computed tomography (CT), and magnetic resonance imaging (MRI), can show the location and type of brain damage.

DISPLAY
5.3   Postneonatally Acquired CP

Metabolic Encephalopathy
Storage disorders
Intermedullary metabolism disorders
Metabolic disorders
Miscellaneous disorders
Toxicity such as alcohol

Infections
Meningitis
Septicemia
Malaria (in developing countries)

Injuries
Cerebrovascular accident
Following surgery for congenital malformations
Near-drowning
Trauma
Motor vehicle accident
Child abuse such as shaken baby syndrome

DISPLAY
5.5   Risk Factors During Pregnancy

Preeclampsia in term infants but not in preterm infants
Multiple pregnancies associated with:
Preterm delivery
Poor intrauterine growth
Birth defects
Intrapartum complications

5.6   Risk Factors During Labor

Likely Causes of Perinatal Asphyxia

Prolapsed cord

Massive intrapartum hemorrhage

Prolonged or traumatic delivery due to cephalopelvic dispro-
portion or abnormal presentation

Large baby with shoulder dystocia

Maternal shock from a variety of causes

Events Associated with Causal Factors

Prolonged second-stage labor

Emergency Cesarean section

Premature separation of placenta

Abnormal fetal position

In Preterm, Can Include:

Meconium-stained fluid

Tight nuchal cord

5.8   Risk Factors for Preterm Infants

Patent ductus arteriosus

Hypotension

Blood transfusion

Prolonged ventilation

Pneumothorax

Sepsis

Hyponatremia

Total parenteral nutrition

Seizures

Parenchymal damage with appreciable ventricular dilatation

Cranial ultrasound is often used for the high-risk preterm infant, as it is less invasive than other imaging techniques. MRI imaging is often preferred, as it provides greater detail of brain tissue and structure.[13] Seventy percent to 90% of children with CP have abnormalities on a brain MRI. The physician should be cautious when interpreting neuroimaging, as the extent of damage to the brain tissue may not correlate directly with physical presentation or functional abilities.[10] When neuroimaging of the brain is unremarkable, other diagnoses that mimic the signs and symptoms of CP may be considered, such as mitochondrial and metabolic disorders and transient dystonia.

Cerebral hemorrhages may be associated with CP. These hemorrhages are labeled as intraventricular hemorrhage (IVH), bleeding into the ventricles; germinal matrix hemorrhage (GMH), bleeding into the tissue around the ventricles; and periventricular intraventricular hemorrhage (PIVH),

bleeding into both areas. Periventricular cyst (PVC) may form in these same areas as the acute hemorrhage resolves.[10] There are known risk factors for hemorrhages including mechanical ventilation and injury during critical periods of brain development. Notably, periventricular white matter is most sensitive to insult and injury between 24 and 34 weeks of gestation.[13,14]

Hemorrhages are graded in increasing severity from I through IV. The grade of bleed alone cannot predict the development or severity of CP.[10] Palmer indicated that cranial ultrasound should be used for low-birth-weight infants to detect grades III and IV hemorrhages, IVH, cystic periventricular leukomalacia (PVL), and ventricular enlargement.[11] After term age, cranial ultrasound and MRI are used to identify cystic PVL and ventriculomegaly, which are associated with subsequent development of CP.[7,11] PVL is the major cause of CP in infants born preterm.[14] The extent and location of white matter damage can lead to different subtypes of CP. Localized damage to the cortical spinal tracts often results in spastic diplegia, and when the lesions extend laterally, quadriplegia is often the result. It is understood that a neurologic examination alone is insufficiently sensitive enough or specific enough for early detection of CP.[11] The quality of an infant's "general movements" (GMs) have been used by doctors and researchers to evaluate brain function.[11,12] Ferrari et al.[11] studied 84 preterm infants at 16 to 20 weeks postterm age and found abnormalities in the GMs. A predominance of cramped synchronous GMs and absence of normal fidgety movements of limbs, neck, and trunk were predictive of CP at 2 to 3 years of age with a sensitivity of 100% and a specificity of 92.5% to 100%. Clearly, abnormal GMs at the fidgety age (2 to 4 months postterm) implies a total absence of the elegant, dancing complexity of fidgety movements and predicts CP with an accuracy of 85% to 98%.[12] GMs can be predictive of later CP and are the best expression of functional motor development. GMs are analogous to later functional motor milestones and may also predict severity, as the earlier the GMs are recognized, the more severe the later limitations in motor function.[11] These

---

5.7   Risk Factors at Birth and Newborn Period

Decreased birth weight

Decreased age at birth (length of gestation is the strongest determinant)

Poor intrauterine growth in moderately preterm but not in the very preterm infant

Low placental weight

Low Apgar scores (scores of 0 to 3 at 5 minutes have an 81-fold increased risk of cerebral palsy)

Neonatal seizures

Sepsis

Respiratory disease

observations and clinical testing warrant referral for therapeutic intervention to improve the infant's later function.[12]

Others have found cognitive abilities to be linked with the severity of CP and to be predictive of many outcomes.[8,15] Blair et al.[16] completed a study in 2001 that indicated that intellectual disability was the single strongest predictor of survival of the child with CP (profoundly mentally retarded children with CP do not live into adulthood) and that the second most important factor impacting life expectancy was the severity of the physical impairments. Katz[8] researched the life expectancy of children with CP and found, from multiple sources, that the causes of mortality related most commonly to the respiratory and circulatory systems, certain cancers, and neurologic complications.

Classification

CP may be classified by the type of movement disorder, anatomical location of the child's impaired motor function, and scope of motor dysfunction. The type of movement disorders can be described as spastic, hypotonic, dyskinetic, or ataxic.[1,17] Traditionally, physicians also classified CP by the anatomical location of the limbs affected. The three most common patterns described are hemiplegia, which involves one arm and one leg on the same side of the body; diplegia, which involves both lower extremities (LEs); and quadriplegia, which refers to involvement of all four limbs as well as back and neck musculature. Once a child is classified by the type of movement disorder and anatomical location of impaired motor function, further differentiation is made on the basis of the severity of motor dysfunction. For example, a child with mild spastic diplegia may walk without an assistive device for community distances, but a child with severe spastic diplegia may require an assistive device to walk household distances. Although commonly classified by their most prominent movement disorder, many children present with a mixed type of movement disorder (i.e., spastic and dyskinetic).

The Gross Motor Function Classification System (GMFCS), created by Palisano and colleagues[18] in 1997, is a classification system based on gross motor function of children with CP (see Display 5.9). Classifying an infant or child according to the severity of the CP can be helpful when looking at prognosis. The GMFCS was developed to fill the need to have a standardized system to measure the "severity of movement disability" in children with CP.[18,19] There are five levels in the test. Level I describes the child with the most independent function, where he or she can perform all the activities of his or her age-matched peers, albeit with some difficulty with speed, coordination, and balance. Level V describes the child who has difficulty controlling his or her head and trunk posture in most positions and in achieving any voluntary control of movement.[18,19] The GMFCS is described in Chapter 3. Beckung and Hagberg[3] described a Bimanual Fine Motor Function Classification

---

System (BFMFCS), which is similar to the GMFCS and has a five-level scale. There is a strong correlation between the GMFCS and the BFMFCS, indicating that the degree of gross and fine motor involvement for a child with CP is often the same.[3] Moreover, a 2006 validation study of the Shriner's Hospital for Children Upper Extremity Evaluation (SHUEE) revealed a fair correlation between the SHUEE and self-care section of the Pediatric Evaluation of Disability Inventory (PEDI).[20]

Spastic

Spasticity occurs in approximately 75% of all children with CP. It is the most common neurologic abnormality seen in children with CP, including those with diplegia, hemiplegia, and quadriplegia.[10,21] A French study in 1997 found the distribution of spastic CP as 40% quadriplegia, 17% diplegia, and 21% hemiplegia.[22] Slightly different distributions were identified for children in North Carolina—44% quadriplegia, 33% diplegia, and 23% hemiplegia.[23] Spasticity is a complex motor abnormality, often difficult to describe, but a common definition is "hypertonia in which resistance to passive movement increases with increasing velocity of movement."[1] The most widely used scale for assessing spasticity is the Modified Ashworth Scale (MAS) (Table 5.1). Spasticity, a hyperactive stretch reflex, is responsive to a variety of treatments, including botulinum toxin, baclofen, selective dorsal rhizotomy, and orthopedic surgery. Detailed descriptions of these treatments can be found later in the chapter. Spasticity causes significant histologic changes, including decreased longitudinal growth of muscle fibers, decreased volume of muscle, change in muscle unit size, and change in muscle fiber type.[10] The muscle changes with

TABLE 5.1	Modified Ashworth Scale
Score	**Description of Muscle Tone**
00	Hypotonia
0	Normal tone, no increase in tone
1	Slight increase in tone manifested by a slight catch and release or minimal increased resistance to joint range of motion
1+	Slight increase in tone manifested by a slight catch and minimal increased resistance to joint range of motion for more than half the joint range
2	More marked increase of tone through most of the whole joint range, but the affected joint is easily moved
3	Considerable increase in muscle tone; passive movement difficult but possible
4	Affected joint is stiff and cannot be moved

spasticity can cause secondary disorders such as hip dislocation, scoliosis, knee contracture, and torsional malalignments of the femur and tibia, amongst others. These changes often have significant effects on function, including effortful gait patterns, difficulty assuming and sustaining seated positioning, and difficulty performing self-care activities such as toileting, bathing, dressing, and self-feeding.

Diplegia

Diplegia is the most common form of spastic CP.[24] A white matter infarct in the periventricular areas caused by hypoxia can lead to spastic diplegic CP.[24] It primarily affects bilateral LEs, resulting in issues with gait, balance, and coordination. In standing, children with diplegia often present with an increased lumbar spine lordosis, anterior pelvic tilt, bilateral hip internal rotation, bilateral knee flexion, intoeing, and equinovalgus foot position (Fig. 5.1). There tends to be a discrepancy between upper extremity (UE) and LE function in children with this form of CP, with the LEs being more affected than the UEs and trunk. Overall, there is a large range in the level of motor involvement for children with diplegia. Gait deficits such as equinus and crouched gait posture tend to be the area of greatest concern for these children (refer to "Gait" section for further details). Owing to bilateral LE spasticity and weakness, energy expenditure is much greater during ambulation, resulting in poor endurance and decreased functional mobility at home and within the community. Children with diplegia generally have normal cognition but may have some social and emotional difficulties. Children with diplegia often require assistive devices such as a posterior walker, or lofstrand crutches. A scooter or wheelchair may be necessary for long-distance mobility.

Hemiplegia

Hemiplegia is a subtype of spastic CP in which the child's upper and lower extremity on the same side of the body are affected. Four main types of brain lesions result in

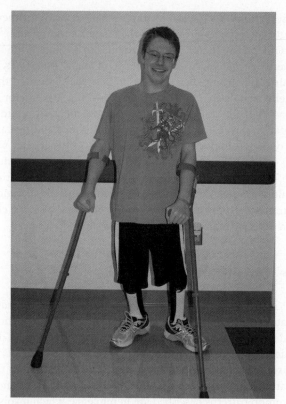

FIGURE 5.1 Child with typical diplegic CP posture.

hemiplegic CP. Periventricular white matter abnormalities have been reported as the most common diagnostic finding in children with hemiplegic CP.[25] Cervical–subcortical lesions, brain malformations, and nonprogressive postnatal injuries have also been identified as the main causes of hemiplegia.[26] The UE is typically more affected than the LE, and both tend to have more distal involvement than proximal involvement. Muscle spasticity on the affected side decreases muscle and bone growth, resulting in decreased range of motion (ROM). Therefore, children with hemiplegia often present with contractures and limb-length discrepancies on the involved side. The affected side of the child with hemiplegia often presents with shoulder protraction, elbow flexion, wrist flexion and ulnar deviation, pelvic retraction, hip internal rotation and flexion, knee flexion, and forefoot contact only due to plantarflexed foot.

Children with hemiplegia tend to achieve all gross and fine motor milestones but not within the typical time frame. For example, children with hemiplegia tend to walk between 18 and 24 months but present with gait deficits. Additionally, acquisition of bimanual hand skills is delayed because of the neurologic impairment of the affected side. For example, children with hemiplegia are able to cut food using a fork and knife, but only after hours of extensive guided practice during occupational therapy and at home. Two widely known standardized assessments are used to evaluate the quality of UE function in children with hemiplegia: the SHUEE[20] and the Assisting Hand Assessment (AHA).[27]

Cognitive function is typically normal in these children, and as adults they are able to work and participate in a variety of professional settings. It should be noted that children with spastic hemiplegia have been found to have social and emotional deficits. These include emotional disorders in 25%, conduct disorders in 24%, pervasive hyperactivity in 10%, and situational hyperactivity in 13%.[15] Overall, children with hemiplegia require minimal equipment or self-care/school accommodations. They may benefit from orthotics, assistive devices such as a cane, adaptive self-care equipment, or accommodations due to visual impairments.

Quadriplegia

Quadriplegia is a subtype of CP in which volitional muscle control of all four extremities is severely impaired. This subtype is also often accompanied by neck and trunk involvement. Like diplegic CP, periventricular white matter lesions are the most frequently observed neuroimaging finding in children with quadriplegic CP. Extensive lesions affecting the basal ganglia or occipital area often lead to visual impairments and seizures, both commonly seen in children with this subtype of CP.[14] Cognition can vary from normal to severely impaired and is unique to each child with quadriplegia. It is important to note that children with quadriplegia who are unable to speak are often regarded as being cognitively impaired. However, once provided a means of effective communication, some are able to express their level of understanding and critical thinking.[17] Gross and fine motor abilities vary widely for children with quadriplegia, from being ambulatory for household distances with an assistive device to being dependent for all care. The equipment needs for these children are considerable through the life span. Common equipment recommendations include mechanical lift systems, wheelchairs, standers, gait trainers/walkers, feeding systems, bath systems, and toileting systems. Home modifications should be considered for children with severe disabilities to maximize the child's independence with transfers and mobility, to ease caregiver strain, and improve safety for the child and caregiver.

Dyskinetic

Dyskinesia and movement disorders result in generally uncontrolled and involuntary movement that includes athetosis, rigidity, tremor, dystonia, ballismus, and choreoathetosis.[8,10,15,21,28] Common abnormalities found in imaging include deep gray matter lesions and, to a lesser extent, periventricular white matter lesions.[24] Athetosis always has involuntary movements that are slow and writhing; abnormal in timing, direction, and spatial characteristics; and are usually large motions of the more proximal joints.[8,10,21] Athetosis is rare as a primary movement disorder and is most often found in combination with chorea.[1] Athetosis is most commonly a secondary movement disorder in conjunction with spasticity. The cortical–basal ganglia–thalamic loop is a sensory and motor feed-forward and feedback circuit and when impaired results in athetosis. Older individuals with athetoid CP are at risk for acquiring devastating neurologic deficits owing to intervertebral disc degeneration and instability in their cervical spines. After a radiologic study of 180 patients, Harada and associates found that disc degeneration occurred earlier and progressed more rapidly in subjects with athetoid CP than in those without CP. Advanced disc degeneration was found in 51% of those studied, which is eight times the typical frequency.[29] Individuals with athetosis typically initiate and attempt control of movement with the jaw and head. This eventually causes musculoskeletal changes such as cervical instability, potential high spinal cord injury, temporomandibular joint dysfunction, and or spinal stenosis. Of note, when athetosis is the primary movement disorder, the cognitive ability of these children tends to be underestimated owing to associated dysarthria. In fact, these children tend to have normal to above-normal intelligence. Rigidity is much less common and is felt as resistance to both active and passive movement and is not velocity dependent.[21] Tremor, a rhythmic movement of small magnitude, usually of the smaller joints, rarely occurs as an isolated disorder in CP but rather in combination with athetosis or ataxia.[10] Dystonia is a slow motion with a torsional element that may involve one limb or the entire body and in which the pattern itself may change over time.[10] Ballismus is the most rare movement disorder and involves random motion in large, fast patterns usually of a single limb.[10] Choreoathetosis involves jerky movement, commonly of the digits and varying in the ROM.[10,15]

Ataxic

Ataxic CP is primarily a disorder of balance and control in the timing of coordinated movements along with weakness, incoordination, a wide-based gait, and a noted tremor.[8,21] This type of CP results from deficits in the cerebellum and often occurs in combination with spasticity and athetosis.[21] The cerebellum is a major sensory processing center, and when impaired, ataxia will result. In contrast to other types of CP, a specific lesion is less common with neuroimaging, and one recent study found lesions in only 39% of children with ataxia.[24] Children with ataxia have difficulty with transference of skills, and may benefit from a specific task-oriented approach to treatment. For example, to master stepping onto and off the school bus, it is most effective to practice the skill using bus steps.

Hypotonic

Hypotonia in a child with CP can be permanent but is more often transient in the evolution of athetosis or spasticity and might not represent a specific type of CP. For example, an infant who presents with generalized hypotonia through the trunk and extremities will often develop spasticity beginning distally and progressing proximally. Hypotonia is typically correlated with congenital abnormality, such as lissencephaly.[10] A common mixed tone pattern is seen in some children with quadriplegia, with spasticity evident in the LEs and severe hypotonia in the trunk and neck.

 ## Assessment of the infant and child with CP

There is disagreement in the literature and in practice regarding how early an infant can be diagnosed with CP. Burns and colleagues[30] believe that a diagnosis of very mild CP should be possible at 8 months of age. Identification depends on a combination of suspicious and abnormal signs revealed during comprehensive assessment of attainment of motor achievements, neurologic signs, primitive reflexes, and postural reactions.

Infants and children with persistent subtle or mild signs should be monitored closely until the possible outcome is clear.[30] Harris,[31] using the Movement Assessment in Infants (MAI), found certain items that can help distinguish the infant with CP from the uninvolved infant at 4 months of age. Items of diagnostic value include neck hyperextension and shoulder retraction, ability to bear weight on the forearms while prone, ability to maintain a stable head position in supported or independent sitting, and the infant's ability to flex the hips actively against gravity.[31,32] Seven of the 17 MAI items that Harris found highly significant predictors for CP are observational items. Both Harris and Milani-Comparetti found that watching the infant move against gravity is of greater diagnostic value than intrusive handling or attempts to stimulate a response.[31,32] Harris[31] compared the diagnostic value of the MAI with the Bayley Scales in infants at 4 months of age and found that the MAI was more sensitive than the Bayley Scales. However, the Bayley Motor Scale was extremely sensitive at 1 year of age. Rose-Jacobs et al.[33] evaluated whether the MAI predicted 2-year cognitive and motor development status measured by the Mental and Psychomotor Scales of the Bayley Scales of Infant Development. They found that the MAI appears to be valid for use with infants born at term who are at risk of developmental delay. This test may be a useful tool to help clinicians make decisions about the provision of intervention services. Nelson and Ellenberg[34] studied children who were diagnosed with CP at 1 year of age who subsequently "outgrew the cerebral palsy." They found that children with mild motor impairment at 1 year of age and those thought to have CP were all free of CP by the age of 7. However, all who were diagnosed with severe CP, and many with moderate CP, still carried the same diagnosis at the age of 7. Those who "outgrew" the CP were likely to have neurologic problems, such as mental retardation, nonfebrile seizures, or difficulty with speech articulation.[34] These findings substantiate the fact that any infant or child who demonstrates neurologic or behavioral abnormalities should undergo follow-up until early school age.

In order to understand the atypical movement and motor control that occurs in children with CP, the therapist must understand the acquisition of motor control against gravity, the development of postural control, and the musculoskeletal development in typically developing children. This information can be found in Chapter 2. Atypical development has been described by multiple authors, including sources cited in this chapter.[35–38]

The purpose of the assessment is to discover the functional abilities and strengths of the child, determine the primary and secondary impairments (compensations used because of the primary impairments), and discover the desired functional and participation outcomes of the child and family. The therapist must use an organized approach to the observation of, interaction with, and handling of the child in order to get an accurate baseline of the child's functional abilities. Display 5.10 is a suggested organization for an assessment according to the Neuro-Developmental Treatment Association Instructors' Group to document the assessment findings and plan of care.[21]

DISPLAY 5.10

Organization for an Assessment of the Infant and Child with CP (based on the Neurodevelopmental Treatment Approach Model of Assessment)

Data Collection
Date of birth
Date of assessment
Chronologic age/adjusted age
Reason for referral
Relevant medical history
Overview of function (a few sentences)
Family and environmental characteristics
Contextual factors (conditions and restraints on function)
Assistive technology/adaptive equipment

Examination
Morphology
Functional skills and the capacity for change
Gross motor control
Communications
Fine motor control
Social skills/control of behavior
Objective test results
Observation of posture and movement
Individual system review related to function
Neuromuscular
Musculoskeletal
Sensory
Respiratory

Cardiovascular

Integumentary

Gastrointestinal

Perceptual/cognitive

Regulatory

Evaluation

List client's competencies

Areas of concern

System impairments

Ineffective posture and movement

Functional limitations

Barriers to participation

Analyze each level and how they interrelate, creating the functional limitations of the client

Analyze the potential for change according to the findings

Plan of Care

Specify the anticipated goals and expected outcomes (long term and short term)

Specify frequency and duration of intervention

Strategies of intervention

Role of client, family, and other medical and educational professionals

Client-centered programs as appropriate

Measures to promote health, wellness, and fitness

Schedule for reexamination

Assessment of Movement

Much information about an infant or child's movement and posture can be observed when the child enters the treatment area. As noted above, the child can also be observed while the therapist takes a history and discusses with the parents the various concerns leading them to seek evaluation.

Observation of the baby or young child being held in the arms or lap of the parent can reveal important information. The following questions may be answered through observation:

1. How does the mother hold the baby? Does she support the head and trunk or does she hold the baby at the pelvis?
2. Are the baby's head and trunk rotated or collapsed consistently to one side?
3. Do the baby's arms come forward to hold the mother or play with a toy in midline? Are the arms held behind the body with the scapulae adducted or are the arms flexed and adducted against the trunk?
4. While being held, does the baby thrust backward into trunk extension or collapse forward into trunk flexion?
5. How are the LEs held: Are they adducted tightly in extension, or are they floppy in flexion and abduction?

6. Is there isolated movement at the toes or ankles, or are the ankles held in plantarflexion or dorsiflexion? Is the foot everted or inverted, and are the toes held loosely or tightly curled?

This type of observational analysis is not limited to the child held in the parent's arms. When the child arrives in a wheelchair, additional questions may add to the baseline information.

1. Did the child propel the wheelchair independently, or was there some assistance?
2. In addition to mobility, does the wheelchair provide total postural support for major segments of the body? If the segments are free of support from the wheelchair, are those segments of the body in good postural alignment and do they move freely?
3. Does the child tend to thrust backward in the chair into trunk extension? Is the pelvis positioned in a posterior or an anterior tilt? If the child assumes these postures, is there similar thrusting and tightness in the extremities?
4. Is the child seated symmetrically, or are there significant asymmetries in the posture?
5. Does the child seem comfortable in the chair?

Children with less severe movement disorders may ambulate into the department, and the following questions will be helpful in assessing the quality of movement of the ambulatory child.

1. Did the child ambulate with or without an assistive device—a walker, cane, or crutches?
2. Did the child need physical assistance from another person while ambulating?
3. Is the child's gait pattern stable, and is the child safe?
4. When assessing spatial and temporal parameters of gait—step length, stance time, swing time, or base of support—is the gait pattern generally symmetric or asymmetric?
5. Does the child's trunk collapse into lateral flexion on weight bearing on one or both legs, or is the trunk maintained in proper antigravity extension?
6. Does the child have a heel–toe gait pattern? Does the child stand on the balls of the feet?
7. Are the hips and knees locked or stuck in extension during stance phase, or are they falling into gravity or pulled into flexion with the child in a crouched position?

In addition to the gross observational assessment of the child as described, the therapist should examine individual aspects of motor function during the evaluation. The therapist should begin with the level of function appropriate to the child's age and functional ability. The following list of positions provides a guideline by which to assess functional antigravity control:

- Supine
- Prone
- Side-lying
- Sitting—short sit, long sit, side sit, ring sit

- Quadruped
- Kneeling
- Half-kneeling
- Standing
- Walking

If the child possesses higher-level skills, the evaluation should be extended to include the following:

- Climbing stairs
- Navigating ramps or curbs
- Unilateral stance
- Running
- Jumping
- Hopping
- Galloping
- Skipping

The child who functions from a wheelchair should be observed for the following parameters:

- Alignment and mobility of body
- Shifting of weight
- Propulsion of wheelchair
- Management of wheelchair and its parts
- Transfer to and from wheelchair

Assessment of Postural Control

Historically, posture was defined through reflex terminology and facilitated through controlled sensory feedback.[39] Infants were evaluated for the presence, absence, and strength of primitive reflexes. The reflexes were thought to "integrate" as the infant developed. Therapists used stimulation of and feedback from optical righting, labyrinthine righting, neck righting, body righting on the head, and body righting on the body to facilitate normal righting and equilibrium responses in the clients.[39] In treatment, lower-level reflexes were inhibited to decrease the abnormal sensory feedback and facilitate the emergence and integration of the righting and equilibrium responses.

According to more recent motor science studies, the human system is no longer thought to function via a hierarchical model. Various systems models are used currently to describe the organization and functions of the nervous system.[39]

In assessing postural control of the infant and child with CP, it is important to understand several concepts. Postural preparations are strategies the child uses before a functional movement and increase stability by changing the base of support or increasing muscle activation around joints.[40] These changes are in anticipation of a specific task learned previously. The child received sensory input (feedback) from having completed the task previously and makes the necessary postural adjustments to complete the task in the most efficient, effective way. For example, the infant, sitting on the floor sees a toy to the side and tries reaching for it. If the object is too far from the base of support, the infant may fall in attempting to reach the toy. On the next attempt, the infant makes adjustments to the base of support and muscle activation to grasp the toy without falling over.

Feed-forward occurs as a result of learning through experience in postural preparations for movement.[39] Postural setting occurs as muscles become active around a joint or joints, without obvious movement, in anticipation of the task. Current motor sciences endorse the importance of anticipation (feed-forward) in movement and postural control.[40] Feed-forward is learned through trial and error, as the example illustrates, and must be child generated and be goal or task oriented. Postural control is learned in a task-specific manner in a variety of environmental conditions.[40] Motor learning occurs when the child is actively involved in the session and advances from using only the feedback responses to feed-forward control.[39] For example, the child experiences the tactile and proprioceptive properties of objects (feedback) when handling and playing with toys. This helps in preshaping the hand in preparation for more refined reach and grasp tasks in the future.

When assessing the child's postural control, find answers to the following questions:

- Does the child have a variety of ways to transition between postures or only stereotypical choices?
- Does the child actively push into the supporting surface with the pelvis or extremities?
- Can the child repeat movements or tasks and make small changes in motor performance?

Assessment of Postural Tone

The clinical term "tone" describes the impairments of spasticity and abnormal extensibility. Abnormally high tone may be caused by spasticity, a velocity-dependent overactivity that is proportional to the imposed velocity of limb movement.[10]

Clinicians tend to use the word "tone" to describe how a muscle or group of muscles feels under their hands when the joints of a body part are moved through a particular range. The sense of abnormally high tone can result from hypoextensibility of the muscle because of abnormal mechanical characteristics.[10] These same muscles can have increased stiffness if they require greater force to produce an expected change in length than is typically expected.

Signs of increased tone include distal fixing (toe-curling or fisting), difficulty moving a body segment through a range, asymmetric posture, retracted lips and tongue, and so on. Signs of decreased tone include excessive collapse of body segments, loss of postural alignment, and inability to sustain a posture against gravity. A child may also have fluctuating levels of stiffness, which is noted as signs of both increased and decreased levels of stiffness. Two more commonly known types of CP exhibiting fluctuating levels of stiffness are athetosis and ataxia.

Musculoskeletal Assessment

Persistent shortening of a muscle or group of muscles without adequate activation of antagonists—resulting from spasticity, increased or decreased stiffness, weakness, or static positioning—places the child at risk for soft tissue contractures and, over time, bony deformity. With an awareness of the sequence usually seen in atypical motor development and with knowledge of the postural and movement consequences, the therapist must be alert for areas at risk for contracture and deformity.

Goniometric Measurements

ROM should be measured with a goniometer at joints with limited motion. The results should be documented clearly for later comparison. Muscles whose influence is exerted across two joints should be examined and elongated over both joints when measurements are taken. Move the child's limb slowly through the range to avoid eliciting a stretch reflex. The first "catch" or tightening of the muscle is the child's functional range for tasks. It is the range that the child can access for function. Therapists can slowly and carefully stretch muscles beyond this point to the second "catch," or what is called the absolute range. This is the actual length of the muscle, but the child cannot actively access the muscle beyond the functional range. The therapist must work with the child and caregivers to bring the two values closer together, approximating the functional range to the absolute range.

Evaluation of the Spine

Mobility of the spine in all planes is necessary for correct alignment; for smooth, symmetric movements of the spine; and for full ROM of the extremities. Evaluation of the child's passive and active movement of the trunk is an essential part of the evaluation. Passive spinal flexion can be evaluated with the child in supine by rounding the spine and putting the child's knees up to his or her chest. Look for the spinous processes to be showing evenly down the child's spine. This is smooth flexion of the spinal column. If an area is flattened—without the spinous processes showing or showing less—it is indicative of a decrease in spinal flexion. Spinal extension, lateral flexion, and rotation are most easily assessed in sitting. The pelvis must be stabilized by the therapist and the trunk taken through the various movements. Note the smoothness of the movement, the end range and end feel, the symmetry in the trunk, and the amount of movement at each joint in the spinal column. Infants and children with CP often have tightness and limitation in length of the capital extensor muscles and lumbar extensor muscles. Movement into thoracic extension can be limited by shortened rectus abdominus and intercostal muscles.

The therapist must document any deviation from normal in the spinal curves. Note scoliosis and excessive kyphosis and lordosis, and whether the curves are structural or functional.

Thoracic Movement

An area of special concern for the child with CP is the coordinated motion of the thorax that occurs during the breathing cycle. In typically developing babies younger than 6 months of age, there is an approximate 90-degree angle between the ribs and the spine. As control of the head and trunk develops typically, and as the baby begins to develop a more upright posture, there is a change in this 90-degree relationship. Owing to both gravity and the forces of the axial musculature in resisting gravity, there is a posterior-to-anterior downward slant to the ribs. As a result of this slant, there is an increased ability to expand the diameter of the thorax in both an anterior–posterior (pump-handle motion) and lateral direction (bucket-handle motion). In addition to this ability to change the inspired volume, the thoracic (external intercostal) and abdominal (obliques) muscles act to fix the ribcage. This fixation facilitates more complete contraction of the diaphragm, thus increasing lung volume. Most children with CP tend to have low levels of stiffness proximally. They also tend to have decreased active balance of trunk flexors and extensors when in an upright position with difficulty sustaining their postural muscles. As a result, there are differences in motion of the chest wall during inspiration. First, the downward slant of the ribs never fully develops, thus minimizing the mechanical advantage of the pump-handle and bucket-handle motions of inspiration. Second, without the muscle tone necessary to stabilize the ribcage, the diaphragmatic fibers, particularly the sternal fibers, serve an almost paradoxic function; that is, they cause depression of the xiphoid process and the sternum during inspiration. The lack of thoracic expansion, in conjunction with the sternal depression, causes shallow respiratory efforts. Vocalizations will be of short duration and will be low in intensity because of poor breath support. Examination of the respiratory excursion of the thorax is a critical portion of the motor assessment for the child with CP. Respiratory function should be assessed with the child in various functional positions. The therapist should develop interventions aimed at increasing postural control throughout the trunk. The therapist must specifically facilitate the postural system muscles, both axial extensor and flexor muscles, particularly the oblique abdominal muscles that aid in the forceful expiration needed for coughing and sneezing.

Evaluations of the Shoulder Girdle and Upper Extremity

The child with CP with excessive axial extension and poor activation of capital flexors and abdominal muscles will likely demonstrate tightness and limitation of the shoulder girdle. Tightness of the pectoralis major muscle persists from infancy as the infant never attains adequate UE weight bearing in prone to lengthen the pectoralis from birth. Dynamic scapular stability fails to develop, and the scapulae become fixed in downward rotation and a forward-tipped position. These fixed positions will restrict motion at the sternoclavicular and acromioclavicular joints.[37] The child with CP is likely to be limited in passive flexion, abduction, and external rotation of the shoulder. Elevation of the shoulder, which is used to stabilize the head, as well as excessive thoracic spine kyphosis, may produce limitations in scapulothoracic movement needed for depression of the shoulder. Moving distally, the therapist often finds limitations in extension of the elbow, supination of the forearm, and extension of the wrist and fingers.

Examination of the Hip and Pelvis

The child with CP, typically with spastic diplegia or quadriplegia, commonly has tightness in the hip flexors, adductors, and internal rotators with resultant limitation in hip extension, abduction, and external rotation. The Thomas test is used to identify a flexion contracture of the hip. Abduction and adduction of the hip should be assessed with the hip and knee extended. Internal and external rotation of the hip should be measured while the infant or child is prone with the hips extended and the knees flexed.

Subluxed or dislocated hips can occur in children with very tight hip flexion, adduction, and internal rotation. Hip subluxation is difficult to assess via physical examination. Hip subluxation/dislocation should be suspected in hip abduction as ROM is limited in young children. The most important measurement for a physical therapist (PT) to consistently track is hip abduction with knee and hip extension. Any child less than 8 years of age with hip abduction of less than 45 degrees on either side should be referred to an orthopedic surgeon for further evaluation.[10] An apparent leg length discrepancy (LLD) may also be noted in a child with suspected unilateral hip subluxation/dislocation. The subluxed or dislocated hip is typically shorter than the more "normal" hip owing to the great majority of subluxations being superior and posterior.[10,41]

Femoral Anteversion

Femoral anteversion is a torsion or internal rotation of the femoral shaft on the femoral neck. Other terms that may be synonymous with femoral anteversion include fetal femoral torsion and persistent fetal alignment of the hip.

At birth, an infant has approximately 40 degrees of femoral anteversion, as measured by the angle between the transcondylar axis of the femur and the femoral axis of the neck. The neonate also has 25 degrees of flexion contracture of the hip due to intrauterine positioning and physiologic flexor tone. In the progression of typical development, hip flexors lengthen as the result of gravitational pull while the child is lying in either a prone or a supine position. Active extension and external rotation of the hip tighten the anterior capsule of the hip joint, thus producing a torque or torsional stress that decreases the anteversion that is present from birth.[42] In addition to the effects of the tightened hip capsule, the hip extensors and external rotators insert near the proximal femoral growth plate. When activated, the extensors and external rotators pull on the plate and help decrease the torsion on the femur. The result of the various forces is that the adult value of 15 degrees of femoral anteversion is reached by 16 years of age.[43,44] Femoral anteversion is determined by biplane roentgenograms. Anteversion may be suspected on the basis of a simple clinical test. Internal and external rotation of the hip are tested with the hip in a position of extension (i.e., with the child in a prone position with knees flexed). Femoral anteversion may be suspected when external rotation at the hip is substantially less than internal rotation.

The infant or child with CP often has overactivity and shortening of the flexors of the hip and poor control of extensors and of external rotators of the hip. Beals,[45] in 1969, studied 40 children with CP and found that the degree of femoral anteversion was normal at birth. However, this study also revealed that the amount of anteversion did not decrease over the first few years of life, as occurs with typically developing children. After 3 years of age, there was no significant change in anteversion with either age or ambulation status. The sample of children with CP had a mean of 14 degrees greater anteversion than the children without CP.[45]

Staheli and associates[46] found greater angles of anteversion of the femur in the involved LE of a group of children with CP than was found in their uninvolved limb. This finding can be easily explained by the consistently poor activation of extensors and external rotators of the hip, preventing the decline in anteversion seen in normal development.

Examination of the Knee

The child with CP may have limited knee flexion or extension as a result of inadequate length of the quadriceps or hamstrings. The length of the medial and lateral hamstrings and the rectus femoris, all of which cross two joints, should be assessed elongating the muscle over the knee and the hip. Passive straight leg raising or measurement of the popliteal angle will indicate the degree of hamstring tightness. If hamstring tightness is excessive, the child may be unable to sit on the ischium with 90-degree flexion of the hip, and stride length may be limited during ambulation.

Tightness of the quadriceps, which limits flexion of the knee, can be identified by looking for a patella that is located more superiorly than typical and by assessing the degree of flexion of the knee with the child in a prone position.

Tibial Torsion

Tibial torsion (tibial version) describes a twist of the tibia along its long axis so that the leg is rotated internally or externally. The specific angle of torsion can be determined in two ways: (1) by the intersection of a line drawn vertically from the tibial tubercle and a line drawn through the malleoli and (2) thigh–foot angle, which is the angle formed by the transmalleolar axis and thigh in prone (Fig. 5.2).

Like the femur, the tibia undergoes developmental torsional changes. The malleoli are parallel in the frontal plane at birth. During infancy and early childhood, the tibia rotates externally, which places the lateral malleolus

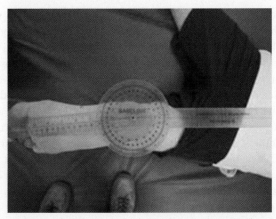

FIGURE 5.2 Thigh–Foot angle (looking down on thigh).

in a posterior position relative to the medial malleolus. The "unwinding" of the tibia, or the progression from relative internal to external tibial torsion, is attributable to changes in force on the tibia arising from the decrease in femoral anteversion that occurs as the child grows. As discussed above, femoral anteversion does not decrease normally with growth, often resulting in compensatory external tibial torsion to maintain the foot facing forward.

Examination of the Foot

Dorsiflexion of the ankle is often limited in the child with CP and must be assessed with the subtalar joint maintained in a neutral position. Neutral alignment will prevent hypermobility of the forefoot while ensuring excursion of the hindfoot.[47]

Midtarsal movement can be assessed stabilizing the hindfoot with one hand while passively supinating and pronating the forefoot with the other. Toes should be straight and mobile with approximately 90 degrees of extension available at the first metatarsophalangeal joint.

With the child standing, the calcaneus should be vertical or slightly inverted in relation to the lower one-third of the leg. Children should begin to show a longitudinal arch at 3.5 to 4 years of age. Depression of the medial longitudinal arch is caused by adduction and plantarflexion of the talus with relative eversion of the calcaneus. This alignment is also associated with internal rotation of the LE. Another mechanism for malalignment during standing occurs in children who have stiffness into extension, including plantarflexion. Their calcaneus is often maintained in some degree of plantarflexion and does not truly participate in weight bearing. The talus stays plantarflexed with "apparent full weight bearing," with pronation achieved through hypermobility into extension through the midtarsal joint.[47,48] These two mechanisms must be examined carefully when considering an orthosis for standing or ambulating.

Discrepancy in Leg Length

Measurement of leg length should be done in supine with the pelvis level in all planes, the hips in neutral rotation and abduction or adduction, and the knees fully extended.

Measurements are taken from the anterior superior iliac spine to the distal aspect of the medial malleolus.

Staheli and associates[46] studied the inequality in leg lengths in 50 children with spastic hemiparesis. Of the 16 children who were older than 11 years of age, 70% had a significant discrepancy in leg length. Ten children had a discrepancy of 1 cm or more, and two children had discrepancies of greater than 2 cm between the involved and uninvolved limbs.

Correction of a discrepancy in the leg length by using a shoe lift is not advocated by some sources.[42] However, children with CP who have asymmetry in tone, muscle activation, posture, and movement are placed at even greater risk for muscle shortening and scoliosis when a discrepancy in leg length exists. Such a child will try to equalize the length by ambulating with the shortened limb in plantarflexion with the heel off the floor, thus maintaining a continually shortened position of the ankle plantarflexors. Leg length in vertical weight bearing should be equalized as early as possible to facilitate equal growth of the child's long bones. When a full-length shoe lift is used to correct the discrepancy in length, the child should be assessed in a standing posture for symmetry of the posterior iliac spines, anterior superior iliac spines, and the iliac crests. When the child wears an orthosis, the shoe lift thickness must take the thickness of the orthosis into account when determining the necessary thickness of the lift. Shoe lifts can be placed inside the shoe or applied to the shoe sole relatively inexpensively.

▶ Gait

One of the questions most frequently asked by parents and caregivers upon being told their child has CP is "When will my child walk?". Walking is one of the most complex human functions, making this prediction very difficult in young children with CP. As per Beckung et al.'s[49] review of 10,000 children with CP in Europe, 54% of children with CP walk without an assistive device, 16% walk with an assistive device, and 30% were nonambulatory. The GMFCS is also helpful to estimate future ambulation potential in children with CP. The GMFCS is a reliable and valid system that classifies children with CP by their age-specific gross motor activity.[50] The GMFCS describes the major functional characteristics of children less than 2 years old, 2 to 4 years old, 4 to 6 years old, and between 6 and 12 years old with CP within each level (see Display 5.9). Rosenbaum et al.[50] used the GMFCS to assist clinicians and caregivers in looking at the infant/child and make predictions for functional mobility on the basis of the findings of the GMFCS. They plotted the patterns of motor development on the basis of longitudinal observations of 657 children with CP and felt that the findings will help parents understand the outlook for their child's gross motor function based on age and the GMFCS level.[50] This may be a more accurate way of predicting future ambulation skills than previously used means such as tracking motor skill acquisitions like sitting independently by 2 years of age.[51]

It is extremely helpful to understand typical gait and how the impairments in the child with CP influence his or her ability to ambulate. Reviewing normal gait is beyond the scope of this chapter, and this author strongly recommends the textbook *Gait Analysis* by Jacquelin Perry and Judith Burnfield.[52] The prerequisites of normal gait in the order of priority are (1) stable lower limb in stance phase, (2) clearance of ground by foot in swing phase, (3) proper positioning of the foot in dorsiflexion in terminal swing, (4) adequate step length, and (5) maximal energy conservation.[52,53] Damage to the central nervous system (CNS) causes loss of selective motor control, abnormal muscle tone, imbalance between muscle agonist and antagonist, and poor equilibrium reactions. As a consequence, many or all of the above prerequisites of normal gait are absent in children with CP.[53]

Observational Gait Analysis

When evaluating the gait mechanics of a child with CP, instrumental gait analysis is the gold standard. The components of a thorough gait analysis include kinematics, kinetics, electromyographic data, measurement of videotape recordings, energy expenditure, and clinical observation.[53] A gait analysis laboratory uses cameras linked to a computer to track reflective markers placed on specific parts of a child's body as the child ambulates down the walkway. The cameras send digitized information to the computer regarding the trajectory of each marker in three dimensions. This data, when analyzed, provides kinematic information such as spatial movement of various joints of the body.[53] Force plates built into the floor of the laboratory record kinetic information such as ground-reaction forces, joint power, and joint moments as the patient walks over them. The information collected from all pieces of the gait analysis is presented as graphic and numerical data for the clinician to interpret and administer appropriate treatment.

Unfortunately, not every therapist has access to a state-of-the-art gait analysis lab, where instrumental gait analysis is performed. Detailed observational gait analysis can be very effective in documenting many of the gait abnormalities described above. When first learning to evaluate gait in the child with CP, a video of the child walking is extremely helpful. Observe gait from the front, back, and each side. The child should be barefoot with shorts to allow visualization of the thigh, knee, lower leg, ankle, and foot. It is best to observe one region of the body at a time through several gait cycles before moving up to the next region. First, observe the foot position at initial contact. Is there heel strike, flat foot, or forefoot contact? When the foot is in midstance, are the toes pointing out or in (referred to as internal or external foot progression angle)? Identify foot alignment at push-off (varus or valgus position) when observing from the front and laterally. Consider the knee/thigh region, and observe the child laterally for degree of knee flexion and extension during swing phase and knee angle/stability during stance phase. Does the knee flex excessively or hyperextend during stance phase? Does the knee flex enough during swing to prevent toe drag? Observe from the front for knee

position during swing and stance phases. Is the knee in valgum during swing and stance phases? Do the medial aspects of the knees touch? Observe the hips from the side, note the amount of hip flexion during late swing, and hip extension at push-off. Does the child achieve hip extension during late stance or stay in flexion? Does the child hyperflex or abduct at the hip during swing? When observing the pelvis and spine, focus on pelvic tilt, pelvic rotation, lordosis, and trunk alignment during all phases of gait. Is there excessive anterior pelvic tilt with increased lumbar lordosis throughout the gait cycle? Does the child have to excessively rotate his or her pelvis and trunk to assist swing of the lower limb? Does the patient elevate the pelvis to prevent the toe from dragging? Lastly, observe the head, arms, and trunk (often referred to as the HAT segment). Does the head and trunk laterally flex to one side when swinging with the opposite side? Do the arms swing normally or remain in a fixed posture? Once completing the observation of each region, watch the body move as a whole without focusing on a particular region to identify other important gait characteristics such as speed, fluidity of movement, stride length, and stride width.

Common Gait Deviations

When discussing gait and gait deviations, it is helpful to understand the link between the primary gait problems and their underlying etiology. Table 5.2 lists the most common gait deviations seen in children with CP and the primary causes of these deviations. Gait deviations in children with CP typically have four main causes: (1) those caused by weakness, (2) those caused by abnormal bony alignment, (3) those caused by muscle contracture, and (4) those caused by muscle spasticity.[53,54] Owing to the overactive stretch response of key walking muscles, spasticity in these muscles can inhibit motion by firing prematurely, resulting in prolonged and inappropriate muscle action.[54] As ambulatory children with CP grow and mature, the abnormal tone and underlying muscle weakness causes skeletal changes that result in abnormal alignment as well as joint contracture. Because most children with CP have both spasticity and weakness in more than one muscle, they typically have multiple gait abnormalities. There are several classic gait patterns that are characteristic of the different types of CP. These classic gait patterns are described in the following section.

Hemiplegic Gait

Almost all children with hemiplegic-pattern CP will walk and the great majority of them will be functional ambulators. In fact, most are independent ambulators without an assistive device by 15 to 24 months.[3] Severe cases of hemiplegic-type CP with involved side abnormalities above the knee and mild increased tone and/or muscle weakness of "noninvolved" side may not ambulate until almost 3 years of age.[10] Beckung et al.[49] found that only 3% of children with hemiplegic CP are not walking by 5 years of age. Severe intellectual impairment was found to be the greatest predictor

TABLE	
5.2	**Gait Deviations and Their Underlying Causes**

Problem	Primary Cause(s)
Pelvis	
Anterior pelvic tilt	Hip flexion contracture/hip extensor weakness
Increased rotation	Decreased push-off from gastrocnemius (gastroc), hip stiffness, hip flexor weakness
Drop of pelvis on swing side	Hip abductor weakness
Hip	
Decreased flexion	Hamstring (HS) or gluteus muscle contractors
	Weak plantarflexors during push-off
	Weak hip flexors
Decreased extension (stance)	Hip flexor contracture; knee flexion contracture
Increased abduction	Weak adductor muscle; abductor contracture
Increased adduction	Adductor contracture/increased tone
Increased internal rotation	Femoral anteversion; increased tone and/or contracture of internal rotators; compensation for external tibial rotation
Increased external rotation	Retroversion of femur; increased tone or contracture of external rotators; compensation for internal tibial torsion
Knee	
Increased flexion at initial contact	Knee flexion contracture; hamstring tone; toe strike due to plantarflexor tone
Decreased flexion at initial contact	Weak hamstrings; weak quadriceps
Genu recurvatum in midstance	Increased gastroc tone; weak gastroc; weak hamstrings
Crouch (stance hip and knee flexion)	Knee joint contracture; HS contracture; hip flexor contracture; poor balance; severe planovalgus feet; ankle equinus
Stiff knee gait	Increased rectus femoris tone; knee stiffness quadriceps contracture; poor push-off from gastroc
Jump knee (knee flex in early stance)	Overactivity of HS
Foot	
Equinus at initial contact	Gastroc/soleus contracture; gastroc overactivity; weak dorsiflexors
Decreased push-off power	Weak gastroc/soleus; severe planovalgus feet
Intoeing (internal foot progression)	Internal tibial torsion; varus feet
Out-toing (external foot progression)	External tibial torsion; severe muscle weakness; poor balance

From Miller F. *Cerebral Palsy*. New York, NY: Springer-Verlag, Inc; 2005:338.

of not being able to walk by age 5, increasing the risk by 56-fold.[49] Before the age of 2, the majority of children with hemiplegic-pattern CP either toe-walk bilaterally or ambulate with a foot-flat, planovalgus gait pattern.[10] Gastrocnemius spasticity is the primary neuromuscular impairment in both these children, and as contracture develops over time, almost all children with hemiplegic CP will walk on their toes without orthotic intervention.[10] Over time, overactivity of the tibialis anterior and posterior will also often cause the foot to turn inward into equinovarus position. When observing a child with hemiplegic CP walking, asymmetrical weight shift to the involved side is the most obvious feature typically noted. Throughout the gait cycle, the involved UE is often positioned in scapular retraction and the pelvis is rotated posteriorly, when compared with the shoulder and the pelvis on the contralateral side. Arm swing also typically occurs only on the uninvolved side, with the involved UE held in shoulder hyperextension and elbow flexion.

LE gait deviations can vary greatly between patients with spastic hemiplegia, but four distinct patterns of gait in children have been described by Winters et al.[55] Type 1, the least involved patient group, presents with drop foot in swing phase of gait, but has normal dorsiflexion PROM (passive range of motion). This group also has increased knee flexion at terminal swing, initial contact, and loading response.

Hyperflexion of hip during swing and increased lordosis are other compensations commonly seen in this group. Treatment for this group typically includes leaf spring or articulating ankle–foot orthosis (AFO) and tibialis anterior strengthening on the involved side. Type 2, the most common subtype, is significant for plantarflexion throughout the gait cycle, full extension or recurvatum of knee in stance phase, as well as hyperflexion of hip and increased lordosis. Contracture of triceps surae prevents the tibia from moving forward on the foot during stance phase, resulting in knee extension or hyperextension in middle and terminal stance phase. As a result, advancement of the trunk is limited; therefore, in order to maintain the center of gravity (COG) over the foot, the child must hyperflex the hip and extend the lumbar spine. Early treatment for these gait deviations includes gastrocnemius stretching, hinged AFOs with an appropriate plantarflexion stop to prevent recurvatum, and botulinum toxin type A (BTX-A) injections into the gastrocnemius.[56] If an achilles contracture develops preventing proper AFO fit, Achilles tendon lengthening in early grade school, with or without articulating AFO use afterward, is the typical treatment for this patient.[10,56] Types 1 and 2 typically have slight LLDs of 1 to 2 cm. This asymmetry should not be corrected with a shoe lift as this will likely cause problems with toe clearance during involved side swing phase.[10]

In addition to the above gait deviations, Type 3 has decreased knee motion, especially during swing phase, due to quadriceps/hamstring co-contraction. Treatment for Type 3 gait dysfunction is similar to Type 2 with the addition of aggressive hamstring stretching, BTX, or muscle lengthening to overactive/contracted hamstring tendons. Type 4, the most involved group, has additional restricted motion of the hip due to hyperactivity of the iliopsoas and hip adductors. This prevents full hip extension at terminal stance phase.[55] It is not uncommon for children in this group to undergo two to three gastrocnemius and hamstring muscle lengthening procedures owing to more significantly increased muscle tone and contractures. These children often develop significant femoral anteversion, requiring derotation osteotomy. It should also be noted that Type 4 children usually have significant LLDs that may require a shoe lift.[10] In addition to Winter et al.'s[55] findings, a more recent analysis of CP gait determined that the most common gait abnormalities found in children with hemiplegic gait include equinus (64%), stiff knee (56%), intoeing (54%), excessive hip flexion (48%), and crouch (47%).[57]

Diplegic Gait

Like the children with hemiplegic-pattern CP, the gait pattern of a child with diplegia can vary greatly depending on the degree of severity of involvement. Generally, children with spastic diplegic-pattern CP ambulate at about half the speed of children without CP.[58] Unlike hemiplegia, there are few children with diplegic CP with only ankle involvement. The great majority of children with diplegic CP have some hip, knee, and ankle involvement. Despite this increased level of involvement, most children with diplegic CP do walk independently, although more severely involved children with diplegic CP require molded ankle–foot orthoses (MAFOs) and an assistive device such as lofstrand crutches or posterior walker to ambulate.

Bony deformities of the long bones of the lower leg and feet are common in children with diplegic CP.[56] Because LE muscles work best when all the bones are in the line of gait progression, muscle effectiveness is reduced when bony malalignment occurs. This dysfunction is often referred to as "lever arm disease."[56]

A common combination of bone deformities in children with diplegic CP that results in lever arm disease is internal femoral rotation (anteversion), lateral tibial torsion, and midfoot collapse.[56] As these bony deformities progress together, the already weak gluteus medius becomes even less effective in controlling hip internal rotation, and the plantarflexors have limited ability to control the progression of the tibia over the foot in stance phase. This causes the hips to internally rotate further and the ankle to drop into excessive dorsiflexion in stance phase as well as increased knee and hip flexion. As a result, the foot drops into a more planovalgus position, which is the most common foot deformity seen in children with diplegic CP.

Like hemiplegic CP, there are several common gait patterns seen in the child with diplegic CP. The most common gait deviations include stiff knee (88%), crouch (74%), excessive hip flexion (66%), intoeing (66%), and equinus (58%).[57] A description of several common gait deviations in this group are described in the next section.

Equinus

When the child with diplegic CP begins to walk, gastrocnemius spasticity commonly causes an equinus gait pattern with the ankle in plantarflexion throughout stance phase with hips and knees extended. Sometimes the child may hyperextend his or her knees to get the heels on the ground, which hides the equinus. BTX-A is often used to decrease spasticity in these children to improve stability in stance. Solid or hinged AFOs are the orthotic management of choice for this population.[56]

Planovalgus

Planovalgus is characterized as equinus of the hindfoot and pronation of the forefoot and midfoot.[59] Planovalgus is primarily caused by plantarflexor muscle weakness, including the tibialis posterior and exacerbated by the "lever arm disease" described earlier in the "Gait" section. Planovalgus malalignment maintains the midfoot and forefoot in an "unlocked" position, decreasing stability in midstance. This often results in excessive loading of the plantar, medial portion of the foot. The force-generating capacity of the already weak tibialis anterior and triceps surae is decreased further by the malalignment of midfoot and forefoot segments. This muscular dysfunction causes the foot to drop into a greater planovalgus position during mid- and late stance and makes effective push-off impossible. Hallux valgus, hindfoot valgus, and external tibial torsion are frequently associated with planovalgus deformity. Planovalgus is also often seen with a crouched gait, which is described below.

Crouch

A crouched gait pattern, with knees and hips flexed throughout the gait pattern, is sometimes seen after growth spurts in child with diplegic CP.[10] Because the muscles of children with CP are weakest in the shortened range, maintaining normal dorsiflexion, hip extension, and knee extension in standing and with ambulation becomes increasingly difficult as children gain weight. Generally, this crouched pattern is initially secondary to overactive hamstrings in stance phase, quadriceps weakness, and triceps surae weakness.[54] In gait, the plantarflexors are of critical importance in maintaining knee extension. During normal gait, the soleus is the only muscle that is active in midstance to control knee extension.[10,52] Because the stance limb is in a closed-kinetic chain, the eccentric activity of the plantarflexors restricts ankle dorsiflexion, maintaining knee extension through a plantarflexion/knee extension couple.[52] Plantarflexor weakness limits the effectiveness of this normal mechanism, allowing the limb to sink into crouch. Plantarflexor control of knee extension is further limited by lever arm disease and stance instability created by planovalgus foot deformity. Increased knee flexion throughout stance phase results in excessive demand on an already weak quadriceps muscle. This causes slow progressive stretching of the quadriceps tendon, resulting in patella alta and later patellofemoral syndrome. This progressive quadriceps dysfunction is a vicious cycle, leading to further crouch. Eventually, this will cause hamstring and hip flexors contracture. Decreased knee extension and decreased stride length results in decreased walking velocity.[54] Aggressive hamstring stretching, quadriceps strengthening, and/or modification of bracing (solid AFO or ground-reaction AFO [GRAFO] to assist plantarflexors in controlling dorsiflexion) is indicated with this gait pattern, but often hamstring lengthening is indicated when contractures develop to improve knee extension at initial contact. Midstance knee flexion of less than 20 degrees is ideal with increased concern as the angle approaches 30 degrees. After 30 degrees of crouch, a weak, overstretched soleus, tight hamstrings, and quickly fatiguing quadriceps make functional ambulation very difficult. During adolescence, weight gain and rapid increase in height can further contribute to increased crouch. Consistent monitoring of hamstring flexibility, weight, strength, and passive knee extension during this period of growth is necessary to prevent rapid worsening of crouch and subsequent impairments/functional limitations.

Jump Knee

The jump knee is another gait deviation commonly seen in children with spastic diplegia with more proximal involvement causing spasticity in the hip flexors, hamstrings, and gastrocnemius.[56] This child presents with anterior pelvic tilt, hip flexion, knee flexion, and ankle equinus.[56] Overactivity of the hamstring muscles produces increased knee flexion in late swing and early stance phases. This child then appears to "jump" due to a strong quadriceps contraction during late stance phase.[60] The ankle does not progress into greater dorsiflexion through stance phase as it does in "crouched" gait, also adding to the appearance of a "jump" during stance phase. Children with this type of gait pattern often require BTX injections to the calf and hamstrings. Orthotic management for children with this gait deviation varies from solid AFOs, hinged AFOs, or GRAFOs, depending on the severity of spasticity/weakness in thigh and ankle muscles.[56]

Stiff Knee

Stiff knee gait is characterized by increased knee extension throughout swing phase, often owing to overactivity of the rectus femoris.[54] Knee flexion in swing is necessary in normal gait to shorten the swing leg and thus allow the foot to swing through without the toes hitting the floor. Decreased knee flexion thus causes a problem with clearing the swing leg foot. This forces the child to compensate with hip circumduction, vaulting (contralateral plantarflexion and/or abduction in swing phase), upward pelvic tilt, and/or pelvic external rotation to prevent toe drag.[54] Other causes of decreased knee flexion in swing include slow overall walking speed and lack of swing limb momentum due to hip flexor weakness or poor push-off.

Recurvatum

Recurvatum gait is described as knee extension in early stance progressing to hyperextension in mid- and late stance phases of gait. The most common cause of equinus is overactivity and/or contracture of the gastrocnemius. Increased spasticity of the gastrocnemius causes the ankle to be in equinus at initial contact and remain in plantarflexion throughout stance phase. This creates an early knee extension movement, causing the knee to be forced into extension. Gastrocnemius weakness and iliopsoas tightness are also possible causes or contributing factors to knee recurvatum.[10] Repeated stress on the posterior structures of the knee leads to stretching of posterior musculature and eventually the posterior capsule of the knee. This can cause chronic, debilitating knee pain in adolescence. Besides the potential for affecting posterior stability of the knee, recurvatum disrupts forward momentum during ambulation, making gait less efficient.[10] Switching to a solid MAFO in patients with weak gastrocnemius or increasing the dorsiflexion angle of a solid or articulating MAFO to 3 to 5 degrees are common changes that often improve back-kneeing.[10]

Idiopathic Toe-Walking versus Mild Diplegic CP

There can be concern and confusion regarding the differentiation between idiopathic toe-walking and spastic diplegic CP. Toe-walking as a toddler is considered a normal variant for new walkers, but is considered abnormal and is classified as idiopathic toe-walking if it persists beyond the first few years of ambulation. Idiopathic toe-walkers typically have normal strength, normal tone, and selective motor control, but still prefer to walk on their toes.[61] Developmental history and physical examination are often helpful in differentiating between idiopathic toe-walking and CP but are not always sufficient. On physical examination, idiopathic toe-walkers typically have only mild gastrocnemius tightness and no hamstring tightness.[61,62] Hicks et al.[62] found that idiopathic toe-walkers typically have increased knee extension in stance and increased external rotation of the foot with increased plantarflexion. Conversely, they found that children with CP had sustained knee flexion at terminal stance and initial contact.[62] Kelly et al. also showed a difference between the two groups with idiopathic toe-walkers having initial motion into dorsiflexion followed by sudden plantarflexion midway through swing phase, causing the foot to land in equinus. It should also be noted that many idiopathic toe-walkers are able to walk with more "normal" gait mechanics when instructed to do so.[63]

Quadriplegic Gait

Most children with quadriplegic CP are not community ambulators, but many do have some ability to ambulate with an assistive device at home or in a therapeutic setting. Many of these children use a gait trainer in early childhood and then transition to a walker with forearm supports years later. The most common gait deviations seen in this type of CP include stiff knee (93%), crouch (88%), excessive hip flexion (78%), intoeing (70%), equinus (68%), and excessive hip adduction/scissoring (63%).[10] In adolescence, some of these children lose their ability to ambulate secondary to weight gain/growth spurt. Even though functional community ambulation throughout life is not a realistic goal for children with this type of CP, encouraging ambulation is very important. Discussion with the patient and family regarding the role of walking is critical early in the therapy process so that the family has time to accept that power mobility will be the best long-term means of mobility from the early school years through the rest of the child's life. Hip subluxation, hip weakness, and osteopenia are all common impairments that can be reduced to some degree with ambulation. Some progress with ambulation can occur up to 12 or 13 years of age in these children.[10] If the child with quadriplegic CP is still using a gait trainer for ambulation at this age, he or she will likely not progress to a posterior walker in adulthood. Discontinuing gait training prior to adolescence is not recommended, as this training will help the child maintain the ability to weightbear with transfers throughout their life. Severe equinovalgus feet, hamstring contractures, hip adductor contractures, hip flexion contractures, and fixed knee flexion contractures are common impairments that limit ambulation in middle childhood and adolescence.[10] Often, these impairments require surgical intervention to prevent the loss of years of ambulation gains. In adulthood, these children should be able to maintain the ambulatory ability they have gained throughout childhood.

Athetotic Gait

The "typical" gait in a child with athetosis is very difficult to describe and even more difficult to address. Athetotic movements are usually first noticed at 2 to 3 years of age. By 3 to 5 years of age, the athetotic pattern is consistent and changes little.[10] Children with milder cases of athetosis have underlying low postural tone that fluctuates to high levels of stiffness. The gait pattern in the LEs is poorly graded and in total patterns of movement. The LE is usually lifted high into flexion and placed down in stance into extension with adduction, internal rotation, and plantarflexion. The hips stay slightly flexed, the lumbar spine is hyperextended, and the thoracic spine is excessively rounded with capital hyperextension, flexion, and rotation of the cervical spine with the jaw jutting forward and rotated to one side. Orthopedic and physical therapy treatments usually have little effect on athetotic movements. Weighted vests and ankle weights are sometimes helpful in improving balance in this group.

Ataxic Gait

The most common features of ataxic gait include general unsteadiness, widened base, irregularity of steps with interjoint incoordination, prolonged stance duration, increased double-limb support duration, slow speed, and large body sways.[64] All gait measurements are highly variable in cerebellar ataxia. Improving gait with physical therapy is not well supported in the literature, but repeated motor training, taping, or light-weighting of the limbs might have some benefit.[64] Owing to profound instability, maintaining balance takes priority over propulsive locomotion, causing several common gait deviations.

 ## Fine motor, adaptive, and self-care skills

Assessment of the fine motor, adaptive, and self-care skills of the infant and child with CP is traditionally one of the main areas of concern for the occupational therapist. If a treatment center or a school does not have an occupational therapist available, the PT should have the basic knowledge to assess these skills and development. A 2011 study conducted by Chen et al. examined quality of life in ambulatory children with CP. This study determined that fine motor functions, including dexterity and visual motor control, "were the most important motor factors associated with health-related quality-of-life" issues.[65] It is valuable for the evaluating PT to be aware of the basic development of self-care, fine motor, and play skills. Knowledge of basic, developmental milestones in self-care and play skills can help the PT more readily identify the need for intervention in specific skill areas. A child following a more typical continuum of self-care skill development will hold a bottle with one or both hands at 4½ to 6 months of age, finger-feed many soft foods at 9 months, pull off his or her socks while seated at approximately 12 months, will hold out arm and push arm through sleeve at 12 months, will bring filled spoon to mouth (messily) at 12 to 14 months, will attempt to put socks on at 24 to 28 months, and will remove unfastened garment at 24 months. It is not until 3½ to 4 years of age that a child will begin to button large buttons on a coat, zip a coat, or attempt to tie shoes. Play skill development is important to understand, as this skill set provides the basis on which more refined fine motor and bimanual hand skills are developed. A child following a more typical continuum of fine motor and play skill development will clap at approximately 7 to 9 months, place toy into open container without support of container's surface at 7 to 8 months, poke an object with index finger at 9 to 10 months, point to object at 11 to 12 months, and demonstrate a fine pincer grasp (small object held between tip of thumb and tip of index finger) at 11 to 12 months of age.[66] The developmental continuum is not a rigid process and is influenced by many factors; therefore, children may master certain skills earlier or later than stated.

Information obtained from parents, caregivers, or teachers may alert the therapist to the needs for intervention related to the infant/child's functional abilities during feeding, dressing, toileting, bathing, and prehensile and manipulation skills for play and school function. Direct clinical observation of a child's performance of basic self-care skills, including removing and replacing socks, shoes, and coat, can be very informative of a child's level of independence in these areas. As the child moves to perform these tasks, the therapist can evaluate sitting balance, mobility and control of head and trunk, weight shifting through pelvis, and use and mobility of the arms. During the evaluation process, the therapist should ascertain the following:

1. How the particular skills are accomplished.
2. The degree of assistance required.
3. At what point assistance was necessary.
4. Whether the child accomplishes the task using compensatory movement that will lead to structural changes and potential deformity.

▶ Speech and language considerations

A comprehensive assessment of speech and language is not within the scope of practice of the PT. However, the PT can offer important information to the speech and language pathologist regarding the speech and language abilities and quality of respiration of the infant and child on the basis of observations made during physical therapy assessment and treatment. In obtaining this information, the PT should consider the following questions:

- Did the infant/child hear your voice or other environmental sounds as noted by becoming quiet or looking in the direction of the stimulus?
- Did the child understand questions asked during the evaluation, and did he or she follow step-by-step directional commands?
- Did the infant/child vocalize or verbalize during the assessment? What types of sounds were made? Did the infant/child repeat or stutter speech sounds?
- If the child was verbal, were the words intelligible? Was breath support adequate for speech or was the child able to speak in only one- or two-word utterances owing to poor control of respiration? Are the expressive language skills delayed for the infant/child's chronologic age?
- If the child was non-vocal, was there another means of communication used (i.e., gestures, sign language, manual language board, electronic communication system)? Did the child use eye localization, pointing, or another means within this alternate system?
- Was the infant/child's communication at a functional level?

The therapist should also ask whether the parents/caregivers or teachers have noted any problems with the infant or child's speech or related functional areas, such as difficulty sucking, swallowing, chewing, feeding, or drinking.

These observations and questions can assist in making a referral to a speech and language pathologist who will perform a more detailed assessment. As appropriate, the speech and language pathologist can institute a therapeutic program that can be augmented during physical therapy sessions.

A comprehensive assessment of the mobility and control of the thorax is essential and will assist the speech and language pathologist in attaining the outcomes established for the child. The mobility of the vertebral column and the ribcage has a great impact on the effectiveness of respiration and breath support for vocalization. It also has an impact on pulmonary hygiene, as improved ribcage mobility and deeper respirations help air to flow in the lungs and can prevent or help cure pneumonia. Ribcage mobility and abdominal support provide a good basis for speech control and voice quality. Cotreatment with the speech and language pathologist can be very beneficial to the child, often resulting in more rapid progress. Addressing the child's musculoskeletal problems will assist the speech and language pathologist in planning therapy for communication and respiration issues.

▶ Establishing functional outcomes

Physical therapy should be aimed at achieving functions identified by the child, the infant or child's parents/caregivers, or specific members of the infant/child's team. A functional outcome may be that the infant will reach for and grasp a toy suspended in front of him or her. The toy must be interesting to the infant to encourage the act of reaching. A child interested in kicking a soccer ball will be more motivated in therapy if the outcome may make the child a better soccer player. "Outcomes" must be functional in nature and should be identified as short-term and long-term outcomes. Each session should be guided by an established outcome, which will usually be related to the identified short-term and long-term outcomes unless the infant or child has a more immediate or unexpected problem. These identified session outcomes will guide the therapist in appropriate treatment strategies for the particular treatment session.

Goals are aimed at changing the child's impairments and are not, in themselves, functional in nature. A few examples of treatment strategy goals are lengthening of the hamstrings, strengthening of a particular muscle or group of muscles, deeper respirations, improved circulation to a body part, symmetric smile, and so on. The therapist will have many treatment goals within a single treatment session that are all aimed toward the successful achievement of the identified session functional outcome. They will address single systems, will merge systems, and should prepare the systems and the client for the accomplishment of the outcome. Each outcome must be observable and measurable, with short-term outcomes often leading to a long-term outcome. Displays 5.11 through 5.13 list examples of measurable and objective long-term and short-term goals for various infants and children.

5.11 Functional Outcomes: Mary, 8 Years Old with Spastic Diplegia

Long-term Outcome (6 months)

Mary will ascend ten of the thirteen 8-inch rise steps in the household staircase leading to the second floor using a step-to pattern and leading with either leg while her right hand is on the railing and the left hand at her side; she will require standby supervision only and complete this task in four of five trials in a 1-week period.

Short-term Outcome (2 months)

1. Mary will safely ascend and descend a 6-inch curb from her sidewalk to the street using forearm crutches and require standby assist only for five of five trials.
2. Mary will walk independently without assistive device and carrying a plastic cup, while wearing her articulating molded ankle–foot orthoses, for 4 feet between the kitchen cupboard and the refrigerator, keeping her head and trunk erect over her vertical pelvis and her other arm free to assist in balance in three out of five trials.

▶ Therapeutic interventions

Several factors help determine the desired treatment approach or treatment technique when working with children with CP. The severity of the child's impairments, their

5.12 Functional Outcomes: Emily, 10 Months Old with a Diagnosis of Moderately Severe Spastic Quadriplegia

Long-term Outcome (6 months)

Emily will sit in a ring on the carpeted floor with her head in midline with a chin tuck and an erect spine over a vertical pelvis, her eyes looking downward to the toy held in her two hands, given full support at her pelvis for 30 to 45 seconds, in two of three trials in a single treatment session.

Short-term Outcomes (2 months)

1. Emily will prop on her extended arms with hands open and wrists in at least 45-degree extension when placed in prone on the floor, keep her head in a vertical position in relationship to the floor to visually scan the environment, and hold the position for 15 to 30 seconds given minimal assistance for stability through her pelvis in two out of three trials.
2. Emily will sit in an adapted chair with tray in place in the therapy room with her hips, knees, and ankles at 90 degrees; her feet touching the surface; head erect over her shoulders; and both arms on the tray for swiping at a cause–effect toy placed in midline on the tray, and sustain postural control for 1 to 2 minutes, twice, by the end of the therapy session.

5.13 Functional Outcomes: Teddy, 6 Years Old with a Diagnosis of Athetoid CP of Minimal to Moderate Severity

Long-term Outcome (6 months)

Teddy will cruise to both sides along a support surface 36 inches in height and 8 feet in length, using bilateral hand support on the surface, keeping his head in neutral extension/flexion position with active rotation to scan the environment, with abduction of the advancing leg in the coronal plane, in his classroom of peers given standby supervision at least two times per day, 5 out of 5 days.

Short-term Outcome (2 months)

Teddy will independently raise his left hand to 80 degrees of shoulder flexion, hand toward the ceiling in 90-degree external rotation, shifting his base of support through his pelvis, while sitting in his classroom chair with his legs in 90-degree hip and knee flexion, both feet flat on the floor with his head, neck, and trunk held in balanced flexion and extension, in response to the teacher's question, two out of three trials.

functional limitations, as well as the child and family's goals all influence the design of an effective treatment plan. This section will highlight therapeutic interventions.

Therapeutic interventions must be guided by the functional or participation outcomes identified upon beginning physical therapy. With the outcome(s) identified, the PT must analyze the function or task that is desired and compare the task analysis to the completed assessment of the infant or child. Answers to the following questions should assist the therapist in selecting and sequencing the appropriate treatment strategies to meet the needs of the client and be successful in the function or task:

- What strengths/competencies does the client possess that will provide a foundation upon which to build toward the functional outcome?
- Which posture and movement behaviors interfere with the successful completion of the functional outcome?
- Which identified impairments are critical to the successful completion of the functional outcome?
- How should these impairments be prioritized with regard to the functional outcome? Place the impairment that most greatly impacts the task first on a list of five or six impairments and continue to place the other four or five impairments in order of importance to the identified outcome.
- What treatment strategies can be utilized to address each of the prioritized impairments?
- Do any of the identified treatment strategies address more than a single impairment? Can they be combined?

- Which of the impairments must be treated in preparation to address any of the other identified impairments?
- In what order must the strategies be sequenced to be most successful?
- How many repetitions are necessary for the client to "own" the task at the end of the treatment session?
- How much assistance is necessary to achieve the desired outcome? Can this be decreased within the treatment session?

Once the session is completed, the therapist should analyze the results of the session and make notes about any necessary changes in treatment strategies, sequencing, amount of assistance or facilitation required, a change in a device used for assistance, or the number of repetitions used within the session. Tieman et al.[67] looked at the capability and performance of mobility in children with CP across the settings of home, school, and outdoors/community that must be taken into account when writing and determining successful completion of the identified functional outcomes. They found that capability and performance of mobility of the children varied across settings. Children tended to perform less well in the higher-demand settings such as school or the community. Since much of the testing in physical therapy occurs in the clinical setting, one must determine whether an outcome is generalizable across different settings.

Documenting and quantifying outcomes for the client is critical to physical therapy. Several authors have discussed the need for outcome research and efficacy studies.[68–70] The Gross Motor Function Measure (GMFM) and the GMFCS have been identified as useful standardized tools to document current status and functional change with intervention provided for children with CP.[19,71] Chapter 3 in this book identifies a variety of assessments and tests of motor development that can quantify change and functional outcomes in children with CP.

Children with CP face a lifetime of functional challenges that can be ameliorated intermittently with physical therapy. The nervous system of the infant and child with CP is impaired in some way, and it is not possible to make that child "normal." Therapists should never allow parents to misunderstand or misinterpret the intent of physical therapy. In general, it is to allow the infant or child to become the most independent in performing functional tasks throughout his or her lifetime. The provision of physical therapy should change in frequency and duration as the infant or child grows and develops, with periods of time when the child does not receive formal physical therapy intervention. Therefore, it is paramount that we identify the most critical times for formal therapy, the times for adjunctive therapies, and the times when an independent program will be adequate.

Anecdotally, bursts of physical therapy have been found to be especially beneficial at our facility after orthopedic surgery, neurosurgery, botulinum toxin injections, and growth spurts that impact the biomechanics of the movement. An unpublished study by Facchin et al. supports an intense burst of therapy and its positive effects on task performance. Long-term follow-up is currently underway to further support this treatment approach. The data to support intensive therapy may influence and alter the current treatment frequency.[72]

There is no singular recommended intervention for any specific category of CP as each infant and child presents a unique array of functional competencies, desired outcomes, functional limitations, and impairments. It is common and necessary to use principles from a variety of treatment approaches for an effective treatment. The therapist must determine the array of methods useful for the patient. Displays 5.14 through 5.17 present the "typical" impairments in four major types of CP. They should be used as references only and not as the "true picture" for that type of CP. Frequently, infants and children will demonstrate impairments from two or more types of CP. For example, an infant or child may have spastic quadriplegia with an athetoid component that involves the UEs more than the LEs. The information included in these tables is derived from numerous sources.[21,36,73–75]

DISPLAY 5.14 "Typical" Impairments of the Infant and Child with Hypertonia

Neuromotor System
Decreased stiffness in neck and trunk

Increased stiffness in extremities, distal > proximal; varies with type, extent, and location of the lesion

Difficulty grading between coactivation (CA) and reciprocal inhibition (RI), times with excessive amounts of either CA or RI

Difficulty initiating certain muscle groups (i.e., hip extensors and triceps)

Difficulty sustaining certain muscle groups (i.e., thoracic extensors and abdominals)

Difficulty terminating certain muscle groups (i.e., hip flexors, adductors, and internal rotators)

Activation of muscles tends to be in small ranges

Difficulty with eccentric control (i.e., quadriceps)

Musculoskeletal System
Limited range of motion of certain muscles (soft tissue shortening)

Other muscles are overlengthened (the antagonists)

Decreased ability to generate force in certain muscles, also in spastic muscles

Strength of poor grade

High risk for scoliosis

At risk for hip subluxation and/or dislocation

(continued)

DISPLAY
5.14
"Typical" Impairments of the Infant and Child with Hypertonia (*continued*)

Sensory/Perceptual System
Decreased tactile and proprioceptive awareness

Difficulty discriminating different kinds of touch

Decreased kinesthesia throughout the body

Decreased vestibular registration

Decreased body awareness

Vision used more in an upward gaze, sometimes asymmetrically

Cardiovascular and Respiratory Systems
Poor cardiovascular fitness due to decreased mobility

Reduced breath support with flared ribs and tight rectus abdominus

Gross Motor Impairments
Limited independent mobility on the floor or in vertical

May use assistive device for mobility

Poor sitting balance with spastic quadriplegia

Poor higher-level balance skills

Fine Motor Impairments
Decreased use of hands due to use for stability and for assistive device for mobility

Poor grasp and release and decreased in-hand manipulation with spastic quadriplegia

Oral Motor Impairments
Usually noted more with spastic quadriplegia

May have drooling, poor articulation

May have difficulty feeding

Discussions and explanations presented in this section include various methods of therapeutic intervention, including therapeutic exercise and strengthening, neurodevelopmental treatment (NDT), therapeutic handling, sensory integration (SI) and sensory processing disorder (SPD), Modified Constraint-induced Movement Therapy (mCIMT), treadmill training and robotic-assisted ambulation, electrical stimulation (ES), aquatics, hippotherapy, and community programs.

Therapeutic Exercise, Strengthening, and Stretching

Therapeutic exercise and strengthening plays an important role in the treatment of the infant or child with CP. Children with CP often present with spasticity, decreased muscle strength, and poor selective muscle control.[76] This muscle weakness may be due to deficits in motor unit activation, decreased muscle volume and alterations in muscle length resulting in loss of muscle force, poor coactivation of antagonist muscle groups, and altered muscle physiology.[77–79] Mobility for children with CP is greatly impacted by both muscle weakness and spasticity. Historically, strengthening was thought to increase spasticity, decrease ROM, and reduce overall function for a patient with CP.[80,81] However, these notions have not held up to careful scrutiny.[81–83] In recent systematic reviews of the literature, the authors have found that strength training can increase muscle strength in CP, and may improve endurance, cardiovascular health, weight management, maintenance of bone mass, self-perception, and gait function.[80–82] Strength training can also improve gait and muscle performance.[84,85] Damiano presents multiple studies that show that strength training improves GMFM scores, gait, and self-perception for a patient with

DISPLAY
5.15
"Typical" Impairments of the Infant and Child with Hypotonia

Neuromotor System
Decreased stiffness throughout the trunk and extremities

Inability to grade the level of stiffness necessary for functional activities

Extension favored over flexion for function

Difficulty coactivating for stability in trunk and in the extremities in horizontal and vertical positions

Muscle activity is initiated in phasic bursts for functional activity

Great difficulty sustaining most muscle groups, especially abdominals and gluteals for proximal stability

Muscles tend to terminate passively

Poor eccentric control of certain muscles (i.e., quadriceps)

Musculoskeletal System
Joints tend to be hypermobile, so the child relies on ligaments for stability

Stability gained through end-range positioning

Contractures develop secondary to positioning of the arms and legs (i.e., pectorals, tensor fascia latae, flexors of the hips and elbows)

Ribcage at risk for becoming flat/ovoid owing to gravity in supine and prone positions

Difficulty generating force throughout the body

Sensory/Perceptual System
Difficulty with tactile and proprioceptive awareness (requires greater input for the sensory information to register)

Decreased kinesthesia and body awareness

May seek increased sensory input, sometimes in unsafe situations

Decreased ability to use both sides together as a wide base is used for stability

Cardiovascular and Respiratory Systems

Decreased breath support and shallow breathing with weak abdominals and diaphragm

Poor cough

Decreased cardiovascular fitness

Gross Motor Impairments

Developmental milestones achieved later

May skip creeping on hands and knees

Uses "W" sitting for stability

Lacks higher-level balance skills

Uses end-range stability without midrange control

Fine Motor Impairments

Lacks shoulder girdle stability and therefore distal strength

Hands without arches

Decreased bimanual skill and in-hand manipulation

Decreased success with independent activities of daily living

Oral Motor Impairments

Decreased strength of oral motor muscles

Breathy voice and short utterances

Decreased rotary chew ability with inability to handle variety of textures

Stuffs mouth due to decreased proprioception

CP. Damiano states that strengthening can improve motor skill or function when the child has some voluntary control in a muscle group.[10,86]

There is little standardization among the studies just noted, many of which were uncontrolled clinical trials. Therefore, some of the reported gains in GMFM scores and functional improvements with strengthening may be overestimated.[78,83] Nonetheless, strength training seems a valuable and effective intervention for patients with CP.[83]

Individuals with CP have poor recruitment of muscle units, inconsistent maintenance of maximal efforts, and considerable weakness, even under the muscles that are spastic. The question to be determined is, "What is the best exercise prescription to produce functional strength gains for CP?" The National Strength and Conditioning Association (NSCA) established strength training guidelines for children and adolescents (Table 5.3).[83] Although not based upon children with CP, these guidelines are a good framework to use as a starting point in protocol development in CP.[83]

To have an effective response to strength training, the child must:

1. comprehend the process;
2. consistently produce a maximal or near-maximal effort;
3. be motivated and be able to attend to the task; and
4. have a family that can support the program and the child.[10]

DISPLAY

5.16 "Typical" Impairments of the Infant and Child with Athetosis

Neuromotor System

Profound global decrease in stiffness, proximal > distal

Poor damping, see high-amplitude and low-frequency oscillations

Difficulty with coactivation, reciprocal inhibition noted much more frequently

Inability to grade initiation or sustaining of muscle activation

Muscle termination tends to be passive

Difficulty with eccentric control of muscles

Musculoskeletal System

Significant asymmetry of the spine and hips

Joints may be hypermobile owing to excessive reciprocal inhibition

Significant hypermobility at C1 and C6–C7 with increasing age, resulting in possible spinal subluxation

Frequent temporomandibular joint problems

Poor ability to generate force

Sensory/Perceptual System

Vision used in upward gaze

Decreased proprioception, tends to be worse in the upper extremities than the lower extremities

Poor body awareness

Poor kinesthesia

Cardiovascular and Respiratory Systems

Respiration fluctuates in rate and rhythm

Poor breath support

Gross Motor Impairments

Developmental milestones achieved later

Limited floor mobility with great difficulty sitting on the floor

Delayed acquisition of ambulation skills

Use of "W" sitting for stability

Fine Motor Impairments

Difficulty using hands for tasks as they are used for stability in vertical and on the floor

Decreased bimanual skill and in-hand manipulation

Decreased success with independent activities of daily living

Oral Motor Impairments

Poor articulation

Breathy voice and short utterances

Prone to temporomandibular joint impairments because of asymmetric use of the facial muscles

Frequent drooling with poor lip closure

DISPLAY
5.17 **"Typical" Impairments of the Infant and Child with Ataxia**

Neuromotor System

Tends to have slight decrease in stiffness in trunk, sometimes in the limbs as well

Poor grading of stiffness

Poor damping, oscillations are of high frequency and low amplitude

Difficulty timing and sequencing initiating, sustaining, and terminating muscle activation

Decreased ability to grade coactivation and reciprocal inhibition

Poor coactivation of trunk, hips, and shoulder girdles

Musculoskeletal System

Difficulty generating force

Tends to rest in end range and rely on ligaments for stability

Sensory/Perceptual System (very significant sensory deficits, which are as restricting as the motor deficits)

Relies on vision for balance and postural alignment; therefore, not free to scan the environment

Visual system with severe nystagmus

Decreased visual perception

Decreased proprioception throughout the body

Increased latency in processing sensory information

Severe postural insecurity; very fearful of movement

Poor vestibular system

Tends to be tactilely defensive with poor discrimination; never gets sustained input

Difficulty generalizing sensory and motor information to perform novel tasks

Cardiovascular and Respiratory Systems

Often fluctuating with poor proximal stability

Limited mobility impacts ribcage development, especially in thoracic expansion

Poor cardiovascular fitness

Shallow and rapid breathing

Gross Motor Impairments

Uses a very wide base to move on the floor independently

Keeps legs flexed in vertical to lower the center of gravity

Pace of development tends to be slower owing to poor balance in upright

Fine Motor Impairments

Poor skills due to an inability to grade precise movements

Difficulty with activities requiring dissociation of the arms

Oral Motor Impairments

Wide range of movement

Difficulty with a variety of textures and tastes

Strength training can be used with children as young as 7 years of age who meet the requirements above. To promote strengthening, one must use high loads with a small number of repetitions (three to eight) arranged in multiple sets with a rest between each set. To improve muscle endurance, the child should have reduced loads but more repetitions (8 to 20) before resting. Loads and repetitions should

be increased with improvement. To date, there is inadequate evidence to support an optimal recommendation for the exercise prescription in CP, but the NSCA guidelines offer a good starting point.[81–83]

A strengthening program can be employed for many reasons. For example, it is beneficial employee a strength training program following invasive procedures such as dorsal rhizotomy, intrathecal baclofen pump insertion, soft tissue and bony surgeries, and Botox injections to maximize functional improvements.[10] Strengthening can occur without weights by carefully selecting activities that require specified muscle groups and closely resemble the goal activity.[76] For example, if the goal is to transition out of the kitchen chair, practicing sit-to-stand transition from chairs of various heights to strengthen the LE can be done in order to reach this goal.

When the infant or child is too weak or has too little postural control to use external weights or even body weight as resistance, the therapist can position the child to (1) eliminate gravity or (2) provide handling and assistance to complete the motion against gravity. An example of progression against gravity is demonstrated for the infant with poor head control. Support the infant in a vertical position with its head aligned over the shoulders so that the infant must balance the head in vertical. The progression is performed by moving the infant slightly off vertical alignment,

TABLE
5.3   NSCA Guidelines for Strength Training Program

Variables of Resistance Training	NSCA Guidelines
Warm-up	5–10 min of dynamic activities
Type	Single- and multijoint exercises utilizing concentric and eccentric contractions
Intensity/volume	1–3 sets of 6–15 repetitions of 50%–85% of 1 RM
Rest intervals	1–3 min
Frequency	2–4 times a week on nonconsecutive days
Duration	8–20 wk
Progression	Increase resistance gradually (5%–10%) as strength improves
Age	7 yr and older

which requires returning the head to vertical and maintaining it there. As strength increases, the infant should improve its ability to return and maintain the head in vertical with eyes parallel to the horizon while the body is taken further toward horizontal. Depending on the severity of the CP, this could happen within a few sessions or over several months or years.

A new area of study uses virtual reality programs to help strengthening. A randomized control trial by Chia-Ling Chen et al.[87] examined the possible benefits of a home-based virtual cycling program for strengthening in children with spastic CP. The results found increases in knee muscle strength but no change in functional outcome scores from gross motor function tests.

Current research and understanding of motor control and motor learning support a strengthening program for all children with CP. Strength training has been found to increase strength and improve activity in children with CP, but the most effective strength training protocols have yet to be determined.[83] Further research is needed to determine optimal strength-training protocols, including mode of activity, intensity, duration, rest between session, severity of CP, and age.

Regular stretching to maintain full ROM and prevent or minimize contractures is also extremely important throughout childhood. Stretching is especially important in children who are not able to move their joints through normal ranges of motion with functional activities. Stretching has been found to reduce severity of tone for several hours in children with CP.[88,89] Also, periods of rapid growth are times to emphasize stretching in therapy and home programs.

Neurodevelopmental Treatment

NDT, also known originally as the Bobath approach, was developed by the Bobaths in England in the early 1940s. The original focus was the treatment of individuals with pathophysiology of the CNS, specifically children with CP and adults with hemiplegia.[90] Dr. and Mrs. Bobath described NDT as a "living concept," and as such, it has continued to evolve over the years. "The Neuro-Developmental Treatment approach is not a set of techniques but more an understanding of the developmental process of motor control and the motor components which make up functional motor tasks."[75] The goal is to have effective carryover from the treatment session to daily life and subsequent treatment sessions. Carryover is actually motor learning, "a relatively permanent change in the capability for responding."[39]

The ultimate goal of NDT is for the child to have the most independent function possible according to age and abilities. Treatment sessions are directed toward a functional outcome and include as much client-initiated movement as possible. The therapist plans for the necessary preparatory work (e.g., muscle elongation) to enable the

client to perform the task and will facilitate and guide the child's movement as needed to decrease or prevent postures and movement behaviors that interfere with functional abilities. "Feed-forward" is developed as the child practices the skill or task with the therapist's guidance. The therapist provides less guidance and assistance as the infant or child anticipates postural and motor requirements.[39] Refer to Display 5.18 for a brief synopsis of key theoretical statements based on NDT.

The neuroscientific basis that reportedly explains NDT has changed over the many decades since Dr. and Mrs. Bobath developed the approach. Currently, the Neuronal Group Selection Theory (NGST) is used to explain how the nervous system changes as a result of experience.[21] This theory emphasizes the concept that development is the result of a complex relationship between genes and the environment. Brain development is fostered by the participation in functional activities within an appropriate environment.[21] Therefore, it is critical that the infant/child engage in activities as much as possible in functionally and developmentally appropriate contexts to generate movement to meet task requirements.[21]

DISPLAY 5.18   **Overview of Neurodevelopmental Treatment Theory**

- Neurodevelopmental treatment is a problem-solving approach to treating infants, children, and adults with CNS deficits for the most independent functional outcomes that are age appropriate and appropriate for the cognitive level.
- Examination and evaluation are integral to the process in prioritizing the impairments and limitations and are continuous throughout the treatment process.
- The functional limitations are changeable with intervention strategies targeting specific impairments within contexts that are meaningful to the client.
- Treatment is directed toward functional outcomes and is active, with the therapist providing the necessary "handling" to guide the movement and assist as necessary toward successful achievement of the identified outcome.
- Handling is used carefully to establish or reestablish the postures and movements that the client needs to become functional in a meaningful way.
- Active carryover by the client and caregivers is essential to successful outcomes.
- Understanding how typical development occurs and how atypical development is a departure from that enables the therapist to anticipate and prevent undesirable postural changes and subsequent decrease in functional abilities.
- Movement and sensory processing are linked. Therapists must address both systems in treatment of the client with CNS dysfunction.
- Neurodevelopmental treatment provides therapists with flexible guidelines for selecting treatment strategies to manage the client according to their individual field of therapy.

Therapeutic Handling

The therapist's hands or a piece of equipment may be used to provide initial support to decrease the infant's impediment of excessive stiffness in order to maintain alignment, initiate weight shifts, support a movement, or aid smooth transitions of movement. This external support should be altered intermittently to provide the infant or child with an opportunity to practice the movement independently.

When there is an absence of body part stability, the therapist may support the body to decrease compensatory stiffness. This external support is thought to facilitate movement. The support can be moved from a proximal point (trunk, shoulder, or pelvis) of greater amounts of support to a more distal point on any of the limbs. By moving the point of support more distally, the therapist expects the child will assume a greater degree of control over the movement at the unsupported joints.

Sensory Integration and Sensory Processing Disorder

SI theory, developed and defined by the work of A. Jean Ayres, PhD, OTR, in the early 1970s, guides the therapeutic approach of SI therapy. Ayres' theory describes SI as "an approach used to enhance the brain's ability to organize sensory input for use in functional behaviors."[91] The interventions provide children with guided sensory input, designed to produce "an adaptive response (i.e., functional behavior) deemed more effective than previously observed behaviors."[91] Strategies for treatment, generated by this theoretical approach, involve methods of helping children achieve and sustain an optimal level of arousal in all environments. This is frequently helpful for the child with a low level of arousal who is difficult to encourage to interact with peers in the classroom or therapist in the treatment session. Conversely, specific strategies will help the child with high arousal to calm and engage in activities of the classroom or purposeful interaction with the environment. In a study conducted by Davies and Gavin in 2007, electroencephalographic (EEG) measures were used to examine brain processing in children with SPD. The study concluded that children with SPD "showed less sensory gating than children who were typically developing," thereby linking inefficient processing of sensory information with unique neurophysiologic findings.[91]

Many infants and children with CP experience difficulty processing sensory input and therefore have even greater difficulty producing a desired motor output. It is necessary to address the infant or child's sensory systems as they specifically affect motor performance and functional activities. The infant or child with CP has difficulty receiving and interpreting sensory information accurately, and is therefore at a disadvantage in responding to the information with appropriate motor output. The therapist must provide the infant or child with sensory information and movement experiences that will help to correctly interpret sensory information and then select a motor output that is functional. When the sensory information or "diet" is supplied throughout the infant or child's day, he or she will more quickly and accurately be able to apply the information in a functional way. It is necessary to educate parents and teachers in ways that will assist the infant or child in learning about sensory information and how it relates to his or her body. Some examples include:

- Use firm pressure when toweling dry after the bath.
- Provide a swinging motion to the infant or child every time you pick him or her up.
- "Dance" with the infant or young child on your shoulder or in your arms when passing between rooms.
- Encourage floor play with rolling over, pushing up, and moving extremities.
- Propose play activities requiring use and strength of the hands such as play dough, silly putty, playing in wet sand, and so on.
- Provide opportunities for "heavy" work such as pushing a laundry basket of clothes or books, pushing the grocery cart or carrying selected "heavier" groceries into the house or pantry, pushing the chair under the classroom table, and replacing the toys that are heavier during classroom clean-up.
- Select equipment on the playground that provides movement to the child such as sliding boards, seesaws, merry-go-rounds, jungle gyms, and so on, according to his or her capabilities and available safety features.

This is presented as a small list of ideas that one can use in the treatment program and within the infant or child's day to promote increased function. There are multiple books available to therapists, teachers, and families that can provide wonderful ideas for incorporating sensory play and a sensory diet into the daily activities of the infant or child.[92–94] When the child's primary impairment is sensory based, it is helpful to refer the child to an occupational therapist who has acquired special training in the sensory systems and perhaps in SI.[92] SI is best used as an adjunct treatment intervention owing to the complex therapeutic needs of a child with CP.

Modified Constraint-induced Movement Therapy

The foundations for this treatment approach are based on work completed by Edward Taub and his coworkers[95] in the mid-1960s. This research highlighted the importance of cortical reorganization and neuroplasticity, which became the theoretical foundations for Constraint-induced Movement Therapy (CIMT).[95,96] There are three major elements that make up CIMT treatment: constraint of the unaffected limb with a cast, massed practice of the affected UE, and intensive shaping techniques used in treatment to train the involved UE.[96,97] The frequency of treatment is also a hallmark of this technique. Traditional CIMT involved constraint of the affected UE 90% of the patient's day, over a 2-week period, with organized intense intervention for 6 hours per day. Boyd completed a systemic review that looked at several randomized control trials studying CIMT use for patients with chronic poststroke symptoms that have shown large functional improvements and carryover into daily activities.[97] These studies have also highlighted the fact that the intensity of training and the massed practice elements of this treatment approach are essential components of the effectiveness of this treatment.[97]

CIMT can be used for children with hemiplegic-pattern CP with certain changes to the typical adult protocols. Modified Constraint-induced Movement Therapy (mCIMT) utilizes less intensive means of constraint such as a glove or a mitten rather than a cast for the affected UE that is easier to manage and better tolerated in children. Treatment time and frequency range from less than 3 hours up to 6 hours of intervention a day, from 1- to 2-week intensive periods of treatment.[72,96]

The body of research for use of mCIMT in children is less robust than for adults following a stroke. There is evidence in children that has shown functional and objective gains; however, most studies have small sample sizes, low statistical power, and variability in methods of constraint and interventions.[72] Taub, DeLuca, and Echols used an mCIMT protocol with 17 children with CP whose unaffected UE was restrained and massed practice of the affected arm for 6 hours a day occurred over 21 days.[98] Improvements were seen in grasp, weight-bearing tolerance, and functional use of the affected UE.[97,98] Charles et al.[99] reported significant treatment influence 3 weeks post-mCIMT and a study by Eliasson et al.[100] reported increased functional use of the affected hand after mCIMT, particularly in those with more severe deficits.

Furthermore, Facchin et al.[72] found that treatment with mCIMT and bimanual intensive rehabilitation treatment had significant improvement in fine grasp of the affected hand, whereas children in the standard treatment group showed minimal or no changes in hand function. Coker et al.[96] studied mCIMT treatment on gait characteristics in children with hemiplegic CP. They theorized that upper and lower extremity benefits could occur simultaneously during mCIMT with cortical reorganization and changes in both UE function and the child's ability to ambulate.[96] Twelve children with hemiplegic CP participated in 5 consecutive days of intensive specific treatment for 6 hours a day wearing a resting hand splint covered by a puppet glove on the unaffected hand. A significant narrowing in heel-to-heel base of support distance, decreased double-limb support time, and increased single-limb support resulted.[96]

Treadmill Training/Robotic Gait Training

Treadmill training is a newer, functional treatment in which patients practice walking on a treadmill to improve their ability to walk at home and in the community. On the basis of the task-specific approach to motor learning, if a child with CP is to improve in the skill of walking, intensive training is necessary. Reciprocal treadmill walking may be partially controlled by the spinal cord and can be stimulated in the absence of higher brain center control.[101] Reciprocal stepping is considered to be largely organized by networks of sensory and motor neurons within the spinal cord called central pattern generators (CPGs).[102] CPGs are likely activated by the brainstem and basal ganglia, which in turn activate the muscles responsible for cyclic and repetitive walking movements.[103] Treadmill use taps into this automatic reciprocal walking mechanism even when higher brain centers have been damaged.[104] Treadmill use as a treatment modality can be split into three major subtypes: (1) partial body weight–supported treadmill training (PBWSTT), (2) robotic-assisted locomotion training (RALT), and (3) treadmill training without support.

With PBWSTT, an overhead harness system is used to support part of the child's body weight while the one or two therapists manually guide the LEs at the foot or lower leg while the patient walks. By supporting a portion of the child's body weight, those with CP can take reciprocal steps without the fear of falling. The optimal percentage of body weight that should be supported by the harness system is unsure, but a recent study suggests that walking with partial body weight support (PBWS) not progressed by decreasing amounts of support is no more effective than traditional overground training without body weight support.[105] Recent studies have shown positive impacts of PBWSTT on gross motor function,[104,106–108] walking speed,[109] and endurance.[110] Owing to common study limitations such as small sample sizes and lack of randomized controlled trials, the evidence that PBWSTT results in improvements in gait and gross motor function for children with CP is not conclusive.[111,112] PBWSTT has clinical limitations. Maintaining patient motivation is often challenging owing to the repetitive nature of this type of training. For example, it is not uncommon for the child to hang from the harness with their feet off the ground, jump, or lean forward on the harness system because of boredom and fatigue.

RALT is another recently developed therapeutic modality with potential to improve gait. The robotic walking system consists of two exoskeletons, several braces to fasten the child to the device, and a harness system for body weight support.[113] This type of robotic treadmill training offers an increase in specificity of gait rehabilitation by allowing a greater amount of stepping practice due to lower patient effort. Gait parameters such as mileage, speed, count steps, guidance forces, and body weight support can be precisely defined for each session, making progression easy to follow.[113] Because RALT maintains a normal physiologic gait pattern while increasing intensity and frequency, some argue that it offers ideal conditions for gait training. A study by Meyer-Heim et al.[113] in 2009 found that children who participated in RALT averaged greater than a 15% increase in gait speed.

PBWSTT harness systems and RALT are available in many rehabilitation centers but are not typically found elsewhere. Basic treadmills are readily available in community centers and schools, making them much more accessible to children with CP. Simple treadmill training without body weight support was recently studied in Greek children with CP and found to have several positive effects.[114] Adolescent children who had treadmill training three times a week for 12 weeks demonstrated significant improvements in walking speed and gross motor function compared with conventional physical therapy.[114]

Electrical Stimulation

ES can be used for pain control, edema reduction, or muscle strengthening. There are several considerations when using this intervention for children with CP. These include the child's age, skin sensitivity, cognitive ability, and tolerance to stimulation. The three methods most extensively used with children with CP are neuromuscular electrical stimulation (NMES), functional electric stimulation (FES), and threshold electrical stimulation (TES).[115–117] Recent research has studied the use of both NMES and FES for atypical gait in children with CP.[117–120] NMES is used for muscle strengthening by applying electric current stimulation of sufficient intensity to elicit muscle contraction. Using stimulation when a muscle should be contracting during a functional activity, such a gait, is referred to as FES.[115] Both NMES and FES can be performed with surface electrodes, footswitches, and, more recently, percutaneous and implanted ES.[120] In a systematic review of current research, Wright et al.[120] discuss the common uses of NMES for gait, including stimulation of the anterior tibialis during swing phase, stimulating the gastrocnemius during stance, or alternating stimulation to the anterior tibialis and the gastrocnemius. One author suggests that greater changes in functional gait measures may be found when stimulating the gastrocnemius with or without stimulation to the anterior tibialis.[117] Further study should determine the most effective electrode placement and duration of treatment for FES during gait.

NMES has been reported to be effective in strengthening the quadriceps of a 13-year-old adolescent with spastic diplegic CP for the development of new skills such as stair climbing.[121] NMES has also been used in conjunction with BTX-A. When NMES is used after BTX-A injection, it may improve ROM in the agonist and strengthen the antagonist muscle group.[120] Lastly, TES is described as a low-level, subcontraction ES applied at home during sleep, proposed by Pape originally to increase the blood flow during a time of heightened trophic hormone secretion resulting in increased muscle bulk.[115,122,123] TES is intended to assist the total management of the child, not to replace primary therapeutic intervention.[123] Pape's research has shown that the child progresses more quickly when TES is used in conjunction with hands-on therapy.[122] To prepare the increased muscle bulk developed with TES for functional use, it must be strengthened and integrated into the child's daily activities. The scarcity of well-controlled trials makes it difficult to support definitively or discard the use of ES in CP.[115,117,120] There appears to be more evidence to support FES and NMES than TES, but the findings must be interpreted with caution owing to the lack of conclusive evidence for or against these modalities. "The age and type of patient most likely to benefit from this intervention and optimal treatment parameters are as yet unknown."[115]

Aquatics

Therapeutic aquatics has been used for millennia for medicinal purposes and is currently pursued for habilation, rehabilitation, health and wellness, and general fitness. The physical properties of water are used to address specified impairments and functional limitations of clients in pursuit of functional outcomes.[10,124] Aquatics and water can be pursued on a participatory level as in swimming or improving ambulation, as competitive swimming such as Special Olympics, or as an individual pursuit. Therapeutic aquatics should be distinguished from adaptive aquatics. In therapeutic aquatics, the therapist examines and analyzes the abilities and limitations of the client, noting the identified goals and functional outcomes. Activities, movements, and exercises can be used in the water to remediate identified impairments and limitations, and a swimming stroke can be taught to ameliorate impairments and strive toward the identified functional outcome. Adaptive aquatics recognizes the client's current abilities and matches the abilities to a stroke for successful swimming. We offer an example of a child with a diagnosis of hemiplegic CP. The stroke of choice by the child will likely be a side stroke with the strong side under the body to propel the child through the water. The *therapeutic* stroke of choice would be a breast stroke so that both arms would be used underwater simultaneously, with a goal of independent use of both arms in the future. In this example, the therapist should facilitate the stroke by assisting the child until the weaker arm has adequate strength to take over the arm pull, more closely resembling the strong arm's pull.[124]

Hippotherapy

Hippotherapy uses a horse for habilation or rehabilitation of an individual as distinguished from therapeutic riding, which focuses on recreation or riding skills for disabled riders.[10,125,126] Hippotherapy has been defined by the North American Riding for the Handicapped Association (NARHA) as the use of a horse as a tool to address impairments, functional limitations, and disabilities in patients with neuromusculoskeletal dysfunction.[10] Hippotherapy may decrease identified impairments in the pursuit of functional outcomes while utilizing the triplanar movement of the horse, which closely resembles the human pelvic motion during gait. The movements of the horse are utilized to promote relaxation, increase ROM, strengthening, proximal control, and so on, toward a functional outcome. Hippotherapy seldom uses a saddle, but rather a blanket so the warmth of the horse can reach the child. Certain contraindications exist, which should be reviewed before selecting this alternative approach.[10] Some stables include the care of the horse and the work of the stable in the routine of the therapy, thereby encouraging cognition, following commands, sequencing activities, memory, and psychosocial elements as well as the sensorimotor elements inherent in the activity. The therapist providing this intervention needs special training, clinical experience, and expertise to help the child with CP realize the identified functional outcomes.[126]

Community Programs

Formal physical therapy should be supplemented in early adolescence and adulthood in those with mild to moderate impairment by alternative activities such as recreational pursuits.[127,128] With the child's age, functional abilities, level of participation, family support, and contextual factors in mind, alternatives to traditional physical therapy to replace treatment for a specified period of time, or to augment the physical therapy, should be considered. These suggestions may be perceived as "nontherapy" by a child tired of going to therapy sessions routinely and may elicit greater cooperation and motivation. Self-esteem rises when the child can participate with friends and can join in the fun. All of the following listed alternative interventions need more research to identify those that are most effective in achieving functional outcomes. Anecdotal evidence is available, but little high-level research has been done to date. These community-based activities include yoga, karate, dance classes, tumbling, swimming, horseback riding, adaptive sports, and music lessons to enhance the child's current abilities and to build on his or her strengths toward new functional skills or enhanced current functional abilities. These alternatives can be very powerful motivators for many children as they perceive that it is only "fun" and not therapy. They can participate in regular classes or classes designed specifically for children with special needs. Involvement in school or community activities is a vital part of any child's development. Participation may at times be supported by skilled physical therapy, such as working on a particular skill like catching a ball, balance for yoga, or shooting a basketball. A transition to community-based activities will help the child incorporate the skills they have gained in therapy and allow them to "make it their own" when using them within their home and community environment.

▶ Adaptive equipment

Adaptive equipment is often a necessary and useful adjunct to treatment of the infant or child with CP. Equipment may offer postural support to the infant or child, or it may aid functional skills and mobility.[10] Any equipment used should be "family friendly" (functional for the family), comfortable,

safe, easy to use, and attractive. Adaptive equipment and its use should coincide with and reinforce functional outcomes for the child. The equipment should be reassessed frequently and adapted as necessary on the basis of the infant's or child's current requirements and growth.

Adaptive seating systems and systems to promote and support standing are the most common pieces of equipment used by infants and children at home and in the classroom to optimize function; to explore the environment and toys; and to interact with siblings, caregivers, and classmates. The majority of this section will focus on these two specific categories of equipment. Chapter 12 deals exclusively with adaptive equipment and environmental aids for children with disabilities, and should be consulted for more detailed information on all equipment available.

Seating and Positioning Equipment

The wheelchair or stroller system is the most important device for nonambulatory children because nonambulatory or marginally ambulatory children with CP lack the necessary postural control and coordination to function in a variety of positions. The concept of a specialized stroller or wheelchair for a child with CP is often difficult for families to accept. Caregivers are often hesitant to discuss seating options because it acknowledges the degree of their child's disability. It may take the family some time to accept the need for a supportive seating system for mobility. It is important for the PT to have open discussions with the family regarding seating, but also be sensitive to the psychological process required for the family's acceptance. Caregivers of children who are ambulatory but lack endurance and strength for functional ambulation are often especially resistant to a wheelchair because they believe that their child will stop making progress with walking. This fear should be discussed with such families. Because of functional limitations while in a wheelchair, many children will continue to ambulate at home and school as often as they had prior to a wheelchair. There is no evidence that the functional ambulation of adults with CP is determined by how much they ambulated as children.[10] In addition to improved efficiency with mobility, an appropriate seating system has been shown to improve UE function,[129,130] enhance respiratory function,[129] improve oral motor function with eating and drinking,[131] and vocalization.[132] When caregivers are given a complete picture of all the advantages of an appropriate seating and mobility system, they eventually become more comfortable with the idea.

When assessing a child for adaptive seating, the PT can gain important information from an assessment out of the chair. Questions to consider include:

- Can the older infant or child sit independently without external support? If so, what is the child's postural alignment?
- How long can the child sit with optimal alignment of the head and trunk?

- Can the infant or child sit by propping on his or her arms, or is he or she dependent on external support to maintain an upright posture?
- Can the child maintain the pelvis in neutral alignment with the trunk and head held in proper alignment?
- Is the infant or child's posture fixed or flexible?

Seating for a child is a multidisciplinary decision that includes the recommendations of the PT, physician, occupational therapist, rehabilitation engineer, and wheelchair vendor. A formal seating clinic allows these players to work with patient and family to help make the best decision for seating and mobility. Seating clinics are typically found in pediatric hospitals and some special education schools. The seating team should discuss the goals of the seating system, the child's current and future functional level, the ability of the seating system to function at home and school, available transportation for the wheelchair or stroller, growth needs of the wheelchair, musculoskeletal deformities, and future surgeries/treatments that may affect posture and alignment. At the end of the evaluation, a prescription for a wheelchair/seating system is generated, and the vendor is responsible for obtaining, building, and adjusting the seating system to the needs of the child.

Seating for the Nonambulator

The age and level of function of the child are the most important factors in deciding on a wheelchair or stroller. The child with severe quadriplegic CP who is dependent for all transfers requires supportive seating from an early age and should be evaluated for their first seating system between 1 and 2 years of age. The first chair is often a tilt-in-space stroller base with solid footrests, trunk laterals, anterior trunk support, and head rest. The tilt in space is necessary so the head has support and will not fall forward onto the chest, thereby overlengthening the posterior neck muscles. A slide-on lap tray should be included for feeding, fine motor, and educational purposes. The second wheelchair, obtained when at school age, is similar in design to the first wheelchair but often on a standard wheelchair base. Power mobility is a consideration at this time for some children with severe athetosis, but practice and careful evaluation of driving controls is necessary to ensure that the child is able to function safely in all environments. Mouth joysticks and sip-and-puff controls are rarely used in children with CP owing to poor oral motor control in these severely impaired children. Many children with severe spastic quadriplegic CP will develop significant skeletal deformities and skin issues as they reach adolescence, thus requiring custom-contoured seating and additional padding. Many of the most severely involved children with CP will develop scoliosis that will require surgical intervention as adolescents. After spinal fusion surgery, many modifications to the wheelchair are required, including raising the backrest and headrest owing to a total back height increase of 1 to 4 inches in the child. Other common adjustments include removal of custom-molded seat backs, adjustments to laterals, adjusted seat depth, and cutouts on seat back at the top or bottom of spinal fusion to prevent pressure.[10]

Seating for the Marginal Ambulator

Children with limited ambulation skills and fair trunk control usually have their first seating and mobility system by 3 years of age. The child with strong UEs and sufficient cognitive ability may benefit from a wheelchair base. If a manual wheelchair is not feasible because of weakness or decreased motor control, a stroller base may help increase the overall chair height, thereby making functional activities easier for the family. Power mobility in very young children has gained in popularity in recent years. Benefits for children to begin power mobility at a young age include reducing the risk of learned helplessness, promoting self-confidence, increasing learning, and allowing visual development.[133] Many young children with CP with minimal walking ability fit the profile of "excellent candidate" for early introduction of power mobility, but several factors must be considered before this important decision. Transportation of the wheelchair, safety in all environments, home setup, and cost–benefit analysis are among serious issues to be considered when power mobility is an option. Power wheelchair is a more appropriate option for these children in later childhood when behavioral maturity, cognitive ability, UE motor control, and caregiver readiness to make the commitment all come together. The Pediatric Powered Wheelchair Screening Test (PPWST) is a valuable tool designed to assist clinicians in determining whether a child with CP has the cognitive skills to be a successful power mobility user.[134] Most children in this group of CP typically use a joystick with the dominant hand for power mobility, but head and leg switches are also useful for more involved children in this group. Seating system needs for these children can vary greatly and may include trunk and thigh laterals supports, chest harness, lap tray, and head support. Swing-away leg rests may be a better choice than solid leg rests if the child can transfer to standing. These children will spend a majority of their waking hours in their seating system, so consistent evaluation of posture and alignment can minimize secondary impairments associated with poor posture.

Seating for the Household and Limited-Community Ambulator

The household ambulator with good trunk control but lacking the endurance to ambulate in the community also requires a mobility device other than an ambulation assist device. Prior to elementary school, these children work hard to improve their functional ambulation and families are typically satisfied with a commercially available stroller for longer trips. Once school aged, most of these children are good candidates for a push wheelchair. Seating system needs for these children are minimal owing to good trunk control and decreased overall use. A solid seat and solid back with seat belt are often all that is required. Older children and adolescents preparing to leave for college often transition to a scooter to allow increased efficiency of movement in the community.

Standers

For older infants or children who are unable to stand independently or for whom sustained standing in proper alignment is indicated, standing systems should be used for external support.[10] A standing program should be initiated by 2 years of age in a child with CP that has not begun standing or ambulating regularly. The potential benefits of a stander include improved weight-bearing tolerance, improved head and trunk control, increased bone density, enhanced hip development and prevention of further LE deformity, sustained muscular stretch of plantarflexors and hip flexors, maintenance of trunk and lower limb PROM, improved coactivation of the LE muscles used for standing, improved respiratory efficiency, improved gastrointestinal motility, improved circulation/decreased decubiti, improved renal function, and improved social interaction with peers. Most of the evidence supporting standers is indirect evidence regarding the negative effects of immobilization.[135] Unfortunately, little research quantifies the necessity of standing to achieve the above-noted benefits of standing.[10,135] Stuberg[135] recommended positioning in standing for 45 minutes two or three times a day to control LE flexor contractures, and for 60 minutes four or five times per week to facilitate bone development. This frequency should by no means be used as an end goal, as many children can safely progress up to a few hours per day in their stander.

Once a decision is made to use a stander, a detailed evaluation should be performed and many factors considered before selecting the most appropriate stander for the child. Information about previous standing equipment, other equipment purchased recently, overall functional level, and expected goals of the stander is extremely important to collect before making the choice of a specific item. This information may move the conversation about equipment in a completely different direction. For example, a common dilemma confronts the child who could benefit from a gait trainer and a stander but owns neither. Usually, third-party payers will only cover the purchase of one of these two types of therapeutic equipment during a specific time frame. If ambulation potential is noted during the evaluation, this must be considered when reviewing standers. A thorough objective assessment with attention to head/trunk control in sitting and standing, posture in sitting and standing, and ROM limitations is the next step in the evaluation process. Overall child height, floor-to-chest height, floor-to-elbow height, leg length, lower-leg length, trunk width, hip width, inseam, and weight must be measured precisely. Like a seating system, the child's age and future growth potential are also an important consideration. Because of the many pros and cons to each type of stander, several standers may have

to be tested before deciding. Besides the obvious benefit of being able to evaluate the posture and alignment of the child during a trial, it is important to determine whether the caregivers can easily and efficiently transfer the child in and out of the stander. Ease of transfer is often the most important factor in compliance with using a stander. After trialling each stander for at least 15 minutes, carefully inspect the skin for pressure areas. Any redness should disappear within 20 minutes of removal from the stander. Once a stander has been chosen, carefully select the accessories required to provide optimal function and that can be removed or adjusted as the child's strength improves.

There are currently four basic stander designs on the market: supine, prone, upright, and sit-to-stand. This section section details the basic differences between these stander types. Please refer to Table 5.4 for more detailed descriptions of each stander's indications and contraindications. Supine standers start in a horizontal or reclined position with the child lying supine. The child can be easily strapped in appropriately while supine and slowly transitioned to a more vertical position. A tilt table is the most basic type of supine stander, but is rarely the best option for children with CP. More sophisticated models of supine standers are available to meet the complex needs of a child with CP. Supine standers can be ordered with components such as trunk and hip laterals, knee pads, hip adduction/abduction support, and head supports. A supine stander is a good option for the younger child with moderate to severe extensor spasticity and poor head control who can be easily transferred via scoop-dependent lift. Children who would benefit from supine standers have poor head control; therefore, optimal tilt should be just short of full vertical to prevent the head from dropping into flexion. Children with extreme extensor spasticity are often not good candidates for this type of stander as the posterior pressure often stimulates their extensor tone. Prone standers provide anterior support to the child and, like the supine stander, is positioned horizontally for ease of transfer. The available components are similar to those of a supine stander with the addition of a chin support to aid in head control and positioning when the child is vertical. Prone standers are not recommended for children with poor head control because they do not provide enough support for the child's head and neck. Traditionally, children in prone standers were placed in a slightly forward flexed position (10 to 20 degrees) to encourage activation of their extensor muscles and improve head control. Because maximum weight bearing and most upright functions occur in the fully vertical position, the forward tilted position is not typically recommended for most children. For the child with fair head and trunk control with the goal of improving head control endurance, the prone stander in a fully vertical position is a better option than the supine stander to achieve optimal weight bearing as well as cervical and trunk alignment. Simple upright standers, or parapodia, are standers into which the child is placed in a standing position. They often do not have support above the pelvis, thus requiring

TABLE

5.4   Guide to Stander Selection

Stander Selection for Children with CP

Type	Indications	Contraindications
Supine 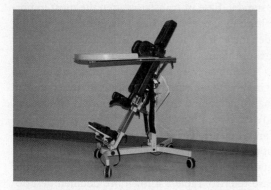	2 yr old to adult Poor head/trunk control requiring head support or reclined position Flexor tone Tracheostomy Unable to tolerate full upright position	Strong extensor tone Good head and trunk control Significant knee and hip flexion contractures Larger patients making transfer difficult for caregiver
Prone 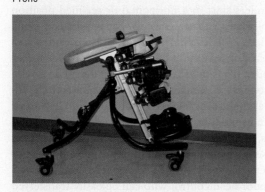	Younger child (often early school–aged) Fair or good head control Fair trunk control Goal is to use upper extremities in standing Goal is to participate in classroom activities while standing Able to tolerate full upright position Dynamic options available allowing mobility for patients with good UE control	Strong extensor tone Uses extensor tone as main means to extend head and trunk to vertical position Poor head control—only phasic activation of cervical extension Larger patients making transfer difficult for caregiver
Upright 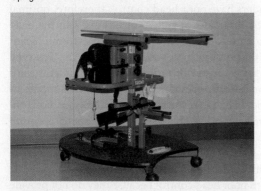	Younger/lighter child Tolerates full upright position for long periods Good head control and endurance Economical choice is important	Poor head control Excessive flexor or extensor tone Hip or knee flexion contractures Large child
Sit-to-stand 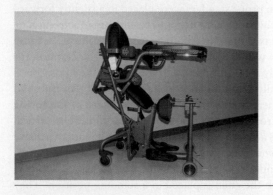	School-age child or adolescent Good head and fair trunk control Mild hip/knee flexion contractures Patient has cognitive and physical ability to transition stander between positions independently	Poor head control Poor posture when stander in sitting

increased trunk and head control. Because most children with CP with good head and trunk control have some ambulatory ability, this type of stander is rarely recommended for children with CP. More supportive upright standers are commercially available and can be a good, economical choice for some children with CP. An upright stander is an acceptable choice for a younger child with good head control, fair trunk control, and poor LE alignment without external support. In the past decade, the sit-to-stand-style stander has become a very popular model for children with CP. Because of its versatility, a variety of nonambulatory or marginally ambulatory children with CP benefit from this type of stander. The child is usually transferred into this stander via stand or sit-pivot transfer. Once properly supported at the knees and trunk in sitting, the child is slowly transitioned to a standing position using a manual hydraulic pump or a power-lift mechanism. This type of stander is an excellent choice for a larger child or adolescent, and the child with mild hip and knee flexion contractures that cannot stand fully upright. For these children, a sit-to-stand stander can provide a low-load, long-duration stretch to the hip flexors, hamstrings, and posterior knee capsule in addition to the other benefits of standing. Some children stay in this style of stander for several hours at a time, alternating between standing and sitting positions. Although this is a great feature of the sit-to-stand models, it is often difficult to adjust the stander to provide optimal posture in both standing and sitting. The caregiver or school aide must therefore be trained in making proper adjustments to the stander after each transition in position.

Ambulation Aids

Many ambulation devices are available to make walking as functional, energy efficient, and least cumbersome as possible. A thorough assessment of the child's functional capabilities in vertical position must be completed before deciding upon the best ambulation aid. Communication with the child's team regarding the child's routines, necessary transitions through the day, and distances to be traveled is important before deciding upon an ambulation device. Rose et al.[136] documented a linear relationship between oxygen uptake and heart rate throughout a wide range of walking speeds for children with and without CP. This study suggested that heart rate be used to evaluate the child's fitness and to measure energy expenditure.[136] This may be a good method to aid in the decision about which assistive device should be used for the child.

Gait Trainers

Gait trainers were developed to improve ambulation skills in children who can take independent or assisted steps but lack the balance and motor control to walk safely with a traditional walker. The use of gait trainers is an area of debate among PTs. Those that support gait trainers argue that walking practice will allow children to strengthen muscles used in ambulation and eventually the child will progress to a less restrictive mobility device such as a walker. Like standers, gait trainers have been promoted to improve bone mineral density, gastrointestinal function, respiratory efficiency, and social interaction with peers. Others argue that children attempting to ambulate in gait trainers have poor posture in the gait trainer, which is counterproductive to gait. They note that many children will choose to sit in the gait trainer with extreme trunk flexion or extension to move the gait trainer forward or backward without significant weight bearing through the LEs. There is no direct evidence currently supporting or refuting the use of gait trainers.

The features of gait trainers vary greatly between models. A four-wheel base and a solid or sling seat that supports the child who cannot maintain standing or who loses balance while walking are common to almost all gait trainers. Some gait trainers, such as the Rifton Pacer by Rifton Equipment, Inc., have many accessories to improve trunk and LE alignment such as trunk supports, forearm prompts, hip guides, and ankle straps to limit abduction (Fig. 5.3). Other gait trainers are more similar to a partial weight-bearing gait training system and use battery power, pneumatic power (Fig. 5.4), or springs to partially unweight the child during ambulation. These devices typically do not have as many accessories to improve LE alignment with ambulation, making it a poor choice for children with alignment issues that cannot be easily corrected with orthoses, such as scissoring due to severe adductor spasticity.

Walkers

Historically, owing to the lack of other options, children with CP had to use the forward walkers commonly prescribed to older adults. Posterior walkers were developed to address many of the postural issues caused by children using anterior walkers and are now considered the walker design of choice for most children with CP. Posterior walkers are more energy efficient for children with CP, and

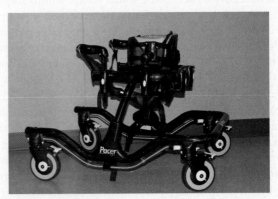

FIGURE 5.3 Rifton Pacer.

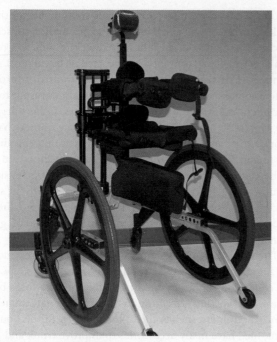

FIGURE 5.4 Up and Go gait trainer.

improve upright posture[137,138] because shoulders are held in greater depression with humeral extension, scapulae tend to be more adducted, leading to greater thoracic extension. The posterior walker may have either two or four wheels. Logan and associates[137] found that the posterior walker with two wheels increased stride length by 41% and decreased double-limb support by 39% over anterior walkers. However, Levangie and colleagues,[138] in their comparison of posterior walkers with four wheels, posterior walkers with two wheels, and anterior walkers, found that the four-wheel posterior walker was more efficient and allowed more significant increases in the child's velocity, right and left stride length, and left step length. The results of the same study found that children walked similarly with anterior walkers and posterior walkers with two wheels.[138] Although this study is important, each child's ambulation abilities and deficits are unique. An evaluation with multiple types of walkers is necessary to determine which walker affords stability and safety while providing for an energy-efficient gait pattern. Several optional accessories are available for posterior walkers such as forearm supports, locking wheels to prevent motion in reverse, swivel wheels, hip guides, and flip-down seats. Forearm supports are common for children with quadriplegic CP because they typically do not have hand, triceps, trunk, and scapular depressor strength to maintain an upright position without forearm supports. Wheels that lock in reverse are often used with children beginning to use a posterior walker who have limited dynamic balance control and trunk stability to prevent the walker from rolling backward with any posterior loss of balance. Swivel wheels should be considered when the child has mastered forward ambulation and would benefit from the increased freedom and speed of turning. Hip guides should be considered when hip abductor strength is insufficient to keep the pelvis in midline as the child walks in the walker. A classic example of a child that would benefit from hip guides is the child whose pelvis is consistently deviated to one side of the walker causing the walker to veer to that side with ambulation. A flip-down seat is an option for the child able to exceed household distances but requires rest breaks for longer walks. For the flip-down seat to be functional, the child must be able to balance briefly with one hand on the walker while rotating the trunk to pull the seat down with the other hand. Consistent reevaluation of a child's ambulation ability is important throughout childhood to determine whether changing these accessories will improve overall function.

Crutches and Canes

Young children with diplegic CP often use upper body strength to substitute for lack of weight-bearing strength of the legs. When taught to ambulate with a posterior walker, this child will frequently rely on the arms for much of the weight bearing and simply "toe-touch" in stance phase or drag the legs. Although functionally mobile with a posterior walker, the walking mechanics are not ideal to promote LE strength, balance, and trunk control for ambulation. For this child, forearm crutches may be a better ambulatory aid as forearm crutches are used primarily to improve balance rather than unweight the LEs. Initially, the child will need assistance to learn to rely on the legs for weight bearing and balance while moving the crutches or canes forward. A four-point gait is initially taught for maximal stability because three points are always in contact with the floor. As the child's coordination and strength improves, a two-point gait pattern and lastly a three-point gait pattern can be recommended to keep up with peers. Although the transition from walker to forearm crutches typically occurs in the early school years for children with spastic diplegia, the slightly more involved older child with spastic diplegia may use a posterior walker for long-distance ambulation. The more involved child may walk with forearm crutches for a shorter distance as the crutches allow for more freedom of movement in the community with fewer architectural barriers than a posterior walker. Some children with mild diplegia or moderate hemiplegia who were independent ambulators in middle childhood may choose one or two forearm crutches in adolescence to minimize falls and increase walking endurance. Axillary crutches are not recommended for children with CP at any point because the children often lack UE control to use them correctly. Children with CP forced to use axillary crutches typically lean forward at the hips and bear most of their weight on the crutches with the axillary pad pressed deep into the axilla. The older child with mild diplegia and normal UE strength may choose a single-point cane as the best long-term device for community-distance ambulation.

▶ Neurologic interventions to treat spasticity

The treatment of spasticity requires a comprehensive evaluation to determine its effects on function, comfort, and ease of care for the child. In addition, treatments for spasticity may prevent secondary problems such as pain, subluxation, and contracture. Of note is that some children have a measure of "control" of their spasticity and learn to use spasticity to assist with standing, transfers, and stepping. In these cases and when treatment will not improve the child's life or ease of care, spasticity treatment should not be considered. Conversely, treatment for spasticity can have a very positive effect on overall function when combined with physical therapy, proper orthoses, and, when appropriate, serial casting.[88] The positive effects from spasticity treatment should not be a substitute for as the benefits will not be realized without proper strengthening, stretching, and functional exercises.

Neuromedical Interventions

Oral Medications

Oral medications are typically used for children with mild or widespread spasticity. Although easy to use, oral medications have side effects such as sedation and may lose their effectiveness within weeks.[10] However, Tilton[88] showed that those sedating effects may improve over several weeks of use. The most commonly used oral spasticity medications for children include diazepam and baclofen. These drugs work by blocking gamma-aminobutyric acid (GABA) in the brain and spinal cord and thereby reduce muscle spasm. Oral baclofen and diazepam both are very sedating, which may impair cognitive functioning of many children who use these medications. Conversely, diazepam taken at night may aid sleep and decrease nightly spasm without daytime carryover of drowsiness.[139] Tizanidine and dantrolene sodium are other oral medications reported to decrease spasticity in children with CP but are not commonly used owing to several negative side effects. There has been little study of the functional effects of any drugs in children, and little is known about optimal dosing, safety, and side effects.

Neuromuscular Blocks

Neuromuscular blocks (also called chemodenervation) are chemicals injected near a peripheral nerve or intramuscularly to prevent nerve–muscle transmission.[88] Phenol and ethyl alcohol were the neuromuscular blocks commonly used to treat spasticity in the 1970s. These chemicals are injected perineurally, causing temporary axonal degeneration, although reinnervation occurred over months to years.[88] Studies have shown improved spasticity with injection of both alcohol[140] and phenol,[141,142] but these chemicals may produce significant pain and dysesthesias after injection, leading to more recent use of botulinum toxin neuromuscular blocks.[143]

Botulinum toxin is a neurotoxin produced by *Clostridium botulinum*, an anaerobic bacteria that typically causes food poisoning and tetanus.[10,88] The botulinum toxin causes temporary muscle paralysis by binding to synaptic proteins at the neuromuscular junctions, thus preventing the junctions from releasing acetylcholine.[10] The binding is irreversible, and the peripheral nerve must sprout a new fiber to form a new neuromuscular junction.[144,145] This process takes approximately 3 to 4 months.[10] Since 1993, BTX-A injections have been used to treat spasticity in those with CP. Because axonal innervation of the neuromuscular junction is eventually reestablished in 3 to 4 months, repeated injections are required to maintain the improvements of the first injections. The injections are separated by at least 12 weeks to decrease the risk of developing neutralizing antibodies.[146] Compared with ethyl alcohol and phenol, Botox has fewer clinical complications, is easy to use, is less painful, can be administered without sedation, and diffuses readily into the muscle; however, it is more expensive with possible shorter-term effects.[143] Kinnette reviewed and analyzed the literature on the actual injections of BTX-A in children and found varying dosing and injection techniques. The total amount of BTX-A injected has increased in the past 10 years without any adverse systemic events reported.[147]

The clinical goals for treating a child with BTX-A often include improved function, prevention or treatment of musculoskeletal complications, increasing comfort, facilitating ease of care, and improving appearance.[146] Benefits from BTX-A include delayed orthopedic surgery, improvement in gait, achieving independent ambulation, improved functional performance in standing and walking, and decrease in spasticity.[143,146,148] These injections must be administered in combination with a therapeutic program of stretching, bracing, and functional exercises to improve the child's maximal level of function.[144–146,149] A recent systematic review assessing Botox injection on walking in CP showed moderate evidence supporting Botox and usual care/physical therapy over physical therapy alone.[150] O'Neil et al. studied physical therapy services to children who received BTX-A injections and found changes in impairments and functional skills. However, she proposed that BTX-A injections are actually adjunctive to the physical therapy and not the reverse, which is commonly accepted. She stated that injections enable the therapist to provide improvement in impairments and function so that goals and outcomes are more easily attained. O'Neil et al.[149] also identified strategies useful in achieving goals and improving outcomes. Fragala et al. studied children's achievements according to the GMFCS after BTX-A injections. She found that children who had higher functional levels at baseline (level I and level II) and had injections in one muscle group versus multiple groups made improvements in ability and the treatment satisfaction level was higher.[145]

Another treatment option is pairing BTX-A injections with periods of serial casting for the injected limb. This combination may prevent contractures and bony deformities, thereby potentially delaying or minimizing the need for multiple orthopedic surgeries later in life. This BTX-A injection/casting combination may achieve joint ROM goals in less time than with casting alone, which may prevent a decrease in ambulation that is sometimes seen after surgical release of the gastrocnemius.[148,151] While several studies have demonstrated advantages using this approach,[148,151–156] other studies have not supported the combination more than casting or Botox alone.[157,158]

Some medical centers use a combination of phenol and BTX-A to treat more muscles in a single episode of anesthesia. Using a retrospective study, Gooch and Patton found that an average of 14 muscles were injected when using the combination. They demonstrated that combined injections reduced muscle tone in the short term, but concluded that further studies are needed to determine optimal dosages and injection sites for both phenol and BTX-A.[159]

Neurosurgical Interventions

Selective Dorsal Rhizotomy

Selective dorsal rhizotomy (SDR), otherwise known as selective posterior rhizotomy (SPR), has been a poorly understood procedure aimed at reducing the spasticity of children with CP.[98,160–163] Patient selection is critical to a good outcome as only two types of patients are appropriate candidates. The first group includes patients who are functionally limited by spasticity but who have sufficient underlying voluntary power to maintain and eventually improve their functional abilities. The second group includes nonambulatory patients whose spasticity interferes with sitting, bathing, positioning, perineal care, and classroom activities.[162,163] The surgery is typically completed across segments L2–S2[160,162] or L2–S1,[163] and only a selected number of dorsal rootlets are sacrificed—those that appear to have the greatest influence on the spasticity and produce abnormal movement patterns.

Intrathecal Baclofen Pump

In addition to being taken orally, baclofen can be delivered to children via a pump surgically implanted subcutaneously or subfacially into the abdomen. A catheter delivers the baclofen from the hockey puck–sized pump to the intrathecal space in the high thoracic region.[164] Many studies have shown the effectiveness of intrathecal baclofen (ITB) in reducing spasticity in children with CP.[165–167] Traditionally, ITB pumps were selected for children with moderately severe spasticity (GMFCS Level IV or V) with the primary goals of decreasing pain/improving comfort, preventing worsening of deformity or function, and improving ease of care.[10,168] In 2011, the results of the largest controlled study of ITB in nonambulatory children with CP determined that ITB decreased tone and spasms, improved comfort and care, but had little impact on function and participation in society 18 months after surgery.[169] Children with minimal or moderate functional limitations were historically not considered candidates for insertion of an ITB pump. A few recent studies, though, have demonstrated improvements in quality of gait[170–172] and improvements of ambulatory status[173–177] in less severely involved children with CP. On the other hand, nonambulatory children are not likely to become ambulatory as a result of ITB pump implantation.[169,178] This has not been proven to be an absolute rule, but realistic goals need to be discussed with the caregivers of nonambulatory children prior to surgery to prevent new ambulation skills from becoming an expectation after surgery. In addition to possible ambulation gains, other studies have shown improvements in overall function as measured by the GMFM in mildly, moderately, and severely involved children with spastic and dystonic CP.[179,180] It should be noted that some children (approximately 12% in two studies[173,176]) showed deterioration of ambulation and transfers after ITB pump implantation, presumably because of decreased ability to use their stiffness and spasticity functionally.[173,176]

The PT has several critical roles before and after ITB pump insertion. The therapist can help to identify clients appropriate for the baclofen pump, assist in the evaluation process to distinguish between spasticity that interferes with function and that which the client is using to function, and assist in setting realistic outcomes prior to surgery. After pump implantation, PTs can assess extremity and trunk tone to assist decision making regarding dosage, help the family and child to become acquainted with bodies that feel and move differently, assess seating for required modifications (such as moving the position of seat belts and trunk supports away from abdominal surgical site), assess new equipment needs, determine rehabilitation service needs, monitor skin integrity, and educate caregivers in postoperative precautions.[168] Postoperative precautions vary among surgeons, but commonly include no hip flexion past 90 degrees, no forced trunk rotation, and lying flat for at least 48 hours after surgery to decrease the incidence of severe headaches secondary to cerebrospinal fluid leaks. Those children with the desired outcomes of increased ease of care and decreased pain will not likely require increased frequency of physical therapy, but those with the goal of functional changes may benefit from a "burst" of therapy starting approximately 1 month after surgery.[168]

▶ Orthopedic interventions

The goal of orthopedic management is to help each individual reach optimal functional ability and prevent deformity

TABLE	
5.5	**Orthopedic Surgery Terms**

Term	Definition
Tendon release/tenotomy	Complete cut of a tendon
Tendon lengthening	Myofascial lengthening of tendon, often via Z-plasty
Percutaneous lengthening	Tendon lengthening involving small cuts into tendon without opening the area for visualization
Recession	Another term used for myofascial lengthening; usually used to differentiate gastrocnemius lengthening only versus entire Achilles tendon lengthening
Osteotomy	Surgical cutting of a bone with the goal of changing the orientation of the bone
Shelf procedure	Refers to a number of pelvic osteotomies that build a shelf superior to the acetabulum to reduce a dislocated hip
Tendon transfer	Involves cutting one end of a tendon and attaching it to another muscle to change or eliminate the presurgical function of that muscle
Arthrodesis	Fusion of at least two bones

through detection at an early stage when simple and more effective treatment options may be instituted.[10,181,182] Physical therapy can help minimize the need for orthopedic surgery, thereby reducing the number of surgeries a child may need. When surgical intervention occurs, the goals of surgery should be to improve function, decrease discomfort, and prevent structural changes that may become disabling.[181]

An understanding of atypical development and movement compensations is necessary to determine how surgery will likely impact the child's future function.

Owing to the fact that children with CP often present with orthopedic impairments at multiple joints, treating only one of these problems may lead to negative consequences at adjacent joints. Therefore, it has become common practice for orthopedic surgeons to perform multiple orthopedic procedures at the same time with the goal of improving overall function. This approach, now commonly known as single-event multilevel surgery (SEMLS), has gained popularity over the past 20 years, especially with access to state-of-the-art comprehensive gait analysis.[183–185] The more common orthopedic problems and surgical procedures involving the spine and LEs will be addressed in the following sections. Refer to Table 5.5 for definitions of surgical terms commonly used and Table 5.6 for common orthopedic surgeries, indications, and postoperative care. General physical therapy interventions are also discussed in the following section. Postoperative protocols can vary greatly depending on the hospital, surgeon, and patient; therefore, the information presented here should be used only as a guide in planning and implementing a therapeutic program.

Spine/Neuromuscular Scoliosis

Spinal deformities are very common in children with CP, with neuromuscular scoliosis being the most common pattern of deformity. Neuromuscular scoliosis is primarily caused by an imbalance between agonist and antagonist muscles in the spine. This imbalance often leads to the development of S-shaped or C-shaped curves in the spine that continue to progress throughout childhood. The incidence of scoliosis is between 20% and 25% in children with CP,[164,186] with the most severe scoliosis typically present in nonambulatory children functioning at Levels IV and V on the GMFCS.[187] Most cases of scoliosis present before the age of 10 years[188] but begin to progress quickly during puberty with curve progression up to 2 to 4 degrees per month.[186] Pelvic obliquity eventually develops owing to the scoliosis extending into the pelvis or hip contracture, which affects the sitting posture in the child's wheelchair. As the curve increases, the adolescent's scoliosis may cause respiratory restriction, pain, pressure sores, and increased difficulty with hygiene management.[187] Unfortunately, neuromuscular scoliosis is not responsive to orthotic management,[186] and there is no evidence supporting the use of stretching, strengthening, joint mobilization, or ES for treatment. The treatment of choice in children older than 10 years with curves greater than 50 degrees and deterioration of functional skills is posterior spinal fusion.[186] This procedure uses a unit rod, a U-shaped rod with a pre-bent pelvic section, that is fixed to the ilium, thereby correcting the pelvic obliquity and scoliosis (Fig. 5.5).[188] It is preferable to delay spinal fusion until the child reaches puberty or has achieved most of the expected growth. The trunk will not be able to grow once the fusion is completed. The complication rate with neuromuscular scoliosis surgery is high, with one study reporting a 68% complication rate. Common complications include pulmonary issues, wounds, hardware failure, curve progression, pancreatitis, and pseudoarthrosis.[189] Despite the high complication rate, caregiver and patient satisfaction rate is high, and the surgery has been shown to significantly improve the quality of life.[187] After surgery, the therapist should evaluate all seating and standing devices as the alteration in alignment can result in skin breakdown and sores if alterations are not completed in a timely manner. There is also increased potential for improvements in respiratory function after surgery as the lungs will generally have more volume for gas exchange and thoracic expansion improves. This should be addressed during postoperative rehabilitation in addition to functional training. A burst of therapy prior to posterior spinal fusion may be beneficial for improving overall spinal mobility as this may decrease the recovery period.

TABLE

5.6	**Common Orthopedic Surgeries for Children with CP**

Surgical procedure	Indications	Complications	Postop Care
Posterior spinal fusion	Neuromuscular scoliosis	Pancreatitis Wound infection	Log rolling only No hip flexion past 90 degrees No forced trunk rotation
Adductor lengthening	Hip subluxation Adductor contracture Scissoring gait Difficulty with perineal hygiene	Reoccurring contracture Heterotopic ossification Overlengthening (rare)	No precautions WBAT
Pelvic osteotomy	Hip subluxation/dislocation	Internal infection Repeat dislocation Loss of fixation	No hip flexion past 90 degrees No forced hip rotation No adduction past midline WBAT
Femoral varus derotation osteotomy	Increased femoral anteversion Hip subluxation/dislocation	Wound infection Femur fracture	No hip flexion past 90 degrees No forced hip rotation WBAT
Iliopsoas release/tenotomy	Hip flexion contracture in nonambulators	Reoccurring contracture Overlengthening	WBAT No precautions
Psoas lengthening	Hip flexion contracture in ambulatory children	Reoccurring contracture Overlengthening	No precautions WBAT
Hamstring lengthening	Hamstring contracture Mild knee flexion contracture	Reoccurring contracture Overlengthening	Knee immobilizer wear 8–12 hr/day
Posterior knee capsulography	Moderate knee flexion contracture	Reoccurring contracture Overlengthening	Strict knee immobilizer use
Rectus femoris transfer	Stiff knee gait	Reattachment of some fibers to quadriceps (rare)	No prone flexion past 90 degrees
Tibial osteotomy	Internal or external tibial torsion	Ankle varus or valgus Compartment syndrome	Short leg cast 6–8 wk WBAT
Tendon Achilles lengthening	Equinus deformity Planovalgus foot	Overlengthening Reoccurring contracture	Short leg casts for 4–6 wk WBAT
Gastrocnemius recession	Gastrocnemius contracture without soleus contracture	Overlengthening Reoccurring contracture	Short leg casts for 4–6 wk WBAT
Subtalar fusion	Severe planovalgus foot	Nonunion Ankle valgus	Short leg casts for 12 wk WBAT
Triple arthrodesis	Severe planovalgus and painful foot	Nonunion Ankle valgus	Short leg casts for 12 wk WBAT
Lateral column lengthening	Planovalgus foot	Reoccurrence of planovalgum	Short leg casts for 12 wk WBAT
Posterior tibialis transfer	Varus foot with tibialis anterior firing throughout swing or stance phase of gait	Over- or undercorrection of varus foot	Casted for 4 wk after surgery WBAT
Anterior tibialis split tendon transfer	Varus foot with tibialis posterior firing throughout stance phase of gait	Over- or undercorrection of varus foot	Casted for 4 wk after surgery WBAT

Hip

A child with CP may require hip surgery for a number of reasons, including to prevent or reduce hip subluxation or dislocation, correct intoeing with ambulation, eliminate scissoring gait, or improve perineal care in a severely impaired child. Hip abnormalities are common in children with CP, with the reported incidence ranging from 2% to 75%.[41]

Femoral Anteversion

Increased femoral anteversion exaggerates hip internal rotation and can severely affect walking by tripping the child when the toe of one shoe catches the opposite shoe during swing. A femoral derotation osteotomy with blade plate fixation (Fig. 5.6), sometimes with medial hamstring release, is the standard surgery for this deformity.[10,190,191] Postsurgical management does not include cast or immobilization,

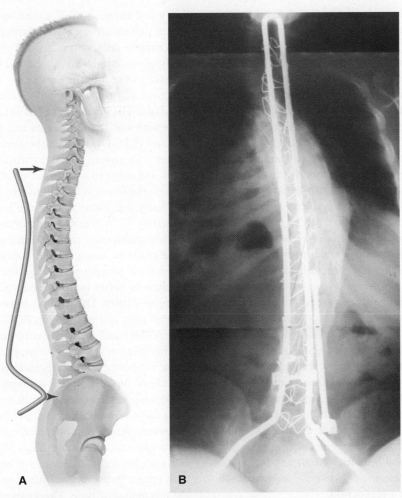

FIGURE 5.5 Posterior spinal fusion: **(A)** Illustration of typical unit pod placement **(B)** Radiograph showing correction of curve with unit rod

and physical therapy begins with PROM on postoperative day 1 or 2. The child is typically transferred out of bed into a wheelchair by day 2. Full weight bearing and assisted ambulation is expected by discharge, which occurs between postoperative days 4 and 7.[10] Physical therapy is directed toward increasing ROM and strengthening the hip muscles for improvement in muscle balance. Functional training is

important for the child to learn new ways of moving with the new hip alignment and possible need for better motor control. Improvement to and beyond presurgical status is expected for up to 1 year.[10] Unilateral hip surgery may result in LLD, which must be considered during treatment and in consultation with the surgeon.

Hip Subluxation/Dislocation

The more severe the neurologic involvement of the child with CP, the greater the chance of hip dislocation or subluxation.[192,193] One study by Soo et al.[193] found that the incidence of hip displacement was 0% for children classified as Level I on the GMFCS and 90% for children classified as Level V on the GMFCS.

To understand the progression of hip abnormalities in children with CP, one must first understand normal hip development. Children with and without CP are born with normal hips that are in an anteverted position. In the normal hip, balanced muscle use during standing and with ambulation promotes development of the acetabulum, femoral head, and remodeling of anteversion. In children with CP, ambulation is key to preventing hip subluxation.

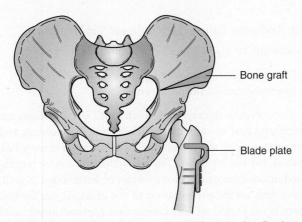

Bone graft

Blade plate

FIGURE 5.6 Pelvic osteotomy with VDRO blade plate fixation.

Children who walk independently by age 5 develop the muscle balance necessary to prevent dislocation. Children using an ambulation aid may develop painless subluxation but seldom require surgical intervention in childhood. The hips of children that do not ambulate may begin to dislocate before age 7.[41] Superior and posterior direction subluxation is the most common pattern of hip subluxation with adductor muscle spasticity being the primary cause of hip subluxation. Passive hip abduction of less than 40 degrees with hips flexed[41] or 45 degrees with hips extended[10] may be indicative of subluxation requiring further evaluation from an orthopedist. Although the adductor longus is the primary offender of the adductor muscles, gracilis and adductor brevis spasticity also contribute to the abnormal forces, resulting in subluxation. The constant cocontraction of the adductors, hamstrings, and hip flexors causes the hips to be held in flexion and adduction and generates excessive forces on the hip. These abnormal and powerful forces usually redirect the femoral head to the superior and posterior aspect of the acetabulum.[41] As subluxation progresses, the femoral head presses up on the lateral edge of the acetabulum, resulting in acetabular flattening and articular cartilage degeneration.[41] In addition to the femoral head changes, the angle of femoral neck inclination remains high and anteversion persists. Electromyography (EMG) studies have implicated spasticity of the medial hamstrings and gluteus medius weakness as the muscle imbalance that leads to the internally rotated position of the hips and persistent femoral anteversion.[41] Left untreated, the femoral head may continue to migrate until it is dislocated. Gamble and coworkers[194] maintain that this process occurs over a 6-year period.

Conservative treatment options to prevent or retard progression of the subluxed hip include neurochemical spasticity interventions and passive muscle stretching of the adductors and hip flexors. ITB can help decrease hip spasticity in moderately to severely involved children, but botulinum toxin is not commonly used owing to the technical difficulty with injections. Proper positioning in a correctly adjusted seating system and consistent standing may slow progression. If progression continues, surgery may become necessary. Surgical management is divided into three basic categories: (1) soft tissue releases to halt early subluxation, (2) soft tissue and bony osteotomies to slow advancing subluxation due to femoral and acetabular dysplasia, and (3) palliative surgery for the painful, arthritic hip.

Postoperative precautions are limited after hip soft tissue releases, which allows for early weight bearing, stretching, and functional strengthening. It is very important to train caregivers to consistently stretch the adductors after surgery to improve the flexibility of the developing scar tissue. Nonadherence to the postoperative stretching protocol will likely reverse hip abduction ROM gains achieved by surgery and further progress the subluxation. Physical therapy must also include muscle strengthening around the hips in order to improve muscular balance between the hip abductors and adductors. Standing activities and gait training with manual

and visual cuing should be used to improve muscle coactivation patterns. For children with progressing subluxation or complete dislocation, femoral anteversion, and acetabular dysplasia, combined muscle and bony surgeries are often necessary to reduce the hip.

Chronic, progressive subluxation leads to acetabular dysplasia. The acetabulum has little potential to remodel, even with soft tissue releases and Varus Derotation Osteotomies (VDROs) to reset the femoral head snuggly in its center.[41] Complete hip reconstruction is indicated in these cases, and refers to a combination of muscle releases, reduction of the femoral head into the acetabulum via VDRO, and lastly, reconstruction of the acetabulum to correct its deformity.[195–198] Acetabular reconstructions, also known as pelvic osteotomies, involve cutting the pelvis and adding bone grafts to create a shelf superior to the acetabulum. These shelf procedures change the orientation of the acetabulum to better hold the reduction of the femoral head after the VDRO. The goal for hip reconstruction is a nearnormal joint and normal hip ROM. Postoperative therapy after VDRO and/or pelvic osteotomies varies depending on the surgeon's postoperative precautions and protocol. Common postoperative precautions after bony osteotomies include no hip flexion past 90 degrees, limited hip rotation ROM, and no hip adduction past neutral. Our facility advocates early mobilization and weight bearing after surgery to prevent skin breakdown, osteopenia, and weakness that occur with immobilization. Typically, the rehabilitation process after hip reconstruction lasts between 6 and 12 months with return to presurgical function usually occurring during this period of time. The focus of postoperative therapy should be on stretching to maintain improved hip abduction ROM, functional strengthening in standing when possible to achieve improved muscle balance around the hips, and proper positioning when seated.

Palliative surgeries for dislocated hips are reserved for children who have failed reconstruction and continue to be painful. Total hip arthroscopy, arthroplasty with a shoulder prosthesis, or resections of the proximal femur are palliative options. The goal of these surgeries is to remove the source of pain and improve function.[10,194,198]

Hip Adductor Contracture without Subluxation

Indications for management of the hip adductors are:

- Improvement in a scissored gait
- Improved care of the perineum

Conservative management such as BTX-A injections are attempted first along with stretching and positioning, and strengthening of the hip abductors to promote muscle balance across the hip joint. The hip adductors can be lengthened in isolation or the iliopsoas can be lengthened as well, depending on the presentation of the child. At our facility, there is no period of immobilization postoperatively and ROM/functional strengthening can be started immediately.[10]

Hip Flexor Contracture

Hip flexion contractures interfere with a standing position because full hip extension becomes impossible. Compensation occurs typically with excessive extension at the thoracolumbar junction, and the knees remain flexed so that body orientation remains vertical. It is difficult to stretch contracted hip flexor muscles because the pelvis rocks forward into an anterior tilt while extension occurs at the thoracolumbar junction. For passive stretching to be effective, the pelvis must be stabilized in either a supine or a prone position. Conservative management includes positioning, typically in prone for activities, while gravity can assist in pulling the pelvis down toward the floor; standing in a stander; and activation and strengthening of the hip extensors, seeking muscle balance across the hip joint. Surgical intervention involves complete cut/resection of the iliopsoas tendon or tendon transfer to the pelvis or hip joint.[10,17,199,200] This procedure is rarely done in isolation but rather as one of multiple surgical sites in a child with greater functional limitations. Physical therapy after surgery should include prone-lying to maximize the lengthening into hip extension and strengthening of the hip extensors and abductors. Facilitation of functional skills should continue, with care taken to prevent a return to the child's previous compensatory patterns of movement.

Knee and Lower Leg

Knee Flexion Contracture

Decreased knee extension ROM is a common finding in children with CP. Despite consistent hamstring stretching, knee flexion contractures often develop. Hamstring contracture may or may not affect function in children with CP and may not require aggressive intervention in all cases.[10] In children with spastic diplegic CP, increased knee flexion in stance phase is often at least partially due to hamstring spasticity and contracture. This flexed knee or "crouched" gait usually includes decreased step length, increased knee flexion in stance, decreased knee extension at terminal swing, increased hip flexion, and increased ankle dorsiflexion in stance. This crouched posture also causes energy inefficiency during gait, partially because of continuous quadriceps firing, which prevents the knee from collapsing into further flexion (see "Gait" section for a more detailed review of crouched gait).[201–203] Persistent knee flexion eventually leads to contracture of the hamstrings and, in more severe cases, knee joint capsule contracture and shortening of the sciatic nerve.[10]

Lengthening tight posterior structures of the knee to prevent further deformity is the goal of treatment for knee flexion contracture. Consistent hamstring stretching is often the first line of defense against contracture. Therapists should teach hamstring stretching before hamstring tightness begins to have an adverse effect on function. BTX-A injection with or without knee immobilizer use is another conservative approach being used with some success to reduce hamstring stiffness. Knee immobilizers can also be used at various times during the day or while the child is sleeping without Botox injections. Providing the child with a standing regimen can also help prevent knee flexion contracture and may help gain length when tightness is not excessive. When conservative management fails, there are three surgical interventions typically available to improve knee extension, depending on the severity of contracture: (1) hamstring lengthening, (2) posterior knee capsulography with hamstring lengthening, and (3) femoral extension osteotomy with hamstring lengthening.

Hamstring lengthening is widely considered to be the surgical procedure of choice for the correction of increased knee flexion.[10,204,205] The hamstrings are usually lengthened distally, and the most common procedures include a combination of Z-plasty/tenotomy of semitendinosus, tenotomy of gracilis, semimembranosus recession/myofascial lengthening, and sometimes biceps femoris recession.[10,203,206] Indications for surgical lengthening of the hamstrings include:

- Severe kyphotic posture in sitting due to shortened hamstrings
- Knee flexion contracture that interferes with walking progression
- Fixed knee flexion contracture greater than 10 degrees
- Popliteal angle of greater than 40 to 50 degrees
- Knee flexion of 20 to 30 degrees at foot contact during gait
- Constant EMG activity of hamstrings during stance and/ or initial swing
- Knee flexion during midstance greater than 20 degrees[10,206–208]

Several studies have demonstrated improvements in knee extension during stance phase after hamstring release, thus decreasing crouch.[209–211] Quadriceps strength at 30 degrees of knee flexion also increases after hamstring lengthening, which is important to prevent progression back into a more crouched posture.[211] Physical therapy begins postop day 1 with knee PROM, bed mobility, weight bearing as tolerated, and family education of knee immobilizer use and stretching. Initially, knee immobilizer use is recommended 2 hours on, 2 hours off during the day and on for the entire night. This wear schedule is eventually weaned down to nighttime only.[10] The importance in teaching the caregivers proper intensity and frequency of hamstring stretching cannot be understated. Following hamstring lengthening, it is recommended that the hamstrings are stretched for 30 seconds three times a day starting postop day 2 and continuing for at least 3 to 4 months after surgery. Careful monitoring of popliteal angle during rehabilitation is used to determine when the frequency can be slowly decreased. Noncompliance with stretching will result in scar formation, with the knee in a flexed position causing a reoccurrence of the original contracture. The outpatient PT should initially focus on improving hamstring flexibility, active/passive knee extension range of motion (AROM/PROM), assisted standing with knees extended (using knee immobilizers and/or AFOs), and strengthening of both knee extensors and flexors (initiated approximately 6 weeks postop) for improved balance across the joint.[10] Despite surgical lengthening, the hamstring muscles have the potential to strengthen to preoperative levels by approximately 9 months after surgery.[205,211] Once lengthened, the hamstring muscle belly recoils, and sacromeres are placed on slack. Over time, the number of sarcomeres in the muscle fibers is reduced to restore optimal filament overlap. This process takes several months and explains the extended time required to increase hamstring strength to the presurgical level. Because the hamstrings cross the knee and hip joints, the therapist must also emphasize ROM and strengthening exercises for the hip musculature. AFOs are often required to control dorsiflexion in standing and with ambulation. Gait training and balance training are often the emphasis of therapy in later phases of rehabilitation, teaching the patient to ambulate and move efficiently in a more upright posture. Functional improvements are not likely to be seen until strength around the knee approximates or exceeds preoperative levels.[205,211]

Although hamstring releases are a relatively simple surgical procedure, there are several noteworthy complications. The most common complication of hamstring lengthening is recurrence of hamstring contracture.[10] This will inevitably lead to return of the crouched/flexed knee gait pattern. In addition to the recurrence of hamstring contracture, crouched gait may return owing to external tibial torsion deformity, quadriceps weakness, or growth spurt.[10,201] Repeat hamstring lengthenings are common due to this functional deterioration, especially if the first surgery occurred in early childhood.[10] Sciatic nerve palsy is also a common complication after hamstring lengthening.[10,203] Hamstring tendon release improves knee extension, but causes the nerves in the popliteal fossa to become taut. These nerves can limit knee extension and can be damaged with aggressive stretching. The PT should evaluate the child for dysesthesias and ability to wiggle the toes immediately after surgery and for the first several weeks after surgery.[203] Foot swelling can also occur in some cases owing to the sympathetic response to the sciatic nerve stretch.[10] Children with postoperative pain managed with an epidural injection are at increased risk for sciatic nerve pain due to the pain medication masking nerve pain and numbness, which allows the patient to tolerate extreme nerve stretches that may lead to prolonged nerve palsy.[203] Genu recurvatum is another complication with hamstring lengthening. Overlengthening results in the hamstring losing the ability to control knee extension in swing phase, thus leading to recurvatum in stance phase.[10,209,210] Knee recurvatum often improves over time, but should be controlled in the short term with a solid or articulating AFO set in slight dorsiflexion.[10]

For more moderate knee flexion contractures (10 to 30 degrees), posterior knee capsulotomy in addition to hamstring release is indicated.[10] Postoperative management is more involved after capsulotomy, with the knees splinted in

extension for 12 to 18 hours per day for 6 weeks and nighttime splinting in extension for up to 6 months.[10] Early knee PROM exercise can prevent knee stiffness, but is much more painful. In addition, the risk for sciatic nerve palsy is greater after posterior knee capsulography, requiring careful grading of hamstring stretching. Severe knee flexion contractures (greater than 30 degrees) are corrected with distal femoral extension osteotomy. Rehabilitation after extension osteotomy is extensive, often requiring therapy for greater than 1 year. Postoperative precautions include knee flexion PROM limited to 90 degrees and knee immobilizer use when not in therapy. Weight bearing may or may not be limited depending on intraoperative fixation.[10]

Stiff Knee Gait due to Rectus Femoris Dysfunction

A stiff knee gait pattern can be caused by several impairments, including decreased hip flexor strength, poor ankle strength, femoral anteversion, tibial torsion, and rectus femoris muscle dysfunction.[10] Rectus femoris transfer is the treatment of choice for decreased knee flexion during swing due to rectus femoris spasticity or inappropriate activation in early to middle swing phase. Botulinum toxin injection prior to surgery can help determine the effect a future rectus transfer may have on gait.

Tibial Torsion

Intoeing or out-toeing due to internal or external tibial torsion are both relatively common in children with CP and typically do not improve with maturity, as seen in children with normal motor control.[17] Like femoral anteversion, internal tibial torsion can cause inefficient gait and tripping. Tibial osteotomy is the only effective surgery to correct internal and external tibial torsion. After surgery, there are usually no precautions or weight-bearing limitations. The lower leg is often casted for 6 to 8 weeks. Rehabilitation is unrestricted after cast removal and should focus on improving walking mechanics and balance. With a more normal foot progression angle, the demands on the plantarflexors and dorsiflexors are changed, requiring specific strengthening to help these muscles handle their new demands.

Ankle and Foot

Equinus Deformity

Equinus, the most common foot deformity in children with CP, results from a muscular imbalance in which the plantarflexors of the ankle are five to six times stronger than the dorsiflexors[10] when there is spasticity around the ankle. In ambulatory children, the hyperactive stretch reflex of the plantarflexors is stimulated during each stance phase, which contributes to the equinus. Spasticity here is manifested as toe-walking, premature heel rise, or premature ankle plantarflexion moment during gait.[10] Children with more severe involvement may have difficulty with foot placement on the pedals of the wheelchair, assisted stand-pivot transfers, and donning of shoes causing a stretch to the triceps surae triggering spastic equinus. Conservative management should include passive stretching, with care taken to "lock" the subtalar joint by slightly inverting the ankle prior to stretching into dorsiflexion; nighttime splinting; and strengthening of the dorsiflexors. A MAFO can help maintain a neutral ankle position, but will neither increase the length of the triceps surae nor allow for any strengthening of the dorsiflexors. If the ankle and foot cannot be brought into a neutral position with the knee in extension, the child will not be able to stand with heels on the ground and will need to compensate in some manner. When an equinus ankle is forced into an orthosis set at 90 degrees, there will be skin breakdown on the heel, or the foot will become hypermobile in the joints distal to the calcaneus. Serial casting offers a conservative method to manage a shortened Achilles tendon, with or without BTX-A injections[144,151,212] (see "Neuromedical Interventions" section). There are a variety of protocols to complete a regimen of serial casting across a joint. Typically, a cast is placed for 1 week with the joint set in the greatest range that does not produce discomfort. The cast should be removed and the child encouraged to play using the mobility at the joint for at least 24 to 48 hours to prevent atrophy of the muscles around the joint and encourage strengthening in the new muscle length that was achieved. The next cast is placed for another week at the new comfortable end range. The number of casts utilized will vary, but the casting trial will continue for 2 to 6 weeks. Care must be exercised to lock the subtalar joint while applying the cast to gain dorsiflexion of the ankle, to ensure stretching of the gastrocnemius/soleus group, and to prevent hypermobility of the subtalar joint.

Tendoachilles lengthening (commonly referred to as TAL) and gastrocnemius recession are the two most common surgical procedures to treat equinus. TAL is most common and is indicated for contracture of both the gastrocnemius and soleus muscle.[10,190,213] For children with normal soleus length and contracture of the gastrocnemius, the surgical procedure of choice is a gastrocnemius recession.[10] The Silverskiod test is often used to determine the difference between soleus and gastrocnemius flexibility (Fig. 5.7A, B) and is used in conjunction with gait analysis to assist with surgical decision making. The gastrocnemius and soleus are two of the most important muscles in ambulation, making the correct amount of lengthening crucial to improving gait mechanics. The goals of lengthening are to decrease triceps surae spasticity, improve heel contact at initial contact, reduce the midstance plantarflexion moment to near normal, and increase power at push-off.[10,214] Reoccurrence or nonimprovement of equinus gait is the most common complication of TAL and gastrocnemius recession with a reported rate of 5% to 40%.[10,214–218] Typically, no more than two total lengthenings are required to treat equinus during childhood. Overlengthening is a less common but much more serious surgical complication, resulting in excessive dorsiflexion in midstance. This gait abnormality

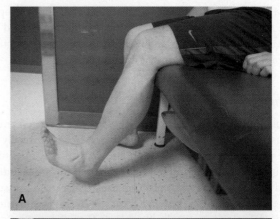

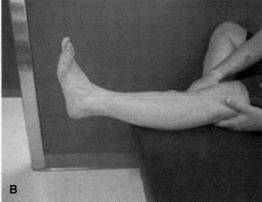

FIGURE 5.7 Silfverskiold test. Measures the difference in flexibility of the gastrocnemius and the soleus muscles. Soleus length is assessed by recording passive range of motion with knee flexed **(A)** and gastrocnemius length is assessed by recording passive range of motion with knee extended **(B)**.

is often referred to as "calcaneal gait"[219] and causes an increased crouched position, which further stretches the plantarflexors and shortens the hip flexors and hamstrings.[10] There is no therapeutic or surgical treatment that can "fix" overlengthening. Long-term and in many cases permanent use of solid AFOs or GRAFOs is often necessary to prevent further progression of crouched gait.

Postoperative care following lengthening or recession requires that a short leg walking cast be worn for 4 to 6 weeks, set in neutral or slight dorsiflexion. Ambulatory children typically are able to tolerate full weight bearing in the walking casts within the first few days after surgery. After removal of the cast, the child's ankle will be quite weak owing to the surgery and weeks of immobilization. It may take several weeks for the child to tolerate standing long periods without the casts. Intermittent solid or articulating AFO use for 3 to 6 months after surgery is recommended to help maintain postsurgical dorsiflexion gains and assist weight bearing with optimal posture. Each child should have an individualized schedule for AFO wear and use the ankle actively when out of the orthosis to facilitate functional strengthening and skill development. It is important to strengthen the entire ankle, especially the dorsiflexors and plantarflexors after surgery. Some clinicians use

NMES or FES to activate the dorsiflexors at the appropriate time. The long-term goal of rehabilitation should be optimal gait mechanics and return to presurgical function approximately 6 to 12 months after surgery.

Planovalgus

A planovalgus foot, also known as a flat foot, is a deformity caused by multiple factors including spasticity (especially of the peroneals or plantarflexors), LE weakness, ligamentous laxity, genetics, and altered biomechanics during standing and walking.[10] This foot position causes increased pressure on the inside of the foot and great toe during ambulation. This deformity is usually flexible at first and can be corrected by reducing the subtalar joint and forefoot to a neutral position with the ankle plantarflexed. In severe cases, the foot eventually turns out so significantly that there is virtually no pressure through the plantar surface of the foot. In most children with CP, though, the planovalgus foot never progresses beyond moderate severity and can be managed with correct triceps surae stretching, ankle strengthening, and orthotic shoe inserts. Three situations contribute to more severe planovalgus deformity: (1) spastic peroneal muscles that change the axis of rotation of the subtalar joint to a more horizontal alignment and abduct the midfoot and forefoot; (2) gastrocnemius/soleus contracture causing plantarflexion of the calcaneus; and (3) persistent fetal medial deviation of the neck of the talus.[42] Most children with CP never require surgical intervention for flat feet,[17] but if the planovalgus deformity causes pain or other functional issues with ambulation, there are several surgical corrections commonly used: (1) lateral column lengthening, (2) subtalar arthrodesis,[190] and (3) triple arthrodesis.[10,190]

Lateral column lengthening (also known as calcaneal lengthening) is usually indicated for the milder, more flexible flat foot. This surgical procedure involves osteotomy of the calcaneus with bone graft used to maintain the osteotomy open after distraction. This osteotomy lengthens the calcaneus with the goal of pushing the foot into a more supinated position.[10] Subtalar motion is moderately restricted after this surgery, but allows greater three-dimensional motion than the subtalar fusion and triple arthrodesis. Postoperatively, the child is placed in short leg walking casts until the osteotomy is healed, which takes approximately 10 to 12 weeks.[17] Subtalar arthrodesis is reserved for more severely planovalgus feet in ambulatory children. Surgery involves inserting bone graft between the talus and calcaneus and then inserting a screw to fuse the bones together in subtalar neutral. Triple arthrodesis is a palliative treatment most often indicated for older children that are nonambulators or marginal ambulators. The surgical procedure involves subtalar fusion surgery as well as fusion of the cuboid to the calcaneus, navicular to the talus, and first cuneiform to the navicular. Postoperative immobilization with a short leg cast after both fusions is also approximately 12 weeks with weight bearing to tolerance. An orthotic will sometimes be used, depending on the results of the surgery and whether the joint(s) require further stability.[10] Owing to joint fusion, the therapist may note joint hypermobility in joints distal to the fusion. This hypermobility should be monitored and may eventually require orthoses to control instability and prevent pain.

Varus Deformity

Varus deformity in the ankle is less common in children with CP and seen mostly in those with hemiplegia and diplegia. It results from imbalance between weak peroneal muscles and spastic posterior or anterior tibialis muscles.[190] The varus foot is very unstable and at risk for inversion ankle sprain. Surgery is often delayed until about 8 years of age. The foot is best managed with splinting, stretching, and strengthening until that time. The indication for surgery is a varus foot in stance or swing phase of gait. Surgical procedures performed for this deformity include lengthening or splitting and transferring of either the posterior or anterior tibialis muscle.[10,190,220–222] Postoperatively, the foot is often casted for 4 weeks in a short leg walking cast in a neutral or slightly dorsiflexed position.[10] After the cast is removed, rehabilitation can be performed without restriction or an orthosis. Therapeutic intervention should emphasize muscle reeducation, particularly when a muscle has been transferred.

▶ Lower extremity orthoses

The decision to use an orthosis and the choice of which orthosis to use should be a collaborative decision between the family, orthopedic surgeon, physiatrist, client, orthotist, and PT. In ambulatory children, the selection should also be based on the understanding of the primary gait deviations.[223] Besides gait observations, the PT's contribution to the team includes assessment of available ROM, passive and active; foot alignment and flexibility during weight bearing and non–weight-bearing situations (structural versus functional deformity); voluntary control of movement in the leg, ankle, and foot; current functional abilities; and the desired functional and participatory outcomes from the device. Because the foot is used for both stability and mobility, the effects of an orthosis on both functions must be considered carefully. It is important to remember that an orthosis will provide stability but will also limit the available movement and any opportunity to strengthen the muscles across the joint being stabilized. Because of this restriction of motion, an orthosis should allow as much motion as possible and only control the undesired movement. There are a variety of options available to allow the medical team to choose the least restrictive and most functional orthoses.

When a child is provided an orthosis, the family should be given a specific wearing schedule to prevent skin breakdown, promote improved function during wearing times, and avoid the atrophy that occurs when a joint or limb is immobilized for an extended period. An orthosis for an infant is rare unless there is a structural deformity that can be influenced by bracing. It is usually when an infant begins consistent weightbearing in standing that a LE orthosis may be considered to manage how the foot contacts the floor.

A common question after fitting a patient with a new LE orthoses is "What type of shoes should we buy?" When answering this difficult question, the therapist must consider the family's resources, the width and intended function of the orthoses and shoes, age of the child, and the environment in which the orthoses will be used. A larger shoe is often required to accommodate the orthosis, but too large a shoe often has a negative impact on gait mechanics. A typical recommendation is not to exceed 1 to 1.5 sizes larger than the shoe size typically worn without the orthosis. Therapist knowledge of shoe brands that are typically wider is helpful in these cases. If the orthoses fit easily into the new shoe when donned for the first time, we recommend trying at least a 0.5 size smaller. An exception to this rule is the nonambulatory child, in which case comfort and ease of donning is of much greater importance than a snug fit. Many LE orthoses today are molded to stabilize the midfoot and forefoot, which reduces the need for a "motion-control" shoe with a good arch support. In general, a low-top, wide shoe with a straight last and an insole that is easily removed may be the best choice for most patients. Shoes are available today that are manufactured specifically for children with LE orthosis, but many common brands of shoes work almost as well.

The following section describes the most common orthoses prescribed for children with CP. Table 5.7 details common indications, contraindications, and special considerations for each type of orthoses, which may also be helpful to therapists for orthoses decision making.

Ankle Foot Orthoses (AFO)

Ankle equinus is the most common joint malalignment in children with CP.[10] For decades, custom-molded AFOs have been the most common method of blocking equinus in children with CP.[224] The modern high-temperature thermoplastics used today for AFOs are able to withstand plantarflexion forces of even the most spastic ankle. Although many variations of AFOs have been studied, there is limited data supporting one type of AFO over another. Figueiredo et al. reviewed the efficacy of AFOs on the gait of children with CP. The authors concluded that AFOs have a positive effect on ankle ROM, gait kinematics and kinetics, and functional activities related to mobility.[225] Unfortunately, as studies with high-quality methods are lacking, it is difficult to conclude which group of children would benefit from which type of AFO.[225] Below, we describe and provide the current evidence supporting the use of the most commonly prescribed AFOs: traditional solid AFOs, articulating AFOs, posterior leaf spring (PLS) AFOs, and ground reaction ankle foot orthoses (GRAFOs). It should also be noted that there are many styles and designs of each type of AFO including the tone-reducing, thin-plastic, wrap-around design commonly used with many children with CP. This design of AFO, commonly referred to as a dynamic ankle–foot orthosis (DAFO), was created and popularized by Cascade DAFO, Inc. Although DAFOs are not a different-"type" AFO, this section will also discuss how this design differs from traditional AFO designs.

Solid Molded Ankle–Foot Orthoses

A solid MAFO with anterior tibial strap and anterior ankle strap is a common orthotic design to provide ankle and foot stability, giving a stable base for children to stand. The thick, high-temperature thermoplastic, absence of an ankle joint, and high calf design of this traditional orthosis allows maximum medial lateral ankle stability and maximum knee stability in standing, and can resist strong plantarflexor spasticity. The solid AFO has also been shown to increase the plantarflexor moment in terminal stance,[226] normalize ankle kinematics in stance,[227] increase stride length,[227,228] and improve the performance of walking/running/jumping skills as measured by the GMFM.[227] A study conducted by Buckton et al.[227] concluded that most children with spastic diplegia would benefit functionally from a solid AFO or PLS-AFO. The solid AFO is also a good choice for the child with severe equinovarus or equinovalgus deformity. Articulating MAFOs, PLS-AFOs, and DAFOs do not control midfoot and forefoot deformity well and would eventually lead to greater foot deformity. Solid AFOs are also commonly prescribed for children who are short-distance ambulators or nonambulators. The short-distance ambulator with significant crouch often requires a more traditional, thicker-plastic, solid AFO to minimize excessive dorsiflexion and knee flexion. The main purpose of an AFO for a nonambulating child with CP is to improve ankle position and prevent contracture. Comfort and prevention of skin breakdown is important, and a simple, well-padded solid AFO is a great choice to improve ankle position, minimize skin issues, and allow easy application for the caregiver. The drawbacks of this orthosis include overall bulkiness of the plastic, making it difficult for caregivers to find shoes that fit this type of brace, decreased distal muscle activation when balancing in standing,[229] and a negative effect on dynamic balance with functional activities such as transitions to standing and stairs. An elastic proximal tibial strap is sometimes used to allow a small amount of passive dorsiflexion, thus making it slightly more dynamic in standing.

Articulating Ankle–Foot Orthoses

An articulating AFO includes an ankle articulation, allowing free dorsiflexion and plantarflexion or free dorsiflexion with a plantarflexion stop. The most frequently prescribed articulating AFO used with children with CP allows free dorsiflexion with a plantarflexion stop. These orthoses inhibit plantarflexion hypertonus while permitting free dorsiflexion, thus giving the child increased ease in rising to stand, negotiating stairs, and ambulating. By allowing free ankle dorsiflexion and some plantarflexion, they also

TABLE 5.7 Guide to Orthoses Selection for Children with CP

Orthoses	Solid Molded Ankle–Foot Orthoses (MAFO)	Dynamic Ankle–Foot Orthoses (DAFO)	Articulated MAFO
Description	Full calf height Proximal tibial strap Dorsal ankle strap	3/4 to full calf height Dorsal ankle strap Forefoot strap With or without proximal tibial strap Thin plastic Full ankle contact with overlapping vamp	Full calf height Proximal calf strap Dorsal ankle straphinge, allowing free dorsiflexion or limited dorsiflexion Plantarflexion stop posteriorly
Indications	Over 1 yr old to adult Moderate to severe ankle plantarflexor spasticity; moderate to severe genu recurvatum with ambulation; mild to moderate crouched gait	At least 1 yr old Moderate to severe ankle plantarflexor spasticity; moderate to severe genu recurvatum with ambulation; better midfoot and forefoot control than solid MAFO	Over 2 yr old to adult Control plantarflexion and allow active dorsiflexion Control of midfoot and forefoot Moderate to severe genu recurvatumNear-normal DF PROM Good hip and knee controlNormal thigh–foot angle
Contraindications	Severe equinus contracture Severe foot deformity Severe crouched gait	Severe equinus contracture Severe crouched gait Large children Severe foot deformities	Severe equinovarus or planovalgus feet No dorsiflexion PROM Crouched gait
Special considerations	Better than DAFO for heavier children/adolescents Good for nonambulatory children for ankle positioning Easy to don	Good choice for younger children with developing standing and ambulation Difficult to don	Good choice for the part-time ambulator with genu recurvatum

Orthoses	Posterior Leaf Spring AFO	Ground-reaction AFO (GRAFO)	Supramalleolar Orthoses (SMO)
Description	Full calf height Plastic trimmed posteriorly above malleoli and sometimes below the malleoli Dorsal tibial strap Ankle and forefoot straps in DAFO model	Solid AFO with proximal anterior plastic Ankle strap	Plastic stops just proximal to malleoli
Indications	Older child, usually more than 10 yrs old, and over 45 lbs, control plantarflexion in swing and stance Plantarflexor tone mild enough to allow ankle to dorsiflex in midstance to terminal stance Controls mild genu recurvatum	Moderate to severe crouched gait Heavier child that solid AFO does not provide enough stability	Over 2 yr old to adult Moderate to severe planovalgus or equinovarus feet
Contraindications	Equinus contracture Foot deformity Crouched gait Thigh–foot angle malalignment Heavy children	Knee flexion contracture more than 10 degrees Severe planovalgus or equinovarus deformity Severe thigh–foot angle malalignment	Ankle equinus Heavier children with severe foot deformity
Other considerations	Must have good hip and thigh control	If lighter than 60 lbs, an AFO with wide proximal strap may be a better choice	Good choice for younger patient who needs a little ankle control during gait development

encourage ankle activation, which may help strengthen the muscles crossing the ankle joint. Significant biomechanical changes were found when the ankle was given freedom to move with an articulating AFO. The benefits included more natural ankle motion during stance, increased stride length, and greater symmetry of segmental LE motion.[226,230–232] Buckton et al.[227] noted that an articulating AFO has a detrimental effect on the gait in some children with diplegic CP, including increased peak knee extensor moment in early stance (leading to recurvatum), excessive ankle dorsiflexion (which would contribute to crouch), and decreased walking velocity. Night splinting with an articulating AFO combined with an adjustable strap attached at the footplate by the toes can be used in some children to increase the length of the gastrocnemius/soleus group by maintaining a prolonged stretch into dorsiflexion (Fig. 5.8). Low-load prolonged stretch of the gastrocnemius is an ideal way to slowly improve dorsiflexion in some children. Lack of comfort and disturbed sleep are common concerns for therapists and families with this type of orthoses. A recent study by Mol et al.[233] refutes that claim and found no statistical significance in sleep disturbances between children using and not using night orthoses.

Posterior Leaf Spring Orthoses

A PLS orthosis is an AFO primarily used for patients with foot drop, but with some stability in stance phase.[234] The PLS-AFO design, with the thermoplastic trimmed posteriorly to the malleoli, is strong enough to prevent plantarflexion during swing and stance but flexible enough to allow some anterior tibial translation and dorsiflexion

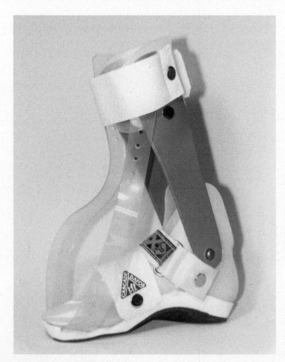

FIGURE 5.8 Nighttime AFO.

from midstance to the beginning of terminal stance. The PLS-AFO is also proposed to have a "spring effect" at pushoff. When the posterior plastic is put on tension as the ankle dorsiflexes, energy is theoretically stored in the plastic and then released to assist plantarflexion during terminal stance. This is reported to decrease fatigue with ambulation in some children with CP. There are multiple strut thicknesses and carbon fiber options available to grade the amount of tibial translation and "spring effect" during ambulation. Thicker plastic posteriorly and/or posterior reinforcement with carbon fiber may be necessary to control more severe crouch in larger children. Ounuu et al.[234] found that the PLS-AFO design improves dorsiflexion during swing and initial contact and allowed normal dorsiflexion in midstance but does not improve the power-generating capabilities of the ankle in children with CP as its name suggests. Careful consideration should be made prior to choosing this AFO design for a child with CP owing to its decreased overall stability and decreased subtalar, midtarsal, and forefoot control. For children with foot deformities, PLS-AFOs can now be combined with a supramalleolar orthosis (SMO) insert to provide the necessary foot stability.

Ground-Reaction Orthoses

The ground-reaction (also known as floor-reaction) AFO is commonly prescribed for ambulatory children who walk with excessive dorsiflexion and knee flexion (crouched gait) during the stance phase of gait.[223] A floor-reaction brace is both a stance and swing control orthosis designed to provide increased resistance to both ankle dorsiflexion and plantarflexion.[223] A DAFO or traditional AFO also helps control crouch in younger children with CP, but as a child's crouched gait approaches 55 degrees, a more supportive floor-reaction orthosis is often required. The floor-reaction AFO is more rigid because of increased plastic thickness, a broad anterior wall (supporting either proximal tibial only or whole length of lower leg), and in some cases carbon fiber reinforcement.[223] This rigidity provides superior resistance to the strong knee flexion and dorsiflexion moment in second rocker of stance phase. To benefit from this type of orthosis, the child must have at least neutral dorsiflexion with the knee extended and less than 20 degrees of internal or external tibial torsion.[10] This orthosis has traditionally not been ideal for children with severe foot malalignments, but newer designs (such as one utilizing an SMO placed within the outer AFO shell) make it an option now for some children with less severe foot deformities. Rogozinski et al. concluded that the best outcomes with floor-reaction orthosis, as determined by peak knee flexion in midstance, occurred when children had knee and hip flexion contractures less than or equal to 10 degrees. The efficacy of the orthosis in controlling peak knee flexion in midstance was poor in children with knee and hip contractures greater than or equal to 15 degrees, thus making the floor-reaction orthosis a poor choice in these children.[223]

Dynamic Ankle–Foot Orthoses

In the past 20 years, inhibitive or DAFOs have become very popular as an alternative to conventional AFOs. DAFOs evolved from inhibitive casts used during the 1970s.[235] Inhibitive casts were purported to decrease spasticity by prolonged stretch and pressure on the tendons of the triceps surae muscle and toe flexors and to inhibit or decrease abnormal reflexes in the LE by protecting the foot from tactile-induced reflexes.[236] The footplate in a DAFO is a custom-contoured plate similar to that used with inhibitive casting. It has built-up areas under the toes, lateral and medial longitudinal arches, and a transverse metatarsal arch with recessed areas under the metatarsal and calcaneal pad areas. These features provide support and stabilization to the arches of the foot and position the midtarsal and subtalar joints in a neutral position.[236] "The footplate is designed to reduce abnormal muscle activity and to effect biomechanical changes, including decreased excessive ankle plantar flexion and improved motions of the lower extremity, pelvis, and trunk during standing and gait."[236] Evidence supporting molding the DAFO footplate with pressure points to inhibit tone is very limited, although this is still commonly used in DAFO designs.[10,237] The DAFO also differs from a traditional AFO in that it provides total contact to the ankle with its wrap-around design. The circumferential design with overlapping vamp may improve proprioception, distribute forces over a larger area of skin, and improve overall alignment, but often makes it more difficult for the child or parent to don the orthosis. Because it requires two hands and considerable strength to open the DAFO, many children may not become independent donning this orthosis. Strapping options on a DAFO include a toe loop to stabilize the first digit, a forefoot strap to control forefoot position, and an ankle strap over the talus that holds the heel down into the heel cup. The DAFO is also made of a thinner, more flexible plastic that allows graded motion unlike the rigid 3/16 inch plastic used in most traditional solid AFOs. This thinner plastic cannot withstand high-stress environments, thus making it ineffective for many patients. The thin, total-contact design also cannot be easily modified if skin problems arise or the child has a growth spurt, limiting the overall life of the orthoses.

The effect of DAFOs on gait mechanics and function has not been extensively studied. Currently, there is conflicting evidence that DAFOs significantly change gait parameters or walking kinematics.[228,232,236,238] Radtka[236] found that both DAFOs with a plantarflexion stop and traditional AFOs increased stride length, decreased cadence, and reduced excessive ankle plantarflexion when compared with no orthoses. Lam et al. demonstrated additional biomechanical gait benefits with the DAFO use compared with the traditional AFO. Specifically, study subjects wearing DAFOs demonstrated increased knee flexion at initial contact compared with traditional AFOs.[228] Carlson et al.,[238] on the other hand, found that neither AFOs nor DAFOs significantly influenced stride length or walking speed. The DAFO also was not found to have much effect on walking kinematics.[238] Romkes and Brunner[232] also concluded in their 2002 study that DAFOs did not improve gait significantly but hinged AFOs did improve gait.

On the other hand, recent evidence suggests that DAFOs have a positive effect on gross motor function and balance in children with CP. Bjornson et al.[239] reported significant improvements in crawling/kneeling, standing, and walking/running and jumping skills as measured by the GMFM 88 and 66 with short-term DAFO use. Burtner et al.[229] investigated balance differences between children wearing solid AFOs and DAFOs. Their study showed that children wearing the more rigid AFO had a decreased ability to respond to balance threats and substitute with an alternate balance strategy. These issues did not occur in the children wearing DAFOs, suggesting that DAFOs are more advantageous for children with spastic CP when balance is perturbed unexpectedly, such as being bumped into by a classmate or standing on a moving object such as a bus that slows down or speeds up suddenly.[229]

Supramalleolar Orthoses

The SMO is typically indicated for the child with good ankle plantarflexion and dorsiflexion control but who needs control of planovarus or planovalgus foot position. The SMO typically has trim lines anterior and superior to the malleoli and a molded footplate providing control at the subtalar joint, midfoot, and forefoot. An anterior ankle strap is occasionally necessary to improve the effectiveness of the SMO.[10] The wrap-around thin-plastic design found in the Cascade DAFO, Inc.–style SMO is often a good option in younger patients, but may not be strong enough to control the foot in larger or adolescent patients.[10] SMOs have been shown to improve balance in children with Down syndrome[240] and those with hemiplegia,[241] but studies on the efficacy of SMO use in children with CP are limited.[242–244]

Foot Orthoses

When the child with CP has control of the ankle joint but requires external support when the foot contacts the floor, a foot orthosis is desirable. For children with CP with good ankle and knee control but poor midfoot and forefoot alignment, a foot orthosis may be beneficial. Foot orthoses include the University of California Berkley Laboratory (UCBL) orthoses and arch supports. UCBL trim lines are inferior to the medial or lateral malleoli, but proximal enough to support the navicular and thus control excessive pronation. The footplate can be proximal or distal to the metatarsal heads, dependent on each child's unique needs. Foot orthoses can be custom-molded or purchased over the counter from a variety of resources.

Use of a shoe insert is indicated for the following:

- Control of the calcaneus, subtalar, and midtarsal joints
- Improved alignment and stability of the LEs and pelvis
- Management of the forefoot for neutral positioning
- Knee pain secondary to foot pathology

Combining Orthoses

A recent trend in orthotics is to order a brace with multiple parts to provide multiple brace options for the child. One such product is the DAFO TURBO (Cascade DAFO, Inc., Bellingham, WA), which is a combination of an SMO and AFO. This can be a great choice for the young child with spastic- or hemiplegic-type CP. The SMO piece can be used for functional activities that require free dorsiflexion/plantarflexion, and the combined orthoses can be used when more ankle stability is required. This combination orthoses is also commonly prescribed for the child with such severe plantarflexor spasticity that donning a traditional DAFO is extremely difficult for the caregiver. This design allows the caregiver to more easily don the SMO piece first without having to worry about maintaining ankle dorsiflexion. Once the SMO piece is donned, it is easily slipped into the AFO piece without worry of plantarflexor tone pushing the heel out of the orthoses.

Home management

A home management program is an essential part of the overall treatment plan for the infant or child with CP, as the ultimate outcome is the most independent function the infant or child can possibly attain over time. The home program should be designed to reinforce movements, positions, and skills that have been practiced in the physical therapy sessions, and to assist in preparing the infant or child for the next session. The therapist must consider the daily routine of the infant/child and family when planning activities for the home and family and the obligations that are inherent in running the household. Perhaps there are siblings, extended family members, and/or multiple generations living in the household who can be facilitators to progress or sometimes barriers, dependent on the demands of the remainder of the household. Siblings can be very valuable in assisting with the home program and incorporating activities and movements into an established routine. "The unique, spontaneous and competitive interaction of siblings offers increased incentives for functional independence."[245]

The household demands will change over time, as will the child's needs, making it mandatory to review and upgrade the home program during each therapy session. Movements, positions, and skills that are incorporated into the activities of daily living and play of the infant/child are more likely to be carried out than a separate, formal exercise regimen. The therapist must also realistically consider the other non–child-related demands placed on the parents/caregivers.

Tetreault et al. studied the compliance of families of children with global developmental delay given a home activity program. The activities given to the parents addressed caring for their child in the home and the actual physical care of the child. This study recommended that the activities be imbedded in the daily routine to promote more practice opportunities and facilitate generalization. They found a compliance rate of 75.6% after 7.5 to 8.5 months.[246]

Therapeutic movement and activity for the infant can be easily incorporated into daily care activities. Therapeutic handling aimed at increasing movement can be done during routine activities, such as diapering, dressing, feeding, bathing, carrying, and lifting the baby from a supported position. A simple way to carry over positioning and hip ROM for an infant or young child is to teach the parents/caregivers specific ways to carry him or her that will add ROM and dissociation of the hips every time the infant is carried. Another idea is to have the young child stand (with or without support) every time the pants are managed, as in dressing, undressing, potty training, and toileting. This reinforces weight bearing through the legs, proprioception, and perception of self as a vertical being. To reinforce proximal strength and balance via routine, the child can be encouraged to sit on a stool or the side of the bed and don a shirt as independently as possible. An ambulatory child should be encouraged to walk to a household event or task such as coming to the dinner table or walking to the bathroom whenever the opportunity presents itself. Ideas such as these are more likely to be maintained as a home program than would be a 30-minute period of PROM and exercise on a daily basis. These are examples only and are not meant to be a child's home program. Each infant or child is a unique entity along with the caregivers and household, and must therefore be treated individually with creativity and understanding. There will be events in the child's life that require a more intensive home program such as postsurgery or during a growth spurt. If the family can manage the routine activities on a regular basis, the times for increased intervention may be less stressful.

For the child who has an interest in other activities, a therapist might recommend taking up a musical instrument, therapeutic horseback riding, therapeutic aquatics, or any other activity that coincides with and reinforces the desired functional outcomes of the child (see "Community Programs" section for the alternative interventions).

School-based therapy

Communication between the school therapist and the child's teacher is essential for appropriate and effective management and education of the child in the classroom. The therapist should obtain information from the teacher regarding the child's daily routine at school. With that information, joint planning for the child can result in an effective and efficient educational program. Major areas of emphasis in school-based therapy services include evaluating any barriers to independence in the classroom or school, evaluating alignment at different times during the day while the child is sitting in their personal wheelchair or classroom seat, and evaluating the opportunities available to stand, and when applicable, ambulate safely. Consistent movement throughout the day, such as standing, walking between activity centers in the classroom, or participating in physical education class, will provide relief from the sitting position. There should be a sharing of the responsibility, assistance, and supervision required between the classroom staff and the child for quantity and quality of position changes and movement. The physical education teacher should be informed of joint movement goals and specific types or patterns of movement that may either be deleterious or beneficial for the child. There should also be a review conducted with teachers for the purpose of and proper use of splints, orthotics, and other assistive or adaptive devices. For full details of enhancing the child's function in the school system, please refer to Chapter 21.

The occupational therapist will share information about the child's fine motor, visual motor, visual perception, visual discrimination, and manipulation skills; attention span; cognition; sensory system modulation; emotional level; and adaptive self-help skills. The speech pathologist will inform the team about the child's speech and language capabilities. This information, along with specific suggestions, should facilitate learning for the child.

Therapists should not expect teachers to handle children therapeutically for the purpose of obtaining postural control. A more realistic expectation would be maintenance of correct alignment, relief from sitting, use of adaptive or assistive devices, and attention to issues regarding safety. The therapist must recognize the teacher as an important ally in the therapeutic arena.

SUMMARY

This chapter explores the unique challenges facing children with CP, as they often present with a wide range of neuromuscular, sensory/perceptual, and cognitive concerns. It is the role of the PT to design a plan of care that focuses primarily on the child's individual needs and desired functional outcomes. To be effective in the assessment, evaluation, and treatment of the infant and child with CP, the PT must consider the complex needs of the child as well as the family. To this end, it is imperative that the PT maintain open communication with the child, the family/caregiver, and the rest of the interdisciplinary team. The ultimate outcome of treatment is to help the child maximize his or her functional independence to become a contributing member of the family and larger community.

CASE STUDIES

CASE STUDY 1 Ella is a 5-year-old girl with a diagnosis of left hemiplegic-pattern CP referred to outpatient physical therapy owing to decreased left LE flexibility, increased gait dysfunction, and poor overall balance. Ella's parents express concern about Ella's safety at school and on the school playground, as she will enter kindergarten in the fall.

Past Medical History

Ella is a bright and happy 5-year-old girl who was diagnosed with left hemiplegia at 3 years of age. She was born full term at 38 weeks' gestation. During the birthing process, a fetal monitor showed frequent fluctuations in Ella's heart rate, indicating distress. For this reason, immediately following her birth, she underwent an MRI to determine whether any cerebral insult occurred. This neuroimaging showed a grade IV intraventricular hemorrhage, enlarged lateral ventricles with the right ventricle larger than the left, increased head circumference, and bulging fontanels. At this time, she also presented with nystagmus. She underwent a shunt placement at 3 months of age owing to congenital hydrocephalus. She was evaluated at 6 months of age by an ophthalmologist who diagnosed her with cortical visual impairment, optic atrophy, and severe visual impairment. An orthopedic surgeon, who gave Ella the diagnosis of left hemiplegia after her third birthday, has also followed her from infancy.

Developmental History

Ella participated in occupational therapy, physical therapy, and speech and language therapy from birth owing to concerns related to overall developmental delay. She was provided all of these services in her home through an early intervention program to address functional concerns that arose from her left hemiplegia, decreased mobility, and decreased vocalizations. At 5 months, Ella was able to roll from supine to prone and vice versa, initiating both transitions by arching through her back and neck. She was able to sit independently at 11 months, but preferred a "W" position. At 18 months, she began creeping with an asymmetrical "bunny hop" pattern. At 21 months, Ella was able to stand independently with right UE support at the family couch and cruise in both directions; however, she preferred to cruise to the right. At 24 months, Ella took her first independent steps, and was walking consistently without an assistive device at 30 months.

Physical Therapy Examination

Precautions: Ventriculoperitoneal (VP) shunt

Pain: According to the Wong Backer Faces Pain Scale, Ella reported a 0/10 pain level related to activities of tasks.

ROM: Right hip, knee, and ankle: within normal limits (WNL); left hip flexion: 100 degrees, left hip extension: 10 degrees, left knee extension: WNL, left popliteal angle: 35 degrees, left ankle dorsiflexion (DF) with knee extension: 2 degrees, left ankle DF with knee flexed: 10 degrees; right shoulder, elbow, and wrist: WNL; left shoulder flexion: 100 degrees, left elbow flexion: WNL, left elbow extension: 10 degrees, left wrist flexion: WNL, left wrist extension: 15 degrees.

Strength: Manual muscle testing (MMT) bilaterally: right hip, knee, and ankle: 5/5; left hip flexion: 3/5; left hip abduction: 2/5; left hip adduction: 2/5; left knee extension: 3/5; left prone knee flexion: 2+/5; left ankle DF: trace.

Tone: MAS: left quadriceps: 1/5; left hamstrings: 2/5; three-beat clonus in left ankle.

Sensation: Intact to light touch, hot and cold, sharp and dull.

Functional mobility: Ella is able to transition from sit-to-stand with increased weight shift to the left. She is able to transition from floor to standing through half-kneel leading with right LE and pulling up on an object using right UE. She is unable to hop on the left foot, but can hop three times in a row on the right. She fatigues quickly and is not able to keep up with her peers on the playground.

Gait/steps: Ella is able to ambulate independently with an asymmetrical gait pattern. She presents with decreased stance time and weight shift on the left in stance phase, has a shortened step length on the left, a retracted pelvis on the left, stiff knee on the left during swing, and initial contact with her forefoot on the left. She is noted to have inconsistent mild knee recurvatum during midstance on the left as well. She is able to ascend standard steps with a step-two pattern holding a railing with her right hand leading with her right foot. When descending steps, she leads with her left foot while holding the railing with her right hand.

Balance: Single-limb stance on the right for 5 to 8 seconds; left less than 1 second.

Equipment: Ella has a solid AFO for her left LE, but parents report that she has not worn them in the past 9 months owing to skin irritation and Ella complaining of pain whenever she wore it.

Physical Therapy Assessment/Prognosis

Ella is a 5-year-old girl with a diagnosis of left hemiplegia. She presented with left LE weakness, decreased ROM, decreased endurance, gait deficits, and difficulty keeping up with her peers. Overall, her prognosis was favorable. She would be able to safely attend her local public elementary school with some necessary accommodations. She would benefit from continued school-based services as well as medical-model therapies to support her following a change in status or other medical interventions. She is also involved in a community dance class, which allows her to interact with her peers as well as work on balance and strengthening in a fun and social setting.

INTERVENTION (Physical therapy one to two times a week)

Stretching: Stretching left hip extensors, left hamstring, left gastrocnemius, and soleus, three repetitions with a 30-second hold for each stretch.

Strength training: Strengthening of left and right LEs was addressed through play skills, as a formal strengthening program was not appropriate due to Ella's age. Activities included side-stepping, transitions on and off the floor and from sit-to-stand, and forward and lateral step-ups.

Therapeutic handling: Therapeutic ball work to address core strengthening, postural control, and left LE strengthening and stretching; facilitation of agonist/antagonist muscle groups during transitions to promote postural alignment and equal weight shifting.

Bracing: After Ella achieved 2 degrees of knee-extended dorsiflexion PROM with regular stretching, an articulating, thin-plastic, total-contact design AFO (Cascade DAFO 2) was recommended for use 6 to 8 hours per day. With her new AFO, Ella almost immediately demonstrated consistent left heel strike, no genu recurvatum, and improved weight shift to the left during stance phase.

Gait training: Gait training focused on improving heel strike at initial contact on the left, weight shifting to the left during stance phase, stride length on the left, and pelvic–femoral mobility due to pelvic retraction on the left.

Patient/parent education: Home program consisted of stretching and strengthening activities associated with the goals that were being addressed during treatment.

Discharge/continuum of care: Ella's parents have been intimately involved in all intervention decisions and have been excellent advocates for all her needs. She has benefited from a variety of interventions at home, in the medical model, and now in school, and within the community. Ella will most likely continue to make progress toward a productive, full life with her family and friends, given the therapeutic and external supports necessary.

CASE STUDY 2   Thomas is a 12-year-old boy with a diagnosis of spastic quadriplegic CP referred to outpatient physical therapy 1 week after extensive surgical interventions including bilateral varus derotation osteotomies, a right Dega procedure, bilateral adductor and hamstring lengthenings, and bilateral lateral column lengthenings.

Past Medical History

Thomas has an extensive medical history. He was born at 29 weeks' gestation and spent 6 weeks in the neonatal intensive care unit (NICU), during which time he was orally intubated for 2 days, then placed on supplemental oxygen via nasal cannula. He had a feeding tube and several other intravenous lines placed during his NICU stay. He underwent cranial ultrasound to determine the extent of his neurologic insult; however, this assessment did not reveal neuroanatomical changes. Thomas had an echocardiogram to rule out cardiac involvement without significant findings. He was discharged from the NICU with an apnea monitor due to respiratory concerns.

Thomas progressed slowly with his gross and fine motor milestones and often used atypical movement patterns to move. At 6 months, he was able to roll from supine to and from prone, but initiated movement with neck and back extension while rolling his body as a complete unit. Thomas was not able to activate his trunk flexors to allow dissociated movement of his UEs from his LEs while rolling. He first attained stability in sitting using a "W" sit pattern, with an anterior pelvic tilt, bilateral hip internal rotation and adduction, knee flexion, and ankle dorsiflexion. Thomas' truncal hypotonicity made sitting without assistance or external support difficult and inefficient. He was able to ring-sit and side-sit with minimal to moderate physical assistance.

By 18 months of age, he was able to maintain ring-sitting with bilateral UE support and close supervision. He attempted to creep; however, owing to poor lower limb dissociation was unable to coordinate the sequence needed to reciprocally creep. He moved around his environment by advancing both arms alternately, then both legs simultaneously using extensor tone to initiate the movement, with poor ability to sustain LE hip flexion.

At 18 months, Thomas underwent his first eye surgery due to retinopathy of prematurity (ROP). This was followed by a second eye corrective surgery when he was 2.5 years old. Following his second eye surgery, his visual perception notably improved during ambulation. Gait training was initiated using a gait trainer with a trunk support, hip guides, bilateral ankle prompts, bilateral forearm prompts, and tilted handgrips to accommodate hand placement. By the time Thomas was 2.5 years old, he had progressed from a gait trainer to a posterior walker with hip guides. He ambulated with poor trunk rotation, increased adduction bilaterally during swing phase causing forefoot to hit heel of stance-phase leg ("scissoring"), decreased terminal knee extension in stance phase due to tight hamstrings (crouched posture), and initial contact at his forefoot/toes due to increased plantarflexor tone and decreased ankle ROM. Owing to his inefficient and effortful gait pattern, Thomas used a manual wheelchair for long distances.

To address the spasticity of his LE, he had two rounds of Botox injections to his hamstrings bilaterally, gastrocnemius, and adductors when he was 3 and 3.5 years old and again when he was 4 years old. He underwent bilateral hamstring lengthenings at age 6. At that time, he also had an adenoidectomy to resolve persistent snoring and difficulty sleeping. At age 8, he underwent a third round of Botox injections to the medial and lateral heads of the gastrocnemius on both legs to address increased plantarflexor tone. This was done in an effort to delay the need for further surgical intervention and improve ambulation ability.

Thomas was involved in therapy from a young age. He participated in home-based early intervention services for the first year of life, received physical and occupational therapies at a children's hospital on an outpatient basis, then moved into weekly school-based services at the age of 5. He had both medically based physical therapy and occupational therapy at a frequency of one to three times a week until the age of 9. Treatment was typically once a week; however, it was increased to two to three times a week following Botox injections and hamstring lengthenings. His family was very involved in his care and was consistent in helping Thomas carry over a home exercise program, which changed as his functional abilities improved. Owing to Thomas' involvement in school activities and his improved functional mobility, medically based physical therapy transitioned to a consultative basis at the age of 9 and was reinitiated following surgery.

Prior Level of Function

Thomas underwent extensive surgical intervention at the age of 12 owing to continued growth, weight gain, increased LE spasticity and contractures, increased crouch gait pattern, pain, poor bony alignment, and decreased ability to move around within his home and classroom.

Functional mobility: Prior to surgery, Thomas was able to transition from sit-to-stand and transition into his walker with close supervision. He was able to transition onto and off the floor by pulling up on a stationary object with minimal physical assistance. He required moderate physical assistance to do so using a half-kneel-to-stand pattern.

Gait/steps: Prior to surgery, Thomas independently ambulated with a posterior walker using a crouched gait pattern with increased adduction across midline during the swing phase and bilateral Cascade Turbo braces. He was able to ambulate household distances and move through his classroom with his walker. He used a manual wheelchair for long distances to minimize fatigue. He was able to manage a curb step given moderate physical assistance.

Bracing: At the age of 12, Thomas was wearing AFOs with SMO inserts, commonly known as TURBO braces made by Cascade. Prior to surgery, he presented with an increased crouched gait pattern.

Physical Therapy Examination

Following surgery, Thomas had an acute inpatient stay at a children's hospital where he received physical therapy for bed mobility, transfer training, and parent education on precautions following surgery. Once he was discharged from the hospital, he returned to undergo an outpatient physical therapy initial examination to determine his postoperative plan of care. The results of this evaluation were as follows.

Precautions: No hip flexion greater than 90 degrees, no forceful hip internal or external rotation, no adduction across midline; knee immobilizers to be worn 2 hours on 2 hours off and throughout the night; weight bearing as tolerated (WBAT) in short leg casts.

Pain: According to the Numeric Pain Scale (0 to 10), Thomas reported a 5/10 pain overall, but reports that left foot is most painful.

ROM: Bilateral hip flexion to 90 degrees, hip abduction to 35 degrees, hip adduction to neutral, popliteal angles: 25 degrees, ankle motion not tested secondary to short leg casts.

Strength: MMT bilaterally: hip flexion: 2+/5; hip abduction: 1/5; hip adduction: 2/5; knee extension: 3/5; prone knee flexion: 2/5; ankle testing not possible secondary to short leg casts.

Tone: MAS: two bilateral adductors and hamstrings.

Sensation: Bilateral LE sensation was intact to light touch, hot and cold, sharp and dull.

Functional mobility: Required moderate physical assistance to perform sit-to-stand transfer; floor-to-stand transfer deferred at this time.

Gait/steps: Ambulates using posterior walker for 10 feet and moderate physical assistance, wearing bilateral knee immobilizers and short leg casts.

Balance: Thomas is able to maintain static standing with both knee immobilizers donned for 5 to 10 seconds *without* bilateral UE support on his walker; able to stand 30 seconds *with* UE support on his walker.

Equipment: Thomas is currently using a manual wheelchair at school, but family notes that his propulsion was slow and inefficient, causing difficulty keeping up with peers. The therapists discussed the advantage of using a power wheelchair with Thomas and his family, and explained that a power wheelchair would provide Thomas energy-efficient mobility for long distances in all environments. Thomas and his family are considering power mobility now that he is older, owing to decreased endurance and his inefficient gait pattern. Thomas repeatedly states that he enjoys school and would like to reserve some energy for academics rather than using it all to get from one class to another. His family is in the process of getting a van modified with a wheelchair lift to accommodate the increased weight and size of a power chair.

Physical Therapy Assessment/Prognosis

Thomas is a 12-year-old young man with a diagnosis of spastic quadriplegic CP. He recently underwent extensive LE surgery to improve hip orientation, increase muscle length, and improve foot alignment. He presents with impairments, including pain, increased LE tone, decreased LE strength, decreased balance, and poor endurance. As a result, he presents with inefficient gait patterns, decreased independence with functional mobility and transfers. The outlook for treatment is good owing to his motivation to walk. Thomas, along with his family and therapists, determined that his long-term goal is to walk 25 feet across a stage at school, then stand for about 5 to 10 minutes using his walker alongside his classmates at the end-of-year celebration.

INTERVENTIONS FOR FIRST 6 MONTHS POSTSURGERY (FREQUENCY: THREE 60-MINUTE SESSIONS PER WEEK POSTOPERATIVELY)

Stretching: Bilateral hip adduction and hamstring stretching, ankle dorsiflexion when casts were removed 8 weeks postop, five reps with a 30-second hold for each stretch.

Strength training: Functional strength training to start including sit-to-stand repetitions from various seat heights and surfaces,

progressing from higher to lower seats with lowest placing hips at a 90-degree angle (using benches, balls, bolsters). Leg strengthening with manual resistance and machines, attention to hip abductors, adductors, extensors and hamstrings, and dorsiflexor strengthening; use of strength training machine with resistance high enough to result in fatigue after one to three sets of 6 to 10 reps (following NSCA strengthening guidelines); core strengthening using medium therapy ball in supine, prone, and sitting.

Therapeutic handling: Functional movement sequences practiced with facilitation to improve coactivation of LE musculature to promote an active base of support while addressing posture and alignment. Such movement sequences include facilitated weight shifting in standing using parallel bars, progressing to walker with facilitation to gluteals and abdominals given visual cues from a mirror; facilitated step-up with input to gluteus medius/maximus and internal/external obliques.

Bracing: Following cast removal, he was fitted for molded solid AFOs to limit crouch and promote good foot alignment.

Aquatic therapy: Casts were removed 12 weeks postop, thereby allowing Thomas to participate in aquatic therapy. Aquatic activities included standing balance and gait training in shoulder-deep water progressing down to waist-deep water, closed-chain functional strengthening, and kicking with kickboard for hip strengthening.

Gait training: Began with stride stance and pregait activities in standing to increase tolerance for weight bearing and preparation for ambulation; progressed to gait training on even surface using personal posterior walker.

Parent/patient education: Review of precautions, transfer training, and home stretching program for hip adductors, hamstrings, and triceps surae (after casts were removed).

INTERVENTION 6 MONTHS POSTOP (PHYSICAL THERAPY: TWO 60-MINUTE SESSIONS PER WEEK, NO POSTOPERATIVE PRECAUTIONS)

Stretching: Continue adductor, hamstring, ankle dorsiflexor stretching, three reps with 30-second hold each to maintain gains achieved.

Strengthening: Progressed resistance with functional closed-chain strengthening as well as focused single-joint strengthening of muscles important to maintaining optimal upright posture such as triceps surae, quadriceps, gluteus medius, and gluteus maximus.

NDT/therapeutic handling: Incorporated primarily into functional activities to address patient/family and therapist-determined goals. Including core strengthening with pelvic weight shifting, flexion rotation and extension rotation activities on ball, foot preparation prior to standing activities, and facilitated weight shifting and balance training with and without UE support on walker.

Gait training: Emphasis on increased walking distance using walker while maintaining optimal posture and alignment to minimize crouch; Partial Body-weight Supported Treadmill Training initiated to increase endurance.

Patient/parent education: Emphasis on ambulation and functional strengthening, family able to decrease frequency of stretching to once a day due to stability of ROM measurements over 8 consecutive weeks.

Discharge/continuum of care One year postoperatively, Thomas reached his personal goal of standing for 5 minutes with his walker and walking across the stage at school to stand alongside of his classmates during the end-of-the-school-year celebration. At this time, he was discharged from a medically based physical therapy program with a home program. The therapists explained that Thomas' therapeutic needs would be best met using an episodic plan of care, and recommended a physical therapy re-evaluation in 6 months' time to determine whether further intervention was needed. Prior to discharge, Thomas' interests were discussed and options for community activities were provided. In view of the time spent in the pool during aquatic therapy, Thomas will attend an adapted swim program at the local YMCA.

▶ Acknowledgments

We would like to thank Jane Styer-Acevedo, PT for her knowledge, inspiration, and contributions to the last three editions of this chapter. We would like to extend our heartfelt gratitude to Dr. Freeman Miller, whose willingness to share his expertise of CP has been critical to our ability to treat our patients effectively and write this chapter. We would also like to thank Gary Mickalowski, CPO and Heather Mickalowski, CPO for assisting with the "Orthoses" section; Chris Church, PT for his assistance with the "Gait" section; and all the therapists at Nemours/AI duPont Hospital for Children who have mentored and supported us. Last but certainly not least, we would like to thank our families for supporting our efforts this past year. This chapter would NEVER have been completed without you.

REFERENCES

1. Rethlefsen S, Ryan D, Kay R. Classification systems in cerebral palsy. *Orthop Clin North Am.* 2010;41:457–467.
2. Rosenbaum P, Paneth N, Leviton A, et al. A report: the definition and classification of cerebral palsy April 2006. *Dev Med Child Neurol Suppl.* 2007;109:8.
3. Beckung E, Hagberg G. Neuroimpairments, activity limitations and participation restrictions in children with cerebral palsy. *Dev Med Child Neurol.* 2002;44(5):309–316.
4. Stiller C, Marcoux BC, Olson RE. The effect of conductive education, intensive therapy, and special education services on motor skills in children with cerebral palsy. *Phys Occup Ther Pediatr.* 2003;23(3):31–50.
5. Niswander KR, Gordon M. The collaborative perinatal project. In: *The Women and Their Pregnancies.* Washington, DC: National Institutes of Health; 1972. DHEW Publication No 73–379.
6. Ellenberg JH, Nelson KB. Cluster of perinatal events identifying infants at high risk for death or disability. *J Pediatr.* 1988;113:546–552.
7. Reddihough DS, Collins KJ. The epidemiology and causes of cerebral palsy. *Aust J Physiother.* 2003;49(1):7–12.
8. Katz RT. Life expectancy for children with cerebral palsy and mental retardation: implications for life care planning. *NeuroRehabilitation.* 2003;18:261–270.
9. SCPE Working Group. Surveillance of cerebral palsy in Europe: a collaboration of cerebral palsy surveys and registers. Surveillance of Cerebral Palsy in Europe (SCPE). *Dev Med Child Neurol.* 2000;42:816–824.
10. Miller F. *Cerebral Palsy.* New York, NY: Springer-Verlag, Inc; 2005.
11. Ferrari F, Cioni G, Einspieler C, et al. Cramped synchronized general movements in preterm infants as an early marker for cerebral palsy. *Arch Pediatr Adolesc Med.* 2002;156(5):460–467.
12. Hadders-Algra M. General movements: a window for early identification of children at high risk for developmental disorders. *J Pediatr.* 2004;145(2 suppl):S12–S18.
13. National Institute of Neurological Disorders and Stroke. Reducing the burden of neurological disease. *Cerebral Palsy: Hope Through Research.* http://www.ninds.nih.gov/disorders/cerebral_palsy/detail_cerebral_palsy.htm#179273104.
14. van Haastert LC, de Vries LS, Eijsermans MJC, et al. Gross motor functional abilities in pretem-born children with cerebral palsy due to periventricular leukomalacia. *Dev Med Child Neurol.* 2008;50:684–689.
15. Liptak GS, Accardo PJ. Health and social outcomes of children with cerebral palsy. *J Pediatr.* 2004;145(2 suppl):S36–S41.
16. Blair E, Watson L, Badawi N, et al. Life expectancy among people with cerebral palsy in Western Australia. *Dev Med Child Neurol.* 2001;43(8):508–515.
17. Miller F, Bachrach S. *Cerebral Palsy: A Complete Guide for Caregiving.* 2nd ed. Baltimore, MD: Johns Hopkins University Press; 2006.
18. Palisano R, Rosenbaum P, Walter S, et al. Development and reliability of a system to classify gross motor function in children with cerebral palsy. *Dev Med Child Neurol.* 1997;39:214–223.
19. Morris C, Bartlett D. Gross motor function classification system: impact and utility. *Dev Med Child Neurol.* 2004;46(1):60–65.
20. Davids J, Peace L, Wagner L, et al. Validation of the Shriners Hospital for Children Upper Extremity Evaluation (SHUEE) for children with hemiplegic cerebral palsy. *J Bone Joint Surg Am.* 2006;88:326–333.
21. Howle JM. *Neuro-Developmental Treatment Approach Theoretical Foundations and Principles of Clinical Practice.* Laguna Beach, CA: The North American Neuro-Developmental Treatment Association; 2002.
22. Rumeau-Rouquette C, Grandjean H, Cans C, et al. Prevalence and time trends of disabilities in school-age children. *Int J Epidemiol.* 1997;26:137–145.
23. Koman AL, Smith BP, Shilt JS. Cerebral palsy. *Lancet.* 2004;363:1619.
24. Krageloh-Mann I, Cans C. Cerebral palsy update. *Brain Dev.* 2009;31:537–544.
25. Wiklund L, Uvebrant P. Hemiplegic cerebral palsy: correlation between CT morphology and clinical findings. *Dev Med Child Neurol.* 1991;33(6):512–523.
26. Cioni G, Sale B, Paolicelli PB, et al. MRI and clinical characteristics of children with hemiplegic cerebral palsy. *Neuropediatrics.* 1999;30(5):249–255.
27. Holmefur M, Krumlinde-Sundholm L, Ellasson AC. Interrater and intrarater reliability of the Assisting Hand Assessment. *Am J Occup Ther.* 2007;61:79–84.
28. Accardo J, Kammann H, Hoon AH Jr. Neuroimaging in cerebral palsy. *J Pediatr.* 2004;145(2)(suppl):S19–S27.
29. Harada T, Erada S, Anwar MM, et al. The cervical spine in athetoid cerebral palsy. A radiological study of 180 patients. *J Bone Joint Surg Br.* 1996;78(4):613–619.
30. Burns YR, O'Callaghan M, Tudehope DI. Early identification of cerebral palsy in high risk infants. *Aust Paediatr J.* 1989;25:215–219.
31. Harris SR. Early neuromotor predictors of cerebral palsy in low birthweight infants. *Dev Med Child Neurol.* 1987;29:508–519.
32. Harris SR. Movement analysis—an aid to diagnosis of cerebral palsy. *Phys Ther.* 1991;71:215–221.
33. Rose-Jacobs R, Cabral H, Beeghly M, et al. The Movement Assessment of Infants (MAI) as a predictor of two-year neurodevelopmental outcome for infants born at term who are at social risk. *Pediatr Phys Ther.* 2004;16(4):212–221.

34. Nelson KB, Ellenberg JH. Children who "outgrew" cerebral palsy. *Pediatrics*. 1982;69:529–535.

35. Bly L. *Motor Skills Acquisition in the First Year: An Illustrated Guide to Normal Development*. Tucson, AZ: Therapy Skill Builders; 1994.

36. Bly L. Abnormal motor development. In: Slaton DS, ed. *Proceedings of a Conference on Development of Movement in Infancy Offered by the Division of Physical Therapy*. Chapel Hill, NC: University North Carolina; May 18–22, 1980.

37. Cochrane CD. Joint mobilization principles: considerations for use in the child with central nervous system dysfunction. *Phys Ther*. 1987;67:1105–1109.

38. Illingworth RS. *The Development of the Infant and Young Child*. 8th ed. New York, NY: Churchill Livingstone; 1983.

39. Bly L. What is the role of sensation in motor learning? What is the role of feedback and feedforward? *NDTA Netw*. 1996;1–7.

40. Cupps B. Postural control: a current view. *NDTA Netw*. 1997;1–7.

41. Valencia F. Management of hip deformities in cerebral palsy. *Orthop Clin North Am*. 2010;41:549–559.

42. Bleck EE. Orthopedic management of cerebral palsy. Philadelphia, PA: WB Saunders; 1979.

43. Shands AR, Steele MK. Torsion of the femur. *J Bone Joint Surg*. 1958;40A:803–816.

44. Michele AA. *Iliopsoas*. Springfield, IL: Charles C Thomas; 1962.

45. Beals RK. Developmental changes in the femur and acetabulum in spastic paraplegia and diplegia. *Dev Med Child Neurol*. 1969;11:303–313.

46. Staheli LT, Duncan WR, Schaefer E. Growth alterations in the hemiplegic child. A study of femoral anteversion, neck-shaft angle, hip rotation, C.E. angle, limb length and circumference in 50 hemiplegic children. *Clin Orthop Relat Res*. 1968;60:205–212.

47. Jordan P. Evaluation and treatment of foot disorders. Presentation at: Neurodevelopmental Treatment Association Regional Conference; May 1984; New York, NY.

48. Calliet R. *Foot and Ankle Pain*. Philadelphia, PA: FA Davis; 1970.

49. Beckung E, Hagberg G, Uldall P, et al. Probability of walking in children with cerebral palsy in Europe. *Pediatrics*. 2008;121:e187–e192.

50. Rosenbaum PL, Walter SD, Hanna SE, et al. Development and reliability of a system to classify gross motor function in children with cerebral palsy. *JAMA*. 2002;288(11):1357–1363.

51. Watt J, Robertson CM, Grace MG. Early prognosis for ambulation of neonatal intensive care survivors with cerebral palsy. *Dev Med Child Neurol*. 1989;31:766–773.

52. Perry J, Burnfield J. *Gait Analysis: Normal and Pathological Function*. 2nd ed. Thorofare, NJ: Slack Inc; 2010.

53. Gage JR, DeLuca PA, Renshaw TS. Gait analysis: principles and applications. Emphasis on its use in cerebral palsy. *J Bone Joint Surg Am*. 1995;77(10):1607–1623.

54. Sutherland DH, Davids JR. Common gait abnormalities of the knee in cerebral palsy. *Clin Orthop Relat Res*. 1993;288:139–147.

55. Winters TF, Gage JR, Hicks R. Gait patterns in spastic hemiplegia in children and young adults. *J Bone Joint Surg Am*. 1987;69:437–441.

56. Rodda J, Graham H. Classification of gait patterns in spastic hemiplegia and spastic diplegia: a basis for a management algorithm. *Eur J Neurol*. 2001;8(suppl 5):98–108.

57. Wren TA, Rethlefsen S, Kay RM. Prevalence of specific gait abnormalities in children with cerebral palsy: influence of cerebral palsy subtype, age, and previous surgery. *J Pediatr Orthop*. 2005;25(1):79–83.

58. Mossberg KA, Linton KA, Fricke K. Ankle-foot orthoses: effect on energy expenditure of gait in spastic diplegic children. *Arch Phys Med Rehabil*. 1990;71:490–494.

59. Davids J. The foot and ankle in cerebral palsy. *Orthop Clin North Am*. 2010;41:579–593.

60. Rodda JM, Graham HK, Carson L, et al. Sagittal gait patterns in spastic diplegia. *J Bone Joint Surg Br*. 2004;86(2):251–258.

61. Westberry D, Davids JR, Davis RB, et al. Idiopathic toe walking: a kinematic and kinetic profile. *J Pediatr Orthop*. 2008;28(3):352–358.

62. Hicks R, Durinick N, Gage JR. Differentiation of idiopathic toe-walking and cerebral palsy. *J Pediatr Orthop*. 1988;8:160–163.

63. Kelly IP, Jenkinson A, Stephens M, et al. The kinematic patterns of toe-walkers. *J Pediatr Orthop*. 1997;17(4):478–480.

64. Mochizuki H, Ugawa Y. Cerebellar ataxic gait [in Japanese]. *Brain Nerve*. 2010;62(11):1203–1210.

65. Chen CM, Chen CY, Wu KP, et al. Motor factors associated with health-related quality-of-life in ambulatory children with cerebral palsy. *Am J Phys Med Rehabil*. 2011;90:940–947.

66. Alexander R, Boehme R, Cupps B. *Normal Development of Functional Motor Skills: The First Year of Life*. San Antonio, TX: Therapy Skill Builders; 1993.

67. Tieman BL, Palisano RJ, Gracely EJ, et al. Gross motor capability and performance of mobility in children with cerebral palsy: a comparison across home, school, and outdoors/community settings. *Phys Ther*. 2004;84(5):419–429.

68. Campbell SK. Quantifying the effects of interventions for movement disorders resulting from cerebral palsy. *J Child Neurol*. 1996;11(suppl 1):561–570.

69. Harris SR, Atwater SW, Crowe TK. Accepted and controversial neuromotor therapies for infants at high risk for cerebral palsy. *J Perinatol*. 1988;8(1):3–13.

70. Palisano RJ, Kolobe TH, Haley SM, et al. Validity of the peabody developmental gross motor scale as an evaluative measure of infants receiving physical therapy. *Phys Ther*. 1995;75(11):939–948.

71. Gorter JW, Rosenbaum PL, Hanna SE, et al. Limb distribution, motor impairment, and functional classification of cerebral palsy. *Dev Med Child Neurol*. 2004;46(7):461–467.

72. Facchin P, Rosa-Rizzotto M, Visona Dalla Pozza L, et al. Multisite trial comparing the efficacy of constraint-induced movement therapy with that of bimanual intensive training in children with hemiplegic cerebral palsy: postintervention results. *Am J Phys Med Rehabil*. 2011;90(7):539–553.

73. Bobath B, Bobath K. *Motor Development in the Different Types of Cerebral Palsy*. London, UK: William Heineman Medical Books; 1982.

74. Finnie NR. *Handling the Young Cerebral Palsied Child at Home*. 2nd ed. New York, NY: Dalton Publications; 1975.

75. Davis S. Neurodevelopmental treatment/Bobath eight week course in the treatment of children with cerebral palsy. Lecture notes. June–July 1997.

76. Scholtes V, Becher J, Comuth A, et al. Effectiveness of functional progressive resistance exercise strength training on muscle strength and mobility in children with cerebral palsy: a randomized controlled trail. *Dev Med Child Neurol*. 2010;52:107–113.

77. McNee A, Gough M, Morrissey M, et al. Increases in muscle volume after plantarflexor strength training in children with spastic cerebral palsy. *Dev Med Child Neurol*. 2009;51:429–435.

78. Scianni A, Butler JM, Ada L, et al. Muscle strengthening not effective in children and adolescents with cerebral palsy: a systemic review. *Aust J Physiother*. 2009;55:81–87.

79. Reid S, Hamer P, Alderson J, et al. Neuromuscular adaptations to eccentric strength training in children and adolescents with cerebral palsy. *Dev Med Child Neurol*. 2010;52:358–363.

80. Lee JH, Sung IY, Yoo JY. Therapeutic effects of strengthening exercise on gait function of cerebral palsy. *Disabil Rehabil*. 2008;30(19):1439–1444.

81. Rogers A, Brinks S, Darrah J. A systemic review of the effectiveness of aerobic exercise interventions for children with cerebral palsy: an AACPDM evidence report. *Dev Med Child Neurol*. 2008;50:808–814.

82. Verschuren O, Ketekaar M, Takken T, et al. Exercise programs for children with cerebral palsy: a systemic review of the literature. *Am J Phys Med Rehabil*. 2008;87(5):404–417.

83. Verschuren O, Ada L, Maltais D, et al. Muscle strengthening in children and adolescents with spastic cerebral palsy: considerations for future resistance training protocols. *Phys Ther*. 2011;91:1130–1139.

84. Pippenger WS, Scalzitti DA. Evidence in practice, what are the effects, if any of lower extremity strength training on gait in children with cerebral palsy? *Phys Ther*. 2004;84(9):849–858.

85. Eagleton M, Iams A, McDowell J, et al. The effects of strength training on gait in adolescents with cerebral palsy. *Pediatr Phys Ther.* 2004;16(1):22–30.

86. Damiano DL, Abel MF. Functional outcomes of strength training in spastic cerebral palsy. *Arch Phys Med Rehabil.* 1998;79:119–125.

87. Chen C, Hsien W, Cheng H, et al. Muscle strength enhancement following home-based virtual cycling training in ambulatory children with cerebral palsy. *Res Dev Disabil.* 2012;33:1087–1094.

88. Tilton A. Management of spasticity in children with cerebral palsy. *Semin Pediatr Neurol.* 2009;16:82–89.

89. Pin T, Dyke P, Chan M. The effectiveness of passive stretching in children with cerebral palsy. *Dev Med Child Neurol.* 2006;48:855–862.

90. Birkmeier K. Curriculum and theoretical base committee update. *NDTA Netw.* 1997;6(4):1–7.

91. Davies PL, Gavin WJ. Validating the diagnosis of sensory processing disorders using EEG technology. *Am J Occup Ther.* 2007;61:176–189.

92. Blanche EI, Botticelli TM, Hallway MK. *Combining Neurodevelopment Treatment and Sensory Integration Principles: An Approach to Pediatric Therapy.* Tucson, AZ: Therapy Skill Builders; 1995.

93. Fisher AG, Murray EA, Bundy AC. *Sensory Integration: Theory and Practice.* Philadelphia, PA: FA Davis; 1991.

94. Ayres AJ. *Sensory Integration and the Child.* Los Angeles, CA: Western Psychological Services; 1979.

95. Taub E, Uswatte G, Pidikiti R. Constraint-induced movement therapy: a new family of techniques with broad application to physical rehabilitation—a clinical review. *J Rehabil Res Dev.* 1999;36(3):237–251.

96. Coker P, Karakostas T, Dodds C, et al. Gait characteristics of children with hemiplegic cerebral palsy before and after modified constraint-induced movement therapy. *Disabil Rehabil.* 2012;32(5):402–408.

97. Boyd RN, Morris ME, Graham HK. Management of upper limb dysfunction in children with cerebral palsy: a systemic review. *Eur J Neurol.* 2001;8(5):150–166.

98. Echols K, DeLuca S, Ramey S, et al. Constraint induced movement therapy in children with cerebral palsy. In: Proceedings of the American Academy of Cerebral Palsy and Developmental Medicine. *Dev Med Child Neurol.* 2001;43.

99. Charles JR, Wolf SL, Schneider JA, et al. Efficacy of a child-friendly form of constraint-induced movement therapy in hemiplegic cerebral palsy: a randomized control trial. *Dev Med Child Neurol.* 2006;48:635–642.

100. Eliasson AC, Krumlinde-sundholm L, Shaw K, et al. Effects of constraint-induced movement therapy in young children with hemiplegic cerebral palsy: an adaptive model. *Dev Med Child Neurol.* 2005;47:266–275.

101. Dimitrijevic MR, Gerasimenko Y, Pinter MM. Evidence for a spinal central pattern generator in humans. *Ann N Y Acad Sci.* 1998;16:360–376.

102. Cohen A, Ermentrout G, Kiemel T, et al. Modeling of intersegmental coordination in the lamprey central pattern generator for locomotion. *Trends Neurosci.* 1992;15:434–438.

103. MacKay-Lyons M. Central pattern generators of locomotion: a review of the evidence. *Phys Ther.* 2002;82:69–83.

104. Mattern-Baxter K, Bellamy S, Mansoor J. Effects of intensive locomotor treadmill training on young children with cerebral palsy. *Pediatr Phys Ther.* 2009;21:308–319.

105. Willoughby KL, Dodd KJ, Shields N, et al. Efficacy of partial body weight-supported treadmill training compared with overground walking practice for children with cerebral palsy: a randomized controlled trial. *Arch Phys Med Rehabil.* 2010;91:33–39.

106. Cherng R, Liu C, Lau T, et al. Effect of treadmill training with body weight support on gait and gross motor function in children with spastic cerebral palsy. *Am J Phys Med Rehabil.* 2007;86:548–555.

107. Day J, Fox EJ, Lowe J, et al. Locomotion training with partial body weight support on a treadmill in a nonambulatory child with spastic tetraplegic CP: a case report. *Pediatr Phys Ther.* 2004;16:106–113.

108. Schindl MR, Forstner C, Kern H, et al. Treadmill training with partial body weight support in non-ambulatory children with CP. *Arch Phys Med Rehabil.* 2000;81:301–306.

109. Dodd KJ, Foley S. Partial body-weight supported treadmill training can improve walking in children with cerebral palsy: a clinical controlled trial. *Dev Med Child Neurol.* 2007;49:101–105.

110. Provost B, Dieruf K, Burtner P, et al. Endurance and gait in children with cerebral palsy after intensive body weight-supported treadmill training. *Pediatr Phys Ther.* 2007;19:2–10.

111. Mutlu A, Krosschell K, Spira DG. Treadmill training with partial body-weight support in children with cerebral palsy: a systematic review. *Dev Med Child Neurol.* 2009;51:268–275.

112. Damiano D, DeJong S. A systematic review of the effectiveness of treadmill training and body weight support in pediatric rehabilitation. *J Neurol Phys Ther.* 2009;33:27–44.

113. Meyer-Heim A, Ammann-Reiffer C, Schmartz A, et al. Improvement of walking abilities after robotic-assisted locomotion training in children with cerebral palsy. *Arch Dis Child.* 2009;94:615–620.

114. Chrysagis N, Skordilis EK, Stavrou N, et al. The effect of treadmill training on gross motor function and walking speed in ambulatory adolescents with cerebral palsy: a random controlled trial. *Am J Phys Med Rehabil.* 2012;91:747–760.

115. Kerr C, McDowell B, McDonough S. Electrical stimulation in cerebral palsy: a review of effects on strength and motor function. *Dev Med Child Neurol.* 2004;46:205–213.

116. Pape KE, Chipman ML. Electrotherapy in rehabilitation. In: Delisa BM, Gans NE, Walsh NE, et al, eds. *Physical Medicine and Rehabilitation: Principles and Practice.* Baltimore, MD: Lippincott Williams & Wilkins; 2004.

117. Seifart A, Unger M, Burger M. The effect of lower limb functional electrical stimulation on gait of children with cerebral palsy. *Pediatr Phys Ther.* 2009;21:23–30.

118. Ho C, Holt KG, Saltzman E, et al. Functional electrical stimulation changes dynamic resources in children with spastic cerebral palsy. *Phys Ther.* 2006;86:987–1000.

119. Durham S, Eve L, Stevens C, et al. Effect of functional electrical stimulation on asymmetries in gait of children with hemiplegic cerebral palsy. *Physiotherapy.* 2004;90:82–90.

120. Wright P, Durham S, Ewins D, et al. Neuromuscular electrical stimulation for children with cerebral palsy: a review. *Arch Dis Child.* 2012;97:364–371.

121. Daichman J, Johnson TE, Evans K, et al. The effects of neuromuscular electrical stimulation home program on impairments and functional skills of a child with spastic diplegic cerebral palsy: a case report. *Pediatr Phys Ther.* 2003;15(3):153–158.

122. Pape KE. Therapeutic electrical stimulation the past, the present, the future. *NDTA Netw.* 1996;1–7.

123. Pape KE, Kirsch SE. Technology–assisted self-care in the treatment of spastic diplegia. In: Sussman MD, ed. *The Diplegic Child: Evaluation and Management.* Rosemont, IL: American Academy of Orthopaedic Surgeons; 1992.

124. Styer-Acevedo JL. Aquatic rehabilitation in pediatrics. In: Ruoti RG, Morris DM, Cole PJ, eds. *Aquatic Rehabilitation.* Philadelphia, PA: Lippincott-Raven; 1997.

125. McCloskey S. Notes from Lecture on Hippotherapy at Arcadia University; April 28, 2004.

126. Casady RL, Nichols-Larsen DS. The effect of hippotherapy on ten children with cerebral palsy. *Pediatr Phys Ther.* 2004;16(3):165–172.

127. Binder H, Eng GD. Rehabilitation management of children with spastic diplegic cerebral palsy. *Arch Phys Med Rehabil.* 1989;70:482–489.

128. Molnar GE. Rehabilitation in cerebral palsy. *West J Med.* 1991;154:569–572.

129. Nwaobi OM, Smith PD. Effect of adaptive seating on pulmonary function of children with cerebral palsy. *Dev Med Child Neurol.* 1986;28:351–354.

130. Reid DT. The effects of the saddle seat on seated postural control and upper extremity movement in children with cerebral palsy. *Dev Med Child Neurol.* 1996;38:805–815.

131. Hulme JB, Shaver J, Archer S, et al. Effects of adaptive seating devices on the eating and drinking of children with multiple handicaps. *Am J Occup Ther.* 1987;41:81–89.

132. Hulme JB, Bain B, Hardin M, et al. The influence of adaptive seating on vocalization. *J Commun Disord*. 1989;22:137–145.

133. Rosen L, Arva J, Furumasu J, et al. RESNA position on the application of power wheelchairs for pediatric users. *Assist Technol*. 2009;21(4):218–226.

134. Furumasu J, Guerette P, Tefft D. Relevance of the pediatric powered wheelchair screening test for children with cerebral palsy. *Dev Med Child Neurol*. 2004;46:468–474.

135. Stuberg WA. Considerations related to weight-bearing programs in children with developmental disabilities. *Phys Ther*. 1992;72:35–40.

136. Rose J, Gamble JG, Medeiras J, et al. Energy cost of walking in normal children and in those with cerebral palsy: comparison of heart rate and oxygen uptake. *J Pediatr Orthop*. 1989;9:276–279.

137. Logan L, Byers-Hinkley K, Ciccone CD. Anterior versus posterior walkers: a gait analysis study. *Dev Med Child Neurol*. 1990;32:1044–1048.

138. Levangie PK, Chimera M, Johnston M, et al. The effects of posterior rolling walkers on gait characteristics of children with spastic cerebral palsy. *Phys Occup Ther Pediatr*. 1989;9:1–17.

139. Verotti A, Greco R, Spalice A, et al. Pharmacotherapy of spasticity in children with cerebral palsy. *Pediatr Neurol*. 2006;34:1–6.

140. Tardieu G, Tardieu C, Hariga J, et al. Treatment of spasticity in injection of dilute alcohol at the motor point or by epidural route. Clinical extension of an experiment on the decerebrate cat. *Dev Med Child Neurol*. 1968;10:555–568.

141. Spira R. Management of spasticity in cerebral palsied children by peripheral nerve block with phenol. *Dev Med Child Neurol*. 1971;13:164–173.

142. Yadav SL, Singh U, Dureja GP, et al. Phenol block in the management of spastic cerebral palsy. *Indian J Pediatr*. 1994;61:249–255.

143. Wong AMK, Chen CL, Chen CPC, et al. Clinical effects of botulinum toxin A and phenol block on gait in children with cerebral palsy. *Am J Phys Med Rehabil*. 2004;83(4):284–291.

144. Sutherland DH, Kaufman KR, Wyatt MP, et al. Injection of botulinum A toxin into the gastrocnemius muscle of patients with cerebral palsy: a 3-dimensional motion analysis study. *Gait Posture*. 1996;4:269–279.

145. Fragala MA, O'Neil ME, Russo KJ, et al. Impairment, disability, and satisfaction outcomes after lower extremity botulinum toxin A injections for children with cerebral palsy. *Pediatr Phys Ther*. 2002;14(3):132–144.

146. Pidcock FS. The emerging role of therapeutic botulinum toxin in the treatment of cerebral palsy. *J Pediatr*. 2004;145(2)(suppl):S33–S35.

147. Kinnette DK. Botulinum toxin A injections in children: technique and dosing issues. *Am J Phys Med Rehabil*. 2004;83(10)(suppl):S59–S64.

148. Bottos M, Benedetti MG, Salucci P, et al. Botulinum toxin with and without casting in ambulant children with spastic diplegia: a clinical and functional assessment. *Dev Med Child Neurol*. 2003;45(11):758–762.

149. O'Neil ME, Fragala MA, Dumas HM. Physical therapy intervention for children with cerebral palsy who receive botulinum toxin A injections. *Pediatr Phys Ther*. 2003;15(4):204–215.

150. Ryll U, Bastiaenen C, De Bie R, et al. Effects of leg muscle botulinum toxin A injections on walking in children with spasticity-related cerebral palsy: a systematic review. *Dev Med Child Neurol*. 2011;53:210–216.

151. Booth MY, Yates CC, Edgar TS, et al. Serial casting vs combined intervention with botulinum toxin A and serial casting in the treatment of spastic equinus in children. *Pediatr Phys Ther*. 2003;15(4):216–220.

152. Boyd RN, Pliatsios V, Starr R, et al. Biomechanical transformation of the gastroc-soleus muscle with botulinum toxin A in children with cerebral palsy. *Dev Med Child Neurol*. 2000;42:32–41.

153. Flett PJ, Stern LM, Waddy H, et al. Botulinum toxin A versus fixed cast stretching for dynamic calf tightness in cerebral palsy. *J Paediatr Child Health*. 1999;35:71–79.

154. Ackman JD, Russman BS, Thomas SS, et al. Comparing botulinum toxin A with casting for treatment of dynamic equinus in children with cerebral palsy. *Dev Med Child Neurol*. 2005;47:620–627.

155. Glanzman AM, Kim H, Swaminathan K, et al. Efficacy of botulinum toxin A, serial casting, and combined treatment for spastic equinus: a retrospective analysis. *Dev Med Child Neurol*. 2004;46:807–811.

156. Hayek S, Gershon A, Wientroub S, et al. The effect of injections of botulinum toxin type A combined with casting on the equinus gait of children with cerebral palsy. *J Bone Joint Surg Br*. 2010;92(8):1152–1159.

157. Corry IS, Cosgrove AP, Duffy CM, et al. Botulinum toxin A compared with stretching casts in the treatment of spastic equinus: a randomized prospective trial. *J Pediatr Orthop*. 1998;18:304–311.

158. Kay RM, Rethlefsen SA, Fern-Buneo A, et al. Botulinum toxin as an adjunct to serial casting treatments in children with cerebral palsy. *J Bone Joint Surg Am*. 2004;86-A:2377–2384.

159. Gooch JL, Patton CP. Combining botulinum toxin and phenol to manage spasticity in children. *Arch Phys Med Rehabil*. 2004;85(7):1121–1124.

160. Peacock WJ, Stoudt LA. Functional outcomes following selective posterior rhizotomy in children with cerebral palsy. *J Neurosurg*. 1991;74:380–385.

161. Guiliani CA. Dorsal rhizotomy for children with cerebral palsy: support for concept of motor control. *Phys Ther*. 1991;71:248–259.

162. Abbott R, Forem SL, Johann M. Selective posterior rhizotomy for the treatment of spasticity: a review. *Childs Nerv Syst*. 1989;5:337–346.

163. Oppenheim W. Selective posterior rhizotomy for spastic cerebral palsy. A review. *Clin Orthop Relat Res*. 1990;253:20–29.

164. Lonstein JE. Cerebral palsy. In: Weinstein SL, ed. *The Pediatric Spine: Principles and Practice*. New York, NY: Ravens Press Ltd; 1994.

165. Albright AL, Cervi A, Singletary J. Intrathecal baclofen for spasticity in cerebral palsy. *JAMA*. 1991;265:1418–1422.

166. Gilmartin R, Bruce D, Storrs BB, et al. Intrathecal baclofen for management of spastic cerebral palsy: multicenter trial. *J Child Neurol*. 2000;15:71–77.

167. Hoving MA, van Raak EP, Spincermaille GH, et al. Efficacy of intrathecal baclofen therapy in children with intractable spastic cerebral palsy: a randomized control trial. *Eur J Paediatr Neurol*. 2009;13:240–246.

168. Barry MJ, Albright AL, Shultz BL. Intrathecal baclofen therapy and the role of the physical therapist. *Pediatr Phys Ther*. 2000;12:77–86.

169. Morton R, Gray N, Vloeberghs M. Controlled study of the effects of continuous intrathecal baclofen infusion in non-ambulant children with cerebral palsy. *Dev Med Child Neurol*. 2011;53:736–741.

170. Brochard S, Lempereur M, Filipetti P, et al. Changes in gait following continuous intrathecal baclofen infusion in ambulant children and young adults with cerebral palsy. *Dev Neurorehabil*. 2009;12(6):397–405.

171. Bleyenheuft C, Filipetti P, Caldas C, et al. Experience with external pump trial prior to implantation for intrathecal baclofen in ambulatory patients with spastic cerebral palsy. *Neurophysiol Clin*. 2007;37:23–28.

172. Shilt J, Reeves S, Lai L, et al. The outcome of intrathecal baclofen treatment on spastic diplegia: preliminary results with minimum of two-year follow-up. *J Pediatr Rehabil Med*. 2008;1:255–261.

173. Gerszen P, Albright A, Barry M. Effect on ambulation of continuous intrathecal baclofen infusion. *Pediatr Neurosurg*. 1997;27:40–44.

174. Conclaves J, Garcia-March G, Sanchez-Ledesma M, et al. Management of intractable spasticity of supraspinal origin by chronic cervical intrathecal infusion of baclofen. *Stereotact Funct Neurosurg*. 1994;62:108–112.

175. Fitzgerald JJ, Tsegaye M, Vloeberghs MH. Treatment of childhood spasticity of cerebral origin with intrathecal baclofen: a series of 52 cases. *Br J Neurosurg*. 2004;18:240–245.

176. Gooch JL, Oberg WA, Grams B, et al. Care provider assessment of intrathecal baclofen in children. *Dev Med Child Neurol*. 2004;46:548–552.

177. Brochard S, Remy-Neris O, Filipetti P, et al. Intrathecal baclofen infusion for ambulant children with cerebral palsy. *Pediatr Neurol*. 2009;40:265–270.

178. Pin TW, McCartney L, Lewis J, et al. Use of intrathecal baclofen therapy in ambulant children and adolescents with spasticity and dystonia of cerebral origin: a systematic review. *Dev Med Child Neurol.* 2011;53(10):885–895.

179. Krach L, Kriel R, Gilmartin R, et al. GMFM 1 year after continuous intrathecal baclofen infusion. *Pediatr Rehabil.* 2005;8:207–213.

180. Motta F, Antonello C, Stignani C. Intrathecal baclofen and motor function in cerebral palsy. *Dev Med Child Neurol.* 2011;53:443–448.

181. Sprague JB. Surgical management of cerebral palsy. *Orthop Nurs.* 1992;11(4):11–19.

182. Dormans JP. Orthopedic management of children with cerebral palsy. *Pediatr Clin North Am.* 1993;40(3):645–657.

183. Thomason P, Baker R, Dodd K, et al. Single-event multi-level surgery in children with spastic diplegia. *J Bone Joint Surg Am.* 2011;93:451–460.

184. McGinley JL, Dobson F, Ganeshalingam R, et al. Single-event multilevel surgery for children with cerebral palsy: a systematic review. *Dev Med Child Neurol.* 2012;54:117–128.

185. Godwin EM, Spero CR, Nof L, et al. The gross motor function classification system for cerebral palsy and single-event multilevel surgery: is there a relationship between level of function and intervention over time? *J Pediatr Orthop.* 2009;29:910–915.

186. Tsirkos A, Lipton G, Chang W-N, et al. Surgical correction of scoliosis in pediatric patients with cerebral palsy using the unit rod instrumentation. *Spine.* 2008;33:1133–1140.

187. Bohtz C, Meyer-Heim A, Min K. Changes in health related quality of life after spinal fusion and scoliosis correction in patients with cerebral palsy. *J Pediatr Orthop.* 2011;31:668–673.

188. Sarwark J, Sarwahi V. New strategies and decision making in the management of neuromuscular scoliosis. *Orthop Clin North Am.* 2007;38:485–496.

189. Comstock CP, Leach J, Wenger DR. Scoliosis in total-body involvement cerebral palsy: analysis of surgical treatment and patient and caregiver satisfaction. *Spine.* 1998;23:1412–1425.

190. Green NE. The orthopedic management of the ankle, foot, and knee in patients with cerebral palsy. Neuromuscular disease and deformities. *Instr Course Lect.* 1987;36:253–256.

191. Moens P, Lammens J, Molenaers G, et al. Femoral derotation for increased hip anteversion. A new surgical technique with a modified Ilizarov frame. *J Bone Joint Surg Br.* 1995;77(1):107–109.

192. Lonstein JE, Beck RP. Hip dislocation and subluxation in cerebral palsy. *J Pediatr Orthop.* 1986;6:521–526.

193. Soo B, Howard JJ, Boyd RN, et al. Hip displacement in cerebral palsy. *J Bone Jont Surg Am.* 2006;88:121–129.

194. Gamble JG, Rinsky LA, Bleck EE. Established hip dislocations in children with cerebral palsy. *Clin Orthop Relat Res.* 1990;253:90–99.

195. Root L, Laplasa FJ, Brourman SN, et al. The severely unstable hip in cerebral palsy. Treatment with open reduction, pelvic osteotomy, and femoral osteotomy with shortening. *J Bone Joint Surg Am.* 1995;77(5):703–712.

196. Brunner R, Baumann JU. Clinical benefit of reconstruction of dislocated or subluxated hip joints in patients with spastic cerebral palsy. *J Pediatr Orthop.* 1994;14(3):290–294.

197. Atar D, Grant AD, Bash J, et al. Combined hip surgery in cerebral palsy patients. *Am J Orthop.* 1995;24(1):52–55.

198. Barrie JL, Galasko CS. Surgery for unstable hips in cerebral palsy. *J Pediatr Orthop B.* 1996;5(4):225–231.

199. Patrick JH. Techniques of psoas tenotomy and rectus femoris transfer: "new" operations for cerebral palsy diplegia—a description. *J Pediatr Orthop B.* 1996;5(4):242–246.

200. Moreau M, Cook PC, Ashton B. Adductor and psoas release for subluxation of the hip in children with spastic cerebral palsy. *J Pediatr Orthop.* 1995;15(5):672–676.

201. Dreher T, Vegvari D, Wolf SI, et al. Development of knee function after hamstring lengthening as a part of multilevel surgery in children with spastic diplegia. *J Bone Joint Surg Am.* 2012;94:121–130.

202. Gage JR. Surgical treatment of knee dysfunction in cerebral palsy. *Clin Orthop Relat Res.* 1990;253:45–54.

203. Karol LA, Chambers C, Popejoy D, et al. Nerve palsy after hamstring lengthening in patients with cerebral palsy. *J Pediatr Orthop.* 2008;28:773–776.

204. Kay RM, Rethlefsen SA, Skaggs D, et al. Outcome of medial versus combined medial and lateral hamstring lengthening surgery in cerebral palsy. *J Pediatr Orthop.* 2002;22:169–172.

205. Abel MF, Damiano DL, Pannunzio M, et al. Muscle tendon surgery in diplegic cerebral palsy: functional and mechanical changes. *J Pediatr Orthop.* 1999;19:366–375.

206. Jones S, Haydar AJ, Hussainy A, et al. Distal hamstring lengthening in cerebral palsy: the influence of the proximal aponeurotic band of the semimembranosus. *J Pediatr Orthop.* 2006;15:104–108.

207. Root L. Distal hamstring surgery in cerebral palsy. In: Sussman MD, ed. *The Diplegic Child Evaluation and Management.* Rosemont, IL: American Academy of Orthopaedic Surgeons; 1992.

208. Gage JR. Distal hamstring lengthening/release and rectus femoris transfer. In: Sussman MD, ed. *The Diplegic Child Evaluation and Management.* Rosemont, IL: American Academy of Orthopaedic Surgeons; 1992.

209. Chang WN, Tsirkos AI, Miller F, et al. Distal hamstring lengthening in ambulatory children with cerebral palsy: primary versus revision procedures. *Gait Posture.* 2004;19:298–304.

210. Gordon AB, Baird GO, McMulkin ML, et al. Gait analysis outcomes of percutaneous medial hamstring tenotomies in children with cerebral palsy. *J Pediatr Orthop.* 2008;28:324–329.

211. Damiano DL, Abel MF, Pannunzio M, et al. Interrelationships of strength and gait before and after hamstring lengthening. *J Pediatr Orthop.* 1999;19:352–358.

212. Mazur JM, Shanks DE. Nonsurgical treatment of tight Achilles tendon. In: Sussman MD, ed. *The Diplegic Child: Evaluation and Management.* Rosemont, IL: American Academy of Orthopaedic Surgeons; 1992.

213. Yngve DA, Chambers C. Vulpius and Z-lengthening. *J Pediatr Orthop.* 1996;16(6):759–764.

214. Kay RM, Rethlefsen SA, Ryan JA, et al. Outcome of gastrocnemius recession and tendo-achilles lengthening in ambulatory children with cerebral palsy. *J Pediatr Orthop B.* 2004;13:92–98.

215. Borton DC, Walker K, Pipiris M, et al. Isolated calf lengthening in cerebral palsy. Outcome analysis of risk factors. *J Bone Joint Surg Br.* 2001;83(3):364–370.

216. Etnyre B, Chambers CS, Scarborough NH, et al. Preoperative and postoperative assessment of surgical intervention for equinus gait in children with cerebral palsy. *J Pediatr Orthop.* 1993; 13:24–31.

217. Gaines RW, Ford TB. A systematic approach to the amount of Achilles tendon lengthening in cerebral palsy. *J Pediatr Orthop.* 1987;7:253–255.

218. Rosenthal RK, Simon SR. The Vulpius gastrocnemius-soleus lengthening. In: Sussman MD, ed. *The Diplegic Child Evaluation and Management.* Rosemont, IL: American Academy of Orthopaedic Surgeons; 1992.

219. Segal LS, Thomas SE, Mazur JM, et al. Calcaneal gait in spastic diplegia after heel cord lengthening: a study with gait analysis. *J Pediatr Orthop.* 1989;9:697–701.

220. Kagaya H, Yamada S, Nagasawa T, et al. Split posterior tibial tendon transfer for varus deformity of hindfoot. *Clin Orthop Relat Res.* 1996;323:254–260.

221. Roehr B, Lyne ED. Split anterior tibial tendon transfer. In: Sussman MD, ed. *The Diplegic Child: Evaluation and Management.* Rosemont, IL: American Academy of Orthopaedic Surgeons; 1992.

222. Green NE. Split posterior tibial tendon transfer: the universal procedure. In: Sussman MD, ed. *The Diplegic Child: Evaluation and Management.* Rosemont, IL: American Academy of Orthopaedic Surgeons; 1992.

223. Rogozinski BM, Davids JR, Davis RB III, et al. The efficacy of the floor-reaction ankle-foot orthosis in children with cerebral palsy. *J Bone Joint Surg Am.* 2009;91(10):2440–2447.

224. Rosenthal R. The use of orthotics in foot and ankle problems in cerebral palsy. *Foot Ankle.* 1984;4:195–200.

225. Figueiredo EM, Ferreira GB, Moreira RC, et al. Efficacy of ankle-foot orthoses on gait of children with cerebral palsy: systematic review of literature. *Pediatr Phys Ther.* 2008;20:207–223.

226. Radtka S, Skinner S, Johanson M. A comparison of gait with solid and hinged ankle-foot orthoses in children with spastic diplegic cerebral palsy. *Gait Posture.* 2005;21:303–310.

227. Buckton CE, Thomas S, Huston S, et al. Comparison of three ankle-foot orthoses configurations for children with spastic hemiplegia. *Dev Med Child Neurol.* 2004;46:590–598.

228. Lam WK, Leong JC, Li YH, et al. Biomechanical and electromyographic evaluation of ankle foot orthosis and dynamic ankle foot orthosis in spastic cerebral palsy. *Gait Posture.* 2005;2:189–197.

229. Burtner PA, Woollacott MH, Qualls C. Stance balance control with orthoses in a group of children with spastic cerebral palsy. *Dev Med Child Neurol.* 1999;41:748–757.

230. Middleton EA, Hurley GR, McIlwain JS. The role of rigid and hinged polypropylene ankle-foot orthoses in the management of cerebral palsy: a case study. *Prosthet Orthot Int.* 1988;12:129–135.

231. Carmick J. Managing equinus in a child with cerebral palsy: merits of hinged ankle-foot orthoses. *Dev Med Child Neurol.* 1995;37(11):1006–1010.

232. Romkes J, Brunner R. Comparison of dynamic and a hinged ankle foot orthoses by gait analysis in patients with hemiplegic cerebral palsy. *Gait Posture.* 2002;15:18–24.

233. Mol EM, Monbaliu E, Ven M, et al. The use of night orthoses in cerebral palsy treatment: sleep disturbance in children and parental burden or not? *Res Dev Disabil.* 2012;33:341–349.

234. Ounuu S, Bell K, Davis R, et al. An evaluation of the posterior leaf spring orthosis using joint kinematic and kinetics. *J Pediatr Orthop.* 1996;16(3):378–384.

235. Hylton N. Dynamic casting and orthotics. In: *The Practical Management of Spasticity of Spasticity in Children and Adults.* Philadelphia, PA: Lea & Febiger; 1990.

236. Radtka SA. A comparison of gait with solid, dynamic, and no ankle-foot orthoses in children with spastic cerebral palsy. *Phys Ther.* 1997;77(4):395–409.

237. Kobayashi T, Leung A, Hutchins, S. Design and effect of ankle-foot orthoses proposed to influence muscle tone: a review. *J Prosthet Orthot.* 2011;23(2):52–57.

238. Carlson WE, Vaughan CL, Damiano DL, et al. Orthotic management of gait in spastic diplegia. *Am J Phys Med Rehabil.* 1997;76:291–225.

239. Bjornson K, Schmale G, Adamczyk-Foster A, et al. The effect of dynamic ankle foot orthoses on function in children with cerebral palsy. *J Pediatr Orthop.* 2006;26(6):773–776.

240. Martin K. Supramelleolar orthoses and postural stability in children with Down syndrome-Martin replies. *Dev Med Child Neurol.* 2005;47:71.

241. Pohl M, Mehrholz J. Immediate effects of an individually designed functional ankle-foot orthosis on stance and gait in hemiparetic patients. *Clin Rehabil.* 2006;20:324–330.

242. Harris SR, Riffle K. Effects of inhibitive ankle-foot orthoses on standing balance in a child with cerebral palsy. A single-subject design. *Phys Ther.* 1986;66:663–667.

243. Ramstrand N, Ramstrand S. AAOP state-of-the-science evidence report: the effect of ankle-foot orthoses on balance—a systematic review. *J Prosthet Orthot.* 2010;22(10):4–23.

244. Kornhaber L, Majsak M, Robinson A. Advantages of supramalleolar orthotics over articulating ankle-foot orthotics in the gait and gross motor function of children with spastic diplegic cerebral palsy. *Pediatr Phys Ther.* 2006;18(1):95–96.

245. Craft MJ, Lakin JA, Oppliger RA, et al. Siblings as change agents for promoting the functional status of children with cerebral palsy. *Dev Med Child Neurol.* 1990;32:1049, 1057.

246. Tetreault S, Parrot A, Trahan J. Home activity programs in families with children presenting with global developmental delays: evaluation and parental perceptions. *Int J Rehabil Res.* 2003;26(3):165–173.

Spina Bifida

Elena Tappit-Emas

Incidence and Etiology
Prognosis
Definitions
Embryology
Hydrocephalus and the Chiari II Malformation
Prenatal Testing and Diagnosis
Fetal surgery
Management of the Neonate
General Philosophy of Treatment
Preoperative Assessment
Management of Hydrocephalus
Physical Therapy for the Infant with Spina Bifida
Overview
Manual Muscle Testing
Range-of-motion Assessment
Postoperative Physical Therapy
Communication with Team Members and Parents
Range-of-motion Exercises
Positioning and Handling
Sensory Assessment
Care of the Young Child
Ongoing Concerns and Issues
Developmental Issues
Handling Strategies for Parents
Physical Therapy for the Growing Child
Developmental Concerns

Infant Devices
Orthotics
Introduction to Bracing
Philosophies of Bracing
General Principles of Orthotics
Children with Thoracic-level Paralysis
Children with High Lumbar Paralysis
Orthotics for Children with Thoracic and High Lumbar Paralysis
Children with Low Lumbar Paralysis
Children with Sacral-level Paralysis
Three-dimensional Gait Analysis
Casting Following Orthopedic Surgery
CNS Deterioration
Hydromyelia
Tethered Spinal Cord
Scoliosis
Latex Allergy
Perceptual Motor and Cognitive Performance
Wheelchair Mobility
Recreation and Leisure Activities
The Young Adult with Spina Bifida
Summary
Case Study
Additional Resources

▶ Incidence and etiology

Spina bifida is one type of neural tube birth defect causing neuromuscular dysfunction. Until recently, the occurrence of spina bifida approached 1 in every 1000 pregnancies, making it the second most common birth defect after Down syndrome. The increased availability of maternal vitamin supplements, more accurate prenatal testing, and pregnancy termination options have greatly reduced the incidence of babies born with this diagnosis in much of the world. In the United States, that number has now stabilized at 3.4 per 10,000 live births. Studies examining the possible causes of spina bifida have evaluated genetic, environmental, and dietary factors that might affect its occurrence. However, no single definitive cause, including chromosomal abnormalities, has yet been identified.[1-3]

Many factors may contribute to a baby being born with spina bifida. The presence of a genetic predisposition may be enhanced by numerous environmental influences. Low levels of maternal folic acid prior to conception have been implicated in several studies. Duff et al. found a significant, though temporary, increase in the number of children born with all types of neural tube defects on the island of Jamaica who were conceived during the months immediately following Hurricane Gilbert in September of 1988. The typical diet of this island is rich in folic acid from fresh fruit and vegetables. The hurricane destroyed much of the island's crops, and for a temporary period, fresh produce was scarce.[4] This study as well as an annotation by Seller proposed a need to fortify commonly eaten foods with folic acid such as orange juice, cereals, flour, rice, and salt.[5]

In 1992, the U.S. Public Health Service made the recommendation that all women receive a daily dose of 400 μg of folic acid during the months prior to conception and 600 μg through the first trimester of pregnancy. With improved education and the support of the medical community, this level of folic acid can be reached through improved diet, dietary supplements, and fortified foods. Folic acid is abundant in dark green leafy vegetables, beans, nuts and seeds, citrus fruits, enriched grains, pasta, bread, and rice.[6] But a diet consistently rich in folic acid can be difficult to maintain, so in 1996, the health departments of both the United States and Canada recommended that all cereal grains be fortified with folic acid to enable women to more easily reach this daily requirement, and 2 years later, fortification was mandated. The U.S. Department of Health and Human Services also set a national objective to reduce by 50% the number of children born with spina bifida by the year 2010.[6-9] The reduction is presently closer to between 26% and 31%, but this improvement is encouraging.[10-12] It appears that the ability of folic acid to significantly reduce the incidence of spina bifida has now pointed researchers to the genes involved with folic acid metabolism and transport as the target of further investigation.[13,14]

Maternal use of valproic acid, an anticonvulsant, is also known to increase the potential for spina bifida. It appears that the developing nervous system is especially sensitive to disruption after exposure to this drug.[14] Maternal use of antidepressants has also been examined and is considered another possible risk factor.[15] Maternal hyperthermia caused by saunas, hot tub and electric blanket use, and maternal fevers during the first trimester of pregnancy were studied, and only the use of hot tubs showed any tendency to increase the risk of spina bifida.[16] But it appears in more recent investigations that this has not attracted wide concern.

In the United States, in past decades, the highest occurrence of spina bifida was seen in families of Irish and Celtic heritage, with as many as 4.5 per 1000 pregnancies. This was thought to be the results of lingering nutritional deficits from the Irish Potato Famine more than 100 years ago, but the true etiology might be the link between a limited diet and an inherent genetic predisposition. Japanese families, with 0.3 per 1000 pregnancies, historically had the lowest occurrence rate. More recently, as the overall number of affected births has decreased for Caucasian women in the United States, there has not been the same level of decrease seen in babies born to African-American women.[17] Also, the number of affected babies born to Hispanic mothers has not decreased as much as in the Caucasian and African-American populations.[18] One suspected factor is a change in diet for Hispanic families. As this group, in the United States, has shifted from rural farms and small towns to large American cities, access to natural folic acid is more difficult. There may also be a genetic resistance to the absorption of folic acid from vitamin supplements, by Hispanic women, compared with the vitamin in its naturally occurring state. There is added concern regarding the effects of language barriers, limited access to prenatal care, reduced compliance with a vitamin regimen, and other negative socioeconomic influences for these women.

In all populations, one cannot disregard the influence of religious practice or personal philosophy on a woman's decision to terminate a pregnancy after a birth defect is identified in the fetus. In a recent multinational study, 63% of women opted to end their pregnancy when spina bifida was diagnosed before 24 weeks of gestation.[19-22]

Lastly, for families in which spina bifida is already present, there is a 2% to 5% greater chance than in the general population of having a second child born with the defect. This introductory section includes a great deal of data primarily to illustrate that the number of babies born with spina bifida has been decreasing in this country and around the world, but for some groups of women, there remain various confounding factors preventing them from experiencing this decrease.

▶ Prognosis

In previous generations, long-term survival of children with spina bifida was reported to range from as low as 1% without treatment to 50% with treatment. A survival rate of more than 90% is now expected when aggressive treatment is provided to the spinal defect and its associated problems. This chapter presents the primary problems affecting this population of children that include hydrocephalus, motor and sensory deficits in the lower extremities, and urologic impairment, as well as the secondary issues such as orthopedic and cognitive/perceptual deficits that are of clinical significance for the physical therapist (PT).

The use of antibiotics to limit infection in the open spine, starting in 1947, and the surgical insertion of ventricular shunts in 1960 to manage hydrocephalus were two major advances in the treatment of spina bifida. Early and consistent use of clean, intermittent catheterization to completely empty the neurogenic bladder has also dramatically improved the survival rate by controlling urinary tract infection and renal deterioration, both of which have been cited as major causes of mortality. These measures, along with the practice of early back closure, continue to improve the chances of survival of children with spina bifida. As the survival rate improved, an increased awareness evolved for the associated problems that were neither immediately evident nor a priority for treatment in the past. The number of severely affected children who have survived has increased. Additionally, an increased number of less severely involved individuals would not have lived without aggressive treatment protocols. Therefore, the full spectrum and complexity of this disability can now be appreciated. Clinicians have the opportunity, not available in previous eras, to work with and learn a great deal from this heterogeneous group.[23,24]

▶ Definitions

The terms myelomeningocele, meningomyelocele, spina bifida, spina bifida aperta, spina bifida cystica, spinal dysraphism, and myelodysplasia are all synonymous. They are used interchangeably by various medical communities throughout the world. We have chosen to use spina bifida for this chapter because it is easy to spell. Spina bifida is a spinal defect usually diagnosed at birth by the presence of an external sac on the infant's back (Fig. 6.1). The sac contains meninges and spinal cord tissue protruding through a dorsal defect in the vertebrae. This defect may occur at any point along the spine, but is most commonly located in the lumbar region. The sac may be covered by a transparent membrane with neural tissue attached to its inner surface, or the sac may be open with the neural tissue exposed. The lateral borders of the sac have bony protrusions formed by the unfused neural arches of the vertebrae. The defect may be large, with many vertebrae involved, or it may be small, involving only one or two segments. The size of the lesion is not by itself predictive of the child's functional deficit.[17,24,25]

Several other congenital spinal defects should be mentioned here. *Spina bifida occulta, myelocele,* and *lipomeningocele* are less severe anomalies associated with spina bifida. *Spina bifida occulta* is a condition involving nonfusion of the halves of the vertebral arches, but without disturbance of the underlying neural tissue. This lesion is most commonly located in the lumbar or sacral spine and is often an incidental finding when imaging is done for unrelated reasons. Spina bifida occulta may be distinguished externally by a midline tuft of hair, with or without an area of pigmentation on the overlying skin. Between 21% and 26% of parents who have children with spina bifida cystica have been found to have an occulta defect. Otherwise, spina bifida occulta has only a 4.5% to 8% incidence in the general population.[17,24,26] Neurologic and muscular dysfunction were previously thought to be absent in individuals with spina bifida occulta. However, a high rate of tethered cord, its associated neurologic problems, and especially urinary tract disorders in these individuals have been found.[27–29] Refer to additional information regarding tethered cord later in this chapter.

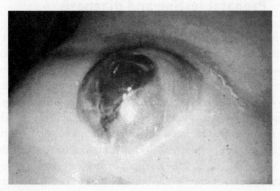

FIGURE 6.1 Spina bifida defect in a newborn infant before surgical repair.

A *myelocele* is a protruding sac containing meninges and cerebrospinal fluid (CSF), but the spinal cord and nerve roots remain intact and in their normal positions. There are typically no motor or sensory deficits, hydrocephalus, or other central nervous system (CNS) problems associated with a myelocele.[25]

Lipomeningocele is a superficial fatty mass in the low lumbar or sacral region of the spinal cord and is usually included with this group of diagnoses. Significant neurologic deficits and hydrocephalus are not expected in patients with a lipomeningocele. However, a high incidence of bowel and bladder dysfunction resulting from a tethered spinal cord has been noted in this population as well as subtle changes in distal leg and foot function, which is usually seen later in childhood or early adolescence, especially after a growth spurt.[30,31]

▶ Embryology

Spina bifida cystica, one of several neural tube defects, occurs early in the embryologic development of the CNS. Cells of the neural plate, which forms by day 18 of gestation, differentiate to create the neural tube and neural crest. The neural crest becomes the peripheral nervous system, including the cranial nerves, spinal nerves, autonomic nerves, and ganglia. The neural tube, which becomes the CNS, the brain, and the spinal cord, is open at both the cranial and caudal ends. Over a period of 2 to 4 days, the cranial end begins to close and this process is completed on approximately the 24th day of gestation.[14] Failure to close results in anencephaly, a fatal condition. The caudal end of the neural tube closes on approximately day 26 of gestation. Failure of the neural tube to close at any point along the caudal border initiates the defect of spina bifida cystica or myelomeningocele. Common clinical signs of spina bifida include an absence of motor and sensory function (usually bilateral) below the level of the spinal defect and loss of neural control of bowel and bladder function. Unilateral motor and sensory loss has been seen and the pattern of loss may also be asymmetric, with a higher motor or sensory level on one side compared with the other. The functional deficits may be partial or complete, but they are almost always permanent.[24,32,33]

▶ Hydrocephalus and the chiari ii malformation

Hydrocephalus and the *Arnold–Chiari malformation* are CNS abnormalities that are closely associated with spina bifida. *Hydrocephalus* is an abnormal accumulation of CSF in the cranial vault. In individuals without spina bifida, hydrocephalus may be caused by overproduction of CSF, a failure in absorption of CSF fluid, or an obstruction in the normal flow of CSF through the brain structures and spinal cord. Obstruction by the *Arnold–Chiari malformation* is considered to be the primary cause of hydrocephalus in most children with spina bifida. This malformation, also known as the *Chiari II malformation*, is a deformity of the cerebellum, medulla, and cervical spinal cord. The posterior cerebellum is herniated downward through the foramen magnum, with brainstem structures also displaced in a caudal direction. The CSF released from the fourth ventricle is obstructed by these abnormally situated structures, and the flow through the foramen magnum is disrupted. Traction on the lower cranial nerves also occurs and is associated with the malformation. Studies using magnetic resonance imaging (MRI) have shown that most children with spina bifida have the Chiari II malformation. Among those with this malformation, the likelihood of hydrocephalus developing is greater than 90%.[34–37]

Theories related to the development of the Chiari II malformation are of interest. At one time, the primary spinal defect was thought to act as an anchor on the spinal cord, preventing it from sliding proximally within the spinal canal as the fetus grew. Traction on the cord was thought to pull down the attached brainstem structures into an abnormally low position. Hydrocephalus was believed to result solely from the hydrodynamic consequence of this blockage.[38] In 1989, McLone and Knepper more closely linked the occurrence of spina bifida, the Chiari II malformation, and hydrocephalus at the cellular level.[39] They theorized that a series of interrelated, time-dependent defects occur during the embryonic development of the primitive ventricular system, causing the Chiari II malformation first and then the resulting hydrocephalus.[40] Their findings indicate that most affected children have a small posterior fossa that is unable to accommodate the hindbrain and brainstem structures, which may influence the abnormal positioning. Significantly, McLone and Knepper found that more than 25% of neonates with spina bifida whom they examined had head circumferences measuring below the fifth percentile. Therefore, neither downward traction from the spinal defect nor pressure from hydrocephalus caused the malformation. They postulated that spina bifida and the accompanying hydrocephalus results from mistimed steps in the development of the ventricular system that is initiated by the failure of the neural tube to close. This explanation has received widespread acceptance among both neuroanatomists and neurosurgeons and should be of interest to PTs who may have wondered about the etiology of the CNS dysfunction that has been observed in many children with spina bifida. Those with spina bifida differ greatly from children who have only hydrocephalus without spina bifida, and they do not resemble patients with acquired spinal paralysis either, two groups with whom they are often compared. The McLone and Knepper theory begins to offer an anatomic rationale for the CNS abnormalities seen in many patients, and offers a viable basis for continued investigation.[39]

Approximately 2% to 3% of children with spina bifida show significant impairment from the Chiari II malformation[40] (Display 6.1). Tracheostomy and gastrostomy may be life-saving measures for the symptoms, which are reported to resolve in many cases as the child grows and the

---

DISPLAY 6.1 — Symptoms Associated with Chiari II Malformation

Stridor—especially with inspiration
Apnea—when crying, or at night
Gastroesophageal reflux
Paralysis of vocal cords
Swallowing difficulty
Bronchial aspiration
Tongue fasciculations
Facial palsy
Poor feeding
Ataxia
Hypotonia
Upper extremity weakness
Seizures
Abnormal extraocular movements
Nystagmus

---

brain matures. In severe cases, vocal cord paralysis, upper extremity weakness, or opisthotonic postures may be seen. Posterior fossa decompression and cervical laminectomy to relieve pressure on the brainstem and cervical spinal structures are accepted courses of treatment, but are associated with varying degrees of success. It is interesting that no correlation has been found between the severity of the Chiari II symptoms and the degree of hydrocephalus seen in the infant, nor has a correlation been found between the child's spinal defect level and these CNS findings. Therefore, attempts to predict which children will experience significant CNS difficulties resulting from the Chiari II malformation have had limited success. Examination by MRI has revealed abnormalities in some children who appear asymptomatic. There is speculation that brainstem auditory-evoked potentials may provide diagnostic assistance. Physicians also believe that there is much to learn at the microscopic level about this abnormality, which may be helpful for further understanding.[17,24,41–44]

▶ Prenatal testing and diagnosis

Increasingly sophisticated and more widely available prenatal testing has allowed for the early diagnosis of spina bifida. Testing provides information that allows a family to make informed decisions about the pregnancy. As prenatal testing has become more the routine than the exception, a significant number of pregnancies are terminated each year when the results have indicated a high likelihood of the fetus having a neural tube defect.[7,45,46] This is a major factor contributing to the decrease in the number of babies being born with spina bifida. For the family that chooses to bring their baby to term, appropriate and coordinated medical care can be arranged in anticipation of the birth.

Alpha -fetoprotein (AFP) is normally present in the developing fetus and is found in the amniotic fluid. AFP levels reach their peak in the fetal blood and in the amniotic fluid from the 6th to the 14th week of gestation. In the presence of spina bifida, after the 14th week, AFP continues to leak into the amniotic fluid through the exposed vascularity of the open spine. Abnormally high levels of AFP in the amniotic fluid provide strong diagnostic evidence for the presence of a neural tube defect. Testing for AFP by amniocentesis and in maternal blood samples has been responsible for the detection of approximately 89% of neural tube defects. But the tests have the potential for both false-positive and false-negative results. Therefore, AFP results are routinely compared clinically with the results of ultrasound imaging before a definitive diagnosis is made.[24,34]

Improved ultrasound equipment and experienced technicians have enabled obstetricians to observe and document several cranial abnormalities that have a high correlation with the presence of spina bifida in the developing fetus. Because a small back lesion may be difficult to detect, clinicians use the presence of the cranial signs as an indication that the fetus may have spina bifida. One example is in the shape of the frontal bones of the fetal skull. They lose their normal convex shape and appear flattened when spina bifida is present, similar to the shape of a lemon. The "lemon sign" can be detected before 24 weeks of gestation. It disappears as the fetus matures and the skull becomes stronger or as hydrocephalus develops and pushes on the flattened skull, reversing its shape into the more typical configuration.[47] Detection of the lemon sign can then be followed by additional ultrasound studies specifically for the purpose of visualizing the back lesion.[48–50]

There has been discussion regarding the best method of obstetric delivery when spina bifida is detected prenatally. A Cesarean section is considered to have a protective effect on the sensitive neural tissue of the neonatal back, thus possibly improving the child's ultimate functional status. Cesarean section reduces the trauma to the exposed nerves of the back that may occur during a vaginal delivery. Moreover, a Cesarean delivery avoids the bacterial contamination of the neonate's open spine during passage through the vaginal canal, reducing the risk of the baby contracting meningitis. A Cesarean section also avoids trauma to the back in the case of a difficult or breech presentation, which could also affect the infant's neurologic function. Finally, with early prenatal detection, it is believed that arrangements for timely back closure surgery at an appropriate hospital can be planned and accomplished more successfully following a scheduled Cesarean section than after an unscheduled vaginal delivery.[51–55]

▶ Fetal surgery

Since 1997, there have been efforts to perform fetal surgery to repair the spinal defect several weeks prior to birth in several institutions. This has not replaced the typical neonatal management for the majority of babies born with spina bifida, but is one methodology that obstetric and neurosurgeons are actively exploring to address the problem, with a selected population of mothers and fetuses. Johnson et al. performed prenatal surgery, between 20 and 25 weeks' gestation and saw a survival rate of 94% with significant reversals in hindbrain herniation, a significant decrease in the need for shunting secondary to hydrocephalus, and improvement in lower extremity function.[56] Two other studies also demonstrated a lessening of hindbrain herniation, a decrease in the need for shunting, and an older median age for the insertion of the first shunt for those infants who did develop hydrocephalus. In these studies, there was no indication that lower extremity motor function improved with fetal surgery.[57,58] In a 2011 study assessing fetal correction of spina bifida performed at three U.S. surgical centers—Vanderbilt University, Children's Hospital of Philadelphia, and the University of California, San Francisco—the outcome for babies who received this surgery between 19 and 25.9 weeks' gestation were generally positive. Known as MOMS (Management of Myelomeningocele Study), the results indicated that by 12 months of age, 30% fewer babies required shunting for hydrocephalus, and the occurrence and severity of hindbrain herniation was reduced by more than 30%. Additionally, at 30 months of age, babies demonstrated better leg movement by as much as two segmental levels as compared with the predicted movement based on the anatomical location of their lesion. The theory that propelled this area of intervention is that the amniotic environment is harmful to the exposed neural tissue and actually has a deteriorating effect on the spinal cord if left unprotected through the months of gestation. When fetal repair is performed, the nervous system of the fetus has additional time to develop in a more normal manner.[3]

All of the prenatal studies pointed out several and significant risk factors for fetal back repair that include an increase in infant mortality, premature births and its associated complications, lowered birth weights, and increased infant morbidity. Maternal complications included preterm labor and placental abruption (premature separation) and thinning of the uterine wall that would impact the success of future pregnancies. But, overall the authors are optimistic that there are significant benefits to be gained by performing fetal surgery and over time, concentrating on improving the surgical procedure and the maternal/fetal selection will reduce the risk factors and diminish many of the negative results.[3,57,58] Dr. David Shurtleff of the Seattle Children's Hospital and other researchers who have been involved in the treatment of children with spina bifida have voiced their concern that larger and more long-range studies are needed before fetal spinal repair can be accepted as the standard of care. At question is whether the initial improvement in motor and neurologic findings will translate into better functional abilities for the older child in the areas of gait, cognitive ability, sexual function, and bowel and bladder control and whether the functional gains will outweigh the risk factors to both mother and child.[3,59–61]

▶ Management of the neonate

General Philosophy of Treatment

Philosophies of treatment for the neonate with spina bifida vary throughout the world and within the United States as well. Because the back lesion was not universally thought to be life threatening, hospitals developed their own protocols for the timing and intensity of treatment for these infants. However, comparing the results of studies in which various initial treatment regimens were used supports the efficacy of early medical intervention. Immediate sterile care of the open spine to prevent infection is essential, and surgical closure of the back within 72 hours of birth is now an accepted goal in most institutions.[17,24,62]

The objective of back surgery is to place the neural tissue into the vertebral canal, cover the spinal defect with surrounding skin and fascia, and achieve a flat, watertight closure of the sac (Fig. 6.2). The open spine provides direct access for infection to the spinal cord and brain. By preventing infection and its associated brain damage, the child's level of function, both physically and cognitively, can be preserved. McLone and associates have shown that babies who suffered gram-negative ventriculitis were less adept intellectually than babies who had no infection. This study is significant in that intellectual function was otherwise not negatively affected by either the presence of hydrocephalus or the level of lower limb paralysis.[17,62-64]

In many institutions, children with spina bifida are treated aggressively with immediate back closure and rapid management of hydrocephalus. Other institutions practice selective treatment. That is, more aggressive management is offered to those children who appear to be less physically involved. In these institutions, the care of the neonate with spina bifida will vary depending on the level of lower extremity paralysis and the presence of other complicating factors. Some of the factors that influence treatment decisions include accompanying abnormalities, such as hydrocephalus, kyphoscoliosis, and renal problems. Still other institutions work to educate parents regarding their baby's status and the long-term implications that spina bifida will have on all of their lives. The parents may then act in a thoughtful manner in combination with support from the medical staff to choose a mutually acceptable course of action. During this period of education and planning, which may last several hours or several weeks, the infant is usually treated to maintain a stable condition and prevent infection.

Regardless of the treatment protocols, this early period provides time for the medical staff to gather information about the child's condition. Discussions can begin about the management of hydrocephalus if it is present or orthopedic deformities that are noted and that may need to be addressed in the coming months. It is important to note that an accurate prediction of the child's functional potential is difficult in these early days even for the baby with seemingly minimal problems. A large number of variables will influence the child's medical condition and cognitive and motor abilities in the coming years. So clinicians must be wary about presenting long-term prognostic information about the child's future. The exception to this may be in the case of a severely impaired child who presents with multiple congenital anomalies as well as spina bifida whose outcome is apparently bleak and for whom aggressive management may not be recommended.[65-67]

Preoperative Assessment

In many centers, the preoperative assessment is done by one physician experienced in the overall care of children with spina bifida. Consults are then requested as needed for specialty services. In other centers, a team of experts will each evaluate the baby and monitor him or her throughout the course of the hospitalization within their individual area of expertise. These professionals may also comprise the team that will be involved in providing the long-term care of the child after initial treatment, discharge, and into the outpatient clinic setting.

The neurosurgeon is concerned initially with the location and extent of the infant's back lesion. Skin grafting may be necessary to gain adequate coverage over a large area. The presence of congenital kyphoscoliosis presents a complication that may lead to impaired wound healing because of excessive pressure at the suture site. This significant spinal deformity may have to be addressed and surgically reduced early in the baby's hospital experience. Congenital scoliosis with accompanying fused ribs at the level of the back lesion may be present and usually predicts a rapid progression of the scoliosis during the growth periods of childhood. The effect of progressive scoliosis on cardiopulmonary function may ultimately be life threatening, even with spinal bracing and surgical intervention. It will impact sitting alignment,

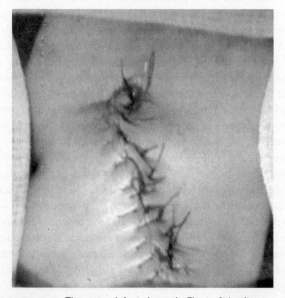

FIGURE 6.2 The same defect shown in Figure 6.1, after surgical repair.

Nutrition and Spina Bifida in Pediatrics

Rebecca Thomas, RD, LDN

Clinical Dietitian, Children's Hospital of Philadelphia

Nutrition-Related Problems	Considerations/Interventions
OBESITY	
After 6 years of age, 50% of people with spina bifida are overweight Children with spina bifida have a higher percentage of body fat, lower total energy expenditure, and reduced physical activity • Increased risk of decubitus ulcers • Increased difficulty with mobility • Decreased social acceptance	Consistent eating pattern/meal schedule Decrease high fat/calorie foods Limit juice/soda Increase intake of fruits/vegetables Encourage lean meats, low-fat dairy products Increase physical activity/physical therapy program Decubitus ulcers/wound healing High-protein diet Additional ascorbic acid and zinc Monitor visceral protein stores Increase physical activity Bone health Encourage weight-bearing activity Ensure adequacy of calcium, vitamin D intake
MALNUTRITION	
Caused by limited variability in intake: limited fruits and vegetables, inconsistent eating patterns, overconsumption of foods/beverages with low nutritional value Abnormal or stunted growth Owing to poor vertebral growth, atrophy of the muscles in the lower extremities; deformities of the spine, hips, and knees; hydrocephalus; renal disease; prolonged hospitalizations • Decreased weight-bearing activity • Decreased bone mineralization	Encourage varied, balanced diet Encourage calorie-dense foods, nutritional supplements if underweight Daily multivitamin
BOWEL CONTINENCE/INCONTINENCE	
Owing to inadequate fiber and fluid in diet and decreased physical activity	Consistent eating pattern/meal schedule Ensure adequate fiber intake via fruits, vegetables, whole grains, nuts/seeds Ensure adequate fluid intake Encourage physical activity

SUGGESTED READINGS

Leibold S, Ekmark E, Adams RC. Decision-making for a successful bowel continence program. *European J Pediatr Surg*. 2000;10(suppl 1):26–30.

Littlewood RA, Trocki O, Shephard RW, et al. Resting energy expenditure and body composition in children with myelomeningocele. *Pediatr Rehabil*. 2003;6(1):31–37.

Nevin-Folino NL, ed. *Pediatric Manual of Clinical Dietetics*. 2nd ed. Pediatric Nutrition Practice Group, American Dietetic Association; 2003.

weight distribution in sitting, and acquisition of upright balance. This anomaly is important to note as a plan of treatment begins to evolve.

A pediatrician or neonatologist may be consulted to assess the general health of the baby and to identify other congenital defects or cardiopulmonary dysfunction that may be present. The urologist can request urodynamic testing during the early neonatal period. Goals of the urologist include minimizing the effects of a neurogenic bladder on the upper urinary tract and producing urinary continence without compromising the health of the system. The bladder may not relax and empty as it should, and residual urine can become a source of chronic infection. Clean intermittent catheterization is widely accepted as the protocol to follow to accomplish the above goals, and although attention to bladder function may not be indicated until after back closure, it is understood that families will better accept intermittent catheterization as a management strategy if it is discussed and taught to them early rather than later in the infant's life. Intermittent catheterization is recognized as one of the most successful methods to preserve kidney function and prevent deterioration that can begin as early as 3 years of age in this population.[68,69]

A comprehensive orthopedic evaluation may not be imperative at this time, but an assessment can offer insight into the severity of any orthopedic problems that are present at birth. The need for early corrective surgery, taping, splinting, or casting and its timing can be discussed and will provide additional information and education to the family and the rest of the medical team. Following the evaluation of the lower extremities and spinal alignment, a plan of orthopedic care can be established for the baby's first months of life. This plan may include other staff, such as the PT, to begin their involvement in the baby's intervention.[17,24,67,70]

Management of Hydrocephalus

After neonatal surgery for back closure, 10% of the infants recover, have their sutures removed, and leave the hospital without further complication. The remaining 90% will begin to develop hydrocephalus. Preoperatively, the open back lesion may act as a natural drain for CSF, and when it is closed, the CSF pressure begins to rise in the cranium. Of the 90% of the infants who develop hydrocephalus, approximately 25% are born with evidence of hydrocephalus and need immediate shunt insertion. Studies show that an additional 55% will develop hydrocephalus within several days of birth. The remaining babies will need shunting within 6 months. The neurosurgeon carefully monitors changes in the baby's head circumference, and studies such as ultrasound, computed tomography (CT), or Magnetic Resonance Imaging (MRI) provide baseline information regarding the size of the lateral ventricles. Later comparisons assist in determining the appropriate time for insertion of a shunt.

Changes in the baby's state often indicate increasing intracranial pressure. As the enlarging ventricles cause the brain to expand within the flexible cranial vault, symptoms of hydrocephalus may be seen singularly or in combination. The most common symptoms are "sunsetting," a downward deviation of the eyes, separation of the cranial sutures, noted on palpation, and/or a bulging anterior fontanelle.

The increasing fluid pressure may stabilize without surgery in some individuals, but it is impossible to predict when this will occur, how great the pressure will become, or how large the head will expand. Vital signs become depressed and respiratory arrest can occur when pressure, from excess CSF on the brainstem structures, becomes too great. Some individuals may survive without treatment for hydrocephalus, but they can be severely impaired as a result.[17,23,67]

Surgical insertion of a shunt will relieve the signs and symptoms associated with increased intracranial pressure. The shunt is a thin, flexible tube that diverts CSF away from the lateral ventricles. It is secured at the proximal and distal ends and is radiopaque for easy location. The ventriculoatrial (VA) shunt moves excess CSF from one lateral ventricle to the right atrium of the heart. Because infections of the VA system can lead to septicemia, ventriculitis, superior vena cava occlusion, and pulmonary emboli, this location is not used as commonly today. The ventriculoperitoneal (VP)

shunt is currently the preferred treatment for hydrocephalus. Although occlusion of this type of shunt may occur more easily than with the VA shunt, complications associated with the VP shunt are far less severe. As it exits the lateral ventricle, the shunt can be palpated running distally down the side of the neck, under the clavicle, and down the anterior chest wall, just below the superficial fascia. The shunt inserts into the peritoneum, where CSF is reabsorbed and the excess excreted (Fig. 6.3).[70,71] An Ommaya reservoir is used in some institutions to siphon excess CSF for a period of time into a superficial well that can be emptied by needle aspiration. It would allow observation for cases in which hydrocephalus might resolve and a shunt would not be indicated, and it will postpone the need for initial shunt insertion until the child is older and more stable.

Although shunt insertion is commonly performed by the neurosurgical team, it is yet another invasive event for the infant who has already had back surgery. In order to spare the infant a second anesthesia, several centers perform simultaneous back closure and shunt insertion. Advocates of this approach believe that healing of the back wound from the inside is compromised when the CSF pressure is permitted to build. Therefore, more rapid healing of the back wound is expected and neither negative sequelae nor increased postoperative complications have been reported by performing the double procedure.[72,73]

After surgery, a plan for physical therapy, based on the infant's condition, can be developed. The priority is for rapid healing, an uneventful recovery, and a speedy discharge to home. Individual surgeons have specific protocols, but at minimum it is appropriate to wait at least 24 to 48 hours postoperatively before initiating physical therapy. In many cases, the extent of hydrocephalus prior to surgery will affect the timing of when the baby may receive oral feedings, position changes, range-of-motion exercises, and normal handling in the upright position. Premature aggressive

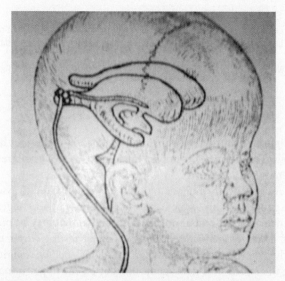

FIGURE 6.3 Location of the lateral ventricles and placement of ventriculoperitoneal shunt.

handling after surgery is not appropriate, particularly for the baby who had significant hydrocephalus. Intracranial pressure can drop dramatically after shunt insertion, and vascular insult can occur if the baby is also held upright, too quickly after surgery.[67]

Physical therapy for the infant with spina bifida

Overview

The role of the PT can begin in the early preoperative period before back closure with an assessment of the neonate's active lower extremity movement. Ideally, the therapist who provides this preoperative evaluation is able to continue treating the baby throughout the hospitalization. It is also helpful if the same therapist can provide the long-term monitoring and parent education as the baby graduates to the outpatient department or specialty clinic. This staffing approach provides consistent support for parents during a stressful period. Also, the importance of staff continuity becomes increasingly evident as the child grows. When changes in function are suspected, the therapist who is familiar with the infant and has a good baseline of observations and documentation can be a valuable resource for the medical team. When a therapist has monitored the baby through the early period of care, the ability to detect even subtle changes is greatly enhanced.[67]

Manual Muscle Testing

A manual muscle test performed by the PT can provide objective information regarding the presence of active movement and the quantity of muscle power present in the baby's lower extremities (Display 6.2). Manual muscle testing should be performed before back surgery whenever possible. Testing may be repeated approximately 10 days after surgery, then at 6 months, and yearly thereafter unless a problem arises, indicating a more frequent schedule. The goal of these early testing sessions is to assist the medical staff to identify the level of the back lesion by assessing the lower extremity movement or lack thereof.[67]

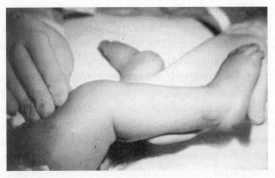

FIGURE 6.4 Palpation and observation of the quadriceps muscle during a preoperative assessment of the active movement in the lower extremities.

Consideration must be given when positioning the baby for this muscle test. Depending on the status of the back lesion or surgical site, the infant may be limited to prone or side-lying. But careful observation and palpation should still allow for identification of most major muscle groups (Figs. 6.4 and 6.5).

A motor level is assigned according to the last intact nerve root found. Lindseth has defined the motor level as the lowest level at which the child is able to perform antigravity movement through the available range.[74] While this degree of certainty may not be possible when testing the infant, preliminary identification of the motor level encourages consistency of communication among professionals involved with the baby. Keep in mind that children assigned the same motor level may still vary widely in their muscle strengths, so it is wise to locate and grade the individual muscle groups as soon as it becomes feasible.

Several factors may influence movement during the infant's first hours of life. The effects of maternal anesthesia, increased cerebral pressure from hydrocephalus, and general lethargy and fatigue from a difficult or long labor may depress spontaneous movements. Conversely, these same factors may render the baby hyperirritable to stimulation. The therapist should tickle or stroke the baby above the level of the lesion or around the neck, face, or shoulder as a stimulus to keep the baby awake and moving. Movement of the

<table>
<tr><td>**DISPLAY**</td></tr>
<tr><td>**6.2**</td><td>**Information Provided by Early Manual Muscle Testing for Children with Spina Bifida**</td></tr>
</table>

Baseline analysis for long-term comparisons
Assessment of existing muscle function
Evaluation of muscular imbalance at each joint
Establishing the degree and character of existing deformity
Preliminary prediction of potential for future deformity
Assistance in determining the need for early splinting
Assistance in determining the need for early orthopedic surgery

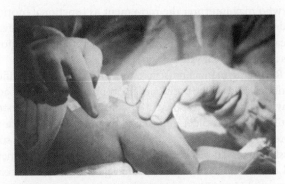

FIGURE 6.5 Stimulation of the infant to elicit movement and palpation during manual muscle testing for the gluteus medius and maximus muscles.

legs can be observed and contractions palpated by stabilizing the limb proximally in order to avoid misinterpreting the origin of a movement. The principles for muscle testing in the infant population are much the same as those for older patients, of course with the exception that the baby cannot follow directions. Gentle resistance to movement at one part of the leg may help increase the strength of a movement at a distal part of the limb, and allowing movement to occur at only one joint at a time will assist in a more accurate interpretation. For example, holding firmly onto the hip and knee in either partial flexion or extension to prevent movement at those joints will enable the therapist to observe and detect weak ankle motion that might otherwise go unnoticed. After locating each movement, the therapist can then assess the general strength of the responsible muscle group. Above all, practice, experience, patience, and ingenuity will improve the accuracy of this early measure of the baby's motor ability.[67,75]

The therapist should note whether or not muscles are functioning, which muscles are strong and can move a joint through its entire range, and which are weak and can move the joint only partially. This distinction will help make determination of the motor level more precise. The ability to distinguish between active and reflexive movement, although sometimes difficult during this early period, will also provide a more accurate identification of the lesion level.[75]

Reflex movement is common in infants with thoracic paralysis. There is usually no active movement at the hip joint, but movement may be noted distally at the knee or ankle. The movement, which may look like fasciculations of the muscle belly or simply a weak, continuous jerking movement of the joint, may be seen when the baby is sleeping or at rest and the other joints of the limb are not moving. Reflex movement is most often observed as flexion of the knee or may be seen at the ankle as either dorsiflexion or plantarflexion. Reflex movement represents sparing of the local reflex arc though cortical control of the movement has been interrupted by the spinal defect. This reflex movement is of concern because of its involuntary nature and because it is usually unopposed by an active antagonist at the same joint. Therefore, this unchecked reflex activity can be a deforming force that often requires intervention. The movement can also be misleading to both staff and family who may interpret the movement as functional motion and think the child's motor level is lower than it is. However, because the movement is not cortically initiated, it seldom has any functional value.[67]

Recording manual muscle testing grades can be modified until the child can be positioned appropriately for gravity and gravity-eliminated responses. Modification is also suggested until the child is older and can be tested with resistance to increase the consistency and reliability of the results. One successful method developed by the physical therapy department at Lurie Children's Hospital of Chicago (formerly Children's Memorial Hospital) uses an "X" to indicate the presence of a strong movement, an "O" for an absent response, a "T" for trace movement when a contraction is palpated but

movement cannot be seen, and an "R" to indicate reflex movement. This scheme of grading, when combined with the existing scale of "0" through "5," or "absent" through "normal" classification, provides significant information about the lower extremities even in these very young patients.

Early manual muscle testing can deduce muscle imbalance around a joint and its potential for deformity. If a deformity is already present, muscle testing can help ascertain whether the cause of the limitation is passive, as a result of in utero positioning, or active, from unopposed muscle movement at a joint, in only one direction. Distinguishing the etiology of joint deformity is helpful for the orthopedic surgeon who may want to consider early surgery to the lower extremities. The surgeon will want to spare potentially useful muscle function while weakening or eliminating movement that will continue to be deforming in nature. Conversely, if the origin of the movement is uncertain, the surgeon may wisely choose to wait until the child is older and a more accurate evaluation is possible before deciding on the type of surgery to perform. Some centers have attempted to use electromyography (EMG) to evaluate lower extremity innervation. EMG studies are interesting from an academic standpoint, but offer little functional information and are not widely used.

There has been poor correlation between early manual muscle testing and the child's ultimate level of gross motor function. So predictions regarding the child's future based on these early assessments must be made carefully. Acquisition of functional skills depends on the innervation and strength of the lower extremity musculature, the child's CNS status, motivation, intellectual capacity, and the family's commitment to long-term compliance, support, and interest. These variables are only a few of the many factors that can influence the functional outcome of the child with spina bifida. Some of these influences are addressed in greater detail in subsequent sections of this chapter.[76,77]

Results of early manual muscle tests should be compared with later tests in order to monitor the child's neuromuscular stability. It is a pleasant surprise to find increased movement and/or strength after back closure, but if a decrease in movement is noted, the neurosurgeon should be alerted. Deterioration of lower extremity motor function may indicate a serious problem and should be brought to the physician's attention.[78]

Range-of-motion Assessment

Preliminary assessment of range of motion (ROM) of the lower extremities can also be performed prior to back closure. Typical, full-term neonates have flexion contractures of up to 30 degrees at the hips and 10 to 20 degrees at the knees, and ankle dorsiflexion of up to 40 or 50 degrees.[79-82] Limitation of ROM in the baby with spina bifida should not be considered an indication for immediate and aggressive stretching. Early limitations in passive flexibility require a safe plan of management executed over several weeks or months. When it becomes apparent that limitations will be both severe and long-lasting, a long-term plan with the orthopedic surgeon can be developed that will likely include a combination of taping, splinting, and/or surgical correction.

There are several common joint limitations seen in the neonate with spina bifida. Extreme tightness of the hip flexors may be evident in the child with a motor level at L-2 to L-3 or L-3 to L-4 owing to the presence of a strong iliopsoas with no opposing force offered from absent hip extensors. Hamstrings, which exert a secondary hip extension force, may also be absent or weak, in which case hyperextension of the knees may also be present along with the hip flexion. Adductor tightness may be seen as a result of innervation of the adductors and absent antagonists, the gluteus medius. If the baby does not have sufficient range of hip extension to safely tolerate prone positioning, the neurosurgeon and nursing staff must be informed in an effort to prevent possible fractures of the femur. Adapted prone positioning in the operating room may be indicated during back closure. One suggestion that has been successful is to elevate the baby on a small, raised, and padded platform or firm stack of towels with both hips safely flexed over one end while the body is supported. Postoperatively, this modified prone position or side-lying will be the safest postures for the baby with limited hip extension. The PT may be the first to note the need for special positioning during the preoperative assessment and can advise the surgical team.[64]

Extreme dorsiflexion at the ankle is another common contracture seen at birth. The child with an L-5 innervation has strong ankle dorsiflexion, provided by the anterior tibialis and toe extensors, but weak or absent toe flexors and lack of plantarflexion from the gastrocnemius/soleus group. Plans may call for serial taping or splinting of the ankle to bring it down to 90 degrees, and in addition, gentle passive exercise often helps reduce this deformity within a short period of time.

Provided that the baby is medically stable and the physician agrees, daily ROM exercise for the lower extremities can begin at bedside as early as a day or two after back closure. Although positioning options are limited after surgery, the prone and side-lying positions are adequate to perform all lower extremity motions needed at this time.[17,67]

Postoperative Physical Therapy

In order for the PT to develop a comprehensive and appropriate program for the infant who has undergone back closure and shunt insertion, consideration must be given to both the neurologic and orthopedic findings, and to be most effective, the therapist should also be sensitive to the state of the family members, who will be more available as they begin to visit their baby on a regular basis.

Communication with Team Members and Parents

In most cases, the family of an infant born with spina bifida will experience a very different and more stressful postpartum period than they had anticipated. Their baby was probably transferred to another facility shortly after birth to receive specialty care. Often, the needs of the recovering mother are superseded by the needs of the baby, so it might be difficult for family members to be as attentive to her as they focus on the infant. Inaccurate information about spina bifida, in general, and their child, in particular, may further compromise the family's coping skills during this physically and emotionally difficult time. It has been reported that parents were told by staff that their child will be mentally disabled, will never walk, and will require around-the-clock care and ultimately institutionalization. These professionals, although well intentioned, are usually not experienced in current methods of evaluation and treatment of children with spina bifida and may only recall information from a previous era in which a bleak outlook for the babies was the norm rather than the exception. This misinformation causes many parents to become confused and frustrated, especially if the specialty team, after assessing the infant, presents what seems to be conflicting information. Therefore, close communication between the therapist and other team members is important. All persons working with the infant should know and understand each other's findings so contradiction does not occur. Information should be provided to the family by the appropriate personnel in an open and honest manner, but also in a sensitive manner.

One objective for the PT should be to reflect a positive and caring attitude during treatment sessions. This approach can help to normalize the involvement of family members with their infant. Teaching portions of a home program to the family can begin immediately. This is a constructive way for the therapist to begin building a relationship with the family and to facilitate their interaction with the infant. The therapist can encourage family members to participate in the infant's care during the hospitalization to prepare them for providing care at home. Waiting until discharge for home instruction will place unnecessary stress on the family members, who have much to learn from many people, in a short period of time. Also, an unexpectedly quick discharge may leave little time for family education, which could have been spread over the entire period of hospitalization. After discharge, follow-up sessions can be scheduled during outpatient or clinic visits to help reinforce the teaching and progress the program. Frequent follow-up appointments with physical therapy may greatly inconvenience a family and may not be as valuable as periodic sessions stretched out over a longer period of time.

Range-of-motion Exercises

Daily sessions for lower extremity ROM exercises can begin after back closure and taught to parents as soon as feasible. Passive ROM exercises should be brief and performed only two or three times each day. It is suggested that parents embed the exercises into a daily routine with their infant, such as during washing and diaper changes, when the baby's

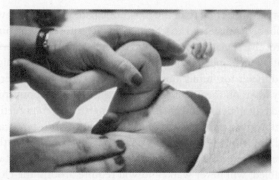

FIGURE 6.6 Exercises for ROM of the lower extremities. Full flexion of one hip and knee is combined with extension of the opposite extremity.

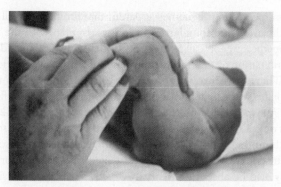

FIGURE 6.7 Placement of the hands close to the joint for range-of-motion exercise of the knee. Note the use of a short lever arm.

legs are normally exposed. The therapist can combine individual leg movements into patterns of movement, so the family only needs to learn three or four patterns for their home program. An example that this author found easy for families to learn is to flex the hip and knee of one leg, while simultaneously stretching the opposite leg into full extension, with the baby in supine. After reversing and repeating this pattern several times, holding both hips and knees flexed, the hips can then be abducted at the same time, leaving only the foot and ankle movements to be done individually (Figs. 6.6 and 6.7).[67]

ROM exercises are performed gently with the therapist's hands placed close to the joint being moved, to use a short lever arm, which prevents stress to soft tissue and joint structures. Several repetitions of each pattern, holding the joint briefly at the end of the range, can maintain and even increase ROM, where there is a mild or moderate limitation. If severe limitations exist, exercise at that joint may require some additional time and repetition. But aggressive stretching should be avoided, regardless of the severity of the contracture.

By participating in the ROM exercises during these early days, parents are encouraged to touch and move their baby's legs while being observed by the therapist. Opportunities to handle their baby with supervision can help alleviate anxiety that many families express about further injuring their infant's back and legs. With the therapist's comforting and supportive words and demonstrations, the exercise program offers a valuable opportunity for the start of positive parent–child interaction.

Passive ROM exercises must continue throughout the child's life. The goal is that the child will eventually learn to perform the exercises independently. Passive exercise is often forgotten by therapists and parents as the child becomes more active and the focus of therapy shifts to concentrate on gross motor activities and gait training. Although one may think these motor activities are adequate for maintaining joint flexibility, they are not. Regardless of how active the child is, only the innervated portions of the limb are being moved, in only some planes of motion, and through only part of the full range of the joint. Therefore, if ROM exercises are discontinued, contractures will develop. For some

children, it may take years before tightness is noted. For others, range is lost in a very short time. Whenever there is loss of flexibility, function will surely be compromised.[17,24,34,67]

Positioning and Handling

Because of our knowledge that babies with spina bifida do not always develop and move the same as their typical peers, the PT can assume responsibility for developing a program of positioning and handling for the hospitalized baby that will also be taught to the parents prior to discharge for continuation at home. Although more positioning options are available as discharge nears, during the first few postoperative days the baby may be limited to prone or side-lying. As the child's medical status stabilizes and tolerance to movement improves, it is advisable that if parents are visiting, they avoid leaving the child immobile for long periods of time when he or she is awake. Handling and carrying strategies can be practiced by the therapist and then recommended to the parents. Finding a comfortable chair is most important, and once seated, the therapist or family member can hold the child prone over their lap, rocking or swaying slowly side to side. This position is restful for the parent and provides novel movement for the infant. The baby may also enjoy a slow walk around the hospital floor while being held up and slightly over the parent's shoulder. This position gives the infant an opportunity to attempt to raise and turn the head. If the supine and sitting positions are contraindicated, parents may gently cradle the infant prone across one forearm. These few position options will provide a small repertoire of acceptable handling strategies when families visit their baby. These positions are also safe for the infant, who needs time to recover and who may not respond well to more aggressive movement and handling. Remember that the primary postoperative goals for the infant is an uncomplicated healing of the back wound, speedy recovery from shunt insertion, and discharge from the hospital.[67]

In many cases, with medical clearance, short periods of supine and supported sitting in the therapist's arms will not affect the course of healing and may be added to the handling repertoire after a few days. This approach will help normalize the baby's experiences during waking hours while being fed or quietly observing the surroundings. It is also useful for the therapist who can note the baby's responses to gravity in each position, feel for changes in muscle tone particularly through the shoulders and neck, and observe any significant asymmetries. Documenting this information will provide a useful baseline against which to compare later developmental findings.[34,67]

Families should first watch, then try to duplicate, the activities recommended for their baby. Be aware that most parents show some hesitation or anxiety on first handling their baby. Lack of hesitation may indicate a poor understanding of the infant's medical condition and may contribute to subsequent poor judgment in other areas of care. Even for families with experience raising older children, some initial level of anxiety can be a healthy sign.

As these teaching sessions proceed, the therapist can begin to "role release" some of the ROM and handling activities, delegating them to the parent. As this transition occurs, the therapist can refocus on other areas of the child's plan of care. The therapist may be asked to repeat the lower extremity manual muscle test prior to the infant's discharge. The therapist can also observe the baby's state, noting changes secondary to hydrocephalus and shunt insertion. Gathering this information may help to identify a later shunt malfunction. When a shunt malfunction begins to occur, in addition to the signs and symptoms presented in Table 6.1, a change in the baby's tone, reaction to movement, and increased irritability during movement may be noted.

TABLE 6.1 Signs and Symptoms of Shunt Malfunction

Infants
    Bulging fontanelle
    Vomiting
    Change in appetite
    "Sunset" sign of eyes
    Edema, redness along shunt tract
Toddlers
    Vomiting
    Irritability
    Headaches
    Edema, redness along shunt tract
School-aged Children
    Headaches
    Lethargy
    Irritability
    Edema, redness along shunt tract
    Handwriting changes
    High-pitched cry
    Seizures
    Rapid growth of head circumference
    Thinning of skin over scalp
    Newly noted nystagmus
    Newly noted eye squint
    Vomiting
    Decreased school performance
    Personality changes
    Memory changes

Family members should also be encouraged to be active in gathering information about their infant. They should be encouraged to play with and observe their baby, not only to foster positive interaction but also to aid the medical staff in assessing the infant's function. Over time, interaction with the medical team becomes less frequent as the child becomes more medically stable and observations by parents can help early identification of problems, such as a shunt malfunction, so that appropriate medical care can be sought.

Sensory Assessment

The PT can perform a sensory assessment on the neonate to determine areas of the infant's lower extremities that react to or are insensitive to touch. By mapping this sensory information, along with the results of muscle testing, the level of the spinal lesion can be more accurately established. This assessment will also identify the areas of intact sensation on the baby's trunk and legs, so stimulation at those spots will make the baby move. It is the novice clinician who strokes the plantar surface of the foot, expecting to make the child react. This technique is successful only when the infant has intact sensation at the sacral nerve roots. Most infants with spina bifida have a higher level of sensory deficit and need to be stimulated on the thigh or somewhere on the trunk. The therapist may find that the level of motor function and sensation is not similar in both legs. Be aware that early results of sensory testing can be inaccurate and incomplete and it is difficult to assess all sensory modalities at this time: light touch, deep pressure, and temperature. A more comprehensive assessment may be indicated when the baby is older.

The information should be shared with the family members, who must become knowledgeable about their child's skin anesthesia. Educating parents about skin care for the baby is often the shared responsibility of the nursing and therapy staffs. It is sometimes difficult for parents to understand the concept that their baby has areas of the lower body and legs that are insensitive to touch. The therapist can help the family discover this information on their own. Using a gentle touch, caress, or tickle, a family member can map out areas of responsiveness when the infant is awake but quiet. The therapist should not use a pin or other sharp object during testing or when demonstrating to parents. The baby's response to a pinprick is no more valid than its response to a gentle touch, and further, seeing staff using a sharp object on their baby may add to the parent's anxieties and concern.

Insensitive areas of the lower extremities will require protection because the child will be unaware of injury to these areas of denervation. For example, families must always test the temperature of bath water prior to immersing the child. They cannot rely on the child's reaction to judge whether the temperature is correct. They must be cautious and not allow their child to play with the faucets and inadvertently add hot water that they will not feel. Open space heaters and radiators need covering or relocation to keep a baby from moving on the floor and resting too close, suffering serious burns. Prior to placing the infant down to play, a search for hidden objects on the floor or in the carpet may prevent an accidental injury from loose tacks or a small sharp toy. The infant's legs and feet should always be covered by tights or socks and pants when playing and crawling on the floor to avoid rug burns and abrasions. Wearing socks or booties will also help prevent problems when children begin to pull their legs up, reach for, mouth, and even bite at their toes, typically at the age of 6 to 8 months.

Skin insensitivity will continue to be a concern throughout the child's life. Wearing new shoes or braces, for example, requires vigilance to avoid pressure areas, sores, and abrasions. Normal sensation keeps the typical person from sitting immobile for long periods of time. Sensory feedback causes individuals to shift around frequently and change their weight distribution, relieving pressure and discomfort. Count the number of times you move and shift your weight during a movie or a dull class. People with areas of insensitivity develop skin problems secondary to prolonged sitting because they do not feel the discomfort and therefore do not shift their weight, change their position, and relieve the pressure. Similarly, when a person with typical sensation feels discomfort from an ill-fitting shoe, they quickly become aware of the problem and are able to readjust their gait to avoid continued abrasion until they can get off their feet or change shoes. For the child without full sensation, such readjustments will not occur, as areas of pressure are not perceived. So, it is important to gradually introduce the use of new orthotics. The brace should be worn for only a few hours at a time, and the skin should be inspected carefully to determine whether there are any pressure areas. When areas of redness last for longer than 30 minutes, an adjustment to the orthosis is indicated. The child should not be permitted to keep wearing the brace in the hopes that the skin will toughen. Rubbing tea bags or alcohol on the site does not help to toughen the skin, as suggested in some home remedies. The accommodation to a new brace is best implemented at home, over a weekend or in the evenings, when regular and frequent skin checks can be made. Unless it is clear that this is more successfully implemented at school, it is not wise to have the child wear a new device for a full day until proper fit and good skin tolerance are ensured. If these issues are not initially addressed and the child experiences skin breakdown, it may lead to extended periods of time out of bracing, infection, possibly the need for hospitalization, and most likely a delay in the progression of the orthotics plan.[24,34,67]

 Care of the young child

Ongoing Concerns and Issues

As the initial phase of intervention for the baby with spina bifida comes to an end, a plan for long-term follow-up care should be developed. Various approaches to the delivery of medical care are seen, but in the best of cases the ongoing care is delivered by specialists located within one institution. When care is divided among several locations, a new role must emerge for parents, and they become their child's case manager, facilitating continuity of care and communication among the professionals. This added responsibility can be a huge burden for some parents and may result in less-than-optimal care for the child. It appears that, because of the multiple specialty areas needed by the child with spina bifida, care is best delivered by experienced professionals who work together as a coordinated team. That is why many pediatric hospitals have organized a multidisciplinary clinic for children with spina bifida and other similar neuromuscular diagnoses, where several specialists working under the same roof can see the child, preferably on the same day. Families are encouraged to continue their child's care at one of these spina bifida clinics if possible. With a team of specialists working together to complement one another, everyone benefits. Communication is facilitated and expedited among professionals, and patient information can be more easily shared to increase learning, maintain a current outlook on interventions, and ultimately provide the best care. Although these clinic appointments can be very long, when problems arise, the necessary personnel are often nearby to address the concern and often without the need for scheduling a return visit. With consistency and coordination by the medical staff, parents can start to develop a sense of trust in their team, which will hopefully decrease their stress, enable them to cope better, and remain focused on addressing the needs of their child.[24,34,65,67]

The child may have to return frequently to the clinic during the first years of life for ongoing follow-up by the various specialists. The neurosurgeon will monitor the status of the back closure, look for the presence of hydrocephalus, determine whether shunt placement is necessary, and check that once a shunt is in place, it is functioning well (Display 6.3).[17,70] The orthopedic surgeon will evaluate spinal alignment and limb flexibility, strength, and joint integrity. Plans are made for lower extremity splints and surgery to prepare the child for standing at the optimal chronologic and/or developmental age (Display 6.4).[24,67] The urologist will monitor bowel and bladder function, assess renal status at regular intervals, and plan a course of care that includes intermittent catheterization and possibly pharmacologic management (Display 6.5). At the appropriate time, a bowel program to attain fecal continence will be implemented that may involve scheduled toileting, diet recommendations, medication, biofeedback, and behavior modification.[67–69,83–85]

As the child's status stabilizes in each of the specialty areas, visits to the clinic will become less frequent. It is not unusual for a child to be seen at 6-month intervals over several years and then yearly if there are no ongoing problems or major concerns. However, more frequent visits may be necessary if a chronic problem requires closer monitoring and intervention.

Developmental Issues

As stated earlier in this chapter, the survival of a greater number of infants born with spina bifida has permitted the clinicians working with these children to gain valuable experience and insight into the full scope of the disability and all of its primary and secondary issues. It is apparent that a significant number of children with spina bifida exhibit CNS deficits, and for some, the effect of these deficits can be more detrimental to the child's function than their lower extremity paralysis. The CNS deficits can have a major impact on the child's acquisition of gross motor, fine motor, perceptual motor, and cognitive skills, and it is critical that the PT understand these problems. The knowledgeable PT can be a resource to other service providers regarding the array of problems they may be observing.

The Chiari II anatomical malformation was identified and studied for years before discussions began regarding how this malformation might relate to the developmental dysfunction that was often seen in children with spina bifida. Using MRI studies, the structural abnormalities have been identified and can be visualized.[31] However, as previously noted, MRI studies are inconsistent in predicting the clinical presentation of a particular child. Up to 85% of children with spina bifida have low tone, with minimal to moderate developmental delay. The most common difficulties are

delayed and abnormal development of head and trunk control and delayed and abnormal acquisition of righting and equilibrium responses, which are all necessary foundation skills for higher levels of movement and functional skills. Interestingly, children who have hydrocephalus without spina bifida do not exhibit the same movement problems with the frequency or severity as children with both spina bifida and hydrocephalus. So when we work with these children, at any age, it is necessary to integrate our background in orthopedics, kinesiology, and orthotics management with concepts of early motor development. While we can only postulate that the Chiari II malformation is a contributor to the movement difficulties we may be seeing, we are still compelled to address all of the child's needs.[24,34,67,69–72]

The earliest problems noted in many infants include prolonged instability of the head and upper body with delayed or weak acquisition of antigravity movement in all positions, balance, and equilibrium responses. The typical baby spends time in various positions right from the beginning of life and experiences the effects of gravity on their head and body in all positions. Typical infants will begin to stabilize their head over their shoulders in the supported upright position in their parent's arms. This early stability occurs well before the baby can lift its head from a prone or supine position. As the baby's head becomes progressively more stable, parents find new and more convenient ways to carry and handle their baby and in less protective manners. This parent–child feedback is most apparent when the baby is held upright in the parent's arms. At first, the parent's hand is placed behind the baby's head to prevent it from falling backward. A few months later, we see this supporting hand only when parents raise or lower the baby from a crib or changing table or when lifting the sleeping baby. In just a few months, almost no guarding of the head is required when the baby is carried in an upright position. The parent has responded to the baby's new skills and has accordingly changed the style of lifting, holding, and carrying, usually without the need for any therapeutic instruction or interventions. For the infant with typical tone, there is physiologic stability of the head and neck. Typical joint proprioception through the cervical spine and the sensitive stretch reflexes of the soft tissue structures of the neck permit the baby's head to fall slowly into gravity, with movement or a position change, but only to a limited degree. The head is held reasonably steady without much active or intentional participation by the infant.

The child with spina bifida who demonstrates poor neck stability may retain a startle response longer than a typically developing infant. Parents respond by continuing to provide the needed head support well past the time the baby should hold his or her head up independently. This begins an abnormal cycle in which the support provided by the parent's hands, while appropriately reacting to the baby's need, actually limits the experiences and opportunities the baby may get to practice and develop better head control, and so the delay is further prolonged. The infant who has low tone lacks the proprioceptive responses to gravity, or the responses may be slow and weak, permitting the head to fall forward or to the side much farther before the stabilizing responses occur. A mechanical disadvantage compounds the problem as the baby grows. The head becomes larger and heavier, so the task of head righting is made ever more difficult by this additional weight and the relatively weak musculature. When an infant with spina bifida is placed in various positions and makes attempts to stabilize his or her head, compensatory patterns of movement can often be seen. Elevation of the shoulders is one pattern noted. This is a developmentally immature alignment for the infant who should have head stability in upright by 4 months of age. Stabilizing the head with this shoulder pattern will act as a block to further development of head-righting skills. The shoulders and upper arms, held elevated and stiff to provide neck stability interferes when the infant should be experiencing and practicing increased freedom of movement and control of the head, separate from the upper extremities.

Compensatory patterns of overusing the arms are seen when the baby attempts to lift his or her head, look around, reach, and play while in the prone position. Side-to-side weight shifting over the hands and arms does not occur easily. When the child lifts an arm to reach for a toy, the prop is removed, stability is lost, and the head and upper chest falls. The child may figure out how to tilt his or her head to one side for a weight shift and let it hang there to unload one arm and reach for a desired object. Once this compensatory pattern is successful, it may not improve without appropriate intervention. As this scenario plays out, months later, the child who did not develop sufficient head and neck strengths and balance reactions will not develop adequate trunk strength and stability to maintain the body in upright positions and may continue to need their upper extremities to prop when placed in sitting. And the child remains stuck, unable to move into or out of the position except in limited, stereotyped ways. To change positions, the child may eventually develop strategies to move but these strategies are usually passive, allowing the body to fall into gravity, involving little muscle activity or control from the neck and trunk. The child may lower his or her head to one side and slowly collapse down to the floor, or may lean forward and crawl out of the sitting position. Getting into and out of sitting from one side or the other requires balance, control,

and strength of the head and trunk, which this child lacks. So getting into and out of the "W" sitting position is usually the easiest. From prone or four-point, the child merely pushes his or her body straight backward with the arms, until the buttocks reach the surface, in between the knees. Using these passive patterns of movement does not help to further improve strength and coordination of the body.

When a typical baby lifts an arm to reach for an object while in prone, a weight shift to one side and back occurs that activates the neck, trunk, hip, and leg musculature to counterbalance and stabilize the baby's position. The baby does not depend on upper extremity support to lift the head and can therefore reach without the head and chest dropping. When the forearms are stabilized on the floor, during typical weight shifting and movement in prone, the arms become more externally rotated while the forearms rotate from pronation into supination, with pressure shifting across from the radial to the ulnar surface of the hands. Increased and varied weight bearing and tactile stimulation across the hands help to reduce the sensitivity of the grasp response. So the typical upper extremity weight-bearing progression aids in opening the baby's flexed fingers and hands. Experiences in the prone position also provide considerable proprioception through the joints of the upper extremities as well as opportunities to increase control and strength.

The child with spina bifida needs coordination and strength of the upper extremities to use assistive devices for ambulation, to perform activities of daily living, and to manipulate paper and pencil for tasks in school. But using the upper extremities in lieu of head and trunk support will limit the baby's motor experiences of the arms and hands. The shoulders remain elevated to continue providing stability for the head. Arms tend to be held in more internal rotation with scapular protraction. The forearms are pronated, and wrist and hand flexion may also be seen. Weight bearing on the hands may remain limited to the radial aspect.

Paralysis of the lower extremities decreases the total amount of tactile, proprioceptive, and vestibular input that the child is receiving from the body. The degree to which this loss affects the individual depends on the remaining movement and sensation available in the legs, the function of the upper body, and the child's CNS status for processing this tactile input. If a child is able to explore the environment actively and independently, knowledge is gained about the body in relation to the environment. A typical baby has a vast number of movement experiences occurring at the same time, and learning is acquired through many sensory modalities. When movement and exploration are limited, learning is ultimately affected. Lower extremity paralysis, in combination with low tone and poor head control, makes gross motor movement, especially against gravity, more difficult for many children with spina bifida, which can also affect the child's motivation and willingness to move. When movement is more difficult, it can become a negative experience, and learning more sophisticated skills will be impacted.

Therapists need to appreciate these impediments on motor learning for children with spina bifida and use this information to facilitate and encourage early handling strategies for parents that will enhance their baby's development and encourage the acquisition of more typical movement patterns.[86–95]

▶ Handling strategies for parents

As mentioned earlier, instruction sessions with parents should begin, when possible, before the child is discharged from the hospital and should continue until the parents are comfortable with their handling and acceptable movement and function of the child is observed. Parents should be aggressive in their involvement, but tempered by the medical status and age of their baby. Teaching sessions should ideally include opportunities for the parents to observe the therapist handling their baby and time to practice with this expert assistance.

Parents often focus on the most conspicuous deficit, their baby's lower extremity paralysis. But the PT has the responsibility of incorporating into the instructional program additional information that will promote the family's understanding of gross, fine, and perceptual motor abilities above the waist. The pace of instruction should be based on the status of the infant and the capacity of the family. Families can be gently alerted, during early treatment sessions, about the developmental delays that may be seen in some children, especially the possible difficulty in developing control of the head and upper body. Parents should not permit the baby to be held or positioned with the head at severe angles. The presence of hypotonus will influence the acquisition of antigravity head control in all directions, and we must alert caregivers to avoid allowing the overstretching of neck muscles and other soft tissue structures. Adapting the car seat with a soft towel roll to maintain erect head alignment is one useful suggestion. Leaning the seat back will also decrease the effect of gravity on the baby's head and neck.

In supine, the infant will be the most asymmetric until active neck flexion is present to maintain the head in midline and the baby may have difficulty turning the head from side to side due to gravity acting on the head. Abnormal compensatory patterns of movement may be seen when the baby tries to turn or the baby may be content keeping the head to one side. The prone position promotes greater symmetry, but may be frustrating if neck and upper trunk extensor strength is poor and the baby cannot easily lift and turn the head. Keeping the head to one side in either prone or supine may tire the infant who may begin to cry. In response, a parent will lift the baby or roll it into a different position. By responding in this manner, the parent unknowingly assumed responsibility for a motor skill that the child should be mastering. Parents should be educated that their good intentions may actually interfere with appropriate muscle development needed for their baby to move in a more acceptable manner and they can be instructed in alternative approaches.

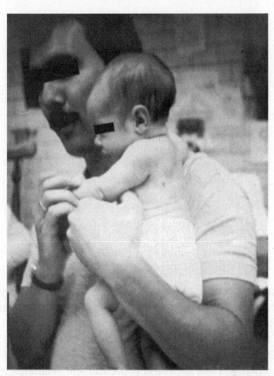

FIGURE 6.8 Typical infant at 6 weeks of age. The infant is stabilizing his head while in an upright position. Note the erect alignment of the thoracic spine in an infant with normal muscle tone.

Extensive literature is available that describes early motor development of the typical child. From this information, as mentioned earlier, we learn that an infant acquires head and neck stability in upright postures before he or she can lift their head from prone or maintain midline control in supine. Gaining the ability to stabilize the head while upright facilitates strengthening of the musculature needed to lift and control the head in the other positions (Figs. 6.8 and 6.9). With these thoughts in mind, the therapist can recommend that parents offer their baby with spina bifida experiences in all positions with a strong emphasis on upright postures.[34,88–93]

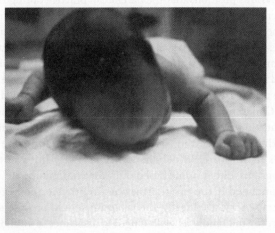

FIGURE 6.9 The same infant as shown in Figure 6.8, barely able to elevate his head to turn it side to side in a prone position.

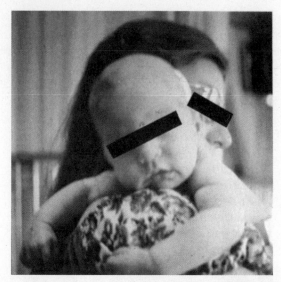

FIGURE 6.10 Infant is being carried high on the adult's shoulder to allow independent movement of the head and an improved position of the upper extremities.

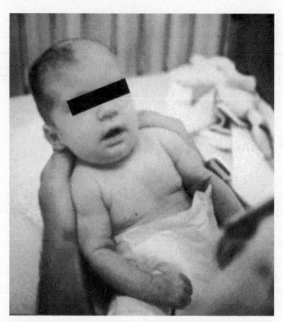

FIGURE 6.11 A suggested position for handling an infant in supine. Note the hand placement of the parent to provide a symmetric midline posture while stimulating the baby in face-to-face play.

Parents can be taught to carry their awake, alert child in ways that will not require support and will facilitate development of antigravity head control without allowing the head to fall suddenly in an uncontrolled manner, eliciting a startle response. Holding the baby high up on the parent's shoulder rather than at the chest level is one position that can be tried (Fig. 6.10). Another useful strategy is for the parent to sit near a table holding their baby in sitting, on the table, facing them, and at eye level. The parent, while engaged in visual play with their child, is providing experiences for practicing independent head control. The infant can be held around the shoulders at first and then lower, at chest level, as head stability and control develops. Providing upright experiences, however, does not mean that the child is placed in an infant seat. More about that, shortly.

Parents can be instructed to observe their infant for prolonged asymmetries. But the therapist should not wait to demonstrate appropriate, symmetric alignment of the baby in various positions that the parent can practice during their normal routines of the day: diaper changes, dressing, meal time, rest, and play (Fig. 6.11). Another position that encourages a more symmetric alignment is with the parent sitting comfortably on a soft chair or sofa, legs elevated with hips and knees partially flexed. The baby can be nestled supine, on the parent's legs, face-to-face, with head and body in midline.

Children with spina bifida often require long-term therapeutic intervention that may be unavailable or inconvenient in the hospital setting. This is especially true for those babies in whom CNS deficits are seen. Early intervention programs, either home based or in the community, are recommended if the program is able to provide the needed therapy services. Ideally, the program should provide support for the family as well. Ongoing assistance is vital once the family leaves the secure environment of the hospital and takes their baby home. The services of a 0-to 3-program should be provided to families whether they are experienced with older children or are first-time parents. It is interesting that some parents, who have other children, may be accustomed to the range of motor development seen in typically developing infants. They may deny or minimize the developmental delays of their child with spina bifida, regardless of the information they are receiving to the contrary. So early and consistent input by the therapist is required to help parents develop a critical eye and an effective approach to address the needs of their child. It is inappropriate to wait until significant delays or abnormalities are seen before referring a child to an intervention program.

▶ Physical therapy for the growing child

Developmental Concerns

A long-range plan of care should be developed by the PT that is acceptable to the neurosurgeon, orthopedic surgeon, and family. The therapy plan for the young child with spina bifida is based largely on the objective findings by the PT integrated with the concerns of the other specialists. Repeated manual muscle tests and careful observation of the child's development enables the therapist to identify the child's strengths and weaknesses. Intervention can then be directed at both the specific issues related to the lower extremities and the child's overall gross motor development (Display 6.6).

Children with spina bifida need to practice activities to improve righting and equilibrium responses of the head and trunk. When the therapist addresses these needs and sees improvement, there is an important secondary benefit. While stimulating the child's automatic balance responses against gravity in all positions, active movement in the trunk and lower extremities can be seen. So these balance responses should become an important part of the child's daily home exercise program because of this two-fold benefit.[67]

Sitting, with movement, stimulates the child's balance, improves head and trunk control, increases the child's visual field, and provides an opportunity for many eye–hand experiences. Head-righting and equilibrium responses in sitting can be tested and improved by holding the child at the shoulders and slowly tilting him or her backward. Beginning conservatively at 20 to 30 degrees, the infant should respond by holding the head steady and then returning the head forward depending on the baby's age and skill level. Next, the therapist brings the infant's body back to midline and repeats the activity to one side, the other side, forward, and to the diagonal directions. If no response occurs in any direction and the child's head hangs, or if the child becomes upset with the activity, the movement may have been too rapid, or the baby was tilted too far. A slower and less challenging movement is used until a response is noted and one can build from there. Changing the position of the supporting hands may also enable a child to react in the direction that was weaker. With the baby positioned on the lap of the handler, gentle downward pressure through the shoulders and thorax or mild bouncing to stimulate and approximate the joint surfaces of the cervical and thoracic spines may also assist. As the child's responses to the tilting become more brisk and strong, the angle of the tilting can be increased. Over time as the child improves, support can be moved distally to the chest and then to the waist, but the activity continues. During this balance and equilibrium routine, especially when the baby is tilted to the diagonal directions, the oblique abdominals as well as lower extremity musculature will contract in response to shifts in the center of gravity and in an attempt to maintain an upright

posture. As equilibrium responses strengthen, active hip flexion, hip adduction and abduction, knee extension, and ankle and foot movements can be seen. There have been instances when children who had limited head and upper body control started working on righting and equilibrium reactions, and over time, a significant improvement was seen not only in these automatic responses, but also in the movement and strength of the legs. Working on developmentally appropriate positions and movement patterns is especially helpful to address the lower extremity needs of young children who cannot follow verbal directions and are unable to intentionally participate in strengthening activities.

When asymmetries in the baby's balance reactions are noted to one or more directions, repetitions can be added in those directions or they can be performed more frequently, but the stronger responses should still be included and not forgotten. For the young child, it is recommended that these sessions of tilting last only about 2 to 5 minutes and stop if the baby becomes tired or upset. It is advisable to help families identify a few opportunities during the child's daily routine and their usual schedule, during which they can practice this activity. For a parent who watches a lot of television, suggest they work with their baby on these exercises during part of each commercial break. They can also work on this equilibrium activity for the amount of time it takes to slowly sing the ABC song, after each time the baby's diaper is changed, trying to keep the baby engaged through the entire song. The song is used as a timing device. While practicing balance and only getting to the letter "G" one day, a parent can aim for more of the song the next time. Identifying specific times when the exercises can be practiced may encourage compliance and enable the responses to strengthen more quickly (Fig. 6.12).

In the prone position, neck and thoracic extensor strengthening is achieved as the child attempts and becomes successful at maintaining the head and thorax up against gravity without the use of his or her upper extremities. Low back extensors, gluteals, quadriceps, and plantarflexors can be activated during prone extension patterns of movement, provided of course that the muscles are innervated. Routine carrying of the infant in the prone position or playing face-to-face with a family member while both are lying on the floor or on a bed will stimulate the baby to hold his or her head erect. As this reaction becomes stronger, the baby can be further challenged with side-to-side weight shifting, which will strengthen the responses and continue to stimulate the muscles of the trunk and lower extremities.

As mentioned earlier, in supine the effects of gravity may cause the child to look the most asymmetric. Strengthening of active neck flexion during sitting and tilting activities will carry over and improve the child's active head control in midline when supine, thus decreasing much of the asymmetry. Spending time in supine facilitates beginning eye–hand coordination and bilateral upper extremity play for the typical child. But if the child with spina bifida remains asymmetric with the head turned to a preferred side, development of these skills will be hampered. Supine also facilitates

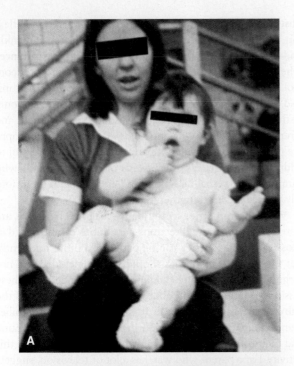

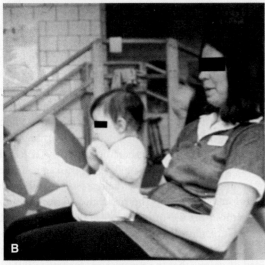

FIGURE 6.12 (A, B) Challenging the child's balance responses to elicit more sophisticated and stronger upper body reactions and strengthening of the lower extremities as they respond.

disassociation of body parts as the child moves into and out of the position while at play. Through rotation of the thorax on the lumbar spine, the lumbar spine on the pelvis, and the lower extremities on the pelvis, a great deal of strengthening and control of these body parts is gained. When the child holds his or her legs up in supine, extending them to kick and play against gravity, neck flexors and abdominal musculature are strengthened as well as the muscles of the lower extremities. Neck and trunk flexors combine with the extensors to provide for good spinal alignment in sitting, which is another goal for the baby as he or she progresses.

A typical infant, held up in their parent's hands, as early as 2 months of age can bear weight on their lower extremities

as a result of the positive support reaction. When this novel response is discovered by parents, it is quickly included into the repertoire of positions that parents use to play with their child. Proprioceptive input through the legs and spine is provided by this weight bearing. The sensory input is important for body awareness and perception of body in space. Standing also provides the baby with a new visual perspective of his or her surroundings. During this early weight bearing, contact between the femoral head and acetabulum, together with muscle contractions around the hip joint, help to stimulate acetabular development, properly seating and stabilizing the hip joint. As the child grows, practice in this position evolves from being reflexive to being volitional. Upright weight bearing continues to challenge and improve extension, control, and balance against gravity and stimulates available muscles in the trunk and lower extremities that will assist with independent sitting and standing.

The family members of a child with spina bifida should be taught to assist their young child to perform brief periods of supported standing several times each day until the child can stand with less assistance, or until a first standing device or bracing is provided for longer periods in upright. Placing the child on a solid table surface, the baby can be supported against the parent's body, and one leg at a time can be stabilized and the body weight lowered onto the leg. The activity does not have to be performed with both legs simultaneously, if this is too difficult (Fig. 6.13). Using a small ball or lowering a child from the parent's shoulder to stand on their lap are two other methods. Many ways can be tried until one is found that is easy and convenient for the parent and success is seen.[34,67]

Returning briefly to general development, as the child with spina bifida becomes more mobile but learns to use his or her arms to compensate for weakness in the trunk and neck, the child may be able to roll over, attain the four-point position, and perhaps pull to stand, if lower extremity function is adequate. But this progression, with increased reliance on the arms, and poor trunk strength will ultimately lead to the child requiring a higher level of bracing than the level of the back lesion might indicate, and the child will also require a more supportive assistive device during gait than would otherwise have been predicted. Therefore, during assessment and treatment, it is not sufficient merely to identify that a developmental milestone has occurred. Rather, it is important to assess the quality of the movement, including such considerations as the child's ability to perform the movement against gravity, whether the movement is typical in appearance, or whether compensatory or abnormal patterns have developed. One can then identify the patterns of movement that need to be enhanced and strengthened as foundations for future skills, as well as the movements that should be avoided or changed.[67] Intervention for the areas of concern can be addressed in a safe and appropriate therapeutic regimen. The physical therapy plan can include activities performed in all positions, the use of gravity to challenge the child, with varied and changing movement

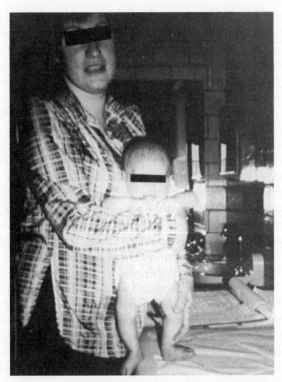

FIGURE 6.13 Brief periods of standing throughout the day will help provide for well-aligned weight bearing in the child without fully innervated musculature of the lower extremities.

experiences to facilitate motor development. By providing these opportunities, there is an increased likelihood that the child's gross, fine, and perceptual motor abilities will be less negatively affected, and the child's gross motor skills will be commensurate with the motor level of the lower extremities.[86–96]

Infant Devices

The issue of infant seats and various baby positioning devices always arises during conversations with parents and should be addressed by the therapist as soon as possible. The available literature is consistent in its insistence that all infants need to be active to acquire the strength and motor control necessary to move against gravity, attain erect sitting and standing postures, and walk. The infant must receive and integrate vast amounts of sensory and motor information to build a foundation of knowledge about his or her body and to develop the ability to function effectively within the environment. Infant walkers, jumper seats, swings, bouncer chairs, and the excessive use of infant seats can have a negative impact on motor development and sensorimotor learning. So the use of these devices will further delay the development of the baby with spina bifida who is already at risk for motor disturbances. (Several of these concerns are explored in greater detail in Chapter 11.)

All infants must experience the upright sitting position because of its influence for mastering many skills. Upright sitting gives the child a new visual perspective of the surroundings and provides the first sensation of the effects of gravity, the weight of the head, and the opportunity to stabilize the head over the shoulders. However, to practice and gain confidence in these early skills, the infant must be stimulated by movement, for example, while being carried in a parent's arms. The experiences of random and varied weight shifting and tilting as the parent moves and walks are physiologically important. Mild bobbing and jerking movements of the head stimulate the stretch reflexes in the joint receptors of the neck, producing muscle contractions that mark the infant's beginning attempts at head control. This stimulation is essential. However, most infant seating devices offer total support, which is unwise for the infant with spina bifida who may be slow to develop head control. Infants with spina bifida need frequent opportunities to participate in activities that challenge the head, neck, and trunk. The infant should be actively moving and turning to see his or her surroundings and to feel and respond to gravity acting on their body parts in different planes. To be seated in a device allows little or no active participation in movement or in the learning process. The device allows the infant to be passive and visually entertained without offering any motor benefits. When the infant tries to move in a seated device, it is common to see an arching or hyperextending of the neck against the back of the device, a pattern that is not conducive to further acquisition of functional skills.

Now consider the child who has sufficient lower extremity function to successfully move around the room in an infant walker. The pelvis and upper body are supported, and the child is often seen with poor alignment, possibly tilted to one side in the walker. Coordinated reciprocal movements of the legs are not necessary to gain momentum in this device, and weight bearing through the legs is often random, momentary, and sporadic. Only a quick, thrusting pattern is necessary to propel the device. It is inappropriate to facilitate and strengthen this pattern because it has no carryover for developing coordinated movements or providing stability to the lower extremities and trunk, both of which are vital components for independent standing and ambulation. Rather, infants should bear weight on their lower extremities while maintaining appropriate, erect alignment of the trunk and upper body over their legs. Parents who are concerned about the "weak" legs of their infant with spina bifida can be guided and encouraged to provide prone, supine, and standing experiences that require more active participation from the child's whole body, as was mentioned in the previous section. Typically, when moving and playing, children use many parts of their body at once. A child who is excited by a bright object or favorite toy will be seen moving his or her arms while also lifting and kicking his or her legs. These movements help strengthen the musculature of the legs and trunk while offering unique sensory stimulation, and parents can be encouraged to play and excite their baby in this manner rather than thinking a device will be helpful.

Parents may initially only plan to use these positioning devices or a walker for short periods of time. But, since most parents strive to be good parents and keep their children happy and content, the time in these devices often increases insidiously. This is especially true if the baby is entertained, further reducing the time the baby spends moving around on the floor. In assessing the use of such devices and the type of instruction a therapist may give a parent, one must consider the lifestyle of the family. Many parents spend long periods of time out of the house, in a car, traveling to appointments, going to the supermarket, shopping center, or other destinations. The infant may go from a car seat into a stroller or shopping cart and back to the car seat. Add this to the time the infant spends sleeping and eating, and it becomes apparent that little time is left for more beneficial activities. However radical the approach may seem, the therapist may find it best to totally discourage the use of all infant devices. Then, if parents must use an infant seat for a brief period of time, for example, during mealtime or to keep the baby nearby while cooking, that parent might be more conscientious and remove the baby as soon as possible. Of course, the exception is in the case of a car safety seat, which must always be used when traveling and whose use should be strongly reinforced.[34,67,86,88,90–92,97]

 Orthotics

Introduction to Bracing

A discussion of orthotics for the young child with spina bifida is most logically approached by grouping the children together who share motor levels that require similar orthopedic and orthotic management. In this chapter, we consider the children with thoracic-level lesions in one group, those with high lumbar L-1 to L-3 lesions in a second group, children with low lumbar L-4 to L-5 lesions in a third group, and those with sacral lesions in a fourth, final group. Early splinting, standing devices, and bracing for initial standing and ambulation will be discussed for each of the groups and a rough plan of progression suggested. One should be aware that within each group the children may have very different patterns of active movement, strengths, and upright function. Thus, the clinician should remember that each child must be evaluated individually and depending on the findings, a management plan specific to that child can be developed, with the information in this section serving as a guide.

Philosophies of Bracing

Some clinics follow a bracing philosophy that preestablishes a plateau of expected maximum function for children on the basis of their lesion level and general gross motor development. Several publications have supported the concept that an ultimate and predictable level of mobility exists for children at each motor level. These approaches advocate establishing reasonable but not unrealistic expectations for each child because much time, effort, and expense can be spent on orthotic management and physical therapy services to teach gait training and maintain upright skills that, for some children, will only be feasible for a short time in their lives. This philosophy is thought to be an efficient, cost-effective method that supports the concept that later functional outcome can be predicted primarily by the child's lesion level at an early age. Institutions that follow this model are often reluctant to brace a child with a thoracic or high lumbar lesion after the early childhood years, since the literature indicates that most adolescents with high-level lesions are mobile only from a wheelchair and have discarded functional ambulation by their teen years. There is, however, opposing research that acknowledges a significant number of variables that affect the level of upright performance of a child, of which lower extremity innervation is only one factor. Interest, commitment, and participation by the family and the child's CNS function, motivation, learning capacity, and the desire for movement are just a few of the factors that should be considered when deciding whether to begin, proceed with, or discontinue an ambulation program. An article from a major clinic in Australia identified that the later the child began to ambulate, the earlier he or she was to abandon it. The article also pointed to rapid growth and weight gain, the need for frequent brace adjustments, and other medical problems as interfering factors that stop a child from ambulation even earlier than might have been expected.[98] An editorial by Dr. Malcolm Menelaus stated that early ambulation is important for a number of physiologic and psychological reasons even if it is abandoned later in the individual's life.[99] Finally, from an ethical standpoint, one might question whether proceeding with or terminating a gait program should be determined by anyone other than the patient as evidenced by his or her abilities, in combination with the family, who is ultimately responsible for their child's program continuity and follow-up care.

The Lurie Children's Hospital in Chicago followed a course of action in which all children who are seen through the myelomeningocele clinic begin a program of early standing and gait training and as the child grows, the medical staff, parents, school personnel, and the child communicate and share their impressions and experiences, so bracing and ambulation can continue for as long as it seems reasonable. When a patient is considered a household or exercise ambulator and uses a wheelchair for primary mobility, this level of gait is still supported and encouraged by the clinic staff.

Adopting this approach means that more time is required to communicate between various institutions and individuals so that everyone is aware of the ambulation goals and is working toward the same end. Because the patient's needs and abilities may be constantly changing, the goals established for mobility also have to be flexible. Changes in medical care for children with spina bifida, as well as advances in orthotics technology and materials, warrant an active and creative approach toward bracing and gait. The end goal is to help each child attain his or her optimal level of performance, regardless of motor level, and to assist the child to maintain this level for as long as is feasible. Consider just one issue: the physical environment of the child and its impact. In this country, in large and small cities, rural and suburban areas, there can be tremendous variations in the style of architecture and the size of homes and apartments. The condition of sidewalks, yards, or driveways, accessibility of schools, access to parks and expanses of space to walk and play, and many other assets or obstacles will influence the child's ability to acquire and maintain gait skills. All information should be considered when helping to develop a gait program, rather than using the child's lesion level as the determining factor.[34,67,81,100,101]

General Principles of Orthotics

Any discussion of bracing raises the fundamental question of whether the child should be braced high and levels of bracing removed as motor control is mastered or whether the child should be braced low, with sections added as the need dictates. Unfortunately, initial orthotic decisions can be imprecise and only become more refined with clinical experience. A brace that is prescribed for a moving, growing, changing child can only be correct for the brief period of time that the child remains exactly as he or she was when evaluated. That period of time may be very short for the 1-to-3-year-old child, longer for the 3- to 5-year old, and longer still for the teenager at 14 to 16 years of age. This means that the younger child who is growing rapidly and is very active may require more frequent brace reevaluations, revisions, and repairs. This is not an indication to become frustrated and give up on the ambulation plan, but rather to be even more diligent and committed to supporting the ambulation process with the patient and family.

Also, in order to make an appropriate brace selection, the CNS function and the effects of CNS dysfunction on the child's ability to move must be considered as well as the motor level of the lower extremities. The orthopedic surgeon, PT, and family should try to gather as much objective information about the child as possible prior to beginning an orthotics program. The PT, having spent time with the child, should have a good impression of the child's motor capabilities. Also, asking parents to share their perceptions of their child's motor function can identify any differences between home and clinic performance. For example, parents can be asked to describe the ways in which their child likes to play, their child's favorite positions, responses to the upright position, degree of assistance needed to change positions, and the method the child uses to move and explore on the floor. The answers to these questions can give the therapist valuable information about how active the child is, even though the child may be sitting quietly in a stroller in the clinic, throughout this conversation. There have also been families who, though excited about the prospects of beginning a bracing and gait program with their child, were able to verbalize that their child did not seem ready to be upright, follow directions, and walk with braces and an assistive device. So the plan was postponed for a few months to enable the child to begin practicing small parts of the gait program, for short periods of time each day, until the child seemed more ready and the parents were agreeable. In specific situations, we may introduce a walker in the house so the child begins to see it as a piece of furniture and is no longer frightened when asked to hold it. Another child may be placed in their braces and allowed to go through their typical day, but nothing more. Or, a child may be braced and propped at the sofa to play, without being asked to move. The ability to break up a process or an activity and introduce it in small portions to the timid or fearful child may make the difference between success and failure.

Once a brace is fabricated for a child, the family should be shown proper donning and doffing. Appropriate leg coverings should be suggested to protect the child's skin. This therapist recommends a long, boy's tube sock for protection or thin, nontextured tights for both girls and boys. Parents should be alerted as to where and how to look for improper fit of a brace and when a brace modification would be indicated owing to poor fit. Pressure along the medial or lateral borders of the feet, ankles, and knees and the bony prominences of hips and legs should be examined. Parents should be included in the plan when a change is being considered, adding or subtracting a section of the brace on the basis of their child's progression or if problems are encountered. Regardless of the brace, families must know whom to call and what action should be taken if the brace does not produce the desired result. They should understand that the problems with the brace do not mean that they or their child are failures or are somehow inadequate. Selecting and fitting the appropriate brace for a child is an ongoing process that may take time to perfect. The need for change to an already existing brace program is often based on sound observations and recommendations from parents, who are living and working with their child each day. Depending on the clinic protocol, when a bracing problem arises, parents should know whom to contact, so that appropriate direction can be given and appointments made. Families should not have braces sitting in a closet for several months, unused, while awaiting a routine clinic appointment to discuss a problem with the therapist or orthopedic surgeon. Likewise, a poorly fitting brace that might cause skin damage should not be worn because the parents want to comply with their home program instructions. Bracing changes that require adding a level of support should not be construed as the child's failure, regression, or lack of progress. Rather, it should be handled as a matter of course for an oftentimes difficult decision that is based on both objective and subjective findings.

Decisions to change the bracing level, unlock joints, or change an assistive device should be made in a thoughtful and considered manner. The child's attitude toward and readiness for gait training plays a large part in the timeliness of these decisions. Generally, the aim is for safe and functional ambulation by 5 or 6 years of age in preparation for mobility in school. But, given the numerous tasks and skills to be mastered, this is not a great deal of time in which to prepare. Parents and therapists may feel rushed when the child is nearing school age, but sufficient time must be allowed for mastery of skills at one stage before progressing to the next. Some families are assertive when expressing their desire to have their child standing and ambulating with as little assistance as possible, as soon as possible. This should not rush the clinician into making a premature decision that might have a negative effect on the child's outcome. The responsible method of practice is to pace the progression of skills slowly to achieve the safest, most secure, and least stressful result for the child and family, while still moving forward. In keeping with this measured approach, only one change at a time should be made to an orthosis or an assistive device. Unlock the proximal joint of the brace or remove a trunk strap, see the outcome and allow some time for the child to adapt, before making the next alteration. Note that the child has progressed nicely with a walker before trying to transition to crutches. Otherwise, diagnosing the etiology of a problem that may arise becomes more difficult if multiple modifications were made at the same time or over too short a period of time.

A well-defined orthotics program should begin as early as the child's first days of life after the initial evaluations are concluded. The PT and orthopedic surgeon can discuss the deformities that are present and those that may likely occur secondary to muscle imbalance or bony deformity around a joint. They can then develop a plan of care, including necessary taping, splinting, and bracing, to address the current and/or anticipated problems. Orthopedic surgery and an early orthotics program can then be coordinated to prepare the child for upright positioning close to the typical developmental age of 12 to 15 months, if possible.[24,67,82]

Children with Thoracic-level Paralysis

The child with no motor control below the thorax has flaccid lower extremities and is at risk for developing a frog-legged deformity. This posture is also commonly seen in the immobile infant who remains in supine for long periods of time. The legs are abducted, externally rotated, and flexed at the hips and knees with the feet in plantarflexion. There is no active leg motion to counteract the effects of gravity and reverse this position. Muscle and other soft tissue structures become increasingly tight over a short period of time without proper attention, and the presence of reflex activity can make the flexed posture more resistant. Prone positioning and daily ROM exercises are advised. Also, gentle nighttime wrapping of the legs in extension and adduction with an elastic bandage can help prevent or minimize the deformity. Flexibility can be gained using these intervention strategies when minimal to moderate tightness already exists, but trying to avoid the problem before it occurs is the primary goal.

As the child grows, a "total-contact" orthosis may be used during nap times and through the night to prevent loss of joint range. Proper fit of the brace will prevent limb movement within the device that can lead to abrasions, and the child should always wear protective tights or long socks. To enable the child to work further on control and strength of the head and trunk, this first orthosis can be adapted with wedged rubber soles so it can be used for brief periods of standing and tilting exercises during the day. During these sessions of standing, the child can practice and become proficient in balance and equilibrium reactions of increasing difficulty (Fig. 6.14). Prone-lying in the splint, while the child is asleep, is recommended to help avoid pressure over the bony prominences, such as the ischial tuberosity, sacrum, and calcaneus. Skin breakdown at these sites is common with persistent supine positioning. Inspection of the skin is also essential after each session with the orthosis, and any red marks that do not fade should be brought to the attention of the orthotist for adjustment.

If the child has moderate to severe limitations in hip ROM, it is inappropriate to use an orthosis to force the limbs into better alignment. This is dangerous and can result in skin breakdown and/or a fracture, especially at the proximal femoral neck. Significant limitations in flexibility are managed best by conservative methods of wrapping and gentle stretching with eventual surgical release of the tight soft tissue structures, including the iliotibial band, hip external rotators, and knee flexors. The orthosis can then be used following surgery to maintain the newly acquired position.

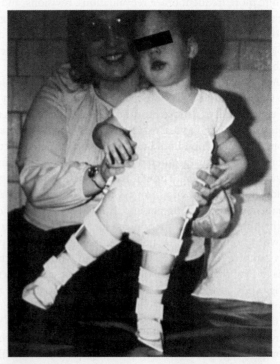

FIGURE 6.14 A total-contact orthosis to be worn at night fitted with wedged soles for periods of standing and weight-shifting activities.

The total-contact orthosis should always include a thoracolumbar section to stabilize the pelvis and lumbar spine. Without this section, the child can move and laterally flex the trunk, causing malalignment of the lower extremities, with adduction of one hip and abduction of the other hip, relative to the pelvis. Contractures at the foot will make later brace and shoe fit difficult, so the total-contact orthosis should also include the lower legs and feet to hold the knees extended and the ankles in a neutral or plantigrade position.

For the older child or adolescent with a high thoracic lesion who may no longer be ambulatory, the total-contact orthosis may be appropriate to use at night, to prevent or minimize contractures that can easily develop in individuals who are sitting all day. Also, a lightweight, foot splint or ankle–foot orthosis (AFO) can be fabricated for use during the day to maintain good positioning and shoe fit for the child who is mobile from their wheelchair.[24,67]

Children with High Lumbar Paralysis

Children with a motor level from L-1 to L-3 will usually exhibit some active hip flexion and adduction, but usually no other strong movements at the hips or knees are present. Weak quadriceps and medial hamstrings may be noted in some children with an L-3 motor level. To prevent flexion/adduction contractures at the hips, the child with a high lumbar lesion can also benefit from the use of the total-contact orthosis. The splint can maintain hip and knee extension with moderate abduction (approximately 30 degrees) and be worn during sleep. It can also serve as the child's first standing device.

Children with this degree of lumbar paralysis will usually require an initial level of bracing that supports the hips and lower legs to stand and walk. Bracing at that level is necessary to stabilize extension at the knees and a 90-degree angle of the ankles and to provide medial–lateral control at the hips and pelvis. A number of children with this level of paralysis who have strong trunk musculature, good sitting balance, and intact CNS function may be able to control the medial–lateral planes of hip movement and ambulate without orthotic control at the hips later in childhood, but they will still require bracing above the knees, as well as some type of assistive device such as a walker or crutches.

Hip subluxations and dislocations are common in children with a high lumbar paralysis owing to the significant muscle imbalance around the hip. It can be either unilateral or bilateral. When hip dislocation is detected, therapists and parents should continue passive ROM exercises, with care, to ensure that there will be no additional loss of joint flexibility or related muscle shortening. There is often fear that more damage to the joint will occur from ROM exercises, but this is not the case. Rather, more harm is done by discontinuing the exercises and allowing additional adductor and flexor tightness to develop. There has been much discussion and debate within the orthopedic community regarding the optimal surgical approach to the dislocated hip in patients

with this level of paralysis. The current consensus is that surgery to relocate either one or both hips is not indicated. This approach avoids many postoperative complications that may be more problematic than the original dislocation. Fractures, pain, and infection can occur as well as a stiff, frozen hip as a result of an open reduction procedure. An immobile hip joint will compromise sitting and standing alignment, and often requires additional surgery, if it can be corrected at all. Redislocation of as many as 30% to 45% of the hips is also common, owing to the lack of dynamic forces around the hip to provide joint stability. Lastly, the hip dislocation does not affect the child's functional abilities in upright. Simple surgical release of soft tissue structures may be decided if the active and unopposed hip flexors and adductors have tightened to the point of restricting range. In the case of a unilateral dislocation, an asymmetric pelvis can result if the involved hip becomes tight. This asymmetric posture creates an uneven foundation for sitting and standing and interferes with proper fit and alignment of braces. Again, addressing the limitation of ROM and achieving a level pelvis without joint surgery is more important than achieving a good radiologic picture. Evaluation for a shoe lift may be necessary for the child with a unilateral hip dislocation in order to equalize leg lengths when the child is upright. Even a small leg-length difference may affect standing alignment and stability of the younger, smaller patient.

When hip surgery is performed, it is appropriate for the PT to be involved with the patient and family for home program instruction when the child leaves with a cast as well as after the cast is removed to assure a flexible hip and a return to the standing or gait program.[24,67,102–107]

Orthotics for Children with Thoracic and High Lumbar Paralysis

When children with T-12 to L-3 motor levels are almost 12 months old and exhibit adequate head control to be positioned upright, they should be considered for the "A frame," also known as the Toronto standing frame. This frame can be used for multiple, short standing sessions during the day in an attempt to duplicate the activities of typical children who pull to stand for short periods of time but are still predominantly mobile on the floor on their hands and knees (Fig. 6.15). The device is easy to don and doff, and a schedule of upright positioning for up to 30 minutes, three to five times each day seems manageable for many parents. The device is freestanding and represents the child's first opportunity to be upright without having hands-on assistance from a parent or using their own upper extremities for support. Engaging the child in finger feeding, block play, and other fine motor activities is ideal during this standing time. Additionally, parents should be instructed to challenge their child while in the device by working on head-righting and balance skills. A recommended activity is to slowly tilt the frame in one direction, watching for the child's righting response of the head and trunk. The frame is returned to midline and then tilted in another

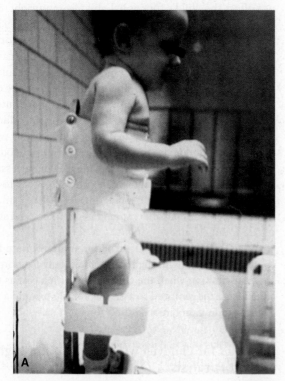

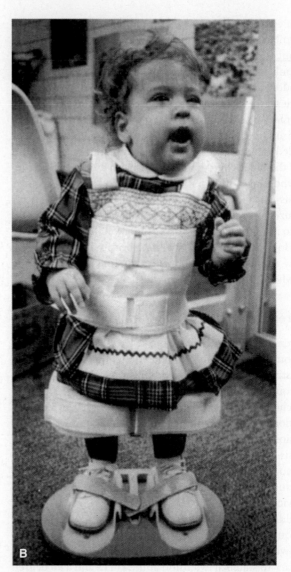

FIGURE 6.15 Toronto A frame showing good alignment for standing. **(A)** Side view. **(B)** Front view.

direction, waiting again for the child's balance response. The frame should be tilted slowly and at a small angle, and all directions should be performed: forward, back, right and left sides, and to the diagonals. This routine is recommended for the first 3 to 5 minutes of each standing session. On the basis of the child's success, further strengthening of the responses and the neck and trunk musculature can be achieved by increasing the angle of the tilt. Again, as mentioned earlier, if asymmetry is seen in the quality of the child's responses, then tilting can be performed more frequently to specific directions to strengthen these weaker reactions. Positioning the child to passively stand in front of the television is not recommended, and unsupervised standing is not advisable because the child's wiggling body can easily topple the device, causing injury.[34,67] As the child progresses in developmental activities, such as rolling, getting into and out of a sitting position, and attempting to crawl, the child may no longer tolerate the immobility of the standing frame. This may indicate a readiness for bracing and ambulation training.

Children with moderate to severe CNS deficits and delayed acquisition of head control and upper extremity function may continue to use the standing frame until they are too tall to properly fit into the frame (at about 6 years of age, depending on the child's height). As the child outgrows the frame, either the parapodium or the Orlau swivel walker may be considered. These are two orthotic options that will provide continued and valuable time in an upright posture while providing adequate support of the upper body to meet the needs of the child with significant motor delay. Both are easy to don and doff, they are simple to size and fit well, and are also freestanding, so require supervision. Regardless of the device chosen, the child should continue an exercise program that includes developmental and preambulation skills to further improve function in the neck, arms, and upper body. While in either device, the child can practice weight-shift activities as described earlier. For the child in a parapodium, a walker or forearm crutches can be introduced at some point to teach forward mobility using a hop-to gait, if the child has sufficient upper extremity strength and coordination. The Orlau swivel walker has a ball-bearing plate at its base that causes a forward progression on smooth level surfaces without the use of an assistive device. Movement of the Orlau walker requires the child to move the head and shoulders in a side-to-side motion that causes the device to unweight on one side and swivel forward. As skills improve, children can progress to different, less supportive and restrictive orthotics, but the child can remain with either of these two devices as long as it will accommodate their growth.[67]

For many years, the standard hip–knee–ankle–foot orthosis (HKAFO) was the only option for the child with a high level of paralysis who had graduated from the standing devices and was ready to ambulate. A thoracic extension could be added to the HKAFO for the child with limited trunk control, but this was very confining and limited the child's potential to walk only as a household or exercise ambulator. Another option, the Louisiana State University Reciprocating Gait Orthosis (RGO), originally developed for the adult with traumatic paraplegia, easily transitioned as a viable option for the child with spina bifida. The RGO uses a system of cables with a dual-action hip joint that flexes one hip while maintaining the opposite hip in locked extension for a stable one-legged stance and a reciprocating pattern of gait. A properly fitted RGO maintains the ankles at 90 degrees with extension at the knee and hip joints and aligns and supports the trunk and pelvis over the legs with lateral thoracic uprights and a strap. Many children who have used the RGO and an assistive device have been able to progress to a more energy-efficient and safer gait pattern than was possible with the HKAFO. As a child's trunk stability improves, the RGO can be modified without decreasing the child's ability. By retaining the cables and dual-action hip joints but removing the chest strap and thoracic uprights, the child can still use the brace mechanism for an assisted reciprocating gait, but with less restriction of the upper body.[108–111]

The isocentric RGO is another device that eliminates the posterior cable system but maintains the same functional properties as the original RGO. Patients and families accustomed to using the original RGO can be switched to the isocentric model when the child grows and a new brace is required or it can be prescribed as the child's first brace.[109]

With hip and knee joints locked, the child ambulating with either of these reciprocating braces and an assistive device performs a lateral weight shift onto one leg and leans slightly back at the shoulders to facilitate the forward flexion of the unweighted leg. Repeating the weight shift and posterior lean produces forward flexion of the opposite leg. This gait pattern requires no active motor function in the lower extremities, but if active hip flexion is present, it can be utilized to flex the limb forward and the weighted leg remains stabilized in extension (Figs. 6.16 to 6.18).[109–111]

When using the standard HKAFO with a pelvic band, locked hip and knee joints, and solid ankle joints, the child can learn either a hop-to or swivel pattern of gait using a walker, later mastering the swing-through pattern with

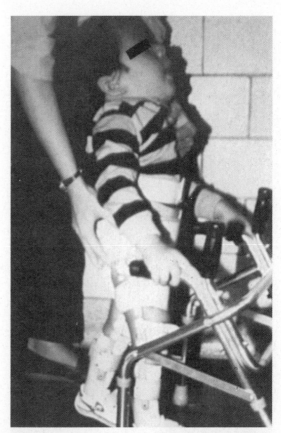

FIGURE 6.16 Gait training with a reciprocating gait orthosis. A lateral weight shift with a slight tilt backward causes the unweighted leg to swing forward.

forearm crutches as arm strength and control increases. The child with active hip flexors can attempt to walk with one or both hip joints unlocked, using a reciprocating gait pattern. In the absence of innervated gluteals however, when both hips are unlocked, the child will jackknife forward. To maintain an erect posture, the child must be able to hyperextend the lumbar spine to shift the center of gravity posterior. The child must also use both upper extremities to remain erect by pushing on the walker or crutches (Fig. 6.19). When unlocking the hip joints of the HKAFO, the pelvic band maintains leg alignment in hip abduction/adduction and medial/lateral rotation, motions the child is unable to actively control. For some children with a high lumbar lesion and an intact CNS, the pelvic band may be removed at some point to allow further freedom for transfers and to permit a faster swing-through gait pattern, when the child progresses to crutches. Arm strength, trunk stability, and the ability to hyperextend the lumbar spine are essential for a stable stance without the pelvic band. When these skills are present, the gait of this child more closely resembles the patient with acquired, traumatic paraplegia.[109,110]

Regardless of the orthosis, most young children and their therapists find that the rollator walker is the most effective assistive device to begin gait training. With four points of stability and two front wheels, this walker provides good support and the child does not have to lift the walker to

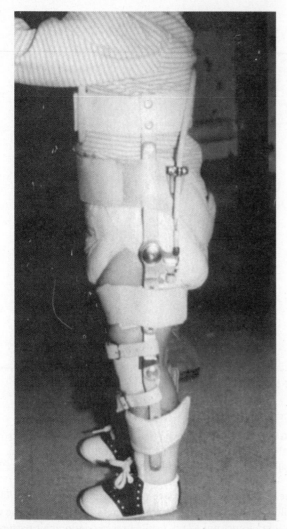

FIGURE 6.17 Alignment and fit of a reciprocating gait orthosis with a thoracic strap and uprights, cable, and dual-action hip joints. Note the use of patellar pad to maintain true knee extension.

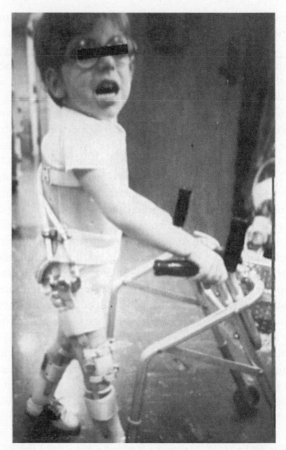

FIGURE 6.18 A reciprocating gait orthosis, fit over a plastic body jacket, to manage scoliosis. Note the erect alignment in this child with paralysis at the T-10 level.

advance it. For this reason, the standard walker is almost never used. An anterior-facing walker also provides better support for children who require bracing above the knee.

Young children can begin the gait program by first learning to hold their walker, often requiring hand-over-hand assistance from an adult. While standing at a low window or mirror, the child is reminded not to let go or move lest they and the walker tilt and fall over. Placing the walker against the wall or mirror stabilizes it in the sagittal plane while the child learns to control the remaining directions. After a few practice sessions, the child may be moved away from the support and shown how to move themselves. If possible, the use of parallel bars should be avoided during initial gait training because they provide too much stability and the young child may develop patterns of leaning and pulling on the bars that will be dangerous when making the transition to a walker that can tilt and fall over. Exceptions to this may be made in cases where a child has difficulty learning to use a walker or is very fearful. But before assuming parallel bars

are the answer, one should first check that the level of bracing is appropriate and not too low so the child feels the need for more support (Table 6.2).

The decision to progress the child from a walker to either axillary or forearm crutches will depend on the child's ability. The child should have a reasonable period of time to walk successfully with the first device before transitioning to another. A typical timeline for progression cannot be easily recommended or predicted, and a degree of experimentation may be necessary. It is best to make the transition by 6 to 8 years of age, when upper extremity strength is sufficient, the child can follow simple cues and verbal directions, and before a child becomes too dependent on the walker or becomes anxious about falling.

A child wearing a body jacket to control scoliosis may find axillary crutches difficult to use. The crutches may be hard to stabilize and may move against the slippery spinal brace. With HKAFO bracing and a truncal addition, axillary crutches can get caught on the lateral uprights. But, axillary crutches encourage a more upright posture and they may work well for the child who does not have good strength or control of the shoulders and needs this added support for a reciprocating gait or hop-to pattern.

The swing-to and swing-through patterns are best accomplished with forearm crutches, and it has been this author's

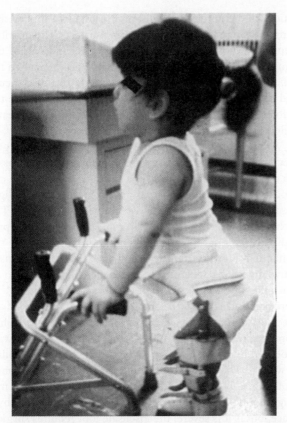

FIGURE 6.19 Hip–knee–ankle–foot orthosis (HKAFO) with hip joints unlocked. The child with an L-4 or L-5 motor level maintains balance with a hyperextended lumbar spine and upper extremity support on the walker. The HKAFO is needed to control medial–lateral instability at the hips due to muscle imbalance.

experience that the vast majority of children with spina bifida who make the transition go from a walker to forearm crutches. However, the child who is using forearm crutches over several years, leaning forward onto the crutches, can develop an upper thoracic kyphosis and tight pectoral muscles that cause elevation and protraction of the shoulders and scapulae. If these postural malalignments begin

to develop, the therapist and family should work together with the child to maintain a flexible, erect thoracic spine and well-aligned shoulders. Prone lifts and exercises for shoulder external rotation and depression, in sitting, prone, and/or supine, will help strengthen the rhomboids and lower trapezius muscles and stretch the tightening pectorals, which may help to minimize any permanent structural changes.

By the time the child, with a thoracic or high-level lumbar paralysis, approaches adolescence, he or she may have already chosen to use a wheelchair as their primary form of mobility to be faster and more competitive with peers. It has been found that girls prefer wheelchair mobility earlier than boys as a result of their earlier puberty and the weight gain and body development that accompanies adolescence. As transition to a wheelchair occurs, children and families may discard the idea of bracing, standing, and walking. The growth spurts and weight gain that are typical of all adolescents make brace management a serious problem for the child with spina bifida. Braces may require more frequent adjustment, repair, and/or replacement. The child might be spending little or no time standing and walking during the school day, so the value of the braces is greatly reduced in their eyes. But spending a full day in a wheelchair increases the likelihood of developing hip and knee flexion contractures and foot deformities. These are common in the non-ambulatory adolescent and can impact the child's wheelchair and transfer skills, bed mobility, and skin integrity. Therefore, when wheelchair mobility is chosen, if possible, children should also maintain a program of positioning and physical activity aimed at avoiding joint contractures and musculoskeletal deterioration. Prone positioning in combination with a standing device, parapodium, or braces can be used during prescribed therapy sessions and for periods of time throughout the week, both at home and at school. Imbedded into the routines of the home, standing in some manner, for homework, meals, relaxation time, etc. will help to maintain the musculoskeletal and physiologic benefits of upright that were discussed earlier in this chapter. Swimming, wheelchair sports and games, wheelchair aerobics, and other

TABLE **6.2**	Ambulation Sequence: T-12 to L-3 Motor Level		
	CNS Status		
	Typical → Mild Deficit	**Mild → Moderate**	**Moderate → Severe**
Preambulation orthosis	Toronto A Frame	Toronto A Frame	Toronto A Frame
Assess	Ambulation bracing at 15–24 mo	Ambulation bracing at 15–24 mo	Continue with A Frame
Ambulation orthosis	HKAFO; locked hips; rollator walker	RGO; thoracic uprights; rollator walker	Orlau swivel walker; no assistive device
Progress	As above, hips unlocked	RGO; remove uprights; rollator walker	RGO; thoracic uprights; rollator walker
Progress	As above, crutches	As above, crutches	
Progress	KAFO, pelvic band removed; crutches	Assess for further changes; consider standard HKAFO or KAFO	Assess for further changes

CNS, central nervous system; HKAFO, hip–knee–ankle–foot orthosis; KAFO, knee–ankle–foot orthosis; RGO, reciprocating gait orthosis.

activities that help weight control and improve cardiovascular function can be a part of the child's activity regimen as well. Maintaining and increasing trunk and arm strength and coordination also remains important for the older child/adolescent so that during these times of growth and weight gain, there is no loss of function.[24,98–100,103,104,112]

Children with Low Lumbar Paralysis

Children with L-4 or L-5 motor function usually have strong hip flexors and adductors. Gluteus medius and tensor fascia lata may be present to contribute to active hip abduction, although the strength of these muscles can vary from a "Poor" to "Good" grade depending on the contribution from the innervated nerve roots. Hip extension power from the gluteus maximus is absent. Children at this level are at risk for flexion contractures as well as early hip dislocation or later progressive subluxation, depending on the relative strengths of the muscles surrounding the hip joint. Inherent ligamentous laxity in the child with low tone also contributes to hip joint instability.

Manual muscle testing around the knee usually shows strong quadriceps and medial hamstrings (semitendinosus and semimembranosus) but absent lateral hamstring function. Kicking and crawling during the early childhood years can produce an internal tibial torsion deformity from the unopposed stimulation by the medial hamstrings on the tibia. This imbalance in muscle forces contributes to a toeing-in posture during standing and gait, which may first be observed when the child pulls to stand and begins to cruise.

Careful manual muscle testing is crucial in children with this lower-level lesion because there is often great variation of motor ability at the ankle and foot (Display 6.7). The anterior and posterior tibialis muscles, long and short toe extensors, peroneus longus and brevis muscles, and toe flexors may be functional, but the strengths in these muscle groups vary greatly. If significant imbalance in strength is found, patients may need to wear splints at night to prevent a progressive loss of flexibility. Splinting may also be recommended to maintain foot flexibility until corrective surgery is appropriate.

With strong dorsiflexors and absent plantarflexors, a calcaneus deformity may have been present at birth, or it may develop through early childhood. An exceptionally high arch, a pes cavus deformity, is caused by the unopposed

action of the anterior tibialis, and results in a foot with a dangerously reduced weight-bearing surface. The distribution of body weight is limited to the heel and ball of the foot, and pressure problems can quickly develop when the child begins walking. Bracing and shoe fit can be difficult, and surgery is often indicated to weaken or eliminate the deforming forces, realign the bones, and provide a greater weight-bearing surface over the entire sole of the foot.[113]

When there is an absence of the plantarflexor (gastrocnemius/soleus) muscles, the various combinations of strengths and weaknesses of the intrinsic musculature can produce additional abnormal ankle, foot, and toe alignment and abnormality of the weight-bearing surfaces. The orthopedic surgeon may consider muscle-lengthening procedures and tendon transfers in an attempt to balance the dynamic forces around the joints or excise the tendons if active muscle balance cannot be reached. The goal is to attain a flat foot that is easy to fit with bracing and shoes.[113,114] Torosian and Dias stated that deformities of the foot are the most common lower limb problem in the spina bifida population. Foot deformities cause pain, interfere with shoe and brace fit, and negatively affect the child's ability to walk.[115] They addressed the management of severe hindfoot valgus, but the principles are universal to all foot malalignment. A mild deformity may be accommodated by a brace, but if it is severe, the insensate foot requires surgical correction because it is highly vulnerable to pressure sores and ulceration.

The clubfoot deformity (talipes equinovarus) is the most common foot deformity requiring surgical correction for children with an L-4 or L-5 motor level (Fig. 6.20). The diagnosis and management of clubfoot has prompted extensive discussion, but most surgeons now follow a protocol that includes gentle manipulation and taping as early as the baby's first weeks of life, followed by application of a well-padded splint, rather than serial casting. Casting had been used extensively in previous years, and the change of approach was in response to the problems that developed from pressure over bony prominences, associated skin irritation, and breakdown. Casting is also not precise in applying the appropriate pressures to a small foot with this multiplane deformity. The clubfoot is often very resistant to conservative treatment, and surgical correction may be inevitable. Recurrence of a clubfoot deformity, secondary to conservative treatment or incomplete surgical correction, can be as high as 68% and may lead to skin problems from a brace and shoe that is difficult to fit.[113] Postoperative gentle passive stretching exercises to maintain flexibility of the foot and a well-padded, properly fitting brace are important, although additional surgery to fully correct the deformity will be necessary in the future. It is reported that when tendon lengthening is used in lieu of excision of the tendons, the deformity is more likely to recur. Since children with this level of motor paralysis will most always need bracing to stabilize the ankle and foot for gait, tendon excision has no functional impact on the child's level of bracing or ambulation potential. The

DISPLAY	
6.7	**Common Foot Deformities in Patients with Spina Bifida**

Pes calcaneus, calcaneovarus, calcaneovalgus
Talipes equinovarus or clubfoot
Pes equines or flatfoot
Convex pes valgus or rocker-bottom foot with vertical talus
Pes cavus, high arch with toe-clawing
Ankle valgus, at the mid- or hindfoot

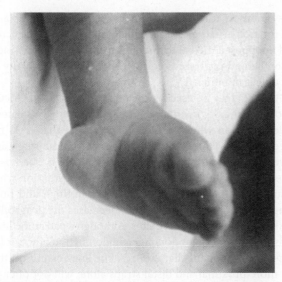

FIGURE 6.20 Talipes equinovarus (clubfoot deformity) in a neonate. She will be treated with serial taping to gently stretch soft tissue structures into a more neutral position followed by surgery.

midfoot of this type of deformity has a prominent medial crease, and the forefoot is adducted. With surgery, the foot lengthens as it becomes better aligned. Prior to surgery, parents can be instructed to perform frequent but gentle stretching of the skin and soft tissue structures, especially of the medial aspect of the foot as well as posterior, at the tight heelcord. This has been found to help prevent wound dehiscence, a complication following surgery, when the skin is stretched thin and taut to cover the longer, corrected foot. The more flexible the soft tissue, prior to surgery, the less likely it is that this will occur.[24,67,116,117]

Regarding hip reduction surgery for the child with an L4 or L5 motor level, the debate continues. When deciding on a course of management, the discussion should focus on the child's motor function, including lower extremity strength and developmental skills and the child's potential to walk with an assistive device versus independently. Surgical correction is considered contraindicated if bracing to the hips and/or assistive devices will always be needed for mobility, because the hip status will not affect these parameters. On the other hand, surgical correction may be considered for the child with good motor control of the trunk and strong quadriceps and gluteus medius musculature. If this child is able to walk with some configuration of AFO or KAFO bracing and no assistive device, a surgeon may choose to address the child's hip(s) to prevent or correct gait deviations that might hamper the child's future unassisted walking. Surgery might also be considered to prevent degenerative changes in the unstable hip. Many surgeons contend that bilateral hip dislocations should never be surgically repaired for fear that postoperative complications could ultimately be more harmful, with minimal functional gains and the greater potential for diminished gait later in life. A unilateral dislocation is usually only corrected in the child with a low level of innervation and intact CNS function who has the potential for ambulation with short bracing and no assistive device.[24,67,118]

It is apparent from this section of the chapter and from the literature that the management of hip dislocations is often a confusing and contradictory subject for the child with a low lumbar lesion. The therapist can play an important role in assisting the physician to identify the child's muscle strengths and weaknesses, skills in the upright position, trunk and pelvic alignment, and overall gross motor ability. This information may then enable the physician to better evaluate the treatment options and decide accordingly. It is widely accepted that function, not X-ray findings, should guide this important decision.

Children with L-4 to L-5 paralysis who have significant CNS deficits may not be able to control their trunk in upright positions or move their legs well. This lack of movement often conveys the impression that a higher level of paralysis exists. The therapist and the family should continue their attempts to remediate the effects of any CNS deficit, by improving coordination and antigravity strength of the head, shoulders, and trunk. An upright program can begin with a Toronto standing frame and progress to a parapodium and then to the RGO for gait training as feasible. These upright devices can offer a psychological and motivational boost for the family and the child who has been slow to acquire gross motor skills. If gait training is performed in a patient and thoughtful manner, some measure of success can be realized. In error, a child with poor trunk stability but a low lumbar paralysis might be fitted for bracing that is too low, based solely on the lower extremity muscle testing. These inappropriate orthotics and the resulting ineffective attempts at gait training can create great frustration for everyone involved. To avoid these situations, use of the RGO seems to provide significant benefits for this group of children who can then be progressed to a lower brace level at some point in the future, as their skills improve.[108–110]

Children who have a lesion level at L-4 to L-5 and without any apparent CNS deficit can be provided with bracing according to their need (Table 6.3). Many children at this level are attempting to stand or can already pull to stand by 10 to 12 months of age, and will not require a standing frame. If the child can control his or her knees while upright, they can go directly to an AFO (Fig. 6.21). Although some children at this motor level will be able to stand and begin to walk without foot support, the AFO will provide ankle stability for stance and gait and assist in normalizing gait parameters, increasing ambulation speed, increasing stride length, decreasing double support time, and decreasing oxygen consumption. The orthosis will also help to control the subtalar joint, preventing heel valgus, and control forefoot adduction/abduction. Care should always be taken that the AFO is set at 90 degrees to give the child a solid foundation for standing and does not permit flexion at the ankle that would translate into compensatory proximal flexion of the knees and hips.[24,67,119] "Twister cables" may be added if tibial or femoral rotation is seen when the child is upright. This is a simple mechanism with a waist band and a cable running laterally down each side, attaching to the proximal lateral aspect of each AFO. They are adjusted to provide the correct amount of rotatory force to better align the foot progression angles of each leg. Internal rotation, emanating from unequal forces at the hip or behind the knee, is very common at this lesion level (Fig. 6.22). However, external rotation of both legs or a combination of internal rotation of one leg and external rotation of the other leg may also be seen. Twister cables can be adjusted to control any of these combinations, and are valuable in aligning the lower leg for a safer and more cosmetic gait. Twister cables should always be attached to both AFOs. They cannot be attached unilaterally. If one leg does not require correction, then the cable on that side can be set at neutral. Twisters can also reduce some of the stance-phase varus or valgus deviations at the knee that are seen in the limb with excessive torsion. Twisters may prevent overstretching of the loose ligamentous structures at the knee if the child were to continue walking with the legs malaligned. Over time, with the help of the twister cables, the child may learn to control minimal rotational deviations independently and avoid surgical correction, but ultimately surgery to derotate the legs will be indicated for most children. Surgery is usually recommended at 6 years of age. The procedure should correct the

bony rotation at its source, either the femur or the tibia. If the rotation is in the lower leg, tendon transfer of the active and unopposed medial hamstrings to a more midline orientation behind the knee is performed so that redeformity of the tibia is minimized.[67]

A KAFO may be used for the child with weak quadriceps who has difficulty maintaining either unilateral or bilateral knee extension when upright. Many braces that cross the knee joint are fabricated with straps across the thigh and lower leg. This author has found that adding a true knee/patellar pad will help maintain better knee extension while reducing the pressure exerted across the thigh and tibial straps. This reduction in pressure decreases the probability of skin breakdown at those sites. Although a pad at the knee adds to the time spent donning and doffing the brace, it is a valuable component that ensures true knee extension that the more proximal and distal straps alone will not offer. In some children who have been ambulatory in bracing with only the thigh and tibial straps, a posterior displacement of the tibia relative to the femur can occur when excessive flexion force is exerted into the tibial strap during standing. The patellar pad prevents this from occurring. One note: if knee flexion is seen on one side when the child stands and walks, prior to considering the KAFO, a possible leg-length discrepancy should first be ruled out, which would cause the longer leg to flex.[24,67]

TABLE 6.3	Orthotic Management for L-4 to L-5 and Sacral Motor Lesions	
	L-4 to L-5	**Sacral**
Muscles present	Hip flexors and adductors	All, with possible exception of gluteus maximus, gastrocnemius/soleus group, and foot intrinsics
	Quadriceps	
	Medial hamstrings	
	Anterior tibialis	
	Some gluteus medius	
	Some foot intrinsics	
Preambulation orthotics	Toronto standing frame (some children may pull to stand, bypassing the frame, and begin with bracing[a])	Usually none needed[a]
Ambulation bracing	RGO if CNS deficits present	AFO with weak gastrocnemius/soleus or crouched gait. Some need no bracing, but shoe insert may help maintain proper foot alignment
	KAFO with weak quadriceps	
	AFO with good truncal balance, with or without "twisters" if torsion is present[a]	
Assistive devices	Start with rollator walker and progress to crutches. An independent gait is possible for some, usually with a gluteus medius lurch and lumbar lordosis	Possibly a walker early on; most progress to an independent gait[a]
Expected functional level	Ambulatory in life unless increased body weight; flexion contractures; poor CNS status; further complications may reduce ambulatory status	Independent gait with moderate to minimal deviations based on patterns of weakness

[a]Control of upper body and CNS status may modify these levels.
AFO, ankle–foot orthosis; CNS, central nervous system; KAFO, knee–ankle–foot orthosis; RGO, reciprocating gait orthosis.

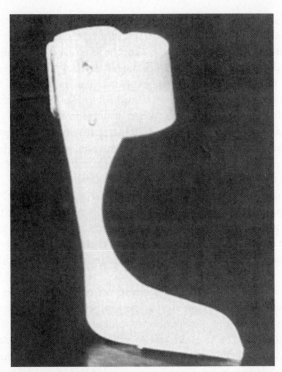

FIGURE 6.21 A plastic ankle–foot orthosis is aligned at 90 degrees or at a neutral position.

Some clinics have used a "floor-reaction" or "anticrouch" orthosis for children who have difficulty attaining knee extension. This orthosis is a standard AFO with an anterior shell that should facilitate knee extension at heel strike. The orthosis is theoretically sound and has been used successfully with other motor disabilities. But problems with excessive pressure across the bony anterior tibia and subsequent skin breakdown have caused some centers to avoid using this brace with the spina bifida population.

A study presented by Hunt et al. explored the use of a hinged AFO that limited mobility at the ankle from 5 degrees of dorsiflexion to 10 degrees of plantarflexion rather than the typical solid ankle. It demonstrated a positive influence on walking velocity; therefore, this brace may warrant further investigation.[120] Allowing dorsiflexion at the ankle that produces consistent knee flexion may have to be monitored by the family and reevaluated at more frequent intervals by the clinicians to avoid development of knee or hip flexion contractures that will limit a child's ambulation skills. Regardless of the orthosis chosen, a careful assessment of the resulting gait pattern should determine the success or failure of a particular device and the need for revision or replacement.

The child with an L-4 or L-5 motor level is often able to begin ambulation with a rollator walker after only a brief demonstration in the clinic. Crutch training for the young child, before the age of 6 years is often more involved and lengthy, and many clinicians believe that crutches are ill-advised until the child has reached a reasonable level of skill

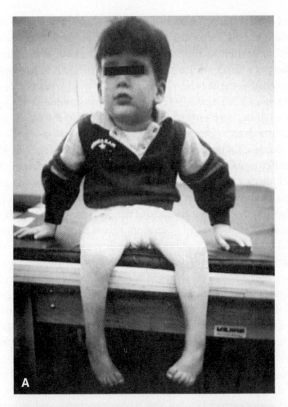

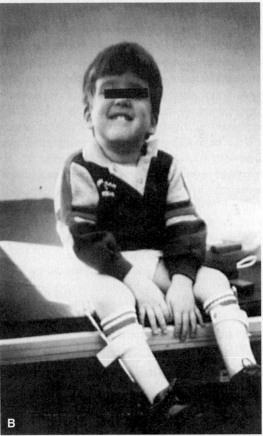

FIGURE 6.22 **(A, B)** A child with an L-4 to L-5 motor level and significant intoeing is portrayed. Twister cables are attached to an ankle–foot orthosis to control rotation or torsion until surgery is indicated.

and self-confidence with a walker. The child must have a sufficient attention span to benefit from short training sessions with crutches without experiencing excessive frustration. The only successful experience this author has had with crutch use earlier than 5 years of age was with a patient whose mother was a PT. She was committed and diligent to have her son enter kindergarten fully ambulatory and independent.

Some children with L-4 to L-5 paralysis will attempt independent, unassisted ambulation. Their gait pattern usually includes a hyperlordotic lumbar spine and a side-to-side gluteus medius lurch that can be quite severe as the child grows. The degree of these deviations depends on the strength of the hip extensors and abductors relative to the hip flexors and adductors as well as the stability and control of the trunk and height of the child. Gait will improve when good back and abdominal strength can assist with holding better alignment of the lumbar spine and pelvis, but some degree of deviation will always be seen when there is weakness and/or muscle imbalance around the hip joints. Secondary external rotation and valgus deformities at the knees and ankles can also occur with unsupported gait. For this reason, therapists should vigorously support the continued use of an assistive device through childhood and adolescence to prevent overstretching of soft tissue structures and arthritic changes to the joints with accompanying pain. Prevention or minimizing of these problems is imperative as they can lead to decreased or total loss of gait skills later in the child's life.

Moderate to severe hip flexion contractures are the single most influential factor leading to the deterioration of ambulation skills in these children. Hip flexion contractures of 20 degrees or more for the child using AFOs and crutches can diminish gait velocity by as much as 65%. For this reason, despite the high degree of activity demonstrated by many children with a low lumbar lesion, ROM exercises remain important. A prone positioning program is also helpful to counteract the hyperlordotic posture of the spine and flexion at the hips that is seen during ambulation. Prone positioning for prescribed periods during the day, as well as through the night, can minimize the development of hip flexion contractures. Activities to maintain spinal mobility and to prevent a fixed lordotic spine should be included. Supine and sitting activities to address abdominal muscle strength, which will influence balance and spinal alignment, are also recommended for a comprehensive long-term program at school and in the home.[77,81,67,105,114,117]

Children with Sacral-level Paralysis

The child with a sacral-level lesion will have a greater degree of muscle function throughout the lower extremities than a child with any other motor level. But, as with other levels, there remains a great deal of variation among the children in this group as well. Muscle forces around the hips and knees are in better balance, with full or partial innervation of the major muscle groups. At the S-1 and S-2 motor levels, strong knee flexors and gluteus medius are expected, while gluteus maximus and gastrocnemius/soleus are present, but may be weak. Children with S-2 to S-3 motor levels have innervation of all musculature of the hips, knees, and ankles, and "Fair" to "Good" strengths can be expected. The incidence of hip subluxation and dislocation is lower in this population than at the higher motor levels. When dislocation does occur, surgical intervention is recommended primarily to avoid later joint pain, reduce lateral trunk flexing, and improve the biomechanics of the child's gait.[106] Significant hip flexion contractures should not develop, and abnormal torsions of the femur and tibia are not as prevalent as with higher-level lesions. Because of the additional musculature available at the proximal joints, through the trunk, hips, and knees, the gait pattern of the child with sacral innervation will more closely resemble a typical gait, although mild to moderate deviations will still be seen.

Manual muscle testing demonstrates that variations in this population are greatest at the foot and ankle with weakness seen in the gastrocnemius/soleus muscle group. Toe flexors may be present and may provide some secondary ankle plantarflexion, but they are usually not strong enough to compensate for a weak gastrocnemius/soleus and stabilize the ankle during stance and through the gait cycle. As a result, AFOs will be indicated for most of these children. If strong plantarflexors are present, external support may not be necessary while the child is young, but close monitoring is necessary, especially during periods of rapid growth and weight gain. The gastrocnemius/soleus may be strong enough to adequately stabilize the tibia of a small child for standing and walking over short distances, but may not be strong enough for the active older, taller, and heavier child. Gait deviations may begin to emerge as the child grows. As the lever arm of the muscle lengthens, a decrease in muscle efficiency may result. The loss of mechanical advantage at the ankle means that additional strength is needed for stabilization, not available in a partially innervated muscle. The gastrocnemius/soleus helps control the forward movement of the tibia over the foot through the components of the stance phase. When strength is inadequate, a crouched gait may develop, because the tibia is permitted to roll too far forward and too rapidly, forcing the foot into dorsiflexion with compensatory hip and knee flexion. Therefore, the child should always be observed both in static standing and in dynamic gait during each physical therapy or clinic appointment. Flexion contractures, though not expected in children with sacral-level lesions, can develop if this flexed posture is not remediated. The added energy expense of walking with a flexion deformity will also reduce ambulation capacity. Surgical lengthening of tight hamstrings is unusual but might be necessary as a result of these changes in gait, and a previously independent ambulator may need an assistive device for support. The crouched gait and its associated problems can be prevented simply by using a fixed ankle AFO as soon as the child demonstrates a need. The child whose posture is maintained by an orthosis can then

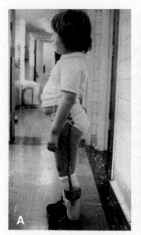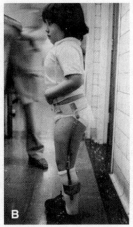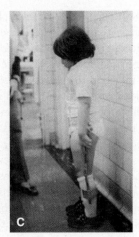

FIGURE 6.23 Nine-year-old girl with an S-1 motor level. **(A)** An independent gait has been achieved with ankle–foot orthoses and twisters. Note the poor alignment and low tone of the trunk, as well as the anterior pelvic tilt with hip flexion. **(B)** Following a long-term program of active exercises for problem areas, she works hard to align the thorax and lumbar spine cortically and improve pelvic alignment. **(C)** Increasing success with correct posture, holding during gait, is next.

go for short periods of time without bracing, to attend a party or special event, without compromising future potential.[67] The child with a sacral motor level is not intact as was once thought before more precise testing and close monitoring by physical therapy was feasible. Though the issues that can develop are not as severe as in the children with higher-level paralysis, these problems are not benign.

As our profession becomes more experienced in addressing foot and ankle problems, the child with a sacral-level lesion may benefit from having molded shoe orthotics placed within the shell of their AFO. This arrangement may more precisely address any of the hindfoot and midfoot malalignments that can arise as the child grows and imbalances of the intrinsic muscles of the foot become more pronounced. AFOs with articulating ankle joints or an AFO fabricated from a more flexible material that permits limited and controlled dorsiflexion with assisted plantarflexion may be indicated for a specific child who will benefit from the opportunity to have a more dynamic gait, thus allowing them to better utilize the active musculature at their ankle and foot.[120,121]

Compared with the child with a higher motor paralysis, the child with a sacral lesion may not appear to need therapeutic intervention. But they may exhibit some mild to moderate gait deviations that can be minimized as they grow and are able to participate in their therapy program. Benefits can be gained from therapy to "fine-tune" the child's gait. This program can be delivered during occasional sessions over a long period of time, with shorter periods of more intense intervention, if deterioration is seen, especially after a growth spurt that may negatively affect the child's alignment. Abdominal strengthening, especially the oblique abdominals as well as the rectus abdominus, and strengthening to the extensors of the trunk and limbs, is recommended. The child should also practice correct alignment of the shoulders, trunk, pelvis, and limbs during standing and ambulation. Tactile, verbal, and visual reinforcement can all be used to help the child learn and maintain proper posture for progressively longer periods of time. Children involved in a program like this may still exhibit their abnormal

gait pattern most of the time, when they are not thinking about how they look. But as the child matures, he or she may desire to walk with a corrected pattern, if even for a short period of time. The child will then have the skill and muscle strength to do so. One patient, with whom this author worked, ran around the playground at school with moderate lateral trunk flexion, severe lumbar lordosis, and bilateral internal rotation of his legs at every step. When entering the clinic area, however, he was able to align his trunk and maintain an erect, symmetric posture with both feet pointing forward, to walk past the team and show off. His mother always commented that she hoped he could walk down the aisle at his wedding looking like that.

It is a pleasure to work with a child who can reach a high level of motor function. The process of working with a child like this is also an educational opportunity for the clinician. The therapist can learn to more closely observe the child, analyze subtle gait deviations, and determine the sources of trunk and limb weakness that contribute to the deviations so an appropriate intervention plan can be made. Is the deviation from muscle paralysis, weakness, low tone, or habitual poor posture? Will addition or modification to bracing or an assistive device solve the problem, and what role will exercise play? The development of careful and critical observational skills ultimately benefits all patients, not only those with spina bifida (Fig. 6.23).

Many of the CNS, biomechanical, and neuromuscular factors that negatively influence the acquisition of mobility skills are not as prevalent in children with sacral-level paralysis compared to children with higher levels of paralysis. Fewer children with sacral lesions have hydrocephalus and require a shunt, and fewer exhibit significant hypotonicity that is pathologic and affects their gross motor development and function. As a result, children with sacral paralysis who present with hip instability or other joint deviations are usually treated aggressively to preserve their potential for life-long community ambulation.[24,67]

The use of a preambulation or standing device may not be necessary for the child at the sacral level if the child is developing strong balance responses in the trunk and exhibits a good quality of movement. The child may already be pulling up to stand by 10 to 12 months of age, as expected for a typical child. A foot splint, commonly fabricated to be worn at night to maintain alignment, may also be used during the day to stabilize a weak ankle, enabling the child to stand while awaiting definitive bracing if the need is seen. With the higher level of functional activity of this group of children, care must still be exercised to monitor the fit of all braces and shoes because sensory deficits, especially in the foot, remain a concern.

For the child who does experience CNS difficulties, one can follow the same course of intervention that would be prescribed for a child with a higher-level lesion. The program should include activities that address flexion and extension strength against gravity through the head and trunk, as well as balance and equilibrium reactions in all positions. The program should also include passive and active exercises for the lower extremities to prevent joint contractures, and a standing and orthotics program based on the skill level of the child.[67,89–93]

Three-dimensional Gait Analysis

The development of increasingly more sophisticated and more readily available gait analysis technology is providing objective information that enables therapists, orthotists, and orthopedic surgeons to visualize and more accurately understand the gait parameters and deviations of the patient with spina bifida. Widely held beliefs and treatment protocols that were developed solely on the basis of anecdotal evidence may now be validated, modified, or discarded by utilizing the three-dimensional information provided by gait analysis. Orthotic prescriptions can be better tailored to the specific needs of the child when the effects of the orthosis can be understood, especially in the sagittal plane kinematics, walking speed, and progression of ground-reaction forces across the foot, and on the three planes of motion of the pelvis, hips, and knees. Vankoski et al. from the gait lab at Lurie Children's Hospital in Chicago found that comparing the gait studies of children with spina bifida to the gait parameters of typical individuals did not provide the most meaningful information to guide and evaluate treatment plans.[122,123] Rather, it was found that children with spina bifida at a given lesion level demonstrate characteristic gait patterns that are reasonably homogenous. These identifiable patterns have become the baseline from which comparisons can be drawn, enabling the clinician to focus on realistic goals for the patient based on his or her motor level and to evaluate more fairly the result of interventions, either conservative or surgical. Ounpuu et al. found that in the absence of the gluteus medius, gluteus maximus, and ankle plantarflexors, certain compensatory movements at the pelvis and hip were consistently noted to enable children to maintain ambulation without an assistive device. This gait pattern of the child with a lumbosacral-level lesion is characterized by exaggerated movement at the pelvis and pelvic obliquity, increased stance-phase hip abduction, increased stance-phase knee flexion, knee valgus, and increased ankle dorsiflexion.[124,125] In another study, Williams et al. reported a 24% incidence of late knee pain in ambulatory patients with a lumbosacral-level lesion. Knee valgus, causing the discomfort, was found to be a result of a combination of internal pelvic and hip rotation and stance-phase knee flexion.[126] The use of gait analysis for early detection of these abnormal knee movements can direct the clinician toward the most appropriate treatment—either surgical intervention such as a tibial derotation osteotomy or the use of KAFOs, to support the knee in extension and avoid pain and joint deterioration. The continued use of crutches was also found to be an important deterrent to arthritic joint changes and pain in this population. Even though the children were able to walk unaided at an early age, continued use of crutches reduced the exaggerated range of movements and joint stress through the lumbar spine, pelvis, hips, and knees, helping to reduce gait deviations and decrease pain in those areas.[121–123] Analysis of the effects of an AFO on gait found that in many of the children examined, there was less stress placed on the knee without the brace than was noted with it. This was especially true for children with L-4 to sacral-level lesions.[127] This study is certainly not an indication to stop using a brace for a child with a lumbar or sacral-level paralysis, because the gait deviations that would arise could be far more disastrous. Rather, this type of analysis may hopefully lead to the development of new orthotics that will provide the needed control at the ankle while avoiding negative influences on the more proximal joints. Three-dimensional gait analysis is clearly moving the focus away from X-ray findings toward the child's functional abilities as a parameter to measure the success of interventions.[107]

Finally, it is interesting to note that even with the high technology of the gait labs in many institutions, the manual muscle test and gross motor assessment provided by the PT remain important components of the child's evaluation for successful development of an orthopedic treatment plan.

▶ Casting following orthopedic surgery

Earlier in this chapter, various deformities commonly associated with different motor levels were mentioned, as were some of the surgical procedures to correct them. After most of these procedures, the child must be immobilized in a cast for a period of time to allow the surgical site to heal undisturbed. The period can vary from 2 to 3 weeks following soft tissue surgery, 6 to 8 weeks for a bony procedure such as a pelvic osteotomy, and even longer. Casts and the associated immobilization should never be considered a benign treatment modality for the child with spina bifida. Pressure and irritation to insensitive skin are always a risk. Fractures, loss of joint flexibility, and loss of gross motor skills are also complications. Even children with minimal or no CNS deficits will exhibit a loss of postural security and antigravity muscle strength following a period of immobilization. Children with significant CNS problems may regress even further. It is troublesome to see children lose skills that they have struggled a long time to acquire.

Most surgeons agree that children with spina bifida should be casted for the shortest possible time needed for adequate healing.[128] Because of problems related to immobility and to minimize the number of hospitalizations and anesthesia, some surgeons will try to perform several procedures at the same time so the child is casted only once. The therapist can assist the child and family to make this period less problematic while supporting the fact that surgery and the subsequent casting period are important parts of the child's program to reduce deformity and ultimately maintain or gain function.[67] Returning the child as quickly and as safely as possible to his or her preoperative status, or to an improved status, should be the objective. Recommendations to manage the child in a cast can be discussed with the family prior to surgery whenever possible so the child's needs are understood and adequate preparation can be made at home for the postoperative period. A child undergoing surgery creates added stress to the normal routine of family life. Important questions are often forgotten when a family first learns that their child will be facing surgery. The therapist may have to anticipate many issues that families will have to face during the time their child will be immobile.

Many children will be in a hip spica cast following pelvic or hip surgery. If unilateral surgery is performed, the full hip spica may still be used to stabilize the pelvis and opposite limb, thereby assuring that no movement will occur at the surgical site. With the surgeon's approval, prone positioning will help prevent skin breakdown at bony sites such as the calcaneus and sacrum, and prone will challenge the child to lift and extend his or her head to watch television, read, or play. Prone positioning in a reclining wheelchair or on a scooter board can provide some mobility if the child can manage self-propulsion. This mobility will also reduce the amount of carrying by family members. Similarly, prone positioning on a padded wagon for trips outdoors may help the family survive this period with less anxiety and frustration because the child is occupied and happy. After several days, the physician may permit the child to stand in the cast, a position that can be easily maintained during mealtime and play. One clever family adapted a hand truck to safely stand and move their taller, heavier preadolescent while she was in a hip spica cast (Fig. 6.24). If the cast is asymmetric, towels can be propped under one foot to level the child, and cast boots will help provide a nonskid surface. To ensure the child's safety, it will be necessary to lean the child forward onto a heavy chair, table, or sofa that will not move. Depending on the child's age and reliability, it may be necessary for a family member to always remain with the child to prevent falling, not merely supervise from a distance. Families living in multilevel homes may have to prepare a temporary bedroom for the child on the first floor. An old crib mattress or a few thick blankets on the floor can be a

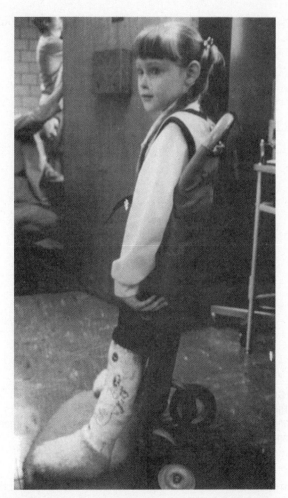

FIGURE 6.24 A parent finds an imaginative and safe way of standing and moving the older child in a hip spica by adapting a commercially available hand truck.

comfortable short-term bed. Care should be taken to avoid abrasion to the toes when the child is prone by allowing the feet to hang over the end of the mattress, or by placing some small towel rolls under the ankles to lift the toes away from the surface. Instruction should be given to family members for safe lifting and turning the child using good body mechanics while also considering the alignment of the child. Even plans to get the child home from the hospital and through the front door of the house may be a challenge.

Regardless of the age of the child in a spica cast, daily exercise periods are important to prevent loss of neck and trunk strength and to maintain the automatic balance responses that will be important when the cast is removed and the child resumes his or her daily activities. Several times each day, the child should perform a routine of exercises with a family member for 10 to 15 minutes that include prone lifts for neck and back extensors, shoulders, and arms. Supine head lifting and partial sit-ups for neck and trunk flexors, and standing with tilting in all directions complete the home program. As the child attempts these activities, muscles are contracting within the cast as well as those muscles that are visible. The muscle activity places stress on the bones of the lower

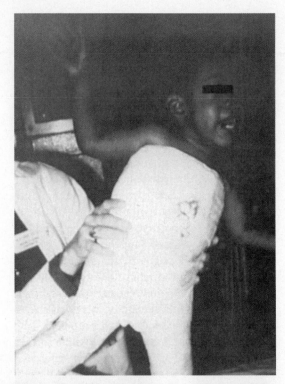

FIGURE 6.25 Child with a hip spica cast after hip reduction surgery. Note how the child is both standing and being tilted. Standing, when the surgeon approves, about 10 days after surgery, is an important aspect of the home care program.

extremities, thereby reducing bone demineralization and the risk of a fracture when the cast is removed. Postural insecurity is diminished as vestibular and proprioceptive stimulation are provided by these challenging antigravity exercises (Fig. 6.25). Families should be warned to avoid propping their child in a half-sitting position for long periods of time that will cause pressure at bony prominences, mentioned earlier, and can contribute to a rounded upper back.

The child may be readmitted for a brief period of intensive therapy once the cast is removed. Whether therapy is provided as an inpatient or outpatient, the goal should be to ensure the child's rapid and safe return to function following cast removal. Lower extremity ROM and strength, especially at the surgical site, are the immediate concerns, along with improvement in balance and equilibrium responses of the neck and upper body. A return to former function can be achieved in a short period of time if the therapist targets all of the child's needs, not only the lower extremity ROM.

If the child has a high-level lesion, surgery might have been performed to gain passive flexibility for better limb alignment and brace fit. For this child, a review of ROM exercises with parents, an orthotic evaluation, and a review of activities to further improve upper body control may be all that is needed after cast removal. The child may then be monitored, until adequate function is achieved, through an outpatient clinic, community facility, or school-based physical therapy program.

The child with a thoracic or high lumbar–level lesion who demonstrates a significant loss of motion at the hip or knee is at risk for fracture. A brief hospitalization may be indicated to regain lost mobility. The child may also be sent home in a bivalved cast or splint to be worn most of the time and removed for a program of frequent ROM exercises and sedentary activities until range is regained, if the family is able to comply. Some children are immobilized in their HKAFOs instead of a cast following soft tissue lengthening or tendon excision to allow parents to gently perform ROM exercises and stand their child during the healing process.

Procedures to relocate or stabilize the hip joint(s) in children with L-4, L-5, or sacral lesions include simple tendon lengthening, femoral or pelvic osteotomy, or the more complex Lindseth procedure, which involves a muscle transfer of a portion of the external obliques to the lateral femur. Candidates for this procedure are those children with the potential for unassisted gait and an intact CNS. Admission to the hospital after cast removal following this procedure may be necessary to ensure that joint mobility and balance skills are again safe and acceptable, and that the child is resuming ambulation without an assistive device. Concentration on trunk strengthening activities helps the transferred muscles regain their role of stabilizing the trunk and pelvis, and the functional goal is to eliminate the excessive lateral trunk flexion during gait that was seen prior to surgery.

Reduced mobility in the lumbar spine and the lower extremities is common after a long casting period. After cast removal, it is often difficult for the child to achieve 90 degrees of hip flexion for good sitting alignment because of adapted shortening of the hamstrings and hip extensors. Hip and low back tightness cause the pelvis to rock posteriorly, with a secondary thoracic kyphosis that requires attention. Gentle activities are indicated to increase pelvic and hip mobility and strength. Working with the child to gradually sit up and maintain active thoracic extension along with active hip flexion will help the child return to and hold a 90-degree alignment. It is safer to help the child work on actively holding a more erect sitting position to gain flexibility than to only move the limbs passively and possibly push too hard on a fragile bone. Care should also be taken to avoid allowing the child to sit with a rounded back for extended periods of time so this poor alignment does not become habitual and compensate for limited range of the hip joints.

Parents should be warned to initially prohibit their child from crawling after a spica cast is removed. Crawling requires hip and knee flexion exceeding 90 degrees. Hip rotation is also required as the child moves into and out of sitting and the four-point position. If the necessary flexibility is not present for these motions when the cast is removed, fractures can occur.[106,107]

Following surgery at the knee or ankle, children may have either one or two long or short leg casts. The family will require instruction to help their child avoid excessive time in supine or sitting. Besides contributing to skin breakdown, development of flexion contractures is always a major concern. Excessive sitting, crawling, and knee walking with short leg casts will increase tightness of the hip and knee flexors. Information regarding alternative positions should be offered to avoid positions that encourage flexion. Prone-lying is the preferred position, with standing and ambulation the preferred activities, when feasible. When ambulation in the cast(s) is permitted, it is achieved quickly when a walker rather than crutches is used as an assistive device for this temporary period. Crutch training is difficult for an inexperienced child because of the additional weight of the cast, potential lack of adequate balance, poor proprioception, and possibly malaligned casts. By comparison, instruction with a walker is usually a faster and safer choice. Brief strengthening exercises can be taught for back, hip, and knee extensors, along with exercises for the trunk to help keep the child mobile during the cast period. With such a multifaceted program, the child will be more likely to rapidly return to his or her previous or improved level of function once the cast is removed.[24,34,128–132]

 CNS deterioration

Throughout life, individuals with spina bifida, their family members, and the professionals involved in their care should be vigilant for any deterioration in function that could indicate hydromyelia or a tethered spinal cord. These neurologic conditions can affect the patient's mobility, gross motor function, urologic function, fine motor skills, and activities of daily living (ADLs). If diagnosed and treated in a timely fashion, the effects can be temporary. If left untreated, the symptoms can worsen, and their effects will be permanent. Therapists must be knowledgeable about these problems because they are often discovered by the clinician during routine appointments, evaluations, manual muscle testing, or in conversation with parents.[24,34,67]

Hydromyelia

Hall et al.[133] conducted a study of patients with spina bifida who exhibited rapidly progressive scoliosis and found that CSF had migrated into the spinal cord. Excess CSF was seen collecting in pockets along the spinal cord that created areas of pressure and ultimately necrosis of the surrounding peripheral nerves, causing the scoliosis. Other symptoms found to be associated with hydromyelia include progressive upper extremity weakness and hypertonus. One point to note: initial examination of the lateral ventricles showed no enlargement and did not indicate that the shunt was malfunctioning. However, revision of the VP shunt produced improvement in the symptoms for those children in whom the diagnosis was made early in this process. Some children required an additional shunt placed at the level of the fluid pockets in the spine to ensure that the excess CSF and its accompanying pressure would be completely eliminated. Lindseth, though an orthopedic surgeon, is a strong advocate for closer

investigation in all cases of rapidly progressive scoliosis, regardless of one's clinical specialty. He stated that it is important to always consider the possibility of CNS complications and not treat scoliosis as a purely musculoskeletal phenomenon. Left untreated, the fluid continues to collect along the spinal cord, causing continued deterioration in both upper and lower extremity function.[24,34,67,133,134]

Tethered Spinal Cord

At approximately 10 weeks of gestation, the vertebral column and spinal cord of the fetus are the same length, and the spinal nerves exit horizontally at their corresponding vertebrae. By 5 months of gestation, the vertebral column has grown more rapidly than the spinal cord, which now ends at S-1. At birth, the cord is at L-3, and by adulthood, the cord is at the L-1 to L-2 vertebral level.

A tethered spinal cord occurs when adhesions anchor the spinal cord at the site of the original back lesion. The child is growing rapidly, but the cord is not free to slide upward and reposition as it should. Instead, it remains bound at the level of the defect. Excessive stretch to the spinal cord causes metabolic changes and ischemia of the neural tissue, with associated degeneration in muscle function. Rapidly progressive scoliosis, hypertonus at one or several sites in the lower extremities, changes in gait pattern, and changes in urologic function may be attributed to this tethering of the spinal cord. Occurrences of increased tone on passive ROM, asymmetric changes in manual muscle testing results, areas of decreasing strength, or complaints of discomfort in the back or buttocks should alert the examiner to consider the presence of a tethered cord.[134,135] Periodic examination by professionals and an alert parent can identify early functional changes associated with this complication so appropriate medical management can be considered (Display 6.8). Petersen suggests, on the basis of his study population, that those children with repaired lesions at levels above L-3 will begin to exhibit symptoms of a tethered cord before age 6 and those with lesion levels below L-4 tend to become symptomatic after age 6. He also found that children with unrepaired back defects exhibit symptoms much earlier, regardless of the location of their lesion level.[136] When tethering is suspected, imaging may be utilized to confirm the diagnosis, and subsequent neurosurgical release can free the cord. After release, the cord may not migrate to its appropriate position, but further growth of the child may proceed without recurrence of the symptoms, and further degeneration in function may be avoided. If the release is performed in a timely manner, permanent neurologic damage can usually be prevented. However, it is becoming clear that total correction of all the symptoms following surgery cannot be assumed.[67] McClone et al. conducted a study of 30 children who exhibited scoliosis as a symptom of cord tethering and who received surgical intervention to release the spinal cord. The children who exhibited the greatest improvement of their scoliosis were

DISPLAY
6.8   **Clinical Findings That May Lead to Diagnosis of Tethered Cord**

Spasticity in muscles with sacral nerve roots
Increased tone in legs with resistance to passive ROM
Sudden increase in lumbar lordosis
Back or buttock pain
Development of scoliosis at a young age
Rapidly progressing scoliosis
Scoliosis above level of paralysis
Change in urologic function
Change in gait pattern
Progressive weakening in leg musculature

those who had spinal curves of less than 50 degrees. During a 2-to-7-year follow-up, 38% of the children began to show progression of their curves owing to the spine retethering, but the remaining children showed a stabilized or improved spinal alignment.[137]

The child who has a thoracic-level paralysis does not have the full complement of active trunk musculature to provide adequate antigravity strength to maintain an erect posture and is always at risk for scoliosis. However, a child with a lumbar or sacral lesion with full innervation of trunk musculature should be evaluated when any curvature develops, especially when it develops over a short period of time. It is recommended that hydromyelia and tethered cord should always be suspected if scoliosis occurs in a child with a motor level below T-12. Clinics that aggressively treat hydromyelia and tethered cord by surgical correction report a reduction in the overall occurrence of scoliosis that will require spinal fusion in their spina bifida population, compared with data from other sites.[138–142]

Scoliosis

The development of a spinal deformity is serious for the child with spina bifida. When scoliosis occurs and trunk alignment is compromised, the child will require additional support to remain erect in upright postures. If the child must lean on his or her upper extremities to stay up, this compensation directly impacts the child's freedom of movement and increases the energy expenditure for all activities. Propelling a wheelchair becomes more strenuous, as the child must work both to maintain the upright position as well as to move the chair. In sitting, a moderate to severe scoliosis creates pelvic obliquity that changes the surface area for weight bearing, causing areas of increased pressure that can quickly lead to skin breakdown. The posterior aspects of the thighs and bony prominences of the ischial tuberosity, greater trochanter, sacrum, and coccyx are especially vulnerable. Gait can become more unstable as truncal alignment and balance are affected. Pelvic and trunk asymmetry will affect the fit of the HKAFO and RGO bracing. When braces do not fit and gait is less efficient, the orthotics may not be worn as frequently

as they should. This can lead to further deterioration of the child's mobility skills.

The use of a spinal brace or body jacket can be useful for the child without trunk stability or to assist in slowing the progression of the curve, but surgical fusion is inevitable for many children. There are numerous methods for and preferred approaches to spinal fusion, and the periods of immobility and restrictions on daily activity vary with each. The type of instrumentation employed and the area and extent of the fusion will also influence the child's functional parameters. If the fusion extends to the sacrum, pelvic mobility is diminished and ambulatory ability can be directly affected. As previously mentioned, gait analysis has shown greater excursion of movement at the pelvis in ambulatory children with spina bifida than in the typical child. Given this information, surgeons have been reluctant to fuse down to the sacrum of an ambulatory child, if this can be avoided. For successful and efficient wheelchair propulsion, upper extremity and trunk movement are both necessary. If flexibility of the distal spine is diminished or absent secondary to fusion, an individual can lose independent wheelchair mobility. So this should also be a consideration when surgery is planned.

Maintaining flexibility and strength in all extremities and preventing skin problems during the postoperative period of immobility, following spinal fusion, should be addressed immediately after surgery, if possible. When a return to full activity is permitted, it is important to reassess the patient to determine whether functional skills have been impacted. The PT should be concerned with the patient's postoperative activity level and assist with resumption of mobility. Spinal fusion can influence the performance of many ADLs in which the child might have been independent, so adaptive strategies may need to be developed in the functional areas that were affected. It is also feasible that once the spine is stabilized the child may have greater freedom of arm movement, and might gain skills that were not possible, while earlier the child had to depend on their arms for support. A comprehensive therapy assessment and intervention program may be indicated to assist this child and their family.[24,34,67]

▶ Latex allergy

Allergic reaction to latex by individuals with spina bifida has become a relatively recent yet serious concern. Latex is a natural rubber used in a wide variety of products that come into contact with human skin and other body surfaces. In the health field, a vast number of commonly used items contain or are made exclusively from latex. Latex has been depended on for its impermeable qualities and strength while still providing sensitivity to touch. This makes it an excellent material for use in sterile gloves, where it provides protection and prevents the spread of illness. It is durable as well as elastic, which accounts for its popularity and wide usage for various types of flexible tubing and in the toy industry (Display 6.9).

Balloons
Pacifiers
Chewing gum
Dental dam
Rubber bands
Elastic in clothing
Beach toys
Koosh balls
Some types of disposable diapers
Glue
Paints
Erasers
Some brands of adhesive bandages
Bulb syringes
Ready-to-use enemas
Ostomy pouches
Oxygen masks
Pulse oximeters
Reflex hammers
Stethoscope tubing
Suction tubing
Vascular stockings
Crutch axillary pads, tips, and hand grips
Kitchen cleaning gloves
Swim goggles
Wheelchair tires
Some wheelchair cushions
Zippered food storage bags

Although it is believed that only 1% of the general population is allergic to latex, the results of various studies point out that 18% to 37% of patients with spina bifida exhibit a significant sensitivity to latex. It was also found that 7% to 10% of health care workers exhibit a latex sensitivity. Allergic reactions may appear as watery and itchy eyes, sneezing, coughing, hives, and a rash in the area of contact. More severe reactions may produce swelling of the trachea, and changes in blood pressure and circulation, resulting in anaphylactic shock. Diagnosis of latex sensitivity is based on a clinical history, observation of a reaction, and immunologic findings following a skin prick allergy test. The cause, to date, is not known, but it is theorized that early, intense, or consistent exposure to latex products results in the development of the sensitivity in many individuals. Some of the more dramatic symptoms were believed to be a result of inhalation of the powder contained in many sterile latex gloves. The powder makes the gloves easy to don and doff, but it can become airborne upon removal of the gloves. Further investigation found that this was not a consistent irritant.

The U.S. Food and Drug Administration (FDA) and the Centers for Disease Control and Prevention (CDC) continue to investigate the problem and support efforts to find the components of latex that are responsible for the allergy,

develop methods of producing safe, nonallergenic rubber, and conspicuously label products that have a latex content. There has been evidence that the latex allergy is also related to a sensitivity to bananas, chestnuts, avocados, and kiwi fruit in some patients, and this relationship is also being investigated. A blood test has been developed that is being used during pre-employment testing for health care workers and for patients with spina bifida to assist them in avoiding the allergen if the test results are positive.

Some believe that children with spina bifida develop a latex allergy because of their high level, right from birth, of exposure to materials containing latex. One study points out that the presence of spina bifida should be considered a risk factor for a latex allergy, and a method employed to prevent latex sensitivity is to practice primary prevention from the first day of life by creating a latex-free environment for the children. In one study employing this strategy for 6 years, the percentage of children sensitive to latex dropped from 26.7% to 4.5%.[143,144]

Advocacy groups are encouraging hospitals to become latex free and asking the FDA to ban latex products in all hospitals. It is recommended that parents, older patients, or other caregivers carry an autoinjectable type of epinephrine that is easy to use in case a patient experiences a serious allergic reaction. All sensitive individuals should wear a Medic Alert bracelet, necklace, or dog tags. Neighborhood paramedic teams, the fire department, and local Emergency Medical Services who might respond to an emergency call should be alerted that the patient has this sensitivity. Keeping a set of nonlatex gloves near the front door for use by emergency personnel, as they enter, is also recommended. Families and patients are encouraged to become familiar with products that must be avoided, and a list of commonly used latex products and alternative nonlatex items is available from the Spina Bifida Association of America. Refer to the end of this chapter for some sources of latex information, latex-free products, and resources that might be shared with parents.[145–153]

▶ Perceptual motor and cognitive performance

The population of children with spina bifida represents a group that is diverse across many domains. Their strengths and challenges are varied, and besides the motor and CNS issues that have already been discussed throughout this chapter, therapists should be aware of possible difficulties that may affect the learning styles and cognitive processing of their patients. This section provides only a brief overview of the vast amount of information that is available regarding perceptual and cognitive performance. Although intervention for these issues may typically fall to the expertise of the occupational therapist or educator, you are encouraged to explore this area because it will directly affect your selection of therapy strategies, teaching methods and your level of success with the child. You can also be a valuable resource for both professionals and families who may be unaware of the link between this diagnosis and the difficulties the child may be experiencing.

Great interest and concern has been expressed regarding the intellectual, sensory, and perceptual motor function of children with spina bifida. Studies have shown that the overall intelligence of the children in this population is unrelated to their anatomic motor level, severity of hydrocephalus prior to shunt insertion, or the number of shunt revisions performed. However, several factors that are considered as influencing cognition include delayed treatment of hydrocephalus, episodes of cerebral infection, and the presence of other CNS abnormalities.[42–64]

Intelligence testing for many children with spina bifida places them within the normal range but below the population mean. Willis and associates found that test scores of their subjects were particularly low in performance IQ, arithmetic achievement, and visual motor integration.[154] When the same children were retested at an older age, their arithmetic achievement and visual motor integration scores declined even further, but reading and spelling abilities did not decline. One conclusion of this study was that a visual–perceptual–organizational deficit was found that influenced the child's ability to solve mathematic and visual–spatial problems.[155] These deficits then become relatively more severe as the child ages when greater accomplishment in math is expected. Standardized assessments reflect the expectation that acquisition of skills will increase with age and educational experience, and therefore the results declined, over time, in the group that was studied. If early foundation skills are not strong, the development of more advanced, intuitive math processing will be limited.

Other research has noted a high degree of attention deficit or distractibility in some children with spina bifida. These problems were especially profound in children who showed poor language development. These same children had poor development of auditory figure-ground, which allows a child to recognize and attend to relevant features in the auditory environment. A child with difficulty in this area may not be able to identify the primary auditory input such as a teacher speaking and giving directions, nor can the child dismiss the irrelevant input such as noise from a truck passing by an open window or another child seated nearby. In a rich auditory environment, extraneous sounds easily distract the child from his or her assigned task. These children may perform better in a quiet, secluded situation, and performance in a typical, busy classroom, for similar tasks, can be poor.

Horn et al. found limited development of language comprehension in many of the children tested.[155] Individual vocabulary comprehension was normal, but comprehension of a story was poor. The children had difficulty identifying and retaining the relevant features of a story while ignoring the unimportant facts. Difficulty learning and memorizing lists of unrelated words has also been noted. However, memory for related facts was better, such as when answering questions about a short story that was read aloud.[155–157]

In all of the studies that are cited, little information was available regarding the early medical treatment of the subjects, methods, and timeliness of interventions or other complications that may have influenced the child. Therefore, it is difficult to hypothesize which factors may have been responsible for the problems. Decreased opportunity to develop and practice fine motor and manipulation skills has been thought to be a factor.[156] Other negative influences might be the limitations of early mobility that affect the child's experiences: exploring the environment, moving his or her body relative to stationary objects, and manipulating and moving those objects. Theoretical rationales for cognitive dysfunction include potential cerebellar abnormalities associated with the Chiari II malformation that would influence the range, direction, force, and rate of voluntary movements of the body and the manner in which movement is interpreted. But, regardless of the cause, the learning difficulties that result are important to note as they will affect many aspects of the child's ability to function and may be a limiting factor for the child's ultimate successes in school and throughout life.

Finally, an interesting study that examined the deficits in conceptual reasoning abilities found many children with spina bifida to be chatty, friendly, and talkative but with repetitive and nonspecific content to their conversations. Many decades before this study was conducted, the term coined for this language style was "Cocktail Party Chatter" for its old school but obvious reasons. There is quantity but little quality to the child's verbalizations, similar to walking through a crowded party and asking how everyone is doing and other niceties, but not processing the answer or going into depth to further a conversation. For the child with spina bifida, it is an organic, processing issue rather than an active behavior or choice that the child is making.[158]

Any discussion of perceptual problems in this population should also address the issue of ocular function. When compared with the typical population, strabismus occurs six to eight times more frequently in children with spina bifida. The lack of conjugate gaze influences spatial relationships, constancy of size, and development of normal visual perception. Visual–spatial problems during manipulation activities have been noted in some children with spina bifida. Other, more frequent ocular problems include nystagmus, poor ocular motility, and other convergence defects. These abnormalities have been attributed to brainstem dysfunction, although there has been no correlation between the severity of the Chiari II malformation and these clinical observations.[159–161]

The consensus seems to be that children with spina bifida need a broad range of movement and learning experiences during their early years. Increased experiences in many areas may help to decrease the negative impact of any one specific area of limitation. Testing with age-appropriate materials and in an environment where the child can focus on the task is critical. Also, eliminating test items that include a motor component may afford a more accurate and valid result (Fig. 6.26).[154–163]

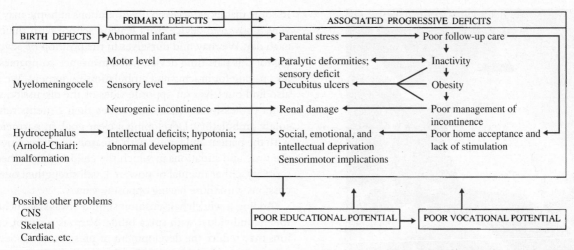

FIGURE 6.26 Primary and progressive deficits in children with spina bifida. (Adapted from *Syllabus of Instructional Courses.* American Academy for Cerebral Palsy; 1974.)

▶ Wheelchair mobility

Much of this chapter has been devoted to bracing and preparing the child for ambulation, but some type of seated mobility must also be considered for the children for whom this is necessary. Any decision to use one of the many devices available should include input from the patient when appropriate, family members, and other professional staff involved with the child. A discussion might first determine the need for and proposed uses of seated mobility. Questions to consider might be whether the device will be primarily for recreation and peer group interaction, for indoor or outdoor use, for use at school, for long family outings, or primarily for family convenience and transport.

A first device for the young child might be a hand-propelled "Caster Cart," "Ready Racer," or "The Wheel," which are all available through medical supply companies or second hand via the Internet. Commercially available electric cars and motorcycles can be modified with a hand switch rather than the usual foot pedal configuration. Imaginative parents have been able to adapt leg positioning and the level of trunk support when necessary, in these items. The devices are relatively inexpensive and low to the ground, facilitating easy transition to the floor or to a standing position. They are cosmetically appealing and are acceptable to both physically challenged and typical children alike. They can be fast and safe when used in the proper environment, and they provide beneficial stimulation and opportunities for recreation and socialization. The child's perceptual skills, upper extremity abilities, and the presence of abnormal tone can guide the therapist in selecting whether a manual or battery-operated device is more appropriate. Excessive upper extremity exertion to propel and maneuver a device may frustrate the child and produce unacceptable changes in tone if CNS dysfunction is present. One study of interest examined young children with otherwise poor independent mobility skills who received instruction in using a motorized wheelchair. Most of the children did very well, and the benefits that were noted included increased curiosity, initiative, motivation, communication, exploration, and interaction with objects in the environment. There were also significant decreases in dependency behaviors. So, rather than limit the child to struggling with a slow ambulation method in environments and situations that might become frustrating, this study supports the idea that, when used appropriately, a wheeled or powered device can be an important addition to the child's mobility program and not have a detrimental effect on motivation for ambulation training.[164]

To include their child in family outings, a stroller can be used until the child is 5 or 6 years of age. Strollers are available in progressively larger sizes, which can accommodate bracing, and can be used in combination with ambulation. For a typical child of that age, it is not unusual to alternate walking and riding in a stroller during a long family outing. But care must be taken not to increase the child's dependency on others for mobility as he or she gets older. It is helpful to know which strollers, travel chairs, or wheelchairs can be safely secured on a school bus and what the local regulations are for appropriate school transport. Seated mobility is helpful for the child who is not ready to ambulate all day in school because of limitations in balance or endurance (Fig. 6.27). A wheelchair can be obtained before the child starts school if boarding, exiting, and safe transportation on the school bus will be an issue for the child not yet fully ambulatory. Excessive distances from the bus loading area into class and to other destinations within the school should also be considered. Other indications for a wheelchair might include the child's lack of efficient mobility, marginally functional or unsafe ambulation, speed of ambulation that is necessary to travel along with peers and/or family, and the child's need for increased recreational activities that would be unavailable solely with ambulation. The child who is ambulatory can be assisted on and off the bus and secured in a car seat or a regular bus seat with a safety belt and/or harness.

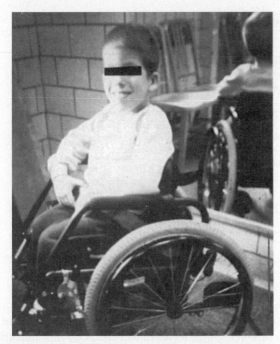

FIGURE 6.27 A lightweight wheelchair is selected for long-distance use in the school and community. This child also uses a reciprocating gait orthosis for shorter distances in the home and school.

The child would then be required to ambulate upon arrival at school and for the remainder of the day. So attendance at school should not universally be contingent on the use of a wheelchair, but must be considered on an individual basis.

The therapist should remember the increased risks for the child in a wheelchair. Scheduling time to use the chair and time out of the chair should be considered. The chance of abandonment of a gait program by family, especially for the child who may have the potential of reaching a high level of efficient ambulation, is always a risk when introducing wheelchair use. Flexion contractures of the hips and knees, skin and pressure problems, and spinal deformity are other issues affecting the seated child that will impact future potential for gait.[132] Therefore, the child should spend time both out of the wheelchair and out of the seated, flexed position every day. Consider periods of time in prone positioning, standing at a standing table or in any of a variety of standers while wearing braces, and opportunities for ambulation.

As the child matures and mobility needs change, a power wheelchair or electric scooter can provide added speed and efficiency. A motorized device, which will conserve energy, may be very important for the individual facing a long and hectic day at school or work. In the area of wheeled mobility, as in many other aspects of care, the skills, imagination, and problem-solving ability of the therapist can be extremely helpful to the individual with spina bifida and his or her family. Developing trusting relationships with dependable vendors and equipment representatives will enable the therapist to remain current in the latest devices that are available, and therefore the child's life can be enhanced.

In some instances, accessibility limitations at home may prevent a powered device from leaving school with the child each day. We may find ourselves in the position of advocating for this part-time device when insurance companies are also paying for bracing and ambulation equipment. We may also find ourselves on opposite sides of the discussion with other professionals who want to see their patients remain solely ambulatory. Developing a clear goal, in partnership with the patient and family, with a reasonable expectation of the time and situations in which the child will use wheeled mobility, either manual or powered, will strengthen our discussions with those having opposing views.

Adding a wheelchair cushion should always be included for the individual with spina bifida. Various types of cushions may reduce the development of pressure sores. Several materials are available, including high-density foams and inflatable types, which can be modified for more even weight distribution when the child exhibits asymmetry. But, regardless of the cushion chosen, activities for pressure relief are still the best means of preventing skin breakdown on the posterior thighs and buttocks and should be performed diligently throughout the day. Frequent wheelchair push-ups, side-to-side weight shifting, and out-of-chair time should be incorporated into the child's daily schedule to provide for regular pressure relief. Also, many methods should be explored that will assist the child to become independent in performing these activities, including reminders from a wristwatch alarm, talking clock, or beeper.[67,165,166]

▶ Recreation and leisure activities

As the child reaches elementary school age, the time available for extended periods of play and movement on the floor may be greatly reduced. Generally speaking, a full-time school curriculum in an integrated or mainstreamed educational setting provides little chance for consistent recreation. Gym class, with an instructor who is imaginative, motivated, and willing to collaborate with a PT, is ideal. Strategies can be developed to include the student with spina bifida into the regular array of activities the rest of the class is performing. Giving the child the opportunity to participate in the regular physical education curriculum, with adaptations or accommodations, may assist the child to find activities in which he or she is able to participate and those which he or she might also enjoy after school hours. It should never be assumed that the child with spina bifida, enrolled in a regular educational program, will automatically be excused from physical education or not be expected to participate in some aspect of an activity that their peer group is performing. The PT can also collaborate with a willing physical education teacher to develop a modification of the grading system that will take into account what the child is doing in class as opposed to what he or she is not able to perform.

The child enrolled in a special education curriculum may have periods of physical education as well as scheduled sessions for the development of recreation and leisure skills along with classmates. Once again, having an innovative and motivated staff will help to provide the child with many experiences that he or she might otherwise have no exposure to and that may become a lifelong hobby or interest.

But, as is true with the population of typical children, the child with spina bifida is most often dependent on the interest, knowledge, and resources of family and friends to provide them with experiences in new, novel, and consistent recreational pursuits. Identifying activities that can be learned and pursued throughout one's life should be considered an important part of the total care plan for the individual with spina bifida. The PT has a valuable role in assisting the patient and his or her family to find appropriate programs that offer wheelchair games and sports or modified programs for the child who is ambulatory, such as adapted/accessible playgrounds, bumper bowling, or T-ball instead of traditional Little League baseball. There are also increasing numbers of teams being formed each season that pair children with special needs with typically mobile children or young adult volunteers to complement everyone's participation. The child with spina bifida should be encouraged to regularly participate in activities that provide cardiovascular challenge, muscle strengthening, improved eye–hand coordination, wheelchair maneuvering skills, and sportsmanship from which all children can benefit. It is not uncommon for the therapist to be asked by families for an opinion or a recommendation regarding adapted bicycles and other home exercise or recreation equipment. Helping to keep the child active, by providing this professional advice to parents, can be a valuable contribution. Often, we cannot stop merely with our recommendation, but may have to provide specific resources, brand names and contact numbers of reliable vendors, and letters to justify the need for the device to insurers, to improve the potential for successful follow-through. Teaming with families and patients is time consuming but ultimately invaluable and highly worthwhile.

The inclusion and expansion of aquatics within the physical therapy profession has resulted in a significant increase in the body of research and information available for the therapist who has the opportunity to add aquatics to his or her clinical repertoire. The interest in health and fitness within the general population has resulted in the building of many more pools that are handicapped accessible and available for both recreation and therapeutic purposes. Providing opportunities to explore and enjoy the benefits of moving in water may assist the child with spina bifida to participate in this recreational activity that is also physically beneficial. Learning water safety and basic swimming skills can be taught to the young child and utilized throughout his or her lifetime. Water competency with or without the use of flotation devices can enable the person with spina bifida to experience a level of independent freedom of movement otherwise unavailable on land. More advanced aquatic skills can also be incorporated into a multifaceted therapeutic program that can be designed for the individual, taught and monitored by the PT who has access to a pool facility.

By utilizing the natural properties of resistance and buoyancy of the water, strengthening the body and increasing cardiovascular efficiency can result. And, it is fun.

This therapist has found that providing therapy sessions in a pool can be an especially useful tool in the rehabilitation program of the child following orthopedic surgery. Children who are already comfortable in the water are easily motivated to work hard on an exercise program with the excitement and novelty of this environment. Mobilizing a child who has been in a cast or in bed recovering from surgery has been achieved more rapidly in the water. Brief, free swim periods can be the rest break that is given in between the therapeutic activities or they can be the reward, at the end of a session, for a child who did a good job. When working on a mat program, taking a rest break usually means the patient is not moving, but the child will continue to move when in the water. Lap swims, races, and in-pool team games such as underwater search and retrieve, basketball, volleyball, or tag are just a few of the many possibilities that will have the child moving significantly more than he or she would in a traditional mat-based therapy session. But, as in all merging of recreation and therapy, the therapist must not compromise the goals that should be addressed or lose sight of their objectives just to have the child happy and playing. Specific exercise routines must be developed, as they would be for any program, so intervention is truly targeting the appropriate areas (Display 6.10).

DISPLAY 6.10 **Examples of Therapeutic Strategies That Can Be Utilized in a Pool Setting**

Provides strengthening to innervated lower extremity musculature, upper extremities, and trunk:

1. Movement of legs in all directions, all planes, with combination patterns of movement not feasible on a two-dimensional gym mat. Can be passive, active, active assistive, and resistive ROMs, depending on need
2. Use of flotation device in deep water with legs in the water, kicking in place against water's resistance
3. Pushing off from side of pool or therapist's hands while prone or supine on water surface to strengthen extension musculature and enjoy the sudden propulsion through the water
4. Swimming laps with only leg motions while holding kickboard or in an inner tube if necessary
5. Lap swims using webbed gloves for added propulsion and resistance and a variety of strokes to address all muscles of shoulders (flotation cuffs can be used around ankles if necessary to prevent legs from dragging on pool floor and provide extension if active gluteal musculature is not present)
6. Resistive swimming with therapist holding legs and preventing forward movement prone or supine
7. Supine, within flotation ring, lifting legs out of water and twisting them side to side for work on all abdominals
8. Ball toss and catch, basketball, newcomb, or volleyball in various water depths, depending on children's ages and abilities

▶ The young adult with spina bifida

Our interest in the patient population with spina bifida should not end when the patient moves on to an adolescent or adult facility for medical care. Although we may not be directly involved with young adults, knowledge about the challenges of this age group can be helpful for the clinician. Knowing the effects of the aging process on patients with this diagnosis, the therapist can gain a perspective that is beneficial for patients of any age. It is also helpful to have an understanding of the long-range effects of various medical, surgical, therapeutic, and intervention decisions. By knowing how they have evolved and how they have influenced the functioning of the older patient, we can attempt to improve our approach with the children. We can modify the existing protocols that were not successful and even discard them while developing new and, hopefully, better strategies that will eventually enhance the lives of our patients at any age.[167]

Selber and Dias in Chicago looked at a population of young adults with sacral-level spina bifida who had been followed at the same medical clinic and by the same staff who employed many of the same protocols since the patients were young children. They were treated aggressively for any symptoms of tethered cord and lower limb deformity. But there were still several complications that many of these individuals shared, including episodes of osteomyelitis, scoliosis, the need for amputations, and a decrease in ambulation function. The patients and their families had many opportunities over the years to receive education for skin care and had long-standing relationships with the clinic staff. The bouts of osteomyelitis may have been the result of many factors besides insensate skin or poorly fitting orthotics and shoes. What is most disturbing is that the problems might have been caused by procrastination in seeking treatment when early skin breakdown was noted, especially in the vulnerable foot and ankle areas. The more severe cases resulted in amputation. Another issue found in the study group was that many individuals maintained their community ambulation status but experienced significant knee pain and had to return to using orthotics, crutches, or canes that had been discontinued, to support and stabilize their gait and reduce joint stress. Recall, earlier in this chapter, that the group of children with sacral-level lesions was thought to be the least affected. These complications should raise an alarm for continued awareness for practitioners, patients, and their families to remain knowledgeable about the complicating factors that can impact function at any point along the life cycle. We can never assume that the intensity of our efforts and interventions can slacken over time, especially when it can potentially have such disastrous results. We may feel like we are unnecessarily repetitive, as I have been in several sections of this chapter, but hopefully the consistent reinforcement of important information may result in a better outcome for the PT student as well as the patient.[168]

Another report that did not specify the lesion levels of the young adults in the study concluded that there was a general disinterest in personal care and poor follow-through on hobbies or areas of interest and commitments. There was also an inability to organize and complete long-range projects specifically related to school activities, assignments, and term papers. And many of the children appeared stubborn and argumentative. Memory problems, poor comprehension of material, deficits in conceptual reasoning, problem solving, and mental flexibility were all identified as weaknesses in the study population.

With typical adolescents and young adults, we expect an evolution of maturity and greater acceptance of responsibility, with increasing ease and compliance in personal care, success at school and in their social lives. But this study demonstrates that the child with spina bifida may have an inherent inability to adapt successfully to these mounting expectations unless they are provided with intervention and supports that focus on remediation of their specific areas of need. It concludes that they should have opportunities to participate in the planning and execution of their own intervention plan to achieve early independence. If the child is actively engaged along with the family, before they have habituated to an excessive level of need and assistance, this action plan has a higher potential for success in the areas in which our population may be specifically limited.[158]

In a study conducted through Riley Children's Hospital in Indiana, the parents of adolescents with spina bifida voiced concerns that centered on lifelong issues affecting their children, such as accessibility, transportation in the community, and independence. The teens, however, were more concerned with the immediate issues of finances, medical care, communication and socialization with friends, and peer acceptance. With the exception of medical care, their issues were, again, not too different from what would be expected of their typical peers. The study concluded that attention should be given to assisting this population with social integration, vocational training, and sexual counseling.[169]

The health risks of poor diet, obesity, reduced physical activity, increased TV watching and other sedentary activities, and substance abuse have been documented as beginning in childhood in the population of typical young adults.[170] In a study of adult patients with spina bifida, Dias et al. found that 80% of their subjects lived with their parents or other relatives and half of those individuals were older than 30 years of age.[171] Although 82% had achieved some level of independence, only 17 patients had married and were living away from family members. Interestingly, the individual's degree of independence was not related to their lesion level or the level of ambulation they had achieved. So it may be inferred that motivational factors may be absent in the cognitive makeup of some individuals with spina bifida that would compel one person to seek increased autonomy versus the other who will live at home with all of the potential isolation and dependency that it may entail.[171]

Dunne and Shurtleff[172] identified some common complaints from adults with spina bifida that included obesity, incontinence, recurrent urinary tract infections, chronic decubiti, joint pain, hypertension, neurologic deterioration, and depression. Urinary incontinence was also a central issue in a self-rating survey completed by a group of adolescent boys and girls with spina bifida. In general, the girls rated themselves lower in physical appearance, athleticism, and global self-worth than the boys. But both the girls and the boys who were continent rated themselves higher than the children who were incontinent. It appeared from this study that urinary continence was more important than the ability to walk for many of these young adults.[173]

Urinary tract infection is the most frequently reported cause of morbidity in the adult population. Patients are very concerned with urinary incontinence and its social implications, and a variety of methods are employed to enable patients to remain dry and infection free. Urinary diversion is a surgical procedure that allows urine to be accessed by catheter from a stoma in the abdomen or collected in an absorbent pad. It was a preferred solution for many patients who did not want to depend on performing intermittent catheterization. When residual urine is permitted to remain in the bladder, it becomes a reservoir for bacteria, resulting in a high rate of infection and potential renal damage. An indwelling Foley catheter was used for some patients, but resulted in a high rate of infection. Other external collecting devices, Valsalva voiding, and diapers were methods commonly tried with varying results and rates of success. It appears that intermittent catheterization performed diligently and on the recommended daily schedule remains the most successful method for adult management of urinary incontinence and was also associated with the lowest risk of infection or renal damage. But, knowing that organizing, compliance, and long-term follow-through may be limited when parents are no longer providing or supervising care, one can see how self-catheterization may be less successful than predicted for the young adult with spina bifida.[174,175]

McClone[176] cited still other problems that were identified by the adult with spina bifida that included a lack of opportunity for job training, lack of viable employment, and decreased ability to achieve psychological and physical independence from family. In two studies, when multifaceted neuropsychological testing was performed on young adults with spina bifida, with and without hydrocephalus, the subjects scored low in areas of verbal learning, verbal recall, and sequencing of complex tasks, and they exhibited a high rate of attention deficit. They were performing in the average range for delayed memory, spatial memory, and visual recognition memory. Almost 50% of the subjects with hydrocephalus in one of the studies exhibited some type of cognitive impairment even though their full IQ fell within the normal range.[177,178] So, one can see how weak verbal recall and sequencing, as well as other areas of challenge mentioned earlier, would significantly impact the patient's ability to experience success in school and learn to take control of and manage the complex responsibilities of their day-to-day lives. Through our interventions with a variety of patients with different learning styles, we are learning to maximize the individual's learning strengths to compensate for their areas of challenge. We are also becoming more adept at incorporating both high- and low-tech adaptations to assist them. So the use of an activity sequencing chart to learn self-catheterization or any multistep procedure seems reasonable. Using photos or pictures for a home exercise program is another adaptation that will avoid having the patient recall lengthy verbal instructions or read and process descriptions on a hand out sheet. Making a video of the patient performing the exercise program that can be watched and followed at home has also been used. Calendars, checklists, or day planners and certainly the use of Tablets, iPads, and other electronic devices may motivate the patient and keep them on track. Although many of these strategies are used with younger patients, the need to continue them with older individuals may mean the difference between success and failure. Family members can also benefit from some of these individualized strategies to aid their compliance as they are expected to remember many different protocols, exercises, and schedules and may require assistance to organize themselves as well.

In some school districts, a special education transition plan is included in the student's yearly educational program when the child is 14 years of age. As a team, the therapists, social worker or counselor, teachers, family, and often the child discuss ideas about what type of educational program might be needed in high school and post–high school, where the child might be able to receive his or her future education, what type of setting would be best, what type of housing might be required when the child no longer lives at home, and what types of job options could be considered. For the population with spina bifida, a preliminary and flexible plan should be developed when the child is much younger than 14 years that includes communication between the medical providers, school, and family, to minimize or prevent some of the long-term problems that have been listed. It appears clear that the adult population has multiple and varied needs and these needs should be addressed as early and consistently as possible by a comprehensive, multidisciplinary team approach that will efficiently identify and address the issues and make referrals to specialists for interventions to help transition the young patient into a more independent adult.

SUMMARY

There are many aspects of care for the PT to consider when treating children with spina bifida. The information presented in this chapter provides both a historic and a contemporary foundation for building a better understanding of this complex birth defect. It also poses some issues that new approaches, technologies, and research may make clearer in the near future. Most often, the role of the PT is defined by the venue in which we work and the age of the children in that setting. Therefore certain sections of the chapter may be more or less relevant than others. Spina bifida is a disability that requires an understanding of the many systems that are affected and how they interact and influence the child's abilities to function across their life span. Concerns and strategies for intervention suggested throughout this chapter reflect the author's humble philosophy that PTs must be knowledgeable about all of the affected body systems that are common to spina bifida and the trends and protocols being applied to their care. The therapist should be aware of the priorities of the families and the other professionals assisting the child. The true challenge to the PT is to integrate these various perspectives into a creative treatment plan that produces the best result for each child. Beginning with a strong basis in anatomy and neurology combined with experimentation and exploration, the PT will discover new and novel ideas for treatment that will not only advance our own clinical abilities to a more sophisticated and successful manner of intervention but, most importantly, will help the child progress to his or her most productive and functional level.

CASE STUDY

Crystal, 9 years old

Significant History

Crystal's back was closed when she was 3 days old, and at 12 days, a VP shunt was inserted to control hydrocephalus. She was discharged to home and had no further complications. She lives with her grandparents and a younger brother and attended an early intervention program from 3 to 5 years of age where she received occupational therapy, physical therapy, and speech services. She did not receive early intervention services until age 3. Crystal entered school 3 years ago and traveled in her personal manual wheelchair, with no bracing.

Present Findings

Crystal has moderate limitations in expressive and receptive language and cognition. She is in a full-time special education classroom for children with similar learning challenges. Crystal is able to follow simple verbal directions. She is the only student in class with a physical disability. Her gross and fine motor skills are her strength, and she enjoys leaving class to push her wheelchair in the hallways, stand, and walk. She is catheterized in the school nursing suite two times daily.

Gross Motor Skills

She is able to transfer, with close supervision for safety, from her wheelchair to her classroom chair and back and to a couch in the nursing suite. She is impulsive and may forget to lock her chair or may be careless moving her legs. She also forgets to position her chair properly, as instructed, and requires cues. Crystal is able to propel her chair very well and steer it without assistance in multiple environments. In her chair, she easily keeps up with her classmates as they transition into and out of the building, to lunch and recess.

Passive Range of Motion

Last year, she had bilateral hamstring releases and was in long leg casts for 6 weeks. When the casts were removed, she remained with a 15-degree knee flexion contracture on the right, but the left knee extended to neutral. When she returned to school following the summer vacation, she had full passive ROM in both legs except for her knees, where she now lacks 40 degrees of extension (R) and 20 degrees extension (L).

Upright Mobility

After her casts were removed, she was fitted with an HKAFO and a butterfly pelvic band to maintain hip extension, and drop locks at the hip and knee joints. The ankles are solid and set at 90 degrees. She was taught to perform a hop-to pattern with all joints locked, using a posterior walker. Her grandparents were instructed in brace donning and doffing at the pediatric hospital where she receives her medical care. She has been coming to school with her walker and her braces and sneakers in a bag to be donned in school for ambulation training. Multiple calls to her family have produced no change in this routine. She and her family report that she is not wearing her braces at home either in the evenings or on the weekends. Crystal's grandmother expresses that donning the brace in the morning is difficult for her owing to lack of time. It is also not reasonable to request that the classroom staff place her in her brace. If the family sent Crystal to school wearing her braces, the school nurse was willing to remove them to perform her late morning catheterizing and put the braces back on her following the afternoon catheterization, but she is resentful that the family will not comply. It is also difficult to get a commitment from Crystal's grandparents that they will help her stand and practice walking after school and/or on weekends.

Crystal receives a weekly physical therapy session in school, and her program consists of transfer training, gait training/practice walking, and a strengthening program for her trunk and upper extremities. Active and active assistive ROM is also performed, with an emphasis on knee extension. She is consistently able to ambulate with close guarding for a distance of approximately 500 yards before becoming tired: She likes to walk to the school nurse for a visit before returning to her class. Crystal's greatest challenge in upright appears to be her excessive right knee flexion contracture, which causes that leg to be relatively shorter than the left. This creates instability when she is upright because her weight bearing is predominantly on the left leg. She must overuse her arms for additional support. She also appears fearful when standing with her posterior walker unless she receives contact guarding for reassurance. Practice with an anterior-facing rollator walker provided the support she needed, and the walkers were switched.

Manual Muscle Testing

She has strong arms and trunk and the following bilateral lower extremity active muscle function: "Fair" hip flexion and adduction; "Poor" knee extension; "Poor" knee flexion; and "Trace" ankle dorsiflexion.

Action Taken

A conference call was held between the school-based PT, the PT staffing the spina bifida clinic, and Crystal's orthopedic surgeon. We decided to experiment, and the pelvic band of the brace was removed. The orthotist also added a 2-inch wedged shoe lift under the right shoe to compensate for her knee flexion and give her a flat surface for standing on her right leg. Crystal's grandmother was called and attended a clinic appointment to again receive instruction on donning and doffing Crystal's braces, and the suggestion to have Crystal wear them daily was repeated by the clinic therapist and physician. The grandmother expressed that the long leg braces (KAFO) were now much easier for her to manage. Additional information was given to alert her that Crystal is nearing adolescence, the time when she will be less likely to gain new upright skills unless her functional walking significantly improves. Crystal's grandmother left that appointment with a renewed commitment.

Results

Crystal is presently coming to school wearing her braces each day. She sits in class with both knees locked, thanks to the assistance of the classroom staff, to stretch her knee flexors on the right and to prevent further tightening on the left. Her legs are propped up on a small box as her wheelchair does not have elevating leg rests. She continues to walk with the therapist each week, and standing has been added to her daily program. She is positioned upright by the classroom staff in a standing box for up to 1 hour each day. It is much easier and quicker for them to lock her knees, and she only requires setup and supervision to pull up to stand. The staff also walks with her from her seat to the standing table and back. The standing box has a tray so she is able to participate in her class activities and desktop work. Because she has active, though weak, hip flexors, she is able to use a reciprocating pattern of leg movement, and the shoe lift has provided a better base of support and reduced her dependence on her arms for support. Her walking endurance has improved. She often switches to a hopping gait that increases her speed. She is able to maintain her trunk erect over her hips and does not flex forward. It is planned that the classroom staff will slowly increase her walking program and she will leave the classroom for longer distances, as they feel more comfortable. The goal is for her to walk twice a day to the nurse for her catheterizations rather than use her wheelchair. The nurse is now able to perform the catheterization without removing Crystal's braces, so it is faster and easier. Finally, a small picture card has been developed and is attached to her chair for easy access, to remind her of the correct sequencing of steps to set up and safely transfer out of her wheelchair. It also serves as a prompt to the staff, who help her. This adaptation has greatly improved her level of safety.

Conclusion

While the pelvic band was initially appropriate for her lesion level and lower extremity strengths, it appeared that its removal was a key to moving her forward in the standing and gait components of her therapy program. The removal of the pelvic band has not impacted her speed, endurance, or pattern of movement in a negative way. The classroom staff is more energized to be involved, and it is easier for them to assist. Her family has also increased their participation and compliance by sending her to school wearing her braces. Crystal is an exercise ambulator, and for the goals of maintaining her upright skills; weight control; leg, trunk, and arm strengthening; and cardiovascular function, this plan has been successful. If she had begun this ambulation program earlier in her life, her strength and motivation to walk might have resulted in a higher level of function. Continued effort will be made by the teacher, school nurse, school PT, and the clinic staff to encourage increased involvement at home, to have Crystal in her braces, and walking on weekends and during extended holiday and summer vacations, at the minimum. If her walking skills improve, additional opportunities to walk longer distances and increased upright time can be added to her daily classroom routine.

REFERENCES

1. Morrisey RT. Spina bifida: a new rehabilitation problem. *Orthop Clin North Am.* 1978;9:379–389.
2. Myers GJ. Myelomeningocele: the medical aspects. *Pediatr Clin North Am.* 1984;31:165–175.
3. Adzick NS, Thom EA, Spong CY, et al. A randomized trial of prenatal versus postnatal repair of myelomeningocele. *N Eng J Med.* 2011;364:993–1004.
4. Duff EM, Cooper ES. Neural tube defects in Jamaica following Hurricane Gilbert. *Am J Public Health.* 1994;84(3):473–476.
5. Seller M. Risks in spina bifida: annotation. *Dev Med Child Neurol.* 1994;36:1021–1025.
6. Share with women: folic acid—what's it all about. *J Midwifery Womens Health.* 2003;48(5):365–366.
7. MMWR Editorial Note. Center for Disease Control and Prevention. MMWR editorial note. 2004;53(17):362–365.
8. Ray JG, Meier C, Vermeulen MJ, et al. Association of neural tube defects and folic acid food fortification in Canada. *Lancet.* 2002;360(9350):2047–2048.
9. Frey L, Hauser WA. Epidemiology of neural tube defects. *Epilepsia.* 2003;44(suppl 3):4–13.
10. Trends in wheat-flour fortification with folic acid and iron—worldwide, 2004 and 2007. *MMWR Morb Mortal Wkly Rep.* 2008;57:8–10. Available at http://www. cdc.gov/mmwr/preview/mmwrhtml/mm5701a4.htm. Accessed November 2012.
11. Periconceptual use of multivitamins and the occurrence of anencephaly and spina bifida. *MMWR Morb Mortal Wkly Rep.* 1988;37:47:727–730. Available at http://www.cdc.gov/mmwr/preview/mmwrhtml/00001309.htm. Accessed November 2012.
12. Mathews TJ, Honein MA, Ericckson JD. Spina bifida and anencephaly prevalence—United States,1991-2001. *MMWR Recomm Rep.* 2002; 51(RR-13):9–11. Available at http://www.cdc.gov/mmrw/preview/mmwrhtml/rr5113a3.htm. Accessed November 2012.
13. Finnell RH, Gould A, Spiegelstein O. Pathobiology and genetics of neural tube defects. *Epilepsia.* 2003;44(suppl 3):14–23.
14. Dias MS, Partington M. Embryology of myelomeningocele and anencephaly. *Neurosurg Focus.* 2004;16(2):E1.
15. Alwan S, Reefhuis J, Rasmussen A, et al. Use of selective serotonin reuptake inhibitors in pregnancy and the risk of birth defects. *N Eng J Med.* 2007;356:2684–2692.
16. Lunsky AM, Ulcicus M, Rothman KJ, et al. Maternal heat exposure and neural tube defects. *JAMA.* 1992;268:882–885.
17. McClone D. Neurosurgical management and operative closure for myelomeningocele. Paper presented at: the Annual Myelomeningocele Seminar; 1982; Chicago, IL.

18. Center for Disease control. Estimating the prevalence of spina bifida. Available at: http://www.cdc.gov/ncbddd/spinabifida/research.html. Accessed September 2012.

19. Smith K, Freeman KA, Neville-Jan A, et al. Cultural considerations in the care of children with spina bifida. *Ped Clin North Am.* 2010;57(4):1027–1040.

20. Canfield MA, Ramadhani TA, Shaw GM, et al. Anencephaly and spina bifida among Hispanics: maternal, sociodemographic and acculturation factors in the national birth defects prevention study, birth defects research (Part A). *Clin Mol Teratol.* 2009;85(7):637–646.

21. Arizona Department of Health Services. Facts about Spina bifida, 1995-2009. Available at: www.azdhs.gov/phstats/bdr/reports/spinabifida.pdf. Accessed July 2012.

22. Johnson CY, Honien MA, Flanders DW, et al. Pregnancy termination following prenatal diagnosis of anencephaly or spina bifida: A systematic review of the literature. *Birth Defects Res A Clin Mol Teratol.* 2012;44(1):857–863.

23. Scarff TB, Fronczak S. Myelomeningocele: a review and update. *Rehab Lit.* 1981;42:143–147.

24. Tachdjian MO. *Pediatric Orthopedics.* Vol 3. 2nd ed. Philadelphia, PA: WB Saunders; 1990:1773–1880.

25. Behrman RC, Vaughn VC, eds. *Nelson's Textbook of Pediatrics.* 11th ed. Philadelphia, PA: WB Saunders; 1979.

26. Wolraich M. The association of spina bifida occulta and myelomeningocele. Paper presented at: the 2nd Symposium on Spina Bifida; 1984;Cincinnati, OH.

27. Fidas A, MacDonald HL, Elton RA, et al. Prevalence of spina bifida occulta in patients with functional disorders of the lower urinary tract and its relation to urodynamics and neurophysiological measurements. *BMJ.* 1989;298:357–359.

28. Warder DE. Tethered cord syndrome and occult spinal dysraphism. American Association of Neurological Surgeons. *Neurosurg Focus.* 2001;10(1):e1.

29. Tubbs RS, Wellons III JC, Grabb PA, et al. Chiari II malformation and occult spinal dysraphism. Case reports and a review of the literature. *Pediatr Neurosurg.* 2003;39(2):104–107.

30. D'Agasta SD, Banta JV, Gahm N. The fate of patients with lipomeningocele. Paper presented at: The American Academy of Cerebral Palsy and Developmental Medicine (ACPDM); 1987; Boston, MA.

31. Kanev PM, Lemire RJ, Loeser JD, et al. Management and long-term follow-up review of children with lipomyelomeningocele. *J Neurosurg.* 1990;73:48–52.

32. Moore KL. *The Developing Human: Clinically Oriented Embryology.* Philadelphia, PA: WB Saunders; 1974.

33. Robbins SL. *Pathologic Basis of Disease.* Philadelphia, PA: WB Saunders; 1974.

34. Umphred DA. *Neurological Rehabilitation.* St. Louis, MO: CV Mosby; 1985.

35. Sharrard WJ. Neuromotor evaluation of the newborn. In: *Symposium on Myelomeningocele.* St. Louis, MO: CV Mosby; 1972.

36. Peach B. The Arnold-Chiari malformation. *Arch Neurol.* 1965;12:165.

37. Peach B. The Arnold-Chiari malformation. *Arch Neurol.* 1965;12:109.

38. McCullough DC. Arnold-Chiari malformation—theories of development. Paper presented at: the 2nd Symposium on Myelomeningocele; 1984; Cincinnati, OH.

39. McLone DG, Knepper PA. The cause of Chiari II malformation: a unified theory. *Pediatr Neurosci.* 1989;15:1–12.

40. Mclone DG, Dias MS. The Chiari II malformation: cause and impact. *Childs Nerv Syst.* 2003;19(7–8):540–550.

41. Lutschg J, Meyer E, Jeanneret-Iseli C, et al. Brainstem auditory evoked potential in myelomeningocele. *Neuropediatrics.* 1985;16:202–204.

42. Hesz N, Wolraich M. Vocal cord paralysis and brainstem dysfunction in children with spina bifida. *Dev Med Child Neurol.* 1985;27:528–531.

43. Hoffman HJ, Hendrick EB, Humphreys RP, et al. Manifestations and management of Arnold-Chiari malformation in patients with myelomeningocele. *Childs Brain.* 1975;1:255–259.

44. Staal MJ, Melhuizen-de Regt MJ, Hess J. Sudden death in hydrocephalic spina bifida aperta patients. *Pediatr Neurosci.* 1987;13:13–18.

45. Biggio JR, Wenstrom KD, Owen J. Fetal open spina bifida: a natural history of disease progression in utero. *Prenat Diagn.* 2004;24(4):287–289.

46. Palomaki GE, Williams JR, Haddow JE. Prenatal screening for open neural-tube defects in Maine. *N Engl J Med.* 1999;340(13):1049–1050.

47. Thomas M. The lemon sign. *Radiology.* 2003;228(1):206–207.

48. Pilu G, Romero R, Reece A, et al. Subnormal cerebellum in fetuses with spina bifida. *Am J Obstet Gynecol.* 1988;158:1052–1056.

49. Benacerraf BR, Stryker J, Frigotto FD. Abnormal ultrasound appearance of the cerebellum (banana sign): indirect sign of spina bifida. *Pediatr Radiol.* 1989;171:151–153.

50. Nyberg DA, Mack LA, Hirsch J, et al. Abnormalities of cranial contour in sonographic detection of spina bifida: evaluation of the "lemon" sign. *Radiology.* 1988;167(2):387–392.

51. Thiagarajah S, Henke J, Hogge WA, et al. Early diagnosis of spina bifida: the value of cranial ultrasound markers. *Obstet Gynecol.* 1990;76:54–57.

52. Bensen J, Dillard RG, Burton BK. Open spina bifida: does cesarean section delivery improve prognosis? *Obstet Gynecol.* 1988;71:532–534.

53. Luthy DA, Wardinsky T, Shurtleff DB, et al. Cesarean section before the onset of labor and subsequent motor function in infants with myelomeningocele diagnosed antenatally. *N Engl J Med.* 1991;324:662–666.

54. Shurtleff DB, Luthy DA, Benedetti TJ, et al. Perinatal management, cesarean section and outcome in fetal spina bifida. Paper presented at: the American Academy of Cerebral Palsy and Developmental Medicine; 1987; Boston, MA.

55. Hogge WA, Dungan JS, Brooks MP, et al. Diagnosis and management of prenatally detected myelomeningocele: a preliminary report. *Am J Obstet Gynecol.* 1990;163:1061–1064.

56. Johnson MP, Sutton LN, Rintol N, et al. Fetal myelomeningocele repair: short term clinical outcomes. *Am J Obstet Gynecol.* 2003;189(2):482–487.

57. Sutton LN, Adzick NS, Bilaniuk LT, et al. Improvement in hindbrain herniation demonstrated by serial fetal magnetic resonance imaging following fetal surgery for myelomeningocele. *JAMA.* 1999;282(19):1826–1831.

58. Buner JP, Tulipan N, Paschall RL, et al. Fetal surgery for myelomeningocele and the incidence of shunt-dependent hydrocephalus. *JAMA.* 1999;282(19):1819–1825.

59. Danzer E, Johnson MP, Adzick NS, et al. Fetal surgery for myelomeningocele: progress and perspectives. *Dev Med Child Neurol.* 2012;54(1):8–14.

60. Verbeek RJ, Heep A, Maurits NM, et al. Fetal endoscopic myelomeningocele closure preserves segmental neurologic function. *Dev Med Child Neurol.* 2012;54(1):15–22.

61. Shurtleff D. Fetal endoscopic myelomeningocele repair. *Dev Med Child Neurol.* 2012;54(1):4–5.

62. Raimondi AJ, Soare P. Intellectual development in shunted hydrocephalic children. *Am J Dis Child.* 1974;127:664–671.

63. McLone DG, Czyzewski D, Raimondi AJ, et al. Central nervous system infections as a limiting factor in the intelligence of children with myelomeningocele. *Pediatrics.* 1982;70:338–342.

64. Ellenbogen RG, Goldmann DA, Winston KW. Group B streptococcal infections of the central nervous system in infants with myelomeningocele. *Surg Neurol.* 1988;29:237–242.

65. Banta J. Long-term ambulation in spina bifida. Paper presented at: the American Academy of Cerebral Palsy and Developmental Medicine; 1983; Chicago, IL.

66. Murdoch A. How valuable is muscle charting? *Physiotherapy.* 1980;66:221–223.

67. Schafer M, Dias L. *Myelomeningocele: Orthopedic Treatment.* Baltimore, MD: Williams . . . Wilkins; 1983.

68. Kaplan G. Editorial: with apologies to Shakespeare. *J Urol.* 1999;161:933.

69. Tanaka H, Katizaki H, Kobayashi S, et al. The relevance of urethral resistance in children with myelodysplasia: its impact on upper

urinary tract deterioration and the outcome of conservative management. *J Urol.* 1999;161:929–932.

70. *An Introduction to Hydrocephalus.* Chicago, IL: Children's Memorial Hospital; 1982.

71. Raimondi AJ. Complications of ventriculoperitoneal shunting and a critical comparison of the 3-piece and 1-piece systems. *Childs Brain.* 1977;3:321–342.

72. Bell WO, Sumner TE, Volberg FM. The significance of ventriculomegaly in the newborn with myelodysplasia. *Childs Nerv Syst.* 1987;3:239–241.

73. Bell WO, Arbit E, Fraser R. One-stage myelomeningocele closure and ventriculo-peritoneal shunt placement. *Surg Neurol.* 1987;27:233–236.

74. Lindseth RE. Treatment of the lower extremities in children paralyzed by myelomeningocele (birth to 18 months). *Am Acad Orthop Surg Inst Course Lec.* 1976;25:76–82.

75. Daniels L, Williams M, Worthingham C. *Muscle Testing: Techniques of Manual Examination.* Philadelphia, PA: WB Saunders; 1956.

76. Strach EH. Orthopedic care of children with myelomeningocele: a modern program of rehabilitation. *BMJ.* 1967;3:791–794.

77. Asher M, Olson J. Factors affecting the ambulatory status of patients with spina bifida cystica. *J Bone Joint Surg Am.* 1983;65(3):350–356.

78. Bunch W. Progressive neurological loss in myelomeningocele patients. Paper presented at: the American Academy of Cerebral Palsy and Developmental Medicine Conference; 1982; San Diego, CA.

79. Coon V, Donato G, Houser C, et al. Normal ranges of hip motion in infants. *Clin Orthop.* 1975;110:256–260.

80. Haas S. Normal ranges of hip motion in the newborn. *Clin Orthop Rel Res.* 1973;91:114–118.

81. Dias L. Hip contractures in the child with spina bifida. Paper presented at: the 2nd Symposium on Spina Bifida; 1984; Cincinnati, OH.

82. Banta JV, Lin R, Peterson M, et al. The team approach in the care of the child with myelomeningocele. *J Prosthet Orthot.* 1989;2:263–273.

83. Lie HR, Lagergren J, Rasmussen F, et al. Bowel and bladder control of children with myelomeningocele: a Nordic study. *Dev Med Child Neurol.* 1991;33:1053–1061.

84. Brem AS, Martin D, Callaghan J, et al. Long-term renal risk factors in children with myelomeningocele. *J Pediatr.* 1987;110:51–55.

85. Anagnostopoulos D, Joannides E, Kotsianos K. The urological management of patients with myelodysplasia. *Pediatr Surg Int.* 1988;3:347–350.

86. Wolf LS. Early motor development in children with myelomeningocele. Paper presented at: the American Academy of Cerebral Palsy and Developmental Medicine; 1984; Washington, DC.

87. Mazur JM. Hand function in patients with spina bifida cystica. *J Pediatr Orthop.* 1986;6:442–447.

88. Anderson P. Impairment of a motor skill in children with spina bifida cystica and hydrocephalus: an exploratory study. *Br J Psychol.* 1977;68:61–70.

89. Dahl M, Ahlsten G, Carlson H, et al. Neurological dysfunction above cele level in children with spina bifida cystica: a prospective study to three years. *Dev Med Child Neurol.* 1995;37:30–40.

90. Bobath B. Motor development, its effect on general development and application to the treatment of cerebral palsy. *Physiotherapy.* 1971;57:526–532.

91. Bobath B. The treatment of neuromuscular disorders by improving patterns of coordination. *Physiotherapy.* 1969;55:18–22.

92. Bobath B. The very early treatment of cerebral palsy. *Dev Med Child Neurol.* 1967;9:373–390.

93. Caplan F. *The First Twelve Months of Life.* New York, NY: Grosset and Dunlap; 1973.

94. Turner A. Upper-limb function in children with myelomeningocele. *Dev Med Child Neurol.* 1986;28:790–798.

95. Turner A. Hand function in children with myelomeningocele. *J Bone Joint Surg Br.* 1985;67:268–272.

96. Agness PJ. Learning disabilities and the person with spina bifida. Paper presented at: the Spina Bifida Association of America Meeting; 1980; Chicago, IL.

97. Cronchman M. The effects of babywalkers on early locomotor development. *Dev Med Child Neurol.* 1986;28:757–761.

98. Williams EN, Broughton NS, Menelaus MB. Age-related walking in children with spina bifida. *Dev Med Child Neurol.* 1999;41(7):446–449.

99. Menelaus M. The evolution of orthopedic management of myelomeningocele. *J Pediatr Orthop.* 1999;18:421–422.

100. Charney EB, Melchionni JB, Smith DR. Community ambulation by children with myelomeningocele and high level paralysis. Paper presented at: the American Academy of Cerebral Palsy and Developmental Medicine; 1989; San Francisco, CA.

101. Beaty JH, Canale ST. Current concepts review. Orthopedic aspects of myelomeningocele. *J Bone Joint Surg Am.* 1990;72:626–630.

102. Dias L. Orthopedic care in spina bifida: past, present, and future. *Dev Med Child Neurol.* 2004;46(9):579.

103. Menelaus M. Hip dislocation: concepts of treatment. Paper presented at: the 2nd Symposium on Spina Bifida; 1984; Cincinnati, OH.

104. Stauffer ES, Hoffer M. Ambulation in thoracic paraplegia [Abstract]. *J Bone Joint Surg.* 1972;54A:1336.

105. Hoffer MM, Feiwell EE, Perry R, et al. Functional ambulation in patients with myelomeningocele. *J Bone Joint Surg.* 1973;55(1):137–148.

106. Swaroop VT, Dias L. Orthopedic management of spina bifida. Part I: hip, knee and rotational deformities. *J Child Orthop.* 2009;3(6):441–449.

107. Swaroop VT, Dias L. Orthopedic management of spina bifida. Part II: foot and ankle deformities. *J Child Orthop.* 2011;5(6):403–414.

108. Yngve D, Douglas R, Roberts JM. The reciprocating gait orthosis in myelomeningocele. *J Pediatr Orthop.* 1984;4:304–310.

109. Dias L, Tappit-Emas E, Boot E. The reciprocating gait orthosis: the Children's Memorial experience. Paper presented at: the American Academy of Developmental Medicine and Child Neurology; 1984; Washington, DC.

110. Douglas R, Larson PF, D'Ambrosia R, et al. The LSU reciprocating gait orthosis. *Orthopedics.* 1983;6:834–839.

111. Center for Orthotics Design, Inc. www.centerfororthoticsdesign. com. Accessed July 5 2007.

112. Williams L. Energy cost of walking and of wheelchair propulsion by children with myelodysplasia. *Dev Med Child Neurol.* 1983;25:617–624.

113. Wright JG. Hip and spine surgery is of questionable value in spina bifida: an evidence based review. *Clin Orthop Relat Res.* 2011;465(5):1258–1264.

114. McDonald CM, Jaffe KM, Mosca VS, et al. Ambulatory outcome of children with myelomeningocele: effect of lower extremity muscle strength. *Dev Med Child Neurol.* 1991;33:482–490.

115. Torosian CM, Dias LS. Surgical treatment of severe hindfoot valgus by medial displacement osteotomy of the os calsis in children with myelomeningocele. *J Pediatr Orthop.* 2000;20(2):226–229.

116. Neto J, Dias L, Gabriel A. Congenital talipes equinovarus in spina bifida: treatment and results. *J Pediatr Orthop.* 1996;16:782–785.

117. Schopler SA, Menelaus MB. Significance of the strength of the quadriceps muscles in children with myelomeningocele. *J Pediatr Orthop.* 1987;7:507–512.

118. Sherk HH, Uppal GS, Lane G, et al. Treatment versus nontreatment of hip dislocations in ambulatory patients with myelomeningocele. *Dev Med Child Neurol.* 1991;33:491–494.

119. Duffy CM, Graham HK, Cosgrove AP. The influence of ankle-foot orthosis on gait and energy expenditure in spina bifida. *J Pediatr Orthop.* 2000;20(3):356–361.

120. Hunt KG, et al. The effects of fixed and hinged ankle-foot orthoses on gait myoelectric activity in children with myelomeningocele. Meeting Highlights of AACPDM. *J Pediatr Orthop.* 1994;14(2):269.

121. Knutson LM, Clark DE. Orthotic devices for ambulation in children with cerebral palsy and myelomeningocele. *Phys Ther.* 1991;71:947–960.

122. Vankoski S, Dias L. Children with spina bifida benefit from gait analysis. *The Standard.* 1997;1:4–5.

123. Vankoski S, Sarwark J, Moore C, et al. Characteristic pelvis, hip and knee kinematic patterns in children with lumbosacral myelomeningocele. *Gait Posture.* 1995;3(1):51–57.

124. Ounpuu S, Davis R, Bell K, et al. Gait analysis in the treatment decision making process in patients with myelomeningocele. In: 8th Annual East Coast Gait Laboratories Conference; May 5–8, 1993; Rochester, MN.

125. Duffy C, Hill A, Cosgrove A, et al. Three-dimensional gait analysis in spina bifida. *J Pediatr Orthop.* 1996;16:786–791.

126. Williams J, Graham G, Dunne K, et al. Late knee problems in myelomeningocele. *J Pediatr Orthop.* 1993;13:701–703.

127. Thompson JD, Ounpuu S, Davis RB, et al. The effects of ankle-foot orthosis on the ankle and knee in persons with myelomeningocele: an evaluation using three dimensional gait analysis. *J Pediatr Orthop.* 1999;19(1):27–33.

128. Porsch K. Origin and treatment of fractures in spina bifida. *Eur J Pediatr Surg.* 1991;1(5):298–305.

129. Drummond D. Post-operative fractures in patients with myelomeningocele. *Dev Med Child Neurol.* 1981;23:147–150.

130. Rosenstein BD, Greene WB, Herrington RT, et al. Bone density in myelomeningocele: the effects of ambulatory status and other factors. *Dev Med Child Neurol.* 1987;29:486–494.

131. Lock TR, Aronson DD. Fractures in patients who have myelomeningocele. *J Bone Jt Surg Am.* 1989;71:1153–1157.

132. Bartonek A, Saraste H, Samuelson L, et al. Ambulation in patients with myelomeningocele: a 12 year follow-up. *J Pediatr Orthop.* 1999;19(2):202–206.

133. Hall P, Lindseth R, Campbell R, et al. Scoliosis and hydrocephalus in myelomeningocele patients: the effect of ventricular shunting. *J Neurosurg.* 1979;50:174–178.

134. Mazur JM, Menelaus MB. Neurologic status of spina bifida patients and the orthopedic surgeon. *Clin Orthop Rel Res.* 1991;264:54–64.

135. Jeelani NO, Jaspan T, Punt J. Tethered cord syndrome after myelomeningocele repair. *BMJ.* 1999;318:516–517.

136. Petersen M. Tethered cord syndrome in myelodysplasia: correlation between level of lesion and height at time of presentation. *Dev Med Child Neurol.* 1992;34:604–610.

137. McClone D, Herman J, Gabriele A, et al. Tethered cord as a cause of scoliosis in children with a myelomeningocele. *Pediatr Neurosurg.* 1990;91(16):8–13.

138. Banta J. The tethered cord in myelomeningocele: should it be untethered? *Dev Med Child Neurol.* 1991;33:167–176.

139. Mazur J, Stillwell A, Menelaus M. The significance of spasticity on the upper and lower limbs in myelomeningocele. *J Bone Joint Surg Br.* 1986;68:213–217.

140. Flanagan RC, Russell DP, Walsh JW. Urologic aspects of tethered cord. *Urology.* 1989;33:80–82.

141. Kaplan WE, McLone DG, Richards I. The urological manifestation of the tethered spinal cord. *J Urol.* 1988;140:1285–1288.

142. Grief L, Stalmasek V. Tethered cord syndrome: a pediatric case study. *J Neurosci Nurs.* 1989;21:86–91.

143. Hochleiter BW, Menardi G, Haussler B, et al. Spina bifida as an independent risk factor for sensitivization to latex. *J Urol.* 2001;166(6):2370–2373.

144. Nieto A, Mazon A, Pamies R, et al. Efficacy of latex avoidance for primary prevention of latex sensitization in children with spina bifida. *J Pediatr.* 2002;140(3):370–372.

145. Centers for Disease Control. Anaphylactic reaction during general anesthesia among pediatric patients, United States. Jan 1990–Jan 1991. *MMWR Morb Mortal Wkly Rep.* 1991;40:437–443.

146. *Allergic Reactions to Latex-Containing Medical Devices: FDA Medical Alert.* Food and Drug Administration; March 29, 1991.

147. Meeropol E, Frost J, Pugh L, et al. Latex allergy in children with myelomeningocele. *J Pediatr Orthop.* 1993;13:1–4.

148. D'Astous J, Drouin M, Rhine E. Intraoperative anaphylaxis secondary to allergy to latex in children who have spina bifida. *J Bone Joint Surg.* 1992;74(7):1084–1086.

149. Meehan P, Galina M, Daftari T. Intraoperative anaphylaxis due to allergy to latex. *J Bone Joint Surg.* 1992;74-A:1103–1109.

150. Lu L, Kurup V, Hoffman D, et al. Characterization of a major latex allergen associated with hypersensitivity in spina bifida patients. *J Immunol.* 1995;155:2721–2728.

151. Medical Sciences Bulletin. Available at: http://pharminfo.com/pub/msb/latex.html. Accessed Jan 2003.

152. Good Latex Allergy Survival Skills. Available at: http://www.net-com.com/~ecbdmd/Glass.html. Accessed Jan 2003.

153. Latex Allergy. Available at: http://www.waisman.wisc.edu/~rowley/sbkids/Sb_latex.html. Accessed Jan 2003.

154. Willis KE, Holmbeck GN, Dillon K, et al. Intelligence and achievement in children with myelomeningocele. *J Pediatr Psychol.* 1990 Apr; 15(2): 161–176

155. Horn DG, Pugzles Lorch E, Lorch RF, et al. Distractibility and vocabulary deficits in children with spina bifida and hydrocephalus. *Dev Med Child Neurol.* 1985;27:713–720.

156. Wolfe GA, Kennedy D, Brewer K, et al. Visual perception and upper extremity function in children with spina bifida. Paper presented at: the American Academy of Cerebral Palsy and Developmental Medicine; 1989; San Francisco, CA.

157. Cull C, Wyke MA. Memory function of children with spina bifida and shunted hydrocephalus. *Dev Med Child Neurol.* 1984;26:177–183.

158. Dise JE, Lohr ME. Examination of deficits in conceptual reasoning abilities associated with spina bifida. *Am J Phys Med Rehab.* 1998;77(3):247–250.

159. Mauk JE, Charney EB, Nambiar R, et al. Strabis-mus and spina bifida. Paper presented at: the American Academy of Cerebral Palsy and Developmental Medicine; 1987; Portland, OR.

160. Lennerstrand G, Gallo JE. Neuro-ophthalmological evaluation of patients with myelomeningocele and Chiari malformations. *Dev Med Child Neurol.* 1990;32:415–422.

161. Rothstein TB, Romano PE, Shoch D. Meningomyelocele. *Am J Ophthalmol.* 1974;77:690–693.

162. Horn DG, Lorch EP, Lorch RF, et al. Distractibility and vocabulary deficits in children with spina bifida and hydrocephalus. *Dev Med Child Neurol.* 1985;27:713–720.

163. Ruff HA. The development of perception and recognition of objects. *Child Dev.* 1980;51:981–992.

164. Butler C. Effects of powered mobility on self-initiated behaviors of very young children with locomotor disability. *Dev Med Child Neurol.* 1986;28:325–332.

165. DeLateur B, Berni R, Hangladarom T, et al. Wheelchair cushions designed to prevent pressure sores. *Arch Phys Med Rehabil.* 1976;57:129–135.

166. Fiewell E. Seating and cushions for spina bifida. Paper presented at: the 2nd Symposium on Spina Bifida; 1984; Cincinnati, OH.

167. Borjeson MC, Lagergren JL. Life conditions of adolescents with myelomeningocele. *Dev Med Child Neurol.* 1990;32:698–706.

168. Selber P, Dias L. Sacral level myelomeningocele: long term outcome in adults. *J Pediatr Orthop.* 1998;18:423–427.

169. Buran CF, McDaniel AM, Brej TJ. Needs assessment in a spina bifida program: a comparison of the perceptions of adolescents with spina bifida and their parents. *Clin Nurse Spec.* 2002;16(5):256–262.

170. Sawin, KJ, Brei TJ. Health risk behaviors in spina bifida: the need for clinical and policy action. *Dev Med Child Neurol.* 2012;54(11):974–975.

171. Dias LS, Fernandez AC, Swank M. Adults with spina bifida: a review of seventy-one patients. Paper presented at: the American Academy of Cerebral Palsy and Developmental Medicine; 1987; Boston, MA.

172. Dunne KB, Shurtleff DB. The medical status of adults with spina bifida. Paper presented at: the American Academy of Cerebral Palsy and Developmental Medicine; 1987; Washington, DC.

173. Moore C, Kogan BA, Parekh A. Impact of urinary incontinence on self-concept in children with spina bifida. *J Urol.* 2004;171(4):1659–1662.

174. Lobby NJ, Ginsburg C, Harkaway RC, et al. Urinary tract infections in adult spina bifida. *Infect Urol.* 1999;12(2):51–55.

175. Campbell JB, Moore KN, Voaklander DC, et al. Complications associated with clean intermittent catheterization in children with spina bifida. *J Urol.* 2004;171(6, pt 1):2420–2422.

176. McClone DG. Spina bifida today: problems adult face. *Semin Neurol.* 1989;9:169–175.

177. Iddon JL, Morgan DJR, Loveday C, et al. Neuropsychological profile of young adults with spina bifida with or without hydrocephalus. *J Neurol Neursurg Psychiatry.* 2004;75:112–118.

178. Barf HA, Verhoef M, Jennekens-Schinkel A, et al. Cognitive status of young adults with spina bifida. *Dev Med Child Neurol.* 2003;45(12):813–820.

ADDITIONAL RESOURCES

Developingchild. Harvard.Edu/topics/understanding intervention (research and topics of interest about the benefits of early intervention).

Scherzer A, Tscharnuter I. *Early Diagnosis and Therapy in Cerebral Palsy.* New York, NY: Marcel Dekker; 1982 (handling strategies for young children).

Williamson GG. *Children with Spina Bifida: Early Intervention and Pre-School Programming.* Baltimore, MD: Brooks Publishers; 1987 (family concerns and PT/OT interventional strategies).

Zabel TA, Linroth R, Fairman AD. The Life Course Model Website: an online transition-focused resource for the Spina Bifida community. *Pediatr Clin North Am.* 2010;57(4): 911–917.

SOURCES FOR LATEX INFORMATION

Food and Drug Administration. www.fda.gov

Spina Bifida Association of America. www.spinabifidaassociation.org

American Latex Allergy Association. http://www.latexallergyresources.org

Traumatic Injury to the Central Nervous System: Brain Injury

Amy Both

Definition

Incidence

Causes of Injury
  Falls
  Motor Vehicle Accidents
  Gunshot Wounds
  Abuse/Assault
  Sports/Recreational Activities

Mechanisms of Injury
  Acceleration–Deceleration Injuries
  Impression Injuries

Primary Brain Damage from Trauma
  Concussion
  Contusion
  Skull Fractures
  Intracranial Hemorrhages
  Diffuse Axonal Injury

Secondary Brain Damage from Trauma
  Cerebral Edema
  Intracranial Pressure
  Herniation Syndromes
  Hypoxic–Ischemic Injury
  Neurochemical Events

Other Consequences from Brain Damage
  Hydrocephalus
  Seizures
  Infections
  Dysautonomia
  Endocrine Disorders

Predictors of Injury Severity and Outcome
  Coma Scales
  Duration of Coma

Depth of Coma
Orientation and Amnesia Assessment
Duration of Posttraumatic Amnesia
Rancho Los Amigos Levels of Cognitive Functioning
Pediatric Rancho Scale
Age
Function
Environmental Influences

Physical Therapy Examination of the Child with Traumatic Brain Injury
  Subjective Examination: Patient History
  Systems Review
  Objective Examination: Tests and Measures

Evaluation, Diagnosis, Prognosis, and Plan of Care
  Evaluation
  Diagnosis and Prognosis
  Plan of Care

Management/Interventions
  Acute Medical Management
  Acute Physical Therapy Management: Prevention
  Low-Cognitive-level Physical Therapy Management: Stimulation
  Midcognitive-level Physical Therapy Management: Structure
  Higher-Cognitive-level Physical Therapy Management: School/Community Reintegration

Prevention
  Bicycle Helmets
  Playground Equipment
  Traffic Behavior
  Car Restraints
  Concussion Screening and Programming

Case Study

▶ Definition

Traumatic brain injury (TBI) occurs when an external, mechanical force either accidentally or intentionally impacts the head.[1–3] It is not associated with congenital injury or degenerative insult. TBI is characterized by a period of diminished or altered consciousness that ranges from brief lethargy to prolonged unconsciousness to brain death.[1,2] According to the *Guide for Physical Therapist Practice*,[4] pediatric TBI falls into one of three preferred practice patterns (see Table 7.1). Symptoms vary greatly depending on the location of the lesion and the extent of underlying brain injury. While approximately 97% of the children who sustain a TBI experience only a mild injury and recover uneventfully,

301

TABLE	
7.1	Preferred Practice Patterns—*Guide to Physical Therapist Practice*, Second Edition

5C	Impaired Motor Function and Sensory Integrity Associated with Nonprogressive Disorders of the Central Nervous System: Congenital Origin or Acquired in Infancy or Childhood
5D	Impaired Motor Function and Sensory Integrity Associated with Nonprogressive Disorders of the Central Nervous System: Congenital Origin or Acquired in Adolescence or Adulthood
5I	Impaired Arousal, Range of Motion, and Motor Control Associated With Coma, Near Coma, or Vegetative State

From American Physical Therapy Association. Guide to physical therapist practice. Second edition. *Phys Ther.* 2001;81(1):1–768.

others are left with partial or total functional disability and/or psychosocial impairment.[5] TBI is also referred to as acquired brain injury, head injury, or closed head injury.

▶ Incidence

In recent years, the number of children who visit the emergency room annually with a suspected head injury has increased to approximately 1,365,000 visits each year.[6] Of those visits, approximately 18% are made by young children between the ages of 0 and 4 years.[6,7] Currently in the United States, the number of new cases of children diagnosed with TBI is estimated at 475,000 per year with 100,000 of those requiring hospitalization.[6,8–10] Overall, brain injury is the leading cause of death and permanent disability in children between 1 and 19 years of age.[8] It is also the third leading cause of death in children less than 1 year of age. In spite of this, the survival rate in children with TBI is better than similarly injured adults.[11,12]

Currently, there are two peak periods of incidence of TBI in children that should be monitored. The first occurs in early childhood (less than 4 years of age) and the second occurs during mid- to late adolescence (15 to 19 years of age).[11,13] In every age group, the incidence of TBI is two times greater in boys than girls, with boys between 0 and 4 years of age having the highest number of hospitalizations and TBI-related deaths.[1,7,9,11,14,15] Premorbid personality and behavior have been found to predispose children to brain injury.[16] Children who are impulsive and hyperactive, and who have difficulty with attention are at an increased risk for injury.[16,17] In addition, there is evidence that once a child sustains a TBI, even a mild TBI, the likelihood of reinjury and a lower threshold for damage to the brain increases.[18,19]

Brain injury and death rates vary considerably by race and socioeconomic status. TBI-associated mortality rates are higher in African Americans, followed by Caucasians and then other races.[5,20] For all races, death rates are inversely related to socioeconomic status.[20] Thus, children of families with low incomes have higher death rates than children of families with upper and middle incomes.

▶ Causes of injury

Falls

Falls account for 35% to 50% of all pediatric TBIs that require hospitalization or result in death.[1,10,11,20,21] Children under 12 months were at the greatest risk of injury from a fall, with 0 to 6 month olds sustaining the highest rate of moderate injury from falls, including falls from a caregiver's arms.[22] Among preschoolers, 51% of the trauma injuries from falls occur while playing on playground equipment.[20] Older children usually escape severe injury in falls from heights of less than 10 feet.[20,23] Although many falls occur accidentally, falls of less than 10 feet bear investigation for potential child abuse.[20,23]

Motor Vehicle Accidents

Motor vehicle accidents (MVAs) account for approximately 25% of all pediatric TBIs and are the most common cause of trauma death in children 5 to 9 years old.[1,2,10,20] Between 4 and 14 years of age, the majority of injuries involving a motor vehicle occur when the child is a bicyclist or pedestrian.[13] In contrast, the majority of motor vehicle injuries sustained during adolescence occur when the adolescent is an unprotected occupant in the automobile.[13] MVAs cause the vast majority of serious injuries and multiple trauma in children, with approximately 70% of the children demonstrating various degrees of coma for some period of time.[20]

Gunshot Wounds

Firearm injuries occur from accidental gun discharges, homicides, and suicides and rank second only to MVAs as the leading cause of trauma death in school-age children and adolescents.[24] The incidence of gunshot wounds among male inner-city youth is extremely alarming, as the children are often both the victims and the perpetrators.[25] More than twice as many children survive their injuries as die, with approximately 25% having permanent sequelae.[26]

Abuse/Assault

Physical abuse in infants and young children is prevalent in children 0 to 4 years old.[10,13] Approximately 80% of the head trauma deaths in children under 2 years of age are due to physical abuse.[13] Abuse frequently results in head injury owing to the vulnerability of the immature brain and the weak supporting neck musculature. Abuse resulting in TBI is characterized by a marked discrepancy between the explanation of how the injury occurred and the nature and severity of the injury. Early identification of abuse is critical to prevent repeated or progressive injury.

Sports/Recreational Activities

Sports and recreational causes account for approximately 29% of the brain injuries to school-age children and

Nutrition for the Child with Traumatic Brain Injury

Susan Boyden, MS, RD, LDN
Clinical Dietitian
The Children's Hospital of Philadelphia

Nutrition-Related Problems	Interventions
UNABLE TO EAT BY MOUTH:	Alternate means of nutrition:
• Impaired gastrointestinal system	Parenteral nutrition
• Comatose/vegetative state	Tube feedings
• Respiratory failure	
• Aspiration risk	
UNABLE TO CONSUME ADEQUATE NUTRITION:	
• Impaired oral motor skills	Dietary modifications:
• Chewing	Modification of food texture/consistency
• Pocketing	Thickened liquids
• Swallowing	High-calorie supplements
• Drooling/leakage	Tube feedings
• Sensory and communication deficits:	
• Unable to see food offered	Ophthalmology evaluation
• Unable to communicate when hungry	Speech therapy referral
• Difficulty communicating at mealtime due to hearing loss	Occupational therapist
• Depression	Audiology evaluation
• Pain issues	Psychology referral
	Medication
	Music therapy
	Child life therapy
INCREASED CALORIE/NUTRIENT NEEDS:	
• Metabolic stress	Nutritional supplements
• Fractures	Tube feedings
• Wound healing	Vitamins/minerals
• Involuntary movements	Parenteral nutrition
Constipation	Adequate fiber and fluids
	Bowel program
	Medications
Gastroesophageal reflux	Small frequent feedings
	Nutrient-dense meals/snacks/formula
	Medication
OBESITY	
• Decreased mobility	Physical therapy program
• Insatiable appetite related to injury to appetite control center	Reduce fat/calories in diet
	Food diary
	Consistent meal schedule

SUGGESTED READINGS

Ekvall SW. Pediatric nutrition in chronic diseases and developmental disorders. In: Cloud H, ed. *Feeding Problems of the Child with Special Health Care Needs.* New York, NY: Oxford University Press; 1993:203–217.

Loan T. Metabolic/nutritional alterations of traumatic brain injury. *Nutrition.* 1999;15:809–812.

adolescents.[20,21] High-risk contact sports, such as football, boxing, and taekwondo, result in up to half of the injuries.[20,21,27] TBI is also seen in other recreational activities when head protection is either not used or forgotten, including diving, baseball, cycling, horseback riding, and rugby.[15]

 Mechanisms of injury

Acceleration–Deceleration Injuries

Acceleration–deceleration injuries are caused when a moving head hits a relatively fixed object, such as the ground or a windshield. The young infant is particularly susceptible to acceleration–deceleration injuries, as there is less restraint of motion in the neck.[28] Therefore, acceleration–deceleration injury in infancy may result in greater differential displacement of the skull and cranial contents.[28] The direction of acceleration injuries may be translational (linear) or rotational (angular). Most TBIs are a result of a combination of both translational and rotational injuries.

Translational Injury

In translational injury, the head in motion strikes a stationary object and responds with lateral displacement of both the skull and the brain. The injury that results from the initial impact of the skull on the brain is known as *coup*. The lesion that occurs in the direction opposite of the initial force is termed *contrecoup*. Contrecoup occurs as the brain decelerates against the bony structures of the skull.

Rotational Injury

Rotational injury occurs when the skull rotates as the brain remains stationary. The effect is angular forces on the brain, surface contusions, lacerations, and shearing trauma. Rotational injury can result in either focal or diffuse brain damage.

Impression Injuries

Impression injuries occur when a solid object, such as a rock or a blunt object, impacts a stationary head. Impression injuries produce skull fracture and a focal lesion at the site of the impact. The presence of skull fracture is associated with an increased risk of intracranial injury; however, the absence of skull fracture does not reliably exclude a significant intracranial injury.[29,30]

 Primary brain damage from trauma

Primary brain damage from trauma is a direct result of the forces that occur to the head at the time of initial impact.[28,31]

Concussion

Concussion is a complex pathophysiologic process affecting the brain characterized by headache, altered awareness and cognitive function, and impaired balance immediately following trauma.[32] Impaired consciousness typically lasts a few seconds to several hours and is related to the transmission of stretching forces to the brainstem as the brain is thrown back and forth in the cranial vault.[33] Concussion can be seen without obvious pathologic changes to the brain; however, it may also be seen with mild diffuse white matter lesions or neurochemical injury.[33] Following concussion, a child may exhibit clinging behavior, disturbances in sleep, irritability, or more distractibility than usual. These behavior changes can last a few days to a few months.[32,33] Children and adolescents may take longer than adults to recover after a concussion.[19]

Contusion

A contusion is a bruising or hemorrhage of the crests or gyri in the cerebral hemispheres. Contusion can be seen following a crush injury or blunt trauma, or during an inertial load injury, such as acceleration–deceleration of the brain within the skull.[34] Contusions occur most commonly in the frontal and temporal lobes of the brain because of bony irregularities in the cranial vault.[33]

Skull Fractures

Skull fractures are seen in both closed head injuries and open, compound head injuries. Linear comminuted fractures result from impact with low-velocity objects, and depressed fractures generally result from impact with higher-velocity objects. Linear fractures can produce contusions, hemorrhage, and cranial nerve damage.[28] Depressed skull fractures of greater than 5 mm are considered significant.[28] Depressed fractures can produce herniation syndromes, contusions, lacerations, and cranial nerve damage.[28]

Intracranial Hemorrhages

Intracranial injury can occur with or without immediate loss of consciousness or skull fracture.[29,30] Two types of intracranial hemorrhage frequently seen following pediatric TBI are extradural and intradural hematomas. Intracranial hemorrhage may not appear initially on clinical examination.[30] The rate of blood collection and the location of the hematoma are related to severity and outcome.[35] Intracranial hemorrhage is a common cause of clinical deterioration and death in patients who experience a lucid interval immediately after injury.

Extradural Hematomas

Extradural or epidural hematomas develop because of the tearing of an artery in the brain, primarily the middle meningeal artery and its branches. In children, epidural hematomas usually follow skull fracture or bending of the skull into the brain.[35] With unilateral epidural hematoma, there is often herniation of the temporal lobe.[36] Coma may ensue and cardiorespiratory arrest is possible.

Intradural Hematomas

Intradural hematomas include subdural and intracerebral hematomas. Acute subdural hematomas occur secondary to injury to veins in the subdural space. Subsequent recovery depends on both the time before hemorrhage evacuation and the extent of damage to underlying brain tissue.[35] Subdural hematomas are frequently seen with inertial injuries and occur commonly in the temporal and frontal lobes.[33] Subdural hematomas are associated with higher mortality rates and poorer functional outcomes.

Intracranial hematomas can result from trauma or rupture of a congenital vascular abnormality.[37] Very severe injuries may cause large intracerebral hematomas that can rupture into the ventricles, causing intraventricular hemorrhage.[33]

Diffuse Axonal Injury

Diffuse axonal injury (DAI) is a microscopic phenomenon not commonly visible on computed tomography (CT) scan. DAI is seen following rotational injury within the cranial vault.[28] The shearing trauma results in diffuse disturbance of cellular structures following TBI. DAI is associated with much of the significant brain damage seen in TBI, including sudden loss of consciousness, extensor rigidity of bilateral extremities, and autonomic dysfunction.[33]

 ## Secondary brain damage from trauma

Secondary brain damage from trauma evolves as a result of the pathophysiologic changes initiated by the primary trauma.[28,31] Research suggests that secondary brain damage from trauma develops over a period of several hours or days.[33] Secondary injuries account for a significant amount of the overall damage that occurs in TBI, and prevention of secondary brain damage is a major goal of the acute management of the child with TBI.[35]

Cerebral Edema

Perhaps the most frequently occurring cause of secondary injuries is cerebral edema. Unchecked cerebral edema accompanied by an increase in intracranial pressure (ICP) can lead to multiple cerebral infarctions, brain herniation, brainstem necrosis, and irreversible coma.[36] Control of brain swelling is often difficult and may require the use of a combination of the following techniques: narcotic sedation, diuretics, barbiturates, systemic neuromuscular paralysis, or hyperventilation.[35,36]

Intracranial Pressure

When a mass, such as a hematoma or cerebral edema, is present following TBI, ICP increases in response to the pressure exerted on the brain. Initial increases in ICP are accommodated by the mechanisms of the ventricular system.[36] However, when the compensatory mechanisms are no longer effective, ICP rises.

In infancy, increases in ICP will cause bulging of the fontanels and separation of the sutures. In children older than 5 years of age, as ICP rises, the contents of the cranial vault are forced downward through the foramen magnum. This causes brainstem compression and may lead to difficulty breathing and even cardiorespiratory arrest.[28] Prolonged increased ICP may lead to the development of posttraumatic hydrocephalus.[28]

Herniation Syndromes

Herniation syndromes result from displacement of the brain by an expanding lesion and cerebral edema. Depending on the location of the lesion, herniation can cause obstructive hydrocephalus, brain shift past midline, or brainstem compression.[33] Herniation can lead to neurologic deterioration of a grave nature, with resultant decreasing levels of consciousness, altered respiration, hypertonicity, hemiparesis, and decorticate posturing.[33]

Hypoxic–Ischemic Injury

The supply of oxygen and nutrients to the brain is dependent on adequate cerebral perfusion. Alterations of cerebral perfusion, raised ICP, or lack of oxygen to the brain may result in hypoxic–ischemic brain damage.[33] Ischemia frequently occurs in the tissue surrounding cerebral contusions or hematomas and ultimately leads to further brain damage. Severe hypoxic injury and diffuse axonal injuries are most likely to cause severe disabilities, including prolonged postcoma unawareness.[33,38]

Neurochemical Events

When trauma occurs to the brain, there is a disruption of the blood–brain barrier and a release of excitatory neurotransmitters and oxygen-free radicals into the blood system.[33] Oxygen-free radicals have an extremely toxic effect on the brain and are damaging to cell membranes and vessel walls.[39] The damage from oxygen-free radicals causes internal disruption of neuronal functioning and further brain damage.[39]

 ## Other consequences from brain damage

Hydrocephalus

Hydrocephalus can be differentiated as either communicating or noncommunicating type. In communicating hydrocephalus, all components of the ventricular system are enlarged and ICP may only be intermittently elevated. Communicating hydrocephalus is seen in the vast majority of posttraumatic cases.[40] Noncommunicating hydrocephalus refers to enlargement of the ventricles of the brain owing to an obstruction of the flow and impaired absorption of cerebrospinal fluid. Children with hydrocephalus may present with changes in mental status, lethargy, nausea/vomiting, headache, gait ataxia, and urinary incontinence.[40] Neurosurgical ventriculoperitoneal shunting procedures are performed in children with hydrocephalus to improve the flow and absorption of cerebrospinal fluid.[40]

Seizures

The occurrence of early posttraumatic seizures is more common in children than adults, with an incidence of approximately 10%.[41] Early posttraumatic seizures in children are frequently of a generalized onset type, such as grand mal and tonic–clonic seizures.[41] Partial or focal seizures and seizures of late onset are uncommon in children.[41] The frequency of seizure activity within the first year after TBI may be predictive of further recurrence.[41] Thus, children who do not experience seizure within the first year following injury are unlikely to develop seizures at a later time.

Infections

Penetrating injuries, such as gunshot wounds and depressed skull fractures, carry inherent risk of brain infection. In addition, neurosurgical procedures to insert ICP monitors and shunts for increased cerebrospinal fluid also carry risk of brain infection. Two common infections following penetrating wounds are meningitis and brain abscess.[40] The physical therapist (PT) can assist the medical team by monitoring for signs of infection such as fever, headache, confusion, neck stiffness, and increased ICP.

Dysautonomia

Dysautonomia, a malfunction of the autonomic system, occurs after brain injury in 13% of children.[42] A combination of hypertension, diaphoresis, and dystonia are the best predictors of a potential diagnosis.[42] Therefore, PTs need to be diligent to monitor the child for signs of dysautonomia in order to alert the medical team and best manage the symptoms noted.

Endocrine Disorders

Although rare, hypopituitarism and precocious puberty are both reported in children following TBI.[41] Linear growth and weight are closely followed so that the need for medical intervention may be determined. The PT should report any concerns of increased weight gain or the development of secondary sexual characteristics to the child's physician.

Predictors of injury severity and outcome

Clinical rating scales are used to standardize the description of patients with TBI, monitor progress, determine a general plan for appropriate medical intervention, predict outcome, and assist with clinical outcomes research.

Predicting recovery and outcome in children with TBI is complex. The rate of recovery following TBI often appears rapid in the first few months but can continue throughout the first year after the accident. After the first year, the incidence of children continuing to demonstrate gains is greater in children with mild TBI; however, in children with severe injury, some improvement is also noted in the second and third years following injury.[43]

Outcome is affected by a number of factors, including location and morphologic characteristics of the injury, complications that occur during the medical stabilization following injury, the age of the child at the time of injury, the length of coma, the duration of posttraumatic amnesia (PTA), the severity of the injury, premorbid psychological and cognitive adjustment, and the family response to the injury. Of all the factors listed above, the duration of coma appears to be the single most consistent predictor of outcome.[18,44]

Coma Scales

Coma is defined as a complete state of unconsciousness in which the child does not open his or her eyes, follow commands, speak, or react to painful stimuli.[45] To assist with determining the level of unconsciousness, Glasgow neurosurgeons Teasdale and Jennett developed a coma assessment scale (Table 7.2), known as the Glasgow Coma Scale (GCS).[45] It is a standardized tool for assessing the neurologic status of a trauma victim and is based on the patient's best response to three categories: motor activity, verbal responses, and eye-opening.

The Pediatric Coma Scale (PCS)[46] has also been found useful in assessment of outcome in children (Table 7.2) and is used in children 9 to 72 months of age.[46] In addition, the PCS developed interpretive norms for several age groups between birth and 5 years (Table 7.3).[28] Children whose coma scores were below the norm for age tended to have poorer outcomes.

Duration of Coma

The duration of coma is directly related to outcome, with outcomes worsening as coma duration increases.[47–49] For the majority of children with mild TBI and loss of consciousness lasting 1 night or less, the results on the long-term outcome measures of cognition, achievement, and behavior are indistinguishable from those of uninjured children.[50,51] In contrast, children with coma lasting more than a few days and moderate to severe TBI experience a variety of physical, cognitive, language, and psychological sequelae that may improve following the injury or result in permanent impairment.

For children with TBI who had a coma with a duration of 1 week or more and survived, it should be noted that a return to regular education is usually not possible. Rarely do young children stay in a persistent state of coma. Ninety percent have been shown to recover to be moderately disabled or better over a 3-year period.[41]

TABLE 7.2 Comparison of Glasgow Coma Scale and Adelaide Pediatric Coma Scale		
	Glasgow Coma Scale (Adults)	Adelaide Pediatric Coma Scale
Eyes open	Spontaneously 4	
	To speech 3	As in adults
	To pain 2	
	None 1	
Best motor response	Obeys commands 6	
	Localizes pain 5	Obeys commands 5
	Withdraws 4	Localizes to pain 4
	Flexion to pain 3	Flexion to pain 3
	Extension to pain 2	Extension to pain 2
	None 1	None 1
Best verbal response	Oriented 5	Oriented 5
	Confused 4	Words 4
	Words 3	Vocal sounds 3
	Sounds 2	Cries 2
	None 1	None 1

From Teasdale G, Jennett B. Assessment of coma and impaired consciousness. A practical scale. *Lancet*. 1974;2(7872):81–84 and Reilly PL, Simpson DA, Sprod R, et al. Assessing the conscious level in infants and young children: a paediatric version of the Glasgow Coma Scale. *Childs Nerv Syst*. 1988;4(1):30–33.

Depth of Coma

In addition to the duration of coma, the depth of coma, as measured by the GCS, is easy to assess and correlates well with prognosis and functional outcome.[49] Using the PCS, a coma score of 3 or 4 is predictive of a poor outcome, while a score of 7 or greater is predictive of a good outcome.[30,52]

Most children who sustain mild brain injury, as determined by the coma scales, are expected to experience a full recovery within several weeks. However, new evidence suggests that following even a mild TBI some children experience problems with balance, response speed, and running agility that persist at discharge.[53] For children who are moderately and severely injured, the degree of initial impairment on a coma scale is related to both the degree of

TABLE 7.3 Age Norms[a]	
0–6 mo	= 9
6–12 mo	= 11
12–24 mo	= 12
2–5 yr	= 13
>5 yr	= 14

[a]For the Adelaide Pediatric Coma Scale Score (from Kaufman BA, Dacey RG. Acute care management of closed head injury in childhood. *Pediatr Ann*. 1994;23:18–28.)

recovery and residual deficit.[51] Strong correlations of depth of coma and outcome severity have been noted, especially in the areas of intelligence, academic performance, and motor performance.[51]

Orientation and Amnesia Assessment

PTA is defined as the interval between injury and the moment at which an individual can recall a continuous memory of what is happening in the immediate environment.[44] Evaluation of PTA in children is challenging, as traditional assessment methods rely on the subject's verbal response. Because standard orientation questions are inappropriate for children owing to their limited cognitive and language skills, the Children's Orientation and Amnesia Test (COAT)[54] was developed. The COAT is reliable for children between the ages of 4 and 15 years.[54] Although the COAT is useful in the age range established, a reliable method of assessing PTA in children under 4 years of age has not been established.[55]

Duration of Posttraumatic Amnesia

In children, the duration of PTA has been found to be more predictive of future memory function than coma scales.[54] The length of PTA has also been used to classify the severity of TBI. In children with PTA of more than 3 weeks' duration, verbal and nonverbal memory was found to be significantly impaired at both 6 months and 12 months postinjury.[54]

Rancho Los Amigos Levels of Cognitive Functioning

The Rancho Los Amigos Levels of Cognitive Function Scale (Rancho Scale)[56] is a descriptive scale of cognitive and behavioral functioning. It is used primarily during inpatient rehabilitation. The Rancho Scale summarizes neurobehavioral function and serves to enhance communication between staff. The Rancho Scale is also useful as a framework for the PT to identify probable treatment issues and to develop treatment strategies on the basis of the current level of cognitive function. The main limitation of the Rancho Scale is that the "phases of recovery" and prediction of discharge functional ratings is often poorly related. In addition, cognitive function and behavior may fluctuate depending on the environment as well as fatigue or stress on any given day (see Display 7.1).

Pediatric Rancho Scale

The Pediatric Rancho Scale[57] is an adapted version of the Rancho Los Amigos Scale that can be used to evaluate young children between the ages of infancy and 7 years. Like the Rancho Scale, the Pediatric Rancho Scale serves to enhance communication of recovery among staff and to

I.   *No response:* Patient appears to be in a deep sleep and is completely unresponsive to any stimuli.

II. *Generalized response:* Patient reacts inconsistently and nonpurposefully to stimuli in a nonspecific manner regardless of stimulus presented. Responses may be physiologic changes, gross body movements, and/or vocalization and are often limited and delayed. Often, the earliest response is to deep pain.

III. *Localized response:* Patient reacts specifically but inconsistently to stimuli. Responses are directly related to the type of stimulus presented. May withdraw an extremity and/or vocalize when presented with a painful stimulus. May follow simple commands such as closing eyes or squeezing hand in an inconsistent, delayed manner. May also show vague awareness of self-discomfort by pulling at nasogastric tube, catheter, or resisting restraints. May show a bias responding to familiar persons. Once external stimuli are removed, may lie quietly.

IV. *Confused-agitated:* Patient is in a heightened state of activity, and agitation is generally in response to own internal confusion. Behavior is bizarre and nonpurposeful relative to immediate environment. Verbalizations frequently are incoherent and/or inappropriate to the environment. May cry or scream out of proportion to stimuli and even after removal, show aggressive behavior, attempt to remove restraints or tubes, or crawl out of bed. Gross attention to environment is very brief; selective attention is often nonexistent. Patient lacks any recall. Has severely decreased ability to process information and does not discriminate among persons or objects; is unable to cooperate directly with treatment efforts. Unable to perform self-care without maximal assistance. May have difficulty performing motor activities such as sitting, reaching, and ambulating on request.

V.   *Confused-inappropriate:* Patient is able to respond to simple commands fairly consistently. However, with increased complexity of commands or lack of any external structure, responses are nonpurposeful, random, or fragmented. Demonstrates gross attention to the environment, but is highly distractible and lacks ability to focus attention on a specific task. With structure, may be able to converse on an automatic level for short periods of time. Verbalization is often inappropriate and confabulatory. Memory is severely impaired; often shows inappropriate use of objects; and may perform previously learned tasks with structure but is unable to learn new information. Responds best to self, body, comfort, and family members. May show agitated behavior in response to discomfort or unpleasant stimuli. Can usually perform self-care activities with assistance. May wander off, either randomly or with vague intentions of "going home."

VI. *Confused-appropriate:* Patient shows goal-directed behavior but is dependent on external input or direction. Response to discomfort is appropriate and is able to tolerate unpleasant stimuli when need is explained. Follows simple directions consistently and shows carryover for relearned/newly learned tasks such as self-care. Responses may be incorrect owing to memory problems, but they are appropriate to the situation. Past memories show more depth and detail than recent memory. No longer wanders and is inconsistently oriented to time and place. Selective attention to tasks may be impaired. May have vague recognition of staff; has increased awareness of self, family, and basic needs.

VII. *Automatic-appropriate:* Patient appears appropriate and oriented within the hospital and home settings; goes through daily routine automatically but frequently robot-like. Patient shows minimal to no confusion and has shallow recall of activities. Shows increased awareness of self, body, family, food, people, and interaction in the environment. Has superficial awareness of but lacks insight into condition; decreased judgment and problem solving. Lacks realistic ideas/plans for the future. Shows carryover for new learning but at a decreased rate. Requires supervision for learning and safety purposes. With structure is able to initiate social or recreational activities.

VIII. *Purposeful-appropriate:* Patient is able to recall and integrate past and recent events and is aware of and responsive to environment. Shows carryover for new learning and needs no supervision once activities are learned. May continue to show a decreased ability relative to premorbid activities, abstract reasoning, tolerance for stress, and judgment in emergencies or unusual circumstances. Social, emotional, and intellectual capacities may continue to be at a decreased level but functional in society.

From Malkmus D, Booth B, Kodimer C. *Rehabilitation of Head Injured Adult: Comprehensive Congitive Management.* Downey, CA: Los Amigos Research and Education Institute, Inc; 1980:2.

assist with developing a framework for treatment management on the basis of cognitive level (see Display 7.2).

Age

The capacity of the brain to guard against and respond to trauma changes with age.[58] Although at one time young children were thought to be spared greater dysfunction following TBI, newer research has demonstrated an increased vulnerability of the young child to the effects of TBI.[58–60]

The age of the child at the time of injury also appears to correlate with increased risk for specific impairments. Young children are more vulnerable to the effects of diffuse injury on memory than older children. Although the plasticity of the developing brain can allow for dramatic recovery of function, the effects of a diffuse insult produced by TBI may ultimately result in greater cognitive impairment in the developing brain than in the mature brain.[58] Children who experience TBI before the age of 5 years exhibit more profound cognitive deficits than those injured later in childhood.[22,61]

DISPLAY
7.2 **Pediatric Rancho Scale**

V. *No response to stimuli:* Complete absence or observable change in behavior to visual, auditory, or painful stimuli.

IV. *Generalized response to sensory stimulation:* Reacts to stimuli in a nonspecific manner; reactions are inconsistent, limited in nature, and often the same regardless of stimulus present. Responses may be delayed. Responses noted include physiologic changes, gross body movement, or vocalizations. First responses are often to pain. Gives generalized startle to loud sounds. Responds to repeated auditory stimulation with increased or decreased activity. Gives generalized reflex response to painful stimuli.

III. *Localized response to sensory stimuli:* Reacts specifically to stimulus. Responses are directly related to the type of stimuli presented. Responses include blinking when strong light crosses field of vision, following moving object passed within visual field, and turning toward or away from loud sound or withdrawing from painful stimuli. Reactions can be inconsistent and delayed. May inconsistently follow simple commands such as "close eyes," "move an arm." May show vague awareness of self by pulling at tubes or restraints. May show a bias by responding to family and not others.

II. *Responsive to environment:* Appears alert and responds to name. Recognizes parents or other family members. Imitates examiner's gestures or facial expressions. Participates in simple age-appropriate vocal play/vocalizations. Gross attention but highly distractible. Needs frequent redirection to focus on task. Follows commands in an age-appropriate manner and is able to perform previously learned tasks with structure. Without external structure, responses may be random or nonpurposeful. May be agitated by external stimuli. Increased awareness of self, family, and basic needs.

I. *Patient is oriented to self and surroundings:* Shows active interest in environment and initiates social contact. Can provide accurate information about self, surroundings, orientation, and present situation as age-appropriate.

From Professional Staff Association of Rancho Los Amigos Hospital I. *Rehabilitation of the Head Injured Child and Adult: Pediatric Levels of Consciousness, Selected Problems.* Downey, CA: Rancho Los Amigos Medical Center, Pediatirc Brain Injury Service and Los Amigos Rsearch and Education Institute, Inc; 1982:5–7.

Moreover, deficits may remain hidden until a time in which the child needs to participate in higher-level academic activities. Clearly, the young child is vulnerable to brain injury.

Function

In spite of improvement in function over time, children with TBI persist in exhibiting lasting differences in balance, gait velocity, stride length, and cadence when compared with healthy peers.[60] Even children with mild TBI have shown problems with balance on the Bruininks Pediatric Clinical Test of Sensory Integration for Balance and the Postural

Stress Test at 12 weeks postinjury.[62] Such information should be taken into consideration when predicting a return to sports and physical activities that require refined balance skills.

Functional limitations and impairments may also be used to predict discharge status for children with TBI.[63,64] The Pediatric Evaluation of Disability Inventory (PEDI) shows promise in being used for classification of recovery of function following TBI, and in the future may assist in facilitating optimal service delivery. During admission to a rehabilitation unit, the recovery of walking is a primary goal for children with TBI.[65] Knowing whether the patient can ambulate by discharge impacts decisions regarding the discharge environment and the equipment needs at discharge. Four factors associated with a nonambulatory status at discharge include prolonged loss of consciousness, lower extremity (LE) injury, impaired responsiveness, and presence of LE spasticity.[65] In addition, low scores on the PEDI Mobility Functional Skills scale and a long length of stay were also associated with nonambulation at discharge.[65]

Environmental Influences

Children with TBI may be particularly vulnerable to the influence of the family dynamics. In families of children between the ages of 6 and 12 years, it has been shown that greater parental distress and burden was associated with poorer fine motor dexterity, behavioral control, and academic performance.[66] The negative consequences of the TBI combined with high levels of family dysfunction make it more difficult for the family to support the child's recovery. PTs need to consider the influence of the home environment on the prognosis for improvement in the child with TBI.[66]

▶ Physical therapy examination of the child with traumatic brain injury

When a child with TBI is referred for treatment, a thorough physical therapy examination is necessary to ensure appropriate physical therapy management. The examination (Display 7.3) should contain, but may not be limited to, information on past medical history, social history and living environment, cognitive/behavioral status, basic sensorimotor status, and functional status. While performing the examination, consideration should be given to the child's tolerance level and attention span, as deficits in either area may limit the PT's ability to complete the examination in one session. The PT may also need to incorporate play into the assessment in an effort to enhance cooperation and obtain a more accurate picture of the child with TBI.

Subjective Examination: Patient History
Medical History

The therapist must thoroughly review the child's past medical/surgical and current condition prior to initiating the physical examination. Information should be gathered

DISPLAY

7.3　**Physical Therapy Evaluation/Assessment Format**

Medical History

Onset and mechanism of injury	Skin integrity
Diagnostic test results (CT scan, MRI, radiographs)	Respiratory status
Medical precautions	Bowel and bladder status
Vital signs	Dysphagia status
Autonomic nervous system function	Medications

Social History and Living Environment

Family and support system	Cultural issues
Educational/prevocational status	Discharge environment

Cognitive/Behavioral Status

Level of arousal	Memory
Orientation	Language/communication
Attention	Executive functions
Behavior/affect	Neuropsychological or psychological assessments

Basic Sensorimotor Status

Hearing/auditory processing
Vision, perception, and visuo-spatial ability
Sensation
Range of motion
Strength
Muscle tone
Abnormal movement patterns, posture, and reflexes
Balance and balance strategies
Praxis and coordination
Speed of movement
Endurance

Functional Status

Bed/floor mobility
Transfers/transitions
Sitting and standing skills
Ambulation on level surfaces
Stair ascension/descension
Ambulation outside/rough terrain
Advanced gross motor skills/sports
Generalization of functional abilities

regarding the mechanism of the injury, severity of damage, and significant changes in the clinical picture over time. Particular attention should be given to reports from CT scans, magnetic resonance imaging (MRI) scans, radiographs, and other diagnostic tests.

Social History and Living Environment

Interviewing the parents, siblings, and/or caregivers of the child with TBI is imperative, as successful therapeutic intervention should be family- and child-centered.[67] The family members are the experts in knowing their child and often can give helpful advice to the therapist regarding the best way to motivate the child in therapy. In addition, information can be gained regarding the conditions and limitations of the home environment. Families should be encouraged to collaborate with the rehabilitation team in the development of an appropriate plan of care and the identification of equipment needs upon discharge. Family or psychosocial information may also be gained by talking to the social worker.

Systems Review

A thorough review of all body systems helps the PT decide which systems will require further testing and often directs the selection of subsequent tests (see Display 7.4). During this review, information that was not noted in the initial history may be obtained and used to inform further examination of concerns.

Objective Examination: Tests and Measures

Children who sustain TBI may experience a complex array of deficits in body structures and functions in physical abilities, emotional development, and cognitive/behavioral functioning (Display 7.5).[66]

Cognitive/Behavioral Status

A comprehensive cognitive examination is beyond the scope of practice of the PT. However, cognition should be grossly assessed by the PT to assist in determining

DISPLAY

7.4　**Sample System Review Questions: Yes/No Answers to a Series of Questions**

Is your patient experiencing any of the following?

General: Fatigue, sleep disturbance, appetite change

Cardiopulmonary: Irregular heart rate or rhythm, blood pressure fluctuations, edema, dyspnea, ventilator use, sputum production

Integumentary: Color changes, abrasion, bruising, decubitus ulcer, infection

Musculoskeletal: Pain, stiffness, swelling, joint limitation

Neuromuscular: Headache, seizures, spasticity, weakness, tremor, gait disturbance, balance loss

Communication, language, affect, and cognition: Inability to make needs known, altered consciousness, disorientation, memory loss, affect changes, behavioral changes

DISPLAY 7.5	Common Clinical Deficits in Body Structures and Functions		
Physical	**Emotional**	**Cognitive/Behavioral**	**Functional**
Headaches	Mood swings	Decreased arousal	Limited bed mobility
Dizziness	Denial	Disorientation	Limited transfers
Visual disturbance	Anxiety	Distractibility	Poor sitting control
Visuospatial impairment	Depression	Inattention	Poor standing control
Hearing loss	Irritability	Impaired concentration	Gait impairment
Sensory loss	Guilt/self-blame	Confusion	Impaired hygiene skills
Cranial nerve injury	Emotional lability	Agitation	Impaired dressing skills
Spasticity	Low self-esteem	Memory deficits/amnesia	Impaired feeding skills
Ataxia/incoordination	Egocentricity	Sequencing difficulty	Fine motor impairment
Balance impairment	Lability	Slowed processing	Sexual dysfunction
Fatigue	Apathy	Impaired judgment	Sleep disorders
Seizures	Impaired problem solving	Speech/language problems	Decreased academic skills

From Taylor HG, Yeates KO, Wade SL, et al. Influences on first-year recovery from traumatic brain injury in children. *Neuropsychology*. 1999;13(1):76–89.

realistic treatment goals and appropriate interventions. Physical therapy examination of cognition should include the following areas: arousal/orientation, attention span and focus, behavior/affect, memory, communication, mental flexibility, problem solving, judgment, and insight.

LEVEL OF AROUSAL/ORIENTATION Trauma that damages the frontal lobe and brainstem may result in impairment of arousal and orientation of the child with TBI. In addition, medications used to diminish spasticity, seizures, or pain may decrease arousal.[36] Impairment in arousal may be expressed as lethargy, drowsiness, or even coma. Decreased levels of arousal will interfere with the child's ability to attend to pertinent stimuli, follow commands, and benefit from feedback in therapy.

ATTENTION Trauma to the frontal lobe may impair attention in the child with TBI. Impairment in attention may affect both the ability to attend to a specific stimulus and the ability to sustain attention over time. Children with TBI who have problems with attention often have difficulty following commands and relearning motor tasks; thus, the impairment may be expressed as distractibility or inattention. This is especially noted when therapy is conducted in busy environments with many distractions. Care must be taken to structure the environment and remove extraneous stimuli as appropriate.

BEHAVIOR/AFFECT After TBI, children may display a wide array of problems in behavior and affect (see Display 7.5). Two common changes in behavior noted during the time of rehabilitation are agitation and confusion. Agitation is characterized by a heightened state of activity and a severely decreased ability to process stimuli from the environment in a useful manner. The child who is agitated may be restless, irritable, and combative. Impulsivity and unsafe behavior may

be observed as the child acts before thinking. Fortunately, agitation in children with TBI does not last as long as the agitated phase of recovery for adults with TBI.[68]

Confusion is characterized by general disorientation and inability to make sense out of the surrounding environment. Confusion may persist through most of the rehabilitative process. When problems with behavior persist and interfere with participation in therapy, it is important for the brain injury rehabilitation team to work together and implement a behavior modification program. Initially, the team must identify the unwanted behaviors and any precipitating factors, including environmental factors, which contribute to the behavior problem. Agitation may be precipitated by factors such as pain, occult fractures, restraints, urinary tract infections, constipation, and overstimulation by staff, family, and friends. Precipitating factors should be addressed prior to the implementation of the behavior modification program and be removed when possible.

Next, rewards and reinforcements for desired behavior and a reward schedule should be determined. The patient's family may be very helpful in identifying rewards that are both motivating and satisfying. The reward schedule must be agreed on by the rehabilitation team to maximize compliance and promote the desired behavior. Once the rewards and schedule have been addressed, the team then moves toward redirecting the child to appropriate actions by praising approximations of desired actions. As the team works together to address the behavior problem in a consistent manner, the incidence of inappropriate actions slowly decreases. Keep in mind that in some cases the environment cannot be modified and behavior management is ineffective. In that case, the managing physician will consider pharmacologic management.

MEMORY Memory impairment is the most common cognitive impairment in children with TBI.[69] Trauma to the temporal lobe commonly affects memory in children with TBI.

Memory includes the ability to learn and recall new information as well as the ability to recall previously learned information. The presence of memory loss, or amnesia, is an indication that a concussion has occurred. The amnesia may be retrograde, involving a period of time prior to the accident, or anterograde, extending from the incident forward in time.

Memory deficits involve verbal recall and visual recognition. They may appear as the inability to remember the sequence of motor tasks from one treatment to another or as unsafe performance of functional skills. The omission of safety-related behaviors when performing functional motor skills, such as transfers and ambulation, can limit independence.

Memory with respect to a child's ability to learn new material is of particular interest to the PT. Although retention of information learned prior to the TBI may remain unharmed, the memory for learning new information may be problematic. The results of a neuropsychological evaluation of a child's memory skills and capacity for new learning will be helpful in the establishment of realistic functional goals and the development of an appropriate rehabilitation program.[37] Working jointly with the child's family and psychologist, the PT may help determine the need for compensatory strategies, assistance, and environmental modification in the rehabilitation setting.

LANGUAGE Language deficits in the child with TBI are addressed in depth by speech and language pathologists. Damage to the temporal lobe may result in expressive or receptive language deficits that will impede communication between the PT and child, thus complicating therapy sessions. Receptive language deficits will impair a child's ability to understand verbal instructions for the performance of a gross motor task. When receptive language impairment exists, determination of the best means of communication will decrease frustration for the child and the therapist. Expressive language disorders impair a child's ability to communicate with others. Although the child with an expressive language disorder may be able to fully comprehend verbally communicated information and form an appropriate response mentally, a breakdown occurs between the formulation of the response and the verbal or gestural execution of what was intended. Once again, the PT's knowledge of the child's most effective mode of communication may lessen the frustration related to the inability to communicate thoughts and feelings.[35]

EXECUTIVE FUNCTIONS Trauma to the prefrontal regions of the frontal lobes results in impairment of executive functions. Executive functions refer to the ability to show initiative, plan activities, change conceptual sets, solve problems, regulate behavior in social settings, and use feedback to initiate behavioral change and monitor success.[35]

Deficits in executive functioning may be demonstrated by impulsive behavior, resulting in failure to observe safety precautions or the inability to recognize when behavior is socially inappropriate.[35] Mental inflexibility may be demonstrated as perseveration on a task or the inability to change activities without becoming disorganized.[35] Difficulty switching conceptual sets may also influence the ability to perform tasks with alternating patterns or reciprocal movements.

Sensorimotor Status

ABNORMAL TONE

Spasticity Because of damage to the cerebral cortex, children with TBI may present with spasticity. The degree of spasticity may range from mild to severe, with distribution that may be either unilateral or bilateral. Children who present with unilateral involvement display motor impairment and dysfunction similar to that of children with hemiplegic cerebral palsy. Children who present with bilateral involvement often have asymmetric distribution and movements dominated by primitive reflex activity. Spasticity is frequently assessed with the Modified Ashworth Scale, but the reliability of the tool is questionable due to its subjective interpretation.[70]

Children with spasticity may also present with abnormal posturing of the extremities or the whole body. The upper extremities typically present with flexor synergy posturing. Flexor synergy posturing interferes with hygiene and functional use of the upper extremity for play, schoolwork, and self-care. The lower extremities commonly present with extensor synergy posturing. Extensor synergy posturing interferes with bed mobility, transfers, and ambulation.

Children with TBI who are severely involved may present with whole body posturing. Whole body posturing can be decorticate (flexion of the upper extremities and extension of the lower extremities) or decerebrate (extension in all extremities) in nature and is frequently seen in the early stages of recovery. As the child improves, whole body posturing is often replaced with more volitional movement, including movement utilizing abnormal synergistic patterns.

Ataxia Because of damage to the cerebellum and basal ganglia, children with TBI may experience ataxia and motor incoordination. The distribution of ataxia can also be unilateral or bilateral. Ataxia may initially be masked by spasticity in the early recovery period. Timing and execution of movement may be difficult, and oscillations during intention may be present and may worsen with task difficulty. Gait in children with ataxia is characterized by a wide base of support and difficulty maintaining static stance. Ataxia is generally not associated with loss of range of motion (ROM) unless combined with spasticity.

Muscle Performance Impairment

STRENGTH LOSS After TBI and loss of consciousness, children may remain in bed for a prolonged period of time. During that time, weakness due to disuse atrophy may be expected and may result in significant reduction in peak torque ability within the first weeks following injury.[71] Weakness is also seen in both the agonist and antagonist muscle groups of a spastic extremity. Standardized manual muscle testing (MMT) may be difficult to perform, as the child with TBI is unable to follow instructions for testing. Therefore, the PT must observe active movement in various tasks and judge the child's ability to dynamically move against gravity and statically sustain weight. As cognitive function begins to return, the therapist can give simple commands and assess the ability to move during tasks such as sitting up on the edge of the bed, rising from a seated position, and reaching overhead. Finally, in children with TBI who are older than 7 years of age and who are able to follow directions, MMT using a handheld dynamometer can yield excellent within-session intrarater reliability for LE strength testing, while precision grip strength testing can be accurately assessed in children older than 5 years of age.[72,73]

IMPAIRED ENDURANCE Children with TBI often present with an overall state of lethargy. Fatigue for a child with TBI may be due to both physical activity and mental activity associated with motor planning. Both impair the child's ability to participate in activities of functional mobility and self-care. Rest breaks within sessions and rest between therapies may help the child with TBI to sustain participation and build endurance.

RANGE-OF-MOTION LOSS Because of the immobilization and stereotypic abnormal movement patterns used, children with TBI who present with spasticity are at risk for loss of active ROM and contracture development. Joints particularly at risk include the elbows, wrists, fingers, knees, and ankle–foot complex. ROM loss can occur quickly and early management is the key to effective prevention.

BALANCE AND POSTURAL CONTROL LOSS After TBI, a loss of balance is present in most children. Postural control may be affected by neurologic impairments, sensory disorganization, or biomechanical constraints. Research has shown that even in children with mild TBI, a loss of balance may prohibit safe participation in preinjury activities for 12 weeks or more postinjury.[74] Care must be taken to thoroughly reevaluate a child for postural control and tolerance of perturbations before allowing the child to safely return to activity. Common functional tools include the Modified Functional Reach test,[75] the Berg Balance Scale,[76] and the Timed Up and Go (TUG) test.[77,78]

Sensory Deficits

HEARING Hearing loss is also common in pediatric TBI.[79] All children with moderate to severe TBI should have a thorough audiologic evaluation to determine the presence of hearing loss. When hearing loss is present, hearing aids, an FM transmitter, or preferential classroom seating may be indicated.[55]

VISION Visual disturbances in children with TBI are common. These deficits may include decreased visual acuity, disturbances of visual pursuit and accommodation, field cuts, reduced depth perception, diplopia, transient cortical blindness, and retinal hemorrhages.[55] When visual problems exist, eye patching, glasses, or preferential classroom seating may help alleviate the difficulty.[55]

Transient cortical blindness lasting no longer than 30 days has been associated with nearly complete recovery of vision.[55] However, cortical blindness lasting more than 30 days generally carries a grave prognosis for children with TBI. Retinal hemorrhages in young children with TBI are strongly suggestive of child abuse.[80]

VISUOSPATIAL SKILLS Problems with vision are also associated with problems of perception and visuospatial function. Such deficits are frequently associated with lesions in the temporal or occipital lobes of the brain. Visuospatial and perceptual deficits may impair gross motor performance and functional mobility skills, thus limiting the potential for functional independence in a child. A figure-ground deficit, or the inability to distinguish a given form from the background, may make noting a change in terrain depth during gait training more difficult. Visuospatial deficits may also make activities of daily living, such as donning an orthosis, more difficult. A child with deficits in visuospatial memory may demonstrate difficulty developing a mental map of his or her environment and consequently may have difficulty moving independently from place to place in the home, school, or community.[35]

Orthopedic Complications

HETEROTOPIC OSSIFICATION Heterotopic ossification (HO), the formation of mature lamellar bone in soft tissue, can occur in children and adolescents following TBI.[81] The risk of incidence of HO is reported to be 20% and identified risk factors include age greater than 11 years and a longer duration of coma.[81] HO commonly occurs at the elbow, shoulder, hip, and knee. Early signs of HO include decreased joint ROM and pain with testing, swelling, erythema, and increased warmth near the involved joint.

The use of physical therapy in the treatment of HO is controversial. Some studies have associated physical therapy and aggressive ROM exercises with HO formation as a result of local microtrauma and hemorrhage to the tissue.[82] In general, gentle but persistent ROM exercises and management of spasticity with medications or nerve blocks are imperative.[82] When HO results in significant functional impairment, surgical excision of the bone from the soft tissue is indicated. HO rarely results in functional impairment in younger children.[81] HO in older children and adults is associated with a poorer functional outcome.[83]

FRACTURES Fractures in the pelvis and lower extremities are commonly associated with the traumatic events causing pediatric TBI, yet surgical repair of fractures may be delayed until the child is medically stable. Postsurgical care may also be complicated by the decreased cognitive status of the child, especially when the child is alert, but confused. Therefore, the child must be closely monitored to ensure that proper alignment and weight-bearing status are maintained during functional activities.

Although radiographs identify major trauma to the extremities, care should be exercised by the PT in evaluating additional musculoskeletal complaints, as there is potential for minor trauma and occult fractures to be identified during the acute recovery phase. Particular attention should be given to persistent complaints and activities that are poorly tolerated.

Functional Measures

Early examination of function is difficult because of the compromised cognitive status of the child with TBI. As the child is more alert and appropriate in interactions in the clinic, the use of standardized measures, especially those that have shown sensitivity in measuring functional change, may be helpful. In infants, the Alberta Infant Motor Scale (AIMS) is useful in noting gross motor function in children 0 to 18 months old,[84] while the Peabody Developmental Motor Scales are useful in assessment of function in toddlers and preschoolers.[85] The WeeFIM (Functional Independence Measure)[86] has been useful for assessing and tracking the development of functional independence in children with disabilities, including TBI, between the ages of 6 months and 7 years. The adult FIM can be used with older children. The WeeFIM measures six domains of function: self-care, sphincter control, mobility, locomotion, communication, and social cognition. The Bruininks–Oseretsky Test of Motor Proficiency[87] is also used to assess gross and fine motor functioning. It is standardized for children from 4.5 years to 14.5 years, but its use in younger children is questionable.

The Gross Motor Function Measure (GMFM) is designed to evaluate changes in motor performance over time. While it is more commonly used in children with cerebral palsy, there is limited evidence to suggest that it may also be used in children and adolescents with TBI with good discriminative capability.[88] As an alternative to the GMFM in children 8 to 17 years of age, early research indicates that the Acquired Brain Injury-Challenge Assessment (ABI-CA) demonstrates challenges in gross motor activities that are beyond what the GMFM examines and can be used in older children.[89] Specific use though has not been validated.

The PEDI[90] has also been developed as a functional assessment tool for children. It measures both capability and performance in the domains of self-care, mobility, and social function. The PEDI can be used in children between the ages of 6 months and 7.5 years. The ABI-specific PEDI subscales were constructed from the mobility, self-care, and caregiver assistance scales of the PEDI and are being used to measure functional change in children with TBI. Initial results revealed that the Caregiver Assistance Self-Care subscale was more sensitive to measuring change than the generic PEDI, but further research is needed to determine the usefulness of the adapted tool.[91] When interpreting changes in scores using the PEDI, it has been noted that change scores of approximately 11% appear to indicate meaningful clinical difference and can be used in interpreting positive changes in group or individual scores on the PEDI.[92]

Children with severe TBI have been reported to exhibit a significantly reduced range of walking speeds (73 to 154 cm/seconds) when compared to typically developing peers (54 to 193 cm/seconds).[93] Periodic assessment of walking speed should be performed during rehabilitation not only to monitor progress, but also to better understand the energy cost of walking at home and in the community. Specific measures such as the 2 minute walk test[94] and the shuttle walk–run[95] assessments are helpful in evaluating children with higher functional levels specifically for endurance during gait.

▶ Evaluation, diagnosis, prognosis, and plan of care

Evaluation

After the examination is complete, the PT must consider all of the data collected and make judgments that will lead to the development of a plan of care. The therapist must weigh the evidence of observed impairments in body structures and function and activity limitations with the knowledge of the pathophysiologic condition of the brain injury and other physiologic processes associated with trauma to better understand the patient's prognosis for expected improvement. In addition, the therapist should consider the environmental and personal factors that impact participations, such as patient's social support and the home environment. Evidence supports the notion that good family support can positively impact recovery and outcome.[56] Finally, the PT should consider the amount of time that has passed since the injury, any interventions received, and progress made during recovery and treatment.

Diagnosis and Prognosis

Using the *Guide to Physical Therapist Practice*[4] as a resource, a physical therapy diagnosis can be determined for the child with TBI. This diagnosis, while not a medical diagnosis, will align the child with a preferred practice pattern and assist with decision making (see Table 7.1). The prognosis of the patient will be affected by predictors associated with severity and outcome as well as complicating factors experienced during the course of recovery. Overall, the incidence of disability in child with TBI is accounted for by mild injury.[96] Those with long acute and rehabilitation stays and low functional gains are associated with greater levels of disability.[97]

In a recent study looking at the recovery of ambulation skills in children and adolescents with TBI, it was noted that LE hypertonicity, brain injury severity, and LE injury combined were critical predictors of ambulation ability after TBI.[98] In addition, dysautonomia in children with TBI is associated with prolonged rehabilitation and less improvement in motor scores during recovery.[42] The PT must consider these factors and the anticipated response to intervention while formulating the prognosis. According to the *Guide*, the expected range of number of visits per episode of care for a child or adolescent with TBI or coma ranges from 5 to 90 sessions.[4]

Plan of Care

On the basis of the physical therapy diagnosis, the PT should determine a plan of care for the child with TBI. The plan of care includes not only the prescribed treatment interventions, but also specific long- and short-term goals designed to help the patient achieve the desired outcomes prior in therapy. Goals should be written on the basis of identified deficits with structure and function that interfere with participation in specific meaningful activities. Goals should be measurable and expressed in behavioral terms. Each short-term goal should be written as a component that leads to the accomplishment of the long-term goal. Time frames in which goals will be achieved are dependent on consideration of the child's cognitive and behavioral status as well as projected length of stay and the care environment.

▶ Management/interventions

Rehabilitation of children with TBI is different from adults with TBI in that the interventions used by the PT must incorporate age-appropriate gross motor challenges at the appropriate level of cognitive function. A number of rehabilitation approaches used in adult stroke, and cerebral palsy populations may be applied to children with TBI. Although the efficacy of various rehabilitation programs is not known, research is indicative of a positive trend in the benefit of rehabilitative services.[99]

Acute Medical Management

Early medical management of the child with TBI focuses on preservation of life, determination of injury severity, and prevention of secondary brain damage.[32] Once the vital signs are stabilized, the child will undergo a general assessment for potential injuries and a neurologic examination. These tests may include radiographic examination of the skull and cervical spine, CT scan of the head, and the use of the GCS. Acute medical intervention for children with TBI may include emergency surgery, the use of mechanical ventilation, and the use of pharmacologic agents. If a subdural or intracerebral hematoma is present, immediate neurosurgery is indicated.[33] A delay in performing the surgery can be life threatening, as it helps decrease ICP and reduce pressure-related secondary brain injuries.[33]

Mechanically assisted ventilation at a rate greater than normal or hyperventilation is used to temporarily reduce ICP.[35] In addition to hyperventilation, pharmacologic agents are also used to decrease cerebral edema and minimize secondary brain damage. Drugs commonly used in the management of edema include mannitol and corticosteroids.[35] Medications may also be used to induce paralysis when the child's body movements interfere with the stability of vital signs and the administration of further medical interventions.[35]

Physical therapy in the acute stage may be deferred to a time in which the child is less medically fragile. Once the child is stable, the PT may use the child's current level of cognitive functioning as a guide in planning interventions. It is important for the PT to remember that the cognitive levels of recovery serve only as a general guideline for recovery. Not all children will experience each level of cognitive recovery or progress through recovery in a strict hierarchical sequence. Either the Rancho Scale or the Pediatric Rancho Scale may assist with identification of current cognitive status and potential concerns for the various stages.

Acute Physical Therapy Management: Prevention

Physical therapy management for children with TBI functioning at low cognitive levels (Rancho Levels I to III and Pediatric Levels V to III) is aimed at the prevention of complications from prolonged inactivity and sensory deprivation. Common complications of prolonged inactivity may include skin breakdown, respiratory complications, and contracture development.

Contracture Management

The importance of preventing soft tissue contractures in the acute recovery phase cannot be overemphasized. Dystonic extensor muscle overactivity is a major contributor to progressive ankle contractures, and the development of contractures will delay functional independence and lead to the need for additional therapy or even surgery later in the rehabilitative phase.[43] In a recent study, ROM, prolonged stretch in a standing frame or tilt table combined with reeducation of functional movement patterns is effective in reducing contractures.[43] In addition to the use of a positioning program, ROM and the application of splints and casts may help improve LE function and prevent soft tissue contractures.[43]

Contractures in prepubertal children who are not forcefully posturing often may be successfully managed with positioning and splinting alone because of the child's smaller size and relative weakness.[54] Coordination of a wearing schedule is a key to enhancing the effectiveness of splinting. Wearing tolerance may be gradual, and the child must be monitored for signs of skin breakdown. In a larger child who is not forcefully posturing, serial casting followed by bivalved fiberglass cast splints may be used to manage contractures.

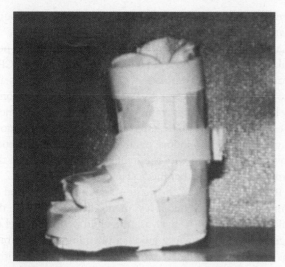

FIGURE 7.1 An example of a bivalved inhibitive cast.

For children with severe extensor posturing who do not respond to a positioning program, splints, or bivalved casts, serial casts are warranted (Fig. 7.1).[54] These casts must be changed initially every 3 to 5 days to prevent skin breakdown.[43,100] Once it is determined that the child will tolerate the casts without skin breakdown, the casts can be worn for up to 2-week intervals until posturing diminishes and volitional control increases. Bivalved fiberglass cast splints may then be used at night to maintain ROM. If used during the day, an alternating schedule may be helpful before discontinuing use.[43,100] Continuous use of serial casts in a child who is alert and moving actively should not exceed 2 months.

Serial casts may be used in conjunction with oral or injectable medications to manage spasticity. Oral medication, such as dantrolene (Dantrium), although useful in decreasing spasticity, is often undesirable because of its sedating properties.[57] Diazepam (Valium) can also be used for treating spasticity but may be associated with increased agitation in children who are emerging from coma.[57] As an alternative, nerve and motor point blocks, such as phenol and Botox A injections, may be more desirable in the management of spasticity in children, as there are no sedating and cognitive side effects.[57] Recent work on the use of Botox injections in children is promising and indicates that Botox may be more effective for maintaining passive ROM of the ankle.[100] When injections are combined with traditional physical therapy, in some cases pain levels decreased and functional gains were also noted in gait, transfers, grasping, and releasing.[100]

Positioning

A positioning program will assist with improving pulmonary hygiene, maintaining skin integrity, preventing contractures, and providing support for body alignment and movement. Positioning should be implemented with the assistance of the nursing staff and the family. Changes in position for the child confined in bed should be made every 2 hours. When the child is sitting, pressure relief procedures should be

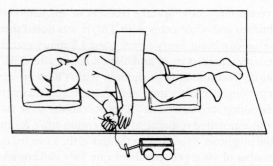

FIGURE 7.2 Child positioned in a side-lyer. Note that the head is maintained in line with the trunk, the upper extremities are in midline, and the lower extremities are dissociated. Gravity is eliminated, and the influence of primitive reflexes is minimized.

performed every 30 minutes. Pressure relief is accomplished by having the child recline on a mat in side-lying or by tilting the wheelchair backward to a semi-supine position.

When designing a positioning program, the PT should take into consideration any orthopedic and neurologic positioning precautions as well as the influence of abnormal tone and primitive reflexes on posture. Positioning in side-lying (Fig. 7.2) may be preferred to positioning in supine or prone as it is helpful to decrease the influence of abnormal primitive reflexes. Positioning in supine should incorporate strategies to reduce the influence of the tonic labyrinthine reflex and extensor tone. Positioning in prone, although allowable, will seldom be carried out at this phase of recovery as it interferes with accessibility for adequately monitoring the child's vital signs and medical status.

Upright positioning, even at an early stage of recovery, may be achieved with the use of an adapted wheelchair (Figs. 7.3 and 7.4). The adapted wheelchair should incorporate either a tilt-in-space or reclining seating system with postural support to assist the child in safely achieving

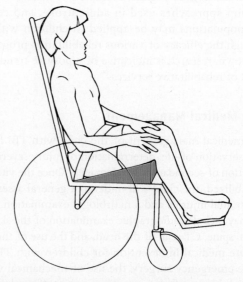

FIGURE 7.3 Child is supported in a wheelchair with a tall back and a seat wedge to maintain hip flexion. The back may be designed to either recline or tilt in space to accommodate fatigue in the child.

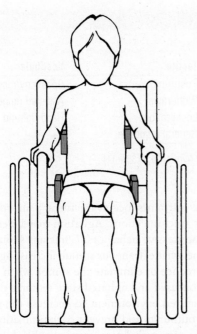

FIGURE 7.4 Child is sitting in a wheelchair with hip blocks and lateral trunk supports for assistance with postural control.

upright while preventing overfatigue. A removable headrest can be used to encourage head control when the child is alert and allow for rest when the child is fatigued.

Low-Cognitive-level Physical Therapy Management: Stimulation

Coma Stimulation Program

Coma stimulation programs were developed on the premise that structured stimulation could prevent sensory deprivation and accelerate recovery. However, controversy exists regarding the efficacy of stimulation used in the care of a comatose child.[101] Sensory input may be provided through the vestibular, visual, tactile, auditory, and olfactory systems (Display 7.6).[102] The rehabilitation team should involve the family in the selection of meaningful items to be used for stimulation to individualize the program. An emphasis should be placed on selecting items that reflect the child's culture, personality, likes/dislikes, hobbies, significant relationships, and pets. In addition, items that are selected should be reevaluated periodically, so ineffective stimuli can be eliminated.

The next step in program development is to determine an appropriate schedule for stimulation. The PT needs to determine the time of day at which alertness is optimal to conduct therapy and modify the child's schedule as necessary. If this is not possible, the PT will need to modify the treatment goals within a given session and attempt to engage the child at the current level of arousal and attention.[35]

Prior to implementation, the PT will need to educate the family on the provision of appropriate levels of sensory stimulation, including the amount of environmental stimulation being provided. Care should be taken to create an environment that is stimulating but not physiologically overstimulating or noxious. Decreasing extraneous auditory and visual activity in the child's room or treatment area may help elicit a response related to specific treatment stimuli.

At the beginning of the session, the PT should orient the child with TBI to who is conducting the session, the surroundings, and the current date and time. Stimulation should be brief and should be implemented using one or two sensory modalities at a time while slowly presenting meaningful items. For the child who is unresponsive or responds only to pain, the initial goal of input is to elicit any type of response to stimuli. The therapist needs to be patient and allow time for the child to respond, as processing of sensory input may be delayed. A variety of responses may occur depending on the stimulation used (Display 7.7).[102] Precautions should be taken to ensure that the child's medical status remains stable following stimulation. Unfavorable responses to stimulation include the development of seizure activity and sustained increases in heart rate, blood pressure, and respiratory rate.[102]

Once the child becomes more alert, the therapist should focus on increasing the consistency, duration, and quality of the child's response. If the vitals are stable, the program should be conducted in a supported sitting or standing to improve alertness. Initial adjustment to upright may require blood pressure monitoring to ensure safe tolerance. As vital signs stabilize, all team members and the family should be encouraged to document the stimuli utilized and the child's response to note progress and assist with carryover.

DISPLAY 7.6	Sources of Sensory Stimulation			
Auditory	**Visual**	**Olfactory**	**Tactile**	**Vestibular**
Verbal orientation	Photographs	Vinegar	Hand holding	Turning
Music	Penlight	Spices	Rubbing lotion	Range of motion
Bells	Familiar objects	Perfume	Heat/cold	Sitting in chair
Familiar voice	Faces	Potpourri	Cotton balls	Tilt table
Tuning fork	Flashcards	Orange/lemon	Rough surfaces	
Clapping	Picture books		Familiar objects	

From Sosnowski C, Ustik M. Early intervention: coma stimulation in the intensive care unit. *J Neurosci Nurs.* 1994;26:336–341.

| DISPLAY | | | | |
| 7.7 | **Common Responses to Stimulation** | | | |

Auditory	Visual	Olfactory	Tactile	Vestibular
Startle reaction	Eye blink	Grimacing	Posturing	Spasticity/movement
Localization	Visual localization	Tearing	Withdrawal	Assisted range of motion
Turn toward sound	Visual tracking	Head turning	Localization	Head righting
Follow commands	Visual attention	Sniffing	General response	

From Sosnowski C, Ustik M. Early intervention: coma stimulation in the intensive care unit. *J Neurosci Nurs.* 1994;26:336–341.

As the child continues to attend to therapy and follow one-step motor commands, the PT can begin to support the development of head and trunk control as well as simple, spontaneous extremity movement patterns, such as reaching or stepping. The therapist should continue to monitor the patient for signs of physiologic overload during treatment and make adjustments accordingly. Response should then be channeled into more purposeful activity and functional skills, such as bed mobility and transfers. At this time, the PT should also begin family education about future recovery phases and possible treatment techniques.

Vegetative State

Some children do not progress following implementation of a coma stimulation program and are in a persistent vegetative state. A vegetative state is characterized by an absence of response to external stimuli and an absence of attempts to communicate needs to others. Children in a vegetative state may have periods of eye-opening, sleep–wake cycles, and primitive reflexive movement of the limbs, but they do not demonstrate a response to pain or have self-awareness.[103,104] Families often have difficulty distinguishing between coma and persistent vegetative state as the outward presentation is similar. Persistent vegetative state is due to primary brain damage; therefore, the focus of care shifts from promoting functional movement to spasticity and contracture management, as noted earlier in acute care management.

Midcognitive-level Physical Therapy Management: Structure

When the child has emerged from coma (Rancho Levels IV and V and Pediatric Level II) and begins to participate in functional activities, other cognitive deficits may become evident. Selection of appropriate activities by the PT should be based on cognitive as well as physical demands, keeping in mind that the progression of cognitive and physical function can proceed at different rates.

The Agitated Patient

Initially, agitation is in response to poor regulation of stimulation and internal confusion. Common factors that may contribute to agitation include overstimulation by staff, parents, and friends; restraints; occult fractures; pain; constipation; and urinary tract infections. Agitation may be expressed as bizarre or aggressive behaviors. Clinicians should attempt to determine what extraneous stimuli increase agitation and attempt to reduce or eliminate the stimuli when possible. A child in a confused and agitated state requires the use of a highly structured environment to decrease the number of behavioral outbursts and prevent overstimulation. The PT may need to give verbal reassurance to the child with TBI as some agitated behaviors can be related to fear. If precipitating factors cannot be successfully reduced or eliminated, then pharmacologic management should be considered.

In the management of agitation, it is important to utilize a team approach that includes the family. Common management strategies include having a quiet room with no television or telephone, limited visitors, and planned rest periods as needed. The child's family may resist suggestions to decrease visitors and stimuli, believing that talking loudly and turning on lights, television, and radio can help to increase the child's alertness and participation in therapy. Staff should reinforce appropriate levels of stimulation during family education.

It is important to protect the child who is agitated from potential injury. Restraints should be removed when possible as they may further agitation. If the unrestrained child is at risk for falling out of bed, it may be necessary to modify the room by placing the mattress on the floor or switch to an enclosed protective bed. Other protective devices include alarm devices, such as sensitized doormats and monitor bracelets used for a child or adolescent who is ambulatory and may wander away from supervision.

During the agitated phase, treatment should be modified to include simple activities that are familiar to the child and well liked to enhance participation and cooperation. Although the child may be able to perform familiar motor activities, the PT should anticipate behavior that is essentially nonpurposeful. Appropriate tasks and activities include ROM exercises to the child's tolerance and functional gross motor activities such as rolling, coming to sit, standing up, and walking. It is important for the PT to work within the child's tolerance level on previously learned skills and to anticipate no carryover for new learning during this phase of recovery.

The child with TBI is often very unpredictable during the agitated phase, so the therapist should be prepared with several activity options. Choices of activities should be offered to the child when possible. When the child is uncooperative with familiar or routine activities, the PT should try to redirect the child to another therapeutic activity. If unsuccessful, the PT may need to resort to involving the child in any activity in which he or she is willing to participate. Therapy of this nature is still beneficial to the child with TBI as it may serve to increase alertness, attention span, and activity level.

For the child who is extremely difficult to manage, cotreatment with other team members and shortened therapy sessions may be necessary until the child tolerates longer interactions. As attention span gradually increases, the PT reinforces longer periods of attention and directs the child with TBI back to more challenging tasks.

The Confused Patient

Although no longer internally agitated, the child with TBI who is confused will require continued behavior management and structure during the therapy session to perform optimally. Structure may include decreasing the complexity of instructions, simplifying the environment, or a motor task (Figs. 7.5 and 7.6). The primary goal of therapy during the confused phase of recovery is to enhance successful participation in functional tasks.

In addition, the PT should give the child as much structure and assistance as necessary to allow for success. In patients with serious deficits, partial weight-bearing locomotion shows promise for establishing an upright posture

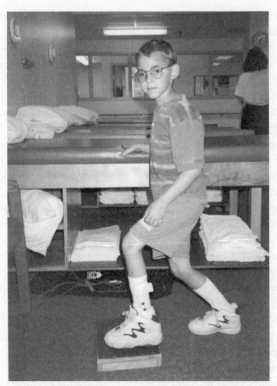

FIGURE 7.6 Lunges on the involved lower extremity enhance balance and may help improve hip and knee control.

during the early stages of gait training.[105] As performance improves, structure can be decreased, and the child can be challenged to perform in a more complex environment.

When the child is confused, it is helpful to work on familiar activities so that the need for verbal instruction is reduced. When giving verbal instruction, the therapist should keep directions simple and allow for delays in processing verbal instructions. In addition, the PT may need to demonstrate new tasks instead of providing the child with verbal explanations to enhance understanding.

Orientation is very important during the confused phase of recovery. The PT should remember to orient the child to his or her surroundings frequently and establish a familiar routine. Thus, the child may begin to work on recall skills and begin to anticipate what is going to happen next in the day. Familiarity and routine are calming and reassuring and may assist with behavior management as well. Items such as a calendar, clock, and schedule card may assist with orientation in an older child. In addition, the therapist may need to assist the child with topical orientation to his or her surroundings.

Encouraging the child to rely on his or her own memory for sequencing of movement or safety rules will challenge the child to become more independent. The use of a therapy journal or verbal rehearsal may help improve the child's memory. However, the therapist should be careful not to frustrate the child who has difficulty remembering. Instead of a continued open line of questioning, the therapist may offer choices and see if the child can recognize the right response. For example, a child who is learning to transfer

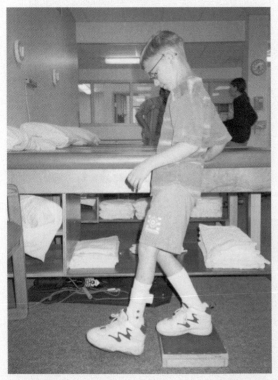

FIGURE 7.5 Stepping down off a small bench facilitates improved eccentric control of the lower extremity during knee extension.

from a wheelchair may be asked whether he or she should scoot forward in the chair or lock the brakes first.

Although new learning is still limited, the PT can begin to integrate principles of motor control and motor learning with principles of therapeutic exercise to treat focal deficits, body structure impairments, and activity limitations. It is the PT's responsibility to select developmentally appropriate functional skills that are motivating and challenging with the correct spatial and temporal demands for the child's abilities. The PT should also focus on selecting functional activities that incorporate the use of both cognitive and physical skills. For example, an activity involving maneuvering a walker through an obstacle course addresses memory for verbal commands, motor planning, and mobility skills.

An essential element in motor learning is the opportunity for practice. The child with TBI should be allowed to experience movement with assistance as necessary, make mistakes, and make corrections as his or her ability levels dictate. Practice should encourage active participation in a meaningful play activity within the current capabilities of the child. Repeated practice will be necessary for the child to learn new or previously mastered gross motor tasks. Current research suggests that the intensity of training is an important consideration in achieving positive outcomes in return of movement and increased PEDI mobility scores.[106] While more intense programs often yield better return and higher scores, this must be balanced with awareness that children with TBI may display reduced endurance and increased fatigue with intense training. The therapist may need to provide rest breaks for the child both within the therapy session and in between therapies to maximize learning.

Determining the type of feedback to be used during therapy is another important consideration in promoting learning. The PT must make choices regarding the timing, precision, and frequency of feedback. In addition, the child's cognitive and sensory function will provide a guideline for determining the appropriate feedback mode. If a child is not aware of one side of his or her body, kinesthetic feedback may not be helpful to enhance learning, while visual and verbal feedback may be more appropriate (Fig. 7.7). Likewise, if a child is aphasic, the therapist will need to facilitate learning using visual and kinesthetic information.

As the child with TBI improves, the PT must modify the task and the environment in order to continue to engage the child actively in therapy. If persistent behavioral problems exist, it may be necessary for the PT to continue to use behavior modification techniques in order to increase compliance in therapy. At this stage of recovery, the child's judgment will be impaired, so it will be important to continue to protect the child from injury.

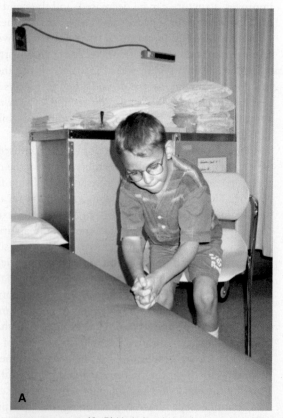
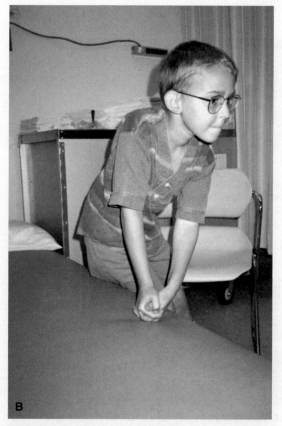

FIGURE 7.7 (A, B) Verbal and visual cues to use hands in midline during transfers may enhance the awareness of the involved side and improve safety during movement.

During both the agitated and the confused phases of recovery, the PT should continue the use of positioning, resting splints, and casting as needed. Orthotics for standing and gait activities may also assist with control for balance and gait. The disadvantages of the orthoses are that they are more difficult to apply and need to be replaced more frequently than standard ankle–foot orthoses (AFOs).

Higher-Cognitive-level Physical Therapy Management: School/Community Reintegration

While research suggests that mobility outcomes achieved during the early stages of recovery are sustained and additional gains may be made within 6 months of returning home, it is important for the PT to remember that not all children will reach a high level of cognitive function (Rancho Levels V to VIII and Pediatric Level I) and have complete physical recovery.[107] Toward the end of the inpatient rehabilitation phase, persistent losses of cognitive and physical function become more apparent, and plans must be made to reintegrate the child with TBI back into the home and/or school setting with continued therapies. The family, medical rehabilitation team, and the school district must work together and jointly plan for reentry into the school setting. The PT may need to evaluate the child for orthotics, assistive devices, and mobility devices necessary for function in the child's home and at school. In addition, the PT may assist with recommendations regarding any environmental modifications to the child's home or school.

For the child with TBI who does reach the higher stages of cognitive recovery, the PT will begin to wean the child from the cognitive cues and structure previously used in order to enhance further independence at home and/or school. Owing to the tendency of TBI to affect vision and hearing, memory, concentration, impulse control, and organizational skills, the classroom environment may be particularly difficult for the child with TBI.[54] Care should be taken not to remove the structure too early as memory retention and generalization of learning in new settings occur at slower rates.

The PT should also continue to focus on treating any residual motor deficits that interfere with functional independence at home or in school. For some children, this will mean continued training with assistive devices and physical assistance for basic motor skills, such as transfers and gait[108] (Figs. 7.8 and 7.9). For others, contemporary treatments may be considered. While some contemporary treatments, such as body weight–supported treadmill training (BWSTT), are quite popular, there is no clear evidence to support their use over conventional gait training in children with physical disabilities.[108,109] However, constraint-induced movement therapy shows promise for improving upper extremity function in children with TBI.[110]

Finally, for children who experience only subtle problems with balance and speed, coordination, timing, and rhythm

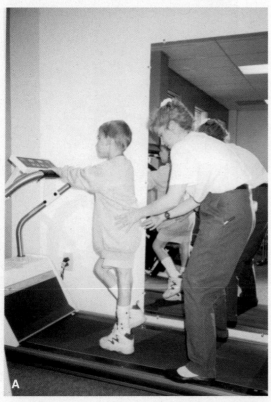
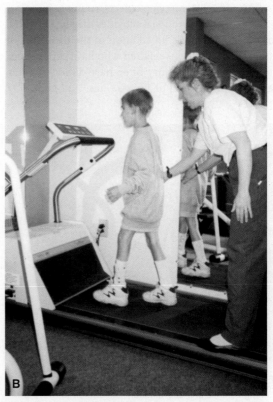

FIGURE 7.8 The use of a treadmill in gait training may facilitate control at various speeds. Training may be performed both with **(A)** and without **(B)** upper extremity support to challenge balance on a dynamic surface.

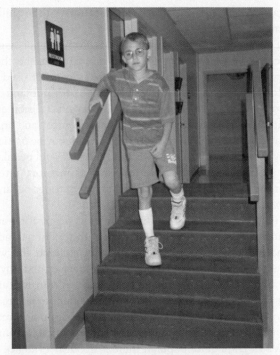

FIGURE 7.9 In gait training on the stairs, note the increased support at the right forearm and the mild internal rotation of the right hip during descent. Verbal cues for upper extremity support and visual cues for lower extremity alignment may improve skill.

of movement, participation in challenging physical activities such as walking exercise on a balance board or therapy ball (Figs. 7.10 and 7.11), carrying objects, running, jumping, hopping, skipping, or recreational activities may be beneficial in improving activity levels. In addition to the problems of motor control and function, children who have experienced moderate or severe brain injury often have difficulty maintaining an appropriate level of fitness (Figs. 7.12 and 7.13).

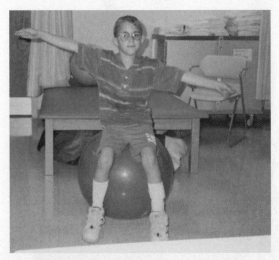

FIGURE 7.10 The therapy ball can be used to challenge dynamic sitting balance and coordination. In addition to moving his arms, the child could also practice alternating forward placement of his feet or move the arms and legs in rhythmic patterns.

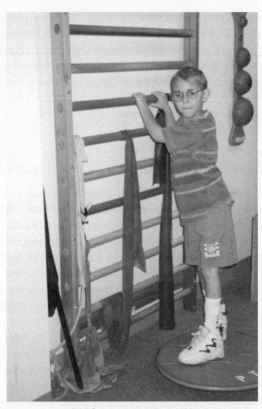

FIGURE 7.11 A BAPS (biomechanical ankle platform system) board can be used to enhance balance and coordination of the lower extremities to maintain balance.

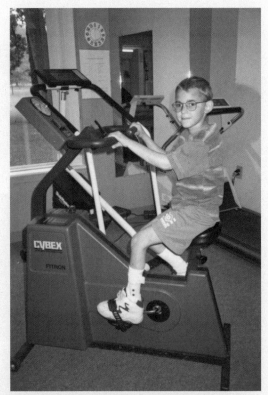

FIGURE 7.12 Bicycling on standard exercise equipment can be used to promote aerobic exercise. It can also be done as part of training before returning to riding a standard child's bike.

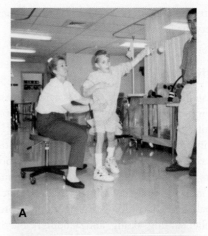

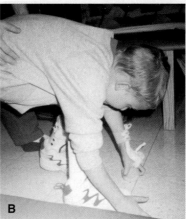

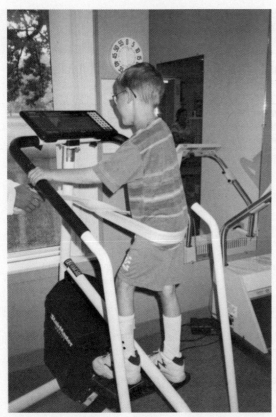

FIGURE 7.13 Exercise on standard exercise equipment may not only improve strength, but may also help improve endurance. The stair stepper improves control in hip extensors and abductors, knee extensors, and ankle plantarflexors. The strap at the hips provides a cue to maintain hip extension and to increase weight bearing on the more involved side.

The PT should design a fitness program that can be continued after discharge from therapy to address wellness and health. The PT can also work with the physical education teacher in designing an adapted physical education program for the child with TBI (Fig. 7.14).

School Issues

The Individuals with Disabilities Education Act recognizes "brain injury" as a separate category of impairment in children, and school curriculum must be adapted for qualifying children with TBI. In addition, the educational services the child receives may provide accommodations and physical assistance for activities of daily living, mobility, and motor tasks, such as writing, in order to assist the child with achieving academic success. A complete discussion of physical therapy in the school system is found in Chapter 19.

▶ **Prevention**

Prevention is the key to decreasing the annual incidence of TBI. Effective prevention involves improving technology to

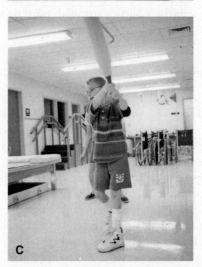

FIGURE 7.14 Sports can be incorporated into therapeutic activities or adaptive physical education to enhance coordination, balance, and motor planning. A game of baseball can incorporate gross motor tasks of **(A)** throwing with the involved arm, **(B)** picking up a ground ball, and **(C)** batting.

decrease the intensity of impact on the brain during collision, increasing awareness and use of safety measures, and mandating protective laws. Children under 12 months are at significant risk for head injury, and much of the risk can be prevented by increased parental supervision or improved home safety devices.[22]

Bicycle Helmets

The consistent use of bicycle helmets can decrease the incidence of injury, as unhelmeted riders are more likely to have a brain injury than helmeted bicyclists.[111–113] Fit of the helmet is important, as poor fit has been associated with an increased risk of TBI in children, especially in boys.[114] Use of helmets can also potentially prevent brain injuries from occurring in sports and recreational activities, including baseball, football, horseback riding, rollerblading, skateboarding, hockey, roller skating, skiing, and sledding.[68] Barriers to helmet use include the lack of awareness of recreational risks and the effectiveness of helmets, cost, and negative peer pressure. Increasing the use of helmets may be accomplished by advocating for educational programs, discount coupons, helmet subsidies, role modeling by parents, and mandatory legislative change.

Playground Equipment

Prevention can also be aimed at preventing falls from playground equipment onto unprotected surfaces. The severity of the injuries can be remarkably decreased if the height of equipment does not exceed 5 feet and materials such as sand, pea gravel, or wood chips are used under the playground equipment.[68] Surface materials must be continually maintained if they are to be effective.

Traffic Behavior

The inability of a child under 11 years of age to assess distances and speeds combined with immaturity and typical levels of impulsiveness results in unsafe traffic behavior. Even after training programs, the majority of young children still exhibit risky behavior, and parents should be cautious of younger children crossing the street alone. More effective community approaches should focus primarily on decreasing the traffic speed, enforcing laws governing pedestrian–motor vehicle interaction, and separating the pedestrian from the traffic[68] (see Case Study).

Car Restraints

The use of occupant seat belt restraints is clearly an effective strategy for preventing injury during a crash. The placement of the child in the back seat of the car and the correct use of car seats can prevent up to 90% of serious and fatal injuries to children under 5 years of age.[68] Unfortunately, misuse of child seats is still a common problem. In older children and adolescents, the use of lap and shoulder belts can prevent approximately 45% of serious and fatal injuries.[68]

CASE STUDY

Justin: Patient Client Management Applied to Preferred Practice Pattern 5C

Element of Patient/Client Management	Application for a Child with Acquired TBI
Examination	*Examples of history:* Age of child, past medical history, prior functional status, medications
	Examples of systems review: Blood pressure fluctuations, abrasion or other problem with skin integrity, inability to make needs known
	Examples of tests and measures: Postural observation, FIM, WeeFIM, PEDI, range of motion, muscle strength testing, gait analysis
Evaluation	*Synthesis* of observed impairments with *interpretation* from functional examination tools commonly used, such as the FIM and PEDI
Diagnosis	Physical therapy diagnosis based on *impairments* and *functional limitations*
Prognosis and plan of care	*80%* of the patients in the preferred practice pattern will achieve the anticipated goals and expected outcomes within *6 to 90 visits per episode of care*
Intervention	*Examples of coordination, communication, and documentation:* Case management, patient/client family meetings, outcome data
	Examples of topics for patient/client-related instruction: Current condition, plan of care, fitness program, risk factors, transitions across settings
	Examples of procedural interventions: Balance training, flexibility exercises, postural stabilization, neuromotor development training, gait training, device and equipment use, biofeedback, passive range of motion
Outcome	Use the *anticipated goals* and *expected outcomes* to assist with monitoring progress and documentation

Justin is an 8-year-old boy who experienced a TBI secondary to a pedestrian–motor vehicle accident. He was unconscious at the scene of the accident and was life-flighted to the nearest pediatric trauma center. On arrival at the emergency room, he had a GCS of 2 and his pupils were fixed and dilated. Justin was in a coma. Diagnostic studies revealed diffuse right intracranial hemorrhage, a right pneumothorax, fracture of the left orbit, and multiple contusions. An ICP monitor, chest tubes, and placement of a tracheostomy tube were required for acute management.

Justin lives at home with his parents and a 6-year-old sister in a two-story home with five steps to enter. His bedroom and bathroom are on the second floor. His past medical history is unremarkable. Justin is a second-grade student at Jones Elementary.

The brain injury rehabilitation team was consulted 3 days after admission, and Justin was determined to be at a Rancho Los Amigos Scale Level II. The brain injury team implemented a coma stimulation program. Caution was taken implementing the program owing to his multiple injuries, monitors, and tube placements. In addition, the PT initiated an inhibitory casting program to manage his left ankle plantarflexion posturing, which was measured at 45 degrees. A resting splint was made to maintain the right ankle in a neutral position. On the basis of the PT's screening, systems review, and examination, Justin's medical diagnosis fits in the physical therapist preferred practice pattern 5C.[4]

Justin slowly emerged from the coma over a period of 2 weeks. Subsequent treatment focused on increasing tolerance to upright on the tilt table, motor control of the neck and trunk during sitting, and contracture management. During the next 2 weeks, Justin's medical condition stabilized, and he progressed to a Rancho Los Amigos Scale Level V. Owing to the severity of his brain injury and the presence of multiple impairments, the acute care team anticipated that Justin would require additional care in an acute rehabilitation setting, an outpatient setting, and additional services at his school setting. His episodes of care would most likely be on the higher end of the range anticipated for preferred practice pattern 5C.

As Justin awoke, his tracheostomy was removed, and he was transferred to a pediatric rehabilitation center. The WeeFIM and the PEDI were used to examine his status upon admission and to determine his projected goals for improvement during his stay. Inhibitory casting was continued for the left ankle plantarflexion contracture, which was now measured at 20 degrees. Justin was given a high-back wheelchair for mobility with a custom-fit modular seating system for postural control. In addition to the previous intervention strategies, Justin also began to work on transfers from supine to sit and from the wheelchair to a mat with moderate assistance. He also engaged in standing activities and gait training. Decreased motor control and hemiplegia on the left were more evident as he increased his activity level. Justin moved in synergistic patterns for both the upper and lower extremities. Strength on the right side of the body was fair. Balance and coordination in upright were poor, and he required maximal assistance for standing activities.

As rehabilitation progressed, Justin's condition improved and he began to follow commands consistently and showed some recall of newly learned tasks. His parents participated regularly in family conferences and family education and were instructed how to assist Justin during tasks of functional mobility as well as how to perform prescribed exercises. At the time of discharge from rehabilitation, Justin was able to propel himself in a regular wheelchair using the right extremities. He was able to transfer from the wheelchair to the mat with supervision and was able to walk short household distances with a forearm crutch on the right. He was still limited in his mobility by the left-sided spasticity. Justin had been evaluated for orthotics and was to receive a left dynamic AFO. Neuropsychological testing was completed prior to discharge and revealed deficiencies in short-term memory, attention span and focus, judgment, and agility to learn new material.

By 4 months after the injury, Justin was transitioning back into his school. His school program was modified for a half-day of inclusion in his regular classroom and a half-day of specialized classroom services. Justin would continue to receive physical therapy through the school setting. He was independent in his transfers and was ambulating with the left forearm crutch and the dynamic AFO more consistently. Justin used the wheelchair only for community mobility.

REFERENCES

1. Keenan HT, Bratton SL. Epidemiology and outcomes of pediatric traumatic brain injury. *Dev Neurosci*. 2006;28(4–5):256–263.
2. Atabaki SM. Pediatric head injury. *Pediatr Rev*. 2007;28(6):215–224.
3. Greenwald BD, Burnett DM, Miller MA. Congenital and acquired brain injury. 1. Brain injury: epidemiology and pathophysiology. *Arch Phys Med Rehabil*. 2003;84(3)(suppl 1):S3–S7.
4. American Physical Therapy Association. Guide to physical therapist practice. Second edition. *Phys Ther*. 2001;81(1):9–746.
5. Langlois JA, Rutland-Brown W, Thomas KE. The incidence of traumatic brain injury among children in the United States: differences by race. *J Head Trauma Rehabil*. 2005;20(3):229–238.
6. Faul M, Xu L, Wald MM, et al. Traumatic brain injury in the United States: national estimates of prevalence and incidence, 2002–2006. *Injury Prev*. 2010;16(suppl 1):A268.
7. Schneier AJ, Shields BJ, Hostetler SG, et al. Incidence of pediatric traumatic brain injury and associated hospital resource utilization in the United States. *Pediatrics*. 2006;118(2):483–492.
8. Kraus JF. Epidemiology of head injury. In: Cooper PR, Golfinos J, eds. *Head Injury*. 4th ed. New York, NY: McGraw-Hill Companies, Inc; 2000:1–25.
9. Marik PE, Varon J, Trask T. Management of head trauma. *Chest*. 2002;122(2):699–711.
10. Guerrero JL, Thurman DJ, Sniezek J. E. Emergency department visits associated with traumatic brain injury: United States, 1995–1996. *Brain Inj*. 2000;14(2):181–186.
11. Faul M, Xu L, Wald MM, et al. *Traumatic brain injury in the United States: emergency department visits, hospitalizations, and deaths*. Atlanta, GA: Centers for Disease Control and Prevention, National Center for Injury Prevention and Control; 2010.
12. Mazzola CA, Adelson PD. Critical care management of head trauma in children. *Crit Care Med*. 2002;30(11)(suppl):S393–S401.
13. Gedeit R. Head injury. *Pediatr Rev*. 2001;22(4):118–124.
14. Koepsell TD, Rivara FP, Vavilala MS, et al. Incidence and descriptive epidemiologic features of traumatic brain injury in King County, Washington. *Pediatrics*. 2011;128(5):946–954.
15. Bazarian JJ, McClung J, Shah MN, et al. Mild traumatic brain injury in the United States, 1998—2000. *Brain Inj*. 2005;19(2):85–91.
16. Brehaut JC, Miller A, Raina P, et al. Childhood behavior disorders and injuries among children and youth: a population-based study. *Pediatrics*. 2003;111(2):262–269.
17. Gerring JP, Grados MA, Slomine B, et al. Disruptive behaviour disorders and disruptive symptoms after severe paediatric traumatic brain injury. *Brain Inj*. 2009;23(12):944–955.
18. Ponsford J, Willmott C, Rothwell A, et al. Cognitive and behavioral outcome following mild traumatic head injury in children. *J Head Trauma Rehabil*. 1999;14(4):360–372.
19. Guskiewicz KM, Valovich McLeod TC. Pediatric sports-related concussion. *PMR*. 2011;3(4):353–364, quiz 364.
20. Kraus JF, Rock A, Hemyari P. Brain injuries among infants, children, adolescents, and young adults. *Am J Dis Child*. 1990;144(6):684–691.
21. Kraus JF, Fife D, Cox P, et al. Incidence, severity, and external causes of pediatric brain injury. *Am J Dis Child*. 1986;140(7):687–693.
22. Crowe LM, Catroppa C, Anderson V, et al. Head injuries in children under 3 years. *Injury*. 2012;43(12):2141–2145.
23. Chadwick DL, Chin S, Salerno C, et al. Deaths from falls in children: how far is fatal? *J Trauma*. 1991;31(10):1353–1355.
24. Factors potentially associated with reductions in alcohol-related traffic fatalities—United States, 1990 and 1991. *MMWR Morb Mortal Wkly Rep*. 1992;41(48):893–899.
25. Kraus JF. Epidemiological features of brain injury in children: occurence, children at risk, causes and manner of injury, severity, and outcomes. In: Bromon SH, Michel ME, eds. *Traumatic Head Injury in Children*. New York, NY: Oxford University Press; 1995.
26. Rivara FP. Epidemiology of violent deaths in children and adolescents in the United States. *Pediatrician*. 1983;12(1):3–10.

27. Koh JO, Cassidy JD. Incidence study of head blows and concussions in competition taekwondo. *Clin J Sport Med.* 2004;14(2):72–79.

28. Kaufman BA, Dacey RG Jr. Acute care management of closed head injury in childhood. *Pediatr Ann.* 1994;23(1):18–20, 25–28.

29. Bonadio WA, Smith DS, Hillman S. Clinical indicators of intracranial lesion on computed tomographic scan in children with parietal skull fracture. *Am J Dis Child.* 1989;143(2):194–196.

30. Hahn YS, McLone DG. Risk factors in the outcome of children with minor head injury. *Pediatr Neurosurg.* 1993;19(3):135–142.

31. Griffith ER, Rosenthall M, Bond MR, et al., eds. *Rehabilitation of the Child and Adult with Traumatic Brain Injury.* 2nd ed. Philadelphia, PA: F.A. Davis; 1990.

32. Almasi SJ, Wilson JJ. An update on the diagnosis and management of concussion. *WMJ.* 2012;111(1):21–27, quiz 28.

33. Marion D. Pathophysiology and initial neurosurgical care: future directions. In: Horn LJ, Zasler ND, eds. *Medical Rehabilitation of Traumatic Brain Injury.* Philadelphia, PA: Hanley & Belfus, Inc; 1996.

34. Kaufmann P, Hofmann G, Smolle KH, et al. Intensive care management of acute pancreatitis: recognition of patients at high risk of developing severe or fatal complications. *Wien Klin Wochenschr.* 1996;108(1):9–15.

35. Kautz-Leurer M, Rotem, H. Acquired brain injuries: trauma, near-drowning, and tumors. In: Campbell S, ed. *Physical Therapy in Children.* Philadelphia, PA: W.B. Saunders; 2012:679–701.

36. Graham DI, Gennarelli TA. Pathology of brain damage after head injury. In: Golfinos J, Cooper PR, eds. *Head Injury.* 4th ed. New York, NY: McGraw-Hill Companies, Inc; 2000.

37. Mysiw JW, Fugate LP, Clinchot DM. Assessment, early rehabilitation intervention, and tertiary prevention. In: Horn LJ, Zasler ND, eds. *Medical Rehabilitation of Traumatic Brain Injury.* Philadelphia, PA: Hanley & Belfus, Inc; 1996.

38. Robertson CS, Contant CF, Narayan RK, et al. Cerebral blood flow, AVDO2, and neurologic outcome in head-injured patients. *J Neurotrauma.* 1992;(9)(suppl 1):S349–S358.

39. Konotos HA. Oxygen radicals in central nervous system damage. *Chem Biol Int.* 1989;72:229–255.

40. Fullerton Long D. Diagnosis and management of intracranial complications in TBI rehabilitation. In: Horn LJ, Zasler ND, eds. *Medical Rehabilitation of Traumatic Brain Injury.* Philadelphia, PA: Hanley & Belfus, Inc; 1996.

41. Weiner HL, Weinberg JS. Head injury in the pediatric age group. In: Golfinos J, Cooper PR, eds. *Head Injury.* Vol 4. New York, NY: McGraw-Hill; 2000.

42. Kirk KA, Shoykhet M, Jeong JH, et al. Dysautonomia after pediatric brain injury. *Dev Med Child Neurol.* 2012;54(8):759–764.

43. Conine TA, Sullivan T, Mackie T, et al. Effect of serial casting for the prevention of equinus in patients with acute head injury. *Arch Phys Med Rehabil.* 1990;71(5):310–312.

44. Katz DI, Alexander, MP. Traumatic brain injury. Predicting course of recovery and outcome for patients admitted to rehabilitation. *Arch Neurol.* 1994;51(7):661–670.

45. Teasdale G, Jennett B. Assessment of coma and impaired consciousness. A practical scale. *Lancet.* 1974;2(7872):81–84.

46. Reilly PL, Simpson DA, Sprod R, et al. Assessing the conscious level in infants and young children: a paediatric version of the Glasgow Coma Scale. *Childs Nerv Syst.* 1988;4(1):30–33.

47. Asikainen I, Kaste M, Sarna S. Predicting late outcome for patients with traumatic brain injury referred to a rehabilitation programme: a study of 508 Finnish patients 5 years or more after injury. *Brain Inj.* 1998;12(2):95–107.

48. Macpherson V, Sullivan SJ, Lambert J. Prediction of motor status 3 and 6 months post severe traumatic brain injury: a preliminary study. *Brain Inj.* 1992;6(6):489–498.

49. Wilson B, Vizor A, Bryant T. Predicting severity of cognitive impairment after severe head injury. *Brain Inj.* 1991;5(2):189–197.

50. Bijur PE. Cognitive outcomes. *J Dev Behav Pediatr.* 1996;17(3):186.

51. Jaffe KM, Fay GC, Polissar NL, et al. Severity of pediatric traumatic brain injury and neurobehavioral recovery at one year—a cohort study. *Arch Phys Med Rehabil.* 1993;74(6):587–595.

52. Lieh-Lai MW, Theodorou AA, Sarnaik AP, et al. Limitations of the Glasgow Coma Scale in predicting outcome in children with traumatic brain injury. *J Pediatr.* 1992;120(2, pt 1):195–199.

53. Gagnon I, Forget R, Sullivan SJ, et al. Motor performance following a mild traumatic brain injury in children: an exploratory study. *Brain Inj.* 1998;12(10):843–853.

54. Ewing-Cobbs L, Levin HS, Fletcher JM, et al. The Children's Orientation and Amnesia Test: relationship to severity of acute head injury and to recovery of memory. *Neurosurgery.* 1990;27(5):683–691, discussion 691.

55. Cockrell J. Pediatric brain injury rehabilitation. In: Horn LJ, Zasler ND, eds. *Medical Rehabilitation of Traumatic Brain Injury.* Philadelphia, PA: Hanley & Belfus, Inc; 1996:171–196.

56. Malkmus D, Booth B, Kodimer C. *Rehabilitation of Head Injured Adult: Comprehensive Cognitive Management.* Downey, CA: Los Amigos Research and Education Institute, Inc; 1980:2.

57. Professional Staff Association of Rancho Los Amigos Hospital, I. *Rehabilitation of the Head Injured Child and Adult: Pediatric Levels of Consciousness, Selected Problems.* Downey, CA: Rancho Los Amigos Medical Center, Pediatirc Brain Injury Service and Los Amigos Rsearch and Education Institute, Inc; 1982:5–7.

58. Anderson V, Jacobs R, Spencer-Smith M, et al. Does early age at brain insult predict worse outcome? Neuropsychological implications. *J Pediatr Psychol.* 2010;35(7):716–727.

59. Kuhtz-Buschbeck JP, Stolze H, Gölge M, et al. Analyses of gait, reaching, and grasping in children after traumatic brain injury. *Arch Phys Med Rehabil.* 2003;84(3):424–430.

60. Kuhtz-Buschbeck JP, Hoppe B, Gölge M, et al. Sensorimotor recovery in children after traumatic brain injury: analyses of gait, gross motor, and fine motor skills. *Dev Med Child Neurol.* 2003;45(12):821–828.

61. Crowe LM, Catroppa C, Babl FE, et al. Executive function outcomes of children with traumatic brain injury sustained before three years. *Child Neuropsychol.* 2013;19(2):113–126.

62. Gagnon I, Swaine B, Friedman D, et al. Children show decreased dynamic balance after mild traumatic brain injury. *Arch Phys Med Rehabil.* 2004;85(3):444–452.

63. Dumas HM, Haley SM, Ludlow LH, et al. Functional recovery in pediatric traumatic brain injury during inpatient rehabilitation. *Am J Phys Med Rehabil.* 2002;81(9):661–669.

64. Williams GP, Schache AG. Evaluation of a conceptual framework for retraining high-level mobility following traumatic brain injury: two case reports. *J Head Trauma Rehabil.* 2010;25(3):164–172.

65. Haley SM, Dumas HM, Rabin JP, et al. Early recovery of walking in children and youths after traumatic brain injury. *Dev Med Child Neurol.* 2003;45(10):671–675.

66. Taylor HG, Yeates KO, Wade SL, et al. Influences on first-year recovery from traumatic brain injury in children. *Neuropsychology.* 1999;13(1):76–89.

67. Rivara JB. Family functioning following pediatric traumatic brain injury. *Pediatr Ann.* 1994;23(1):38–44.

68. Rivara FP. Epidemiology and prevention of pediatric traumatic brain injury. *Pediatr Ann.* 1994;23(1):12–7.

69. Levin HS, Eisenberg HM. Neuropsychological outcome of closed head injury in children and adolescents. *Childs Brain.* 1979;5(3):281–292.

70. Clopton N, Dutton J, Featherston T, et al. Interrater and intrarater reliability of the Modified Ashworth Scale in children with hypertonia. *Pediatr Phys Ther.* 2005;17(4):268–274.

71. Bloomfield SA. Changes in musculoskeletal structure and function with prolonged bed rest. *Med Sci Sports Exerc.* 1997;29(2):197–206.

72. Katz-Leurer M, Rottem H, Meyer S. Hand-held dynamometry in children with traumatic brain injury: within-session reliability. *Pediatr Phys Ther.* 2008;20(3):259–263.

73. Golge M, et al. Recovery of the precision grip in children after traumatic brain injury. *Arch Phys Med Rehabil.* 2004;85(9):1435–1444.

74. Aitken ME, Jaffe KM, DiScala C, et al. Functional outcome in children with multiple trauma without significant head injury. *Arch Phys Med Rehabil.* 1999;80(8):889–895.

75. Bartlett D, Birmingham T. Validity and reliability of a pediatric reach test. *Pediatr Phys Ther.* 2003;15(2):84–92.

76. Franjoine MR, Gunther JS, Taylor MJ. Pediatric balance scale: a modified version of the berg balance scale for the school-age child with mild to moderate motor impairment. *Pediatr Phys Ther.* 2003;15(2):114–128.

77. Williams EN, Carroll SG, Reddihough DS, et al. Investigation of the timed 'up & go' test in children. *Dev Med Child Neurol.* 2005;47(8):518–524.

78. Zaino CA, Marchese VG, Westcott SL. Timed up and down stairs test: preliminary reliability and validity of a new measure of functional mobility. *Pediatr Phys Ther.* 2004;16(2):90–98.

79. Fligor BJ, Cox LC, Nesathurai S. Subjective hearing loss and history of traumatic brain injury exhibits abnormal brainstem auditory evoked response: a case report. *Arch Phys Med Rehabil.* 2002;83(1):141–143.

80. Forbes BJ, Rubin SE, Margolin E, et al. Evaluation and management of retinal hemorrhages in infants with and without abusive head trauma. *J AAPOS.* 2010;14(3):267–273.

81. Hurvitz EA, Mandac BR, Davidoff G, et al. Risk factors for heterotopic ossification in children and adolescents with severe traumatic brain injury. *Arch Phys Med Rehabil.* 1992;73(5):459–462.

82. Djergaian RS. Management of musculoskeletal complications. In: Horn LJ, Zasler ND, eds. *Medical Rehabilitation of Traumatic Brain Injury.* Philadelphia, PA: Hanley & Belfus, Inc; 1996.

83. Johns JS, Cifu DX, Keyser-Marcus L, et al. Impact of clinically significant heterotopic ossification on functional outcome after traumatic brain injury. *J Head Trauma Rehabil.* 1999;14(3):269–276.

84. Piper MC, Pinnell LE, Darrah J, et al. Construction and validation of the Alberta Infant Motor Scale (AIMS). *Can J Public Health.* 1992;83(suppl 2):S46–S50.

85. Darrah J, Magill-Evans J, Volden J, et al. Scores of typically developing children on the Peabody Developmental Motor Scales: infancy to preschool. *Phys Occup Ther Pediatr.* 2007;27(3):5–19.

86. Rice SA, et al. Rehabilitation of children with traumatic brain injury: descriptive analysis of a nationwide sample using the WeeFIM. *Arch Phys Med Rehabil.* 2005;86(4):834–836.

87. Deitz JC, Kartin D, Kopp K. Review of the Bruininks-Oseretsky Test of Motor Proficiency, second edition (BOT-2). *Phys Occup Ther Pediatr.* 2007;27(4):87–102.

88. Linder-Lucht M, Othmer V, Walther M, et al. Validation of the Gross Motor Function Measure for use in children and adolescents with traumatic brain injuries. *Pediatrics.* 2007;120(4):e880–e886.

89. Ibey RJ, Chung R, Benjamin N, et al. Development of a challenge assessment tool for high-functioning children with an acquired brain injury. *Pediatr Phys Ther.* 2010;22(3):268–276.

90. Feldman AB, Haley SM, Coryell J. Concurrent and construct validity of the Pediatric Evaluation of Disability Inventory. *Phys Ther.* 1990;70(10):602–610.

91. Kothari DH, Haley SM, Gill-Body KM, et al. Measuring functional change in children with acquired brain injury (ABI): comparison of generic and ABI-specific scales using the Pediatric Evaluation of Disability Inventory (PEDI). *Phys Ther.* 2003;83(9):776–785.

92. Iyer LV, Haley SM, Watkins MP, et al. Establishing minimal clinically important differences for scores on the pediatric evaluation of disability inventory for inpatient rehabilitation. *Phys Ther.* 2003;83(10):888–898.

93. Katz-Leurer M, Rotem H, Keren O, et al. The effect of variable gait modes on walking parameters among children post severe traumatic brain injury and typically developed controls. *NeuroRehabilitation.* 2011;29(1):45–51.

94. Katz-Leurer M, Rotem H, Keren O, et al. The relationship between step variability, muscle strength and functional walking performance in children with post-traumatic brain injury. *Gait Posture.* 2009;29(1):154–157.

95. Vitale AE, Jankowski LW, Sullivan SJ. Reliability for a walk/run test to estimate aerobic capacity in a brain-injured population. *Brain Inj.* 1997;11(1):67–76.

96. Rivara FP, Koepsell TD, Wang J, et al. Incidence of disability among children 12 months after traumatic brain injury. *Am J Public Health.* 2012;102(11):2074–2079.

97. DeWall J. Severe pediatric traumatic brain injury. Evidence-based guidelines for pediatric TBI care. *EMS Mag.* 2009;38(9):53–57.

98. Dumas HM, Haley SM, Ludlow LH, et al. Recovery of ambulation during inpatient rehabilitation: physical therapist prognosis for children and adolescents with traumatic brain injury. *Phys Ther.* 2004;84(3):232–242.

99. Kramer ME, Suskauer SJ, Christensen JR, et al. Examining acute rehabilitation outcomes for children with total functional dependence after traumatic brain injury: a pilot study. *J Head Trauma Rehabil.* 2013;28(5):361–370.

100. Verplancke D, Snape S, Salisbury CF, et al. A randomized controlled trial of botulinum toxin on lower limb spasticity following acute acquired severe brain injury. *Clin Rehabil.* 2005;19(2):117–125.

101. Lombardi F, Taricco M, De Tanti A, et al. Sensory stimulation for brain injured individuals in coma or vegetative state. *Cochrane Database Syst Rev.* 2002(2):CD001427.

102. Sosnowski C, Ustik M. Early intervention: coma stimulation in the intensive care unit. *J Neurosci Nurs.* 1994;26(6):336–341.

103. Ashwal S. The persistent vegetative state in children. *Adv Pediatr.* 1994;41:195–222.

104. Latour JM. Caring for children in a persistent vegetative state: complex but manageable. *Pediatr Crit Care Med.* 2007;8(5):497–498.

105. Seif-Naraghi AH, Herman RM. A novel method for locomotion training. *J Head Trauma Rehabil.* 1999;14(2):146–162.

106. Dumas HM, Haley SM, Carey TM, et al. The relationship between functional mobility and the intensity of physical therapy intervention in children with traumatic brain injury. *Pediatr Phys Ther.* 2004;16(3):157–164.

107. Dumas HM, Haley SM, Rabin JP. Short-term durability and improvement of function in traumatic brain injury: a pilot study using the Paediatric Evaluation of Disability Inventory (PEDI) classification levels. *Brain Inj.* 2001;15(10):891–902.

108. Brown TH, Mount J, Rouland BL, et al. Body weight-supported treadmill training versus conventional gait training for people with chronic traumatic brain injury. *J Head Trauma Rehabil.* 2005;20(5):402–415.

109. Damiano DL, DeJong SL. A systematic review of the effectiveness of treadmill training and body weight support in pediatric rehabilitation. *J Neurol Phys Ther.* 2009;33(1):27–44.

110. Karman N, Maryles J, Baker RW, et al. Constraint-induced movement therapy for hemiplegic children with acquired brain injuries. *J Head Trauma Rehabil.* 2003;18(3):259–267.

111. Kiss K, Pinter A. [Are bicycle helmets necessary for children? Pros and cons]. *Orv Hetil.* 2009;150(24):1129–1133.

112. Coffman S. Bicycle injuries and safety helmets in children. Review of research. *Orthop Nurs.* 2003;22(1):9–15.

113. Cassidy JD, Carroll LJ, Peloso PM, et al. Incidence, risk factors and prevention of mild traumatic brain injury: results of the WHO Collaborating Centre Task Force on Mild Traumatic Brain Injury. *J Rehabil Med.* 2004;(43)(suppl):28–60.

114. Rivara FP, Astley SJ, Clarren SK, et al. Fit of bicycle safety helmets and risk of head injuries in children. *Inj Prev.* 1999;5(3):194–197.

Traumatic and Atraumatic Spinal Cord Injuries in Pediatrics

Heather Atkinson and Elena M. Spearing

Examination
   History
   Systems Review
   Tests and Measures
Evaluation, Diagnosis, and Prognosis
Intervention
   Medical Intervention
   Therapeutic and Functional Interventions
Coordination, Communication, and Documentation
   Education
   Discharge Planning
   School Reentry
Illness Prevention and Wellness
   Fitness
   Circulation

Dysreflexia/Hyperreflexia
Growth Abnormalities
Anticipatory Planning
Outcomes
   Vocational Outcomes
   Psychological Outcomes
   Life Satisfaction Outcomes
Future Directions
   Prevention
   Research
Summary
Case Studies

As with all pediatric conditions requiring care from a physical therapist (PT), working with a child poses special challenges. Treatment of a child with traumatic or atraumatic spinal cord injury not only demands attention to their current age-specific needs, but also requires special consideration of their physical, cognitive, and emotional development. Spinal cord injury (SCI) is a lifelong disability, and PTs have the responsibility to anticipate the variety of changes a child will encounter as he or she grows and develops over his or her lifetime. A catastrophic illness or injury such as an SCI has profound effects on both the child and his or her family. A PT has the unique opportunity to be not only a teacher, a guide, and an advocate, but also a coach who empowers his or her clients to live life to its fullest potential.

The National Spinal Cord Injury Association (NSCIA) defines pediatric SCI as an acute traumatic lesion of the spinal cord and nerve roots in children from newborn through 15 years of age.[1] According to the NSCIA, there are an estimated 12,000 new cases of SCI per year. In the United States, there are currently 236,000 to 327,000 people living with SCI. The average age of injury is 41 years, with 53% of injuries occurring between the ages of 16 and 30.[2,3] The overall incidence of pediatric SCI is 1.99 injuries per 100,000 children in the United States.[4] Approximately 80% of adult

SCI are male, and in children, males are twice as likely to be affected than females.[2,4]

General mechanisms of traumatic spinal injury for adults include flexion/extension, axial loading, burst, and compression fractures. A child's spine, however, does not fully mature until between the ages of 8 and 10 years and therefore can lend itself to a different mechanism of injury. These immature features can predispose a child under 11 years of age to an upper cervical spine injury at the level of C-3 or above.[5] Ligamentous laxity, disproportionately large head size, and relatively horizontal facet joints can create a fulcrum for a sagittal force and allow a large amount of translatory movement. A child over 11 years of age has a greater tendency toward injury to the lower cervical spine (C-3 and below) as opposed to the adult population.[5] Thoracolumbar injuries in young children are also unique on account of anatomic differences between children and adults. Specifically, the ring apophysis in the growing pediatric spine can slip or separate into the spinal canal from an axial traumatic force and mimic the symptoms of a herniated intervertebral disk.[5] Finally, the ligamentous laxity in the pediatric spinal column can allow the vertebra to stretch and recoil during a force to the spine or head; however, this action also causes the relatively inflexible spinal cord inside to stretch as well. This stretching can cause distraction or ischemia to delicate neuropathways and cause an invisible SCI that is not picked up on radiographic assessment as there is no obvious fracture or dislocation. This phenomenon is known as spinal cord injury without radiographic abnormality (SCIWORA) and can present as a complete or incomplete injury. SCIWORA is a prevalent manifestation, and has been reported in 19% to 34% of all children who experience SCI.[6] All children who have experienced a trauma should have both head injury and SCIWORA ruled out, owing to the increased potential for neurologic devastation. SCIWORA can also have a delayed onset, so all medical staff, including the PT, should carefully monitor the child's clinical presentation.

Additional causes of traumatic SCI include motor vehicle accident, violence, falls, and sports. The causes of SCI that are unique to pediatrics include birth trauma, child abuse, and motor vehicle lap belt injuries.[5] Motor vehicle restraints are designed to dissipate force over bony areas of the body to prevent injury during a crash. Small children are often improperly positioned in a car with the lap belt riding higher than the pelvis, causing a fulcrum of force in the thoracic or lumbar spine and severe pressure on the abdomen. Children with this type of injury often have a burn mark across the abdomen and may have significant visceral injury as well.[5,7]

Atraumatic SCI includes all other spinal cord dysfunction such as myelopathies, cancer, and stroke. Clinically, atraumatic SCI often presents similarly to either a complete or incomplete SCI. Myelopathies include both compressive and inflammatory disorders. Compressive myelopathies are often caused by an underlying structural abnormality (stenosis, spondylolisthesis) combined with some antecedent trigger such as a fall or car accident with resultant compression on the spinal cord. Chiari malformations and protruding disks also have the potential to cause compression on the spinal cord. Inflammatory myelopathies include an entire spectrum of neuroinflammatory disorders, including acute transverse myelitis (ATM), Guillain–Barré syndrome (GBS), multiple sclerosis (MS), acute disseminated encephalomyelitis (ADEM), and neuromyelitis optica (NMO).[8]

ATM affects both children and adults and has the potential to be significantly disabling.[9] The cause of transverse myelitis is not clearly defined, although more information is becoming available about its neuropathology and possible treatments. An underlying systemic inflammation or autoimmune disorder can trigger the development of any inflammatory myelopathy, including transverse myelitis.[8,10] In addition, infection is also considered in these disorders and may initiate the cascade of events resulting in spinal cord dysfunction. There is some documentation relating the onset of transverse myelitis with vaccination, although the benefits of vaccination still far outweigh the risks.[8,10] There is also a high incidence of an antecedent infection (respiratory, gastrointestinal, systemic) prior to the development of transverse myelitis. It is thought that this antecedent infection initiates a cascade of cellular and immune-mediated events that ultimately result in attack of the spinal cord. A specific protein byproduct in this cellular reaction (interleukin-6) has a unique affinity for the spinal cord and has been demonstrated to kill spinal cord cells. Additionally, the spinal cord itself responds differently from other internal organs in how it responds to autoimmune dysfunction.[8,10] Although it is still unknown why a specific transverse segment of the spinal cord is targeted, increased knowledge about the immunopathogenesis of transverse myelitis is leading to better treatment options. These options will be discussed later in this chapter.

Atraumatic SCI can also be caused by cancer. This may be a primary tumor with focal dysfunction, or it could be in the form of metastases with more diffuse dysfunction. Nonetheless, the physical effects can include sensory and motor abnormalities as well as spasticity and bowel and bladder dysfunction.[11]

Another form of atraumatic SCI is stroke. This can be caused by arterial or venous ischemia, watershed infarct, arteriovenous malformation (AVM), or a dural arteriovenous fistula. Onset can be either sudden or gradual, depending on the type of bleed. The overall course of recovery may vary as well.[12]

Although traumatic and atraumatic injuries can present similarly, understanding the exact nature of the injury can assist the clinician in formulating a hypothesis that will guide the examination, evaluation, diagnosis, prognosis, intervention, and ultimately outcome that the child achieves.

▶ Examination

History

The PT begins with a thorough history taken from all available resources. This may include any or all of the following.

History of Present Illness

- Mechanism and date of injury
- Any loss of consciousness at the time of injury or potential brain injury
- Any acute medical treatment received (spinal stabilization, steroids, etc.)
- Description of onset and progression of symptoms if atraumatic
- Any medical tests, labs, procedures, or films relating to the injury (specifically neuroimaging tests such as magnetic resonance imaging [MRI] that have been correlated with prognosis)
- Any complications or comorbidities apparent during hospital course
- Medications for current or any other condition

Medical History

- All other pertinent medical information, including hospitalizations or procedures
- Birth history if applicable to mechanism or onset of injury

Developmental History

- Developmental history, including prior level of function
- Any previously owned adaptive equipment

Social History

- Cultural beliefs and behaviors
- Primary caregivers, family, and community resources
- Learning style of client and caregivers
- Current living situation, including living environment, community characteristics, and projected discharge destination
- Social interactions, activities, and support systems
- Current and prior school situation (services received, individualized education plans)
- Leisure activities/sports/dreams for the future

Systems Review

Guided by the history and initial information, the PT proceeds to examine the patient system by system.

Cardiovascular/Pulmonary

Vital signs such as blood pressure, heart rate, and respiratory rate are taken before, during, and after activity. Evaluating tolerance for the upright position can sometimes be a slow process as patients with SCI are at risk for orthostatic hypotension. Compression stockings and abdominal binders are helpful to aid in vascular support. Patients with a lesion above T-6 are also at risk for autonomic dysreflexia (Display 8.1).

Patients with neuromuscular weakness also have decreased respiratory efficiency. Quality of cough, breathing pattern, and chest and diaphragmatic excursion measurements should be taken. Access to medical tests such as vital capacity and forced expiratory volume are also helpful. For patients on ventilators, parameter settings should be noted. Collaboration with medical, nursing, and respiratory staff can help in assessing respiratory potential. These measurements may need to be repeated, especially if the child is weaning ventilatory support. In some practice settings,

---

DISPLAY 8.1 Autonomic Dysreflexia

Autonomic dysreflexia is the body's response to lack of sympathetic input during noxious stimuli. The noxious stimulus may include kinked catheter tubing, constipation, muscle spasm, ingrown toenail, or even ROM exercises. Symptoms vary but most often include elevated blood pressure, diaphoresis, headache, and bradycardia and require immediate attention. Treatment requires removal of the noxious stimulus, positioning to decrease blood pressure, and pharmacologic intervention if needed. If left untreated, autonomic dysreflexia may progress to a life-threatening situation.

DISPLAY 8.2 Nutrition

It is important for any person with a new SCI to have a full nutritional workup in order to ensure that caloric intake is meeting new energy demands and that there is a healthy balance between intake and output. Patients with SCI are at risk for lowered immunity and decreased nutritional status.[52] Unfortunately, both of these issues can delay wound healing, so it is important for the PT to discuss the nutritional status with the child's physician and nutritionist if there is any disruption in skin integrity. The PT may also refer a child with an SCI to a nutritionist at any point along the continuum of care to promote a healthy and balanced diet that is individualized for that child's unique needs.

PTs have an active role in airway clearance interventions. Therefore, a complete examination of the pulmonary system is necessary.

Integumentary

The skin of a child with an SCI must be fully assessed. This includes color, integrity, bruising, and the presence of any scar formation. Neurovascular signs such as pulses, skin temperature, and edema should also be assessed regularly. Decubitus ulcers can be a chronic problem for children with SCI, and vigilant pressure relief and proper skin care are the only way to prevent this problem. Education regarding position changes and pressure relief should begin during the initial examination (Displays 8.2 through 8.4).

Musculoskeletal System

Range of motion (ROM), tone, strength, symmetry, and posture are assessed. In the acute phase, tone may initially be flaccid and ROM full, but special precautions are required

---

DISPLAY 8.3 Latex Allergy

Patients with significantly increased exposure to latex products, such as children with myelomeningocele or SCI, can develop an allergy to latex. To decrease their exposure to latex, products that are latex free should be used whenever possible. Owing to the need for catheterization supplies and gloves, over the course of a lifetime, many institutions now advocate a "latex-free" environment in which health care workers and other caregivers utilize latex alternatives to provide care. Many products commonly found in both the home and hospital environment contain latex and have the potential to cause a reaction in the client. Care must be taken to ensure that the client does not encounter latex if he or she already has an allergy to it or to prevent one from occurring. Products that contain latex include Thera-Band, Ace wraps, catheters, many toys, balloons, and even Band-Aids. Many companies offer a latex-free substitute for therapeutic modalities.

to prevent loss of flexibility. Spasticity can begin quickly and interfere with the child's flexibility goals. ROM assessment should be performed with overall diagnosis and prognosis in mind. For example, shortening of certain structures (long finger flexors, low back extensors) may be desirable in some situations. Similarly, overlengthening of certain muscle groups such as the hamstrings and shoulder internal rotators may be desirable depending on the expected functional outcomes.

Spasticity assessment is most widely performed using the modified Ashworth scale while noting any clonus or spasms (Displays 8.4 and 8.5).[13] Other assessment tools include the visual analog scale, the Wartenberg pendulum test, and the Penn Spasm Frequency Scale. Surface electromyography and isokinetic dynamometry are also used to assess spasticity in spinal cord–injured patients.[13] It is important to remember that spasticity may vary throughout the day or with different activities and may even be useful in some functional situations. For example, someone with significant lower extremity weakness may rely on his or her spasticity for stability in weight bearing for transfers or ambulation. Some patients can even learn to trigger a spasm in order to help their lower extremity move in a certain way. Conversely, excessive spasticity can lead to problems with ROM, positioning, or comfort. For incomplete SCIs and

those experiencing neurologic recovery, spasticity can mask underlying neuromuscular recovery; however, it may be necessary for functional activities. A thorough knowledge of the child's spasticity and movement patterns will assist the therapist in understanding the child's process of recovery. It will also allow the therapist to make valuable contributions to the medical team. Medical management often requires a balance between decreasing and increasing spasticity based on the child's goals and functional needs. Therapists should have a thorough understanding of the medical management of spasticity in order to provide educated recommendations to the physician.

For strength assessment in the pediatric population, performing manual muscle testing can provide valuable information if the child is able to fully participate in the examination. Games such as "Simon Says" can be useful in helping the child understand the task. For the very young or those with cognitive impairments, strength testing can be performed with observation, noting whether the child has the ability to move against gravity or against any resistance (i.e., reaching for a toy in different planes of movement or lifting/kicking against something with force). In the case of SCI, the therapist should note both gross and individual muscle strength and prevent substitution by the patient. It is important for the PT to assess motor abilities of all spinal levels as this information will have significant impact for the physical therapy diagnosis and prognosis. Strength assessment should be performed on a regular basis in the early phases of recovery as the period of spinal shock can produce different results.

Sensory examination includes a thorough screen of all sensory spinal tracts and further individualized testing when warranted. Light touch, temperature, pinprick, and proprioception are important indicators of spinal function. The clinician can further pinpoint where the breakdown occurs using a dermatomal chart indicating spinal level.

The presence or absence of any sensory or motor function in the lowest sacral segment is an indication of prognosis, and should not be overlooked in the examination process. Often this information is obtained by the examining physician; however, in some practice settings, a PT may also perform this assessment.

Position, posture, and alignment must be assessed in children with SCI. Children with muscular weakness and imbalances are at risk for developing spinal deformities and scoliosis. Proper positioning is a crucial component to maintaining proper alignment. Radiographic films of the bones and joints can assist the therapist in determining the child's skeletal alignment (Display 8.6).

Neuromuscular System

In the neuromuscular system, the PT examines all functional movements. Movements can be isolated or synergistic during functional activity. Functional movements are related to available ROM, tone, and strength. While the therapist

Patients with upper motor neuron lesions such as SCI are at risk for the development of heterotopic ossification (HO). Primary areas affected are large joints such as the hip, shoulder, knee, and elbow. Patients are most at risk during the first 1 to 4 months after injury. There is no acute treatment for the pediatric population since medications that are used for the prevention of HO in adults have not been approved for use with the pediatric population. HO can be surgically excised, but only after the abnormal bone formation is completely mature, usually 1 to 2 years after onset. Current best practice advocates the use of gentle ROM to affected joints and avoiding immobilization or aggressive ROM.[18,19] The entire team should be vigilant in screening for the development of HO since it can be a major setback for the child.

may strive to assist the client to achieve the most "normal" movement pattern, it may be more important to the client to be able to perform the activity in any way possible. Neuromuscular assessment also includes gross coordinated movements, including functional mobility, transfers, locomotion, balance, and coordination. In the acute stages of a new SCI, functional movement may be limited to bed mobility and sitting balance on the edge of the bed. When the injury is no longer acute or during reexamination, the client may be able to withstand more rigorous examination. For those with SCI, this portion of the examination also includes wheelchair mobility and skills. In these cases, the wheelchair is considered as an extension of the person's body.

The PT also examines the client's communication, affect, cognition, language, and learning style. This includes the client's level of consciousness; orientation to person, place, and time; ability to make his or her needs known; expected emotional and behavioral responses; and learning preferences (for both the child and the caregiver). If the child has sustained either a mild or more severe traumatic brain injury as a result of the accident, the PT should also consider examination techniques outlined in Chapter 7 (Display 8.7). A knowledge of normal cognitive development will assist the therapist in determining what may be a new cognitive deficit versus a deficit that was present prior to the onset of the SCI.

Because of the high velocity and trauma often associated with SCI, there is an increased risk of associated traumatic brain injury, which may be as high as 24% to 59%.[22] Consequently, cognition should always be screened, and neuropsychological testing may be indicated with any person who has sustained an SCI in order to rule out any mild deficits.

Tests and Measures

The PT has a wide variety of tests and measures to further characterize and quantify the information gathered during the examination. These include, but are not limited to:

- Aerobic capacity and endurance
- Anthropometric characteristics
- Assistive and adaptive devices
- Arousal, attention, and cognition
- Circulation
- Cranial and peripheral nerve integrity
- Environmental, home, and work (job/school/play) barriers
- Ergonomics and body mechanics
- Gait, locomotion, and balance
- Integumentary integrity
- Joint integrity and mobility
- Motor function (motor control and motor learning)
- Muscle performance (including strength, power, and endurance)
- Neuromotor development and sensory integration
- Orthotic, protective, and supportive devices
- Posture
- ROM (including muscle length)
- Reflex integrity
- Self-care and home management (including activities of daily living [ADLs] and instrumental ADLs [IADLs])
- Sensory integrity
- Ventilation and respiration
- Work (job/school/play), community, and leisure integration or reintegration (including IADLs)

▶ Evaluation, diagnosis, and prognosis

During the evaluation process, the PT synthesizes the information that was discovered during the history, systems review, and tests and measures. He or she then formulates a physical therapy diagnosis and prognosis. In the case of SCI, the type and severity of the injury is central to establishing a prognosis and a plan of care.

Standards for neurologic and functional classification of SCI were identified by the American Spinal Injury Association (ASIA) in 1982.[14] This multidisciplinary group of experts established common terminology and a standard classification system for the medical field. It was last revised in 2011 and is now entitled "American Spinal Injury Association: International Standards for Neurologic Classification of Spinal Cord Injury (ISNCSCI)."[15] This document serves to standardize the examination of myotomes and dermatomes among clinicians. Using the information from the examination and the guidelines set forth on the ISNCSCI form, the clinician can determine a sensory and a motor diagnostic level for both the right and left sides of the body. Furthermore, this classification scheme states whether the injury is complete or incomplete. The clinician

A = Complete. No sensory or motor function is preserved in sacral segments S-4 to S-5.

B = Incomplete. Sensory but not motor function is preserved below the neurologic level and extends through the sacral segments S-4 to S-5.

C = Incomplete. Motor function is preserved below the neurologic level, and the majority of key muscles below the neurologic level have a muscle grade <3.

D = Incomplete. Motor function is preserved below the neurologic level, and the majority of key muscles below the neurologic level have a muscle grade ≥3.

can then assign an ASIA level of impairment (Display 8.8) for classification. Some spinal cord lesions present as a clinical syndrome, as described in Display 8.9, and this terminology can also be used universally when discussing the client's presentation with other health care professionals. Although the ASIA has not yet published a specific worksheet for children and youth, current study supports the use of the tool in children older than 6 years who can follow the directions for pinprick and light touch when applied to their cheek.[16,17]

Physical therapy diagnoses for this population may include the following: decreased strength, decreased ROM, decreased endurance, decreased airway clearance and respiratory efficiency, decreased functional mobility, and decreased independence in the home, school, or community due to SCI.

After establishing a physical therapy diagnosis, the clinician can prognosticate the optimal level of function the child may achieve. The amount and intensity of physical therapy services required to achieve that level of function can be

Central cord syndrome: presents with greater weakness in the upper extremities than the lower extremities and presents with sacral sparing
Brown–Sequard syndrome: presents with ipsilateral proprioceptive and motor loss and contralateral loss of pinprick and temperature
Anterior cord syndrome: presents with variable loss of motor function and sensation to pinprick and temperature and has sparing of proprioception
Conus medullaris syndrome: may present with areflexic bladder, bowel, and lower extremities or may show preserved bulbocavernosus and micturition reflexes
Cauda equina syndrome: presents with areflexic bladder, bowel, and lower extremities

discussed as well as future episodes of care that may be needed over the course of the child's lifetime. Formulating a physical therapy prognosis incorporates information from the examination and should be based on evidence from current scientific literature. The PT is also guided by the medical prognosis in developing goals that the child may be able to achieve. Prognoses for someone with a complete injury and someone with an incomplete injury can be very different based on neurologic potential for recovery. Studies suggest that some individuals with SCI may skip to the next level on the ASIA Impairment Scale during the period of neurologic recovery.[18-20] Ongoing reassessment of the patient using the ASIA Impairment Scale is critical not only to understand the patient's current status and potential ability, but also to monitor for possible change. The most significant recovery is expected in the first year after injury, but some patients show improvement for up to 5 years.[21]

Although the principles of examination, evaluation, and diagnosis are similar to those of clients with traumatic injuries, atraumatic SCIs can be more unpredictable in their outcomes. Transverse myelitis can have varying functional outcomes. Approximately 30% of those afflicted have full recovery, 30% have partial recovery, and another 30% have little to no recovery.[22] There are some medical factors that help prognosticate recovery, including speed of onset, amount of paralysis, and speed of recovery in the first month, but these are never certain, as the Case Study at the end of this chapter will illustrate. Early treatment with corticosteroids is considered the first-line treatment and has been shown in case studies and research with patients with MS to improve the functional outcome.[23] Published research also demonstrates that a high level of interleukin-6 in the cerebrospinal fluid (CSF) correlates with a poor functional outcome.[10,14] The potential for a large amount of neurologic recovery can alter the entire focus of physical therapy from goals of learning to compensate with the remaining intact musculature to a goal for recovering lost function. Atraumatic SCI caused by a tumor may present with similar clinical symptoms to a traumatic SCI, but cancer treatment such as radiation and chemotherapy can have profound effects on the child's functioning, physical therapy treatment, and the family as a whole. This can greatly impact the child's prognosis.

When considering the child's prognosis, the clinician should keep in mind both the child's potential for neurologic recovery and the functional outcomes that can be realistically achieved. The accepted outcome measures used for adults with SCI include the Modified Barthel Index (MBI), the Functional Independence Measure (FIM), the Quadriplegic Index of Function (QIF), and the Spinal Cord Independence Measure (SCIM).[24] These outcome measures have not been standardized in the pediatric population. Although no standard functional outcome measure for pediatric clients with traumatic or atraumatic SCI has been documented, the clinician can identify anticipated functional outcomes on the basis of both the adult SCI literature and myelodysplasia

TABLE 8.1	Functional Expectations by Level of Involvement		
Level of Injury	**Mobility**	**Transfers**	**Activities of Daily Living**
C-1–C-4	• Sipping or blowing to independently control a power wheelchair, power-tilt mechanism, and environmental controls	• Dependent for all transfers	• Dependent for dressing, bathing, and bowel and bladder management
C-5: addition of biceps and deltoids	• Can propel a manual wheelchair with hand rims for short distances on level surfaces • Power wheelchair for longer distances	• Able to assist with transfers and bed mobility	• Able to assist with feeding, grooming with adaptive equipment and setup • Dependent for dressing and bathing
C-6: addition of pectorals	• Able to independently use manual wheelchair with projections on the hand rims	• Independent with self-care with equipment • Independent with upper extremity dressing, assists with lower extremity • Independent with bowel program, needs assistance with bladder program • Can drive with a specially adapted van	• Assists with sliding board transfers
C-7–T-1: addition of triceps	• Able to independently propel a manual wheelchair on level surfaces	• Independent with adaptive equipment • Can drive a car with hand controls	• Independent transfers with or without sliding board
T-4–T-6: addition of upper abdominal	• Can ambulate with RGOs for short distances with a walker	• Independent for grooming, bowel and bladder, dressing and bathing	• Independent transfers with or without sliding board
T-9–T-12: addition of lower abdominals	• Household ambulation with RGOs or HKAFOs and assistive device	• Independent for grooming, bowel and bladder, dressing and bathing	• Independent transfers with or without sliding board
L-2–L-4: addition of gracilis, iliopsoas, and quadratus lumborum	• Functional ambulation with KAFOs with crutches	• Independent for grooming, bowel and bladder, dressing and bathing	• Independent transfers with or without sliding board
L-4–L-5: addition of hamstrings, quadriceps, and anterior tibialis	• Able to ambulate with AFOs with or without assistive device	• Independent for grooming, bowel and bladder, dressing and bathing	• Independent transfers with or without sliding board

AFO, ankle–foot orthosis; HKAFO, hip–knee–ankle–foot orthosis; KAFO, knee–ankle–foot orthosis; RGO, reciprocating gait orthosis.

literature. A discussion of general functional expectations by level of involvement is discussed in Table 8.1.[16]

Understanding the child's prognosis for functional outcomes leads the clinician to develop a plan of care that includes specific interventions and the frequency, intensity, and duration of those interventions. It also incorporates anticipated goals, expected outcomes, and discharge plans. When working in an interdisciplinary model, the plan of care may involve other health care professionals in both establishing interdisciplinary goals and providing the intervention to achieve them. For example, a child working on transfers in the hospital should have the opportunity to practice these transfers in a variety of environments and situations that incorporate the family, nurses, and other therapists and to help simulate the situations the child will encounter after discharge.

Standardized outcome measures performed prior to and after physical therapy intervention are useful in measuring the progress the child has made over the course of an episode of care. Some outcome measures used in pediatrics include the WeeFIM (Functional Independence Measure),

Pediatric Evaluation of Disability Inventory (PEDI), and Gross Motor Function Measure (GMFM).[25] Creativity may sometimes be useful in modifying existing outcome measures for a patient with paralysis. For example, the 9-minute walk/run can be modified into a 9-minute "wheelchair run" to measure endurance. The PT should be familiar with all available outcome measures in order to choose the most appropriate one for the client. Standardized outcome measures can help the therapist pinpoint weaknesses as well as focus and modify the plan of care.

▶ Intervention

Medical Intervention

Surgery

MUSCLE TRANSFERS Recent advances in surgical techniques have allowed for the transfer of muscle function from one group to another. If there is sufficient remaining muscle strength in two or more muscle groups that work together to perform a movement, one of the muscles can be transferred biomechanically to perform another movement. There is little or no adverse effect on the original motion. Most commonly, elbow extension is achieved by transferring the posterior deltoid to the triceps. There are, however, promising results with a biceps-to-triceps transfer for elbow extension to achieve overhead function.[26] Similarly, wrist extension is achieved by transferring the brachioradialis to the extensor carpi radialis. Active grasp is achieved by transferring the brachioradialis and using it as a thumb flexor.[27]

Processes such as tenodesis, arthrodesis, tendon lengthenings, rerouting, releases, and tendon transfers have the capacity to restore function to persons with tetraplegia. All these surgeries require not only careful surgical technique, but also comprehensive postoperative physical and occupational therapy. There is an abundance of literature on these procedures in the adult population. Although there are fewer studies performed on children, the results are similar.[27]

SPASTICITY Spasticity is the clinical manifestation that accompanies upper motor neuron disease. A muscle displays an increased resistance to passive motion that results from the hyperactivity of the spinal and brainstem reflexes. In SCI, acutely, there is usually flaccidity, then flexor spasticity presents, and then finally extensor spasticity. Options for this population are similar to those with central nervous system dysfunction. Oral baclofen, intrathecal baclofen, botulinum toxin, and neurologic and orthopedic surgery are options when spasticity interferes with daily function.

The medical management of spasticity with movement can be conservative and include removing the noxious stimuli, stretching, positioning, using orthotics, biofeedback, and electric stimulation. All these, however, have short-term effects. When that is not enough, there are other agents that have been shown to reduce muscle spasticity.[28] Pharmacologically, baclofen acts as a γ-aminobutyric acid (GABA) analog at the site of the spinal cord. A common side effect, however, is that baclofen can cause drowsiness, fatigue, and weakness.[28] Baclofen administered intrathecally acts directly on the spinal cord with less risk of drowsiness and weakness than oral baclofen. There is risk of infection with the pump insertion.[28] Dantrolene sodium acts on the muscle to inhibit the release of calcium from the sarcoplasmic reticulum. This medication carries the same effects of drowsiness and fatigue and can damage liver function. Clonidine via the oral route or patch acts centrally as an α-agonist. Clonidine can lead to hypotension; however, side effects are limited to dry mouth and drowsiness. Diazepam (Valium) acts on the limbic system. Adverse reactions can include drowsiness and fatigue, and its use can lead to drug dependency.[28]

Chemical nerve blocks work at the motor point. Lidocaine is a short-acting agent. Phenol can last up to 6 months. Botulinum toxin is so specific that it goes straight to the muscle.[28]

PAIN The adult literature has shown that patients with SCI experience many different complaints of pain.[28–30] Studies of chronic pain reported by children are few, but do report the same results. They report that pain associated with pediatric-onset SCI is common. Reports of nociceptive pain were greater than neuropathic pain.[31] Data suggest that although it is common, chronic pain in childhood SCI has a significantly smaller impact on daily activities than that reported in the literature for adult-onset SCI.[31]

Studies have looked at multiple interventions for pain, including medications, physical therapy, psychotherapy, and spinal cord stimulators. There is consistency in the reports of pain in patients with SCI; the reports of pain continue through the postacute stage, with 60% of patients with an SCI reporting pain at 6 and 12 months postinjury.[28] The International Association for the Study of Pain has proposed a scheme for characterizing SCI. It classifies pain into two types: neuropathic and nociceptive. Nociceptive pain is musculoskeletal and visceral. Neuropathic pain is classified as above the level, at the level, or below the level of injury. Nociceptive pain is characterized by dull, aching, movement-related pain that is eased by rest and responds to opioids. Neuropathic pain is usually described as sharp, shooting, burning, and electrical with abnormal sensory responsiveness (hyperesthesia or hyperalgesia). Antidepressants and anticonvulsants are usually used for SCI; however, neither is particularly effective for SCI pain. Recent reports have shown promise for opioids and α-adrenergic antagonists, as well as baclofen, a GABA-b agonist, when there is spasticity interfering with function.[28]

Sodium channel blockers such as lidocaine and tetracaine hydrochloride have shown decreases in allodynia (pain from a stimulus that is not usually painful). Opioids have been demonstrated to help neuropathic pain as well as nociceptive pain. Intrathecal clonidine in combination with morphine had an analgesic effect in patients with SCI.[28]

SURGICAL PROCEDURES Surgical procedures such as cordectomy, cordotomy, and myelotomy are most effective for spontaneous lancinating or shooting pain. They are not effective for burning or aching pain. Complications associated with these procedures include contralateral pain, bowel and bladder dysfunction, loss of sexual function, and development of spasms.[28]

SPINAL CORD STIMULATORS Spinal cord stimulators were first used in the 1970s to manage severe pain such as reflex sympathetic dystrophy (RSD). Spinal cord stimulators inhibit spinal transmission of pain through electrical stimulation via the gate control theory. One to two leads are placed in the epidural space of the spinal cord, and a small electric current is sent through the electrodes. A receiver or battery pack is placed under the skin in the abdomen.[32] Results have been mixed; some subjects have reported decreased pain. It has been shown to be most effective in patients with incomplete pain or postcordotomy pain,[28] and less effective in patients with complete injury. Complications may include infections, allergic reaction, electrode migration, CSF leak, and bleeding. Deep brain stimulation was also used in the 1970s and 1980s; however, it has not been used recently because the Food and Drug Administration (FDA) has not approved it for any pain indications.[28]

Therapeutic and Functional Interventions

When working with a child or adolescent with an SCI, physical therapy interventions are similar to those used with adults with SCI, but the approach may be different.

The PT provides interventions that consist of a variety of procedures and techniques that are individualized for each client. These will produce changes in the client's overall function and help make progress toward the identified goals. The therapist should always be reassessing the patient's response to interventions and modifying them as needed. There are some differences when working with children with SCIs, which will be highlighted here. Interventions will be discussed as generalizations, though some specifics to the type and level of SCI will also be mentioned.

Therapeutic Exercise

Therapeutic exercise should include ROM for specific areas of limitations. Special attention should be given to the areas where tone is abnormal. Hamstrings, heel cords, and adductors often develop contractures early. In some cases, however, contractures are necessary to improve function. As mentioned previously, examples of this include maintaining a shortening of the long finger flexors to achieve finger flexion when the wrist is extended (Fig. 8.1). Some children can use this active tenodesis for a functional grip. There are other situations where excessive ROM is necessary. For example, having increased hamstring flexibility will allow a patient with an SCI to be able to perform lower extremity dressing independently.

The implementation of therapeutic exercise in children is similar to that with other populations, with a few

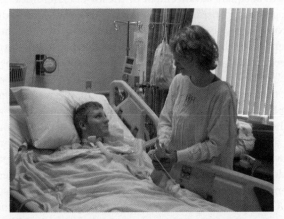

FIGURE 8.1. Physical therapy begins in the intensive care unit with positioning, passive and active range of motion, and family education.

exceptions. Some muscle groups may not be able to be strengthened or improved owing to complete denervation. In contrast, some muscle groups may require greater than normal strength to compensate for other muscle groups that are no longer functioning. When considering pediatric clients, age-appropriate interventions will likely provide greater success. For example, it is unlikely that a 4-year-old will perform biceps curls with a free weight as instructed; however, he or she may engage in pulling against resistance in a tug-of-war activity. Therapeutic exercises can often be incorporated into play, but it is imperative to remain focused on the goals being worked toward. In other situations, a child may perform traditional sets of strengthening exercises but may need to be rewarded with a fun and equally therapeutic play activity such as shooting basketballs with wrist cuff weights. Other therapeutic interventions to provide include:

- Aerobic and endurance conditioning or reconditioning
- Balance, coordination, and agility training
- Body mechanics and postural stabilization
- Flexibility exercises
- Gait and locomotion training
- Relaxation
- Strength, power, and endurance training for head, neck, limb, pelvic-floor, trunk, and ventilatory muscles[33,34]

Therapeutic exercises as described above can be performed in a land or aquatic environment. Aquatic therapy can be very useful as the buoyancy of the water can assist in neuromuscular reeducation in clients with neurologic disorders who have several muscle groups with $\frac{3}{5}$ or less strength.[35] An aquatic environment can also be fun for children, and they often perform more work while having more fun.

Functional Training in Self-Care and Home Management (Including Activities of Daily Living and Instrumental Activities of Daily Living)

Devices and adaptive equipment for children with SCI include wheelchairs, standers, braces, and ADL devices. The PT may provide the following types of interventions:

- ADL training
- Devices and equipment use training
- Functional training programs
- IADL training
- Injury prevention or reduction

For an adult, IADLs include caring for dependents, home maintenance, household chores, shopping, and yard work. For children, IADLs include participation in school and play activities. Play is an integral part of a child's life and is necessary for development and maturation. Training a child to utilize new movement patterns in playing an age-appropriate game or sport is very important in a child's life. Other IADLs may include performing basic household chores depending on family desire and eventually prevocational and vocational

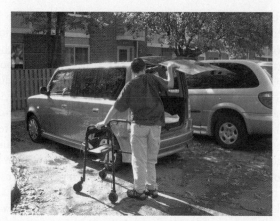

FIGURE 8.2. Adolescents can attend special automobile driving classes for people with disabilities and learn what modifications they may need to safely drive a vehicle.

training. ADL or IADL training might include collaboration with an occupational therapist.

Adaptations for driving make it possible for some people with SCI to operate a vehicle. Adolescents who are candidates for driving should be referred to rehab centers for driving assessment and training (Fig. 8.2).

MOBILITY A wheelchair may be the primary means of locomotion for a child with an SCI. Children as young as 18 to 24 months can independently propel a wheelchair.[36] Evaluation for the appropriate wheelchair should take place as part of a team assessment. There are many options to allow children to function independently in a wheelchair. Reclining-back wheelchairs can be used to accommodate braces when sitting at a right angle is difficult. Seating principles such as distribution of weight, propulsion, and environmental controls should be considered with children with SCI (Fig. 8.3).

Braces and Ambulation

RECIPROCATING GAIT ORTHOSES VERSUS HIP–KNEE– ANKLE–FOOT ORTHOSES The reciprocating gait orthosis (RGO) is a bracing system composed of a bilateral hip, knee, and ankle orthosis with the right and left sides connected by a cable. More recently, a version has been designed to be cableless (isocentric RGO [IRGO]).[37] The cableless connection allows one side of the orthosis to flex when the other extends. The user biomechanically extends one side by weight shifting onto one side while extending his or her trunk. This unweighting mechanism allows the opposite side to flex. Repeating this action on the contralateral side simulates the gait pattern. Some IRGO models allow hip abduction to occur for the purpose of self-catheterization. Physical therapy and rehabilitation training for RGOs involves assessment for appropriateness.[38]

There are many things to consider when recommending RGOs. In order to use RGOs, patients should have lower limb weakness with the inability to control the knees and

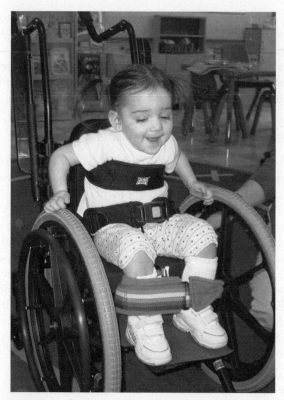

FIGURE 8.3. Beginning wheelchair mobility training as early as possible allows the child to experience a sense of freedom and explore his or her environment for learning opportunities.

hips. Additionally, children need to have sufficient upper extremity strength for weight bearing and advancing an assistive device. Patients must be free of lower extremity contractures and be able to sit comfortably with hips and knees flexed to at least 90 degrees. Children should also be cognitively able to follow directions and be motivated to do activities that will allow them to use the RGO system. Prior to the RGO fitting, special attention should be paid to upper extremity strengthening and stabilization activities, especially in the upright position. With RGOs, weight shifting is key to adequate advancement of the lower extremities. This weight shift consists of a diagonal weight shift, push-down through upper extremities, and unweighting of the contralateral side while extending the trunk. No active hip flexion is required to use RGOs. Training for RGO use begins in the parallel bars. Mirrors can help provide visual feedback for this motion. Hands-on facilitation of the weight shifting by the PT can provide mechanical and tactile feedback to help the child learn the movement. The therapist should be aware of any substitutions, particularly lateral trunk movement and the urge to pull the limbs through using the abdominals. This is usually very typical for those patients who have learned a swing-through pattern prior to using RGOs or for those who have sustained spinal cord pathology after they were independently ambulating. In addition to ambulation, other functional skills must be learned such as donning and doffing the braces, coming to and from

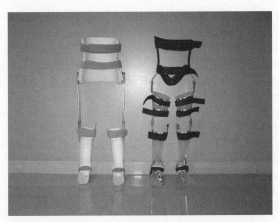

FIGURE 8.4. Braces. **(A-Left)** Reciprocating gait orthoses. **(B-Right)** Hip–knee–ankle–foot orthoses.

standing to sitting, and negotiating all levels and uneven surfaces, elevations, and inclines.

Learning to ambulate with RGOs requires intensive rehabilitation. Therapy should occur daily until independent ambulation is achieved. At that time, the child should be given the opportunity to practice the ambulation skills within the context of everyday activities. It is important to establish realistic goals with the patient, family, therapists, orthotist, physician, and other members of the health care team (Figs. 8.4 and 8.5, Display 8.10).

There is evidence to support the decision-making process when determining the appropriate brace system. When

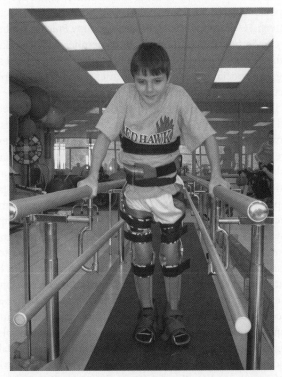

FIGURE 8.5. Ambulation training requires excellent upper body strength and endurance and begins in the parallel bars until the child is ready to progress to an assistive device.

DISPLAY

8.10 **To Walk or Not to Walk, and Family-Centered Care**

One of the first questions a child or caregiver will ask when first faced with a SCI is, "Will I/he/she ever walk again?" Although many PTs will defer to the physician on this difficult topic, the therapist inevitably will discuss walking at some point with the client and should be well prepared to answer the question before it is asked. For some clients with SCI, walking *is* a possibility. This "walking" may require long leg bracing, implantable electric stimulation, and/or assistive devices; however, it may not be the type of walking the child is expecting. The PT should always be honest in what current best practice can achieve, and the child and family can then make an informed decision about whether walking is a goal they want to pursue. Walking as exercise, even with bracing and assistive devices, has benefits that are not only physical but emotional.[68] Walking can also improve the quality of life for children as they can be on an eye-to-eye level with their peers. Many studies have been performed looking at energy expenditure with ambulation and wheelchair use in the myelodysplasia population, but little research has been done on the pediatric SCI population. Generally, as a child grows and becomes larger, it becomes increasingly difficult to keep up with peers while ambulating. Often, the child ends up choosing a wheelchair as his or her primary means of mobility. The most important concept is that the child is choosing that means of mobility for him- or herself.

During the process of rehabilitation, it is the PT's responsibility to help the client deal with his or her body in its current condition, and to help the child achieve the highest level of independence possible. Striving for independence also requires reintegration back into the community and bridging the client with others in the community. One of the most valuable things a therapist can give his or her client is to put him or her in a situation that challenges him or her to think and solve problems. The therapist can show the patient all the things that he or she can do—the way he or she is now—and provide support as the patient goes through the emotions of losing the way he or she used to be.

A therapist can also provide hope for the future. For a child with an incomplete or atraumatic injury, the period of recovery can last up to 5 years. Being realistic while allowing some hope can help focus and motivate the patient and sustain him or her through this difficult period. The child should come to understand that even though something is not probable does not always mean it is not possible. A child with a complete injury should learn all of the skills necessary as though he or she is going to be a primary wheelchair user. The opportunity for ambulation with an assistive device should be provided if the patient and family desire and if there is potential. To walk or not to walk is not an easy question. It requires careful consideration of the child's diagnosis and prognosis, the known functional potentials based on the literature, and input from the child and family. Being realistic while hopeful and working with the child and family on establishing goals together is the essence of family-centered care.

ambulation was compared between RGOs and hip–knee–ankle–foot orthoses (HKAFOs) for thoracic-level injury, the oxygen cost for ambulating with the HKAFOs was higher than for the RGOs. However, there was no significant difference in oxygen cost with a high lumbar–level injury. Additionally, velocity of ambulation was faster for RGOs than HKAFOs for thoracic-level patients.[39] Again, there was no difference in the high lumbar–level patients. In this study, seven out of eight patients preferred RGOs to HKAFOs.[39]

LOCOMOTOR TRAINING Locomotor training for patients with SCI has received significant attention and acceptance in the rehabilitation community in recent years. By utilizing the concept of activity-based plasticity and automaticity, locomotor training creates a stimulus for the spinal cord network below the level of the lesion to experience repeated sensory input with the goal of generating a learned response in spinal cord circuitry to take steps.[40–42] The Christopher and Dana Reeve Foundation NeuroRecovery Network (NRN)[43] has led the way for large multisite trials exploring the effects of locomotor training in persons with SCI, and the results thus far have been compelling.[43,44] By using repeated practice stepping on a treadmill with both body weight support and manual facilitation with progression to overground training, some persons with SCI have demonstrated significant changes in functional ability, including gait speed and balance.[42,44,45] The NRN offers continuing education for clinicians interested in learning the parameters and techniques of locomotor training utilized in the multisite trial.

FUNCTIONAL ELECTRIC STIMULATION For those children and adolescents with SCI resulting in C-4 tetraplegia, active functional upper extremity movement is limited to shoulder shrug. Assistive technology such as joysticks and head arrays assist these patients with communication and mobility. Options for self-care are limited for those with this level of injury. There are robotic devices, but these are expensive and cumbersome. Some patients who have retained shoulder retraction may be able to use mobile arm supports; however, these have shown little promise for those with cervical injury due to decreased control of the glenohumeral joint.[46] Functional electrical stimulation (FES) uses surface electrode stimulation to produce functional movement. Grasping, wrist flexion, extension, and elbow extension have been used with voice activation systems.[47] Intramuscular stimulation systems have also been used to achieve flexion and extension with sip-and-puff-control activators.[47] The literature also describes a system of using FES and stimulating hand grasp and release, elbow movement, and arm abduction by using proportionally controlled movement of the contralateral shoulder with glenohumeral joint stability achieved by a suspended sling.[47] Researchers at Shriners Hospital have shown that the combination of FES and surgical reconstruction provided active palmar and lateral grasp

and release in a laboratory setting. The study also showed that FES systems increased pinch force, improved the manipulation of objects, and typically increased the independence in six standard ADLs as compared with pre-FES hand function. Subjects also reported preferring the FES system for most of the ADLs tested.[46]

Patterns of home use for electric stimulation have described a persistent but sporadic pattern of FES use that was influenced by the patient's perception of standing as a separate but occasional activity performed for an increased sense of fitness and well-being.[48] Studies have shown that the FES system generally provides equal or greater independence in seven mobility activities as compared with long leg braces, provided faster sit-to-stand times, and was preferred over lower leg braces in a majority of cases.[48]

FES during cycling is also being explored as a therapeutic intervention for children with chronic SCI.[49] Preliminary results suggest that children with SCI who receive electrically stimulated exercise can experience changes in muscle strength and/or muscle hypertrophy, which could lead to various health benefits such as improved cardiovascular health and decreased risk of diabetes.[49] Other potential benefits from FES cycling may include a slower rate of bone mineral density loss, but more study is warranted.[50]

 ## Coordination, communication, and documentation

Coordination, communication, and documentation are very important when working with a child with an SCI. Practice Pattern 5H in the *Guide to Physical Therapy Practice* outlines specific important components to remember when working with children with an SCI. Specifically, the child's school setting and special education requirements should be emphasized when planning for discharge.

The PT plays an integral part in the health care team and may assist in coordinating care between disciplines or between care settings. One of the goals of family-centered care is to ensure a smooth transition for patients and families across professionals and institutions. Communication is critical to coordinating a child's care, and the PT often participates in case conferences, patient care rounds, and family meetings when in an interdisciplinary setting. The therapist may need to make referrals to other sources and communicate with other providers if practicing in an ambulatory or school setting. The PT must manage admission and discharge planning and coordinate this with other professionals when necessary. Discharge planning also includes the need to communicate a patient's care and needs among equipment suppliers and community resources. Discharge planning also requires the therapist and the team to use available funding wisely, and to assist the family in procuring charitable funds if needed. Planning for reentry into the school and the community requires ongoing open communication and

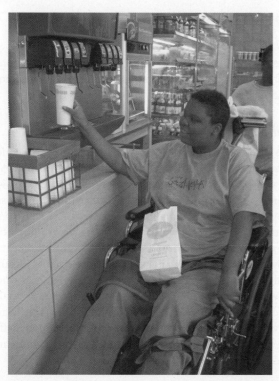

FIGURE 8.6. Therapists can focus their plan of care to assist their clients in returning to activities enjoyed prior to their injury.

coordination of care (Fig. 8.6). Documentation should follow the American Physical Therapy Association's Guidelines for Physical Therapy Documentation as described in the *Guide to Physical Therapist Practice.* It is imperative for the profession as a whole to have a consistent and reliable means of documenting patient status, changes in function, changes in interventions, elements of patient/client management, and outcomes of intervention.

Education

Caregiver instruction is as important when working with children as the patient education itself. Caregivers must be independent with all aspects of the home program recommendations so as to be able to facilitate their child's independence.

The primary focus for all physical therapy intervention should be patient and family education. Incorporating the family goals, the therapist establishes the plan of care and seeks to educate the child and family according to their learning style to help them make progress toward their goals, with the ultimate goal being discharge and reintegration into the community. Education begins in the earliest stages of rehabilitation and includes basic education about the client's diagnosis, the role of physical therapy, the prognosis, the plan of care, and what is needed for the family to help the child achieve his or her goals. Tasks such as performing ROM, bed and wheelchair positioning,

pressure relief maneuvers, and donning/doffing splints and equipment begin in the acute phases of treatment. Often, the family members are thankful to be able to start doing something for their child. It is important for the client and his or her family to receive education about skin integrity, autonomic dysreflexia, and stretching multiple times over the course of the admission since these are issues that the child will face over his or her lifetime. As the child advances through the phases of rehabilitation, he or she and his or her family change from being less active participants to becoming more active participants. Families must learn and demonstrate all aspects of patient care, and the child needs to learn how to teach others how to care for him or her. Caregivers of children with an SCI often need support to prevent "burnout" in these types of cases. The PT may be the health care professional referring the caregiver to a support group or mental health professional. Some children perform better in physical therapy when family members are present, but other children may not. In cases when caregivers are asked to step out of a session to enable the child to become a more active participant, the therapist will follow up with a brief education session and explain what the child was able to do and what they can practice together that night. Children often demonstrate increased motivation for their personal exercise programs if there is some sort of reward associated with it. Parents and pediatric psychologists can be extremely useful in helping to determine a plan to increase desirable behaviors and active participation by the child to help support his or her physical therapy goals.

Discharge Planning

Education of the child, the parent, and the child's teacher is critical prior to discharge planning. School visits by the team may be helpful. Medical issues must be stressed with the school, including neurogenic bladder, bowel and skin integrity, autonomic dysreflexia, orthostatic hypotension, and thermoregulation.

School Reentry

All children are entitled to a free and appropriate education.[51] Related services include transportation, developmental, corrective, and other supportive services to assist the child with a disability to benefit from special education. Children with SCI and mobility impairments may need extra time between classes or the use of a peer buddy system to help them manage their school challenges. Community resources include counseling, respite care, financial support, legal rights, and advocacy. There are also national, state, and local government agencies, some of which include the NSCIA, the National Parent Network on Disabilities, and the Family Resource Center on Disabilities.

▶ Illness prevention and wellness

Fitness

It is important for the child with an SCI to remain active (Fig. 8.7). Lack of activity can lead to a child becoming overweight, and children with an SCI are at increased risk for becoming overweight.[52] Aerobic and endurance conditioning should be performed to improve cardiorespiratory status. Patients with lower extremity paralysis can perform upper extremity activity with ergometers, arm bikes, and seated yoga and dance. There are also various wheelchair sports such as track and field, basketball, tennis, etc. Studies support that physical training has a positive influence on respiratory muscle strength and thoracic mobility, as well as quality of life, especially in subjects with quadriplegia.[53]

Circulation

Although deep vein thrombosis and pulmonary embolism are rare in children, in order to prevent circulatory problems, children with SCI are often placed on prophylactic blood anticoagulation agents. Precautions against injury should be maintained as these children may be at risk for increased bruising.

Dysreflexia/Hyperreflexia

For patients with an SCI above T-6, interventions to prevent and monitor for autonomic dysreflexia are extremely important. It is important to teach patients who are at risk for autonomic dysreflexia to identify its signs and symptoms as well as educate others about its treatment.

Studies show that there is a similar prevalence of dysreflexia in children with pediatric-onset SCI compared with adult-onset SCI. Dysreflexia is diagnosed less commonly in infants and preschool-aged children, and these two populations may present with more subtle signs and symptoms.[54]

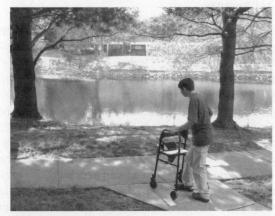

FIGURE 8.7. Teens with a spinal cord injury often have to problem-solve how to access things that they enjoy.

Growth Abnormalities

Hip Subluxation

There is a high incidence of hip subluxation/dislocation in children with SCI.[55] The rate is significantly higher among children with onset of injury before 10 years of age.

Scoliosis

The incidence of progressive paralytic scoliosis subsequent to acquired SCI has been reported to range from 46% to 98% in patients injured before their adolescent growth spurt.[56] Other studies have revealed that more severe scoliosis is related to a younger age at onset of paralysis. Age at injury has been shown to be a critical factor influencing the development of paralytic scoliosis. Some studies have shown that early bracing in patients whose curve is less than 20 degrees may decrease or prevent surgery. Patients whose curve ranges from 20 to 40 degrees should undergo a trial of bracing with the goal to delay surgery. In patients with large curves greater than 41 degrees, the use of bracing is ineffective and may actually lead to skin breakdown and hindrance of ADLs.[56]

Renal Disease

Good bowel and bladder management is important for prevention of renal disease.[57] Urogenic hygiene education is very important as well. There are many traditional options for handling bowel and bladder incontinence. There is reflex voiding and pressure voiding, where voids are timed and facilitated manually by increasing external pressure on the bladder. Catheterization is another means of emptying the bladder. There are indwelling catheters, but these are not without problems. External condom-type catheters and pads are also options.

Nurses, physicians, and occupational therapists work together to afford children and young adults as much independence as possible. Readiness for this includes having the necessary cognitive abilities. A child must also have the fine motor skills to be able to independently use the equipment for self-catheterization. The typical age a child begins to understand is around 2 to 3 years. Total independence is expected by 5 years of age whether or not the child has SCI.

There are also surgical procedures such as FES and urologic diversion surgeries. The overall goal for these is to avoid infection and to use antibiotics sparingly owing to the development of resistant organisms.

The goal for bowel continence is to control constipation, be convenient, and allow independence. Diets rich in fiber with adequate fluid and exercise are the best way to achieve these goals. Training the bowels is done by habitual voids (every other day). Digital stimulation and the use of suppositories and enemas can assist with the process. For bowel and bladder incontinence, it is important that orthoses do not interfere with the ability to self-catheterize. Some brace options allow for abduction to eliminate the need for donning and doffing the braces for catheterization.

Skin Integrity

The importance of skin inspection and pressure relief is increased in those with decreased sensation. Children can be taught to do independent pressure relief, which may include wheelchair tilts, sitting push-ups off the seat, or unweighting each side in the wheelchair.

Bone Density

Owing to decreased weight bearing, patients with an SCI are at risk for osteoporosis, especially thoracic- and lumbar-level–injured patients. Patients who have spinal cord neoplasm may also suffer from osteopenia owing to their chemotherapy regimes. Standing programs are the best way to maintain strong bones. Care should also be taken when performing ROM, positioning, and sometimes transfers and ambulation because of the potential for fractures due to osteopenia and osteoporosis. Additionally, there is some support for the improvement in bone density of children with and without disability with the use of lower extremity cycling with and without the use of electrical stimulation.[58]

Anticipatory Planning

This intervention involves planning for things that a child or adolescent may encounter in life. Often these are normal things that are encountered by children and adolescents even without an SCI.

Sex Education/Reproduction

Teenagers with SCI often have questions about their fertility, and they must be educated about this. Boys should learn about fertility options. Females should understand that they are still able to conceive and bear a child with the proper medical care and should understand the implications of potential pregnancy. Male fertility significantly decreases after SCI owing to the inability to ejaculate and poor sperm quality. There are options for those males who want to father a child, including intravaginal and intrauterine insemination and in vitro fertilization. In a female with an SCI, fertility is not affected.[59]

Higher Education/Job Training

When an adolescent begins to think about his or her life goals, there are many things to consider. Attending college in a manual chair may not be the best option for a patient, even if the upper extremities are not involved. There is an increased risk of upper extremity dysfunction and overuse syndromes with clients who have paraplegia in college and the workforce. Additionally, those entering the workforce need to understand their rights under the Americans with Disabilities Act.

▶ Outcomes

When determining what the appropriate adult outcomes are, one must determine what the important milestones are in the life of an adult. In this Anglo-American culture, these milestones for young adults include moving away from parents, achieving an education or training, obtaining a job, becoming financially independent, establishing significant relationships, and forming a family.[60]

Overall, it is a young adult's goal to keep pace with his or her peers and achieve these outcomes at the same rate. Other indicators are the ability to move around the community and integrate within it. Some argue that the measure of the means is the individual's satisfaction and quality of life.

One study that looked at outcomes of pediatric-onset SCI showed that adults with pediatric SCI are not equivalent to their peers.[61] When compared with the general population of the same age, those with SCI have equivalent education levels but demonstrate lower levels of community involvement, employment, income, independent living, and marriage. They also report lower life satisfaction and perceived physical health. Additionally, there are reports that despite similar education, there is difficulty for adults with SCI to obtain jobs. When they do obtain a job, they are not paid similarly to their peers.[61] This presents a challenge for health care providers to work toward transitioning their patients to adult roles.

There is also evidence that adults who were injured as children have better outcomes than adults who were injured as adults. The assumption is that those who were injured at a younger age are enabled to develop the career goals and educational preparation that facilitated their entry into the adult workforce. The most highly correlated items to a positive outcome were education, functional independence, and decreased number of medical complications.[60,61]

Vocational Outcomes

A long-term follow-up study of adults who sustained SCIs as children or adolescents showed that there was a high rate of unemployment as compared with the general population. Predictive factors of unemployment included education, community mobility, functional independence, and decreased medical complications. The variables that were positively associated with employment included community integration, independent driving, independent living, and higher income and life satisfaction. Although studies have identified the importance and positive impact of returning to work after sustaining an SCI, only 38% of individuals return to work after SCI.[62] This provides insight into areas to target during rehab.[60]

Refining the vocational rehabilitation process to include individual placement and follow-up and increasing the number of suitable jobs are ways to improve the employment outcomes.[63]

Psychological Outcomes

Patients with SCI often experience frustration, loss, and depression. This is especially important to remember with children with SCI because they are in the midst of developing their personality. Adolescent control, anger, fear, and loss of dignity all contribute to psychological implications for the child with an SCI.[64]

Life Satisfaction Outcomes

In a study of long-term outcomes and life satisfaction of adults who had pediatric SCIs, life satisfaction was associated with education, income satisfaction with employment, and social and recreational opportunities. Life satisfaction was inversely associated with some medical complications. Life satisfaction was not significantly associated with level of injury, age at injury, or duration of injury.[64]

 Future directions

Prevention

There is currently no cure for SCI, traumatic or atraumatic. Prevention and public awareness are clearly the best means to avoid the lifelong disability associated with SCI. Many accidents involving SCI can be avoided with knowledge and education. Along with car seat guidelines for infants and toddlers, the National Highway Traffic Safety Administration (NHTSA) recommends that children from ages 4 to 8 and under 57 inches tall be placed in a booster seat until they can be properly positioned with a passenger seat belt. The shoulder harness and lap belt together provide the safest protection for passengers and have decreased the incidence of SCI caused by lap belt alone. Other prevention measures include protective gear in sports and the prohibition of certain full-contact maneuvers such as "spearing" that carry more risk for SCI. Fall prevention for children can include window and stair guards as well as avoidance of wheeled baby walkers and trampolines. Violence prevention has taken on many forms in public education as well as legislation on both the community and federal levels. Education about prevention can be found extensively on the Internet and can be focused toward children, teenagers, parents, or teachers. Vehicle safety, water and diving safety, bike safety, playground and sports safety, and gun safety play a large role in avoiding injury (Display 8.11).

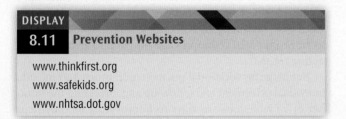

DISPLAY

8.11   Prevention Websites

www.thinkfirst.org

www.safekids.org

www.nhtsa.dot.gov

Research

Although there is no cure at the present time, there is hope for the future. There are a number of experimental therapies in human clinical trials that offer promise for improving outcomes in SCI. These include the administration of therapeutic agents such as minocycline, riluzole, and magnesium. Also, systemic hypothermia has gained public attention.[65] Similarly, improved knowledge about the neuropathology of transverse myelitis has given physicians clues about what medications to administer during certain points of the cascade of events. While this is not yet curative, it may help the final outcome. It is important to note that most of these clinical trials are with adults.

One of the most exciting areas of research is the use of stem cells for spinal cord regeneration in both traumatic and atraumatic injuries.[66] In motoneuron-injured adult rats, stem cells have been shown to not only survive in the mammalian spinal cord, but to also send axons through spinal cord white matter toward muscle targets.[67,68]

With the addition of certain factors and developmental cues, Deshpande et al. have shown these axons to not only reach their muscle targets, but also to form neuromuscular junctions and become physiologically active, allowing partial recovery from paralysis in adult rats. This groundbreaking research is the first time scientists have shown that stem cell axons can form neuromuscular junctions and synapses within a living body's overall neural circuitry.[69] Further research will continue to expand upon these principles with the ultimate goal to one day become a successful treatment for humans with paralysis.[66] The complexity of the original nervous system will unlikely be completely recreated, but rather the new-growth axons will find their way to muscle in a more primitive manner. Therefore, the plasticity and self-regulation of the nervous system will likely prune and select advantageous motor pathways that will allow for function. This selection process requires appropriate external stimulation such as instructed activities and exercise.[70] Physical therapy will play a key role as stem cell studies advance toward human trials and will be instrumental in this revolution of knowledge, treatment, and possibilities.

SUMMARY

This chapter has detailed the examination, intervention, evaluation, prognosis, and care planning for children who have acquired an SCI. Specific attention was given to functional implications in both evaluation and treatment. It is important to keep in mind that although there are common themes that emerge with all patients, each child and family is unique and individual. Keeping a family-centered approach to treatment will ensure the most optimal outcomes for each and every child.

CASE STUDIES

CASE STUDY 1 **Mark** is a 15-year-old boy who developed transverse myelitis of his cervical spine (C-2 to C-5) with full quadriplegia and ventilator dependency within the first 24 hours. Over the course of the first month of hospitalization, Mark made very little recovery and could only demonstrate trace to poor movement in the right wrist and right ankle. He was transferred to an inpatient respiratory rehabilitation unit with the goal of providing family education for a safe discharge home. Prior to his illness, he lived alone with his mother in a two-story condominium. His father recently died from cancer and there was no other family nearby to provide support. Mark was an honor student and wanted to become a pilot for the U.S. Air Force. His past medical history was significant for depression.

Examination

Mark initially presented with $0/5$ strength throughout except minimal right ankle dorsiflexion and minimal right wrist extension. Sensation was absent from the neck down, and he was dependent for all mobility. He was unable to tolerate sitting out of bed in a chair owing to anxiety and discomfort, and was unable to hold up his head. His tone was flaccid from the neck down and ROM was within normal limits throughout. He was dependent on a ventilator for all breathing, and he was unable to produce a cough.

Evaluation

Mark presented with the following problems: decreased strength, decreased mobility, decreased airway clearance, and respiratory insufficiency. In addition, he had immense needs for caregiver education. His initial goals for physical therapy included tolerating out of bed in a wheelchair for 8 hours to prepare for return to school, power mobility on level surfaces with supervision, and caregiver education regarding all aspects of dependent care.

Physical Therapy Diagnosis

Impaired strength and decreased functional mobility due to transverse myelitis.

Physical Therapy Prognosis

Good potential to achieve the above goals with caregiver assistance. Ambulation not likely due to medical prognostic factors of quick speed and severity of onset, slow rate of neurologic recovery, and complicating factors such as ventilator dependency. Mark did have good potential to use a power wheelchair with a head array or sip-and-puff mechanism in the community.

Physical Therapy Interventions and Reexamination

Interventions were initially aimed at maintaining ROM and skin integrity through positioning, pressure relief, and family education. Out-of-bed tolerance was increased with the use of a tilt-in-space wheelchair with elevating leg rests, an abdominal binder, and compression stockings to provide vascular support. Strengthening of available muscle groups was performed using traditional therapeutic exercises as well as biofeedback and neuromuscular electric stimulation (NMES).

As the weeks went on, Mark began to experience neurologic recovery, and it was crucial to reexamine and reevaluate and adjust goals and interventions as necessary. A time line is provided below to illustrate the highlights of his medical and physical therapy course in rehabilitation:

September: Onset of illness, full quadriplegia, and vent dependency in first 24 hours

October: Interventions as above; began standing program using a tilt table, sitting edge of mat with maximal assistance; development of grip on right upper extremity, development of increased tone (modified Ashworth scale 2 to 3) throughout all extremities

November: Began stand-pivot transfers; developed gross flexion/extension of right leg, minimal right elbow flexion (brachialis) and bilateral elbow extension

December: Began ambulation training in partial weight-bearing walker (knee immobilizer and molded ankle–foot orthosis on left lower extremity); developed right biceps strength; started weaning from the ventilator; received power wheelchair for mobility

January: Began walking with platform rolling walker, rolling supine to prone independently; moved left leg for first time (knee flexion/extension, great toe extension); tracheostomy capped during the day and bilevel positive airway pressure (BiPAP) at night

February: Decannulated with no external support and was transferred from the respiratory rehab service to the neurorehab service to achieve new goals of increasing independence with transfers and ambulation

March: Started performing bed mobility, sit to stand, and transfer board transfers with supervision only; ambulating with walker and no bracing and supervision only; starting to propel manual wheelchair with minimal assistance; received Botox injections to bilateral adductors and left hamstrings

April: Ambulating with forearm crutches; stood with quad cane for 30 seconds; moved left ankle for first time; discharged from inpatient setting to outpatient therapies

Currently: Primary power wheelchair user in community; uses walker at home and for short distances; Mark is now working toward long-term goal of independent ambulation in the community

Owing to Mark's unexpected but definite neurologic recovery, it was crucial to constantly reexamine and reassess his goals and interventions. It was also important to communicate his changes with the family and the team and to advocate for more time in intensive rehab. Finally, it became very important to Mark, his mom, and the team to return Mark to home and school before the end of the school year to get assimilated back into the community and to re-form peer relationships before the summer, when he would have a bigger chance of isolation.

A constant theme during his physical therapy course included the constant reexamination of strength in upper and lower extremities and the neck and trunk. This also required careful assessment and a good working knowledge of Mark's fluctuating spasticity and subsequent communication with the medical team who adjusted his antispasticity medication. Interventions were progressed to work on Mark's current strengths and to challenge his weaknesses. Gait training and orthotic and assistive device assessment was also everchanging and constant, and a variety of bracing options were tried to correct his left knee. Mark was able to flex and extend his left hip and knee, but he felt unstable in late stance. An articulating ankle–foot orthosis (AFO) did not achieve the stability he needed, so he trialed a stance-control knee–ankle–foot orthosis on loan from a local vendor. He had difficulty making the mechanism work properly for him, so he continued on with the current program and continued to use only an articulating AFO on his left ankle. Another constant theme in his physical therapy course was the consideration of the disablement model (Display 8.12).[71] While addressing Mark's impairments and functional limitations was critical in the achievement of his goals, considering the impact of disability and handicap in his life was also very important to him. Physical therapy played a definite role in assisting Mark and his mother to become advocates for themselves, both to his school and to the community.

DISPLAY 8.12   Using the ICF Framework for Patients with Spinal Cord Injury

The World Health Organization describes health and functioning using the *International Classification of Functioning, Disability, and Health* (ICF).[71] The ICF incorporates body, individual, and societal perspectives of function and shifts the focus from disability to positive capabilities. It integrates the interplay of health condition, body structures/functions (impairments), activities (abilities and limitations), participation (abilities and restrictions), and also considers the positive and negative influences a person's internal and external environment may have on their overall functioning. Evaluating and integrating all of these factors help to create patient and family-centered goals and identify areas of prioritization.

For patients with spinal cord injury, the health condition includes the original pathology discussed in this chapter and is useful during examination, evaluation, and determining goals for treatment. Most often physical therapy interventions are aimed at impairments and activity limitations, but a truly holistic approach considers the participation and environmental factors as well. While improving impairments and activity limitations were important to help Keith become more independent, becoming involved in an activity such as sled hockey helped him to overcome some of the participation restrictions that he faced. Giving him and his mom the tools and community resources to start a team in their area taught them valuable lessons in advocacy that they can continue to use throughout their lifetime. For Mark, finding ways to contribute to society was a primary goal for him. Independence in power mobility was the first step that physical therapy could help him with, and accessing favorite activities in the environment is an ongoing collaborative effort. Considering all aspects of the ICF model will enable the physical therapist to ensure best practice and family-centered care.

Currently, 18 months after his initial diagnosis, Mark remains a primary power wheelchair user in the community and uses a walker at home and for short distances. He is now working toward his long-term goal of independent ambulation in the community and is beginning to take independent steps with a quad cane. Socially, he is active in extracurricular activities and is on the honor role at his school. He currently works for an airplane museum, where he is able to enjoy his love of aviation. He continues to work hard and is looking forward to attending college for technical engineering.

This case is an example of the vast diversity PTs encounter in patient populations. Although all factors indicated a poor outcome, Mark's immense determination and constant hard work helped him to achieve goals no one dreamed possible. PTs have an awesome responsibility to balance being realistic about expected outcomes while also challenging their patients to achieve their fullest potential. Working together as a team with patients and families, amazing and life-changing things can be accomplished.

CASE STUDY 2   Keith is an 11-year-old boy who was involved in a motor vehicle accident. He was an unrestrained rear-seat passenger and was ejected from the car when it struck a tree. He had loss of consciousness and was intubated at the scene. In the emergency room, he was noted to have no movement in both lower extremities, and computed tomography revealed a T-6 fracture with spinal cord infarct. Other injuries included left epidural hematoma, occipital fracture, bilateral pulmonary contusions, and right iliac fracture with retroperitoneal hematoma. During this time, he received acute-care physical therapy to address ROM, positioning, elevating the head of the bed to increase upright tolerance, and caregiver education. Once Keith was extubated and stabilized, he was admitted to an inpatient rehabilitation program. Socially, he lived with his mother and two younger siblings in a two-story house with his bedroom and bathroom on the second floor and two steps to enter. His father was the driver of the vehicle, and his parents were in the process of a divorce. He attended the local public school and was extremely involved in athletics.

Examination

Keith presented with 4 ± 5 strength above the level of T-6 and $\%5$ strength and no sensation below that level. He was wearing a thoracic–lumbar–sacral orthosis (TLSO) for fracture stabilization and was not yet cleared for lower extremity weight bearing. His tone was grossly 2 on the modified Ashworth scale throughout his lower extremities, with three beats of clonus in each ankle and occasional flexor spasms in his left lower extremity when touched. His passive ROM was within normal limits throughout, with bilateral straight leg raise to 90 degrees. He was able to roll with minimal to moderate assistance using bed rails and transferred wheelchair to a level surface with a transfer board, push-up blocks, and moderate assistance. He required minimal assistance to sit upright and moderate assistance to reach outside his base of support.

Evaluation

Keith presented with decreased strength, decreased endurance, decreased flexibility, decreased bed mobility, decreased transfers, decreased functional mobility, and need for family education. Goals established at that time to be achieved during the inpatient rehabilitation admission included:

1. Roll independently supine to prone without a bed rail
2. Side-lying to sit with minimal assistance for lower extremities only
3. Transfer to level surfaces with a transfer board and contact guard assistance
4. Transfer to uneven surfaces with a transfer board and minimal assistance of one
5. Transfer floor-to-wheelchair with assistance only for lower extremities
6. Stand in parallel bars with bracing as needed and contact guard for 5 minutes with vital signs stable
7. Ambulate 25 feet with a walker and bracing as needed and contact guard assistance
8. Independent wheelchair mobility on level surfaces for 3000 feet without fatigue
9. Ascend and descend a 2-inch curb in his wheelchair with a spotter
10. Independence with wheelchair push-ups for pressure relief every 30 minutes
11. Patient independent with self-ROM
12. Caregiver independent with passive ROM, knowledge of skin checks, safeguarding for all levels of functional mobility, and all adaptive equipment management

Physical Therapy Diagnosis

Decreased strength and functional mobility due to ASIA A T-5 SCI.

Physical Therapy Prognosis

Excellent potential to achieve above goals due to current physical status, motivation, and family support. On the basis of the evidence, Keith has the potential to ambulate household distances with bracing and an assistive device but will most likely be a primary wheelchair user in community.

Interventions

INCREASING UPRIGHT TOLERANCE

Utilized compression stockings, abdominal binder to help prevent orthostatic hypotension. Increased time out of bed in wheelchair and on tilt table using knee immobilizers and solid AFOs for stability in the weight-bearing position.

INCREASING STRENGTH

Worked with interdisciplinary team on increasing arm strength throughout the day. Activities included progressive resistive exercises, trunk strengthening, and upper extremity dynamic activities.

INCREASING FLEXIBILITY

Performed ROM and stretching exercises to the lower extremities, which were carried out by family members as a bedside exercise program under the supervision of nursing staff. Keith was eventually taught to perform self-ROM. Special care was taken to allow enough hamstring flexibility to allow future floor-to-chair transfers and to maintain length in hip flexors and heel cords to allow for standing and assistive ambulation.

INCREASING BALANCE

Keith initially worked on improving sitting balance and reaching outside his base of support with his TLSO, but later learned to sit without the TLSO when it was discontinued owing to fracture stability and healing.

INCREASING ENDURANCE

Worked on increasing periods of aerobic activity, including dynamic activities, wheelchair propulsion, and recreational activities, which will be described later.

MAINTAINING SKIN INTEGRITY

Keith was instructed in performing wheelchair push-ups to provide adequate pressure relief. He was also instructed in performing daily skin checks to all insensate areas. He maintained a positioning program in bed and used a gel cushion on his wheelchair.

IMPROVING BED MOBILITY AND TRANSFERS

Keith was instructed in the head–hips relationship and was taught how to move his body without creating shear forces along his bottom. He initially used a transfer board to perform transfers, but eventually was able to transfer with no equipment and use a transfer board only for car transfers. He was also trained in techniques for floor-to-chair transfers, scooting along the floor, and bumping up and down steps.

AMBULATION

Keith initially began standing in the parallel bars using knee immobilizers, temporary solid ankle orthoses, and his TLSO. He attempted to learn how to hang on his Y ligaments, but this was very difficult with the TLSO. Once the TLSO was no longer necessary for fracture stabilization, Keith was able to align and position himself in a standing position in the parallel bars. He was extremely motivated to walk using any assistive device or bracing necessary despite the knowledge of its difficulties. He started with a pair of RGOs, and after much practice preferred to swing through rather than utilize the reciprocating mechanism, which he thought was slower and made him feel more fatigued. He was ordered and received a pair of lightweight single upright THKAFOs (trunk–hip–knee–ankle–foot orthoses) and was trained in donning, doffing, and ambulation.

IMPROVING WHEELCHAIR SKILLS

Keith was trained in propulsion, wheelies, ascending and descending curbs and ramps, and wheelchair recoveries. He was also trained in basic wheelchair maintenance.

EQUIPMENT

Keith received multipodus boots to wear in bed, molded AFOs to wear while in his wheelchair, THKAFOs for standing and walking, forearm crutches, a rigid-frame wheelchair, a transfer board, a commode, and bath equipment.

FAMILY EDUCATION

Keith's mother was trained and independent with safeguarding for all levels of functional mobility, all adaptive equipment management, and coaching Keith with his home exercise program.

Keith was independent in pressure reliefs, skin checks, his home exercise program, and training others how to safely assist him when needed. With the aid of the interdisciplinary team, Keith and his family were provided with basic knowledge of SCI in general and living with a disability.

Reexamination

Keith was reexamined during several points of his admission, but most notably when he had a change in medical status. Once his spinal fractures were adequately healed and he no longer required the use of the TLSO for fracture stabilization, Keith's entire center of gravity changed, and he needed to learn to use his body in a different way. He was also fully reexamined at the time of discharge from the inpatient setting, and he still had several physical therapy needs that were to be taken care of on an outpatient basis.

The Interdisciplinary Team

As is the case with most inpatient rehabilitation settings, Keith had a full team of professionals working closely on his case to achieve his family goal of safe discharge back to home. Although various disciplines have specific roles in caring for a child with an SCI, the team must communicate and work closely together. There is often overlap between professionals, and all team members should carry over the teaching of others to provide optimal family-centered care. Keith had a rehabilitation doctor overseeing his medical course with consulting medical services as needed such as orthopedics and urology. He also had nurses who primarily focused on skin, education, bowel and bladder program, and carrying over day-to-day skills such as ADLs and transfers. Psychosocial support came from a psychologist, child life staff, social worker, and the hospital chaplain. Educational needs were covered by the education coordinator, teacher, and neuropsychologist. He received speech therapy initially to work on increasing speaking volume and intensive occupational therapy to achieve goals of independence in ADLs. Physical therapy, occupational therapy, and nursing worked closely together so that Keith had the opportunity to practice new skills in a variety of environments. Together, the team, Keith, and his mother were able to achieve his family goal of successful reintegration back to home, school, and the community.

Discharge Planning

In order to ensure successful reintegration back to home, school, and the community, discharge planning began from the first day of admission. His family learning styles and needs were assessed and barriers to successful reintegration into the world were identified. First, owing to Keith's mild traumatic brain injury, he was fully assessed by the hospital education staff and neuropsychologist to identify any new cognitive or learning needs upon return to school. Several meetings were set up with the staff at his school to problem-solve and determine an appropriate educational plan and to remove any physical barriers. To prepare Keith to go home, the physical and occupational therapists performed a home evaluation with both Keith and his mother present. Measurements were taken and the basic layout was assessed in order to make appropriate home modification recommendations, but Keith

and his mom also had the opportunity to practice transfers and mobility under the direction of the therapists. The therapists were then able to identify any new physical or occupational needs and what still required more practice in the hospital environment prior to discharge home. Child life and psychology were instrumental in working with Keith's psychosocial issues regarding transition back into the community, but physical therapy played a large role in helping Keith to identify what types of leisure activities he may enjoy. Previously an athlete, Keith was very interested in pursuing adaptive sports, including wheelchair basketball. Physical therapy introduced him to the idea of sled hockey, and Keith soon found it to be his favorite activity. The therapist had a loaner roller sled for Keith to try out while still an inpatient and helped him and his mom connect with community resources so that he could join a team upon discharge. Keith was thrilled at the idea of playing sports again, making contacts with peers and adult athletes with SCIs, and stated that his new goal was to play sled hockey for the U.S. Paralympic team. This illustrates the importance of considering the entire disablement spectrum in order to treat patients holistically. Follow-up services were established, and Keith had a series of scheduled appointments with physicians trained to follow the needs of a person with SCI through the life span. Keith and his mom were given the tools needed to be advocates for themselves in both the health care and school systems as well as community resources to provide help along the way.

The Continuum of Care

Keith was recommended to be followed by outpatient physical therapy closer to his home to continue work on progressing wheelchair and ambulation skills to achieve his ultimate long-term goal of becoming as independent as possible. A recent study noted that patients with SCI who achieve a higher level of independence have improved quality of life and smoother transition to adulthood.[72] Keith may present with new pathologies, impairments, functional limitations, or disabilities as he grows and develops throughout his lifetime and may require future episodes of care from a PT. Emphasis should be placed on resolving those new problems and returning the patient to self-sufficiency, wellness, and a healthy lifestyle (Fig. 8.8).

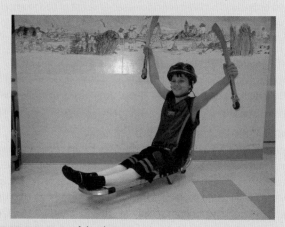

FIGURE 8.8. Adaptive sports such as sled hockey can help fulfill a child's need for peer interaction and participation in the community.

REFERENCES

1. The National Spinal Cord Injury Association (NSCIA). Spinal cord injury statistics. http://www.spinalcord.org/. Accessed March 27, 2013.
2. National Spinal Cord Injury Statistical Center. *Spinal Cord Injury: Facts and Figures at a Glance*. Birmingham, England: The University of Alabama at Birmingham; 2012.
3. Parent S, Mac-Thiong JM, Roy-Beaudry M, et al. Spinal cord injury in the pediatric population: a systematic review of the literature. *J Neurotrauma*. 2011;28(8):1515–1524.
4. Parent S, Dimar J, Dekutoski M, et al. Unique features of pediatric spinal cord injury. *Spine (Phila Pa 1976)*. 2010;35(21)(suppl): S202–S208.
5. Segal LS. Spine and pelvis trauma. In: Dormans JP, ed. *Pediatric Orthopedics and Sports Medicine: The Requisites in Pediatrics*. St. Louis, MO: Mosby; 2004.
6. Buldini B, Amigoni A, Faggin R, et al. Spinal cord injury without radiographic abnormalities. *Eur J Pediatr*. 2006;165(2):108–111.
7. Shepherd M, Hamill J, Segedin E. Paediatric lap-belt injury: a 7 year experience. *Emerg Med Australas*. 2006;18(1):57–63.
8. Kerr DA, Ayetey H. Immunopathogenesis of acute transverse myelitis. *Curr Opin Neurol*. 2002;15(3):339–347.
9. Borchers AT, Gershwin ME. Transverse myelitis. *Autoimmun Rev*. 2012;11(3):231–248.
10. Kerr DA, Calabresi PA. 2004 Pathogenesis of rare neuroimmunologic disorders, Hyatt Regency Inner Harbor, Baltimore, MD, August 19th 2004–August 20th 2004 [Congresses]. *J Neuroimmunol*. 2005;159(1–2):3–11.
11. Pollono D, Tomarchia S, Drut R, et al. Spinal cord compression: a review of 70 pediatric patients. *Pediatr Hematol Oncol*. 2003;20(6):457–466.
12. Meisel HJ, Lasjaunias P, Brock M. Modern management of spinal and spinal cord vascular lesions. *Minim Invasive Neurosurg*. 1995;38(4):138–145.
13. Alexander MS, Anderson K, Biering-Sorensen F, et al. Outcome measures in spinal cord injury: recent assessments and recommendations for future directions. *Spinal Cord*. 2009;47(8):582–591.
14. Kirshblum S, Burns SP, Biering-Sorensen F, et al. International standards for neurological classification of spinal cord injury (revised 2011). *J Spinal Cord Med*. 2011;34(6):535–546.
15. Kirshblum SC, Waring W, Biering-Sorensen F, et al. Reference for the 2011 revision of the International Standards for Neurological Classification of Spinal Cord Injury. *J Spinal Cord Med*. 2011; 34(6):547–554.
16. Chafetz R, Gaughan JP, Vogel LC, et al. The international standards for neurological classification of spinal cord injury: intra-rater agreement of total motor and sensory scores in the pediatric population. *J Spinal Cord Med*. 2009;32(2):157–161.
17. Mulcahey MJ, Gaughan JP, Chafetz RS, et al. Interrater reliability of the international standards for neurological classification of spinal cord injury in youths with chronic spinal cord injury. *Arch Phys Med Rehabil*. 2011;92(8):1264–1269.
18. Linan E, O'Dell MW, Pierce JM. Continuous passive motion in the management of heterotopic ossification in a brain injured patient. *Am J Phys Med Rehabil*. 2001;80(8):614–617.
19. Van Kuijk AA, Geurts AC, Van Kuppevelt HJ. Neurogenic heterotopic ossification in spinal cord injury. *Spinal Cord*. 2002;40(7):313–326.
20. Smith JA, Siegel JH, Siddiqi SQ. Spine and spinal cord injury in motor vehicle crashes: a function of change in velocity and energy dissipation on impact with respect to the direction of crash. *J Trauma Inj Infect Crit Care*. 2005;59(1):117–131.
21. Kirshblum S, Millis S, McKinley W, et al. Later neurologic recovery after traumatic spinal cord injury. *Arch Phys Med Rehabil*. 2004;85(11):1811–1817.
22. Sommer JL, Witkiewicz PM. The therapeutic challenges of dual diagnosis: TBI/SCI. *Brain Inj*. 2004;18(12):1297–1308.
23. Fronmon E, Dean W. Transverse myelitis. *New England J Med*. 2010;363:564–572.
24. Anderson K, Aito S, Atkins M, et al. Functional recovery measures for spinal cord injury: an evidence based review. *J Spinal Cord Med*. 2008;31(2):133–144.
25. Lollar DJ, Simeonssonn RJ, Nanda U. Measures of outcomes for children and youth. *Arch Phys Med Rehabil*. 2000;81(12)(suppl 2):S46–S52.
26. Kozin SH, D'Addesi L, Chafetz RS, et al. Biceps top triceps transfer for elbow extension in persons with tetraplegia. *J Hand Surg Am*. 2010;35(6):968–975.
27. Mulcahey MJ, Betz R, Smith B. A prospective evaluation of upper extremity tendon transfers in children with cervical spinal cord injury. *J Pediatr Orthop*. 1999;19(3):319–328.
28. Burcheil KJ, Hsu FP. Pain and spasticity after spinal cord injury: mechanisms and treatment. *Spine (Phila pa 1976)*. 2001;26(24) (suppl):S146–S160.
29. Warms C, Turner J, Marshall H. Treatments for chronic pain associated with spinal cord injuries. Many are tried, few are helpful. *Clin J Pain*. 2002;18(3):154–163.
30. Yap EC, Tow A, Menon EB, et al. Pain during in-patient rehabilitation after traumatic spinal cord injury. *Int J Rehabil Res*. 2003;26(2):137–140.
31. Jan F, Wilson P. A survey of chronic pain in the pediatric spinal cord injury population. *J Spinal Cord Med*. 2004;27(suppl 1):S50–S53.
32. Forest DM. Spinal cord stimulator therapy. *J Perianesth Nurs*. 2006;11(5):349–352.
33. Sheel AW, Reid WD, Townson AF, et al. Effects of exercise training and inspiratory muscle training in spinal cord injury: a systematic review. *J Spinal Cord Med*. 2008;31(5):500–508.
34. Roth EJ, Stenson KW, Powley S, et al. Expiratory muscle training in spinal cord injury: a randomized controlled trial. *Arch Phys Med Rehabil*. 2010;91(6):857–861.
35. Kelly M, Darrah J. Aquatic exercise for children with cerebral palsy. *Dev Med Child Neurol*. 2005;47(12):838–842.
36. Tefft D, Duerette P, Furumasu J. Cognitive predictors of young children's readiness for power mobility. *Dev Med Child Neurol*. 1999;41(10):655–670.
37. The Center for Orthotics Design. Isocentric RGO. http://www.centerfororthoticsdesign.com. Accessed October 9, 2006.
38. Vogel LC, Lubicky JP. Ambulation in children and adolescents with spinal cord injuries. *J Pediatr Orthop*. 1995;15(4):510–516.
39. Katz D, Haideri N, Song K. Comparative study of conventional hip-knee-ankle-foot-orthoses versus reciprocal-gait orthoses for children with high level paraplegia. *J Pediatr Orthop*. 1997;17(3):377–386.
40. Behrman AL, Harkema SJ. Locomotor training after human spinal cord injury: a series of case studies. *Phys Ther*. 2000;80:688–700.
41. Roy RR, Harkema SJ, Edgerton VR. Basic concepts of activity-based interventions for improved recovery of motor function after spinal cord injury. *Arch Phys Med Rehabil*. 2012;93(9):1487–1497.
42. Harkema SJ, Hillyer J, Schmidt-Read M, et al. Locomotor training: as a treatment of spinal cord injury and in the progression of neurologic rehabilitation. *Arch Phys Med Rehabil*. 2012;93(9):1588–1597.
43. Christopher & Dana Reeve Foundation. NeuroRecovery Network (NRN). http://www.christopherreeve.org/site/c. ddJFKRNoFiG/b.5399929/k.6F37/NeuroRecovery_Network.htm. Accessed March 18, 2013.
44. Harkema SJ, Schmidt-Read M, Lorenz DJ, et al. Balance and ambulation improvements in individuals with chronic incomplete spinal cord injury using locomotor training-based rehabilitation. *Arch Phys Med Rehabil*. 2012;93(9):1508–1517.
45. Buehner JJ, Forrest GF, Schmidt-Read M, et al. Relationship between ASIA examination and functional outcomes in the NeuroRecovery Network Locomotor Training Program. *Arch Phys Med Rehabil*. 2012;93(9):1530–1540.
46. Smith B, Mulcahey MJ, Betz RR. Development of an upper extremity FES system for individuals with C-4 tetraplegia. *IEEE Trans Rehabil Eng*. 1996;4(4):264–270.
47. Mulcahey MJ, Betz R, Smith BT. Implanted functional electrical stimulation hand system in adolescents with spinal injuries: an evaluation. *Arch Phys Med*. 1997;78(6):597–607.

48. Moynahen M, Mullin C, Chohn J, et al. Home use of a functional electrical stimulation system for standing and mobility in adolescents with spinal cord injury. *Arch Phys Med Rehabil.* 1996;77.

49. Johnston TE. Modlesky CM. Betz RR, et al. Muscle changes following cycling and/or electrical stimulation in pediatric spinal cord injury. *Arch Phys Med Rehabil.* 2011;92(12):1937–1943.

50. Lai CH, Chang WH, Chan WP, et al. Effects of functional electrical stimulation cycling exercise on bone mineral density loss in the early stages of spinal cord injury. *J Rehabil Med.* 2010;42(2):150–154.

51. Individuals with Disabilities Education Act (IDEA). 20 U.S.C. 1400.

52. Liusuwan A, Widman L, Abresch RT, et al. Altered body composition affects resting energy expenditure and interpretation of body mass index in children with spinal cord injury. *J Spinal Cord Med.* 2004;27(suppl 1):S24–S28.

53. Moreno MA, Samuner AR, Paris JV, et al. Effects of wheelchair sports on respiratory muscle strength and thoracic mobility of individuals with spinal cord injury. *Am J Med Rehabil.* 2012;91(6):470–477.

54. Hickey K, Vogel L, Willis K, et al. Prevalence and etiology of autonomic dysreflexia in children with spinal cord injuries. *J Spinal Cord Med.* 2004;27(suppl 1):S54–S60.

55. McCarthy J, Chavetz R, Betz R. Incidence and degree of hip subluxation/dislocation in children with spinal cord injury. *J Spinal Cord Med.* 2004;27(suppl 1):S80–S83.

56. Mehta S, Betz R, Mulcahey MJ. Effect of bracing on paralytic scoliosis secondary to spinal cord injury. *J Spinal Cord Med.* 2004;27 (suppl 1):S88–S92.

57. Merenda L, Brown JP. Bladder and bowel management for the child with spinal cord dysfunction. *J Spinal Cord Med.* 2004;27 (suppl 1):S16–S23.

58. Lauer RT, Smith BT, Mulcahey MJ, et al. Effects of cycling and/or electrical stimulation on bone mineral density in children with spinal cord injury. *Spinal Cord.* 2011;49(8):917–923.

59. Deforge D, Blackmer J, Garrity C. Fertility following spinal cord injury: a systematic review. *Spinal Cord.* 2005;43(12):693–793.

60. Anderson CJ, Vogel LC, Betz RR, et al. Overview of adult outcomes in pediatric-onset spinal cord injuries: implications for transition to adulthood. *J Spinal Cord Med.* 2004;27(suppl 1):S98–S106.

61. Anderson CJ, Vogel LC. Employment outcomes of adults who sustain spinal cord injuries as children or adolescents. *Arch Phys Med Rehabil.* 1998;79(12):1496–1503.

62. Lidal IB, Huynh TK, Biering-Sørensen F. Return to work following spinal cord injury: a review. *Disabil Rehabil.* 2007;29:1341–1375.

63. Sinden KE, Ginis KM, SHAPE-SCI Research Group. Identifying occupational attributes of jobs performed after spinal cord injury:implications for vocational rehabilitation. *Int J Rehabil Res.* 2013;36(3):196–204.

64. Vogel LC, Klaas SJ, Lupicky JP. Long-term outcomes and life satisfaction of adults who had pediatric spinal cord injury. *Arch Phys Med Rehabil.* 1998;79(12):1496–1503.

65. Kwon BK, Sekhon LH. Emerging repair, regeneration, and tranlational research advances for spinal cord injury. *Spine.* 35(215):263–270.

66. Mothe AJ, Tator CH. Advances in stem cell therapy for spinal cord injury. *J Clin Invest.* 2012;122(11):3824–3834, 67.

67. Harper JM, Krishnan C, Darman JS, et al. Axonal growth of embryonic stem cell-derived motoneurons in vitro and in motoneuron-injured adult rats. *Proc Natl Acad Sci USA.* 2004;101(18):7123–7128.

68. Kerr DA, Llado J, Shamblott MJ, et al. Human embryonic germ cell derivatives facilitate motor recovery of rats with diffuse motor neuron injury. *J Neurosci.* 2003;23(12):5131–5140.

69. Deshpande DM, Kim YS, Martinez T, et al. Recovery from Paralysis in adult rats using embryonic stem cells. *Ann Neurol.* 2006;60(1):32–44.

70. Ramer LM, Ramer MS, Steeves JD. Setting the stage for functional repair of spinal cord injuries: a cast of thousands. *Spinal Cord.* 2005;43:134–161.

71. *International Classification of Functioning, Disability and Health.* Available at: http://www.who.int/classifications/icf/en. Accessed December 5, 2013.

72. Anderson CJ, Vogel LC, Willis KM, et al. Stability of transition to adulthood among individuals with pediatric-onset spinal cord injuries. *J Spinal Cord Med.* 2006;29(1):46–56.

73. Bohannon RW, Smith MB. Inter-rater reliability of a modified Ashworth scale of muscle spasticity. *Phys Ther.* 1987;67:206–207.

Neuromuscular Disorders in Childhood: Physical Therapy Intervention

Alan M. Glanzman and Jean M. Flickinger

Introduction
Duchenne Muscular Dystrophy
  Diagnosis
  Pathophysiology
  Clinical Presentation and Progression
  Treatment
  Physical Therapy Examination
  Review of Systems
  Tests and Measures
  Physical Therapy Intervention

Myotonic Dystrophy
Limb-Girdle Muscular Dystrophy
Congenital Myopathy
Congenital Muscular Dystrophy
Spinal Muscular Atrophy
Charcot–Marie–Tooth Disease
Case Study

Introduction

Children with neuromuscular disorders have a lifelong challenge to maintain function. That challenge can be met with the help of a knowledgeable physical therapist. In this chapter, the term *neuromuscular disease* refers to disorders whose primary pathology affects any part of the motor unit from the anterior horn cell out to the muscle itself. Common to all of these disorders is muscle weakness, which may be produced by pathology at any part of the motor unit. When characterizing neuromuscular disorders and their pathology, it is convenient to consider the various anatomic divisions of this motor unit: the anterior horn cell, the peripheral nerve, the neuromuscular junction, and the muscle.

Neuromuscular diseases of the muscle may be either hereditary or acquired and are variously classified as a myopathy or dystrophy, in which the cause of the muscle weakness is attributable to pathology confined to the muscle itself. Similarly, neuropathy, in which the muscle weakness is secondary to an abnormality of either the anterior horn cell or peripheral nerve, can be characterized based on a particular disorder's primary impairment of either the axon or axonal myelination.

The term *muscular dystrophy* describes a group of muscle diseases that are genetically determined and have a steadily progressive degenerative course and characteristic degenerative features on microscopic examination of the muscle. Further classification of the muscular dystrophies is based on their clinical presentation, including the distribution of weakness, mode of inheritance, and pathologic findings. In the past two decades, much has been discovered in the area of molecular biology to help us better understand and classify the childhood muscular dystrophies. After the cloning of the gene for Duchenne muscular dystrophy (DMD) in 1987,[1,2] we have learned more about the relationship between the different dystrophies and how they relate to the dystrophin–glycoprotein complex (DGC), found within the muscle cell membrane (Fig. 9.1). The DGC is a group of proteins that links the subsarcolemmal cytoskeleton and extracellular matrix with the contractile apparatus of the muscle and gives stability to the muscle cell membrane.[3] When different proteins in the DGC are deficient or made incorrectly, structural abnormalities in the muscle can be identified and different corresponding muscular dystrophies become phenotypically apparent. For example, when dystrophin is deficient, the result is Duchenne or Becker muscular dystrophy (BMD). When one of the sarcoglycan proteins is deficient, other limb-girdle muscular dystrophies (LGMDs) result. A deficiency of Merosin results in one specific type of congenital muscular dystrophy (CMD).

Some of the above dystrophies are categorized by the deficiency of proteins which characterize and often name the

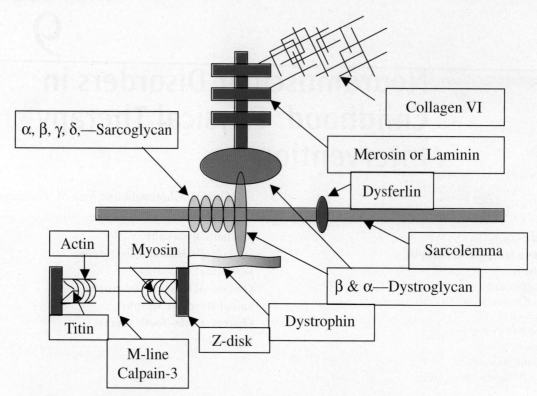

FIGURE 9.1 Muscle cell membrane and associated protein complexes implicated in muscle disease.

corresponding disorder. DMD and BMD are also known as *dystrophinopathies* because dystrophin is deficient in these conditions. Some of the LGMDs are also known as *sarcoglycanopathies* because one of the sarcoglycan proteins is deficient in these conditions. Similarly Merosin negative congenital muscular dystrophy is the result of a deficiency of Merosin.

The term *spinal muscular atrophy (SMA)* refers to neurogenic disorders whose underlying pathology affects sensory neurons and spinal interneurons and as a result the anterior horn cell,[3a,3b,4] as in the spinal muscular atrophies. The term *motor neuropathy* refers to neurogenic disorders whose underlying pathology affects the peripheral nerve, as in Charcot–Marie–Tooth (CMT) disease. Further classification of CMT is based on clinical presentation and mode of inheritance.

The neuromuscular disorders vary significantly in their presentation, pathology, and progression but are linked with regard to physical therapy intervention by their common characteristic of muscle weakness leading to loss of function and physical deformity. A physical therapist with an understanding of these disorders can help identify, predict, intervene, and possibly prevent unnecessary complications throughout the course of each disorder. The purpose of this chapter is to provide an overview of select neuromuscular diseases, including clinical presentation, pathology, diagnosis, disease progression, medical treatment, and physical therapy intervention.

Because Duchenne muscular dystrophy (DMD) is one of the most common and best known of the dystrophies affecting children, much of this chapter is devoted to a discussion of this disorder. Physical therapy interventions and principles that apply to the management of weakness and

deformity in patients with DMD are also applicable to other neuromuscular diseases that present with similar symptoms and complications with the exception of strengthening strategies. Knowledge of the various disorders will allow appropriate decisions to be made about the suitability and timing of various physical therapy interventions. Other neuromuscular diseases that are reviewed in this chapter include BMD, myotonic dystrophy (MTD), LGMD, congenital myopathy, CMD, SMA, and CMT disease.

Duchenne muscular dystrophy

DMD, also known as pseudohypertrophic muscular dystrophy or progressive muscular dystrophy, is one of the most prevalent and severely disabling of the childhood neuromuscular disorders, occurring in approximately 1 in 3500 live male births.[2] It is a dystrophinopathy in which the child becomes weaker and usually dies of respiratory insufficiency and/or heart failure due to myocardial involvement in the second or third decade of life.[5] There is an X-linked inheritance pattern to DMD whereby male offspring inherit the disease from their mothers, who are most often asymptomatic. Advances in molecular biology has shown the defect to be a mutation at Xp21 in the gene coding for the protein dystrophin.[1,6]

Diagnosis

The clinical presentation gives the first clues to the diagnosis, which is confirmed by the results of laboratory studies.

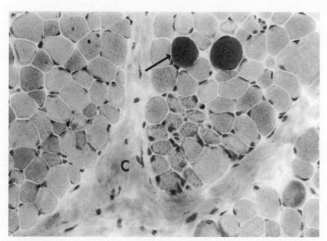

FIGURE 9.2 Dystrophic changes include a marked variability in fiber size; dark, "opaque" fibers (*arrow*); and abnormal quantities of fibrous connective tissue (*C*). (Trichrome, ×300) (From Maloney FP, Burks JS, Ringel SP, eds. *Interdisciplinary Rehabilitation of Muscular Dystrophy and Neuromuscular Disorders*. Philadelphia, PA: J.B. Lippincott; 1984:203.)

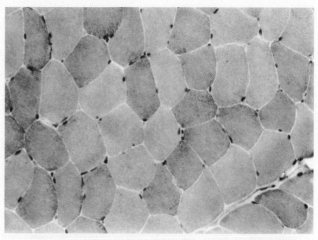

FIGURE 9.3 Normal adult muscle. Muscle fibers are cut in a plane transverse to their long axis and appear to have polygonal tightly packed appearance. One or more darkly stained nuclei are seen at the edge of most fibers. (Trichrome, ×300) (From Maloney FP, Burks JS, Ringel SP, eds. *Interdisciplinary Rehabilitation of Multiple Sclerosis and Neuromuscular Disorders*. Philadelphia, PA: J.B. Lippincott; 1984:202.)

Laboratory findings include an abnormally high serum creatine kinase (CK) level, which is 50 to 200 times the normal level[7] and usually ranges from 15,000 to 35,000 IU/L (normal less than 160 IU/L).[8] Electromyogram (EMG) findings show nonspecific myopathic features with normal motor and sensory nerve velocities and no denervation. A muscle biopsy may be performed to confirm the diagnosis and shows degenerating and regenerating fibers, inflammatory infiltrates, and increased connective tissue and adipose cells (Fig. 9.2), which can be seen when compared to normal muscle (Fig. 9.3). Immunohistologic staining of the tissue reveals the absence of dystrophin along the muscle cell membranes.[9]

Advances in genetic testing have allowed diagnosis by the type of mutation present in DMD and BMD. With the decrease in the cost of genetic analysis, this is often the first line of testing when the phenotypic presentation and high CK is consistent with that of DMD or BMD. Approximately 65% of patients with DMD and BMD have gross deletions of the dystrophin gene, which results in either the complete absence of dystrophin in DMD or some levels of truncated protein in BMD.[10] One-third of DMD cases are caused by very small point mutations that are not detectable by the first line genetic analysis techniques and a two-step process is needed first evaluating for the presence of gross deletion and following up with a more sensitive test to determine the presence of point mutations or other genetic rearrangements.[10] There is also a high frequency of new mutations occurring in approximately one-third of the cases of DMD, which may in part be secondary to the very large size of the dystrophin gene.[2] With the availability of genetic analysis, all male family members may be screened for the disorder and all female family members may be screened for their carrier status once a mutation is identified in the proband.

Pathophysiology

The absence of dystrophin leads to a reduction in all of the dystrophin-associated proteins in the muscle cell membrane and causes a disruption in the linkage between the subsarcolemmal cytoskeleton and the extracellular matrix. The exact cause of muscle cell necrosis is unknown. However, lack of dystrophin is thought to cause sarcolemmal instability and an increase susceptibility to membrane microtears, which may be exacerbated by muscle contractions. This causes increased calcium channel leaks, and an increase in reactive oxygen species. The increase in reactive oxygen species is activated through a pathway driven by mechanotransduction by the microtubule cytoskeleton of the cell. The activation of this signaling pathway results from membrane stress and ultimately impacts calcium signaling and results in an increase in which raises intracellular calcium levels, leading to muscle cell necrosis.[2,11]

The following describes the clinical features of DMD. BMD also follows a similar pattern of muscle degeneration, but at a much slower and variable rate.

Clinical Presentation and Progression

The onset of the disorder is insidious, usually resulting in symptoms between 2 and 5 years of age; however, symptoms may not be noticed for months or years, and the disease may be misdiagnosed for years.[7]

Earliest symptoms may include a reluctance to walk or run at appropriate ages, falling, and difficulty getting up off the floor, toe-walking, clumsiness, and an increase in the size of the gastrocnemius muscles. This "pseudohypertrophy," is marked by a firm consistency of the muscle when palpated (Fig. 9.4).

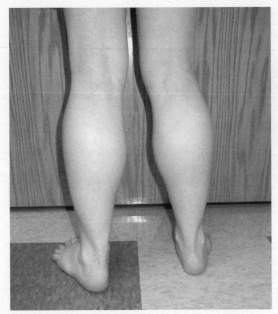

FIGURE 9.4 Ten-year-old with Duchenne dystrophy. Pseudohypertrophy of the calf.

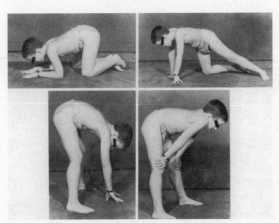

FIGURE 9.6 Gower's sign. This series of maneuvers is necessary to achieve an upright posture, and it occurs with all types of pelvic and trunk weakness. The child "climbs up the legs" when rising from the floor. (From Lovell WW, Winter RB, eds. *Pediatric Orthopaedics*. 2nd ed. Philadelphia, PA: J.B. Lippincott; 1986:265.)

The weakness is steadily progressive with proximal muscles tending to be weaker earlier in the course of the illness and to progress faster (Fig. 9.5). Weakness of the hip and knee extensors often results in an exaggerated lumbar lordosis that is characteristic of the early stages of disease. The lordosis occurs in response to the attempt to align the center of gravity anterior to the fulcrum of the knee joint and posterior to the fulcrum of the hip joint. This realignment gives

maximum stability at both joints. The child attempts to broaden the base of support during walking and thus develops a gait that resembles waddling. The child may develop iliotibial band (ITB) contractures, which are made worse by this wide-based stance. As the weakness progresses, the child rises from the floor by "climbing up the legs." This maneuver, known as Gowers sign, is indicative of proximal muscle weakness (Fig. 9.6).

As the disease progresses, there is a tendency to develop contractures. These contractures typically result in

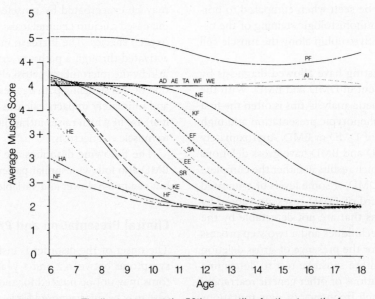

FIGURE 9.5 The lines represent the 50th percentiles for the strength of individual muscles plotted against age. AD, ankle dorsiflexor; AE, ankle evertor; AI, ankle invertor; EE, elbow extensor; EF, elbow flexor; HA, hip abductor; HE, hip extensor; HF, hip flexor; KE, knee extensor; KF, knee flexor; NE, neck extensor; NF, neck flexor; PF, plantarflexor; SA, shoulder abductor; SR, shoulder external rotator; TA, thumb abductor; WE, wrist extensor; WF, wrist flexor. (Courtesy of the Collaborative Investigation of Duchenne Dystrophy [CIDD] Group).

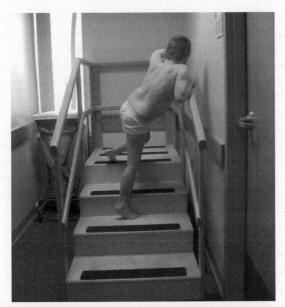

FIGURE 9.7 Ten-year-old with SMA type III. Notice the use of the upper extremities to assist climbing the steps. This posture or use of a hand to extend the knee are the two most typical patterns noted with proximal weakness.

plantarflexion at the ankle, with inversion of the foot being the earliest contractures to develop and flexion at both the hips and knees typically becoming more noticeable with the onset of wheelchair dependence.

This early loss of range of motion (ROM), noted in the hamstrings, hip flexors, ITBs, and heel cords, limits stance and

ambulation and patients find it difficult to achieve the mechanical alignment necessary to hold themselves in an upright posture using their weak musculature. As these boys spend more time sitting, an increasing degree of contracture is seen at the hips and knees, and upper extremity contractures begin to develop in the elbows, shoulders and long finger flexors.

Functional activities may be performed more slowly by children with DMD than by typically developing children, but most of those affected are able to walk, climb stairs (Fig. 9.7), and stand up from the floor without too much difficulty until 6 or 7 years of age. At this time, a relatively rapid decline in function has been documented, which generally results in a loss of unassisted ambulation at 9 to 10 years of age. By convention for a child to fit the DMD categorization of a dystrophinopathy, loss of ambulation should be by the age of 13 after which the patient would be considered to have either BMD or an intermediate phenotype. Some children will choose to use long-leg braces and continue to walk as an exercise ambulator for an additional year or so but will need help getting to and from standing.[12] A partial weight-bearing walker may also be used at this stage. A graphic representation of the ages at which the children have increasing difficulty with various functional activities is presented in Figure 9.8. These functional activities are considered to be "milestones" and represent significant points in disease progression. The arm grades awarded were developed by Brooke and associates[12] (Table 9.1), whereas the leg grades are based on a scale proposed by Vignos et al. (Table 9.2).[13]

As is demonstrated by the range and distribution of percentiles in Figure 9.8, the clinical course of disease progression in individual children is not homogeneous.

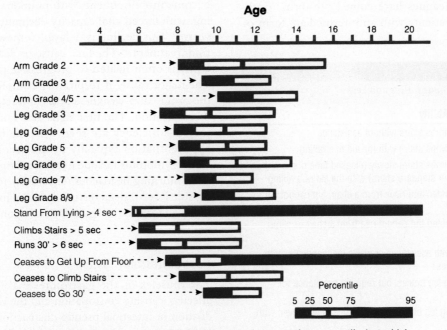

FIGURE 9.8 Graphic representation of the ages (expressed as percentiles) at which children with DMD have increasing difficulty with functional tasks. (Courtesy of the Collaborative Investigation of Duchenne Dystrophy [CIDD] Group.)

TABLE 9.1 Functional Grades: Arms and Shoulders	
Grades	**Functional Ability**
1	Standing with arms at the sides, the patient can abduct the arms in a full circle until they touch above the head.
2	The patient can raise the arms above the head only by flexing the elbow (i.e., by shortening the circumference of the movement) or by using accessory muscles.
3	The patient cannot raise hands above the head, but can raise an 8-oz glass of water to the mouth (using both hands if necessary).
4	The patient can raise hands to the mouth, but cannot raise an 8-oz glass of water to the mouth.
5	The patient cannot raise hands to the mouth, but can use the hands to hold a pen or to pick up pennies from a table.
6	The patient cannot raise hands to the mouth and has no useful function of the hands.

The mildest of the X-linked progressive dystrophies resulting from abnormalities of dystrophin has been termed Becker muscular dystrophy. This classification applies to individuals who maintain independent ambulation until 16 years of age. The type of mutation on the dystrophin gene causing BMD allows for some dystrophin to be produced. The dystrophin produced is insufficient in quantity and quality, causing muscle breakdown to occur at a slower rate than in DMD. Boys with BMD will usually present with symptoms between 5 and 15 years of age, although onset is variable and may not occur until as late as the third or fourth decade.[2] The course of BMD is much less predictable than that of DMD; however, patients with BMD usually live at least until their fourth or fifth decade.[2]

Brooke and colleagues have coined the term "outliers"[12] to describe patients with an intermediate form of

TABLE 9.2 Functional Grades: Hips and Legs	
Grades	**Functional Ability**
1	Walks and climbs stairs without assistance
2	Walks and climbs stairs with the aid of a railing
3	Walks and climbs stairs slowly (elapsed time of more than 12 sec for four standard stairs) with the aid of a railing
4	Walks unassisted and rises from a chair, but cannot climb stairs
5	Walks unassisted but cannot rise from a chair or climb stairs
6	Walks only with assistance or walks independently with long leg braces
7	Walks in long leg braces, but requires assistance for balance
8	Stands in long leg braces, but is unable to walk even with assistance
9	Is in wheelchair
10	Is confined to bed

dystrophinopathy when describing the population of boys who, when compared with the DMD population's usual pattern of disease progression, fall outside the usual limits. These outliers by convention are classified by the fact that they retain the ability to ambulate until age 13 but lose this ability by 16 years of age.[2] Antigravity neck flexion is also relatively preserved early on in the disease process in these patients[2] as well as in BMD while one of the earliest signs of weakness in the untreated DMD population is neck flexor weakness. Investigators are studying genetic heterogeneity with regard to DNA mutations and the resulting dystrophin expression in an attempt to better understand the varying levels of clinical severity associated with DMD.[14,15]

Scoliosis

Scoliosis develops as the age of the untreated child with DMD increases; significant curves are generally not noticed until wheelchair independence after 11 years of age.[16] This scoliosis tends to progress as the back muscles become weaker and as the child spends less time standing and more time sitting, resulting in a positional scoliosis, which, over time, becomes fixed. Treatment with corticosteroids decreases the likelihood that scoliosis will develop to the point of needing surgical correction[17] and treatment with bracing has not been shown to be effective in this population.[18,19,20]

Respiratory Involvement

In addition to the voluntary muscles, DMD affects other organs also. As the respiratory musculature atrophies, coughing becomes ineffective and pulmonary infections become more frequent, with pulmonary function declining, with forced vital capacity declining a mean of 5% per year.[20a] This decline is delayed somewhat by corticosteroid treatment.[21] The final cause of death in patients with DMD is often related to progressive pulmonary decline. The major cause of respiratory complications in DMD is the progressive weakness and contracture of the muscles of respiration. The first signs and symptoms of respiratory insufficiency are seen with the onset of nocturnal hypoventilation typically in the second decade of life. These symptoms include excessive fatigue, daytime sleepiness, morning headaches (secondary to increased carbon dioxide levels), sleep disturbances (nightmares), or feeling the need to strain to "gulp for air" upon arousal during the night.

Gastrointestinal System

The muscles of the gastrointestinal (GI) tract are also affected, causing constipation and the risk of acute gastric dilation or intestinal pseudo-obstruction, which can cause sudden episodes of vomitting, abdominal pain, and distention. If not treated properly, this requires medical attention and can lead to death.[3]

Cardiac Issues

Heart muscle is also affected by a deficiency of dystrophin, resulting in dilated cardiomyopathy, arrhythmia, and congestive heart failure.[22] In DMD, the posterobasal portion of the left ventricle is affected greater than other parts of the heart. In DMD, heart muscle involvement generally occurs later than skeletal muscle involvement and may not present until the late second decade.[23] In BMD and female carriers of the dystrophin mutation, cardiac involvement can occur later and may sometimes require heart transplantation.[23] Monitoring of these patients should begin early in the second decade for DMD and BMD and for female carriers of the dystrophin mutation in the third decade.[23]

Motor and sensory neurons are undamaged, and fortunately Bowel and bladder control typically remains intact despite impaired motility

Cognition

A high rate of intellectual impairment[24] and emotional disturbance has been associated with DMD.[25] Although intelligence may be reduced among some children with DMD, most children are cognitively normal and any existing deficit is not progressive and is not related to the severity of disease.[26] IQ scores fall approximately one standard deviation below the mean[25] and affect verbal scores greater than performance scores however some children are not cognitively delayed and function at age appropriate levels.[2] When cognitive delay is noted this is not progressive, but this intellectual deficit may hinder the child's development and may make a physical evaluation of the child difficult.

Treatment

Although definitive treatment is lacking, proper management[27] can prolong the maximum functional ability of the child. This program of management begins once the diagnosis is established, and it is initiated concurrently with referral for parental counseling in an attempt to mitigate the guilt, hostility, and fear commonly experienced by the parents should this be desired.

The clinician can propose a positive approach on the basis of the following: (1) some of the complications which magnify the functional disability of DMD are predictable and preventable; (2) an active program of physical therapy may prolong ambulation and more closely approximate the normal independence of later childhood; and (3) if a specific treatment ever becomes available, those in optimal physical condition are most apt to benefit.[28]

Medical Treatment

There is no pharmaceutical cure for the genetic abnormality in DMD, but corticosteroids[29,30] including prednisone and deflazacort increase strength and improve functional ambulation from 6 months to up to 2 years in patients with DMD.[31,32] Further investigation has shown that prednisone, despite its many side effects, keeps those affected by DMD "stronger for longer."[33,34] Adverse effects of prednisone include excessive weight gain, cushingoid appearance, behavioral abnormalities, and excessive hair growth.[31] Deflazacort has similar effects with a slightly different side effect profile and may result in less weight gain and bone demineralization but perhaps a higher risk of cataracts with equivalent strength and functional benefits to prednisone.[30]

Creatine monohydrate, a naturally occurring substance, often used by body builders to increase muscle performance, is sometimes recommended for boys with DMD.[35] When healthy subjects take oral creatine for 1 to 4 weeks, the result is increases in muscle levels of creatine and improvements in maximal exercise performance and recovery from exercise.[36] Boys with DMD showed increases in fat-free mass (FFM), strength, and subjective reports of improvement after creatine supplementation.[35]

Since the discovery of the genetic defect and identification of the dystrophin protein there has been a significant interest in the development of medical therapies for children with DMD. These efforts fall into a number of broad groups that include: gene therapy, cell therapy, mutation specific medication, modulation of utrophin expression, modulation of blood flow to the muscle, and treatments to address fibrosis.[37] To date there is not an approved therapy to cure the disease.

Orthopedic Treatment

Spinal fixation is generally recommended for boys with DMD if their scoliosis begins to progress rapidly and their spinal curve becomes greater than 30 degrees, usually once boys are wheelchair-bound.[38] The goals of spinal surgery should include providing a stable spine, maximally correcting scoliosis, correcting pelvic obliquity, and providing sagittal-plane alignment for improved comfort and function.[38,39] Spinal stabilization should be segmental from T2 or T3 at the upper end and attaching into the body of the ilium or sacrum at the lower end, and should attempt to correct pelvic obliquity and provide a lumbar lordosis.[39] The above surgery allows for immediate post-op mobilization often without an orthosis. Timing of surgery is critical as the risks of surgery become greater as the disease progresses. The decision for spinal stabilization should be viewed in the context of the patient's pulmonary function since this relates to the patient's ability to tolerate the rigors of surgical correction. Vital capacity (FVC) below 30% or 35% is related to higher complication rates.[20] Failure of extubation following surgery is also an important post op risk and some centers will use bilevel positive airway pressure (BiPAP) as a way to transition following extubation immediately after surgery should this be necessary.

Other orthopedic surgeries include Achilles tendon or gastroc-facial lengthening, Yount fasciotomies, tibialis posterior transpositions, and percutaneous tenotomies in an attempt to increase joint ROM for prolongation of ambulation. Besides surgery, orthopedic intervention is required in the event of a fracture. There is an increased risk of low energy fractures in boys diagnosed with DMD and BMD as well as in patients with SMA types II and III compared to controls. Many lower extremity fractures lead to a permanent loss of function resulting in loss of ambulation. Some have recommended aggressive therapy with early remobilization in lower-limb fractures where ambulation is fragile. Use of partial weight-bearing support treadmills and gait trainers as well as aquatic therapy can be utilized in the rehabilitation process to allow earlier mobilization in a safe environment once cleared by the orthopedic physician for weight bearing.

Pulmonary Treatment

A child with DMD will need to be followed by a pulmonologist beginning in the second decade of life for regular monitoring of pulmonary status initially focusing on evaluation for nocturnal hypoventilation. If the history and pulmonary function test results suggest that the lungs are not being adequately ventilated, the pulmonologist will need to discuss options for assisted ventilation. Nasal bilevel positive pressure (BPAP) ventilation may be used at night to assist breathing and to provide a rest for overworked respiratory muscles.[40] An adjustment period is often necessary when this type of ventilation is used, but after a period of time, the patient often derives the benefits of improved sleep and increased energy and alertness in the daytime. Ventilatory assistance might be required both day and night for children with advanced respiratory failure.[41] Ventilators are typically compact, battery-driven devices that can be attached to an appropriately modified wheelchair and breaths can be delivered by tracheostomy or by a mouth piece that can be held in the mouth when it is needed. The pulmonologist can also recommend various airway clearance techniques and medications to improve pulmonary health including procussion and postural drainage during illness and the use of a coughalator for airway clearance and to maintain ribcage and lung flexibility.

Cardiac Treatment

Regular cardiac echocardiogram (ECHO) and electrocardiogram monitoring by a cardiologist is necessary for boys with DMD, BMD, and female carriers. Cardiac medications for arrhythmias and ventricular function may be necessary. Patients with BMD also may eventually need heart transplantation for dilated cardiomyopathy.

Gastrointestinal/Nutrition

A GI specialist can help with constipation issues as well as monitor for intestinal pseudo-obstruction. A nutritionist can help prevent weight gain and assist with diet recommendations in the early years and with weight loss and nutritional support in later life when self feeding becomes difficult and aspiration becomes more of a risk.

Physical Therapy Examination

The role of the physical therapist in treating DMD and BMD is an important one and requires a solid understanding of both the unique features and the natural history of the disease in addition to a delicate approach to the issues related to treating a progressive and fatal disorder. When discussing examination and treatment of the child with DMD, it is helpful to categorize the disease into three general life stages: the early or ambulatory stage, the transitional phase during loss of ambulation, and the later/wheelchair stage when the child or young adult is wheelchair dependent for most of his functional activities.

Each child with DMD should undergo a physical therapy examination. Such an examination involves the gathering of information that contributes to the development of a plan of care.[42] That care plan will be based largely on the functional significance of the therapist's findings in the context of the natural history of the disease.

History

A thorough history should be taken and should include: family history; birth and developmental history; a review of systems, including cardiac, pulmonary, GI, integumentary, and musculoskeletal systems; functional mobility; social history,environmental barriers; and current durable medical equipment. The primary concerns of the child and family should also be understood prior to examining the child.

Family History

Understanding the child's family history is important. The child and family may already know someone with the disease and may have a different perspective than someone diagnosed with no family members with the disease who is unfamiliar with the characteristic phenotypic course. If the child's mother or sisters are carriers, they will need to understand both their risks of cardiomyopathy as well as implications for future family planning.

Developmental History

The physical therapist should gather information regarding the child's birth and development. Often, boys with DMD are late walkers, may never gain the ability to jump, and lag behind their peers in gross motor skills. Parents often report frequent falling or clumsiness as boys develop weakness. It is common for boys to have a lower IQ, and they may have learning disabilities that need to be addressed in school however this is only a subset of the population and many boys are cognitively normal.

Review of Systems
Pulmonary

A good pulmonary history is required to determine whether the child has any pulmonary issues that require treatment or referral to a pulmonologist. Does the child have a strong cough, is it productive cough? Can the child clear his own secretions? Does the family currently perform percussion and postural drainage with intercurrent illness or use any devices to aid in airway clearance to maintain pulmonary health? Does the child exhibit any symptoms of respiratory insufficiency or nighttime hypoventilation? If the child demonstrates these symptoms, the child must be referred to a pulmonologist for evaluation for nocturnal hypoventilation.

Other systems, including cardiac, GI, integumentary, and musculoskeletal systems will also need to be reviewed to determine whether referral to a specialist is necessary.

Tests and Measures

Functional Ability

Systematic and serial recording of standard tasks shows that the child with DMD is in one of two general phases: stable performance or declining performance. During the stable phase, which may continue for several years, the child may demonstrate normal performance of various tasks during the serial evaluations, despite a continuing decline in strength. A discrepancy exists in the age at which the aforementioned tasks are failed, as illustrated in Figure 9.8.

The use of timed testing during examinations in the clinical setting is useful for monitoring patient function as well as for predicting loss of ambulation. Activities that are frequently timed include: transferring from supine to standing, running or walking a distance of 10 m, transferring from sitting to standing, and climbing up four steps. Qualitative description along with timing adds useful information in monitoring function and level of fatigue. For example, it is helpful to note during the floor-to-stand transfer whether a Gowers maneuver is present and whether the child requires the use of one or both hands on knees to complete the transfer. When climbing the steps, it is helpful to describe how many rails are required, the pattern or sequence of steps used (reciprocal versus marking time), and whether use of upper extremities is required to push on knees or to pull up on the rail to ascend steps.

Timed function tests can be useful in predicting loss of ambulation. When the time to ambulate 10 meters is greater than 9 seconds, this is predictive of loss of ambulation within 2 years. A 10 meter timed test of greater than 12 seconds is predictive of loss of ambulation within 1 year. When a child is no longer able to attain standing from floor, it is predicted that loss of ambulation is likely to occur within 2 years.[43]

It has been[44,45] demonstrated that, although functional ability appears to remain at a constant stage in many children during the plateau phase, while actual muscle strength declines, walking speed continues[46] to remain stable even when compared to normative data. Brooke and coworkers[47] and Florence and associates[48] have presented a clinical evaluation protocol for DMD—assessing strength, pulmonary function, and functional tasks in combination—that has been demonstrated to be reliable in documenting the disease course in patients with DMD.[12] In addition, the protocol is able to detect not only the therapeutic effect of pharmaceutical intervention, but the time course and differences in various dose levels of such intervention.[29] However, many centers also use the six minute walk test and instrumented strength measurement such as hand held myometry (HHM) in combination with a gross motor assessment designed for DMD such as the North Star Ambulatory Assessment.[49]

Muscle Testing

Measurement of muscle strength by way of manual muscle testing (MMT) remains a valid approach to assessing the progression of disease in children with DMD.[48] MMT has been shown to be both reliable[32] and sensitive to changes in strength in patients with DMD.[50]

Because muscle weakness is characteristic of muscle disease, MMT must be a routine part of the physical therapy evaluation of the child with a dystrophy or a myopathy. The longitudinal results of MMT in children with DMD show linearity in the decline of muscle strength.

By the time the child reaches 7 years of age, or with serial strength scores recorded for 1 year, it is possible to estimate the rate of progression as either rapid (10% deterioration per year), average (5% to 10% deterioration per year), or slow (5% deterioration per year). There is a variation in the rapidity of progression, and MMTDynamo me trylong with performance of functional tasks, helps determine when bracing or wheelchairs will be needed.

Handheld myometry has been used to better quantify muscle strength in boys with DMD.[51,52] HHM and grip and pinch dynamometers can be useful in obtaining more objective and specific muscle strength data. HHM and dynamometry has been found to be reliable and valid in people with weakness.[53–55]

Range of Motion

Standard assessment of joint motion with goniometry should be done periodically. Loss of full ankle dorsiflexion, ankle eversion, knee extension, and hip extension, with resultant contractures, occurs commonly in patients with DMD. Measurement of ankle dorsiflexion, knee extension, hip extension, and ITB tightness are probably the most important aspects of goniometric testing. Measurement of the popliteal angle is useful in monitoring hamstring flexibility. Special tests, including Thomas test and Ober test,[56] can also be useful in monitoring hip flexor and ITB tightness.

Physical Therapy Intervention

The primary problems encountered by children with DMD include the following:

1. Weakness
2. Decreased active and passive ROM
3. Ambulation dysfunction

4. Decreased functional ability
5. Decreased pulmonary function
6. Emotional trauma—individual and family
7. Progressive scoliosis
8. Pain

After a physical examination of the patient, the physical therapist can identify current problems and, on the basis of a thorough understanding of the natural history of the disease process, should be able to predict the trajectory of functional decline. On the basis of the specific areas of concern for each family, it is possible to identify five major goals of management common to all children with DMD:

1. Prevent deformity.
2. Prolong functional capacity.
3. Improve pulmonary function.
4. Facilitate the development and assistance of family support and support of others.
5. Control pain, if necessary.

As the preceding five goals are accomplished, we fulfill our general goal for all individuals with neuromuscular disease: helping them be as independent and comfortable as possible within the limits of their disability.

ROM exercises and stretching, orthotics and splinting, assessment and management of adaptive equipment,and appropriate positioning. Prolonging functional capacity of ensuring safety while functioning may require the prescription of specific orthotics or adaptive equipment can all be helpful in addressing the goals of preventing deformity and prolonging function.

Support for the family may be aided by good rapport with the medical personnel; family education in regard to the disease process and its implications; referral to the Muscular Dystrophy Association (MDA), where they would have access to other families facing similar problems; and the educational, social, financial, and medical care opportunities offered by the MDA. The child and family may be aided by appropriate timing of referral to other associated medical personnel, including orthotist, occupational therapist, nutritionist, adaptive equipment clinic, social worker, or medical specialists, including orthopedic surgeon, pulmonologist, GI specialist, or cardiologist.

Pain control may or may not be necessary and is often dependent on how successful stretching and bracing strategies were in the child's earlier years. Appropriate stretching, fit and positioning in wheelchairs, cushions, alternating pressure pads, or specialized mattresses and hospital beds can go a long way in assisting the control of discomfort in these children.

Home Program

Because much of the responsibility for daily treatment must be assumed by the family or friends of the patient with DMD, an effective program of care at home is essential. Although sustaining enthusiasm and adherence with the home program may be difficult, the likelihood of success can be improved by giving simple instructions, requesting a limited number of exercises and repetitions each day, and offering extensive feedback and positive reinforcement to people in the support system. Outpatient physical therapy once or twice each week at times may be indicated with the primary goal of instructing family members in an appropriate home program, providing safe guidelines for exercise, and monitoring of orthotic or splinting needs. Out-patient physical therapy as well as aquatic therapy may also be indicated in the event of a fracture. Early intervention physical therapy may be indicated for the younger child if diagnosed early, with a transition to physical therapy in the school setting when the child reaches school age. Periodic reevaluation, retraining, and motivation sessions for parents are recommended.

Preventing Deformity

The tendency for development of plantarflexion contractures is usually the earliest problem. Daily stretching of the Achilles tendons should slow down the development of this deformity. The use of night splints in combination with heelcord stretching has been shown to play a significant role in preventing the equinovarus deformity associated with DMD.[16] Use of night splints has been shown to be more effective in preventing deformity of the Achilles tendon than stretching alone.[57] Boys with DMD who used night splints early on (prior to the loss of ambulation) walked independently longer than boys who did not use splints.[58]

No studies are available on which to base a passive stretching prescription, but the regimen often prescribed is between 10 and 15 reps, holding at least 15 seconds, performed at least once, and preferably twice, daily.[59] As soon as the physical therapist sees any change in the length of the hamstring muscles during a periodic evaluation, hamstring stretching is added to the home program. The ITB, hip flexors, and ankle inverters are other structures that must be monitored carefully for loss of ROM, which usually occurs in all these structures as a result of either weakness or static position.

If plantarflexion contractures and the resultant knee, ITB, and hip flexion contractures are allowed to continue unchecked, the child will progress much sooner than necessary to the late ambulation stage and will lose the ability to ambulate at an earlier age than with intervention. At least 2 to 3 hours of standing or walking is recommended daily in addition to stretching to help prevent contracture formation.[59] Therefore, a stander may be considered to aid in the prevention of contractures once ambulation becomes tenuous.

Serial casting to manage plantar flexion contractures has also been used successfully without loss of function in ambulatory boys with DMD,[60] however, careful selection of appropriate candidates and monitoring of functional tasks between cast changes is imperative.

Minimizing Spinal Deformity

As the child's sitting time increases, so does kyphoscoliosis. Previous clinical observations have documented that the convexity will likely be toward the dominant extremity.[61] Because of this relationship, it has been recommended that the child with adequate bilateral manual skills have the wheelchair drive moved from side to side periodically. Many boys, however, are resistant to this idea for practical reasons and preferences and it has not been shown in controlled trials to have an impact.

A lateral support and viscous fluid filled or air cushions in wheelchairs have been used in an attempt to provide appropriate pressure relief and spinal positioning while the patient is seated in the wheelchair, but no studies are available to prove their clinical efficacy. Typically, spinal orthoses are not used in patients with DMD since they have not been shown to delay the development of the spinal curve and might increase work of breathing.

The increasing sophistication of spinal instrumentation within the field of orthopedics has made spinal fixation an option for children with DMD. Physical therapy plays an important role in getting these children "up and moving" within days after surgery, depending on their medical status. Additional post operative concerns specifically for the physical therapist to consider relate to the rigidity of the trunk following fusion. Patients will be taller and entrance into their van as well as other areas need to be considered. Difficulty with self feeding resulting from the limitation in trunk flexibility also needs to be considered. Many patients will benefit from a preoperative evaluation for a mobile arm support so that they can continue be independent with self feeding following surgery. The other concern is seating and positioning. The head rest and back of the wheelchair will need to be adjusted following surgery to accommodate the increased trunk length and if surgical correction results in a pelvic obliquity and asymmetric weight bearing, accommodation within the wheelchair cushion might be necessary. Typically an air filled cushion with special set up to control pressure in different areas of the cushion is optimal however some will find the instability that comes with this type of cushion unacceptable and an asymmetric base below a pressure relieving viscous fluid filled cushion might be preferable. Typically foam or gel cushions provide insufficient pressure relief in this population.

Initially, referrals for spinal stabilization were attempts to improve or stabilize a patient's respiratory function to alleviate the mechanical disadvantage the kyphoscoliosis placed on the already weak respiratory muscles, as well as to prevent the potentially deleterious effect of this scoliosis on respiratory function. Recent studies have demonstrated no salutary effect of segmental spinal stabilization on respiratory function based on either short- or long-term follow-up, but all studies have documented improved sitting comfort, appearance, and stabilization, or improvement of kyphoscoliosis.[62–64]

Activity Level/Active Exercise

Normal, age-appropriate activities for a young boy with DMD are encouraged. The family should be instructed to allow the child to self-limit his activities and allow rests when needed. Care should be taken to avoid overusing muscles and causing fatigue. Signs of overuse weakness include feeling weaker 30 minutes postexercise or excessive soreness 24 to 48 hours after exercise.[65] Other signs include severe muscle cramping, heaviness in the extremities, and prolonged shortness of breath.[65] In general, eccentric muscle activities such as walking or running downhill and closed chain exercises such as squats should be avoided if possible as they tend to cause more muscle soreness. Resistive muscle strengthening is not recommended in boys with DMD because of the risk of contraction-induced muscle injury.

Strengthening

Strength training in boys with DMD has been a subject of controversy. Research on strength training and exercise programs in human subjects with DMD has been limited and has had mixed outcomes. There are few well-controlled, randomized studies, and most have had heterogeneous groups of subjects that include different forms of muscular dystrophies with very different pathologies and clinical presentations. Most of the studies looked at short-term strength gains in individual muscles, but few looked at long-term effects and functional benefits after exercise regimens.

In an early study in 1966, Vignos and Watkins found improvements in weight-lifting capacity in subjects with various forms of muscular dystrophy over a 1-year training period. The strength benefits plateaued in the subjects with DMD after approximately 4 months, and results were less sustainable than in patients with other dystrophies.[66,67] Little functional benefits were found in the subjects with DMD, although greater strength gains and functional benefits were found in subjects with limb-girdle and fascioscapulohumeral forms of muscular dystrophy.[66] In 1979, de Lateur and Giaconi found that isokinetic submaximal strength training minimally improved strength in four boys with DMD without negative side effects.[68] Scott et al.[69] also found absence of deterioration with mild to moderate exercise in the short term. Most of the researchers recommended that exercise programs should be started early on in the course of the disease as individuals with the least amount of muscle impairment benefited the most from training programs.[67,70] There is very little research on exercise in nonambulant patients with DMD.[70]

There is no evidence in humans that increased activity or resistive exercise caused physical deterioration[70]; however, there are ethical issues related to studying this in boys since studies of the mdx mouse, a dystrophin-deficient mouse, have indicated damage to muscle cell membranes, which increases during exercise.[71] Eccentric exercise, in particular, may induce muscle cell damage as was demonstrated in a downhill treadmill running protocol with mdx mice.[72]

Connolly et al. showed 40% to 45% fatigue when comparing the first two and last two pulls when measuring repetitive grip strength of mdx mice.[73] Various other mdx mice studies have contributed to the theory of contraction-induced muscle cell damage. Lack of dystrophin increases susceptibility to muscle cell damage. Microtears in the muscle cell membrane increase with muscle contractions and cause an increase in calcium leak channel activity, which in turn causes an increase in intracellular calcium. This increase causes calcium-dependent proteolysis, which eventually leads to cell death.[71,74]

Endurance exercise such as swimming has been found to be beneficial in mdx mice by increasing the resistance to fatigue in muscles by increasing the proportion of type I (slow oxidative) fibers.[75]

Care must be taken in interpreting and transferring data from the mdx mouse model to humans. The muscle sizes and forces experienced by muscle groups vary, and the stance of the mouse is quite different from humans. In addition, the natural history of the mdx mouse is different than the course of DMD in humans.[70]

More research is needed in the area of strength training; however, given the current research on mice and humans, general recommendations can be made. Avoidance of maximal resistive strength training and eccentric exercise is recommended in boys with DMD. Submaximal endurance training such as swimming or cycling may be beneficial, especially in the younger child with DMD.[76,77]

Prolonging Ambulation

As patients with DMD become weaker, their gait pattern is altered in an attempt to improve stability during walking. Stride length decreases, and the width of the base of support increases to provide a more stable base. The ITB accommodates to the new, shortened position associated with the wider base of support. Weakness in the gluteus medius becomes more pronounced, and the child assumes the typical waddling gait associated with a compensated trendelenberg.

The lordotic curve increases with progressive weakness of the gluteus maximus. As that muscle weakens, the child attempts to increase stability, moving the center of gravity posterior to the fulcrum of the hip joint by pulling the arms back and by exaggerating the lordosis. Stability at the hip joint during standing is now provided passively by structures anterior to the hip joint, primarily the iliofemoral ligament. The presence of a mild knee flexion contracture or the application of an ankle–foot orthosis (AFO) with its angle set in too much dorsiflexion would make ambulation difficult or impossible because of the impact of the weight line and position of the joint axis of the child.

Treatment programs combining passive stretching and lower extremity bracing at night have demonstrated a reduction in the rate of progression of lower extremity contractures and have prolonged ambulation.[58,78] Various surgical interventions—including Achilles tendon lengthening and Yount fasciotomies,[79] tibialis posterior transpositions,[80] and percutaneous tenotomies[81,82]—in combination with vigorous physical therapy and orthotic intervention (bilateral KAFOs), have been reported to improve and prolong ambulation.[83–85]

Whatever the surgical methods, a vigorous postoperative physical therapy program should aim to get the patient up and standing and walking as soon as possible. Active joint stretching will help maintain, and may even increase, ROM at those muscles that have been released. The goal of the postoperative physical therapy program is independent ambulation with a minimum of 3 to 5 hours per day of standing and/or walking. Even when no steps are possible, the child is asked to stand at least 1 hour a day (in a stander if necessary). Optimal stance is with the back in extension so that the center of gravity falls behind the hip joint.

Before any lengthening surgery is considered, families must thoroughly weigh the benefits and risks involved with surgical intervention. When patients are still ambulatory, an overcorrection of a heel-cord contracture may result in immediate loss of ambulation[59] (McDonald, 1998) or may result in ambulation with long leg braces only, which may be cumbersome and not very functional. With the increased use of corticosteroids, many boys are reaping the benefit of prolonged ambulation without the risks of surgical intervention, and many centers do not recommend orthopedic intervention uniformly for all patients with DMD.[27] An alternative to surgical correction for those patients with contractures at the ankle that are limiting ambulation is serial casting. This is best reserved for patients that have developed early contractures and are still good ambulators and able to rise from the floor independently. It is vital to assure that the patient is able to ambulate in the cast, and the casts should be changed either weekly or twice a week to assure that the period of casting is as short as possible.[60]

Wheelchair Use

When ambulation becomes more difficult, falling becomes more frequent, and the child with DMD is unable to get to the places he needs without undue fatigue, it is time to consider the use of a wheelchair for a primary means of mobility. Ideally this will be in advance of a total loss of ambulation and the child will be able to use the chair for longer distances initially. Because of the rapid decline in function and the fatigue induced by pushing a manual wheelchair, a power wheelchair or scooter is generally recommended for a first wheelchair option. Because of the time it takes to order and get insurance approval for a power wheelchair, the therapist will need to estimate when a child will no longer be able to ambulate. According to clinical guidelines developed by Brooke et al (1989)[16] for predicting loss of ambulation, ambulation ceased 2.4 years (range = 1.2 to 4.1 years) after the patient could no longer climb four standard (6-inch) steps in less than 5 seconds and 1.5 years (range, 0.6 to 2.2 years) after more than 12 seconds were needed.[86]

Some boys with DMD and their families initially resist a powered wheelchair and feel a powered scooter is more acceptable socially; however, most scooters do not provide sufficient seating support later in the course of the disease and can be difficult to transport on a bus compared with power wheelchairs. Most school buses are able to transport a wheelchair, but not a scooter. A scooter can be a nice transitional piece of equipment to be used while the child is still ambulatory but requires assistance for longer distances. It is important to consider the timing of this purchase, however, since most insurance companies only reimburse for power mobility every 3 to 5 years. A boy with DMD can quickly decline in function and strength and may require a more supportive wheelchair before funding is available again. It is important to discuss these factors to help patients and their families through the decision-making process.

Initially, a power wheelchair with a conventional joystick and pressure relieving cushion is usually sufficient to meet the needs of the first-time wheelchair user. As scoliosis develops, a lateral support on the convexity of the scoliotic curve is recommended. Bilateral lateral supports are often not used as this may limit the child's ability to shift weight and perform functional tasks in the chair. Patients with DMD often use neck and trunk motions to compensate for trunk weakness in their daily activities; therefore, a seating device that is too stable may restrict a person's ability to perform these maneuvers.[87] A proper pressure-relieving seat cushion is also recommended. Potential pressure areas and/or areas of pain or discomfort can vary depending on the type of spinal deformity present.[87] In patients with scoliosis or kyphoscoliosis, patients complained of pain on the lateral thoracic area and ischial area on the convex side of the curve. In patients with extended spines, pain was reported on bilateral posterior aspects of thighs and bilateral ischial areas. In patients with kyphotic spines, pressure was felt on the sacrum.[87] This should be considered when selecting a pressure-relieving seat cushion.

Once a child undergoes a spinal fusion, some adaptations to the wheelchair and seating components are usually indicated as the child will in effect become taller and less able to compensate for antigravity upper extremity movements. The spinal deformity will now be corrected partially and pressure areas may change as a result. Adjustments in the fit and placement of laterals, headrests, and footrests may need to be made as well as modifications made to the seat cushion. An adjustable mobile arm support may be indicated to support the upper arm in a position to allow the elbow to move in a gravity-eliminated plane to assist with activities such as eating or brushing teeth as the child will no longer be able to compensate for weakness with trunk flexion Success with this type of device is often dependent on the child's ability to overcome the antigravity assist provided and pull the arm down.

As the disease progresses, power tilt-in-space capability will be necessary to provide pressure relief and relaxation as neck and trunk musculature weaken. This may also be required for pressure relief following spinal fusion if a residual pelvic obliquity is present. Additional features such as ventilator adaptations will need to be added on as respiratory status declines. As hand strength becomes more markedly impaired, a change in the power control may be indicated with the first choice for adaptation being a proportional mini joystick.

In a recent study by Pellegrini et al., adults with DMD who had lost their ability to drive a power wheelchair without restriction using a conventional joystick were able to regain unrestricted driving once they changed to an alternative control system including mini-joystick, isometric mini-joystick, finger joystick, or pad.[88] In some drivers, the position of the control needed to be modified as well as the device, such as using an isometric mini-joystick with the chin or lips. The study also found that restricted ability to drive a power wheelchair correlated significantly with a decrease in key pinch strength.[88]

Power mobility, although often resisted initially, can provide boys with DMD a positive sense of independence and important means of independent mobility. Careful discussion of power mobility options and provision of adapted mobility early on in the disease process for long distances, while the boy is still ambulating, can help boys with DMD and their families come to accept the positive aspects of power mobility with confidence when the need for such assistance arises.

Weight Control

The need to guard against obesity is especially important now that the use of corticosteroids in patients with DMD has become more prevalent, as weight gain is a significant side effect. Weight management for the ambulatory child is now equally as important as it is for the child who is limited to a wheelchair. Despite good use of transfer techniques and proper body mechanics by others, excessive weight gain can reduce the child's ability to get transferred and may restrict both mobility and social activity. Moreover, excessive weight gain in the child with neuromuscular disease may not only reduce mobility, but may also have a deleterious effect on self-esteem, posture, and respiratory function.

Edwards and associates have demonstrated that controlled weight reduction in obese children with DMD is a safe and practical way to improve mobility and self-esteem.[89] However, it is probably easier to prevent excessive weight gain in the young, ambulatory child than to initiate dietary restriction in an obese, seated adolescent. It has been proposed that this philosophy of weight control be promoted early for children with neuromuscular disease (taking into account the need for fat intake in early development). Normal growth charts make no allowance for the progressive loss of muscle in DMD, so if the child continues to gain weight according to normal standards, accumulation of fat tissue may occur since there is muscle wasting in boys with DMD. Typically many boys with DMD are overweight at the outset of their teen years and by the end of their teenage years a large portion are underweight as a result of feeding and GI difficulties.[90] Griffiths and Edwards studied the relationships between body composition and breakdown products of muscle which provides data on ideal weight guidelines for weight control in boys with DMD.[91] The physical therapist can play a major role in promoting this weight control philosophy with the child and family. Despite efforts focused on weight control, often boys become too big for their parents to lift and use of a hydraulic lift becomes necessary. One or more family members must be trained in the safe and proper use of such a lift that ideally allows the divided leg sling to be removed following the transfer so adequate pressure relief can be attained from the wheelchair cushion.

Facilitating Sleep

Air or memory foam mattresses or commercial flotation pads often improve sleeping comfort for children with advanced deterioration who have difficulty positioning themselves or changing position at night. These devices also provide relief for family members who might otherwise be up three to five times per night to turn the child. A hospital bed may be useful in the later stages of disease to assist with positioning and transfers, as well as to elevate the head of the bed.

Activities of Daily Living

The physical therapist should routinely assess the child's ability to perform activities of daily living (ADLs). The patient's ability to feed himself, turn pages in a book, and do necessary personal hygiene tasks must all be assessed periodically. The physical therapist may choose to request an occupational therapy consultation. A home visit is most helpful in assessing adaptive equipment needs and accessiblity.

Respiratory Considerations

The physical therapist's role in the pulmonary care of patients with DMD will vary depending on each individual practice setting. All physical therapists working with boys with DMD, however, should be aware of the importance of maintaining good pulmonary health, whether directly or indirectly involved with their respiratory care.

As the diaphragm, trunk, and abdominal muscles weaken, tidal volume and the ability of the patient to effectively clear secretions decreases. Spontaneous periodic deep breaths, as occurs with sighs and yawns, which help to reinflate atelectic zones and spread surfactant, become absent.[92] A good history and periodic sleep studies and pulmonary function testing with the child in both the seated and supine positions are the most effective means of monitoring respiratory insufficiency. In addition, family members should be trained in the techniques of bronchial drainage, chest percussion, and cough assist.[93]

Use of inspiratory and expiratory aids has been shown to prolong survival as well as decrease hospitalizations

significantly when following an intensive protocol.[94] In this study by Bach et al., patients with DMD used noninvasive intermittent positive pressure ventilation (IPPV), manually assisted cough, and mechanically assisted cough (using mechanical insufflation–exsufflation cough assist). They used the above techniques when needed as indicated by an oximeter, to maintain oxyhemoglobin saturation (SaO_2) greater than or equal to 95%. The protocol patients required fewer hospitalizations and days in the hospital when were compared to patients conventionally managed with tracheostomy and IPPV alone.[94] Pulmonary function after the performance of inspiratory muscle training has been shown to improve in boys with DMD.[95] Wanke et al. found improvements in respiratory muscle strength in 10 out of 15 boys with DMD, and improvements remained at 6 months after inspiratory muscle training had ended. The five subjects that did not show improvements after 1 month of training had less than 25% predicted vital capacity; therefore, the authors concluded that inspiratory muscle training was beneficial in the early stage of DMD.[96] In a study of the long-term effects of respiratory muscle training (RMT) in 21 subjects with DMD and SMA type III, the authors concluded that despite the rapidly reversible RMT-induced strength benefits, long-lasting improvements in respiratory load perception persisted after 12 months.[97]

Facilitating Family Support

The physical therapist plays an important role in providing support, motivation, and training of the patient with DMD and his family members. Successful family support depends on the early involvement of the physical therapist to help the family understand the natural history and opportunities that exist to impact progression of the disease with a home program that is monitored and adapted appropriately. Assessment of the social situation and compliance of the family should be part of each visit.

The mild to moderate intellectual impairment found in some of these young boys often imposes both educational and emotional stressors, in addition to the obvious physical changes accompanying DMD. The child learns that the disease will continuously erode the quality and quantity of his existence, and the resultant reliance and dependence on others frequently give rise to stress within the family. Although not a psychotherapist, the physical therapist must be aware of the emotional factors involved with the illness and must provide strong emotional support to optimize the patient and families ability to function as a team with the goal of optimizing the boys function and quality of life. A healthy emotional environment for the family and the child with DMD is at least as important to the child as the prevention of contractures.

Management of Pain

Most of the pain that occurs in these disorders is of three types. First some boys complain of muscle pain which is often reflective of overuse and delayed muscle soreness. Second some older children will develop an impingement syndrome at the shoulder from being lifted for transfers. Finally when the ability to perform independent pressure relief diminishes some children have pain related to pressure either in the wheelchair or in bed at night. If pain becomes a problem, routine methods of treatment aimed at addressing the cause of the pain may be helpful. Sometimes making the patient aware of the cause of muscle aches will allow them to self limit. Other times medical treatment with creatine can be helpful. Instruction in lifting techniques and proper positioning of the hands so as not to over stress the shoulder during lifting or support the arm in the wheelchair properly can be helpful. Finally proper wheelchair and bed positioning can aid in adequately distributing the pressure and diminishing the pain.

Summary

A successful treatment program focused on maintaining flexibility and ameliorating functional limitation through the use of assistive technology should optimize quality of life and maintenance of the maximal functional independence allowed by the child's level of strength (See Case Study A.M., 10-year-old Caucasian with Duchenne Muscular Dystrophy).

 ## Myotonic dystrophy

Myotonic dystrophy type I (DM1) is an autosomal dominant disorder whose gene location is on chromosome 19[97] with the myotonic dystrophy Type II gene being found on the 3rd chromosome.[98] Myotonic Dystrophy presents with a continuum of severity from the severe congenital presentation to parents that are identified only because their children present with weakness[98] and are identified. In the most typical form of DM1, the symptoms are first noticed during adolescence and are characterized by myotonia, a delay in muscle relaxation time, and muscle weakness. The typical presentation to the clinic is with complaints of weakness and stiffness. Stiffness, which is often the major complaint, is characteristic of the myotonia. Patients often have a characteristic physical appearance that includes a long, thin face with temporal and masseter muscle wasting; frontal balding; and weakness and wasting of the sternocleidomastoids. The pattern of weakness in DM1 presents first with distal wasting and weakness, manifested by a foot drop and difficulty opening jars while type II myotonic dystrophy presents primarialy with a phenotype of proximal weakness. In type I, proximal muscle weakness occurs in the later stage of the disease. The most severe form of DM1 is congenital and is associated with generalized muscular hypoplasia, mental retardation, and a high incidence of neonatal mortality. Children with congenital DM1 are typically born to mothers afflicted with the disorder and DM1 demonstrates

anticipation with each generation being more severely affected than the prior generation. Because DM1 is inherited in an autosomal dominant pattern, an individual with the disease has a 50/50 chance of each offspring having the disease. The severe congenital form of DM1 is characterized by maternal transmission only. This group is often plagued with mental retardation, speech disturbances, delayed motor milestones, distal weakness, and spinal deformities. With survival to adulthood, these individuals follow the pattern of the classic course of the disease, in which cataracts and cardiac conduction abnormalities are common. There is involvement not only of skeletal muscle, but also smooth muscle and cardiac conduction defects are often seen, particularly first-degree heart block. There may be associated infertility, decreased respiratory drive, and numerous endocrine problems. Currently, there is no treatment for the disorder, and the etiology of the genetic defect is unknown. There is no curative pharmacologic treatment, although some medications may be used to ameliorate the symptoms of myotonia. The objectives of current therapeutic intervention are to reduce the distal wasting and weakness and control the spinal deformities.

Death in these individuals is usually caused by heart block or problems secondary to decreased respiratory drive. The respiratory complications may be severe and once mechanically ventilated, these patients are very difficult to wean. The congenital forms of DM1 may be accompanied by severe developmental delays, in which case intervention that employs various motor development approaches may be beneficial.

Limb-girdle muscular dystrophy

Limb-girdle muscular dystrophy (LGMD) is the term used to refer to a group of progressive muscular dystrophies that primarily affect the proximal musculature. The initial presentation can be quite variable, extending from early childhood into adulthood. Unlike DMD, the underlying pathology of LGMD is quite heterogeneous. There is an ever growing list of distinct LGMD genes identified (Table 9.3). These have been labeled 1A through H representing the dominant forms and 2A through Q representing the recessive forms.[99] With the elucidation of the underlying genetic and biochemical defects that can cause LGMD, it has become apparent that each of these defects is associated with specific phenotypic patterns. It is beyond the scope of this chapter to discuss all of the forms of LGMD here; however, we will discuss the ones that present typically in childhood and may present for treatment in pediatric practice.

The sarcoglycanopathies (LGMD C, D, E, and F) represent those forms of LGMD that most closely resemble the progression of Duchenne. The sarcoglycanopathies are recessively inherited, with a significant number of cases presenting sporadically.[100] These four forms of LGMD are caused by a deficiency of a group of muscle membrane

TABLE 9.3	Limb-girdle Muscular Dystrophy[165,166]	
Disease Name	**Gene, Inheritance**	**Protein Product**
LGMD2A Calpainopathy	15q15.1 Recessive	Calpain-3
LGMD2B Dysferlinopathy	2p13.2 Recessive	Dysferlin
LGMD2C γ-Sarcoglycanopathy	13q12.12 Recessive	γ-Sarcoglycan
LGMD2D α-Sarcoglycanopathy	17q21.33 Recessive	α-Sarcoglycan
LGMD2E β-Sarcoglycanopathy	4q12 Recessive	β-Sarcoglycan
LGMD2F δ-Sarcoglycanopathy	5q33.3 Recessive	δ-Sarcoglycan
LGMD2G Telethoninopathy	17q12 Recessive	Telethonin
LGMD2H	9q33.1 Recessive	TRIM32
LGMD2I KRP	19q13.32 Recessive	Fukutin-related protein (FKRP)
LGMD2J Titinopathy	2q24.3 Recessive	Titin
LGMD2K Disorder of Glycosilation	9q34.13	O-mannosyltransferase 1
LGMD2L	11p14.3	Anoctamin 5
LGMD2M Disorder of Glycosilation	9q31.2 Recessive	Fukutin
LGMD2N Disorder of Glycosilation	14q24.3 Recessive	O-mannosyltransferase 2
LGMD2O Disorder of Glycosilation	1p34.1 Recessive	O-mannose beta-1,2-N-acetylglucosaminyl transferase
LGMD2P	3p21.31 Recessive	Dystroglycan 1
LGMD2Q	8q24.3 Recessive	Plectin 1f
LGMD1A Myotilinopathy	5q31.2 Dominant	Myotilin
LGMD1B Laminopathy	1q22 Dominant	Lamin A/C
LGMD1C Caveolinopathy	3p25.3 Dominant	Caveolin-3
LGMD1D (OMIM) (HUGO: LGMD E)	2q35 Dominant	Desmin
LGMD1E (HUGO: LGMD E)	7q36.3 Dominant	DNAJ/HSP40 homolog, subfamily B, Member6
LGMD1F	7q32.1–32.2 Dominant	
LGMD1G	4p21 Dominant	
LGMD1H	3p25.1–p23 Dominant	

proteins (Fig. 9.1). The sarcoglycan proteins are coded for on four different chromosomes: γ-sarcoglycan at 13q12, α-sarcoglycan at 17q21.1, β-sarcoglycan at 4q12, and δ-sarcoglycan at 5q33. A deletion of any one of these proteins as the primary defect results in problems incorporating the entire complex or portions of the complex into the membrane. In almost half the cases, this results in incomplete incorporation of dystrophin in the membrane.[100] As a result, there is a great degree of phenotypic overlap between these muscular dystrophies in addition to a similarity between the sarcoglycanopathies and DMD.

Findings on medical evaluation include elevated serum CK to anywhere from 5 times to 100 times normal.[101] The EMG examination is marked by myopathic findings similar to those seen in DMD. Muscle biopsy is typically needed to determine the diagnosis, although this is changing with the advent of inexpensive genetic panels. Muscle biopsy should show a variation in fiber size, degenerating and regenerating fibers, and central nuclei. When stained by immunohistochemical techniques with monoclonal antibodies to the specific sarcoglycan proteins, the specific pathologic basis of the impairment can often be identified. When biopsy is able to identify the protein abnormality genetic testing can also be used to finalize the diagnosis.[102]

Patients with sarcoglycanopathies have an increased risk of dilated cardiac myopathy. Politano et al.[101] found a 40% rate of presymptomatic cardiomyopathy in these patients in addition to signs of hypoxic myocardial insults. The patients with dilated cardiomyopathy had primarily γ- and δ-sarcoglycanopathies, and those with hypoxic damage had β-, γ-, and δ-sarcoglycanopathies.

These four proteins, α-, β-, γ-, and δ-sarcoglycan, are closely associated with dystrophin, the defective protein in DMD. LGMD, in general, and sarcoglycanopathies, in particular, can present with a similar albeit somewhat more variable phenotype when compared with DMD. The distribution of muscle weakness is marked by a proximal-to-distal gradient, and in sarcoglycanopathies the abductors and extensors of the hip are the most severely and first involved. Other muscles of the upper extremity that become involved include the deltoids, pectoralis major, rhomboids, and infraspinatus, and a significant number of patients demonstrate a progressive lordosis and anterior pelvic tilt.[100]

A second form of LGMD, type 2A or calpainopathy, is also recessively inherited and is caused by the absence of calpain-3 that results from a deletion on chromosome 15q15.1–15.3.[103] Calpain-3 is the first enzyme that was identified as the causative defect of a progressive muscular dystrophy. Calpain-3 is part of a larger group of calpain molecules whose exact function is still not entirely clear but may be involved in the modulation of cytoskeletal proteins. Calpain-3 can also be reduced in patients with LGMD2B and 2J because presumably calpain acts together with dysferlin and connectin (titin) in the membrane repair process and are the primary protein defects in these forms of LGMD (Fig. 9.1).[104]

Clinical presentation of LGMD2A includes a typically elevated CK and muscle biopsy findings with degenerating and regenerating fibers, central nuclei, and a variation in fiber size. The EMG will have typical myopathic features. Patients show no intellectual deficits, and cardiac defects have not been reported at increased rates in LGMD2A.[105] Unlike other muscular dystrophies, there seems to be no direct correlation between the amount of protein identified on biopsy and the severity of clinical presentation,[104] and the age at presentation does not necessarily provide guidance for the timing of ambulation loss.[106] However, patients with in-frame genetic defects on both alleles tend to have a later onset of symptoms and a later diagnosis as compared with those with heterozygous or homozygous null mutations. Ambulation typically continues throughout childhood, with the average child loosing ambulation in the late teens or early 20s; however, there can be a significant variability between patients, with some continuing to ambulate into middle age and others loosing ambulation in early childhood.[105]

LGMD2A has a wide variation in the severity of presentation and in the course of the disease. Typically, the presentation is in the second decade of life initially with proximal atrophy. This is most commonly expressed as scapular winging. Weakness of the elbow flexors can also be present. The wrist extensors are typically weaker than the flexors, and the hip adductors are more affected, while the abductors are preserved long into the disease process. The knee extensors typically remain stronger than the flexors, and the ankle evertors are typically weaker than the invertors. Contractures are typically found in the calf muscles along with atrophy of this muscle in most European patients; however, in Brazilian patients hypertrophy can be found in the calf. Finger-flexion and elbow-flexion contractures may also be present early on in the disease process. These muscle imbalances correspond with a typical standing posture of hip abduction, knee hyperextension, and inversion at the ankle that is preserved long into the disease process. Patients with LGMD 2A typically remain able to stand with support far into the disease process because of this pattern of contracture and muscle involvement.[105,106]

The last form of LGMD that will be discussed here is LGMD 2I. LGMD 2I is recessively inherited and caused by a mutation in the fukutin-related protein gene (FKRP). This gene is also the cause of some forms of CMD, which we will discuss later. The gene is found on chromosome 19q13.3,[107] and the encoded protein FKRP is a glycosyltransferase that aids in the O-glycosylation of α-dystroglycan and a as a result of its absence α-dystroglycan does not form properly.[108] α-dystroglycan is located in the extracellular space and is associated with the dystrophin complex that spans the membrane and proper glycosylation is required for its association with Laminin-α2.[109]

Diagnosis is established first by clinical presentation which is marked by weakness. EMG shows a typical myopathic pattern and an elevated serum CK which is typically is in the thousands. Muscle biopsy is typically characterized

by a variation in fiber size with type 1 predominance, degenerating and regenerating fibers, an increase in central nuclei, and increased connective tissue.[107] Immunohistochemistry in these patients can be variable, with the most common finding being a reduction of laminin α-2; reductions in α-dystroglycan can also be found.[110]

Clinical presentation of patients with LGMD2I can vary somewhat, with initial onset of symptoms typically in the first two decades of life. A significant number of patients present with a Duchenne-like phenotype. In these patients, onset is typically in the preschool years. The pattern of weakness is similar to that of Duchenne, with proximal weakness predominating and gastroc/soleus contracture and hypertrophy most pronounced. However, in the more severely involved patients, the shoulder girdle is more involved than the pelvic girdle. In the milder patients, the opposite is true. In the more severe patients, respiratory function can become an issue as the disease progresses; however, this appears to progress at a slower rate than Duchenne. Most patients with LGMD 2I typically maintain fairly good respiratory function throughout the first two decades of life.[111,112] Cardiac defects are a common characteristic of LGMD2I.[113] Male patients with heterozygous mutations are at increased risk for developing dilated cardiac myopathy when compared with female patients or those with homozygous mutations[112] and as a result these patients need to be monitored more closely by their physician.

Clinical care for patients with LGMD revolves around anticipating the development of contractures and conservative management with the use of dynamic or static resting splints to maintain muscle length. ROM exercises and exercise to optimize muscle endurance such as swimming can be considered, but because this is a dystrophic process, strengthening exercise, especially of the eccentric variety should be avoided.

▶ Congenital myopathy

Congenital myopathy describes a group of diseases, including nemaline myopathy, central core myopathy, and centronuclear (myotubular) myopathy. The three broad categories are based on the microscopic appearance of the muscle; centronuclear myopathy is marked by an abnormal predominance of central nuclei as compared to the normally peripherally placed nuclei of the muscle cell, central core myopathy is marked by the presence of central clearing, or cores, within the cytoplasm, and nemaline myopathy is characterized by nemaline rods which can be seen by electron microscopy. These as well as the other congenital myopathies typically result from abnormalities of the sarcomeric proteins. These diseases are characterized by weakness and muscle atrophy that typically presents at birth. There are, however, forms that can present later in life. The congenital myopathies represent a group of disorders that are less well characterized when compared with the other disorders we have discussed thus far. The broad diagnostic classifications are based on morphologic characteristics found on muscle biopsy, with subtyping based on clinical features. In each broad category, there are a number of genetic mutations that can be the predisposing factor; however, there is significant clinical variability that can be seen. Here we will discuss two of the most common congenital myopathies, nemaline myopathy and central core myopathy.

Nemaline myopathy has a wide range in the severity of clinical presentation as well as heterogeneity of genetic causes.[114] Nemaline is a genetically heterogenous myopathy with mutations in the genes that code for either actin, nebuline, or tropomyosin (β-2 and 3)as well as other proteins. The inheritance pattern is most often sporadic but can also be dominant or recessive. Pathologically, on muscle biopsy there are cytoplasmic inclusions visible on light microscopy and called either rods or nemaline bodies seen by electron microscopy that represent deposits of z-line proteins.[115–117]

Nemaline myopathy has been divided into seven different forms on the basis of severity and other factors by the European Neuromuscular Center. These types include the typical or classic form, the severe form, the intermediate form, the mild form, and the adult-onset form. In addition, there is a severe Amish type with neonatal onset and a category for other forms. The typical form of nemaline myopathy presents at birth or early infancy with respiratory insufficiency being an issue, especially at night. These patients often become ambulatory; however, some will need wheeled mobility. The severe form is characterized by weakness from birth. Often, in this type of nemaline myopathy, no spontaneous movement is evident. These patients can have arthrogryposis and fractures at birth. Lack of respiratory effort and the resulting respiratory insufficiency and ventilator dependence often lead to death in the first year of life. The intermediate form presents in infancy or at birth. Patients are able to breath on their own by a year and either do not ambulate at all or progress and develop contractures over time and loose the ability to ambulate by 11 years of age. The mild form presents in childhood, often with a history of normal developmental milestones. This form is often slowly progressive, and in the later stages this form can be clinically indistinguishable from the classic or typical presentation. The adult form tends to be more progressive and can also demonstrate inflammatory change on biopsy as well as cardiomyopathy.[118,119] The most common form is the classic or typical form representing 43% of cases in one series.[120] The intermediate and severe congenital forms represent 20% and 16%, respectively, with the less severe form with childhood and adult-onset representing the remaining cases.

Central core myopathy is named for the appearance of the presence of histological cores on muscle biopsy. If the cores appear centrally and are large, the name *central core myopathy* is used, and if there are multiple small cores, the term *multiminicore myopathy* is used. Despite the use of these two terms, these only represent a pathologic description and

may represent different stages in the same disease process in some cases. Family members with presumably the same disease process may have both central and multiminicores, and the same patient first with multiminicores may later in the disease process present with central cores.[116] These cores are areas within the muscle that contain no mitochondria, are negative for oxidative enzymes, and contain a collection of proteins that include many of the proteins that have been identified in other muscle diseases as well as many other proteins. One of the most common genes identified as being responsible for central core disease is found on 19q13; it codes for the ryanodine receptor 1 protein (RYR1) and controls the release of calcium from the sarcoplasmic reticulum.[116,121,122]

Clinically, central core myopathy can be relatively static or mildly progressive over long periods and phenotype/genotype correlations are emerging surrounding the specific calcium channel abnormality that a given mutation yields with some variability also being based around the existence of dominant vs. recessive inheritance.[123] The pattern of weakness typically includes facial weakness, neck flexor weakness, and proximal weakness with the legs being more involved than the arms.[124] There is a spectrum of patients with central core myopathy, and more severe forms have been noted. The other clinical feature of patients with RYR1 mutations is the susceptibility to malignant hyperthermia, which is a severe reaction to anesthesia.

Centronuclear (myotubular) myopathy is the other main category of congenital myopathy and results primarily from an abnormality in the MTM1 gene which codes for the protein myotubularin however other genes also contribute to a portion of this population. Clinical presentation typically is more severe with ventilator and wheelchair dependence being common. Myopathic facial muscles with opthalmoplegia are a common occurrence.[114]

▶ Congenital muscular dystrophy

CMD can be divided into those CMDs with CNS involvement and those without CNS involvement. Fukuyama CMD, Walker–Walburg syndrome, and muscle–eye–brain disease represent the group of CMDs with CNS involvement and all typically demonstrate muscle, brain, and eye abnormalities. The typical brain abnormalities include a cobblestone lissencephaly with cerebral and cerebellar cortical dysplasia secondary to a neuronal migration abnormality. Eye and vision abnormalities span a wide range of possible abnormalities and vary from one disease to the other, but may include structural abnormalities of the eye as well as myopia and retinal detachment.[125] The muscle abnormalities are based on abnormal glycosylation of α-dystroglycan resulting from the absence of various enzymes that facilitate the process of glycosylation. Glycosylation is the addition of glycans to a protein to form a glycoprotein. As a result of the common pathophysiology, there is significant overlap in the clinical presentation of these diseases and the pathologic findings encountered during the diagnostic workup. All present congenitally in the typical case although there are also milder limb girdle phenotypes. Walker–Warburg syndrome is the most severe of the CMDs, and children typically die by 3 years of age. Muscle–eye–brain disease has a variable clinical picture and presents in infancy. The more mildly involved patients may ambulate for a period of time during childhood; however, their functional abilities are limited by spasticity and ataxia resulting from the brain abnormalities as well as the muscle weakness. Most patients with Fukuyama CMD will achieve standing, and some can take steps in early childhood. Typically, in the second decade, respiratory failure becomes a problem, beginning with nocturnal hypoventilation. This can progress, limiting the life expectancy of these patients to the third decade of life. Cardiomyopathy is also a feature commonly seen in these patients, and they should be periodically followed by cardiology.

Merosin (laminin)-negative CMD (also known as LAMA2 related CMD or MDC1A) is the most common CMD, representing half of all cases of CMD. The absence of merosin in the muscle (Fig. 9.1) results from an abnormality of the LAMA2 gene found on chromosome 6q2. Merosin-negative CMD also shows CNS involvement in the form of abnormalities of the periventricular and subcortical white matter. To better anticipate the clinical course it is important to subdivide the group by the presence of total absence of Merosin and partial absence, with complete absence predicting a more severe phenotype. The clinical course of this disorder is characterized by severe weakness at birth or in early infancy and the development of contractures, particularly at the ankle and eventually at the knee and elbow. The severe weakness can improve over time, and most patients will sit by 2 or 3 years of age and upwards of 25% will stand or walk with bracing. Muscle strength can be stable over time; however, nocturnal hypoventilation may be a problem for many of these patients, typically by the second or third decade of life, and a third may have seizures or cardiac abnormalities.[126,127]

Ullrich CMD results from the abnormalities of collagen VI. Collagen VI is composed of 3 associated proteins which form a triple helix. Abnormalities of Collagen VI can result from mutations of any of the 3 subunits COL6A1, A2, or A3. COL6A1 is located on 21q22.3, COL6A2 is located on chromosome 22q23.3, and COL6A3 is located on chromosome 2q37.[128] Collagen VI is found in the extracellular matrix (Fig. 9.1) and presumably acts to transmit force from the muscle to the bone and tendon. Ullrich CMD is typically recessively inherited; however, dominant negative inheritance represents a significant minority of these patients.[129] A dominant negative exists where the affected gene product negatively impacts the nonaffected alleles protein production. The milder form of collagen VI abnormality, Bethlem myopathy, is typically dominantly inherited and although historically they were viewed as separate conditions the phynotype is one of a continuous spectrum and there is a movement toward referring to these disorders as

COL6 related myopathy. On muscle biopsy, findings can range from mild myopathic findings to dystrophic in the more severe patients; however, it is rare to see necrotic and regenerating fibers. Classically, findings include variation in fiber size and infiltration of the muscle by fatty and fibrotic tissue. Patients with Ullrich CMD typically have weakness at birth in all but the mildest cases. There is an increased risk of congenital hip dislocation as well as torticollis and arthrogyposis, the latter two of these typically improve with stretching. Gross motor skills are typically delayed; however, there are improvements seen in motor skills in the first few years of life, and patients typically gain the ability to sit independently and stand with bracing. A significant number of patients also gain the ability to ambulate independently. Contractures of the hips, knees, and elbows are typical and are combined with hyperlaxity of the distal joints in addition to laxity at the shoulders and hips. In patients that achieve ambulation, the ability to walk, is most often limited by progressive knee flexion contractures or planovarus contracture at the ankle. Respiratory insufficiency can be a problem for the more severely affected patients as they age and can be found in patients who are still ambulatory.[127]

Physical therapy intervention in CMD and congenital myopathy needs to take into account the natural history of the specific disorder, and realistic goals need to be planned on the basis of the natural history of the disease. A focus on the maintenance of flexibility with stretching and appropriate bracing or serial casting as needed is important. Bracing may be needed for nighttime positioning, for standing or ambulation, as well as for those who are not ambulatory. Standers and wheelchairs as well as bathroom adaptations may provide practical assistance. Even in those patients who have some household ambulation, power mobility may be necessary for community mobility or for longer distances at school and in the community.

▶ Spinal muscular atrophy

SMA is a disorder that is manifested by interneuron abnormality and a loss of anterior horn cells. This results in a phenotypic spectrum of disease states that have been divided into three types of SMA on the basis of a functional classification system.

Three categories of SMA occur in childhood:

1. SMA type I (Werdnig–Hoffman disease)
2. SMA type II
3. SMA type III (Kugelberg–Welander disease)

The classification of a child with SMA into one of the above types of SMA is based solely on the child's maximal functional abilities. The child that is so weak that they have never learned to sit is diagnosed with SMA type I. Those children that learn to sit but never learn to walk without an assistive device have type II SMA and the children that walk independently are diagnosed with SMA type III.

Genetics

SMA is inherited as an autosomal recessive disorder. The underlying genetic defect is located on chromosome 5q13, where the survival motor neuron (SMN) gene is located and the SMN protein is coded for.[129,130] In this region of the chromosome, there are two homologous genes, SMN1 and SMN2, that code for the SMN protein. Typically, there is one copy of SMN1 and multiple copies of SMN2. SMN1 produces most of the protein that the body uses, and when the gene is affected it produces no protein and the SMN2 gene must be relied on to produce the SMN protein. Most (85% to 90%) of the SMN protein that SMN2 produces is not functional. The total amount of SMN produced in patients with SMA, therefore depends on how many copies of SMN2 the patient has. The number of SMN2 copies also correlates with how severe the phenotypic presentation of the disease is.

Pathophysiology

SMN plays a role in the function of all cells, mediating the assembly of a set of proteins that associate with RNA and function as part of the splicing machinery in every cell. The alpha motor neuron and interneurons are most impacted by the diminished levels of SMN although there is some recent data that other tissues are affected as well[131] the phenotype of SMA is dictated by motor neuron loss and patients with SMA as a result have a portion of their alpha motor neurons undergo apoptosis.

As a result of the loss of motor neurons, EMG results will be characterized by diminished compound motor unit action potentials (CMAP) that are often of short duration; the diminished CMAP will track the course of the disease. Positive sharp waves and fibrillations are also found, and typically conduction velocities and sensory studies are normal.[132] The number of motor units are also diminished in children with SMA. The number of remaining motor units can be estimated by EMG using motor unit number estimation (MUNE). The MUNE reflects the number of lower motor neurons that innervate a given muscle. In addition to CMAP, the MUNE can be used to monitor the progress of the underlying pathologic process affecting the motor neuron.[133]

Typically, the histopathology found on muscle biopsy is characterized by groups of small atrophic fibers interspersed with groups of large hypertrophic fibers (Fig. 9.9). This type of grouped atrophy is characteristic of a neurogenic process. The groups of atrophic fibers are the result of lack of innervation to that motor unit. All three types of SMA have an underlying pathology that affects the interneuron and anterior horn cell; as a result, they share some common clinical features. All children with SMA will demonstrate some degree of weakness, albeit to varying degrees, depending on the type of the disease. Patients with SMA will typically have absent deep tendon reflexes; however, this is not completely

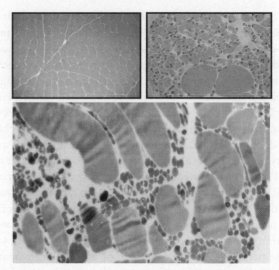

FIGURE 9.9 Neuropathic changes associated with SMA as compared with normal (upper left). Note the hypertrophic changes and grouped atrophy.

uniform. About half of patients will have fasciculations that can be seen in the tongue as spontaneous small muscle contractions[134]; these can be seen on muscle ultrasound at times even if they are not visible in the tongue. Since only the lower motor neuron is affected, sensation is typically intact as is cognitive function in patients with SMA. Since this is a lower motor neuron disease, no upper motor neuron signs should be noted.

SMA Type I (Werdnig–Hoffman Disease)

SMA Type I is almost always noted within the first 3 months of life. However, the diagnosis may not be made for a number of months. Depending on severity, decreased movement may be noted during pregnancy or within the first weeks or months after birth. Axial hypotonicity is often the first symptom noted and difficulty feeding is often a concern shortly after the onset of weakness. Muscle wasting is often severe, and spontaneous movements are infrequent and of small amplitude. On examination, the infant with SMA type I will present with a head lag on pull-to-sit and will drape over the examiner's hand when a landau is performed. The infant will be dominated by gravity, and in supine the legs will be abducted and flexed, and the arms will move primarily with the elbows on the surface, and if they can be brought to midline, this will be with difficulty. In the most severely affected infants, axial strength will be so diminished that in supine the head will not be able to be maintained in midline. Prone position is poorly tolerated due to respiratory limitation and prone skills will be similarly limited. Infants with SMA Type I will not be able to prop and typically cannot turn their heads from side to side in prone. In vertical, some infants will demonstrate tenuous head control, while most will not be able to maintain their heads erect.

Infants with SMA Type I typically develop significant oral motor weakness that makes feeding progressively more difficult. These infants have difficulty taking in sufficient calories to gain weight and thrive. Medical options for supplemental feeding in these patients include nasogastric feeding or the surgical placement of a gastrostomy tube with Nissan fundoplication to diminish the potential for gastro-esophageal reflux.

Patients with SMA Type I also have limited respiratory function and develop an abnormal paradoxical pattern of breathing, with the diaphragmatic muscles playing the primary role in ventilation. In these infants, inspiration is diaphragmatically initiated, and as negative pressure develops in the thoracic cavity, the intercostals and other thoracic muscles that typically stabilize the ribcage fail and the ribcage collapses with each breath. Typically, the belly also rises as the diaphragm lowers. In the weakest infants, the chest and the abdomen will be directly out of phase. In the infants who are a bit stronger, the chest will stabilize or expand briefly with the abdomen prior to collapsing, this is in contrast to the normal condition of almost simultaneous abdominal and thoracic expansion. Pulmonary infections are common in infants with SMA Type I and pulmonary management is an important facet of care for these patients. Both the inability to take a deep breath and the lack of an effective cough can cause serious respiratory complications, including atelectasis and pneumonia. Percussion and postural drainage should be recommended for use when the infant has upper respiratory infections to move the secretions from the small airways. These infants may also be treated with a mechanical in-exsufflator or coughalator that delivers a positive pressure insufflation followed by an expulsive exsufflation that simulates a cough as an additional means of airway clearance[135] and as a way of maintaining flexibility of the lungs and ribcage. Approximately half of the children with infantile SMA do not survive beyond 2 years of age without the assistance of mechanical ventilation.[136] For those that do choose to have tracheostomies or use noninvasive ventilation, the life span can be extended significantly beyond this with half of children with SMA type 1 surviving to 10 years of age in one trial with aggressive respiratory management and nutritional support.[8,136]

Children with SMA Type I have such severe weakness that it is difficult for them to participate in play activities. Switch toys are appropriate for those children that survive past 8 months (when cause and effect begins to develop) to allow the child access to play. In addition, younger infants may benefit from a sling-and-spring setup that can be made from theraband tubing and velfoam cuffs attached to the infant carrier to aid in antigravity shoulder movement and to promote access to toys. The approach to physical therapy for these children must be aimed at quality of life for both the child and the family.

SMA Type II

Type II SMA also affects infants but is less severe than SMA Type I. Initial presentation is typically later in the first year of life when the child is noted to not be pulling to stand. These children are characterized by proximal weakness and wasting of the extremities and trunk musculature. Fasciculations are common on examination of the tongue in these patients. There is also often a fine resting tremor when the child attempts to use the limbs. This is not an intention tremor, but has been referred to as a minipolymyoclonus.[8]

In children with SMA type II, there is a delay in the acquisition of motor skills that is somewhat variable between children. Approximately one-third of children with SMA type II will sit by the normal time of 6 months, and 90% will be able to sit by their first birthday.[137] Some children may continue to gain skills throughout the second year, but there is typically a peak after which a slow decline in skills ensues, the rapidity of which depends largely on the underlying disease severity. Of those children that become independent sitters, and are diagnosed with SMA type II, 75% will remain independent sitters until 7 years, and half will remain sitting at 14 years of age.[138] Motor skills that employ a long lever arm are most difficult for these patients, and as a result, prone and quadruped skills are most delayed because it is difficult to maintain head control in these positions. Transitions to and from sit will also be difficult because of the weight of the head during the transition. Despite a slow overall decline in function as these children grow up, there are often long periods of relative functional stability spanning years. Despite what one would anticipate on the basis of the decline in function, there is not a detectable loss in strength over time in children with SMA.[139] However, this data represents a group of patients over the age of 4 years, since younger children cannot be reliably tested.

The pattern of weakness seen in the extremities is most notable for the relative strength in the distal muscles as compared with the proximal muscles. On average, strength in patients with type II and III SMA falls between 20% and 40% of predicted based on age. Quadriceps strength tends to be the most diminished, averaging 5% of normal. However, in patients with SMA that ambulate, the variation in quadriceps strength can be threefold as compared with patients that do not ambulate.[140,141]

Contracture formation is also an issue in the management of patients with SMA type II. Limitations of the knee flexors and ankle plantarflexors are frequently the most significant contractures in the lower extremity, and contractures of the elbow flexors and wrist flexors are the most significant in the arm. For the hands, resting hand splints are appropriate for night use, and for the legs, knee–ankle–foot orthosis (KAFO), as discussed in the next section, will aid in maintaining ROM. In addition, a daily stretching program will help maintain the patient's flexibility.

By definition, these children do not ambulate independently; however, some of these children may learn to walk with bracing or an assistive device.[142] However, the ambulation is often not functional. Nonetheless, it is important to encourage standing in patients with SMA type II. Standing

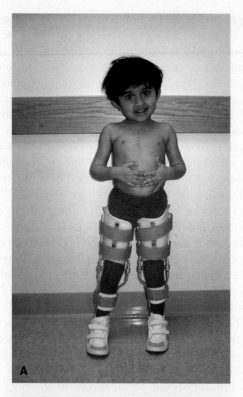

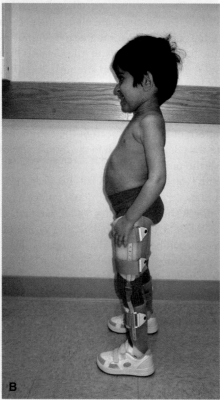

FIGURE 9.10 Anterior–posterior **(A)** and lateral view **(B)** of 3-year-old with type II SMA wearing ischial weight-bearing knee–ankle–foot orthoses.

will act to maintain joint mobility, maintain bone stock, prevent problems associated with long-term wheelchair sitting, and attempt to keep the patient's back as straight as

possible for as long as possible. These patients often require KAFOs for standing, and as they become weaker, the addition of a pelvic band or the use of a stander or parapodium may be necessary. The proximal portion of the KAFO may be shaped for ischial weight bearing to improve comfort and control of the proximal femur (Fig. 9.10). During the school-age years when the child becomes too heavy to lift into standing, a transition to a more traditional stander becomes appropriate if contactures allow and bracing may be only necessary to stabilize the foot and ankle. For those children who can continue in a standing program, there are a number of options, some that will accommodate flexion contractures and others that assist in the transfer, alleviating some of the burden on the parent.

Feeding and swallowing difficulties are seldom a problem early in the course of the disease, but many children do not gain weight well, and some require supplemental feeding as they get older to maintain optimal body weight.

These children often survive into adulthood, but are vulnerable to pulmonary infection and may require mechanical ventilation either at night secondary to nocturnal hypoventilation or full time. The use of a mechanical in-exsufflator in this population is also helpful in airway clearance, as is percussion and postural drainage during intercurrent illness, since these patients also lack the muscle strength to produce a strong cough and clear secretions that develop with illness.[135]

Children with SMA type II are predisposed to kyphoscoliosis, similar to that which affects other children with neuromuscular weakness. Spinal bracing has been characterized as not preventing progression of the spinal curve,[143] and when spinal bracing is worn, pulmonary function is limited by the external restriction as compared with pulmonary function without bracing.[144] However, as a practical matter for patients who have pain or postural instability as well as scoliosis, a soft spinal orthosis can provide support for the trunk and allow improved tolerance in sitting for those patients who choose not to have a fusion. Typically, scoliosis in this population and in patients with type III SMA has been treated surgically with segmental spinal fusion. This prevents the inevitable progression of the curve, which can be more rapid once the patient is in a wheelchair full time.[145] However, there is a downside to spinal fusion. Fusion can also be associated with some loss of functional skill. When the flexibility of the spine is taken away, some tasks can become more difficult, especially in the weaker patients. Ambulatory patients (with SMA type III) are also at risk of functional decline following a fusion since spinal and pelvic flexibility is diminished and a fusion that maintains pelvic mobility might be preferable in this population.[146] Despite this, typically the benefits of preventing the inevitable progression of the scoliosis and the associated pulmonary and functional decline outweigh the risks associated with the surgery, and patients typically report improved comfort and sitting balance following surgery.[147]

SMA Type III (Kugelberg–Welander Disease)

SMA type III is characterized by symptoms of progressive weakness, wasting, absent reflexes and fasciculations. Age of presentation can vary from the toddler years into adulthood, the latter of which some would classify as type IV. Proximal muscles are usually involved first, and because of the age and pattern of presentation, this disease may be confused with the muscular dystrophies. Deep tendon reflexes are decreased, but contractures are unusual, and progressive spinal deformities are uncommon as long as the child remains ambulatory. Diagnosis is established on the basis of the clinical picture and the results of diagnostic laboratory studies, including an EMG and muscle biopsy, which show denervation as in the other forms of SMA. In addition, genetic testing will show a deletion of the SMN gene on the fifth chromosome.

Prognosis in patients with SMA type III can be aided by a good developmental history. Patients who have symptoms that begin prior to 2 years of age have a relatively poorer prognosis when compared with patients who have symptoms that begin after the age of 2. Russman et al. followed 159 patients with SMA and found that in patients with SMA type III, if symptoms begin after 2 years of age, on average patients continued to ambulate until 44 years of age while in those who began to have symptoms prior to 2 years of age, ambulation was maintained until an average of 12 years of age.[138]

Treatment from a physical therapy standpoint is focused primarily on the maintenance of function and flexibility. Patients need to be braced appropriately while they are still ambulating and for standing after they stop ambulating. Once patients become more difficult to handle in braces for standing, standers, where the patient is aided which aid patients to standing from a sitting position, can be helpful to maintain flexibility and bone stock by allowing weight bearing through the long bones.

▶ Charcot–Marie–Tooth disease

CMT disease, also known as hereditary motor and sensory neuropathy (HMSN), is a slowly progressive neuropathy that affects peripheral nerves and causes sensory loss, weakness, and muscle wasting primarily in the distal musculature of the feet, lower legs, hands, and forearms. It is the most frequently inherited peripheral neuropathy affecting 1 in 2,500 persons.[148] There are four different types and many subtypes of CMT, depending on the specific gene defect, inheritance pattern, age of onset, and whether the primary defect results in an abnormality of the myelin or axon of the nerve. CMT1, a demyelinating form, is the most common form of CMT and often is characterized by an autosomal dominant inheritance and the typical onset of symptoms is in childhood or adolescence.[149,150] In the most common subtype, CMT1A, a duplication of the PMP22 gene or peripheral myelin protein 22 gene on chromosome 17 is

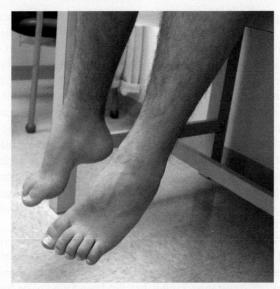

FIGURE 9.11 Sixteen-year-old with CMT. Notice the high arch and hammertoes on both feet as well as the varus position of the ankle.

present.[151] CMT2 shares the inheritance pattern and time of onset of CMT1; however, it primarily affects the axon of the nerve.[149] CMT1 and CMT2 share the same clinical features as noted above. CMT3, also known as Dejerine–Sottas disease (DS), is often not used as a separate category any longer[152] and had been used to define an autosomal dominant congenital hypomyelinating neuropathy with onset in infancy and more severe weakness.[65,150] CMT4 is autosomal recessive and may also be referred to as AR-CMT2.[153] There are other forms of CMT, including an x-linked form (CMTX) and a mild congenital form.

CMT is diagnosed by physical exam, genetic testing, electromyography (EMG), and nerve conduction velocity (NCV) tests. Symptoms of weakness usually begin in the feet and ankles, as is characteristic of length dependent neuropathies, with a foot drop. Later in the course of the disease weakness of the hands and forearms can be appreciated. Many people with CMT develop contractures in the feet causing cavovarus deformity involving the forefoot, hindfoot, midfoot, and toes (Fig. 9.11).[151] Contractures in the long finger flexors may also develop. Decreased sensation to heat, touch, pain and most prominently vibration is also present distally.

A physical therapy program can benefit individuals with CMT by improving strength, ROM, and functional activities.[154] Orthotic assessment and prescription can greatly improve the gait and functional mobility of a person with CMT by preventing contracture formation and providing a more stable base for ambulation.[155–157] It has also been proposed that Custom braces may also improve aerobic performance and decrease energy expenditure in patients with CMT.[158] There is not a lot of data to guide the specific choice of brace type in CMT but the therapist should be guided by a few underlying principals in selecting appropriate bracing. First given that patients have significant weakness the brace weight is an important issue and a lighter brace will decrease the tendency for the patients gait pattern to be dominated by poor lower leg deceleration at the end of swing. Carbon fiber braces with a posterior leaf spring design to prevent foot drop often provides sufficient dorsiflexion assist for the more mild cases where there is not significant fixed deformity. However, these provide limited deformity accommodation or control and may require the use of a foot orthotic insert or if greater control is required an articulating ankle foot orthosis can be used and a varus control strap added. Stretching, night splints, and serial casting can also improve ROM, but if a fixed deformity develops, orthopedic surgery to correct the deformity may be necessary to produce a plantigrade foot.[59]

A resistance training program can improve strength[159] and ADLs in patients with CMT. The addition of creatine monohydrate has been investigated as an adjunct to exercise.[160,161] Resistance training has also been found to be helpful with respect to strength and function with improvement noted after a home-based strengthening program.[162,163,164]

 ## Summary

The disorders discussed in this chapter are all characterized by weakness and wasting of the skeletal musculature, progressive deformity, and increasing disability. The physical therapist plays an important role in the management of these disorders. The therapist's roll centers on the maintenance of function, both through the management of what is often a progressive process and the provision of assistive technology to compensate for functional limitations. This may be as simple as recommending bath equipment to make transfers more manageable or as involved as prescribing power mobility to compensate for the loss of ambulation. The therapist is also in a position to provide teaching surrounding the natural history and act as a resource for outcome measurement both for monitoring of individual patients and as part of a clinical trial team. Finally the therapist can work together with the psychosocial members of the team to facilitate the necessary emotional support for the affected child and family.

CASE STUDY

A.M., 10-Year-Old Caucasian with DMD

A.M. is a 10-year-old Caucasian boy with a diagnosis of DMD. He was diagnosed at 4 years of age when it was noted that he was slow getting up off the floor after story time at preschool and appeared unable to keep up with his school mates. He has been followed periodically by physical therapy since that time for family education in ROM and active stretching exercises and for monitoring the status of his muscle strength, function, and joint contractures.

At 4 years of age, the family had been instructed in stretching of the heel cords to be performed on a daily basis and A.M. had been fitted with night splints to maintain a neutral position at his ankles during sleep. (He was encouraged to wear his "moon boots" throughout the night, but if it was only 2 to 3 hours at neutral before he took them off, this shorter period was considered beneficial.) A.M. was started on prednisone by his neurologist and became somewhat stronger and was able to run better. These functional gains, however, came with a price. A.M. initially gained some weight, but since his parents knew to watch for this, his weight gain was not as great as it could have been. In addition, A.M. was somewhat more active and inattentive in school. Despite the side effects, his parents chose to keep him on the medication because they felt the benefits outweighed the side effects. At 5 to 6 years of age, the stretching of hip flexors and iliotibial bands had been added to the daily stretching regimen because he had developed mild flexion and abduction contractures.

At this time, A.M. comes to physical therapy with the chief complaint of an increased number of falls (approximately four per day), increased difficulty rising from a chair and ascending and descending stairs, and no longer being able to get off the floor without the use of "furniture" along with his Gower's maneuver.

Strength in the upper extremities (UE) graded in the "good" range (4 out of 5), with the lower extremities (LE) grading "fair" (3 out of 5) to "poor" (2 out of 5) in the proximal muscle groups. Measurements of joint contractures revealed hip flexors that measured –10 degrees bilaterally, iliotibial bands at 0 degrees bilaterally, knees at neutral, and –10 degrees at the right ankle and –8 degrees on the left. In the UE, ROM was within normal limits bilaterally and functionally still independent.

Stretching exercises were reviewed and emphasized with the family. Contracture releases were also discussed with the family as an option and a future referral to the orthopedic surgeon was discussed. A.M. and his family were instructed to return to physical therapy in conjunction with being fitted by the orthotist with the long leg braces should they opt for surgery. The need for a wheelchair, only to be used for long-distance transport and on uneven terrain, was addressed, and since it had been discussed at previous visits, they were ready to order this and chose a power wheelchair. They had a "buggy" that they used for long distances, but it was clear that this did not provide the independence that A.M. wanted, especially outdoors with his friends.

Contact was made with the treating physical therapist in the school district for his or her suggestions or comments regarding power mobility, and issues related to home and school accessibility were discussed with the family and therapist, in terms of both transport and access.

A.M. became a full-time wheelchair user at 12, and despite the lateral support on his chair, he developed scoliosis, which required fusion when it reached 40 degrees. Following the fusion, A.M. had trouble feeding himself and was ordered a mobile arm support and also began to use the tilt feature on his most recent power chair not only for pressure relief, but also to clear the door while entering his adapted van since he grew 3 inches following the surgery.

As A.M. got older, the focus of therapy shifted to maintaining hand function, and resting hand splints and ROM for the long finger flexors and elbow flexors were taught.

At 22, A.M. was having increasing difficulty driving his chair. He was unable to drive in reverse and could no longer reposition his arm when he went over bumps. In addition, through further discussion, it became apparent that he had been having trouble accessing his computer and had not discussed this at previous clinic visits. A.M. was ordered a mini-joystick to drive his wheelchair and a mouse emulator so he could access the computer with his wheelchair control. In addition, he was referred for evaluation for an on-screen keyboard word prediction software and a dictation program.

REFERENCES

1. Koenig N, Hoffman EP, Bertelson CJ, et al. Complete cloning of the Duchenne muscular dystrophy (DMD) cDNA and preliminary genomic organization of the DMD gene in normal and affected individuals. *Cell.* 1987;50:509–517.

2. Tsao CY, Mendell JR. The childhood muscular dystrophies: making order out of chaos. *Semin Neurol.* 1999;19:9–23.

3. Mendell JR, Sahenk Z, Prior TW. The childhood muscular dystrophies: diseases sharing a common pathogenesis of membrane instability. *J Child Neurol.* 1995;10:150–159.

3a. Francesco L. An SMN-dependent U12 splicing event essential for motor circuit function. *Cell.* 2012;151(2):440–454.

3b. Wendy I. SMN is required for sensory-motor circuit function in Drosophila. *Cell.* 2012;151(2):427–439.

4. Roselli F, Caroni P. A circuit mechanism for neurodegeneration. *Cell.* 2012;151(2):250–252.

5. Melancini P, Vianello A, Villanova C, et al. Cardiac and respiratory involvement in advanced stage Duchenne muscular dystrophy. *Neuromusc Disord.* 1996;6:367–376.

6. Hoffman EP, Brown RH, Kunkel LM. Dystrophin: the protein product of the Duchenne muscular dystrophy locus. *Cell.* 1987;51:919.

7. Crisp DE, Ziter FA, Bray PF. Diagnostic delay in Duchenne's muscular dystrophy. *JAMA.* 1982;247:478–480.

8. Behrman RG, Kleigman R, Jenson HB. *Nelson Textbook of Pediatrics.* 16th ed. Philadelphia, PA:WB Saunders; 2000.

9. Brooke MH. *Clinicians' View of Neuromuscular Disease.* 2nd ed. Baltimore, MD:Williams & Wilkins; 1986:117–159.

10. Blake DJ, Weir A, Newey SE, et al. Function and genetics of dystrophin and dystrophin-related proteins in muscle. *Physiol Rev.* 2002; 82:291–329.

11. Khairallah RJ, Shi G, Sbrana F, et al. Microtubules underlie dysfunction in duchenne muscular dystrophy. *Sci Signal.* 2012;5(236):ra56.

12. Brooke MH, Fenichel GM, Griggs RC, et al. Clinical investigations in Duchenne dystrophy: Part 2. Determination of the "power" of therapeutic trials based on the natural history. *Muscle Nerve.* 1983;6: 91–103.

13. Vignos PJ, Spencer GE, Archibald KC. Management of progressive muscular dystrophy of childhood. *JAMA.* 1963;184:89–96.

14. Magri F, Govoni A, D'Angelo MG, et al. Genotype and phenotype characterization in a large dystrophinopathic cohort with extended follow-up. *J Neurol.* 2011;258(9):1610–1623.

15. Tuffery-Giraud S, Béroud C, Leturcq F, et al. Genotype-phenotype analysis in 2,405 patients with a dystrophinopathy using the UMD-DMD database: a model of nationwide knowledgebase. *Hum Mutat.* 2009;30(6):934–945.

16. Brooke MH, Fenichel G, Griggs R, et al. Duchenne muscular dystrophy: patterns of clinical progression and effects of supportive therapy. *Neurology.* 1989;39:475–481.

17. Dooley JM, Gordon KE, MacSween JM. Impact of steroids on surgical experiences of patients with duchenne muscular dystrophy. *Pediatr Neurol.* 2010;43(3):173–176.

18. Colbert AP, Craig C. Scoliosis management in Duchenne muscular dystrophy: prospective study of modified Jewett hyperextension brace. *Arch Phys Med Rehabil.* 1987;68(5 pt 1):302–304.

19. Cambridge W, Drennan JC. Scoliosis associated with Duchenne muscular dystrophy. *J Pediatr Orthop.* 1987;7(4):436–440.

20. Karol LA. Scoliosis in patients with Duchenne muscular dystrophy. *J Bone Joint Surg Am.* 2007;89(suppl 1):155–162.

20a. Sonia K, Ramirez A, Aubertin G, et al. Respiratory muscle decline in duchenne muscular dystrophy. *Pediatr pulmonol.* 2013; doi: 10.1002/ppul.22847.

21. Machado DL, Silva EC, Resende MB. Lung function monitoring in patients with duchenne muscular dystrophy on steroid therapy. *BMC Res Notes.* 2012;5(1):435.

22. Judge DP, Kass DA, Thompson WR, et al. Pathophysiology and therapy of cardiac dysfunction in Duchenne muscular dystrophy. *Am J Cardiovasc Drugs.* 2011;11(5):287–294.

23. McNally EM, Towbin JA. Cardiomyopathy in muscular dystrophy workshop. 28–30 September 2003, Tucson, Arizona. *Neuromusc Disord.* 2004;20:1–7.

24. Nardes F, Araújo AP, Ribeiro MG. Mental retardation in Duchenne muscular dystrophy. *J Pediatr (Rio J).* 2012;88(1):6–16.

25. Leibowitz D, Dubowitz V. Intellect and behavior in Duchenne muscular dystrophy. *Dev Med Child Neurol.* 1981;23:577–590.

26. Prosser JE. Intelligence and the gene for Duchenne muscular dystrophy. *Arch Dis Child.* 1969;44:221–230.

27. Bushby K, Finkel R, Birnkrant DJ, et al. Diagnosis and management of Duchenne muscular dystrophy, part 2: implementation of multidisciplinary care. *Lancet Neurol.* 2010;9:177–189.

28. Ziter FA, Allsop K. The diagnosis and management of childhood muscular dystrophy. *Clin Pediatr.* 1976;15(6):540–548.

29. Brooke MH, Fenichel G, Griggs R, et al. Clinical investigation of Duchenne muscular dystrophy. Interesting results in a trial of prednisone. *Arch Neurol.* 1987;44:812–817.

30. Angelini C, Peterle E. Old and new therapeutic developments in steroid treatment in Duchenne muscular dystrophy. *Acta Myol.* 2012;31(1):9–15.

31. Manzur AY, Kuntzer T, Pike M, et al. Glucocorticoid corticosteroids for Duchenne muscular dystrophy. *Cochrane Database Syst Rev.* 2004;(2):CD003725.

32. Drachman DB, Tokya RV, Meyer E. Prednisone in Duchenne muscular dystrophy. *Lancet.* 1974;2:1409–1412.

33. DeSilva S, Drachman D, Mellits D, et al. Prednisone treatment in Duchenne muscular dystrophy. Long-term benefit. *Arch Neurol.* 1987;44:818–822.

34. Fenichel G, Florence J, Pestronk A, et al. Long-term benefit from prednisone therapy in Duchenne muscular dystrophy. *Neurology.* 1991;41:1874–1877.

35. Banerjee B, Sharma U, Balasubramanian K, et al. Effect of creatine monohydrate in improving cellular energetics and muscle strength in ambulatory Duchenne muscular dystrophy patients: a randomized, placebo-controlled 31P MRS study. *Magn Reson Imaging.* 2010; 28(5):698–707.

36. Chetlin RD, Gutmann L, Tarnopolsky MA, et al. Resistance training exercise and creatine in patients with Charcot-Marie-Tooth Disease. *Muscle Nerve.* 2004;30:69–76.

37. Fairclough RJ, Bareja A, Davies KE. Progress in therapy for Duchenne muscular dystrophy. *Exp Physiol.* 2011;96(11):1101–1113.

38. Bentley G, Haddad F, Bull TM, et al. The treatment of scoliosis in muscular dystrophy using modified Luque and Harrington-Luque instrumentation. *J Bone Joint Surg Br.* 2001;83(1):22–28.

39. Miller F, Moseley CF, Koreska J. Spinal fusion in Duchenne muscular dystrophy. *Dev Med Child Neurol.* 1992;34:775–786.

40. Leger P, Jennequin J, Gerard M, et al. Home positive pressure ventilation via nasal mask for patients with neuromuscular weakness or restrictive lung or chest-wall disease. *Respir Care.* 1989;34:73–79.

41. Bach J, O'Brien J, Krotenberg R, et al. Management of end-stage respiratory failure in Duchenne muscular dystrophy. *Muscle Nerve.* 1987;10:177–182.

42. Florence J, Brooke M, Carroll J. Evaluation of the child with muscular weakness. *Orthoped Clin North Am.* 1978;9(2):421–422.

43. McDonald CM, Abresch RT, Carter GT, et al. Profiles of neuromuscular diseases. Duchenne muscular dystrophy. *Am J Phys Med Rehabil.* 1995;74(5)(suppl):S70–S92.

44. Ziter FA, Allsop KG, Tyler FH. Assessment of muscle strength in Duchenne muscular dystrophy. *Neurology.* 1977;27:981–984.

45. Allsop KG, Ziter FA. Loss of strength and functional decline in Duchenne dystrophy. *Arch Neurol.* 1981;38:406–411.

46. Henricson E, Abresch R, Han JJ, et al. Percent-predicted 6-minute walk distance in duchenne muscular dystrophy to account for maturational influences. Version 2. *PLoS Curr.* 2012;4:RRN1297.

47. Brooke MH, Griggs R, Mendell J, et al. Clinical trial in Duchenne dystrophy. I. The design of the protocol. *Muscle Nerve.* 1981;4:186–197.

48. Florence JM, Pandya S, King W, et al. Clinical trials in Duchenne dystrophy. Standardization and reliability of evaluation procedures. *Phys Ther.* 1984;64:41–45.

49. Scott E, Eagle M, Mayhew A, et al. Development of a functional assessment scale for ambulatory boys with Duchenne muscular dystrophy. *Physiother Res Int.* 2012;17(2):101–109.

50. Griggs R, Moxley RT 3rd, Mendell JR, et al. Prednisone in Duchenne dystrophy. A randomized, controlled trial defining the time course and dose response. *Arch Neurol.* 1991;48:383–388.

51. Stuberg W, Metcalf W. Reliability of quantitative muscle testing in healthy children and in children with Duchenne muscular dystrophy using hand held dynamometers. *Phys Ther.* 1988;68(6):977–982.

52. Brussock C, Haley S, Munsat T, et al. Measurement of isometric force in children with and without Duchenne's muscular dystrophy. *Phys Ther.* 1992;72(2):105–114.

53. Kilmer DD, McCrory MA, Wright NC, et al. Hand-held dynamometry reliability in persons with neuropathic weakness. *Arch Phys Med Rehabil.* 1997;78:1364–1368.

54. Hyde SA, Steffensen BF, Fløytrup I, et al. Longitudinal data analysis: an application to construction of a natural history profile of Duchenne muscular dystrophy. *Neuromuscul Disord.* 2001;11(2):165–170.

55. Mathur S, Lott DJ, Senesac C, et al. Age-related differences in lower-limb muscle cross-sectional area and torque production in boys with Duchenne muscular dystrophy. *Arch Phys Med Rehabil.* 2010;91(7):1051–1058.

56. Magee DJ. *Orthopedic physical assessment.* 2nd ed. Philadelphia, PA:WB Saunders; 1992.

57. Hyde SA, Floytruuup I, Glent S, et al. A randomized comparative study of two methods for controlling Tendo Achilles contracture in Duchenne muscular dystrophy. *Neuromusc Disord.* 2000;10:257–263.

58. Scott OM, Hyde SA, Goddard C, et al. Prevention of deformity in Duchenne muscular dystrophy. *Physiotherapy.* 1981;67:177–180.

59. McDonald CM. Limb contractures in progressive neuromuscular disease and the role of stretching, orthotics, and surgery. *Phys Med Rehabil Clin N Am.* 1998;9:187–209.

60. Glanzman AM, Flickinger JM, Dholakia KH, et al. Serial casting for the management of ankle contracture in Duchenne muscular dystrophy. *Pediatr Phys Ther.* 2011;23(3):275–279.

61. Johnson E, Yarnell S. Hand dominance and scoliosis in Duchenne muscular dystrophy. *Arch Phys Med Rehabil.* 1976;57:462–464.

62. Miller F, Moseley C, Koreska J, et al. Pulmonary function and scoliosis in Duchenne dystrophy. *J Pediatr Orthop.* 1988;8:133–137.

63. Miller R, Chalmers A, Dao H, et al. The effect of spine fusion on respiratory function in Duchenne muscular dystrophy. *Neurology.* 1991;41:37–40.

64. Alexander WM, Smith M, Freeman BJ, et al. The effect of posterior spinal fusion on respiratory function in Duchenne muscular dystrophy. *Eur Spine J.* 2013;22(2):411–416.

65. Carter GT. Rehabilitation management in neuromuscular disease. *J Neurol Rehabil.* 1997;11:69–80.

66. Vignos P, Watkins M. The effect of exercise in muscular dystrophy. *JAMA.* 1966;197:121–126.

67. Ansved T. Muscle training in muscular dystrophies. *Acta Physiol Scand.* 2001;171:359–366.

68. de Lateur B, Giaconi RM. Effect on maximal strength of submaximal exercise in Duchenne muscular dystrophy. *Am J Phys Med.* 1979;58:26–36.

69. Scott OM, Hyse SA, Goddard C, et al. Effect of exercise in Duchenne muscular dystrophy. *Physiotherapy.* 1981;67(6):174–176.

70. Eagle M. Report on the muscular dystrophy campaign workshop: exercise in neuromuscular diseases Newcastle, 2002. *Neuromusc Disord.* 2002;12:975–983.

71. McCarter GC, Steinhardt RA. Increased activity of calcium leak channels caused by proteolysis near sarcolemmal ruptures. *J Membrane Biol.* 2000;176:169–174.

72. Brussee V, Tardif F, Tremblay J. Muscle fibers of mdx mice are more vulnerable to exercise than those of normal mice. *Neuromusc Disord.* 1997;7:487–492.

73. Connolly AM, Keeling RM, Mehta S, et al. Three mouse models of muscular dystrophy: the natural history of strength and fatigue in dystrophin-, dystrophin/utrophin-, and laminin α2-deficient mice. *Neuromusc Disord.* 2001;11:703–712.

74. Alderton JM, Steinhardt RA. How calcium influx through calcium leak channels is responsible for the elevated levels of calcium-dependent proteolysis in dystrophic myotubes. *Trends Cardiovasc Med.* 2000;10:268–272.

75. Hayes A, Lynch GS, Williams DA. The effects of endurance exercise on dystrophic mdx mice I. Contractile and histochemical properties of intact muscles. *Proc Biol Sci.* 1993;253:19–25.

76. Markert CD, Ambrosio F, Call JA, et al. Exercise and duchenne muscular dystrophy: toward evidence-based exercise prescription. *Muscle Nerve.* 2011;43:464–478.

77. Markert CD, Case LE, Carter GT, et al. Exercise and duchenne muscular dystrophy: where we have been and where we need to go. *Muscle Nerve.* 2012;45(5):746–751.

78. Harris SE, Chérry DB. Childhood progressive muscular dystrophy and the role of physical therapy. *Phys Ther.* 1974;54:4–12.

79. Archibald DC, Vignos PJ Jr. A study of contractures in muscular dystrophy. *Arch Phys Med Rehabil.* 1959;40:150–157.

80. Spencer GE. Orthopaedic care of progressive muscular dystrophy. *J Bone Joint Surg Am.* 1967;49:1201–1204.

81. Roy L, Gibson DA. Pseudohypertrophic muscular dystrophy and its surgical management: review of 30 patients. *Can J Surg.* 1970;13:13–20.

82. Siegel IM. Management of musculoskeletal complications in neuromuscular disease. Enhancing mobility and the role of bracing and surgery. In: Fowler WM Jr, ed. *Advances in the Rehabilitation of Neuromuscular Diseases: State of the Art Reviews.* Vol 4. Philadelphia, PA: Hanley & Belfus; 1988:553–575.

83. Ziter FA, Allsop KG. The value of orthoses for patients with Duchenne muscular dystrophy. *Phys Ther.* 1979;59:1361–1365.

84. Heckmatt JZ, Dubowitz V, Hyde SA, et al. Prolongation of walking in Duchenne muscular dystrophy with lightweight orthoses. Review of 57 cases. *Dev Med Child Neurol.* 1985;27:149–154.

85. Vignos PJ. Management of musculoskeletal complications in neuromuscular disease: limb contractures and the role of stretching, braces and surgery. In: Fowler WM Jr, ed. *Advances in the Rehabilitation of Neuromuscular Diseases: State of the Art Reviews.* Vol 4. Philadelphia, PA: Hanley & Belfus; 1988:509–536.

86. Bach JR, Campagnolo DI, Hoeman S. Life satisfaction of individuals with Duchenne muscular dystrophy using long-term mechanical ventilatory support. *Am J Phys Rehabil.* 1991;70:129–135.

87. Liu M, Kiyoshi M, Kozo H, et al. Practical problems and management of seating through the clinical stages of Duchenne's muscular dystrophy. *Arch Phys Med Rehabil.* 2003;84:818–824.

88. Pellegrini N, Guillon B, Prigent H, et al. Optimization of power wheelchair control for patients with severe Duchenne muscular dystrophy. *Neuromusc Disord.* 2004;14:297–300.

89. Edwards RHT. Weight reduction in boys with muscular dystrophy. *Dev Med Child Neurol.* 1984;26:384–390.

90. Martigne L, Salleron J, Mayer M, et al. Natural evolution of weight status in Duchenne muscular dystrophy: a retrospective audit. *Br J Nutr.* 2011;105(10):1486–1491.

91. Griffiths R, Edwards R. A new chart for weight control in Duchenne muscular dystrophy. *Arch Dis Child.* 1988;63:1256–1258.

92. Perez A, Mulot R, Vardon G, et al. Thoracoabdominal pattern of breathing in neuromuscular disorders. *Chest.* 1996;110:454–461.

93. Birnkrant DJ, Bushby KM, Amin RS, et al. The respiratory management of patients with duchenne muscular dystrophy: a DMD care considerations working group specialty article. *Pediatr Pulmonol.* 2010;45(8):739–748.

94. Bach JR, Ishikawa Y, Kim H. Prevention of pulmonary morbidity for patients with Duchenne muscular dystrophy. *Chest.* 1997;112(4):1024–1028.

95. Topin N, Matecki S, Le Bris S, et al. Dose-dependent effect of individualized respiratory muscle training in children with Duchenne muscular dystrophy. *Neuromuscul Disord.* 2002;12(6):576–583.

96. Wanke T, Toifl K, Merkle M, et al. Inspiratory muscle training in patients with Duchenne muscular dystrophy. *Chest.* 1994;105:475–482.

97. Gozal D, Thiriet P. Respiratory muscle training in neuromuscular disease: long-term effects on strength and load perception. *Med Sci Sports Exerc.* 1999;31(11):1522–1527.

98. Udd B, Krahe R. The myotonic dystrophies: molecular, clinical, and therapeutic challenges. *Lancet Neurol.* 2012;11(10):891–905. doi: 10.1016/S1474-4422(12)70204-1.

99. Kirschner J, Bonnemenn CG. The congenital and limb-girdle muscular dystrophies: sharpening the focus, blurring the boundaries. *Arch Neurol.* 2004;61:189–199.

100. Khadikar SV, Singh RK, Katrak SM. Sarcoglycanopathies: a report of 25 cases. *Neurol India.* 2002;50:27–32.

101. Politano L, Nigro V, Passamano L, et al. Evaluation of cardiac and respiratory involvement in sarcoglycanopathies. *Neuromusc Disord.* 2001;11:178–185.

102. Ferreira AF, Carvalho MS, Resende MB, et al. Phenotypic and immunohistochemical characterization of sarcoglycanopathies. *Clinics (Sao Paulo).* 2011;66(10):1713–1719.

103. Richard I, Roudaut C, Saenz A, et al. Calpainopathy-a survey of mutations and polymorphisms. *Am J Hum Genet.* 1999;64:1524–1540.

104. Han R. Muscle membrane repair and inflammatory attack in dysferlinopathy. *Skelet Muscle.* 2011;1(1):10. doi: 10.1186/2044-5040-1-10.

105. Zatz M, de Paula F, Starling A, et al. The 10 autosomal recessive limb-girdle muscular dystrophies. *Neuromusc Disord.* 2003;13:532–544.

106. Pollitt C, Anderson LVB, Pogue R, et al. The phenotype of calpainopathy: diagnosis based on a multidisciplinary approach. *Neuromusc Disord.* 2001;11:287–296.

107. Driss A, Amouri R, Hamida B, et al. A new locus for autosomal-recessive limb-girdle muscular dystrophy in a large consanguineous Tunisian family maps to chromosome 19q3. 3. *Neuromusc Disord.* 2000;10:240–246.

108. Brockington M, Blake DJ, Prandini P, et al. Mutations in the fukutin-related protein gene (FKRP) cause a form of congenital muscular dystrophy with secondary laminin α-2 deficiency and abnormal glycosylation of α-dystroglycan. *Am J Hum Genet.* 2001;69:1198–1209.

109. Alhamidi M, Kjeldsen Buvang E, Fagerheim T, et al. Fukutin-related protein resides in the Golgi cisternae of skeletal muscle fibres and forms disulfide-linked homodimers via an N-terminal interaction. *PLoS One.* 2011;6(8):e22968. doi: 10.1371/journal.pone.0022968.

110. Poppe M, Cree L, Bourke J, et al. The phenotype of limb-girdle muscular dystrophy type 2I. *Neurology.* 2003;60:1246–1251.

111. Mercuri E, Brockington M, Straub V, et al. Phenotypic spectrum associated with mutations in the fukutin-related protein gene. *Ann Neurol.* 2003;53:537–542.

112. Poppe M, Bourke J, Eagle M, et al. Cardiac and respiratory failure in limb-girdle muscular dystrophy 2I. *Ann Neurol.* 2004;56:738–741.

113. Pane M, Messina S, Vasco G, et al. Respiratory and cardiac function in congenital muscular dystrophies with alpha dystroglycan deficiency. *Neuromuscul Disord.* 2012;22(8):685–689. doi: 10.1016/j.nmd.2012.05.006.

114. Nance JR, Dowling JJ, Gibbs EM, et al. Congenital myopathies: an update. *Curr Neurol Neurosci Rep.* 2012;12(2):165–174. doi: 10.1007/s11910-012-0255-x.

115. Clarkson E, Costa CF, Machesky LM. Congenital myopathies: diseases of the actin cytoskeleton. *J Pathol.* 2004;204:407–417.

116. Goebel HH. Congenital myopathies at their molecular dawning. *Muscle Nerve.* 2003;27:527–48.

117. Bönnemmann CG, Laing NG. Myopathies resulting from mutations in sarcomeric proteins. *Curr Opin Neurol.* 2004;17:1–9.

118. Sanoudoud, Beggs AH. Clinical and genetic heterogeneity in nemaline myopathy-a disease of skeletal muscle thin filaments. *Trends Mol Med.* 2001;7:362–368.

119. Wallgren-Pattersson C, Laing NG. Report of the 70th ENMC International Workshop: Nemaline Myopathy 11–13 June 1999, Naarden, the Netherlands. *Neuromusc Disord.* 2000;10:299–306.

120. Ryan MM, Schnell C, Strickland CD, et al. Nemaline myopathy: a clinical study of 143 cases. *Ann Neurol.* 2001;50:312–320.

121. Zhang Y, Chen HS, Khanna VK, et al. A mutation in the human ryanodine receptor gene associated with central core disease. *Nat Genet.* 1993;5(1):46–50.

122. Quane KA, Healy JM, Keating KE, et al. Mutations in the ryanodine receptor gene in central core disease and malignant hyperthermia. *Nat Genet.* 1993;5(1):51–55.

123. Jungbluth H, Sewry CA, Muntoni F. Core myopathies. *Semin Pediatr Neurol.* 2011;18(4):239–249. doi: 10.1016/j.spen.2011.10.005.

124. Quinlivan RM, Muller CR, Davis M, et al. Central core disease: clinical, pathological, and genetic features. *Arch Dis Child.* 2003;88:1051–1055.

125. Muntoni F, Voit T. The congenital muscular dystrophies in 2004: a century of exciting progress. *Neuromusc Disord.* 2004;14:635–649.

126. Voit T. Congenital muscular dystrophies: 1997 update. *Brain Dev.* 1998;20:65–74.

127. Bertini E, D'Amico A, Gualandi F, et al. Congenital muscular dystrophies: a brief review. *Semin Pediatr Neurol.* 2011;18(4):277–288. doi: 10.1016/j.spen.2011.10.010.

128. Demir E, Ferreiro A, Sabatelli P, et al. Collagen VI status and clinical severity in Ullrich congenital muscular dystrophy: phenotype analysis of 11 families linked to the COL6 Loci. *Neuropediatrics.* 2004;35:103–112.

129. Baker NL, Morgelin M, Peat R, et al. Dominant collagen VI mutations are a common cause of Ullrich congenital muscular dystrophy. *Hum Mol Genet.* 2005;14:279–293.

130. Guillian T, Brzustowicz L, Castilla L, et al. Genetic hemogeneity between acute and chronic forms of spinal muscular atrophy. *Nature.* 1990;345:823–825.

131. Hamilton G, Gillingwater TH. Spinal muscular atrophy: going beyond the motor neuron. *Trends Mol Med.* 2013;19(1):40–50. doi: 10.1016/j.molmed.2012.11.002.

132. Dumitro D. *Electrodiagnostic Medicine.* Philadelphia, PA: Hanley and Belfus; 1995.

133. Lomen-Hoerth C, Slawnych MP. Statistical motor unit number estimation: from theory to practice. *Muscle Nerve.* 2003;28(3):263–272.

134. Iannaccone ST, Brown RH, Samaha FJ, et al. DCN/SMA Group. Prospective study of spinal muscular atrophy before age 6 years. *Pediatr Neurol.* 1993;9:187–193.

135. Miske LJ, Hickey EM, Kolb SM, et al. Use of the mechanical in-exsufflator in pediatric patients with neuromuscular disease and impaired cough. *Chest.* 2004;125:1406–1412.

136. Oskoui M, Levy G, Garland CJ, et al. The changing natural history of spinal muscular atrophy type 1. *Neurology.* 2007;69(20):1931–1936.

137. Rudnik-Schoneborn S, Hausmanowa-Petrusewicz I, Brokowska J, et al. The predictive value of achieved motor milestones assessed in

441 patients with infantile spinal muscular atrophy types II and III. *Eur Neurol*. 2000;45:174–181.

138. Russman BS, Bucher CR, Shite M, et al. DCN/SMA Group. Function changes in spinal muscular atrophy II and III. *Neurology*. 1996;47:973–976.

139. Iannaccone AT, Russman BS, Browne GH, et al. Prospective analysis of strength in spinal muscular atrophy. DCN/Spinal Muscular Atrophy Group. *J Child Neurol*. 2000;15:97–101.

140. Merlini L, Bertini E, Minetti C, et al. Motor function-muscle strength relationship in spinal muscle atrophy. *Muscle Nerve*. 2004;12:561–566.

141. Koch BM, Simenson RL. Upper extremity strength and function in children with spinal muscular atrophy type II. *Arch Phys Med Rehabil*. 1992;73:241–245.

142. Granata C, Cornelio F, Bonfiglioli S, et al. Promotion of ambulation of patients with spinal muscular atrophy by early fitting of knee-ankle-foot orthoses. *Dev Med Child Neurol*. 1987;29(2):221–224.

143. Shapiro F, Specht L. Current concepts review. The diagnosis and orthopaedic treatment of childhood spinal muscular atrophy, peripheral neuropathy, Friedreich ataxia, and artrogryposis. *J Bone Joint Surg Am*. 1993;75A:1699–1714.

144. Tangsrud SE, Lodrup Carlsen KC, Lund-Petersen KC, et al. Lung function measurements in young children with spinal muscle atrophy; a cross sectional survey on the effect of position and bracing. *Arch Dis Child*. 2001;84:521–524.

145. Rodillo E, Marini ML, Heckmatt JZ, et al. Scoliosis in spinal muscular atrophy: review of 63 cases. *J Child Neurol*. 1989;4:118–123.

146. Tsirikos AI, Chang WN, Shah SA, et al. Preserving ambulatory potential in pediatric patients with cerebral palsy who undergo spinal fusion using unit rod instrumentation. *Spine (Phila Pa 1976)*. 2003;28(5):480–483.

147. Phillips DP, Roye DP, Farcy JPC, et al. Surgical treatment of scoliosis in a spinal muscular atrophy population. *Spine*. 1990;15:942–945.

148. Chetlin RD, Gutmann L, Tarnopolsky M, et al. Resistance training effectiveness in patients with Charcot-Marie-Tooth Disease: recommendations for exercise prescription. *Arch Phys Med Rehabil*. 2004;85:1217–1223.

149. Shy ME, Blake J, Krajewski K, et al. Reliability and validity of the CMT neuropathy score as a measure of disability. *Neurology*. 2005;64:1209–1214.

150. Muscular Dystrophy Association. Charcot-Marie-Tooth Disease and Dejerine-Sottas Disease. www.mdausa.org. Accessed May 1, 2005.

151. Azmaipairashvili Z, Riddle EC, Scavina M, et al. Correction of cavovarus foot deformity in Charcot-Marie-Tooth Disease. *J Pediatr Orthop*. 2005;25:360–365.

152. Patzkó A, Shy ME. Update on Charcot-Marie-Tooth disease. *Curr Neurol Neurosci Rep*. 2011;11(1):78–88.

153. Shy ME, Patzkó A. Axonal Charcot-Marie-Tooth disease. *Curr Opin Neurol*. 2011;24(5):475–483. doi: 10.1097/WCO.0b013e32834aa331.

154. El Mhandi L, Millet GY, Calmels P, et al. Benefits of interval-training on fatigue and functional capacities in Charcot-Marie-Tooth disease. *Muscle Nerve*. 2008;37(5):601–610; doi: 10.1002/mus.20959.

155. Phillips MF, Robertson Z, Killen B, et al. A pilot study of a crossover trial with randomized use of ankle-foot orthoses for people with Charcot-Marie-tooth disease. *Clin Rehabil*. 2012;26(6):534–544.

156. Ramdharry GM, Day BL, Reilly MM, et al. Foot drop splints improve proximal as well as distal leg control during gait in Charcot-Marie-Tooth disease. *Muscle Nerve*. 2012;46(4):512–519.

157. Guillebastre B, Calmels P, Rougier PR. Assessment of appropriate ankle-foot orthoses models for patients with Charcot-Marie-Tooth disease. *Am J Phys Med Rehabil*. 2011;90(8):619–627;doi: 10.1097/PHM.0b013e31821f7172.

158. Bean J, Walsh A, Frontera W. Brace modification improves aerobic performance in Charcot-Marie-Tooth Disease: a single subject design. *Am J Phys Med Rehabil*. 2001;80:578–582.

159. Sackley C, Disler PB, Turner-Stokes L, et al. Rehabilitation interventions for foot drop in neuromuscular disease. *Cochrane Database Syst Rev*. 2009;8(3):CD003908.

160. Chetlin RD, Mancinelli CA, Gutmann L. Self-reported follow-up post-intervention adherence to resistance exercise training in Charcot-Marie-Tooth disease patients. *Muscle Nerve*. 2010;42(3):456; doi: 10.1002/mus.21705.

161. Chetlin RD, Gutmann L, Tarnopolsky M, et al. Resistance training effectiveness in patients with Charcot-Marie-Tooth disease: recommendations for exercise prescription. *Arch Phys Med Rehabil*. 2004;85(8):1217–1223.

162. Burns J, Raymond J, Ouvrier R. Feasibility of foot and ankle strength training in childhood Charcot-Marie-Tooth disease. *Neuromuscul Disord*. 2009;19(12):818–821. doi: 10.1016/j.nmd.2009.09.007.

163. Lindeman E, Spaans F, Reulen J, et al. Progressive resistance training in neuromuscular patients. Effects on force and surface EMG. *J Electromyogr Kinesiol*. 1999;9(6):379–384.

164. Kilmer DD. The role of exercise in neuromuscular disease. *Phys Med Rehabil Clin N Am*. 1998;9(1):115–125.

165. Mitsuhashi S, Kang PB. Update on the genetics of limb girdle muscular dystrophy. *Semin Pediatr Neurol*. 2012;19(4):211–218.

166. Neuromuscular Disease Center. Limb-Girdle Muscular Dystrophy (LGMD) Syndromes. http://neuromuscular.wustl.edu/musdist/lg.html#lgmd1f. Accessed February 22 2013.

Intellectual Disabilities: Focus on Down syndrome

Dolores B. Bertoti and Mary B. Schreiner

Introduction
Historical Review
Definition
Incidence
Diagnosis
  Assessment of Intellectual Functioning
  Assessment of Skill Level
Classification
  Educational Classification
  Medical Classification
Etiology and Pathophysiology
Primary Impairments
  Neuromotor Impairments
  Learning Impairment
Physical Therapy Evaluation and Intervention Principles
  Key Elements of Assessment
  Sensory Assessment and Intervention
Key Elements of Physical Therapy Intervention
  General Principles
  Learning Characteristics
  Intervention to Limit Cognitive Impairment
  Intervention to Limit Physical and Functional Impairments
  The Importance of Focused Intervention

The Team Concept and Collaboration
A Management Model for Physical Therapists for the Child with Down syndrome
  Definition
  History and Incidence
  Pathophysiology and Associated Impairments of the Child with Down syndrome
  Neuropathology
  Sensory Deficits
  Cardiopulmonary Pathologies
  Musculoskeletal Differences
  Additional Physical Characteristics
Physical Therapy Assessment and Intervention for the Child with Down syndrome
  Learning Differences
  Associated Motor Deficits
  Developmental Delay
  Physical Therapy Evaluation and Intervention Implications
  Musculoskeletal Problems
  Cardiopulmonary Fitness
  Physical Therapy Life Span Evaluation and Intervention Implications
The Person with Intellectual Disabilities Moving into and through Adulthood: Key Management Issues
Summary
Case Study

Introduction

The physical therapist (PT) plays a challenging and important, multifaceted role in the management of children with intellectual disabilities. This challenge is inherent within the clinical presentation of such a child who exhibits simultaneous and interactive impairments in the neuromotor, musculoskeletal, developmental, cognitive, and affective domains. The PT must be able to not only accurately assess the child, but must also innovatively develop, implement, modify, and share with parents and other providers of service an accurate plan of care. In this chapter, we offer an approach to assist the entry-level PT with assessment, intervention, and management of the child with intellectual disabilities. The strategy presented is from a functional perspective, delineating the interactive effects of common impairments associated with such disabilities and the role of the PT in managing these impairments to promote maximum best function of the child within his or her environment. Physical therapy management for the child with Down syndrome is outlined as a model strategy (Fig. 10.1).

Historical review

The history of society and its treatment of people with intellectual disabilities have had an intriguing, interesting, and still unfolding interactional relationship. As societal trends followed a path of increased education and understanding, the quality of these interactions wandered along a pathway from severe humiliation, to tolerance and

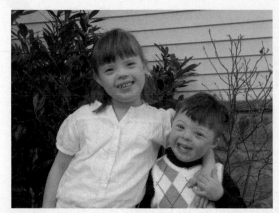

FIGURE 10.1 Introducing Angelo and Juliana, siblings with Down syndrome. Julianna was adopted by her family when Angelo was 3 years old.

protection, to understanding and acceptance, and now evolving onto a pathway that promotes full inclusion and self-determination. In the earliest of recorded interactions between the two groups, people with intellectual disabilities were ignored, received little or no care, or were even left to die.[1] Spartan society believed in survival of only the fittest, and many people, including the physically and mentally impaired, were left to perish.

Conversely, in ancient Rome and during the Middle Ages, it was not uncommon for wealthy people to keep a "fool" or "court jester" in return for the amusement these people provided for the household and its guests.[1] Artistic work of the Middle Ages shows people who depict the physical characteristics of what we now identify as Down syndrome serving as clowns and jesters.[2] In the later Middle Ages, particularly in Europe, superstitious beliefs led to the execution of many people who were considered to be "witches and warlocks." People with intellectual and other disabilities were undoubtedly included in these groups.[1] This idea that people with disabilities were social menaces persisted throughout the 19th century, with the eventual trend away from execution but still toward punishment, imprisonment, and isolation.[3]

In the early 20th century, there was a publicly perceived need to shelter and protect people with intellectual disabilities from the misunderstanding, abuses, and wrath of society. Consequently, people perceived as having a mental deficiency were isolated in asylums, shelters, and farm communities. These communities, however, rapidly became overcrowded. The goal of this public effort was clearly housing rather than provision of services or education.

Interest in providing services to assist people with intellectual disabilities had a difficult beginning. In the early 1800s, Jean Marc Itard, a French physician, became intrigued with an intellectually challenged youngster whom the physician had captured in the forests of Aveyron in France. Acting on his then-revolutionary premise that intellectual performance could be affected by environmental stimulation, Itard succeeded in teaching this "Wild Boy of Aveyron." Although Itard's work helped the boy improve over a 5-year period,

the gains were not sufficient for acceptance of the boy into Parisian society at that time. Society frowned on the child, and Itard believed he had failed.[4]

In 1840, Johann Jacob Guggenbuhl established a center in Switzerland for a then-innovative approach involving group teaching for children with intellectual disabilities. His work received worldwide acclaim as a major reform. This reform influenced the work in Europe and in the United States of Edouard Sequin, who was a world leader in the development of educational and residential services for people with intellectual disabilities. In 1876, Seguin was made president of the newly formed Association of Medical Officers of the American Institutions for Idiotic and Feeble-Minded Persons. This association later (1876) became the American Association of Mental Deficiency (AAMD), which renamed itself in 2006 as the American Association on Intellectual and Developmental Disabilities (AAIDD).[5]

In the United States, the social organization accompanying the Industrial Revolution reinforced this concept of group care of children, as well as stimulating a sense of social responsibility.[1] Throughout the 1800s, small gains fluctuated with a sense of frustration and futility, and there was a large-scale movement to house the "incurables" in large, overcrowded facilities in isolated areas.[2] As such, education first promoted for use with individuals with severe disabilities, including those with intellectual disabilities, was generally provided in large institutions designed as much to protect persons with disabilities from the public as to protect the public from them.

During the mid-19th century, an interesting development began, referred to as "special education." The notoriety of famous people like Samuel Gridley Howe and Horace Mann publicized the educational experiences of Laura Bridgman, a child who was blind and came to be educated at a school for the blind then housed at the Perkins Institute in Massachusetts. Howe's description of the processes used at the Institute with Bridgman were further distributed in reports written by Charles Dickens. Dickens' articles were widely read, aided by his popularity at that time, and helped give fuel to the special education movement.[6,7]

This treatment model, delivered in large, segregated settings, persisted through the end of World War II, when the emphasis for care of people with intellectual disabilities evolved to include "programming." This shift to a plan of activity was mainly the result of efforts by the National Association for Retarded Citizens (NARC) and other parent or professional advocacy groups.[2] Increasing awareness of the negative effects of residential segregation and the limitations of existing programs led to a critical reappraisal of existing kinds of care available for people with intellectual disabilities. Influenced by the Civil Rights Movement, the 1960s represented a time of expansion in program legislation and funds allocation for all persons with disabilities. Discrimination against and segregation of people with intellectual disabilities were finally recognized as negative and undesirable.[2]

In the early 1970s, American visitors to Scandinavian countries encountered the concept of "normalization," which was defined as the principle of educating persons with handicaps to the maximum extent feasible within the "normal" environment of the nonhandicapped.[8] This process obviously required major development and use of community support systems. This era became known as the era of "deinstitutionalization." As an example, in 1972 the Association for Retarded Citizens won a landmark decision against the Commonwealth of Pennsylvania that provided access to public education for children with intellectual disabilities. This decision stated that "It is the Commonwealth's obligation to place each mentally retarded child in a free, public program of education and training appropriate to the child's capacity . . . placement in a regular school class is preferable to placement in a special public school class and placement in a special public school is preferable to placement in any other type of program of education and training."[8] Similar landmark cases were happening in states across the country. This deinstitutionalization movement continued into the 1980s, and public interest was further stirred by a series of investigations and publications of the conditions of several institutions. Televised broadcasts "exposed abuse, neglect, and lack of programming at Willowbrook, a state institution for persons with intellectual disabilities on Staten Island."[9] This spurred the interest of Jacob Javits, a state senator from New York, to propose legislation to regulate practices in institutions.[8] Since that time, many changes have occurred as a result of public interest and educators. Most of the nation's institutions serving the population with intellectual disabilities have closed, and other types of educational facilities and housing have been developed. Living arrangements in the community have now become the norm for the long-term care and support of people with intellectual disabilities.

The most current approach to programming in the field of intellectual disabilities is a functional, integrated model. Society as a whole, and therefore the countless legislatures and service providers of today's society, view intellectual disabilities along a changing paradigm, with a more functional definition and a focus on the interaction between the person, the environment, and the intensities and patterns of needed supports. The term readers will hear most frequently now is "support," including needed level of support for maximum function of the individual with intellectual disabilities in the environment.[9]

▶ Definition

Intellectual disabilities have been defined by the American Psychiatric Association (2013) in the Diagnostic and Statistical Manual of Mental Disorders (5th ed.) using three criteria (10). The first of the three is that of deficits in general mental abilities, measured only partially in terms of IQ that typically falls at least two standard deviations below the norm; that is,

a score of less than 65-75 on an individualized, standardized, culturally appropriate, psychometrically sound test.[11] More specifically, this deficit in mental ability is reflected in functional challenges in "reasoning, problem solving, planning, abstract thinking, judgment, learning from instruction and experience and practical understanding".[10] Second, an individual with intellectual disabilities will concurrently have deficits in adaptive functioning, which are "how well a person meets community standards of personal independence and social responsibility, in comparison to others of similar age and sociocultural background".[10] Finally, both of these criteria must be in evidence during childhood or adolescence, considered a person's developmental period.[10]

This definition reflects a continued emphasis on the adaptive behavior dimensions, but differs from earlier definitions by adding that these limitations result in the need for ongoing support. For example, an individual with an intellectual disability may require intermittent, limited, extensive, or pervasive support to function competently in their daily routines of life.[12] Intellectual disabilities are generally regarded as a condition existing in an individual that is described by the specific performance of the individual not due to a specific trait, although it is influenced by certain characteristics or capabilities of the individual. Rather, intellectual disabilities describe a performance *state* in which functioning is impaired. This distinction is central to understanding how the present definition broadens the concept of intellectual disabilities and how it shifts the emphasis from measurement of traits to understanding the individual's actual functioning in everyday living. For any individual with intellectual disabilities, the description of its current state of functional behavior requires knowledge of the individual's capabilities as well as an understanding of the behavior within the structure and expectation of the individual's personal and social environment.

▶ Incidence

Using the identifier of two or more standard deviations below the mean as part of the definition, about 3% of the population of the United States is assumed to have intellectual disabilities, but actual prevalence is closer to 1%, with severe intellectual disability occurring approximately in six out of 1000. 10 Overall, males are diagnosed more frequently than females especially in the mild range (a ratio of 1.6:1)[11], but this ratio varies within some sex-linked genetic syndromes.

▶ Diagnosis

A diagnosis of intellectual disabilities is based on the criteria embodied within the definition reflecting intellectual functioning level, adaptive skill level.

Assessment of Intellectual Functioning

The determination that a child's intellectual functioning is significantly below average is arrived at through the administration of a standardized intelligence test, usually administered by a psychologist. Fulfillment of this criterion for diagnosis of intellectual disabilities is made on the basis of two or more standard deviations below an IQ of 100 considered "normal, or an IQ of 70 or 75 or below.[5,11] The instruments most commonly used for the assessment of intellectual functioning in children are the Stanford–Binet Intelligence Scale,[13] one of the Wechsler Scales, such as Wechsler Intelligence Scale for Children-IV[14] or Wechsler Preschool and Primary Scale of Intelligence-III,[15] and the Kaufman Assessment Battery for Children.[16] These tests are usually administered by a trained school or clinical psychologist.

Assessment of Adaptive Skill Level

Impairments in adaptive functioning, rather than low IQ, are usually the presenting symptoms in individuals with intellectual disabilities.[11] Adaptive skills are those skills considered to be central to successful life functioning and are frequently related to the need for supports for persons with intellectual disabilities. The adaptive areas in which limitations are specifically exhibited are in the following areas: communication, self-care, home living, social skills, community use, self-direction, health and safety, functional academics, leisure, and work. To fulfill the diagnostic criteria for intellectual disabilities, deficits in two or more areas of adaptive functioning must be present, thus showing a generalized limitation in adaptive skill level.[5,11] To address the level of adaptive behaviors, the practitioner must perform a functional assessment of the child's behavior across all environmental settings. Several scales are available to measure adaptive functioning, such as the Vineland Adaptive Behavior Scales[17] and the American Association on Intellectual Disabilities Adaptive Behavior Scale.[19] Table 10.1 describes the general adaptive behavior characteristics of children and adults with different levels of intellectual disabilities.[19]

Classification

In keeping with contemporary disablement models,[20–22] the key elements defining intellectual disabilities include *capabilities, environment, functional limitations,* and *participation restriction.* Current classification carries with it an application of the new diagnostic criteria directly correlated with need for support. Needed supports will vary along a number of dimensions: (1) support may be necessary in some areas of adaptive skills but not in others; (2) support requirements may be time-limited or ongoing; and (3) the intensities of the supports required, the types of support resources, and the support functions will be specific to the individual and the life cycle. It is important to note that the need for supports may vary across environments as well as across the life span. There are basically four intensities of support: intermittent, limited, extensive, and pervasive. Support services may come to the child with intellectual disabilities from four sources: the individual child (e.g., ability to make choices), other people (e.g., parent, teacher), technology (e.g., assistive devices), or habilitation services (e.g., physical therapy, occupational therapy, speech therapy).[5]

Educational Classification

Current special education practices are shaped by both the definition of intellectual disabilities and the need for supports. Contemporary educational placement terms follow a more functional approach, highlighting the need for support and thereby being descriptive of the child's needs for

TABLE 10.1	Adaptive Behavior Characteristics of Persons with Intellectual Disability		
Chronologic Age of the Person with Intellectual Disability			
IQ	Preschool	School-aged	Adult
50–55 to 70	Often appears unimpaired; develops functional social and communication skills	Academic skills of sixth grade are possible; special education support is needed for secondary school	Can learn social and vocational skills
35–40 to 50–55	Impaired social skills; can communicate; may need supervision	Can develop up to fourth grade academic skills with special training/modification	Unskilled or semiskilled vocation
20–25 to 35–40	Severely impaired communication; impaired motor skills	May learn to communicate; basic personal health habits; limited academic skills	Needs complete support and supervision for any self-support activity
<20–25	Requires full support; dependent for care; limited sensorimotor development	Some motor development; continues to be dependent for care; limited success with training	Limited motor ability and communication; continued dependency for care

Updated by authors from original source.[19]

TABLE 10.2 Etiologic Classification of Intellectual Disabilities	
Prenatal Onset	**Examples**
1. Chromosomal disorder	Down, Turner, or Klinefelter syndrome
2. Syndrome disorders	Neurofibromatosis, myotonic muscular dystrophy, Prader–Willi, tuberous sclerosis
3. Inborn errors of metabolism	Phenylketonuria, carbohydrate disorders, mucopolysaccharide disorders (e.g., Hurler type), nucleic acid disorders (e.g., Lesch–Nyhan syndrome)
4. Developmental disorders of brain formation	Neural tube closure defects (e.g., anencephaly), hydrocephalus, porencephaly, microcephaly
5. Environmental influences	Intrauterine malnutrition, drugs, toxins, alcohol, narcotics, maternal diseases
Perinatal Causes	
6. Intrauterine disorders	Placental insufficiency, maternal sepsis, abnormal labor or delivery
7. Neonatal disorders	Intracranial hemorrhage, periventricular leukomalacia, seizures, infections, respiratory disorders, head trauma, metabolic disorder
Postnatal Causes	
8. Head injuries	Intracranial hemorrhage, contusion, concussion
9. Infections	Encephalitis, meningitis, viral infections
10. Demyelinating disorders	Postinfectious and postimmunization disorders
11. Degenerative disorders	Syndromic disorders (e.g., Rett syndrome), poliodystrophies (e.g., Fredreich ataxia), basal ganglia disorder, leukodystrophies
12. Seizure disorders	Infantile spasms, myoclonic epilepsy
13. Toxic-metabolic disorders	Reye syndrome, lead intoxication, metabolic disorders (e.g., hypoglycemia)
14. Malnutrition	Protein-calorie, prolonged IV alimentation
15. Environmental deprivation	Psychosocial disadvantage, child abuse/neglect

From American Association on Intellectual Disabilities (AAID) and International Classification of Functioning, Disability and Health (ICF). Geneva, Switzerland: World Health Organization; 2001.

educational success. This descriptive terminology for educational programs through which many children with intellectual disabilities may be served, depending on the child's priority needs, includes support described as follows:

- Autistic support
- Learning support
- Life skills support
- Emotional support
- Visual support
- Hearing support
- Speech and language support
- Physical support
- Multiple disabilities support[23]

Physical therapy in the educational setting is considered a related service to special education, and is discussed in another chapter of this text.

Medical Classification

In the past, medical classification had been closely correlated with IQ scores but more recently, professionals are recognizing that "IQ measures are less valid in the lower end of the IQ range" (APA, 2013, p.33). Instead, classification occurs using levels of support needed by an individual, using a range of mild, moderate, severe, and profound 11,24-25.

 Etiology and pathophysiology

Over 350 etiologies for intellectual disabilities have been identified.[26,27] These can be broadly categorized into prenatal, perinatal, and postnatal causes. Etiologic causes with examples are depicted in Table 10.2. Movement disorders are associated with some etiologies more than others. Many children also present with a variety of associated disorders such as visual, hearing, or additional medical problems. In approximately 30% to 40% of individuals with intellectual disabilities seen in educational or clinical settings, no clear etiology can be determined despite extensive evaluation efforts.[11]

 Primary impairments

Neuromotor Impairments

Many types of intellectual disabilities have associated neuromuscular, musculoskeletal, and cardiopulmonary impairments. Table 10.3 details the most common intellectual disabilities conditions and their associated neuromotor impairments.[28–43] Most neuromuscular impairments are present as a result of primary pathology in the central nervous system (CNS). Secondary impairments then

TABLE 10.3 Neuromuscular, Musculoskeletal, and Cardiopulmonary Impairment Associated with Selected Conditions of Intellectual Disability			
Condition	**Neuromuscular**	**Musculoskeletal**	**Cardiopulmonary**
Cri-du-chat syndrome[28]	Hypotonia in early childhood, sometimes later hypertonia	Minor upper extremity anomalies, scoliosis	Congenital heart disease is common
Cytomegalovirus[29] (prenatal infection)	Hypertonia, seizures, microcephaly	Secondary to neuromuscular problems	Mitral stenosis, pulmonary valvular stenosis, atrial septal defect
De Lange Syndrome[30,31]	Spasticity, seizures, intention tremor, microcephaly	Decreased bone age, small stature, small hands and feet, short digits, proximal thumb placement, clinodactyly fifth digit, other hand and finger defects, limited elbow extension	Neonatal respiratory problems, cardiac malformations, recurrent upper respiratory tract infections
Down syndrome[32,33]	Hypotonia, low muscle force production, slow postural reactions, slow reaction time, motor delays increasing with age	Joint hyperflexibility, ligamentous laxity, foot deformities, scoliosis, atlantoaxial instability (20%)	Congenital heart disease (40%), lung hypoplasia with pulmonary dysplasia
Fetal alcohol syndrome[31,34]	Fine motor dysfunction, visual-motor deficits, weak grasp, ptosis	Joint anomalies with abnormal position or function, maxillary hypoplasia	Heart murmur, often disappears after first year
Fragile X syndrome[35,36]	Hypotonia, poor coordination and motor planning, seizures	Hyperextensible finger joints, prominent jaw, scoliosis	Mitral valve prolapse
Hurler syndrome[27,31]	Hydrocephalus	Joint contractures, claw-like deformities of hands, short fingers, thoracolumbar kyphosis, shallow acetabular and glenoid fossae, irregularly shaped bones	Cardiac deformities such as cardiac enlargement due to right ventricular hypertension, death frequently due to cardiac failure
Lesch–Nyhan syndrome[37]	Hypotonia followed by spasticity, chorea, and athetosis/dystonia; compulsive self-injurious behavior	Secondary to neuromuscular problems	
Prader–Willi syndrome[38,39]	Severe hypotonia and feeding problems in infancy, excessive eating and obesity in childhood, poor fine and gross motor coordination	Short stature, small hands and feet	May be associated with cor pulmonale (most common cause of death)
Rett syndrome[40–43]	Hypotonia in infancy, then gradually increasing hypertonia and lack of acquired skill; ataxia, apraxia, choreoathetosis and/or dystonia, progression from hyperkinesia to bradykinesia with age, slow reaction time, stereotypic hand movements (clapping, wringing, clenching) drooling, involuntary rhythmic tongue movement/deviation, seizures	Scoliosis, kyphosis, joint contractures, hip subluxation or dislocation, equinovarus deformities	Immature respiratory patterns, breathing irregularities, such as hyperventilation, apnea
Williams syndrome[31,34] (elfin facies)	Mild neurologic dysfunction, poor motor coordination	Hallux valgus	Variable congenital heart disease

Adapted with permission from McEwen I. Intellectual disabilities. In: Campbell SK, ed. *Physical Therapy for Children*. 4th ed. Philadelphia, PA: WB Saunders; 2011.

include deficits typically of concern to the PT such as deficits in motor control, coordination, postural control, force production, flexibility, and balance.[44] Physical therapy assessment and treatment of these impairments for children with intellectual disabilities are similar to those procedures used in any pediatric setting. Use of Table 10.3 can guide the pediatric PT in anticipating typical management concerns associated with common intellectual disabilities or disorders. The intellectual disabilities themselves, viewed as an additional or confounding impairment, require some adaptation in evaluation and treatment application because of the specific cognitive limitations presented by the child.

Learning Impairment

Learning is impaired in children with intellectual disabilities who demonstrate an impaired ability to utilize advanced cognitive processes, manage simultaneous or multiple demands, and successfully organize complex information, with subsequent effects on task performance and task mastery.[45] Poor memory, limited generalization (i.e., the inability to perform a learned task across different environments), and poor motivation also may impair the learning of a child with an intellectual disability.[46] Memory impairment is seen with difficulty recalling multistep directions or steps to complete a task. When an individual cannot generalize, a change in settings may be extremely challenging. Finally, the slow learning rate and frequent failure to learn experienced by individuals with intellectual disabilities can produce a low level of motivation and self-determination in the acquisition of many necessary life skills.

PTs must be able to adapt assessment and intervention approaches to accommodate the impaired intellectual functioning. Clearly, the range of cognitive deficit and ability found in children with intellectual disabilities is indicative of variant levels of performance, functioning, and potential.[47] It is the task and the challenge of the therapist to assist the child to maximize his or her potential for optimum functioning and participation across environments.

Physical therapy evaluation and intervention principles

Key Elements of Assessment

Meaningful assessment always focuses on the child's functioning. A successful and effective physical therapy assessment of the child depends largely on the therapist's approach to the child. Four important elements should facilitate the process of assessment.

First, throughout the assessment, the therapist must analyze both what the child can do and the *processes underlying the observed skills and behaviors*.[48] Thus, the therapist must determine not only the tasks the child can accomplish, but also why the child can do those specific tasks and not others. Movements must be broken down into components, and basic mental, physiologic, and physical processes must be analyzed in relation to those tasks.

Second, evaluative procedures used for children, particularly children with intellectual disabilities, often differ from the more rigid clinical procedures used for adults. As in all of pediatrics, much information can be gathered by interacting with the child through observation and during play. Standard evaluative tests and procedures may be used as rapport is established, depending on the functional level of the child. Owing to the attention deficits and associated problems of the child with intellectual disabilities, the evaluation should be done serially and be ongoing. Consistent with the functional approach to curriculum and intervention planning, the PT should perform an evaluation with as many *functional aspects*, using age-appropriate materials, as is reasonable.

The third important element necessary for appropriate assessment is related to the basic orientation of the therapist. As with other areas of physical therapy, but more importantly with the child with multiple disabilities, the therapist must be able to identify not only the disability but also the child's abilities, however minimal. The skilled therapist will identify even the smallest of abilities and effectively communicate the importance of those abilities to the child, parents, and other professionals working with the child. A major focus of intervention involves attempts to increase

those abilities. This *"positive" orientation and approach* will have a beneficial effect on the child's self-image and on those people working with the child.[49] If our actions suggest a true concern and expectation for progress, however limited that progress may be, the effect of this attitude should encourage the child, the teachers, and the family to strive toward goals that have been identified.[49]

The fourth important element in evaluation is that the therapist must always concurrently assess *sensory processes and attention*. Children experience their world through their senses and the feedback received from sensory input and their attempts at interaction with the world. They assimilate the information; they take action; and they consequently modify subsequent actions. The therapist must understand by what means—or even whether—the child perceives the world, including you, the evaluator, before continuing with the evaluation.

Sensory Assessment and Intervention

The therapist must determine the basic responsiveness of the child before deciding on an appropriate interaction strategy for the rest of the evaluation. An early educator, Kinnealy, distinguished two broad categories of behaviors typical of children with intellectual disabilities on the basis of their reactions to various sensory stimuli or environmental input.[50] She described one group as having difficulty monitoring the intensity of sensory input and, therefore, difficulty in modulating the response. The other group was described as having reduced perception of the incoming stimuli. This group required more intense input for arousal or elicitation of a response. This initial difference in perception of sensory stimulus is a critical point of departure that the therapist must ascertain during the first attempt at interaction with the child.

Visual

When assessing the child's visual sense, the therapist should note the ability of the child to orient to, focus on, and track a visual stimulus. Notable responses include difficulty in tracking across the midline and noting the presence or absence of resting eye movements (nystagmus). During intervention and integration into classroom activities, visual stimulation activities can be used to provide practice in both focusing and tracking. Children who have poor head control may have an inadequate base of support for eye movements. Intervention aimed at improving postural mechanisms may improve visual skill.[48] Adaptive aids to ensure proper body positioning should be used as needed. Vestibular input may also improve visual focusing and processing because vestibular reflexes, in combination with optic and tonic neck reflexes, maintain a stable image on the retina while the head and body are in motion.[48] The vestibulo-oculomotor pathways contribute to skilled movements of the eyes that can be used for educational skills, including reading and writing[5] (Fig. 10.2).

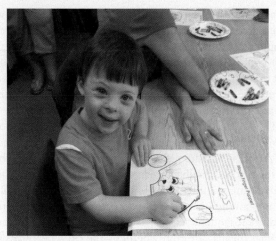

FIGURE 10.2 Angelo engaged in visual-motor and fine motor activity.

Auditory

The child's response to auditory stimuli may range from an absence of response, to simple orientation to and movement toward the stimulus, to a startle response.[48] Although it is difficult to assess hearing loss in a child with intellectual disabilities or multiple handicaps, referral for a complete audiologic evaluation is indicated whenever there is a possibility of a hearing loss. Audiologic testing can be used to identify a hearing loss, to differentiate between conductive and sensorineural loss, and to quantify the degree of loss. Tympanometry (an objective measure of eardrum function) helps identify a conductive loss when behavioral testing is unreliable. Testing for brain stem–evoked response traces the passage of an auditory stimulus from the ear to the brain stem. Central or cortical deafness describes a lack of interpretation of auditory information due to brain damage.

Vestibular stimulation is a component of intervention aimed at enhancing auditory integration. Although the vestibulocochlear nerve (cranial nerve VIII) has been described as comprising two separate entities (vestibular and auditory), it developed phylogenetically as a unit, and its portions appear to be related functionally.[48] There is clear clinical evidence that difficulties in hearing interfere with equilibrium responses. Vestibular input may not only improve equilibrium reactions, but may also sometimes enhance auditory attention and integration.[51,52]

Tactile

The tactile system is the largest sensory system, and it plays a major role in both physical and emotional behavior.[53,54] The tactile system develops earliest in utero, and the ability to process tactile input is important for neural organization. The sensation of touch is, in fact, the "oldest and most primitive expressive channel" and is a primary system for making contact with the external environment.[54,55] When

threatened, there is a predominant response of increased alertness and increased affect. When not challenged, however, the person is free to explore and manipulate the environment.[56,57] Many children with developmental disorders have a disordered tactile system. With neurologic impairment, many children demonstrate an aversive response to some types of tactile stimulation. This aversion to tactile stimuli, called *tactile defensiveness*, is often manifested by such behavior as hyperactivity or distractibility.[56] Children who demonstrate tactile defensiveness may display avoidance reactions around the hands, feet, and face. This behavior has obvious implications for the manner in which a child explores the environment, appreciates tactile sensation, and thus learns. Tactile defensiveness in the oral area may cause the child to reject textured or flavored food in preference to smoother, blander foods.

Tactile defensiveness may reflect a generalized "set" of the nervous system by which the child interprets stimuli as "danger."[56] Tactile functions were among the first means by which the child received information about his or her environment in order to adapt appropriately. Developmental disorder may produce behavior that appears to be less sophisticated and less discriminatory than normal. Tactile defensiveness or overresponsiveness may be present as poorly developed mechanisms for the interpretation of information. Clinically, the child may appear anxious, emotionally labile, or threatened and unable to cope. Compensatory behavior may be characterized by withdrawal, irritability, or distractibility.[56] Ayres has suggested various intervention approaches designed to facilitate increased organization of the tactile system and increased integration of this subsystem into effective environmental interaction. The proprioceptive system plays a cooperative role in this functional scheme.[56,57] The PT can easily incorporate appropriate activities for both the tactile and the proprioceptive systems into intervention. Heavy touch or weight bearing are excellent activities for decreasing tactile hypersensitivity and promoting proximal joint stability. Light touch or stimuli that tickle or irritate the child should be avoided in favor of activities that offer deep pressure and stability.

The response of the child with intellectual disabilities to tactile input must be observed and monitored during assessment and intervention. The therapist must note whether the child responds to the stimulus (i.e., the touch of the therapist's hand), and if so, the therapist must identify the type of response. If the input is noxious, does the child respond with a grimace, or does the child move actively to avoid the stimulus? One might surmise that the child who actively removes or withdraws from the noxious stimulus is not only aware of the stimulus but also has some proprioceptive sense by which to locate and remove the stimulus. Conversely, the therapist must be aware of the child who is so totally unaware of sensory input that the therapist is unable to penetrate and reach the child by any means.

Knowing the child's level of awareness will direct the therapist through subsequent stages of the evaluation and intervention process.[46]

Vestibular

Along with the tactile system, the vestibular system is one of the earliest developing sensory systems. The tracts within the vestibular system are fully myelinated by 20 weeks of gestation.[56] Information from the vestibular system tells us our position exactly in relation to gravity, whether or not we are moving, and our speed and direction of movement.[53] The vestibular system is so sensitive that changes in position and movement have a powerful effect on the brain, which can change with even the most subtle adjustments of movement or posture.[56]

The vestibular system has a strong effect on muscle tone and movement. This influence is mediated through the lateral and medial vestibular nuclei and affects efferent transmission to both intrafusal and extrafusal muscle fibers. Vestibular influence usually exerts a facilitatory effect on the gamma motoneuron to the muscle spindle and may influence the alpha motor neurons supplying skeletal muscle. By activating the gamma efferent to the muscle spindle, the afferent flow from the spindle is maintained and regulated for assistance with motor function. This basic role in muscle function and mobility gives the vestibular system an important role in the development and maintenance of body scheme that depends on interpretation of movement.[56,57] Impulses ascending to brain stem and cortical levels synapse with tactile, proprioceptive, visual, and auditory impulses to provide both perception of space and orientation of the body within that space.[53] Vestibular input seldom enters conscious thought or awareness except when the stimulus is so intense that we are rendered dizzy. It is important to know whether the child overreacts to or is threatened by movement, or has difficulty in attending to and assimilating movement experiences.[58] With a knowledge of the child's response to vestibular stimulation, activities can be chosen to improve balance, simulate experience of movement, activate muscle contraction, promote awareness and eye contact, and increase spatial awareness and perception. Examples of equipment used in these movement activities include swings, barrels, and scooter boards.

Self-Stimulation

Self-stimulation is an area of concern for some children with intellectual disabilities. This behavior can take many forms, including self-abuse. Examples of self-stimulation include constant mouthing of objects or the hand, spinning, head banging, hand or arm flapping, teeth grinding, rocking, and self-biting. Evaluation of the sensory status of the child may identify the reason for self-stimulation. The child may be performing self-stimulation to fulfill a basic sensory need, or he or she may be overly stimulated and may be reacting out of frustration or an inability to cope with sensory overload.[47]

In educational programs, the tendency is to discourage self-stimulation, especially when the stimulation is abusive or socially unacceptable. An appropriate sensory input must be substituted or the child may substitute another form of self-stimulation. A child who cannot cope with the sensory stimuli in the environment and is being overstimulated needs to have sensory input graded to tolerance.[47] As in all other areas of evaluation and intervention, the therapist must look beyond the behavior to the processes that are initiating it. Underlying sensory abnormalities or deficiencies must be recognized and intervened with before a change in behavior can be expected.

The manner in which the child provides self-stimulation can suggest strategies that may improve or eliminate the behavior. Slow, rhythmic rocking may be the distractible child's method of calming himself or herself, whereas violent, irregular rocking may be the hypotonic child's method of providing sensory input that will increase muscle activation and alertness. The type of behavior must also be considered in relation to the developmental age of the child. Constant mouthing of objects and hands is socially unacceptable for a school-aged child. If, however, that child is functioning at a lower developmental and functional level than age would dictate, oral exploration is a primary component of the learning process.[47] Rather than restricting such oral exploration and stimulation, the child must be provided means of oral stimulation, such as toothbrushing and foods of various textures, to help facilitate progression to the next developmental and functional level.

To summarize, the PT assessing the child with intellectual disabilities must have various skills and must approach the evaluation with a flexible but organized strategy. Assessment must include developmental testing, functional assessment, musculoskeletal assessment, posture, and strength and assessment of the sensory systems. Because the main goal of intervention is to enhance developmental skill attainment and to improve function, there must be a thorough examination of all sensory and motor components of development. It is challenging and rewarding to evaluate such a complex group of skill areas and still have a concise picture of the whole child.

▶ Key elements of physical therapy intervention

General Principles

Intervention with and management of the child with intellectual disabilities must be directed toward the development of the child's full potential in all areas of learning: motor, cognitive, and affective. The child's ability to respond appropriately and effectively in terms of movement, intellectual function, and attitudes and feelings serves as the major long-range goal of intervention. This concept of intervention applies to the total function of the child. A deficit in one type of behavior may influence all other types. The child who needs motor stability may also benefit from psychological stability. Influences used to change the former may also have an effect on the latter and vice versa.[49,60]

There are several important elements to remember when designing effective intervention programs for children with intellectual disabilities. The therapist must recognize the importance of choosing activities that accommodate the mental age of the child but are also as age-appropriate as possible. Activities in the intervention program should be interesting, fun, and meaningful. Because children with intellectual disabilities often have a poor attention span, therapeutic activities should be chosen that most effectively and efficiently meet the identified goal. Rather than asking a child to do a standard exercises for strengthening, the necessary therapeutic activities can be translated into a functional task or social game, often including other family members. This approach not only sustains interest, cooperation, and enthusiasm, but it emphasizes carryover into activities of daily living. It may also promote achievement of goals in other areas, such as social, emotional, self-help, and cognitive skills. The therapist must be imaginative and should integrate many different approaches to develop an effective intervention approach for a particular child in a particular situation (Fig. 10.3).

Repetition and consistency are crucial aspects of any program in which learning is expected. The therapist must design several activities that teach the same component task but do so in different ways. For example, if the goal is to improve extension strength of the trunk, the therapist may use activities such as a basketball drop or scooter board games. These activities are varied but enjoyable methods of attaining the same goal. This approach to program planning ensures not only the necessary repetition of activities, but also offers the dimensions of interest and fun for a child with limited comprehension or attention.

One of the most important yet most difficult skills for the therapist to master is the ability to delineate priorities for intervention and to establish effective and appropriate

long-term plans. It is easy for the therapist to become overwhelmed when the therapist is challenged by a child with numerous deficits in many areas of development. When developing intervention plans, it is important to consider the child as a whole person. All pieces of the assessment puzzle should merge to provide the therapist with a composite picture of how the child is or is not functioning within the child's world. The priorities for programming should become clear by looking at the child's overall development in this functional sense.[59]

Learning Characteristics

Differences in the Child with Intellectual Disabilities

An overview of cognitive development is necessary to understand the cognitive limitation of the child with intellectual disabilities and to design effective treatment programs to overcome those cognitive limitations.

Piaget's Theory of Intellectual Development

Jean Piaget, in order to explain normal and abnormal intellectual development, divided the developmental process into four stages: the sensorimotor period (0 to 18 months); the preoperational stage (2 to 7 years); the stage of concrete operations (7 to 12 years); and the period of formal operations (12 years and older).[61] The delineations offered by Piaget's stages provide a basis for understanding the sequence of normal development and the limitations that are typical at each stage of cognitive development. Utilizing Piaget's theory of development can be useful in understanding the various degrees of cognitive impairment seen in intellectual disabilities.

Children learn mainly through exploration of the senses and through movement during the sensorimotor stage, which Piaget explained as an equilibration process. The unknown is presented as a confrontation with the unexplained and less understood, and the child learns by his or her attempts to manipulate the environment with strategies with which to create new understandings, called accommodations. The inability to coordinate sensorimotor activity to reach certain goals is displayed by children with behaviors reflective of seriously impaired cognitive abilities, many of whom have coexisting physical and sensory impairments. Children thought to be functioning at this early stage explore their environment through much experimentation, which may even be repeated over and over. Accommodations to manage the environment when not routinely understood cannot be generalized to new situations. In fact, most learning involves discoveries made by trial and error. The preoperational stage is characterized by the development of language and the beginnings of abstract thought. Children at this stage can use symbols to represent objects that are not present, and may be able to classify and group objects, although not proficiently. A child with an IQ between 35 and 55 may not develop beyond this stage.[61]

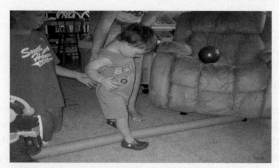

FIGURE 10.3 Two-year-old Angelo navigating his way around environmental obstacles and refining his postural control and balance, guided by his family.

During the concrete operations stage, the ability to order, classify, and relate experience to an organized whole begins to develop.[61] The child can solve some mathematical problems and can read well. The child can generalize learning to new situations and can begin to recognize another person's point of view. There is still an inability to deal with hypothetical or abstract problems. Persons with mild cognitive impairments often remain at this level of development.[61]

Piaget's final stage—formal operations—normally begins at 12 years of age and continues throughout life. The abilities to reason and hypothesize are characteristic of this stage. The child with intellectual disabilities seldom reaches this level of development. Cognitively, these children have characteristically limited memory, general knowledge, and abstract thinking, all combined with a slower learning rate.[24]

Intervention to Limit Cognitive Impairment

Concrete Concepts Compared with Abstract Concepts

Children with intellectual disabilities are less able to grasp abstract concepts than concrete concepts. When working with children with intellectual disabilities, the therapist must present concepts using meaningful, concrete directions. Activities are best understood when demonstrated, done passively first, or translated into familiar functional activities pertaining to daily life. Using step-by-step examples and pictures to represent activities would be useful to building understanding of the expectations. The child learns from the telling, the retelling, the demonstration, the practicing, and ultimately the actual performing in the "real" environment. Therapists need to understand the performance level in order to plan and direct the intervention plan.

Memory

The ability of the person with intellectual disabilities to remember is related to the type of retention task involved. Use of short-term memory is consistently difficult for the child with intellectual disabilities.[62–64] There is a high level of distractibility caused by external, irrelevant stimuli associated with these short-term memory deficits. However, this short-term memory problem can be overcome by repetitions to enhance the use of long-term memory, an area that tends to be a relative strength for children with intellectual disabilities. With this knowledge in mind, some of the following strategies can be used during physical therapy sessions.

- Remove irrelevant, distracting material from the activity area. Do not work with the child in distracting surroundings, even if room dividers or curtains must be used to separate a small space from a larger, busy area.
- Present each component of the task clearly and separately.
- Begin with simple tasks and then progress to more difficult tasks.
- Explain your expectations of the child at each stage of the intervention.

- Try to support the tasks with visual aids, or model the task repeatedly.
- Give immediate and consistent positive reinforcement.
- Repeat directions as often as necessary.
- Check the accuracy of performance frequently.
- Keep the child informed of progress, and give the child an opportunity to demonstrate or practice the new skill independently.

Most educators agree that practice, review, and overlearning help the child with intellectual disabilities with long-term retention of skills. The therapist can promote learning and retention by repeating both the directions and the steps needed to complete the intended skill. It is important to provide ample opportunity to practice and use the newly learned material. PTs inform parents and teachers of a child's progress and should encourage practice of the newly learned task at home or in the classroom. Learning cannot occur or be retained when the physical therapy sessions are an isolated segment of the child's day. Here again, the use of pictures and examples to extend the learning could be developed for the child to use in the home or community. Extended practice and communication with other team members are both vital.

Transfer of Learning

Transfer of learning is the ability to apply newly learned material to new situations having components that are similar to those of the material that was newly learned.[63] The Piagetian term for this process is assimilation. The learning challenge has been understood and the child has invented new strategies that are found to be useful in performing within the environment. The literature on transfer of learning suggests that two factors, in particular, be considered when formulating a plan for intervention.

Meaningfulness is an important element in transfer of learning for the child with cognitive impairment. A meaningful task is both easier to learn at the outset and easier to transfer to a second setting than one that has no meaning for the learner. This concept strongly supports the use of functional activities during physical therapy as opposed to meaningless "splinter skills."

Moreover, learning can be transferred best when both the initial task and the transfer task are *similar*. If, for example, the therapist is working on the ability to push rather than to pull on an assistive device, all of the therapy tasks, such as pushing in a prone position, sitting push-ups, and other tasks, can be transferred more readily to the task of pushing on the assistive device. *Consistency* also helps the child see the connection between therapy tools and their function.

Knowledge of basic learning concepts and an understanding of cognitive development are crucial for the PT working with a child who is intellectually impaired. The utility of the Piagetian theories to the understanding of good therapy practices is clear: learning is supported through the challenge stage while the child is learning to apply the strategy.

The process is enhanced through repetitions and the use of visual aids, with demonstrations of the usefulness of the habilitation skill, all of which support the accommodation, the understanding, and thus fosters generalization of the skill. Physical therapy is a learning situation, and some modifications in approach will be necessary to accommodate the differences in performance seen in the child with intellectual disabilities.

Intervention to Limit Physical Impairments and Functional Limitations

Pediatric PTs traditionally have focused their efforts on interventions designed to reduce musculoskeletal, neuromuscular, and cardiopulmonary impairments; decrease functional limitations; and prevent secondary impairment.[44] Early identification of these musculoskeletal, neuromuscular, and cardiopulmonary problems, and anticipation of their recognition as associated within specific diagnoses, gives the therapist an insight into appropriate life-span management of the child with intellectual disabilities. A glance again at Table 10.3 gives the therapist familiarity with some of the specific musculoskeletal, neuromuscular, or cardiopulmonary risks associated with common types of intellectual disabilities. Within this chapter, a focus on physical therapy management for the child with Down syndrome will offer the entry-level therapist a strategy for applying this management model to any child with any type of intellectual disabilities diagnosis. The child's needs change throughout the life span and will determine the level of support intervention required by physical therapy. Although this text is a pediatric physical therapy resource, this author will discuss life-span management issues relevant to the client with developmental disabilities as he or she moves into and through adulthood.

The Importance of Focused Intervention

Interventions designed by the therapist should be directed by the results of the multifaceted assessment and guided too by the findings of the functional assessment. Together, these assessments will provide the therapist and the intervention team direction to design focused interventions to develop skills that can be applied in varied environments.

To ensure the desired learning, the therapist is encouraged to design discrete tasks that reflect the child's participation within the current environments and to set goals that increase the participation levels. This will address the child's need for meaningful, purposeful, and concrete activities to more naturally provide the motivation to learn. As mentioned earlier, children with cognitive impairment learn better through multimodal teaching. Therapists are encouraged to use these techniques while teaching new tasks and practicing those previously introduced. To do this, we encourage the use of the "Practitioner's P's" methodology: *Plan, Present, Picture, Practice,* and *Perform.* First, it is

important to *Plan* the procedures for learning in specific discrete steps. Next, the therapist needs to be *Present* in ways that are understood by the child, being aware of any communication needs uncovered during the assessment stages. Following the presentation of the tasks to be learned during the session, the *Picture* of the task to be performed should be presented as well. This can be done through the use of pictures taken of the specific skill performance, through the use of available commercially produced stick-figure diagrams, or by showing a video clip. Another form would be the therapist modeling the task in step-by-step fashion. The fourth step is to have the child *Practice* the task. In this portion of the session, the therapist guides the child through the steps of the task using the hand-over-hand methodology. The fifth and final P is for the child to *Perform* the task. Using these five P's, the therapist will be encouraged to use the multimodal methods more routinely.

▶ The team concept and collaboration

When working with the child with intellectual disabilities, PTs must view themselves and their intervention goals as part of a total management plan. A transdisciplinary team is the standard approach for children with special needs. The current inclusion model offers strong support for the team concept. One of the main values of a transdisciplinary approach is the pooling of knowledge so that a composite and relevant course of action can be made. Because the child with intellectual disabilities will have delays in many areas of development, the skills of many professionals can be used. No single profession has the necessary scope of expertise or the resources to effectively provide care and education throughout the life of the child with intellectual disabilities.

In order to be effective, each professional on the team must understand the periodic shift of authority and emphasis during different stages of development. Physical therapy will sometimes be of paramount importance, whereas at other times, the PT may play a consultative or advisory role. Success of the team in helping the child achieve the maximum potential depends on each professional offering the needed expertise to alleviate specific problems when appropriate. Communication among team members and respect for one another's unique knowledge and skills are keys to making the team process truly collaborative and therefore effective.

Team members must ensure that consistency and reinforcement are present throughout the child's total program. For example, if certain sounds are being taught in speech therapy, these sounds can be reinforced during physical therapy sessions. The PT and special education teacher must work in partnership with the child. The therapist is uniquely qualified to assist the teacher in understanding the impact of impaired sensorimotor function on the achievement of cognitive milestones. For example, consider the child with

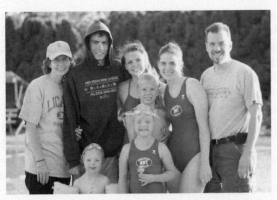

FIGURE 10.4 A family engaged in common fun physical activity, inclusive of Angelo and Julianna's interests and capabilities.

severely impaired movement control, average head control, and preferred movement patterns dominated by poor motor control patterns and strong tonic reflex patterns. Knowledge of normal development of movement control is invaluable to the teacher when working on a cognitive skill with the child. A simple suggestion from the therapist that the child be side-lying rather than supine could enable the child to reach for and manipulate the toy or utensil. Such a cooperative approach both facilitates the child's accomplishment and reduces the frustration of the teacher. The PT must communicate and work with all members of the team when appropriate. The present-day model of inclusion certainly facilitates this collaborative team concept.

PTs must recognize the importance of the parents as part of the therapeutic team because program carryover into the home is important for maximum effectiveness. The parents must be taught to work effectively with the child to help achieve goals of the program for all areas of intervention and education. When asking parents to participate in a home program of care, PTs must assess the abilities of the parent and identify potential problems or conditions in the home that may limit the successful participation of the parents. Referral to appropriate agencies may help parents alleviate or resolve those problems or conditions. The long-term nature of problems associated with intellectual disabilities and management of those problems requires a major commitment from the family (Fig. 10.4).

 A management model for physical therapists for the child with down syndrome

Definition

Down syndrome is a chromosomal disorder resulting in 47 chromosomes instead of 46.[65] Commonly called trisomy 21, Down syndrome results from faulty cell division affecting the 21st pair of chromosomes, either owing to a nondisjunction (95%), translocation (3% to 4%), or, least commonly, as a mosaic presentation (1%).[65]

History and Incidence

Down syndrome is the most common cause of intellectual disabilities and is encountered frequently by pediatric PTs. Approximately 4000 infants with Down syndrome are born annually in the United States at a rate increasing with maternal age, from 1 in 2000 when the mother is age 20, to 1 in 10 when the mother reaches the age of 49, with an overall incidence of 1 in 800 to 1 in 1000 live births.[66]

Evidence of Down syndrome dates to anthropologic records stemming from excavations in the seventh century of a Saxon skull that had many of the structural changes associated with Down syndrome.[67] Artwork throughout the Middle Ages depicts children with the now-recognized facial characteristics of Down syndrome. Despite these early historical conjectures, there are no published documented reports of Down syndrome until the 19th century. This lack of evidence may be because of the prevalence of infectious diseases and malnutrition that overshadowed research into genetic problems. Also, until beyond the mid-19th century, many children born with Down syndrome probably died in early infancy.[67]

In 1846, Edouard Sequin described a patient with features suggestive of Down syndrome. In 1866, John Langdon Down published a description of the characteristics of the recognizable syndrome, which has since borne his name.[67] It was not until the mid-1950s that methods to visualize chromosomes allowed more accurate studies of human chromosomes, leading to Lejeune's discovery that an alteration in the 21st chromosomal pair, leading to a trisomy of this pair, is the hallmark of Down syndrome.[68]

Pathophysiology and Associated Impairments of the Child with Down syndrome

Down syndrome results in neuromotor, musculoskeletal, and cardiopulmonary pathologies, which all require management by pediatric PTs. As with any etiology of intellectual disabilities, an awareness of the pathologies and impairments indigenous to that specific etiology will offer the practicing therapist a model for life-span management for the child.

Neuropathology

The primary CNS neuropathology in children with Down syndrome is due to several well-documented abnormalities. Overall brain weight in individuals with Down syndrome is 76% of normal, with the combined weight of the cerebellum and brain stem being even smaller—66% of normal. There is also microcephaly, and the brain is abnormally rounded and short with a decreased A-P diameter, specifically called microbrachycephaly.[69] The number of secondary sulci is reduced, resulting in a simplicity of convoluted patterns in the brains of children with Down syndrome.[70] Several cytologic distinctions of the brain include a paucity of small neurons, a migrational defect involving small neurons, and decreased synaptogenesis owing to altered synaptic morphology.[70] There are also structural abnormalities in the dendritic spines in the pyramidal tracts of the motor cortex that may underlie the motor incoordination so often seen in children with Down syndrome.[71] There is evidence of a lack of myelination with a delay in the completion of myelination between 2 months and 6 years of age. These abnormalities may explain the overall developmental delay typically seen in children with Down syndrome.[72] Some studies claim that up to 8% of children with Down syndrome also have a seizure disorder.[73]

Sensory Deficits

Visual and hearing deficits, and speech impairments are common in children with Down syndrome and must be identified on physical therapy assessment and intervention. Visual deficits include congenital as well as adult-onset cataracts, myopia (50%), farsightedness (20%), strabismus, and nystagmus.[73] Other ocular findings of less clinical significance include the presence of Brushfield spots in the iris and the classic presence of epicanthal folds.

Many children with Down syndrome (60% to 80%) have a mild to moderate hearing loss.[73] Otitis media often contributes to intermittent or persisting hearing loss in children with Down syndrome.[65]

Cardiopulmonary Pathologies

Forty percent of children with Down syndrome are born with congenital heart defects; most commonly, atrioventricular canal defects and ventriculoseptal defects.[65] Although usually repaired in infancy, heart defects not corrected by age 3 are highly associated with greater delays in motor skill development.[74]

Musculoskeletal Differences

Children with Down syndrome demonstrate many musculoskeletal differences of concern to the PT. Linear growth deficits are observed, including a decrease in normal velocity of growth in stature, with the greatest deficiency between 6 and 24 months of age,[75–77] leg-length reduction,[78] and a 10% to 30% reduction in metacarpal and phalangeal length. Muscle variations may also be present, including an absent palmaris longus and supernumerary forearm flexors. There is also a lack of differentiation of distinct muscle bellies for the zygomaticus major and minor and the levator labii superior, which may account for the typical facial appearance of the child with Down syndrome.[79]

The most significant musculoskeletal differences, however, are due largely to the hypotonia and ligamentous laxity characteristic of this disorder. Ligamentous laxity is thought to be due to a collagen deficit and commonly results in pes planus, patellar instability, scoliosis (52%), and atlantoaxial instability.[75,80,81] Atlantoaxial subluxation with risk for atlantoaxial dislocation is caused by laxity of odontoid ligament, with possible excessive motion of C1 on C2 (12% to 20% incidence).[82] Hip subluxation is also common in children with Down syndrome.

Generalized hypotonia, found in all muscle groups, is a hallmark feature in children with Down syndrome and is a major contributing factor to developmental motor delay.[32] Grip strength, isometric strength, and ankle strength have all been found deficient in studies on school-age children with Down syndrome.[83,84]

Additional Physical Characteristics

The back of the head is slightly flattened (brachycephaly), and the fontanels are frequently larger than normal and take longer to close. There may be areas of hair loss, and the skin is often dry and mottled in infancy, rough in the older child. The face of the child with Down syndrome has a somewhat flat contour, primarily because of the underdeveloped facial bones, facial muscles, and a small nose. Typically, the nasal bridge is depressed and the nasal openings may be narrow. The eyes are characterized by narrow, slightly slanted eyelids, with the corners marked by epicanthal folds. The mouth is small, the palate narrow, and the tongue may take on a furrowed shape in later childhood. Dentition is often delayed and may be spotty. The abdomen may be slightly protuberant secondary to hypotonia, and the chest may take on an abnormal shape secondary to congenital heart defect. More than 90% of children with Down syndrome develop an umbilical hernia. Hands and feet tend to be small, and the fifth finger is curved inward. In about 50% of children with Down syndrome, a single crease is observed across the palm on one or both hands (simian crease). The toes are usually short, and in the majority of children with Down syndrome, there is a wide space between the first and the second toes, with a crease running between them on the sole of the foot.

▶ Physical therapy assessment and intervention of the child with down syndrome

Physical therapy assessment of the child with Down syndrome should view the child from multiple perspectives. The therapist must be aware of coexisting medical problems and remain especially alert to those typically associated with Down syndrome such as cardiac status, atlantoaxial stability, hearing and visual status, and the presence of seizure disorders. Speech difficulties may be present, and therapists may find effective communication difficult during assessment and subsequent intervention. The therapist must also integrate the child's cognitive capabilities into the evaluation process, including discussion of formal intelligence tests as appropriate and interviews with parents, and the therapist may perform a brief cognitive assessment as part of a comprehensive developmental test battery. Evaluation includes any or all of the following measures as appropriate for the age and setting within which the child is evaluated: comprehensive developmental testing, component testing of gross and fine motor skills including qualitative observational assessment of movement, musculoskeletal assessment, assessment of automatic reactions and postural responses, and ultimately, a functional assessment. These pediatric evaluation procedures are discussed elsewhere in this text. Evaluation of the child with any type of intellectual disabilities disorder, including Down syndrome, additionally encompasses assessment of the musculoskeletal, neuromotor, and cardiopulmonary impairments associated with the specific diagnosis (Table 10.3), and knowledge of the coexistence of the cognitive deficit associated with intellectual disabilities and how that affects physical therapy assessment and intervention.

Learning Differences

Generally, children with intellectual disabilities such as Down syndrome have been found to:

1. be capable of learning,
2. benefit from frequent repetitions in order to learn,
3. have difficulty generalizing skills,
4. need more frequent practice sessions in order to maintain learned skills,
5. need extended time to respond, and
6. have a more limited repertoire of responses.[85]

The levels of cognitive impairment seen in children with Down syndrome vary, from profoundly to mildly impaired, with a mild to moderate impairment being most common. As with any child with coexistent visual or hearing deficits, therapists must adapt interaction, assessment, and teaching to accommodate these coimpairments. Children with Down syndrome typically have attention deficits and difficulties with information processing. Research also shows a myriad of specific cognitive problems encountered in children with Down syndrome, including difficulties in sequential verbal processing, social–cognitive skills, auditory memory, and motor planning.[47,86–88] Children with Down syndrome appear to have significant impairments in verbal–motor interactions, with learning least proficient when the mode of response or reception calls for auditory or vocal skill.[89] Therapists should employ frequent visual demonstration, practice and rehearsal, and multimodal sensory approaches to best interact with the child. The child may benefit from hand-over-hand demonstrations to aid in movement pattern development. The child with Down syndrome is more likely to remember the rules and patterns of a new activity if he or she is presented with input over many modalities—visual and kinesthetic as well as verbal.

Associated Motor Deficits

The ligamentous laxity and generalized muscular hypotonia associated with Down syndrome contribute the most to the motor delays and secondary musculoskeletal impairments that are of utmost concern to pediatric PTs. The degree to which muscular hypotonia is present will vary, but most investigators agree that it is the most frequently observed characteristic in children with Down syndrome.[32] Hypotonia is distributed to all major muscle groups, including neck, trunk, and all four extremities.

Developmental Delay

Clinically, muscular hypotonia has been highly correlated with developmental delay, including delay in attainment of gross and fine motor milestones,[74,90] and delay in other areas of development such as speech acquisition and cognitive development.[91,92] A slower rate of development of postural reactions has been noted in children with Down syndrome.[93] Additional studies by Harris and Rast and Shumway-Cook also demonstrated difficulties in postural control, antigravity control, deficits in postural response synergies when balance perturbations were introduced, and, consequently, the development of compensatory movement strategies as children with Down syndrome attempted to learn to move and stabilize themselves.[33,93,94] These investigators attribute the movement deficiencies seen in children with Down syndrome primarily to disturbances in postural control and balance.

In addition to developmental delay, there is evidence to suggest that muscular hypotonia, ligamentous laxity, and postural difficulties contribute to some movement differences observed in children with Down syndrome. Examples include "W" sitting, where the child will characteristically spread his or her legs to a full 180-degree split while in prone and then advance to a sitting posture by pushing up with his or her hands into sitting.[95] Gait acquisition is delayed and immature, characterized by a persistent wide-based gait and out-toeing.[95,96] These differences in movement qualities are likely caused by muscular hypotonia, ligamentous laxity, and a resultant lack of trunk rotation. Hypotonia is thought to contribute to slower reaction time and depressed kinesthetic feedback. Children with motor impairments are at subsequent risk for secondary impairments because of their restricted ability to explore the environment, which may impair cognition, communication, and psychosocial development.[97–99]

Physical Therapy Evaluation and Intervention Implications

Evaluation should include administration of a comprehensive or component test to measure and track the developmental delay. Qualitative assessment of movement will alert the therapist to movement differences and possible emerging compensatory strategies. Intervention must include an understanding from a functional, dynamic systems perspective: the control parameters most likely to cause a responsiveness shift when attempting to influence developing motor strategies.[100] The general goal is to anticipate gross and fine motor delay and provide interventions to minimize it by:

- teaching the caregivers appropriate positioning and handling activities to use throughout early infancy and childhood to promote antigravity control and weight bearing,
- designing activities to encourage the development of antigravity muscle strength in all positions,
- emphasizing trunk extension and extremity loading, which tend to increase axial muscle tone,
- encouraging the emergence of righting and postural reactions through use of rotation within and during movement,
- encouraging dynamic rather than static exploration of movement,
- facilitating the emergence of developmental milestones when chronologically appropriate, including supported sitting and standing, when trunk control and alignment are able to be established (Fig. 10.5),
- anticipating the delay in postural control responses and providing functional opportunities to enhance development in areas of cognition, language, and socialization, and
- teaching parents and other team members activities and position choices that will enhance the child's overall development.[101]

Musculoskeletal Problems

In addition to generalized muscular hypotonia, ligamentous laxity is a hallmark musculoskeletal characteristic of Down syndrome and commonly results in pes planus, patellar instability, scoliosis (52%), and atlantoaxial instability.[75,80,81]

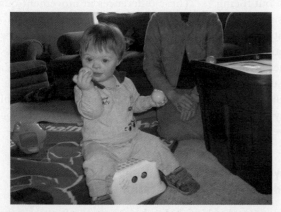

FIGURE 10.5 Incorporating play within the natural home environment as Angelo develops and practices balance and postural control.

The previously noted atlantoaxial relationship is identified by sagittal-plane radiographs of the cervical spine in three different positions: flexion, neutral, and extension.[102–104] A joint interval of 6 to 10 mm is considered symptomatic. A joint interval of more than 4.5 mm carries precautions with it. Early signs of atlantoaxial dislocation include gait changes, urinary retention, reluctance to move neck, and increased deep tendon reflexes (DTRs).[82] In cases of dislocation with symptomatic atlantoaxial instability, posterior arthrodesis or fusion of C1 and C2 is recommended.[102] In addition to atlantoaxial instability, thoracolumbar scoliosis is also an associated vertebral column musculoskeletal impairment frequently seen in children and adolescents with Down syndrome, usually defined as of a mild to moderate degree.[81]

In the lower extremities, hip instability, patellar instability, and foot deformity are the most common musculoskeletal concerns for the PT managing the child with Down syndrome. Hip subluxation is secondary to developmental acetabular dysplasia and long, tapered ischia that result in decreased acetabular and iliac angles as well as laxity of ligamentous support.[80] Pes planus and metatarsus primus varus are the major foot deformities seen in children with Down syndrome.[81]

Ligamentous laxity makes any joint less resistant to trauma, malalignment, or uneven forces. Alignment and support are crucial. The atlantoaxial joint is less resistant especially to superimposed flexion, where the joint interval is already widened. Therapists should avoid exaggerated neck flexion, extension, rotation, and positions or movements that may cause twisting or undue forces. With caution, joint approximation or compression of the cervical spine should be performed gently with all children with Down syndrome, but these activities are contraindicated in children with identified atlantoaxial instability. Therapists should also use caution when placing a child in the inverted position or in other positions that increase risk of a fall onto the head.[82] In the infant and child under the age of 2 years, a radiograph will not reliably detect atlantoaxial instability. Extreme caution must be taken, and any activity that may result in cervical spine injury should be avoided. PTs must closely monitor children with Down syndrome for changes in neurologic status and be vigilant in assessing the risk of atlantoaxial instability. Parent education should include discussion of atlantoaxial instability, symptoms of neurologic compromise, periods and activities that may carry increased risk, and activities to avoid if instability is identified.[82]

The Committee on Sports Medicine of the American Academy of Pediatrics recommends an initial set of cervical spine radiographs at 2 years of age and follow-up radiographs in grade school, at adolescence, and adulthood.[102] Contact sports and physical activities that may result in cervical spine injury may be contraindicated.[105] The following activities are considered to be restricted for children with even asymptomatic atlantoaxial intervals of greater than 4.5 mm: gymnastics (somersaults), diving, high jump, soccer, butterfly stroke in swimming, exercises that place pressure on the head and neck, and high-risk activities that involve possible trauma to the head and neck.[102–106]

Screening for scoliosis should be a routine part of life-span management of the child with Down syndrome, especially during periods of increased risk such as growth spurts, puberty, and throughout adolescence. Parents should be taught to perform routine screening for scoliosis. Activities and exercises should promote symmetry and alignment.

Musculoskeletal assessment should also include biomechanical assessment of the lower extremity and orthotic management, if indicated, for pes planus. In the infant, assessment of hip stability is a routine part of a physical therapy evaluation with referral for orthopedic assessment if hip instability is suspected. Supported standing in a stander should not be instituted unless hip stability and proper alignment has been established.

The general goal is to maintain alignment and encourage normal movement forces to promote optimal biomechanical forces for best musculoskeletal development and prevention of anticipated malalignment and instabilities. Suggestions include:

1. use of aligned compression or weight-bearing forces to stimulate longitudinal bone growth as well as thickness and density of the bone and shaft,
2. aligned, supported weight bearing to promote joint stability and formation, and
3. facilitation of muscular cocontraction, force production, and increased muscle tone.

In summary, the impact of these associated motor deficits upon the child's development and overall functioning often requires physical therapy. Most of these movement problems have their basis in CNS pathology or primary musculoskeletal differences. These motor deficits often lead to secondary impairments in flexibility, stability, force production, coordination, postural control, balance, endurance, and overall efficiency. The specific intervention used will depend on the identified problems and on the consequences that can be predicted and perhaps prevented.

Neuromuscular Impairments	Functional Implication
Hypotonia, low force production	Motor delay, poor contraction
	Movement paucity
Slow automatic postural reactions	Balance limitations
	Slow reaction time
	Decreased speed
Joint hypermobility	Instability, movement anxiety
Atlantoaxial instability, scoliosis, foot deformities	May preclude access to activities or limit participation level in activity

Cardiopulmonary Fitness

General physical fitness is often below desired levels in children with intellectual disabilities, and specifically, in children with Down syndrome.[107] Children with Down syndrome are at risk for restrictive pulmonary disease with concomitant decreased lung volumes and a weak cough, because of generalized trunk and extremity weakness.[108–110] Reduced cough effectiveness may contribute to high incidence of respiratory infections. Decreased lung volumes, including vital capacity and total lung capacity, may contribute to a deficiency of the pulmonary system to oxygenate the mixed venous blood or remove the carbon dioxide from the same blood.[111] If there is a reduction in the maximum amount of oxygen available for transport, the energy available for activities is lowered, leading to a reduced level of physical fitness.

Physical Therapy Life Span Evaluation and Intervention Implications

The implications for life-span management of the child with Down syndrome are obvious.

There needs to be greater emphasis on physical fitness that may increase cardiopulmonary endurance and muscular strength. Programming should begin with children of primary school age in order to prevent a slowing of activity and the subsequent onset of obesity and long-term atherosclerotic risk profiles.[107] Knowledge of improvement reported from training programs for children with Down syndrome supports the ability of these children to respond to early intervention.[112,113] PTs play an important role in the cardiopulmonary fitness arena through direct intervention or in consultation with special educators or physical/recreational educators. The general goals are to encourage cardiopulmonary endurance, overall physical fitness, and parent/caregiver/client education. Participation in sports and recreational activities such as swimming, dancing, and martial arts should be encouraged and supported from early childhood and onward (Fig. 10.6).

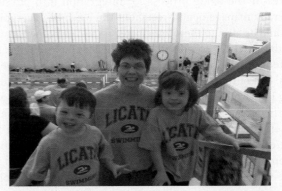

FIGURE 10.6 Mom encouraging participation in group recreational activities, such as swimming, for the multiple benefits of physical fitness and socialization.

▶ The person with intellectual disabilities moving into and through adulthood: key management issues

Intellectual disabilities and Down syndrome both represent types of developmental disabilities. The Developmental Disabilities Assistance and Bill of Rights Amendment of 1987 defines a "developmental disability" as a severe and chronic disability that manifests before age 22, is attributable to a mental and/or physical impairment, results in substantial functional limitations in three or more major life activities, and reflects a need for a combination and sequence of special, individualized services that are of extended duration or lifelong.[114,115] With increased sensitivity to life-span issues and the recent availability of both retrospective reviews and good clinical case reports, the recent literature documents typical life-span management concerns. Concurrently, the current practice of physical therapy focuses attention on wellness and preventative management. It is imperative that the practitioners of today integrate a proactive, wellness-focused preventative bias into a client's management plan. Because persons with intellectual disabilities, including Down syndrome, typically begin intervention in childhood, the PT is likely to be the clinician to follow that client into and through adulthood. This section will highlight some of the typical challenges for persons with intellectual disabilities and/or Down syndrome as they grow older.

These persons can now expect an increased life expectancy and will experience the same age-related changes that occur in the general population.[116,117] The aging process appears to start earlier in persons with intellectual disabilities, perhaps as early as age 35, and generally at around age 55.[117-120] The onset and the impact of the age-related changes are influenced by the severity of the person's existing disabilities and are likely to have a more significant effect if the person has multiple coimpairments.[116]

A review of the literature reveals several pertinent features of the aging process for integration into physical therapy management throughout the life span. Therapists should be alert to these anticipated issues: early menopause with the related secondary effects, such as increased risk for osteoporosis, thyroid dysfunction, obesity, diabetes mellitus, late onset of seizure disorder, increased visual or hearing impairment, cardiac disease, depression, dementia, and Alzheimer disease.[121-125] Physical therapy evaluation and intervention should include preventative management for the early onset of any number of these disorders. Evaluation methods may require that standardized tests be modified for use with the cognitively impaired individual.[126] As emphasized throughout this chapter, a main focus of assessment and intervention is to preserve safe, independent function or caregiver assistance, as required. Therapists need to use an individualized and multidimensional approach to meet these wide-ranging needs of adults with developmental disabilities.[127]

SUMMARY

The PT is challenged to use various skills in the management of the child with intellectual disabilities. The many complex and persistent difficulties encountered by children with intellectual disabilities often require innovative methods of physical therapy evaluation and intervention. It is easy to understand that PTs may feel overwhelmed by the complexity of this population.

This chapter has attempted to give therapists a "user-friendly" strategy for physical therapy management, including evaluation and intervention, for *any* child with a diagnosis of intellectual disabilities. Therapists are reminded to view the intellectual disability itself as only a partial description of that child's learning impairment. The total learning impairment may vary in severity with a mild to a profound influence on that child's functional learning capabilities. This may be compounded by other concomitant sensory deficits, including visual, hearing, or sensory organizational problems. Physical therapy evaluation and intervention must incorporate not only the basic principles of pediatric physical therapy but also an understanding of the principles of teaching and learning related to the child with intellectual disabilities.

There are at least 350 known etiologies for intellectual disability. The therapist can easily investigate any of those specific etiologies to become knowledgeable with any commonly associated neuromuscular, musculoskeletal, or cardiopulmonary impairments. This investigative approach will focus the therapist's assessment skills and alert the PT to the presence of likely coimpairments or associated medical problems. An understanding of the primary pathology and associated motor deficits readily assists the therapist in establishing treatment goals and priorities. Effective physical therapy management of the child through the life span can anticipate secondary deformities and risks for that child, which should be shared with parents and other team members. This chapter illustrated the application of this investigative strategy to the physical therapy management of a child with Down syndrome. This same strategy can be applied to any intellectual disabilities diagnosis encountered in pediatric physical therapy practice.

Communication of the changing needs of children with intellectual disabilities to parents and other professionals requires not only technical expertise on the part of the therapist but also the ability to be a sensitive listener and creative teacher. Through an effective transdisciplinary approach to the child and his or her family, we can strive to help the child with intellectual disabilities to function at his or her best in society.

CASE STUDY

By Ann Marie Licata, PhD, assistant professor of education, Alvernia University, and parent of children with Down syndrome

This case study will summarize the use of physical therapy with two children with Down syndrome in the same family:

"Heel, toe, let's go," I heard our son, Vincent, echo as he helped his younger brother Angelo take strides along the path to the mailbox, a scene typical for our family as we work together in an effort to help Angelo and Julianna, the two youngest members of our family. Angelo and Julianna were born with Trisomy 21, more commonly known as Down syndrome. While two of our six children have the same medical diagnosis, each is an individual, possessing a charm-like quality that wins the hearts of their family members and those whom they encounter. Like their personalities, Angelo and Julianna's unique stories of development are vastly different, providing for a rich contrast and heartwarming account that gives greater depth to our family experiences and is a testament to the individuality of all persons, with or without Down syndrome (Fig. 10.7).

Our story begins on a beautiful October day in the early afternoon when our fifth child, a little boy, whom we named Angelo, was born. As an older mother, I carefully counted his ten toes and fingers and pronounced him "perfect." His Apgar score was strong, and we were elated to now be parents of three boys and two girls. It was not until later that day that we were quite surprised to learn that our "perfect" little boy had Down syndrome. As a professional educator who had worked in different capacities throughout my career and had supported many children with disabilities and their families, I had never imagined that I would be a mother to a special needs child.

Once we were over the initial surprise that news of this nature often delivers, we began to immediately discern the supports that Angelo would need. Children born with Down syndrome tend to have more related health concerns with their heart, eyes, and ears. Within the first 24 hours of his life, Angelo's heart was examined and found to be normal. Several days later, Angelo's hearing was also found to be within the normal range. While we knew Angelo's vision must be assessed, that task happened 3 months into his short life, again with a positive affirmation that he had normal vision. With these initial physical concerns addressed, we then quickly moved on to considering the overall developmental supports that Angelo would need. At 2 weeks of age, we telephoned the office of Early Intervention, seeking an evaluation to determine the need for supportive services. We did not know at the time that Angelo's medical diagnosis of Down syndrome automatically qualified him for the therapies that he would need.

By Angelo's fifth week of life, he had been assessed by a team and found to be in need of two services, including physical therapy. A selection process allowed us to choose the person whom we would grow to trust, Angelo's PT, Nancy. With very limited knowledge of the adventure on which our family was about to embark, Nancy began Angelo's weekly 1-hour therapy sessions in our home, initiating the process with a formal plan for his development, an individual family services plan (IFSP). We did not realize the hours of effort that it would take to help Angelo achieve the developmental tasks that we take for granted, such as rolling over, sitting independently, crawling, and walking. Because of Angelo's low muscle tone and motor delays, we were coached by his PT on how to teach or train his muscles to become strengthened so that they could support and move him as he wanted to move (Fig. 10.8).

We had confidence that he would accomplish these tasks, knowing that his delays in motor development were impacting his cognitive growth. Nancy had explained that Angelo's delay in crawling and walking would also slow his ability to explore the world around him. We knew he would reach these developmental milestones that would support his overall development, but the question that plagued us was "when?"

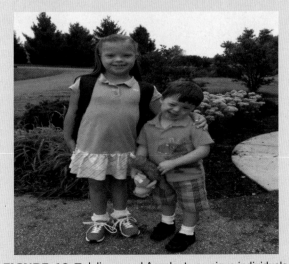

FIGURE 10.7 Julianna and Angelo, two unique individuals.

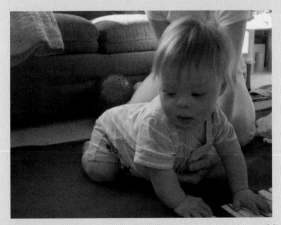

FIGURE 10.8 Angelo actively investigates and navigates his home environment as the therapist uses that natural environment to facilitate development.

Being a professional educator and mother of four other children who all displayed typical development, I thought I understood how children grew and matured. It was only when Angelo began to crawl and later walk initially at over 2 years of age that Nancy's subtle reminders helped us to realize that typical development was truly a miracle. How could I have missed this fact all these years? This revelation was cause for celebration, and celebrate we did. Angelo's attainments of the developmental milestones were viewed as huge victories—a realization of much greater joy than I had ever experienced or appreciated for my four older children. Even now, at age 5, we commemorate the small wins along the way, as Angelo has recently learned the skill of jumping and, yes, even running and playing soccer (Fig. 10.9).

Helping us to recognize the joys and celebrations of achievement were a part of what Angelo's therapists did naturally—by building a relationship with not just Angelo, but with all members of our family, Nancy gave us the confidence that we needed as parents of a child born with Down syndrome. She encouraged our interactions, connected us with resources, and used us as resources for other families who needed support. She frequently sought out opportunities to include Angelo's brothers and sisters in his therapy sessions, recognizing the significance of the support that he needed and the enduring bond that Angelo had made with each one of us. These weekly interactions, while not designed for this purpose, helped the members of our family grow closer to one another, forming a single family unit, stronger than we could have imagined (Fig. 10.4).

Nancy's friendly demeanor and genuine interest in not just Angelo and his development, but our entire family extended beyond the scheduled 1-hour therapy sessions. Frequently, she brought newspaper clippings of the older children's swimming achievements, building rapport and establishing a relationship that would last for a long time. Nancy, like Angelo's other therapists, gave us support and encouragement as parents. She helped us to recognize the strengths that we had as a family and that my husband Kenny and I shared as parents.

During the first 2 years of Angelo's life, we were blessed with many competent caring individuals who supported us along the way. What Angelo also helped us to realize was that there were others like him in this world who needed a mom and dad, especially because of their disabilities. Angelo helped us to conquer our fears when considering the possibility of helping another child to find a family—our family. After much thought, prayer, and many sleepless nights, our family began the international journey shortly before Angelo's second birthday to adopt Julianna, our daughter who was born with Down syndrome. Nine months later, we brought our 8-year-old daughter home to her five siblings. Her homecoming was another opportunity for our family to celebrate.

Unlike Angelo, Julianna had no therapeutic intervention as a baby. She had lived initially in a baby house orphanage and was later sent to a mental institution in her home country. Despite her lack of educational experiences, Julianna was amazingly physically coordinated, drop-kicking a ball better than most of her typically developing peers. Julianna quickly taught herself many of the developmental skills that she may have missed, including how to alternate feet while descending stairs, snap her fingers, and swing. As parents, we observed firsthand that no two individuals with Down syndrome are alike; their strengths and needs were very different (Fig. 10.10).

Angelo continues to receive physical therapy, as well as other supportive services that meet his needs at this stage of his life. Julianna too receives services, and continues to thrive in the physical domain, playing soccer on an age group club team and swimming competitively. Their abilities differ, as do their personalities. It is so true that no two individuals are the same regardless of the conditions or labels that they might share.

As the members of our family continue to grow older, we become closer to one another, supporting each other along the

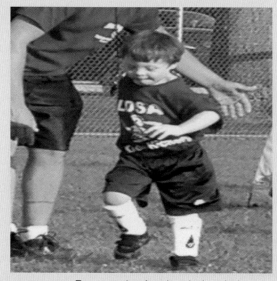

FIGURE 10.9 Team member Angelo enjoying playing soccer!

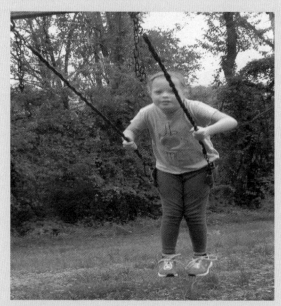

FIGURE 10.10 Julianna learns how to propel *herself* on a swing!

journey. An appreciation for each other's strengths and differences has become the norm in our home, noting what make each of us uniquely special. Our life experiences with one another have given us a connection that cannot be broken. The therapeutic terms, jargon, and skills that have been acquired through our experiences, initially with Angelo and now with Julianna, help us all to be grateful for the simple joys in life, acknowledging that not only are our lives a gift, we are each a gift to one another.

Acknowledgments

We would like to thank all of those individuals with an intellectual disability who have offered us the privilege of working with you and getting to know you. You have taught us far more than we could ever hope to have taught you! With deep humility, we acknowledge the strength, unconditional love, and devotion that the families of children with intellectual disability model for all of us. Most especially, we are deeply humbled and grateful for the contribution of our colleague Ann Marie Licata, as she shares her family's story in the case study in this chapter. Their family story offers inspiration for countless families and therapists.

REFERENCES

1. Nichtern S. *Helping the Retarded Child.* New York, NY: Grosset and Dunlap; 1974.
2. Sebelist RM. Intellectual disabilities. In: Hopkins HL, Smith HD, eds. *Willard and Spackman's Occupational Therapy.* 9th ed. Philadelphia, PA: JB Lippincott; 1996.
3. National Institute on Intellectual disabilities. *Orientation Manual on Intellectual disabilities.* Ontario, Canada: York University; 1981.
4. Itard J. *The Wild Boy of Aveyron.* Englewood Cliffs, NJ: Prentice-Hall; 1962.
5. American Association on Intellectual Disabilities (AAID). 1719 Kalorama Road, NW, Washington, DC: 2009–2683.
6. Sorrells AM, Rieth HJ, Sindelar PT. *Critical Issues in Special Education: Access, Diversity, and Accountability.* Boston, MA: Pearson Education Inc; 2004.
7. Winzer MA. A tale often told: the early progression of special education. *Remedial Spec Educ.* 1998;19(4):212–219.
8. PARC v. Commonwealth of pennsylvania, 1972. In Heward WL. *Exceptional Children.* Upper Saddle River, NJ: Merrill Prentice Hall; 2003.
9. http://www.National Disability Rights Network. Protection & Advocacy for Individuals with Disabilities. About/Our History (Willowbrook)
10. American Psychiatric Association. DSM-5 development. Intellectual Disability. Retrieved from http://www.dsm5.org/Pages/Default .aspx.
11. Website for proposed DSM-5 definition. http://www.dsm5org/ Proposedrevision/Pages?proposedrevision.apex?rid=384.
12. Luckasson R, Coulter DL, Polloway EA, et al. *Mental Retardation: Definition, Classification, and Systems of Supports.* Washington, DC: American Association on Mental Retardation; 1992.
13. Roid GH. *Stanford-Binet Intelligence Scale.* 5th ed. Itasca, IL: Riverside; 2003.
14. Wechsler D. *Wechsler Intelligence Scale for Children-IV.* San Antonio, TX: Psychological Corp; 2003.
15. Wechsler D. *Wechsler Preschool and Primary Scale of Intelligence III.* San Antonio, TX: Psychological Corp; 2002.
16. Kaufman AS, Kaufman NL. *Kaufman Assessment Battery for Children.* Circle Pines, MN: American Guidance Service; 2003.
17. Sparrow SS. *Vineland Adaptive Behavior Scales.* Circle Pines, MN: American Guidance Service; 1984.
18. Adams GL. *Comprehensive Test of Adaptive Behavior.* Columbus, OH: Merrill; 1984.
19. Sloan W, Birch JW. A rationale for degrees of retardation. *Am J Ment Defic.* 1955;60:262.
20. Jette AM. Toward a common language for function, disability, and health. *Phys Ther.* 2006;86:5:726–734.
21. World Health Organization. *International Classification of Functioning, Disability, and Health.* Geneva, Switzerland; 2001.
22. National Institutes of Health. *Draft V: Report and Plan for Rehabilitation Research.* Bethesda, MD: National Institutes of Health, National Center for Rehabilitation and Research; 1992.
23. Chinn PC, Drew CJ, Logan DR. *Intellectual Disabilities: A Life Cycle Approach.* St.Louis, MO: CV Mosby; 1979.
24. Algozzine B, Ysseldyke J. *Teaching Students with Mental Retardation: A Practical Guide for Every Teacher.* Thousand Oaks, CA: Corwin Press; 2006.
25. Brown I, Percy M. *A Comprehensive Guide to Intellectual and Developmental Disabilities.* Baltimore, MD: Paul H Brookes Publishing Company; 2007.
26. *International Classification of Diseases* (ICD). Ann Arbor, MI: World Health Organization; 1992.
27. Leonard H, Xingyan W. The epidemiology of mental retardation: challenges and opportunities in the new millennium. *Ment Retard Dev Disabil Res Rev.* 2002;8:117–134.
28. Nyhan WL, Sakati NO. *Genetic and Malformation Syndromes in Clinical Medicine.* Chicago, IL: Year Book Medical Publishers; 1976.
29. Baraitser M, Clayton-Smith J, Donnai D. *Clinical Dysmorphology.* Philadelphia, PA: Lippincott, Williams and Wilkins 2011.
30. Liu J, Krantz I. Cornelia de Lange syndrome, cohesin, and beyond. *Clin Genet* [serial online]. 2009;76(4):303–314. Available from: Academic Search Premier, Ipswich, MA. Accessed September 28, 2012.
31. Jones KL. *Smith's Recognizable Patterns of Human Malformation.* 5th ed. Philadelphia, PA: WB Saunders; 1996.
32. Harris SR, Shea AM. Down syndrome. In: Campbell SK, ed. *Pediatric Neurologic Physical Therapy.* 2nd ed. New York, NY: Churchill Livingstone; 1991.
33. Shumway-Cook A, Woollacott MH. Dynamics of postural control in the child with Down syndrome. *Phys Ther.* 1985;65(9): 1315–1322.
34. Bloom AS, et al. Developmental characteristics of recognizable patterns of human malformation. In: Berg JM, ed. *Science and Service in Intellectual Disabilities: Proceedings of the Seventh Congress of the International Association for the Scientific Study of Mental Deficiency* (LASSMD). New York, NY: Methuen; 1985.
35. Keenan J, Kastner T, Nathanson R, et al. A statewide public and professional educational program on fragile syndrome. *Ment Retard.* 1992;30(6):355–361.
36. Rinck C. Fragile X syndrome. *Dialogue on Drugs, Behavior and Developmental Disabilities.* 1992;4(3):1–4.
37. Anderson LT, Ernst M. Self-injury in Lesch-Nyhan disease. *J Autism Dev Dis.* 1994;24:67–81.
38. Aughton DJ, Cassidy SB. Physical features of Prader-Willi syndrome in neonates. *Am J Dis Child.* 1990;144(11):1251–1254.
39. Dykens EM, Cassidy SB. Prader-Willi syndrome: genetic, behavioral and treatment issues. *Child Adolesc Psychiatric Clin N Am.* 1996;5:913–927.
40. Guidera KJ, Borrelli J Jr, Raney E, et al. Orthopaedic manifestations of Rett syndrome. *J Pediatr Orthop.* 1991;11(2):204–208.
41. Holm VA, King HA. Scoliosis in the Rett syndrome. *Brain Dev.* 1990;12(1):151–153.
42. Nomura Y, Segawa Y. Characteristics of motor disturbance in Rett syndrome. *Brain Dev.* 1990;12(1):27–30.
43. Stewart KB, Brady DK, Crowe TK, et al. Rett syndrome: a literature review and survey of patents and therapists. *Phys Occup Ther Pediatr.* 1989;9(3):35–55.

44. McEwen I. Intellectual disabilities. In: Campbell SK, ed. *Physical Therapy for Children.* 4th ed. Philadelphia, PA: WB Saunders; 2011.

45. Detterman DK, Mayer JD, Canuso DR, et al. Assessment of basic cognitive abilities in relation to cognitive deficits. *Am J Ment Retard.* 1992;97(3):251–286.

46. Turnbull A, Turnbull HR, Wehmeyer ML, et al. *Exceptional Lives.* Boston, MA: Pearson; 2013.

47. Horvat M, Croce R. Physical rehabilitation of individuals with intellectual disabilities: physical fitness and information processing. *Crit Rev Phys Rehabil Med.* 1995;7(3):233–252.

48. Montgomery PC. Assessment and treatment of the child with intellectual disabilities. *Phys Ther.* 1981;61:1265–1272.

49. Shields N, Bruder A, Taylor N, et al. Influencing physiotherapy student attitudes toward exercise for adolescents with Down syndrome. *Disabil Rehabil.* 2011;33(4):360–366.

50. Kinnealy M. Aversive and nonaversive responses to sensory stimuli in mentally retarded children. *Am J Occup Ther.* 1973;27:464–472.

51. deQuirds JB. Diagnosis of vestibular disorders in the learning disabled. *J Learn Disabil.* 1976;9:50–58.

52. Moore J. Cranial nerves and their importance in current rehabilitation techniques. In: Henderson A, Coryell J, eds. *The Body Senses and Perceptual Deficit.* Boston, MA: Boston University; 1973:102–120.

53. Ayres AJ. *Sensory Integration and the Child, 25th Anniversary Edition.* Los Angeles, CA: Western Psychological Services; 2005.

54. Collier G. *Emotional Expression.* Hillsdale, NJ: Lawrence Erlbaum Associates; 1985.

55. Royeen CB, Lane SJ. Tactile processing and sensory defensiveness. In: Fisher AG, Murray, EA, Bundy AC, eds. *Sensory Integration: Theory and Practice.* Philadelphia, PA: FA Davis Company; 1991.

56. Ayres AJ. *Sensory Integration and Learning Disorders.* Los Angeles, CA: Western Psychological Services; 1973.

57. Clark RG, Gilman S, Wilhaus-Newman S. *Essentials of Clinical Neuroanatomy and Neurophysiology.* 10th ed. Philadelphia, PA: FA Davis; 2002.

58. Westcott SL, Lowes LP, Richardson PK. Evaluation of postural stability in children: current theories and assessment tools. *Phys Ther.* 1997;77:629–645.

59. Batshaw NL. *Children with Disabilities.* 3rd ed. Baltimore, MD: Paul H. Brookes; 2013.

60. Harvey B. Down's syndrome: a biopsychosocial perspective. *Nursing Standard.* 2004;18(30):43–45.

61. Piaget J. Part I: Cognitive development in children-Piaget development and learning. *J Res Sci Teaching.* 2003;40(suppl 1):S8–S18.

62. Bird EKR, Chapman RS. Sequential recall in individuals with Down syndrome. *J Speech Hearing Res.* 1994;37:1369–1381.

63. Hale CA, Borkowski JG. Attention, memory, and cognition. In: Matson JL, Mulick JA, eds. *Handbook of Intellectual Disabilities.* New York, NY: Pergamon Press; 1991.

64. Urban M. Early observations of genetic diseases. *Lancet* [serial online]. 1999;354:SIV21.

65. Dykens EM, Hodapp RM, Finucane BM. *Genetics and Mental Retardation Syndromes.* Baltimore, MD: Paul H Brookes Publishing Company; 2000.

66. Website for incidence of Down syndrome given by the National Down syndrome Society. http://www.ndss.org/en/About-Down-Syndrome/Incidences-and-Maternal-Age.

67. Pueschel SM. Cause of Down syndrome. In: Pueschel SM, ed. *A Parent's Guide to Down Syndrome: Toward a Brighter Future.* Baltimore, MD: Paul H Brookes Publishing Co; 1990.

68. Lejeune J, Gauthier M, Turpin R. Les chromosomes humain en culture de tissus. *CR Acad Sci (D).* 1959;248:602.

69. Penrose LS. *Down's Anomaly.* London, UK: Churchill Livingstone; 1966.

70. Scott BS, Becker LE, Petit TL. Neurobiology of Down's syndrome. "Progress in neurobiology." *Prog Neurobiol.* 1983;21(3):199–237.

71. Marin-Padilla M. Pyramidal cell abnormalities in the motor cortex of a child with Down's syndrome. *J Comp Neurol.* 1976;67:63.

72. Wisniewski KF, Schmidt-Sidor B, et al. Postnatal delay of myelin formation in brains from Down's syndrome. *Clin Neuropathol.* 1989;6(2):55.

73. Pueschel SM. Medical concerns. In: Pueschel SM, ed. *A Parent's Guide to Down syndrome: Toward a Brighter Future.* Baltimore, MD: Paul H Brookes Publishing Co; 1990.

74. Zausmer EF, Shea A. Motor development. In: Pueschel SM, ed. *The Young Child with Down Syndrome.* New York, NY: Human Sciences Press Inc; 1984.

75. Shea AM. Growth and development in Down syndrome in infancy and early childhood: implications for the physical therapist. In: *Touch Topics in Pediatrics.* Lesson Alexandria, VA: American Physical Therapy Association; 1990.

76. Castells S, Beaulieu I, Torrado C, et al. Hypothalamic versus pituitary dysfunction in Down's syndrome as a cause of growth retardation. *J Intellect Disabil Res.* 1996;40:509–517.

77. Cronk CE, Crocker AC, Pueschel SM, et al. Growth charts for children with Downsyndrome: 1 month to 18 years of age. *Pediatrics.* 1988;81(1):102–110.

78. Rarick GG, Seefeldt V. Observations from longitudinal data on growth and stature and sitting height of children with Down syndrome. *J Ment Defic Res.* 1974;18:63–78.

79. Bersu ET. Anatomical analysis of the developmental effects of aneuploidy in man: the Down syndrome. *Am J Med Genet.* 1980;5:399.

80. Dummer GM. Strength and flexibility in Down's syndrome. In: *American Association for Health, Physical Education, and Recreation: Research Consortium Papers: Movement Studies,* vol 1. book 3. Washington, DC: American Association for Health, Physical Education and Recreation; 1978.

81. Diamond LS, et al. Orthopedic disorders in patients with Down's syndrome. *Orthop Clin North Am.* 1981;12(1):57.

82. Gajdosik CG, Ostertag S. Cervical instability and Down syndrome: review of the literature and implications for physical therapists. *Pediatri Phys Ther.* 1996;8:1:31–36.

83. Morris AF, Vaughan SE, Vaccaro P. Measurements of neuromuscular tone and strength in Down syndrome children. *J Ment Defic Res.* 1982;26(pt 1):41–47.

84. MacNeill-Shea SH, Mezzomo JM. Relationship of ankle strength and hypermobility to squatting skills of children with Down syndrome. *Phys Ther.* 1985;65(11):1658–1661.

85. Orelove FP, Sobsey D. Designing transdisciplinary services. In: Orelove FP, Sobsey D, Silberman RK, eds. *Educating Children with Multiple Disabilities: A Transdisciplinary Approach.* Baltimore, MD: Paul H Brooks; 1991.

86. Marcel MM, Armstrong V. Auditory and visual sequential memory of Down syndrome and non-retarded children. *Am J Ment Defic.* 1982;87(1):86.

87. Edwards JM, Elliott D, Lee TD. Contextual interference effects during skill acquisition and transfer in Down's syndrome adolescents. *Adapt Phys Act Quart.* 1986;3(3):250.

88. Elliott D, Weeks DJ. A functional systems approach to movement pathology. *Adapt Phys Act Quart.* 1993;10:312.

89. Griffiths MI. Development of children with Down's syndrome. *Physiotherapy.* 1976;62:11–15.

90. Harris SR. Relationship of mental and motor development in Down's syndrome infants. *Phys Occup Ther Pediatr.* 1981;1:13.

91. Canning CD, Pueschel SM. Developmental expectations: an overview. In: Pueschel SM, ed. *A Parent's Guide to Down syndrome: Toward a Brighter Future.* 2nd ed. Baltimore, MD: Paul H Brookes Publishing Co; 2001.

92. Cicchetti D, Sroufe LA. The relationship between affective and cognitive development in Down's syndrome infants. *Child Dev.* 1976;47:920.

93. Haley SM. Postural reactions in children with Down syndrome. *Phys Ther.* 1986;66(1):17–31.

94. Rast MM, Harris SR. Motor control in infants with Down syndrome. *Dev Med Child Neurol.* 1985;27(5):682–685.

95. Lydic JS, Steele C. Assessment of the quality of sitting and gait patterns in children with Down's syndrome. *Phys Ther.* 1979;59(12): 1489–1494.

96. Parker AW, Bronks R. Gait of children with Down syndrome. *Arch Phys Med Rehabil.* 1980;61(8):345–351.

97. Hays RM. Childhood motor impairments: clinical overview and scope of the problem. In: Jaffe KM, ed. *Childhood Powered Mobility.* Washington, DC: RESNA; 1987:1–10.

98. Affoltier FD. *Perception, Interaction and Language: Interaction of Daily Living: The Root of Development.* New York, NY: Springer-Verlag; 1991.

99. Kermonian R, et al. Locomotor experience: a facilitator of spatial cognitive development. *Child Dev.* 1988;59:908–917.

100. Ulrich BD, Ulrich DA, Collier DH, et al. Developmental shifts in the ability of infants with Down syndrome to produce treadmill steps. *Phys Ther.* 1995;75:20–29.

101. Long TM, Cintas HL. *Handbook of Pediatric Physical Therapy.* 2nd ed. Baltimore, MD: Williams & Wilkins; 2001.

102. American Academy of Pediatrics, Committee on Sports Medicine. Atlantoaxial instability in Down syndrome. *Pediatrics.* 1984;74(1): 152–154.

103. Pueschel SM, Scola FH. Atlantoaxial instability in individuals with Down syndrome: epidemiologic, radiographic, and clinical studies. *Pediatrics.* 1987;80(4):555–560.

104. Singer SJ, Rubin IL, Strauss KJ. Atlantoaxial distance in patients with Down syndrome: standardization of measurement. *Radiology.* 1987;164(3):871–872.

105. Giblin PE, Micheli LJ. The management of atlanto-axial subluxation with neurological involvement in Down's syndrome: a report of two cases and review of the literature. *Clin Orthop Relat Res.* 1979;(140):66–71.

106. Cooke RE. Atlantoaxial instability in individuals with Down syndrome. *Adap Phys Act Q.* 1984;1:194–196.

107. Dichter CG, Darbee JC, Effgen SK, et al. Assessment of pulmonary function and physical fitness in children with Down syndrome. *Pediatr Phys Ther.* 1993;5(1):3–8.

108. Polacek JJ, Wang PY, Eichstaedt CB. *A Study of Physical and Health Related Fitness Levels of Mild, Moderate, and Down syndrome Students in Illinois.* Normal, IL: Illinois State University Press; 1985.

109. DeCesare J. Physical therapy for the child with respiratory dysfunction. In: Irwin S, Tecklin JS, eds. *Cardiopulmonary Physical Therapy.* 3rd ed. St. Louis, MO: Mosby–Yearbook; 1995.

110. Connolly BH, Michael BT. Performance of retarded children, with and without Down syndrome, on the Bruinicks Oseretsky Test of Motor Proficiency. *Phys Ther.* 1986;66(3):344–348.

111. Ruppel G. *Manual of Pulmonary Function Testing.* 3rd ed. St. Louis, MO: CV Mosby; 1982.

112. Skrobak-Kaczynski J, Vavik T. Physical fitness and trainability of young male patients with Down syndrome. In: Berg K, Eriksson BO, eds. *Children and Exercise IX.* Baltimore, MD: University Park Press; 1980.

113. Weber R, French R. *The Influence of Strength Training on Down syndrome Adolescents: A Comparative Investigation.* Texas, TX: Texas Women's University.

114. Herge E, Campbell JE. The role of the occupational and physical therapist in the rehabilitation of the older adult with mental retardation. *Top Geriatr Rehabil.* 2004;13(4):12–22.

115. Amadio AN, Lakin KC, Menke JM. *1990 Chartbook Services for People with Developmental Disabilities.* Minneapolis, MN: Center for Residential and Community Services; 1990.

116. Nochajski SM. The impact age-related changes on the functioning of older adults with developmental disabilities. *Phys Occupat Ther Geriatr.* 2000;18:5–21.

117. Lubin RA, Kiley M. Epidemiology of aging in developmental disabilities. In: Janicki MP, Wisniewski HM, eds. *Aging and Developmental Disabilities: Issues and Approaches.* Baltimore, MD: Paul H. Brookes Publishing Co; 1985:95–113.

118. Connolly BH. General effects of aging on persons with developmental disabilities. *Top Geriatr Rehabil.* 1998;13(3):1–18.

119. Campbell JE, Herge E. Challenges to aging in place: the elder adult with MR/DD. *Phys Occupat Ther Geriatr.* 2000;18:75–90.

120. Seltzer MM, Seltzer GB. The elderly mentally retarded: a group in need of service. *J Gerontol Soc Work.* 1985;8:99–119.

121. Gill CJ, Brown AA. Overview of health issues of older women with intellectual disabilities. *Phys Occup Ther Geriatr.* 2000;18:23–36.

122. Rapp C. Improved lifespan for persons with Down syndrome: implications for the medical profession. *Excep Parent.* 2004;34:70–71.

123. Finesilver C. Down syndrome. *RN.* 2002;65:43–49.

124. Platt LS. Medical and orthopaedic conditions in special Olympics athletes. *J Athlet Train.* 2001;36(1):74–80.

125. Post SG. Down syndrome and Alzheimer disease: defining a new ethical horizon in dual diagnosis. *Alzheimer Care Quart.* 2002;3(3): 215–224.

126. Bruckner J, Herge E. Assessing the risk of falls in elders with mental retardation and developmental disabilities. *Top Geriatr Rehabil.* 2003;19:206–211.

127. Hotaling G. Rehabilitation of adults with developmental disabilities: an occupational therapy perspective. *Top Geriatr Rehabil.* 1998;13:73–83.

Autism Spectrum Disorders and Physical Therapy

Anjana Bhat, Deborah Bubela, and Rebecca Landa

Defining ASDs

Classification or Subcategories of ASDs

Incidence

Etiology and Risk Factors

Neuropathology of ASDs

Diagnosis and Prognosis

Impairments

Cognitive Impairments

Sensory-perceptual Impairments

Motor Impairments

Examination

History Taking

Observations of Naturalistic Play

Cognitive Assessment

Sensory-perceptual Assessment

Motor Assessment

Evaluation Synthesis

Intervention

Team Approach to ASD Treatment

Sensorimotor Treatment Approches for Children with ASD

Physical Therapy in Early Intervention

Physical Therapy in School Systems

Recreational Activities and the Use of Technologies

Conclusions

Case Study

T he broad objectives of this chapter are to increase awareness among physical therapists (PTs) about the various multisystem impairments of autism spectrum disorders (ASDs), including motor impairments; propose assessments that will increase our understanding of the child with ASD; and propose possible motor interventions for infants, children, and adolescents with ASDs that are supported by available evidence.

Defining ASDs

ASDs are a neurodevelopmental disorder in which persons present with a range of impairments in social interaction, verbal and nonverbal communication, as well as restrictions in behaviors and interests.[1] Additionally, the majority of the children with ASDs may have significant perceptuo-motor impairments that deserve assessments and interventions.[2,3]

Classification or subcategories of ASDs

The diagnostic criteria outlined in the American Psychiatric Association's Diagnostic Statistical Manual–IV, Text Revision (DSM-IV TR)[1] classify ASDs into three subtypes on the basis of symptom severity: autism, pervasive developmental disorders–not otherwise specified (PDD-NOS), and Asperger

syndrome (Table 11.1). *Autism* is characterized by marked abnormalities in social interaction and communication as well as the presence of stereotypies and unusual interests, with symptoms emerging prior to 3 years of age within the domains of social communication development and imaginative play. Qualitative social impairments mainly include impairments in nonverbal behaviors such as eye gaze, facial expressions, body postures, and gestures during social interactions. Additional hallmarks of autism include a failure to develop peer relationships, the lack of spontaneous sharing of interests and enjoyment, and the lack of social or emotional reciprocity. Communication impairments include a delay or lack of spoken language, impaired ability to initiate or sustain a conversation with others, use of repetitive or idiosyncratic language, as well as lack of spontaneous, pretend play. Restricted repetitive and stereotyped behaviors and interests include one or more stereotyped patterns of interest, inflexible adherence to routines and rituals, stereotyped and repetitive motor mannerisms, and persistent preoccupation with parts of objects. The diagnosis of *PDD-NOS* is identified when the child presents with fewer symptoms of the aforementioned characteristics of autism. The entire range of intelligence quotient (IQ) is represented in children with autism or PDD-NOS, and the level of functioning varies from one child to another. *Asperger syndrome* is characterized by a significant impairment in social interaction and the presence of repetitive behaviors and restricted and unusual

TABLE

11.1   Prevalence and Key Diagnostic Impairments for the Various Subcategories of Individuals with ASDs as well as Early Symptoms in Infants at risk for ASDs.

Broader Autism Phenotype (BAP)
Prevalence: 25% to 50% of infant siblings of children with ASDs present with BAP symptoms.

Symptoms: Verbal and nonverbal communication delays, social delays, motor delay, and/or unusual sensory interests. These symptoms are not severe enough nor present across enough developmental systems simultaneously to meet diagnostic criteria for ASDs.

Infants and Toddlers with ASDs
Prevalence: 20% of infant siblings of children with ASDs and 1 in 110 children in the general population will present with ASD.

Symptoms: Verbal and nonverbal communication delays and social delays that meet diagnostic criteria for ASDs as early as 14 months of age. Motor delays/abnormalities may be present, but are not diagnostic.

Children and Adults with Autism
Prevalence: Fombonne and Tidmarsh offer a conservative prevalence estimate of 10 per 10,000 children with ASDs may develop autism.[99]

Diagnostic criteria: Marked impairment in social interaction, communication along with restricted behaviors and interests that emerges prior to 3 years of age.

Children and Adults with PDD-NOS
Prevalence: Prevalence estimates are unknown for PDD-NOS. This category is considered a catch all when other two diagnoses are not suggested so the rest of the children may fall under this subcategory.

Diagnostic criteria: Marked impairment in social interaction, communication, and restricted behaviors and interests. Fewer specific behavioral features are required for a diagnosis of PDD-NOS.

Children and Adults with Asperger syndrome
Prevalence: 2 per 10,000 children with ASDs present with Asperger syndrome.[99]

Diagnostic criteria: Significant impairment in social interaction and restricted behaviors and interests that is typically detected after three years of age. In addition, there are no clinically significant delays in expressive language or cognitive development.

Adapted from Bhat A, Landa R, Galloway J. Perspectives on motor problems in infants, children, and adults with autism spectrum disorders. *Phys Ther.* 2011;91(7):1116–1129 with permission from American Physical Therapy Association. This material is copyrighted, and any further reproduction and distribution requires written permission from APTA.

interests. Individuals with Asperger syndrome do not exhibit clinically significant delays in acquisition of expressive language or in cognitive development. It is important to note that the recently released DSM-V has eliminated the aforementioned diagnostic subcategories and here on clinicians are expected to provide a broader diagnosis of "Autism Spectrum Disorder", possibly making it easier for all individuals to receive services. Clinicians and researchers critical of these changes are afraid of the impact it may have on individuals who currently have a diagnosis of Asperger or PDD-NOS. Overall, the long-term impact of these changes in diagnostic criteria remain to be seen.

▶ Incidence

According to the latest report from the Centers for Disease Control, 1 in 110 children in the general population will be diagnosed with ASDs, an incidence significantly greater than the 1 in 150 reported in 2000.[4] The incidence of ASDs is five times more common in boys (1 in 54) than girls (1 in 252).[4] ASDs have become the most commonly diagnosed pediatric

condition in the United States, with 36,500 new cases per year, adding to a total of 730,000 cases.[4] Families of children with ASDs incur an average of $3.2 million in lifetime costs with an estimated $34.8 billion in societal costs for all families having individuals with ASDs.[5] Specifically, average medical expenditures for individuals with an ASD were 4.1 to 6.2 times greater than for those without an ASD. In addition to medical costs, intensive behavioral interventions for children with ASDs could cost up to $40,000 to $60,000 per child per year.[6] Taken together, the rising incidence and the growing costs of treating ASDs are an urgent call for clinicians to diagnose and treat this disorder early to improve the future outcomes of individuals with ASDs.

▶ Etiology and risk factors

The neuropathology of autism begins during the prenatal or perinatal period of development.[7] Although there is no clear etiology, twin studies point to genetics as one of the risk factors.[8] Twin studies have shown that among identical twins, the occurrence of ASD in one child increases the chance of the other having ASD by 36% to 95%.[8] Among siblings, if one child has ASD, then the other child has a 31% risk of developing ASD.[8] Furthermore, siblings of children with ASDs are reported to have a 25% to 50% risk of developing other developmental delays that warrant intervention, for example, social, language, sensory, or motor delays or abnormalities.[9] For this reason, researchers often conduct a prospective follow-up of infant siblings of children with ASDs to understand the early development of infants at risk for ASDs.[9] Other populations at risk for developing ASDs include infants who were born prematurely,[10] were born to older parents,[11] or who were exposed to prescription medications such as valproic acid and thalidomide during gestation.[12]

Neuropathology of ASDs

Brain development in individuals with ASDs typically goes through three stages: (1) overgrowth in infancy and early childhood; (2) slowing and arrest of growth in late childhood; and (3) degeneration in preadolescence and adulthood.[13–15] Head circumference of 1- to 2-year-old children who later developed autism was significantly greater than typically developing children.[13–15] Head size is near normal at birth, thus indicating that brain overgrowth may occur in the first 2 years of life. Brain overgrowth continues into early childhood and is observed in children with autism with a mean age of 4 years.[16] The brain overgrowth period mainly affects the frontal lobes, temporal lobes, and amygdala. In particular, there is an overconnectivity in the short-range neuronal fibers and an underconnectivity of the long-range neuronal fibers.[17] The lack of long-range connectivity within the brain leads to the poor integration of sensorimotor, social communication, and cognitive functions. These neuroanatomical findings align with the complex information processing theory of autism in that basic associative learning or simple motor tasks are intact in children with ASDs, whereas complex cognitive functions such as executive functioning (EF) or complex motor planning is impaired.[18] In addition, a recent functional magnetic resonance imaging (fMRI) study revealed that children with autism showed persistent frontal lobe activation and reduced cerebellar activation during a finger-tapping task.[19] In contrast, typically developing peers had increased cerebellar activation compared with frontal lobe activation once the motor pattern was learned and became automated.[19] This lack of transition in neural activation from the prefrontal regions to the cerebellum could be attributed to the lack of long-range neuronal connections between the cortical and subcortical regions and may be the neural basis for incoordination and related motor difficulties observed in children with autism.[18,19] Other researchers have reported deficits in basal ganglia functioning in individuals with Asperger syndrome, as seen by the shorter step length and higher cadence during walking.[20–22] Lastly, children with ASDs may have impaired mirror neuron systems found in the frontoparietal cortices of the brain.[23,24] Mirror neuron systems are a group of neurons that activate during action production as well as action observation and may play a role in observation-based motor learning.[23] These impairments may explain why children with ASDs have poor imitation skills and difficulties learning motor and social skills through observation of others.[24]

Diagnosis and prognosis

The developmental history of a child with ASD will differ on the basis of diagnostic classification. Children who develop autism or PDD-NOS will present with language delays anytime between the second and third years of life.[25] However, parents often report other perceptuo-motor or language delays earlier in life.[26–29] A child with Asperger syndrome will usually present with typical to near-typical development until around 5 to 6 years of age. Parents may later report difficulties in social interaction in spite of typical language and average to above-average intellectual capacity.

Trained clinicians are able to diagnose ASDs using the gold-standard tool called the Autism Observation Schedule (ADOS)[30] and the companion parent interview called the Autism Diagnostic Interview–Revised (ADI-R).[31] The ADOS is a 45-minute to 1-hour standardized qualitative assessment that evaluates a child's social reciprocity, nonverbal and verbal communication, as well as stereotypical behaviors and interests using various play-based activities with an adult tester. The ADOS can be administered to individuals from 12 months of age to adulthood. For each coding item within the three domains of interest (social, communication, and repetitive behaviors), a child is given scores ranging from 0 to 3, with 0 signifying typical or near-typical performance. A diagnostic algorithm is developed on the basis of a subset of coding items. For example, in verbal children the sum of 10 social communication items and 4 repetitive behavior items provides a total score ranging from 0 to 28. A score of 9 and above is termed autism and a score from 7 to 9 is termed autism spectrum. Recently, comparison scores have been developed to describe the symptom severity of a child with autism. Comparison scores have prognostic value as they can help evaluate long-term improvements following treatment.

Other differential diagnoses that should be considered for children who present with a range of social, communication, and sensorimotor difficulties include Rett disorder, childhood disintegrative disorder (CDD), and fragile X syndrome. Rett disorder is a neurological disorder with defined genetic origin involving the grey matter of the brain leading to decelerated brain growth between 5 months to 4 years of age.[32] It occurs only in females and leads to loss of hand function and emergence of stereotypical arm movements within the first year of life.[1,32] Poor whole body coordination and balance, impaired language skills, and poor psychomotor development are also observed. In contrast, CDD presents as ASD with typical development until developmental regression occurs with sudden loss of language skills before 10 years of age.[1] Lastly, fragile X syndrome is a clearly defined genetic disorder found in males with clinical presentation similar to ASDs with the exception that the etiology can be confirmed through genetic testing.[1,33] Important physical features associated with fragile X syndrome include large body size, forehead, face, and ears as well as low muscle tone and increased joint laxity.

 Impairments

In this section, we describe the cognitive, social communication, sensory-perceptual, and motor impairments found in infants and children with ASDs.

Cognitive Impairments

Attention and Other Social Skills

Children and adults with ASDs have attentional impairments such as difficulty disengaging attention and increased focus on objects.[34,35] These impairments may contribute to social functional deficits such as lack of or delayed response to name and/or delays in joint attention (the ability to shift attention to the attentional focus of a social partner).[36] Theories of social impairment suggest that children with autism may prefer nonsocial cues over social cues and may avoid eye contact and looking at faces owing to the complexity of social stimuli.[37,38] These basic attentional preferences may give rise to complex social deficits such as difficulties in understanding others' mental states (emotions, intentions, and desires) and lack of empathy.[39] During development, children with ASDs show delays in responding to attentional bids of others. Spontaneous sharing of attention with others continues to be deficient until late childhood.[39]

Language

Language is clearly affected in children with autism, with some children never acquiring functional speech.[40–42] Language impairments include impaired pragmatic language such as poor use of nonverbal cues such as gaze, facial expressions, turn-taking, and body language during communication with others, poor prosody (i.e., rhythm, stress, and intonation during speech), poor phonology (i.e., word articulation), and atypical linguistic forms such as echolalia (i.e., immediate or delayed imitation of words).[41,42]

Executive Functioning

EF is defined as the ability to maintain a problem-solving set related to a goal that requires skills such as planning, impulse control, response inhibition, organized search, and flexibility in thought process.[43] In terms of perceptual inflexibility, children with ASDs may show resistance to distraction and an inability to shift attention between activities or stimuli.[34] In terms of motor inflexibility, children with ASDs may show repetitive behaviors or have difficulty inhibiting movements.[1] In terms of inflexibility in social communication, children with ASDs will show a lack of reciprocity

leading to one-sided conversations and lack of turn-taking during nonverbal and verbal communication.[1]

Sensory-perceptual Impairments

Sensory-perceptual processing impairments can be categorized into sensory modulation disorders and atypical sensory perception.

Sensory Modulation Disorders

Sensory modulation disorders are difficulties in regulating and organizing the nature and intensity of responses to specific sensory inputs, including tactile, olfactory, visual, auditory, proprioceptive, and vestibular inputs.[44] Children with ASDs can be "underresponsive" such that they are slow to respond or may fail to respond to name or react to pain.[44] "Overresponsive" children may have exaggerated or prolonged responses to sensory inputs such as covering of ears to loud sounds or background noise.[44] Sensation-seeking children may crave for sensory input for extended periods by performing stereotypical movements of body rocking or arm flapping, etc.[44] Various parent questionnaires have been used to report sensory modulation issues, for example, the Short Sensory Profile or the Infant and Toddler Sensory Profile.[45] The severity of sensory modulation impairments appears to directly correlate with overall symptom severity and level of functioning of children with autism.[46] Recently, mixed patterns of sensory processing have also been reported in children with ASDs between 3 and 10 years of age: (1) "inattention/ excessive attention"; (2) "atypical tactile/smell sensitivity"; and (3) "atypical movement sensitivity/low energy and weak motor responses."[47] These subgroups include underresponsive and overresponsive children with ASDs within specific sensory domains. The third subgroup included children with ASDs who had clear motor impairments. For example, children with "atypical movement sensitivity" are usually overresponsive to proprioceptive and vestibular input, whereas children with "low energy/weak motor responses" may present with fine and gross motor difficulties.[47] Therefore, children who perform poorly on the "movement sensitivity/low energy" sections of the Sensory Profile questionnaire may be at a greater risk for motor delays and long-term motor impairments.

Atypical Visual and Auditory Perception

Children with ASDs show enhanced local processing compared with global processing of perceptual information.[48] They are unable to understand the interelement relationships between the parts of a complex presentation of stimuli and are hence unable to understand the overall context and meaning of a complex picture or a piece of music. The enhanced local processing may contribute to their heightened perception of visual and auditory information. For example, during visual search tasks involving several similar-looking objects, typically developing children use a serial search strategy to find the odd object, whereas children with ASDs will encounter a pop-out phenomenon where they perceive each individual object in parallel and immediately identify the outlier.[49] Similarly, children with ASDs have heightened pitch perception, greater pitch discrimination, and better memory of musical pitch; however, they may lack emotion perception within the musical content.[50,51] Interestingly, evidence indicates that these perceptual skills can be developed with age and may be intact in adults with ASDs. It is not surprising that music education and music therapy are often used as training tools to facilitate social communication skills in children with ASDs owing to their advanced musical abilities.[52,53]

Motor Impairments

While social communication impairments are considered hallmarks of ASDs, there is substantial evidence to consider motor impairments as a core deficit of ASDs owing to its widespread prevalence and its correlation with other social communication impairments.[3,54,55] For example, the large effect sizes calculated in a recent meta-analysis on motor impairments in individuals with ASDs suggested that this group has significantly greater motor impairments compared with healthy controls.[55] Moreover, recent reviews indicate clear impairments in arm motor functions, bilateral coordination, gait and balance, as well as praxis/motor planning in young and older children with ASDs.[3,54,55] A comprehensive listing of motor impairments is provided in Table 11.2.

Motor Stereotypies

Children and adolescents with autism may show several different motor stereotypies, including repetitive behaviors such as whole body rocking, twirling, jumping, bouncing, and arm flapping. Object-related behaviors such as poking, rubbing, or spinning objects are also commonly demonstrated by children with ASDs.[56] Children with ASDs may show covering of eyes or ears because they are "overresponsive" to certain visual and auditory inputs from a very young age.[56,57] Individuals with ASDs may also show resistance to change and compulsive behaviors such as inflexible routines during their daily activities.[31,56] Motor stereotypies often correlate with level of functioning and autism severity with a greater presence of stereotypies in the more affected children.[31,58] Repetitive behaviors are often clearly present by 2 years of age because of the difficulty of distinguishing them from typical motor stereotypies of infants within the first year of life.[55,57] Specifically, toddlers who later developed autism showed more atypical hand and finger movements and more stereotypical object play, such as excessive banging or preoccupation with spinning objects or with part of an object, compared with toddlers with milder forms of ASDs such as PDD-NOS.[59] Interestingly, reduced spontaneous movement exploration or limited change in body postures are often present in infants at risk for ASDs.[60] Repetitive behaviors may also be considered as a child's means of obtaining different forms of visual or kinesthetic stimulation and may be a function of the sensory modulation impairments found in children with ASDs.[44]

TABLE 11.2	Motor Impairments in Children and Adults with Autism	
Motor Impairments/ Motor Delays	**Impairments in School-aged Children and Adults with ASDs**	**Delays in Infants at risk for ASD, and Toddlers and Preschoolers with ASDs**
Gross motor coordination	Poor upper and lower limb coordination, including bilateral coordination and visuomotor coordination.	Gross motor delays in supine, prone, sitting skills in the first year of life. Delayed onset of walking in the second year of life. Gross motor delays are present in preschoolers recently diagnosed with ASD.
Fine motor coordination	Poor fine motor coordination such as performance on manual dexterity tasks, for example, Purdue pegboard task.	Reaching and grasping delayed in infants at risk for ASDs. Fine motor delays persist in the second and third years of life.
Motor stereotypies	Motor stereotypies are common in older children and adults with ASDs.	Motor stereotypies such as repetitive banging of objects or unusual sensory exploration may appear in the first year of life, but most often emerge in the second year of life.
Postural	Feed-forward as well as feedback control of posture is affected in children and adults with ASDs. Overall, deficient postural control persists in adults with ASDs.	Postural delays in rolling, sitting, etc. Unusual postures may be held for brief to long periods in infants who later developed ASDs.
Imitation and praxis	Imitation impairments are present during postural, gestural, and oral imitation. Performance of complex movement sequences is poor during imitation, on verbal command, and during tool use, suggesting generalized dyspraxia not specific to imitation.	

Adapted from Bhat A, Landa R, Galloway J. Perspectives on motor problems in infants, children, and adults with autism spectrum disorders. *Phys Ther.* 2011;91(7):1116–1129 with permission from American Physical Therapy Association. This material is copyrighted, and any further reproduction and distribution requires written permission from APTA.

Motor Coordination and Arm Function

School-age children and adolescents with ASDs often show impairments in running speed and agility, bilateral co-ordination, manual dexterity, and ball skills, as based on various standardized motor measures.[61–64] Past studies reported greater motor deficits in children with low IQ compared with children with average and above-average IQ.[63,64] However, recent studies recognize that motor impairments are observed across the spectrum, including children with ASDs with low and high IQ.[2] Coordination impairments are also observed during functional activities such as walking, reaching, writing, and gestural communication.[20,22,65–67] Poor use of hand and body gestures such as pointing, showing, and reaching out to caregivers is in fact one of the core social impairments in autism.[1] Furthermore, lack of associated gestures during story telling leading to asynchrony between hand gestures and language production is coded for within the ADOS administration, the diagnostic tool for ASDs.[30]

Motor Delay

Motor incoordination in children with ASDs may emerge as early as infancy. Retrospective and prospective studies tracking the motor development of high-risk infants who later developed ASDs or language delays have reported gross motor and fine motor delays as early as 6 months of age.[26,27,68–70] For example, infants who later develop ASDs may show delays in gross motor milestones such as head holding, rolling, sitting, crawling, and walking.[26–28] Infants who later developed ASDs were also reported to have early motor delays in reaching, banging, clapping, block stacking, scribbling, pointing, and turning door knobs.[70] In addition, these early manual-motor skills of children with autism correlated with their later speech fluency at school age.[70] Fine motor delays have been more thoroughly studied than gross motor delays owing to their relationships with nonverbal communication. There is recent evidence that preschoolers diagnosed with ASDs have comparable impairments in fine and gross motor performance.[70] Therefore, it is extremely important to assess early motor performance of infants and toddlers at risk for autism, including infant siblings of children with autism or preterm infants.

Gait and Balance

Walking patterns of children with ASDs have been described as "ataxic" owing to the inconsistency between strides or "parkinsonian" shuffling nature of steps and lack of alternating arm swing.[20,22] Toe-walking is often reported by clinicians, although it is not well studied by researchers. On the basis of standardized testing, static and dynamic balance is found to be affected in children with ASDs.[61,71] Moreover, deficits in feedback (responding to postural perturbations) and feed-forward (anticipatory postural adjustments) mechanisms have been reported in individuals with ASDs, which may account for the poor balance observed during clinical assessments.[72] Furthermore, infants who later develop ASDs show delays in acquiring advanced postures such as standing and sitting compared with typically developing infants.[28,60] Delayed onset of walking was one of the first gross motor delays observed in toddlers who developed language delays later in life.[25] It has been reported that some at-risk infants who showed delayed onset of autism symptoms did not present with motor delays within the first year.[73] The delayed onset of autism symptoms may present as a developmental regression in the second and third years of life.[73] Therefore, it would be important to monitor motor development as well as social communication development over the first 3 years of life in infants at risk for ASDs.

Motor Planning, Praxis, and Imitation

Praxis refers to one's ability to plan, coordinate, and execute complex movement sequences.[74] Children with ASDs often present with dyspraxia (difficulty with planning, coordinating, and executing movement sequences) during oromotor, fine motor, and gross motor activities.[75] These deficits typically represent more complex processing and are not simply related to basic motor abnormalities such as abnormal tone or muscle weakness. Individuals with ASDs usually acquire the ability to perform simple motor tasks, for example, fundamental motor milestones, walking, and reaching skills, although delays may be experienced. However, complex motor tasks such as complex sports, handwriting, daily living skills such as dressing and tying shoe laces, or other movement sequences associated with broader goals persist for school-age children with ASDs. Praxis is often measured during gesture production, in response to verbal command, on imitation, or during tool use.[76] Children with ASDs showed similar errors within each of these conditions, indicating a generalized praxis impairment that is not limited to movement imitation.[76] Studies of imitation of oromotor, fine motor, and gross motor actions in this population have verified that children with ASDs have difficulties with various forms of imitation from early on in life.[75,77–79] Poor imitation skills put children with ASDs at a clear disadvantage when learning daily living skills from their peers and caregivers.

Strength and Tone

The only study evaluating muscle strength in children with ASDs reported that hand muscle strength was poor in children with ASDs compared with typically developing children.[80] The presence of abnormal reflexes has been reported in infants who later developed ASDs.[81] Tonal abnormality resulting in toe-walking has also been observed in children with ASDs.[81] Hypotonia is also often reported in retrospective studies of infants who later developed ASDs and is often observed in school-age children with ASDs.[81,82] In fact, clinicians often report postural muscle hypotonia in children with ASDs.

Endurance and Physical Activity Levels

Children and adults with ASDs are at a high risk of developing obesity in view of their low physical activity levels and poor cardiorespiratory endurance.[83,84] Two different retrospective analyses of survey databases conducted in the United States reported that 23.4% of older children and adolescents with ASDs were obese (body mass index [BMI] greater than 95th percentile), 19% were overweight (BMI greater than 85th percentile), and 35.7% were at risk for overweight.[85] It is reported that obesity is either equally likely or three times more likely in children with ASDs than the general population.[85] While there is little known about factors leading to obesity in children with ASDs, it is suggested that less time spent in physical activity programs and more time spent in sedentary activities such as working at a computer may be contributing factors.[84,86,87] This pattern could be directly related to the social impairments of children with autism and to their preference to engage in solitary, technology-based activities such as watching television or playing video games. Unusual dietary patterns in children with ASDs may occur owing to restricted food habits, which is also a function of the ASD diagnosis.[84,85] Long-term use of antiseizure medications such as valproate has been implicated for obesity in children with developmental disorders.[88] While there is significant evidence for delayed motor development and motor incoordination in children with ASDs, no study has directly correlated motor skill performance or the lack of participation in organized sport or physical activity with obesity in children with ASDs. Taken together, there is a clear need to enhance endurance and physical activity levels in children and adults with ASDs to improve their quality of life.

 Examination

The components of an examination for a child with autism will vary on the basis of the child's age, level of functioning, and range of impairments. In this section, we offer ideas for appropriate history taking as well as nonstandardized and standardized assessments.

History Taking

After obtaining basic identifying information, including date of birth, age, gender, height, weight, and handedness, one should collect birth history, including prenatal, perinatal, and postnatal history, family history, developmental history, medical history, treatment history, as well as the child's current level of functioning and expectation of the caregiver and/or child. Prenatal, perinatal, and postnatal history may provide some insight into the etiologies of the diagnosis (see "Etiology and Risk Factors" section). When obtaining family history, ask for presence of ASD diagnosis in other family members such as siblings or relatives. When obtaining developmental history, ask about the child's overall development, for example, whether motor and communication milestones were achieved at appropriate ages. Specifically, onset ages for motor milestones such as

reaching, sitting, crawling, standing, and walking are important in identifying the degree and length of motor delay. In addition, onset ages for communication milestones such as production of vowel sounds, consonant sounds, variegated babbling, first words, two- to three-word phrases, and complex language are important. As part of the medical history, ask when the diagnosis was obtained, any medications the child may be taking, presence of motor stereotypies, and any dietary modifications. Children with ASDs may have food allergies for which gluten-free and casein-free diets may have been recommended. This is especially important to know if use of edible treats is considered for rewards. In terms of treatment history, it is important to know about the other services the child has received or is receiving (e.g., behavioral therapies, social skills training, speech or occupational or music therapy), including their intensity, frequency, and duration, as this will directly affect the family's ability to engage in physical therapy. It is important to identify the child's current level of functioning in performing activities of daily living, including the level of caregiver support throughout the day. It is important to ask about the child's present communication, cognitive, and sensorimotor abilities and difficulties. Last but not the least, ask the caregiver's expectations for their child and the child's expectations for himself or herself, when the child has adequate communication.

Observations of Naturalistic Play

Children often need time to warm up to strangers, and allowing a 10-to-15-minute period where the child explores the toys within the examination space would be a nice icebreaker for the child. During this period, the examiner could complete history taking and move onto observing the child's play for nonverbal and verbal communication, repetitive behaviors, and motor performance. In terms of nonverbal communication skills, observe the child's use of gestures, reciprocal interactions and turn-taking, the use of spontaneous versus responsive communication with the caregiver or tester, as well as rapport between the child and the caregiver. Gestures could be "instrumental" such as showing, pointing, and giving, or "descriptive" such as actions describing verbs or adjectives within a sentence. In terms of verbal communication skills, collect a language sample to understand the level of verbal communication: specifically, the number of words used within phrases and the appropriateness of the language based on the child's developmental level. Review of the speech evaluation can provide more specific insight into the child's level of language.

The complexity and variability of the child's play should be considered. Is the child using objects for their intended purpose and demonstrating any imitation within the play schemes? Alternately, does the child only focus on the mechanical characteristics of play objects? For example, a typically developing child playing with trains may build tracks and pretend to bring cargo to the station, while a child with

ASD may become preoccupied with the spinning of the train wheels. The evaluator should also consider whether the child demonstrates curiosity and variability within play activities offered by the environment.

In terms of motor skills, observe the child's ability to perform those motor tasks expected of his or her age with attention to movement control and sophistication of movement patterns. Observe the child's fine motor skills such as reaching, transfers, use of two hands for symmetrical and asymmetrical activities, as well as gross motor skills such as basic walking patterns, balancing on one leg (static balance), and balancing while walking on narrow surfaces (dynamic balance). Complex motor skills such as clapping, marching, jumping, skipping, galloping, hopping, etc (dual and multi-limb coordination) provide insight into the child's bilateral coordination abilities. For low-functioning children, it might be best to observe them during functional tasks such as climbing stairs and kicking a ball in order to infer balance and coordination skills. Simple instructions such as "can you do this" within an imitation game could offer appropriate visual cues to complete the task. Note: if some of the activities are part of a standardized assessment, then they do not have to be repeated here.

Cognitive Assessment

Intellectual abilities of children with ASDs are evaluated using various cognitive assessments, typically administered by clinical psychologists or educators. For example, the Stanford–Binet Intelligence Test (SBIT) can be administered to individuals between 2 and 85 years of age to assess nonverbal and verbal IQ. The Kaufman Brief Intelligence Test (KBIT) is often administered in individuals between 4 and 90 years of age and within school settings because various professionals can administer it. The Wechsler Intelligence Scale for children (WISC) offers similar information for children between 6 and 16 years of age. While the KBIT is used widely across professions and is a quick IQ measure, it is considered unreliable when assessing IQ in nonverbal children. To understand a child's verbal and nonverbal abilities, it would be valuable to obtain reports on IQ measures, when available. However, in the absence of these measures, instructing the child to follow simple one-step or two-step commands to bring something to you or the child's conversational abilities can offer you information on the child's current abilities. Secondly, observe for inattention and hyperactivity during the child's play because it will dictate the amount of time the child can actively engage with you during assessment and treatment sessions.

Sensory-perceptual Assessment

First, rule out hearing and vision impairments by asking the caregiver during history taking, and by reviewing medical and speech and language evaluation reports. The child's records may include hearing tests such as the brain stem auditory-evoked response audiometry (BAER) or pure tone testing conducted by audiologists. Secondly, obtain caregiver reports on whether the child has sensory modulation issues such as hypo- or hyperresponsiveness to various sensory stimuli. Some children may be using noise-canceling earphones to reduce the noise levels in their environment. Parent questionnaires such as the Infant and Toddler Sensory Profile or the Short Sensory Profile can be used.[45] A detailed Sensory Integration and Praxis Test (SIPT)[89] is typically administered by the occupational therapist (OT) on the team, and reviewing that report would offer ideas for supporting the child's sensory responses during therapy sessions.

Motor Assessment

Motor performance can be assessed by obtaining parent responses through motor questionnaires, by administering standardized and/or developmentally appropriate measures of motor performance, and through observation of the child's current levels of motor functioning during functional activities of daily living as well as standardized functional assessments. Table 11.3 provides a full listing of questionnaires and assessment for children with ASDs.

Motor Questionnaires/Parent Interviews

Motor-related instruments include the Movement Assessment Battery for Children (ABC)–questionnaire version or the Developmental Coordination Disorders Questionnaire (DCDQ).[90] A typical administration lasts about 15 to 30 minutes. These questionnaires provide therapists with the parent's and/or teacher's impressions of what the child can do in terms of fine motor and gross motor skills, as well as static and dynamic activities occurring in home and school environments. Other factors that might affect a child's motor performance, such as attention, anxiety, etc., are also considered within these instruments. The DCDQ allows one to compare a child's motor performance with that of children with developmental coordination disorders to assess the severity of the motor impairment. The Children's Assessment of Participation and Enjoyment (CAPE)[91] is a useful measure to examine how children between 5 and 21 years of age participate in everyday activities outside of the mandated school activities. The measure assesses whether the child has opportunities and interest to engage in any of the 55 different activities including information on: (1) whom they typically do the activity with (e.g., parent, friend), (2) where they do the activity (e.g., home, at a friend's house), and (3) how much they enjoy doing the activity. Each activity is presented to the child/youth on a card with a drawing of the activity and a phrase (in words) describing the activity. Overall, motor questionnaires are a reflection of the caregiver and child about the child's motor abilities and interest and could be a useful measure to determine activity themes that would be relevant and motivating to the child.

TABLE

11.3 Reliability and Validity Data on Motor Assessments for ASDs

Motor Assessments	
For young and older children	**For infants and toddlers**
Movement Assessment Battery for Children (MABC) Concurrent validity with Bruininks Test: 0.76 Interrater reliability: 0.96 Test–retest reliability: 0.77	Gross and fine motor subtests of Mullen Scales of Early Learning (MSEL) Validity: 0.5 or higher Reliability: 0.65 or higher
Bruininks–Oseretsky Test of Motor Proficiency (BOTMP) Concurrent validity with MABC: 0.88 Reliability: 0.90	Alberta Infant Motor Scale (AIMS) Concurrent validity with PDMS-2: >0.9 Interrater reliability: 0.99 Test–retest reliability: 0.99
Peabody Motor Developmental Scales (PDMS)-2 Concurrent validity with BSID: high to very high Test–retest reliability: 0.73–0.89 across subtests	
	AOSI has a motor control component that predicts ASDs at 3 years of age Interrater reliability: 0.7–0.9 Test–retest reliability: 0.7
Praxis and Imitation Batteries Modified Florida Apraxia Battery Interrater reliability: 0.85–0.95 Sensory Integration and Praxis Testing Concurrent validity: 0.46–0.71 for some subtests Interrater reliability: moderate to high	

Adapted from Bhat A, Landa R, Galloway J. Perspectives on motor problems in infants, children, and adults with autism spectrum disorders. *Phys Ther.* 2011;91(7):1116–1129 with permission from American Physical Therapy Association. This material is copyrighted, and any further reproduction and distribution requires written permission from APTA.

Standardized Assessment

There are multiple measures of overall motor performance such as the Peabody Developmental Motor Scales, Movement ABC, or the Bruininks–Oseretsky Test of Motor Performance (BOTMP), which include subtests to quantify the child's performance within various motor domains, including fine and gross motor coordination, balance, strength, etc.[55] The typical administration time is about 1 to 1.5 hours to complete the full assessment. For example, the BOTMP-2 has eight subtests: running speed and agility, balance, bilateral coordination, strength, upper limb coordination, response speed, visual-motor control, and upper limb speed and dexterity.[92] It provides raw, standard, and percentile scores for the subtests as well as the overall assessment. A short-form version of the full assessment is also provided to conduct an initial assessment of motor performance in about a half-hour.

Motor impairments are observed in children with ASDs with various levels of cognitive functioning; hence, one clear limitation of all motor assessments is that we are unable to discern whether poor motor performance is reflective of primary motor impairment or an artifact of poor comprehension. This is especially true for children with ASD who not only have known verbal comprehension limitations, but also present with difficulties in imitating actions. There is a clear need to further develop observational motor measures during functional tasks for children who are nonverbal and low functioning.

Developmental Screening

Children who are screened for ASDs under 3 years of age receive screening for developmental delays and autism-specific signs. Screening tools take about 15 minutes to complete and may include general parent questionnaires such as the Ages and Stages Questionnaire (ASQ)[93] or the autism-specific parent questionnaires such as the Modified Checklist for Autism in Toddlers (MCHAT).[94] Recently, researchers have developed a multisystem observational tool called the Autism Observation Schedule for Infants (AOSI) in young infants at risk for ASDs, and it is inclusive of a motor component.[95]

Developmental Assessments

Multidomain developmental assessments such as the Bayley Scales of Infant Development (BSID)[96] or Mullen Scales of Early Learning (MSEL)[97] could be used to obtain the child's overall cognitive and motor performance. A single domain may take about 15 to 20 minutes to complete, and a full assessment could be well over 1 hour. The BSID can be used for children from birth to 3 years of age and the MSEL is normed from birth to 5 years of age. Both have subdomains for gross motor, fine motor, visual reception, receptive, and expressive language. Raw scores, scaled scores, composite scores, and percentile scores can be calculated for each subtest as well as overall development. Single-domain assessments such as the Alberta Infant Motor Scale may also be used to assess gross motor delays using raw subscale scores or overall percentile scores. The Vineland Adaptive Behavior Scale (VABS)[98] is a caregiver interview and observational measure or a parent/caregiver questionnaire to help evaluate individuals across the gamut of functional skills from preschool to 18 years of age. This measure assesses adaptive behaviors, including the ability to cope with environmental changes, to learn new everyday skills, and to demonstrate independence. The test measures five domains: Communication, Daily Living Skills, Socialization, Motor Skills, and Maladaptive Behavior. The Communication Domain evaluates the receptive, expressive, and written communication skills of the child. The Daily Living Skills Domain measures personal behavior as well as domestic and community interaction skills. The Socialization Domain covers play and leisure time, interpersonal relationships, and various coping skills. The Motor Skills Domain measures both gross and fine motor skills.

Praxis and Imitation Assessment

Imitation and praxis can be measured using the Modified Florida Apraxia Battery[99] or subtests of the SIPT.[89] Both these measures typically assess praxis at three levels: during imitation, following verbal command, or during tool use. Gestures or actions range from fine motor to gross motor, simple to complex, meaningful to meaningless. The child's motor responses are scored for spatial, temporal, and reversal errors. Furthermore, SIPT is a standardized and normed measure for examining various sensorimotor skills, including motor coordination, sensory integration, and praxis in children between 4 and 9 years of age. Specifically, subtests of postural praxis, praxis on verbal command, sequencing praxis, bilateral motor coordination, and kinesthesia might be relevant. Note that among the standardized measures for imitation, SIPT is the only one that is normed.

Strength and Tone Assessment

Abnormal tone is often reported in infants who later developed ASDs and in children with ASDs. For example, hypotonia has been reported in young infants who later developed autism and is often found in children with autism. It most often affects posture and balance of the child with autism and is assessed during observation of the child's posture and movement. For example, observe for slouched or swayback postures, hyperextended knees or elbows, toe-walking, etc. Strength is not often assessed in children with autism. Only one study has reported muscle weakness in hand muscles of children with autism[80]; hence, it is important to consider measuring pinch and grip strength using hand and finger dynamometry, especially when the child has significant fine motor difficulties such as poor handwriting.

Physical Activity Level Assessment

These could be measured subjectively using activity diaries or self-report surveys, or objectively using pedometers, accelerometers, etc. Parents will need to record the information for children or those children who are not capable, and self-report may be reliable for adolescents. While subjective measures are prone to errors owing to recall bias, the objective measures are expensive and could be bothersome to children with ASDs who have associated sensory issues.

Functional Assessment

Functional performance can be measured using the Pediatric Evaluations of Disability Inventory (PEDI)[100] or the School Functional Assessment (SFA).[101] The PEDI is a standardized measure to assess functional capabilities and performance in the areas of self-care, mobility, and social function. It is designed to assess young children between 6 months and 7 years or older children who present with functional abilities lower than those of a typically developing 7-year-old. Scores are assigned on the basis of observation or parent/caregiver report. The PEDI allows calculation of both standard and scored performance scores. Results of the PEDI can be used to monitor a child's performance over time and develop intervention plans. The SFA[101] is a criterion-referenced instrument used to quantify and monitor a child's performance of nonacademic activities within the elementary school setting—kindergarten through sixth grade. The educational team members familiar with the child complete the scoring in three areas: participation, task supports, and activity performance. This instrument yields criterion cutoff scores that help establish eligibility for special education services and monitor a child's performance while promoting team collaboration.

Evaluation Synthesis

a. Convey evaluation instructions in a manner the child can comprehend. Use picture schedules, simplify verbal commands, hand-on-hand instruction, visual models, breaks, and rewards to ensure that the child complies, understands your instructions, and demonstrates what is asked of him or her (see Table 11.4 for specific strategies).

b. Identify cognitive impairments that govern the motor activities planned. For example, level of focus (i.e., overfocused attention or inattention), presence of hyperactivity, and intellectual level (i.e., nonverbal, verbal but delayed, verbal/hyperverbal, and age-appropriate).

c. Identify sensory modulation impairments that will affect the child's engagement in the intervention plan.

d. Identify the child's key motor impairments: coordination, balance, praxis, etc, and plan for activities that are comprehensive. Prioritize goals depending on the child's and family's highest need. Most likely, the family has been asked to participate in multiple therapies and has little time to focus on a range of motor activities.

TABLE 11.4	Strategies for Structuring Physical Therapy Treatment Sessions for Children with Autism

Principles	Specific Strategies
1. Structuring the environment	1. Use just the right amount of space for the motor activities to be performed. 2. Use the same space to ensure predictability. 3. Limit the materials to the ones required for the session. 4. Remove or cover the other distractors in the room. 5. Put up rules sheet, listing of activities, or picture schedules to describe the expectations from the child and the structure of the sessions, whenever appropriate. 6. Follow a predictable routine. You could vary the routine of the child if that is a treatment goal. Begin with small (versus large) changes to the routine. When these changes are made, be sensitive to its effects on the child. 7. Promote transitions with the use of picture schedules or predictable verbal or gestural commands, for example, "a good job and a hi-five at the end of each trial." Within a session, if the activities break up into warm-up, whole body, and walking themes, then use pictures to define those activities, and have the child either move the picture schedule off the board or have him or her check off the activity from an available list. This helps the child keep track of the session.
2. Instructions for the activity	Use the various means of communication available to the child. For example, for a verbal child, verbal instructions are appropriate. However, for a nonverbal child, sign language/gestural communication, visual picture schedules, and short verbal commands may be needed.
3. Prompting/modeling/ feedback	1. Models could be the PT, peers, paraprofessionals, or caregivers who join the child. Your child may benefit from parallel and/or mirrored motions, so you will need to determine what works best for your child and for the actions being practiced. 2. When possible, use group activities because they are valuable for learning social monitoring. This may also reduce the child's anxiety because he or she is not put on the spot. On the other hand, distracting peers may increase the anxiety in some children. It is important to judge what will meet the individual needs of the child. Both group and individual activities provide different important experiences for the child. 3. Make sure that the child is attending to you before you begin your instructions. He or she may use foveal/ peripheral vision to attend to you. 4. First say, "Child's name, do this?" then show the action. If he or she did not move correctly, then hand-on-hand feedback could be provided. Determine whether this helps the child's performance by asking them to repeat the action on their own. Some children may not like "hand-on-hand" feedback or may not improve performance with such feedback. 5. Use external props to clarify the goals of the activity.
4. Repetition	1. Practice is important for motor learning and should be encouraged within a session but also across sessions. 2. Caregivers should practice the same activities between the two physical therapy sessions. 3. Generalization to a different space and a different caregiver will be facilitated through such practice.
5. Active engagement	1. It is important to allow for free movement and improvisational activities. 2. Waiting is critical for the child to explore spontaneously and actively problem-solve. After the initial instructions are provided, allow the child to move freely (without excessive prompting). 3. Prompting could be used in the second trial of the same activity. For low-functioning children, more prompting will be required. 4. Allow the child to choose a theme or a set of activities for the session. Encourage them to move differently than you. Promote movement creativity and spontaneity.
6. Progression	1. In terms of progression, it is important to create the just-right challenge for the child. It is important to allow for success. You could choose to increase the complexity of activities across sessions or within a session for a given activity. Note that trial-and-error learning is important, so the child does not have to achieve 100% success. If the child is not discouraged by his or her motor performance, then adding complexity to the activity is okay. However, if the child is easily frustrated by failure, then it is important to create a safe environment for the child that allows for success and avoids excessive feedback and prompting. 2. Look out for negative behaviors such as tantrums, noncompliance, and self-injurious behaviors. If these are observed, then ask the child to communicate in appropriate ways—verbalizing or signing that the activity be stopped. This will imply that the task is difficult for the child and should be simplified.
7. Reinforcement/rewards	1. Various rewards could be provided. 2. Verbal and gestural reinforcement in the form of "good jobs" and "hi-fives." 3. Breaks from activity to do favorite sensory activities—spinning, containment, or deep pressure or free play. 4. Stickers or small toys. Provide if the aforementioned ideas do not seem to work. 5. Edibles. Provide if the aforementioned ideas do not seem to work. This may be more appropriate for low-functioning children. It is important for the snack to be healthy; otherwise, it will affect the overall health and wellness of the child.

▶ Intervention

While motor performance is relatively spared compared with social communication skills, the multiple motor impairments listed in the earlier sections may significantly contribute to the functional limitations of children with ASDs. The early motor delays, the continued motor deficits later on in life, and their long-term ramifications deserve the attention of motor specialists such as PTs who can contribute to the overall treatment programs of children with ASDs. It is difficult to separate the dynamic interplay of movements, sensory processing, communication, and social interaction as a child interacts with his or her environment and caregivers. Bhat, Landa, and Galloway have suggested that motor impairments will lead to reduced movement exploration, difficulties in keeping up with peers during playtime, and missed opportunities during social interactions.[55] Together, these problems will limit the initiation and maintenance of social relationships and will ultimately contribute to delayed social skills and long-term social impairments.[55]

Despite the implicit and explicit relation of motor abilities and overall development, the majority of autism interventions are focused on enhancing the social communication and academic skills of children with ASDs. Over the years, various interventions have evolved to address the sensory and motor needs of children with ASDs. Although these interventions are frequently practiced, relatively few empirical studies support the use of these interventions to enhance sensorimotor performance, social engagement, and long-term quality of life.[55,102] The majority of the sensorimotor intervention studies involve small sample sizes or single cases or case series. Moreover, research in this population is also challenged by the variability among the children with ASDs and the complexity of the multiple factors that affect treatment outcomes.

Team Approach to ASD Treatment

Children with ASDs present with multiple, complex developmental variations that are best addressed through a team approach. Given the variability of presentation within the autism spectrum, individualized programs with different types of therapies are imperative to meet the unique needs of each child with ASD. Family members provide essential information about the child's behavior, current level of functioning, and areas of interest that can be utilized in program development. The family along with the trained professionals identifies skills and behaviors to be developed. Special educators and psychologists help understand and address the cognitive and behavioral challenges demonstrated by children with ASDs. Speech and language pathologists will help the child with ASD to communicate with family, educators, and caregivers through verbal or alternative means and to gain nonverbal and verbal communication skills. OTs and PTs can provide insight and programming to address sensory-perceptual processing and enhance motor

performance. Other medical personnel can provide information about the child's health that is critical to program planning. Coordinated efforts of these trained professionals along with the family and other caregivers can provide structured and consistent interactions for the child with ASD that will promote positive and meaningful social engagement as well as learning of important skills.

Sensorimotor Treatment Approaches for Children with ASD

The standard of care treatment approaches for children with autism include the Applied Behavioral Analysis (ABA),[102,103] the Treatment and Education of Autistic and related Communication-handicapped Children (TEACCH),[104,105] the Picture Exchange Communication System (PECS),[106] and the Sensory Integration (SI) therapy[107] as well as some others that lack substantial research evidence to support their use.

Applied Behavioral Analysis

ABA is the current intervention standard for children with autism, and is accepted as an effective means for reducing negative behaviors while improving appropriate communication and prosocial behaviors, and teaching new skills to children with ASDs.[102,103] The broader goals of ABA programs are to reinforce desirable behaviors and reduce those that are undesirable. This is accomplished by breaking down a complex task into a series of simple steps and providing positive reinforcement in a predictable manner in response to the child successfully meeting the criteria established for each step. Traditional ABA practices of discrete trial training are performed in a 1:1, controlled setting using a blocked practice format using adult-developed materials and tasks with several repetitions.[108,109] These traditional approaches have received significant criticism because they do not promote naturalistic interactions involving child-preferred and child-centered activities. More contemporary ABA models such as incidental teaching approaches promote spontaneity during motivating contexts that involve natural rewards within naturalistic environments.[110,111] These approaches promote child-preferred and child-selected activities to increase repetition and to sustain engagement. Principles of ABA are typically applied to academic, social, communication, and vocational skills. PTs could incorporate the principles of task analysis, repetition, and positive reinforcement using contemporary approaches to promote acquisition of specific motor skills, activities of daily living, or specific vocational skill sets. Communication among all team members is important to establish acceptable criteria, use of reinforcements, and reinforcement scheduling.

In this section, we compare ABA strategies to motor learning principles that are often used within physical therapy interventions. Specifically, principles of task analysis, repetition/practice, feedback, reinforcement, and generalization are similar across the two treatment approaches;

however, the value for trial-and-error learning and self-produced behaviors may differ. First, task analysis is a critical component of both ABA and motor learning.[102,112] Both approaches promote breaking down complex activities into simpler parts and practicing each part as well as the whole. Children with ASDs are capable of learning simple cause-and-effect relationships[38] as well as simple motor skills in an implicit manner using a "learning-by-doing" approach.[113,114] For example, if a child is practicing jumping jacks, you can break up the activity into multiple steps and practice it in parts. The repetition with active engagement inherent in the contemporary ABA programs is equivalent to the high levels of self-produced practice promoted by the current motor learning theories. Repetition is critical for mastering skilled behaviors. Both approaches also promote the use of positive reinforcement upon successful task completion. While motor learning theories limit reinforcement to verbal and gestural reinforcers, traditional ABA programs also promote the use of materialistic reinforcers such as toys and edibles. However, contemporary ABA approaches promote the use of "access to desired activities" as the reinforcement and discourage the use of materialistic reinforcers. For example, improved proficiency while doing jumping jacks could be a naturally occurring reinforcement and an intrinsic motivation for the child. Activities designed must create the appropriate level of challenge so that the child experiences success. The intervention program can gradually include more complex activities based on the child's skill level and can be practiced in varying environments to maximize generalization. Activities should be not only developmentally appropriate, but also intrinsically motivating, tailored to meet the functional needs of child and family, and able to serve a lifelong purpose.

Prompting or providing feedback is also common to both ABA and motor learning approaches. Motor learning theories propose that actions are reinforced when the end goal is emphasized through immediate visual, kinesthetic, or verbal feedback.[112] While ABA programs promote the use of graded prompting, including visual, verbal, and hand-on-hand instruction, motor learning theories promote the use of both internal (self-produced) and external feedback (provided in the environment/by the caregiver). Children with ASDs are able to use both proprioceptive and visual feedback, but it is unclear whether they have a preference for one or the other.[115] Glazebrook et al. (2009) indicated that children with ASD took longer to process information presented through visual rather than proprioceptive channels.[115] These findings may indicate that physical guidance through an action, if tolerated by the child, may be more effective than providing visual feedback. There is some evidence that visual modeling using two-dimensional maps of each step or computerized video feedback may also promote skill development.[116] For example, you could either show the components of a jumping jack action sequence in parts, or offer key verbal cues for the missing components, or take the child through the action manually. Children

with ASDs also have difficulty understanding movement goals.[117] Therefore, it is important to couple the feedback provided with the appropriate end goal of the task to promote motor learning. For example, for the two key postures within a jumping jack sequence, you could use verbal cues such as "pencil" for hands down and feet together posture and "rocketship" for hands up and feet apart posture. This would help improve the child's understanding of what is expected of him or her.

One tenet that clearly differs between ABA and motor learning approaches is the value placed on trial-and-error learning. Our observations of school-based ABA programs suggest that they promote predominantly errorless, prompted teaching. In contrast, motor learning principles promote active, self-produced exploration wherein errors are allowed and spontaneity is encouraged. In fact, trial-and-error learning is considered vital for greater generalization of motor skills. Therefore, PTs must be careful to allow opportunities for spontaneous movement exploration such as free, unprompted movement because that is often lacking in children with ASDs. The dynamical systems theory of motor control reminds clinicians that the child with ASD, with his or her unique qualities, is embedded within an environment that can be molded to reduce or increase the complexity of motor activities. Once you use the environment to create the just-right challenge for the child, remember to wait for the child to respond spontaneously before beginning prompting or providing feedback and reinforcement. Specific recommendations for implementing ABA strategies within a physical therapy treatment session are provided in Table 11.4.

Sensory Integration Therapy

Sensory-perceptual information, including tactile, visual, and auditory stimuli created in the child's environment, can have profound effects on the child with ASD. A child who is experiencing a fight-or-flight response will not be open to learning. Hence, it is important that the child feel safe and comfortable within the treatment environment. Children with ASD are known to process sensory stimulation differently than typically developing children, with atypical patterns emerging as early as within the first year of life.[46,68] Sensory modulation disorders of hyper- or hyposensitivity are often present in children and adults with ASD.[46] A variety of SI therapy techniques have been proposed to address the sensory impairments of children with ASDs.[46] First, the classic SI therapy purports to focus directly on the neurologic processing of sensory information by providing somatosensory and vestibular activities sought out and controlled by the child to allow the child to better modulate, organize, and integrate environmental stimuli.[118] Empirical studies investigating this treatment method have consisted of case or case series design with weak evidence for efficacy.[119] This form of treatment has come under criticism with a call for greater evidence-based treatment.[107] Second, the "Sensory Diet" provides more adult-structured, passively applied, and cognitively focused sensory-based activities than traditional SI therapy to meet the individual needs of a child.[119,120] The "diet" may include activities such as brushing with a surgical brush, joint compression, and deep pressure. However, there is weak empirical evidence to support the use of sensory diets in children with ASDs.[119,120] Third, specific sensory stimulation techniques have been used to promote positive behaviors, reduce stereotypies, and to modulate arousal. Deep pressure is commonly used to elicit a calming effect, with delivery through therapeutic touch or devices such as the Hug Machine (a deep pressure–generating device), pressure garments, or weighted vests.[121,122] However, there are a limited number of studies to support their use. Children receiving touch therapy at a frequency of 15 minutes per day, 2 days per week for 4 weeks showed improvements in responsiveness to sounds and social communication.[121] Investigation of the Hug Machine twice weekly for 20 minutes per session over a 6-week period showed a statistically significant decrease in scores on a tension scale and marginal reduction of anxiety.[122] When implementing such sensory techniques, especially those that are adult-guided, it is important to monitor the child's stress levels as a means of assessing the effects of such programs.[46,119]

Treatment and Education of Autistic and Related Communication-handicapped Children

TEACCH emphasizes a very structured organization of the environment along with an activity sequence that allows some flexibility within a predictable routine.[105] Specifically, the space of the teaching environment is uniquely organized, the activity schedules are used to increase organization and predictability, individual workstations are used to promote independent and goal-directed activities, and appropriate visual cues are offered for successful task completion. A controlled trial found that children who participated in a TEACCH-based program for 4 months along with their typical day program demonstrated significantly greater improvements than their peers who participated in day programs only.[104] Specific ideas on structuring the environment within a physical therapy treatment session are provided in Table 11.4.

The Picture Exchange Communication System

PECS facilitates communication using elaborate picture exchange techniques. It is often used to provide visual cues for word learning and also helps structure a child's daily schedule.[106] Specifically, picture schedules can be used throughout the day or within an activity to inform the child of the activities as well as transitions between activities. Evidence suggests that the use of PECS increases the duration of spontaneous nonverbal and verbal communication and facilitates skill generalization in children between 18 months and 12 years.[71,123] More specifics on how to incorporate picture schedules within a physical therapy treatment session are provided in Table 11.4.

Other Approaches

There are other approaches that promote the development of sensorimotor skills; however, there is weak evidence to support their use.[71,124] Greenspan and Wieder's "floortime" play is intended to enhance social–emotional relationships and cognitive growth.[71] Gutstein and Sheely's relationship development intervention (RDI)[125] and Mahoney et al.'s responsive teaching (RT) address auditory processing, language, motor planning, sequencing, and sensory modulation and visual processing impairments in children with ASDs.[124,126] Currently, there is limited empirical research being done to support claims for these interventions.[127]

Physical Therapy in Early Intervention

The Infant Sibling Research Consortium confirms the lack of evidence to guide optimal programming in infancy and toddlerhood. They recommend the use of caregiver-facilitated, reciprocal social play contexts, particularly infant-initiated social interactions that require the child to actively engage with the caregiver.[128] They too recommend promoting social communication and motor systems of the at-risk infant. Moreover, they advocate individualized interventions based on the delays observed in the infant. Given these recommendations, a multisystem approach through caregiver handling is recommended. Infants at risk for ASDs can receive a variety of social, object-based, and postural experiences that facilitate general and specific movement patterns, positive affect, as well as verbalizations.[55] In the first half-year of life, parents can provide cues through verbal reinforcement as well as physical handling of the infant.[129] Similarly, object-based cues can be provided by cause-and-effect toys.[129,130] Parents should encourage hands and feet reaching by offering objects near the infant's arms or legs as well as age-appropriate locomotor and object exploration skills. During object-based interactions, caregivers must incorporate triadic contexts wherein relevant social behaviors like joint attention, that is, sharing of object play with caregivers, are encouraged.[38] Postural experiences can be provided by passively placing or by actively moving the child within the postures that appear to be delayed in the infant.[131]

If the child is diagnosed with ASD or presents with concerns leading to that diagnosis prior to age 3, early intervention should be recommended. Early intervention is typically conducted in the home or other natural environment with family-directed goals outlined on the Individualized Family Service Plan. Such a model of intervention is centered on functional activities and maximizes the likelihood of generalizing to naturally occurring situations.

Physical Therapy in School Systems

The public school system is responsible for children who carry the diagnosis of ASD at 3 years of age and older who require special education services. In addition to the family, the educational team may consist of the regular education teacher, special education teacher, speech-language pathologist, psychologist, OT, PT, and school nurse, depending on the child's needs to engage in the educational program. The goals of the program will be developed by the team specifically for that student and outlined on the Individualized Education Plan (IEP). Direct and/or consultative physical therapy service is appropriate for many students with ASD.

The Individuals with Disabilities Education Act (IDEA) requires that students receive educational program in the least restrictive environment. Because of the range of abilities and behavior, appropriate settings for children with ASD range from specialized programs and self-contained classrooms to full inclusion in regular classrooms. As with other students receiving special education services, transition planning for students with ASDs formally begins as early as 14 years of age, and by age 16 a formal plan must be included in the IEP. The student, parents, educators, and all involved community agencies should be involved in developing a comprehensive transition plan that may include preparation for secondary education or competitive, supported or sheltered employment depending on the student's interests, abilities, and behavior.[127] All members of the educational team may play a role in preparing the student with ASD to enter the community as independently as possible.

Recreational Activities and the Use of Technologies

While there is little empirical evidence to support alternative therapies such as music therapy,[53] hippotherapy,[132] aquatic therapy,[133] and yoga[134] specifically for children with ASDs, these activities may be considered as a means of community involvement and preparation for lifelong fitness activities for some children with ASDs. Community-based yoga, music, dance, and martial arts may serve as other alternatives for physical activities if necessary modifications and accommodations can be made to create a positive learning environment. Special consideration should be given to the child's safety, interest, ability level, and tolerance to environmental stimuli. Therapists may be helpful in making recommendations to promote positive experiences in these alternative activities.

Children with ASDs have a predilection for using advanced technologies; hence, these have been used in meaningful ways to promote social, communication, and motor skills in children with ASDs.[135] Specifically, computer technologies such as Wii boards,[135] Dance Dance Revolution,[135] as well as robotic technologies[136,137] could be used to facilitate social and motor skills, as well as physical fitness in children with ASDs. Evidence to support their use is currently limited. But, when appropriate, these technologies could be employed in home and school environments to provide the required practice, generalization to other environments, to standardize the activities, and to intrinsically motivate a child during the activity.

▶ Conclusions

In this chapter, we have offered evidence for qualitative and quantitative differences in motor development among children and adolescents with ASDs as compared with those without autism. Significant impairments in motor coordination, postural control, imitation, and praxis are present in individuals with ASDs. These areas of need can be addressed using fundamental principles of current motor learning and dynamical systems theories, along with ABA, TEACCH, and PECS principles through direct intervention and/or consultation with family, caregivers, and educators. We have also provided clinicians with specific strategies to implement various treatment approaches within a physical therapy session. Given the heterogeneity of presentations of children with ASD, each child must be considered individually with respect to motor abilities, sensory responses, social communication, and cognition. The PT can make a valuable contribution to the team working with the child with ASD by providing information about the child's sensorimotor abilities, recommending activities to address the individual's unique motor needs, and suggesting modifications to promote the child's ability to learn in his or her typical environments, school, and home. Suggestions may take the form of changing expectations, modifying classroom activities to minimize negative sensory responses and address motor challenges, teaching compensatory strategies, and promoting more active engagement with the caregivers within various learning situations.

CASE STUDY

Chris—a 4-year-old boy with autism

Chris is a 4-year-old boy who lives with his parents in a midsized home in a suburban area. He attends the preschool program of his local elementary school, where he receives special education support services. He was diagnosed with autism at 30 months of age.

History

Chris' mom reported having a full-term pregnancy and a delivery that was without any notable problems. However, there is a family history of ASD because his uncle had the same diagnosis. Chris sat independently by 9 months, walked without assistance at 16 months, and would often fall while walking for several months. When Chris was 20 months old, his mother prompted evaluation by their pediatrician, and eventually a specialist, because she was concerned that Chris appeared to have a language delay and behaved "differently" than her friend's children. While he did not always attend to people calling his name or talking with him, Chris seemed very sensitive to sounds such as kitchen timers, constructions sounds, etc., as demonstrated by tantrums when such sounds occurred. He would sit watching moving objects for extended time periods, such as the fan, so much so that it was difficult for him to stop that activity. At 20 months, he had not produced words, but grunted, growled, or cried to convey distress. He would not convey his needs or his feelings through gestures such as pointing to something he wanted or showing the toys that he played with. When they went to play dates with other children, Chris did not interact and would often remove himself from where the other children were playing, sometimes hiding behind the couches. He would repeatedly activate toys with flashing lights. His mother was very concerned because Chris would eat only macaroni and cheese and applesauce, and would refuse to even try most other foods.

Birth-to-three programming began shortly after the diagnosis was made. Educational, speech, and occupational therapy services were provided on a regular basis until Chris' third birthday. Interestingly, his parents insisted on physical therapy services for the overt gross motor issues they observed; hence those services were later added to his program. The early intervention staff provided the family with strategies to promote social communication and motor skills, modulate his sensory responses, engage Chris in the family's routine, and plan transition into the preschool program.

Current status

Chris is currently enrolled in the morning preschool program at the local elementary school. On the basis of birth-to-three recommendations and initial assessment by the educational team, Chris receives specialized educational instruction, including one-on-one paraprofessional support, along with direct speech and language, occupational, and physical therapy services infused in the typical preschool activities. His individualized educational program addresses receptive and expressive language, social interaction, sensorimotor development, and self-help skills. The parents and the educational team meet once monthly to discuss Chris' progress and to coordinate efforts to maximize consistency of expectations and interactions.

Language and social interaction

Chris demonstrates echolalic speech, that is, he repeats a few words uttered by adults or on television shows. All staff model appropriate verbal responses to situations clearly with emphasis and praise Chris when he imitates the correct response. He has very little spontaneous interaction with his peers and tends to engage in activities that do not involve interaction with others. Teachers and therapists have paired him with the least threatening peers for play and academic activities with favorable results. Chris does enjoy his time with the other children. He is able to stay in the desired location and concentrate on the task at hand with support. Chris demonstrates signs of anxiety (increased stereotypies and raised vocalizations) during transitions between activities and locations. A picture schedule is used to help Chris orient to his daily schedule. All classroom and related services are represented on the schedule. Pictures are also available to represent activities within each center and to allow choices. He consistently looks toward the picture schedule to determine the next step in his routine, and he seems to make transitions more

easily in response to prior notification through pictures than if no or little warning is provided. A similar picture system is used for the different home routines. Chris has recently begun spontaneously pointing to pictures of objects he would like on occasion. When Chris successfully performs the desired behavior, those involved with programming provide rewards that have been agreed upon by parents and educators. Each team member is aware of the plan and provides the reinforcement for a job well done and additional wagon time (Chris' preferred activity) for successful completion of the activities asked of him.

Sensorimotor development

Chris has developed stereotypic behavior of rocking and occasionally spinning. He flaps his hands and watches them at times. He continues to become distressed with loud sounds; he often covers his ears and increases rocking motion. Such responses also occur if adults or peers touch him. He prefers to play with the computer and toys that have lights.

He will sit in circle time for only a few minutes before he wants to get up and move quickly about the classroom. On the playground, he enjoys activities that provide movement such as the swings, slides, and rotary equipment. It is sometimes a challenge for Chris to end such activities. In physical education, Chris typically runs around the space, behavior escalates, and he sometimes tries to hide under the mats that are stacked against the wall.

Chris is ambulatory without physical assistance around the interior and exterior of the school; he needs supervision and cuing for safety and direction. His gait pattern is usually characterized by toe-walking. He is able to run and change directions, but his motor planning is clearly affected. He is unable to perform actions involving multiple steps required for using the stepper, scooter, or the bicycle. He has not demonstrated multilimb actions such as galloping, skipping, or maintaining one-leg stance, and he usually does not respond to the request of copying the demonstrations of the PT/OT. He cannot ascend and descend stairs without the support of a railing and appears to lack balance in situations that require a narrow base of support. He presents with slightly diminished muscle tone as demonstrated by joint laxity and difficulty maintaining antigravity positions for extended periods.

Chris' performance on the Movement ABC indicated that he functions in the 9th percentile for Manual Dexterity, 5th percentile for Aiming and Catching, and 1st percentile for Balance. Using the Sensory Profile, parents and educators provided information about Chris' responses to sensory stimuli. On the basis of their responses, definite differences with hypersensitivity were identified in the following areas: Tactile Sensitivity, Taste/Smell Sensitivity, Auditory Filtering, and Visual/Auditory Sensitivity.

On the basis of observations throughout the school day, input from all team members, and results of standardized testing, the PT and OT have collaboratively made recommendations for strategies to help regulate sensory responses and promote gross and fine motor development. The OT and paraprofessional have found that Chris tends to sit longer in the circle activities when deep pressure input is provided. Use of a weighted lap blanket also seems to lengthen periods of quiet sitting. Chris tends to be more engaged in the physical education activities when the lesson is conducted in a room smaller than the gymnasium. The staff is currently in the process of collecting data about time-on-task and signs of anxiety when wearing a weighted vest with special attention to performance during physical education.

A designated time is now built into Chris' routine to use the swing on the playscape. Since adding this opportunity for Chris to get vestibular input, the rocking and flapping stereotypies have diminished. A rocking chair is available in the listening/story center, and Chris is usually allowed to use it for short time periods as a reward for completing his therapeutic/academic activities. A rocking horse is occasionally included as a gross motor option at recess. He has a cart that he loads with various objects that he pushes at home and at school. The parents and school staff have developed a plan for after-school hours that allows Chris to play on his swing set and run in the yard with supervision shortly after he comes home.

The speech and occupational therapists are currently working closely with the parents to systematically introduce textures and flavors into Chris' diet to expand his food choice repertoire. Chris' mother follows through by sending in snacks of various textures that can be trialed under the supervision of the trained related service providers.

The PT recommended a trial of wearing high-top work boots to help improve Chris' gait pattern with positive results; consistent foot-flat and occasional heel strike have been noted. Balance, coordination, and gross motor planning are being addressed within his physical therapy program. He is encouraged to walk on different ambulation surfaces that vary by texture, size, pitch, compliance, and stability. On more challenging surfaces, Chris' performance is enhanced if the PT provides some manual support for him to hold onto gently and guards him. As carryover, the paraprofessional walks with Chris along the railroad ties surrounding the playscape each day during recess while providing guarding and some manual support.

Motor planning is addressed by engaging in throwing and catching through the use of beanbags and balls that vary in size, texture, and compliance. Targets have been chosen that will yield activation of lights or motion when successfully reached. Similar activities are done at school and during play at home. He is also learning to use exercise equipment such as a stepper and a tricycle, but needs significant instruction and physical support to complete the activity. The paraprofessional is typically supporting the PT during these activities.

Self-help skills

Chris requires assistance to manage dressing and toileting at school and at home. He uses pull-ups as he does not indicate when he needs to use the toilet. He is able to use his hands or utensils to feed himself, and he is able to independently use a cup with a spout to drink. His diet is limited to a few preferred food choices.

The PEDI was done with observation and report by parent and educational staff, yielding normative standard scores for self-care of less than 10 (Caregiver Assistance less than 10), Mobility 20.4 (Caregiver Assistance 60.7), and Social Function less than 10 (Caregiver Assistance less than 10).

The family identified washing and bathing as being particularly challenging as Chris seems genuinely fearful. The school staff plans to perform the SFA when Chris enters kindergarten.

Family and educators identified hand washing and toileting as priorities. The special educator, the OT, and the PT broke each task into concrete steps and developed specific instructions for each step. The steps were described using a picture schedule placed at a location near the sink where he washes his hands. Everyone in school and at home who assists Chris with the hand washing and toileting go through the picture schedule in the specified manner using the same terminology, provide praise along the way, and reward him when he successfully completes the task. Proper participation in self-help skills is also reinforced through stories that are part of the preschool curriculum.

Collaborative input and efforts of the family, educators, caregivers, and medical personnel are imperative to optimize the programming for a child with ASD. The likelihood of the child acquiring important lifelong functional skills is enhanced when:

a. The activities are meaningful to the child and family and serve a long-term function.

b. The activities are individualized to the child's ability level.

c. The program accounts for and is respectful of the child's ability to take in information from the caregivers within the child's environment.

d. The people who interact with the child with ASD are consistent in their expectations and implementation of the program.

REFERENCES

1. Association Psychiatric Association. *Diagnostic and Statistical Manual of Mental Disorders (DSM-IV-TR)*. 4th ed. Washington, DC: 2000.

2. Jansiewicz E, Goldberg M, Newschaffer C, et al. Motor signs distinguish children with high functioning autism and Asperger's syndrome from controls. *J Autism Dev Disord*. 2006;36(5):613–621.

3. Fournier K, Hass C, Naik S, et al. Motor coordination in autism spectrum disorders: a synthesis and meta-analysis. *J Autism Dev Disord*. 2010;40(10):1227–1240.

4. Centers for Disease Control. Prevalence of autism spectrum disorders—Autism and Developmental Disabilities Monitoring Network (ADDM), United States, 2006. *MMWR Surveill Summ*. 2009;58(10):1–20.

5. Ganz M. *Understanding Autism*. Boca Raton, Florida: Taylor & Francis; 2006.

6. Centers for Disease Control and prevention. Facts about ASDs. http://www.cdc.gov/NCBDDD/autism/facts.html. Accessed 2012.

7. Bauman M, Kemper T. Neuroanatomic observations of the brain in autism: a review and future directions. *Int J Dev Neurosci*. 2005;23(2–3):183–187.

8. Sumi S, Taniai H, Miyachi T, et al. Sibling risk of pervasive developmental disorder estimated by means of an epidemiologic survey in Nagoya, Japan. *J Hum Genet*. 2006;51(6):518–522.

9. Zwaigenbaum L, Thurm A, Stone W, et al. Studying the emergence of autism spectrum disorders in high-risk infants: methodological and practical issues. *J Autism Dev Disord*. 2007;37(3):466–480.

10. Guinchat V, Thorsen P, Laurent C, et al. Pre-, peri-, and neonatal risk factors for autism. *Acta Obstet Gynecol Scand*. 2012;91(3):287–300.

11. Sandin S, Hultman C, Kolevzon A, et al. Advancing maternal age is associated with increasing risk for autism: a review and meta-analysis. *J Am Acad Child Adolesc Psychiatry*. 2012;51(5):477–486.

12. Narita M, Oyabu A, Imura Y, et al. Nonexploratory movement and behavioral alterations in a thalidomide or valproic acid-induced autism model rat. *Neurosci Res*. 2010;66(1):2–6.

13. Courchesne E, Redcay E, Kennedy D. The autistic brain: birth through adulthood. *Curr Opin Neurol*. 2004;17(4):489–496.

14. Dementieva Y, Vance D, Donnelly S, et al. Accelerated head growth in early development of individuals with autism. *Pediatri Neurol*. 2005;32(2):102–108.

15. Dawson G, Munson J, Webb SJ, et al. Rate of head growth decelerates and symptoms worsen in the second year of life in autism. *Biol Psychiatry*. 2007;61(4):458–464.

16. Sparks B, Friedman S, Shaw D, et al. Brain structural abnormalities in young children with autism spectrum disorder. *Neurology*. 2002;59(2):184–192.

17. Casanova M, Buxhoeveden D, Switala A, et al. Minicolumnar pathology in autism. *Neurology*. 2002;58(3):428–432.

18. Williams D, Goldstein G, Minshew N. Neuropsychologic functioning in children with autism: further evidence for disordered complex information processing. *Child Neuropsychol*. 2006;12(4–5):279–298.

19. Mostofsky S, Powell S, Simmonds D, et al. Decreased connectivity and cerebellar activity in autism during motor task performance. *Brain*. 2009;132(pt 9):2413–2425.

20. Hallett M, Lebiedowska M, Thomas S, et al. Locomotion of autistic adults. *Arch Neurol*. 1993;50(12):1304–1308.

21. Rinehart N, Bradshaw J, Brereton A, et al. A clinical and neurobehavioural review of high-functioning autism and Asperger's disorder. *Aust N Z J Psychiatry*. 2002;36(6):762–770.

22. Vilensky J, Damasio A, Maurer R. Gait disturbances in patients with autistic behavior: a preliminary study. *Arch Neurol*. 1981;38(10):646–649.

23. Cattaneo L, Rizzolatti G. The mirror neuron system. *Arch Neurol*. 2009;66(5):557–560.

24. Dapretto D, Pfeiffer P, Scott A, et al. Understanding emotions in others: mirror neuron dysfunction in children with autism spectrum disorders. *Nat Neurosci*. 2006;9(1):28–30.

25. Landa R, Garrett-Mayer E. Development in infants with autism spectrum disorders: a prospective study. *J Child Psychol Psychiatry*. 2006;47(6):629–638.

26. Bhat A, Galloway J, Landa R. Relationship between early motor delay and later communication delay in infants at risk for autism. *Infant Behav Dev*. 2012;35(4):838–846.

27. Flanagan J, Landa R, Bhat A, et al. Head lag in infants at risk for autism: a preliminary study. *Am J Occup Ther*. 2012;66(5):577–585.

28. Ozonoff S, Young G, Goldring S, et al. Gross motor development, movement abnormalities, and early identification of autism. *J Autism Dev Disord*. 2008;38(4):644–656.

29. Paul R, Fuerst Y, Ramsay G, et al. Out of the mouths of babes: vocal production in infant siblings of children with ASD. *J Child Psychol Psychiatry*. 2011;52(5):588–598.

30. Lord C, Rutter M, DiLavore PC, et al. *Autism Diagnostic Observation Schedule (ADOS)*. Los Angeles, CA: Western Psychological Services; 1999.

31. Lord C, Rutter M, Le Couteur A. Autism diagnostic interview-revised (ADI-R): a revised version of diagnostic interview for caregivers of individuals with pervasive developmental disorders. *J Autism Dev Disord*. 1994;24(5):659–685.

32. Genetics Home Reference. Rett syndrome. http://ghr.nlm.nih.gov/condition/rett-syndrome. Accessed 2011.

33. Genetics Home Reference. Fragile X syndrome. 2007; http://ghr.nlm.nih.gov/condition/fragile-x-syndrome. Accessed June 8, 2012.

34. Townsend J, Harris N, Courchesne E. Visual attention abnormalities in autism: delayed orienting to location. *J Int Neuropsychol Soc*. 1996;2(6):541–550.

35. Wainwright J, Bryson S. Visual-spatial orienting in autism. *J Autism Dev Disord*. 1996;26(4):423–438.

36. Mundy P, Thorp D. *New Developments in Autism: The Future is Today*. London, England: Jessica Kingsley Publishers; 2007.

37. Dawson G, Webb S, McPartland J. Understanding the nature of face processing impairment in autism: insights from behavioral and electrophysiological studies. *Dev Neuropsychol*. 2005;27(3):403–424.

38. Bhat A, Galloway JC, Landa R. Visual attention patterns during social and non-social contexts of learning in infants at risk for autism and typically developing infants. *J Child Psychol Psychiatry*. 2010;51(9):989–997.

39. Mundy P, Sigman M. Joint attention, social competence, and developmental psychopathology. *Dev Psychopathol*. 2006;1:293–332.

40. Mundy P, Sigman M, Kasari C. A longitudinal study of joint attention and language development in autistic children. *J Autism Dev Disord*. 1990;20(1):115–128.

41. Eigsti I-M, de Marchena A, Schuh J, et al. Language acquisition in autism spectrum disorders: a developmental review. *Res Autism Spectrum Disord*. 2011;5:681–691.

42. Tager-Flusberg H, Paul R, Lord C. *Language and communication in autism*. In: Cohen D, Volkmar F, eds. *Handbook of Autism and Pervasive Developmental Disorders*. 3rd ed. New York, NY: John Wiley & Sons Inc; 1997:195–225.

43. Ozonoff S, Pennington B, Rogers S. Executive function deficits in high-functioning autistic individuals: relationship to theory of mind. *J Child Psychol*. 1991;32(7):1081–1105.

44. Ben-Sasson A, Hen L, Fluss R, et al. A meta-analysis of sensory modulation symptoms in individuals with autism spectrum disorders. *J Autism Dev Disord*. 2009;39(1):1–11.

45. Tomchek S, Dunn W. Sensory processing in children with and without autism: a comparative study using the short sensory profile. *Am J Occup Ther*. 2007;61(2):190–200.

46. Baranek G, Parham L, Bodfish J. *Sensory and motor features in autism: assessment and intervention*. In: Volkmar FR, Paul R, Klin A, et al., eds. *Handbook of Autism and Pervasive Developmental Disorders*. Hoboken, NJ: Wiley; 2005:831–857.

47. Lane A, Young R, Baker A, et al. Sensory processing subtypes in autism: association with adaptive behavior. *J Autism Dev Disord*. 2010;40(1):112–122.

48. Bölte S, Holtmann M, Poustka F, et al. Gestalt perception and local-global processing in high-functioning autism. *J Autism Dev Disord*. 2007;37(8):1493–1504.

49. Gernsbacher M, Stevenson J, Khandakar S, et al. Why does joint attention look atypical in autism? *Child Dev Perspect*. 2008;2(1):38–45.

50. Heaton P. Pitch memory, labelling, and disembedding in autism. *J Child Psychol Psychiatry*. 2003;44(4):543–551.

51. Bhatara A, Quintin E, Levy B, et al. Perception of emotion in musical performance in adolescents with autism spectrum disorders. *Autism Res*. 2010;3(5):214–225.

52. Whipple J. Music in intervention for children and adolescents with autism: a meta-analysis. *J Music Ther*. 2004;41(2):90–106.

53. Wigram T, Gold C. Music therapy in the assessment and treatment of autistic spectrum disorder: clinical application and research evidence. *Child Care Heatlh Dev*. 2006;32(5):535–542.

54. Dzuik M, Gidley Larson J, et al. Dyspraxia in autism: association with motor, social, and communicative deficits. *Dev Med Child Neurol*. 2007;49(10):734–739.

55. Bhat A, Landa R, Galloway JC. Perspectives on motor problems in infants, children, and adults with autism spectrum disorders. *Phys Ther*. 2011;91(7):1116–1129.

56. Bodfish J, Symons F, Parker D, et al. Varieties of repetitive behavior in autism: comparisons to mental retardation. *J Autism Dev Disord*. 2000;30(3):237–243.

57. Loh A, Soman T, Brian J, et al. Stereotyped motor behaviors associated with autism in high-risk infants: a pilot videotape analysis of a sibling sample. *J Autism Dev Disord*. 2007;37(1):25–36.

58. Walker D, Thompson A, Zwaigenbaum L, et al. Specifying PDD-NOS: a comparison of PDD-NOS, Asperger syndrome, and autism. *J Am Acad Child Adolesc Psychiatry.* 2004;43(2):172–180.

59. Chawarska K, Klin A, Paul R, et al. Autism spectrum disorder in the second year: stability and change in syndrome expression. *J Child Psychol Psychiatry.* 2006;48(2):128–138.

60. Nickel L, Thatcher A, Iverson J. Postural development in infants with and without risk for autism spectrum disorders. Paper presented at: 9th Annual International Meeting for Autism Research; 2010; Philadelphia, Pennsylvania.

61. Ghaziuddin M, Butler E. Clumsiness in autism and Asperger syndrome: a further report. *J Intellect Disabil Res.* 1998;42(pt 1):43–48.

62. Green D, Baird G, Barnett A, et al. The severity and nature of motor impairment in Asperger's syndrome: a comparison with specific developmental disorder of motor function. *J Child Psychol Psychiatry.* 2002;43(5):655–668.

63. Miyahara M, Tsujii M, Hori M, et al. Brief report: motor incoordination in children with Asperger syndrome and learning disabilities. *J Autism Dev Disord.* 1997;27(5):595–603.

64. Szatmari P, Archer L, Fisman S, et al. Asperger's syndrome and autism: differences in behavior, cognition, and adaptive functioning. *J Am Acad Child Adolesc Psychiatry.* 1995;34(12):1662–1671.

65. Mari M, Castiello U, Marks D, et al. The reach–to–grasp movement in children with autism spectrum disorder. *Philos Trans R Soc Lon B Biol Sci.* 2003;358(1430):393–403.

66. Glazebrook CM, Elliott D, Lyons J. A kinematic analysis of how young adults with and without autism plan and control goal-directed movements. *Motor Control.* 2006;10(3):244–264.

67. Fuentes C MS, Bastian A. Children with autism show specific handwriting impairments. *Neurology.* 2009;73(19):1532–1537.

68. Baranek G. Autism during infancy: a retrospective video analysis of sensorymotor and social behaviors at 9-12 months of age. *J Autism Dev Disord.* 1999;29(3):213–224.

69. Bryson S, Zwaigenbaum L, Brian J, et al. A prospective case-series of high-risk infants who developed autism. *J Autism Dev Disord.* 2007;37(1):12–24.

70. Gernsbacher M. Infant and toddler oral- and manual-motor skills predict later speech fluency in autism. *J Child Psychol Psychiatry.* 2008;49(1):43–50.

71. Greenspan SI, Wieder S. Developmental patterns and outcomes in infants and children with disorders in relating and communicating: a chart review of 200 cases of children with autistic spectrum diagnoses. *J Dev Learn Disord.* 1997;1:87–141.

72. Minshew N, Sung K, Jones B, et al. Underdevelopment of the postural control system in autism. *Neurology.* 2004;63(11):2056–2061.

73. Landa R, Gross A, Stuart E, et al. Developmental trajectories in children with and without autism spectrum disorders: the first 3 years. *Child Dev.* 2013;84(2):429–442.

74. Dewey D. What is developmental dyspraxia? *Brain Cogn.* 1995;29(3):254–274.

75. Demyer M, Hingtgen I, Jackson R. Infantile autism revisited: a decade of research. *Schizophr Bul.* 1981;7:388–451.

76. Mostofsky SH, Dubey P, Jerath VK, et al. Developmental dyspraxia is not limited to imitation in children with autism spectrum disorders. *J Int Neuropsychol Soc.* 2006;12(3):314–326.

77. Charman T, Baron-Cohen S. Brief report: Prompted pretend play in autism. *J Autism Dev Disord.* 1997;27(3):325–332.

78. Rogers SJ, Bennetto L, McEvoy R, et al. Imitation and pantomime in high-functioning adolescents with autism spectrum disorders. *Child Dev.* 1996;67(5):2060–2073.

79. Stone W, Yoder P. Predicting spoken language level in children with autism spectrum disorders. *Autism.* 2001;5(4):341–361.

80. Kern J, Geier D, Adams J, et al. Autism severity and muscle strength: a correlation analysis. *Res Autism Spectr Disord.* 2011;5(3):1011–1015.

81. Teitelbaum P, Teitelbaum O, Nye J, et al. Movement analysis in infancy may be useful for early diagnosis of autism. *Proc Nat Acad Sci.* 1998;95(23):13982–12987.

82. Adrien J, Lenoir P, Martineau J, et al. Blind ratings of early symptoms of autism based upon family home movies. *J Am Acad Child Adolesc Psychiatry.* 1993;32(3):617–626.

83. Tyler C, Schramm S, Karafa M, et al. Chronic disease risks in young adults with autism spectrum disorder: forewarned is forearmed. *Am J Intellect Dev Disabil.* 2011;116(5):371–380.

84. Curtin C, Anderson S, Must A, et al. The prevalence of obesity in children with autism: a secondary data analysis using nationally representative data from the National Survey of Children's Health. *Br Med Counc Pediatr.* 2010;10(1):11.

85. Bandini L, Anderson S, Curtin C, et al. Food selectivity in children with autism spectrum disorders and typically developing children. *J Pediatr.* 2010;157(2):259–264.

86. Matson M, Matson J, Beighley J. Comorbidity of physical and motor problems in children with autism. *Res Dev Disabil.* 2011;32(6):2304–2308.

87. Chen A, Kim S, Houtrow A, et al. Prevalence of obesity among children with chronic conditions. *Obesity.* 2009;18(1):210–213.

88. Rimmer J, Yamaki K, Lowry B, et al. Obesity and obesity-related secondary conditions in adolescents with intellectual/developmental disabilities. *J Intellect Disabil Res.* 2010;54(9):787–794.

89. Ayres J. *Sensory Integration and Praxis Tests (SIPT).* Los Angeles, CA: Western Psychological Services; 1996.

90. Henderson SE, Sugden DA. *Movement Assessment Battery for Children.* London, UK: Psychological Corporation; 1992.

91. King G, Law M, King S, et al. *Children's Assessment of Participation and Enjoyment (CAPE) Manual.* San Antonio, TX: Hartcourt Assessment; 2004.

92. Bruininks R. *The Bruininks-Oseretsky Test of Motor Proficiency (BOTMP) Manual.* Circle Pines, MN: American Guidance Service; 1978.

93. Squires J, Bricker D. *Ages & Stages Questionnaires, Third Edition (ASQ-3).* Baltimore, MD: Brookes Publishing; 2009.

94. Robins DL, Fein D, Barton ML, Green JA. The modified checklist for autism in toddlers: an initial study investigating the early detection of autism and pervasive developmental disorders. *J Autism Dev Disord.* 2001;31(2):131–144.

95. Bryson S, Zwaigenbaum L, McDermott C, et al. The autism observation scale for infants (AOSI):scale development and reliability data. *J Autism Dev Disord.* 2008;38(4):731–738.

96. Bayley N. *Bayley Scales of Infant and Toddler Development—Third Edition.* San Antonio, TX: Pearson Assessment; 2005.

97. Mullen E. *Mullen Scales of Early Learning.* Circle Pines, MN: American Guidance Service; 1995.

98. Volkmar F, Sparrow S, Goudreau D, et al. Social deficits in autism: an operational approach using the Vineland adaptive behavior scales. *J Am Acad Child Adolesc Psychiatry.* 1987;26(2):156–161.

99. Rothi L, Gonzalez R, Heilman K. Limb praxis assessment. In: Hove E, ed. *Apraxia: The neuropsychology of action.* Erlbaum, UK: Psychology Press/Taylor & Francis; 1997:61–73.

100. Haley SM, Coster WJ, Ludlow LH, et al. *Pediatric Evaluation of Disability Inventory (PEDI).* San Antonio, TX: Psychological Corporation; 1992.

101. Coster W, Deeney T, Haltiwanger J, et al. School function assessment (SFA). San Antonio, TX: The Psychological Corporation; 1998.

102. Landa R. Early communication development and intervention for children with autism. *Ment Retard Dev Disabil Res Rev.* 2007;13(1):16–25.

103. Sallows G, Graupner T. Intensive behavioral treatment for children with autism: four-year outcome and predictors. *Am J Ment Retard.* 2005;110(6):417–438.

104. Ozonoff S, Cathcart K. Effectiveness of a home program intervention for young children with autism. *J Autism Dev Disabil.* 1998;28:25–32.

105. Mesibov GB, Shea V, Schopler E. *The TEACCH Approach to Autsim Spectrum Disorder.* New York, NY: Kluwer Academic/Plenum; 2005.

106. Bondy A, Frost A. Communication strategies for visual learners. In: Lovaas OI, ed. *Teaching Individuals with Developmental Delays: Basic Intervention Techniques.* Austin, TX: Pro-Ed; 2003:291–304.

107. Bundy AC, Murray EA. Sensory integration: a Jean Ayre's theory revisited. In: Bundy AC, Murray EA, Lane S, eds. *Sensory Integration: Theory and Practice*. Philadelphia, PA: FA Davis; 2002.

108. Lovaas OI. Behavioral treatment and normal educational and intellectual functioning in young autistic children. *J Consul Clin Psychol*. 1987;55:3–9.

109. McEachin JJ, Smith T, Lovaas OI. Long-term outcome for children with autism who received early intensive behavioral treatment. *Am J Men Retard*. 1993;97:359–372.

110. Stahmer A, Ingersoll B. Inclusive programming for toddlers with autistic spectrum disorders: outcomes from the children's toddler school. *J Positive Behav Interven*. 2004;6(2):67–82.

111. Pierce K, Schreibman L. Increasing complex social behaviors in children with autism: effects of peer-implemented pivotal response training. *J Appl Behav Anal*. 1995;28(3):285–295.

112. Shumway-Cook A, Woollacott M. *Motor Control: Translating Research in Clinical Practice*. 3rd ed. Philadelphia, PA: Lippincott Williams & Wilkins; 2007.

113. Gidley Larson JC, Bastian AJ, Donchin O, et al. Acquisition of internal models of motor tasks in children with autism. *Brain*. 2008;131(11):2894–2903.

114. Mostofsky SH, Bunoski R, Morton SM, et al. Children with autism adapt normally during a catching task requiring the cerebellum. *Neurocase*. 2004;10(1):60–64.

115. Glazebrook C, Gonzalez D, Hansen S, et al. The role of vision for online control of manual aiming movements in persons with autism spectrum disorders. *Autism*. 2009;13:411–433.

116. Maione I, Mirenda P. Effects of video modeling and video feedback on peer-directed social language skills of a child with autism. *J Positive Behav Interven*. 2006;8:106–118.

117. Fabbri-Destro M, Cattaneo L, Boria S, et al. Planning actions in autism. *Experiment Brain Res*. 2009;192(3):521–525.

118. Miller L, Anzalone M, Lane S, et al. Concept evolution in sensory integration: a proposed nosology for diagnosis. *Am J Occup Ther*. 2007;61(2):135–140.

119. Baranek G. Efficacy of sensory and motor interventions for children with autism. *J Autism Dev Disord*. 2002;32(5):397–422.

120. Stagnitti K, Raison P, Ryan P. Sensory defensiveness syndrome: a paediatric perspective and case study. *Aust Occup Ther J*. 1999;46:175–187.

121. Field T, Lasko PM, Henteleff T, et al. Brief report: autistic children's attentiveness and responsivity improve after touch therapy. *J Autism Dev Disord*. 1997;27:33–339.

122. Edelson SM, Goldberg M, Edelson MG, et al. Behavioral and physiological effects of deep pressure on children with autism: a pilot study evaluating the efficacy of Grandin's Hug Machine. *Am J Occup Ther*. 1999;53:143–152.

123. Yoder PJ, Stone WL. Randomized comparison of two communcation interventions for preschoolers with autism spectrum disorders. *J Consul Clin Psychol*. 2006;74(3):426–435.

124. Mahoney G, Perales F. Relationship-focused early intervention with children with pervasive developmental disorders and other disabilities; a comparative study. *J Dev Behav Pediatr*. 2005;26:77–85.

125. Gutstein SE, Sheeley RK. *Relationship Development Intervention with Children, Adolescents, and Adults*. New York, NY: Jessica Kingsley; 2002.

126. Mahoney G, McDonald J. *Responsive teaching: Parent-mediated developmental intervention*. Baltimore, MD: Paul H. Brookes; 2003.

127. Myers SM, Johnson CP. Management of children with autism spectrum disorders. *Pediatrics*. 2007;120:1162–1182.

128. Zwaigenbaum L, Bryson S, Lord C, et al. Clinical assessment and management of toddlers with suspected autism spectrum disorder: insights from studies of high-risk infants. *Pediatrics*. 2009;123(5):1383.

129. Heathcock J, Lobo M, Galloway J. Movement training advances the emergence of reaching in infants born at less than 33 weeks of gestational age: a randomized clinical trial. *Phys Ther*. 2008;88(3):1–13.

130. Lobo MA, Galloway JC, Savelsbergh GJP. General and task-related experiences affect early object interaction. *Child Dev*. 2004;75(4):1268–1281.

131. Lobo M, Galloway J. Experience matters: The relationship between experience, exploration, and the emergence of means-end performance. *Child Dev*. 2008;79(6):1869–1890.

132. Bass M, Duchowny C, Llabre M. The effect of therapeutic horseback riding on the social functioning of children with autism. *J Autism Dev Disord*. 2009;39:1261–1267.

133. Pan C. The efficacy of an aquatic program on physical fitness and aquatic skills in children with and without autism spectrum disorders. *Res Autism Spectr Disord*. 2011;5(1):657–665.

134. Koenig K, Buckely-Reen A, Garg S. Efficacy of the get ready to learn yoga program among children with ASDs: a pretest-posttest control group design. *Am J Occup Ther*. 2012;66(5):538–546.

135. Getchell N, Miccinello D, Blom M, et al. Comparing energy expenditure in adolescents with and without autism while playing nintendo—Wii Games. *Games Health J*. 2012;1(1):58–61.

136. Diehl JJ, Schmitt LM, Villano M, et al. The clinical use of robots for individuals with autism spectrum disorders: a critical review. *Res Autism Spectr Disord*. 2011;6(1):249–262.

137. Robins B, Dautenhahn K, te Boekhorst R, et al. *Effects of repeated exposure to a humanoid robot on children with autism*. Paper presented at: Universal Access and Assistive Technology; 2004; Cambridge, UK.

Adaptive Equipment and Environmental Aids for Children with Disabilities

Emilie J. Aubert

Role of Adaptive Equipment
Precautions When Using Adaptive Equipment
  Misuse
  Poor Planning
  Equipment Use Compared with Facilitation of Function
  Safety Issues
  Psychosocial Issues
Determining a Child's Equipment Needs
  Evaluation and Assessment of the Child
  Assessment of the Family, Home, and School
Equipment Selection
  Purchasing Equipment
  Renting or Borrowing Equipment
  Fabricating Equipment
Equipment for Positioning
  Sitting
  Standing
  Side-lying
  Overall Considerations for Positioning
Mobility Equipment
  Scooter Boards
  Prewheelchair Device

  Wheelchairs
  Tricycles
  Bicycles
  Gait Trainers or Support Walkers
  Other Mobility Aids
Transporting Children with Disabilities
Equipment for Infants and Toddlers
  Hospitalized Children
  Infants and Toddlers without Physical
    Impairments
Activities of Daily Living
  Toileting and Bathing
  Feeding
  Playing
Access Technologies
  Communication Systems
  Environmental Controls
Universal Design
  Tablet Computers, iPads, Androids,
    and Similar Devices
Summary

The ability of a person to function in daily life does not occur in a vacuum. Functioning relies on context. Functioning, as defined by the World Health Organization (WHO) in the International Classification of Functioning, Disability and Health (ICF), is the result of the interaction of an individual with the physical and social environment.[1] Furthermore, disability, the inability to perform a skill in a given setting, is a "universal human experience."[1(p3)]

Children with disabilities often need help interacting with their environments. This help may come from family members, teachers, peers, and health care professionals such as physical and occupational therapists. Physical and occupational therapists are able to teach a child to function in a variety of environments and to transfer functional skills to newly encountered environments through direct treatment and consultation, often incorporating adaptive equipment into the plan of care. The use of adaptive equipment is an intervention strategy that is known to improve function and to mitigate negative environmental or contextual elements that can be barriers to the child's participation.[2]

Physical therapists have many products at their disposal to help children with disabilities with positioning, mobility, activities of daily living (ADLs), and interacting with various environments. These devices are generally referred to as adaptive equipment.

Most adaptive equipment can be classified as assistive, alternative, or augmentative technology.[3] Assistive technology includes devices that are used to increase the ease of performing a certain function, improve a function, or maintain a function.[4] Devices such as modified eating utensils that are easier to grip with a hand that has limited range of motion, reachers that allow access to items that are out of reach for a variety of reasons, and orthotic devices that stabilize a particular joint(s) to allow for safe and energy-efficient ambulation are examples of assistive technology.

Alternative technology provides a substitute means toward the same end function, such as using a wheelchair for mobility in the community instead of walking.

An augmentative device supplements an inadequate function, but child's unaided function remains, as would be the case for a child with dysarthria whose family can understand his speech yet who needs a speech-generating device to be understood by people unfamiliar with him.[3]

Adaptive equipment can also be classified as low technology (low-tech), mid-tech, or high-tech.[3,5] Examples of low-tech devices are pencil grips or eating utensil grips and communication boards with head pointers or mouth sticks; mid-tech equipment includes switches, computers, word scanners, and powered toys. High-tech equipment uses complex electronic devices and microcircuits and includes note-taking devices, computers with talking software, electronic communication devices that use eye gaze to elicit digital speech, and power wheelchairs.[3,5-7]

Many new commercially available products made from a variety of materials are being developed every year in an attempt to meet the equipment needs of children with disabilities, and customized equipment can be fabricated to meet individual specifications for a given child. The great variety of products and materials available and the constantly changing and expanding market present a challenge to the therapist who tries to give parents useful suggestions regarding equipment. How can students, recent graduates, or physical therapists inexperienced in treating children acquaint themselves with these products, to feel confident in guiding families who need adaptive equipment for their children? What conditions should be evaluated before making decisions regarding adaptive equipment? What is the true role of adaptive equipment for children with physical disabilities and are there particular dangers or contraindications with adaptive equipment? These questions are addressed in this chapter, the main goal of which is to provide the student and the therapist who is inexperienced in pediatrics with a theoretical construct to facilitate decision making about adaptive equipment, regardless of familiarity with any particular piece of equipment. Common types of equipment such as prone standers, side-lyers, and wheelchairs are discussed, along with approaches to practical clinical decision making. While there are some scientific and objective guidelines on which to base a decision about adaptive equipment, the selection of adaptive equipment for children is often more art than science. As physical therapists, the goal is to try to meet the needs of children with disabilities by using a critical approach to document successes and failures, in the hope of eventually transforming this art into more of a science.

Role of adaptive equipment

Adaptive equipment is becoming increasingly necessary as an adjunct to direct treatment. No child can realistically receive the constant handling needed throughout the day to prevent abnormal movement patterns and postures or support more independent function. Although the physical therapist may teach families, day care providers, and teachers about methods of handling the child to encourage optimal development and function, the child must be allowed time to move, explore, and relax without constant help. The increased cost of direct care and the increasing number of children needing therapeutic intervention suggest a need for alternatives to direct patient handling.

One alternative is the judicious use of adaptive equipment to facilitate correct positioning during a child's free, independent time. Adaptive equipment can also provide reinforcement of and use of positions, movements, and skills introduced to the child during treatment sessions. Similarly, abnormal or undesirable positions or movements can often be prevented by use of correct equipment.

Known benefits of using adaptive equipment include improved function, increased functional independence, increased control over one's environment, improved sense of autonomy and self-determination, increased motivation, enhanced social interactions, enhanced visual attention and perception, improved cognition, and improved ability for parents, other caregivers, and teachers to assist the child with function.[8] Adaptive equipment can facilitate the performance of skills that a child might otherwise be unable to accomplish, thereby promoting motor, sensory, cognitive, perceptual, emotional, and social development.[8-13] Adaptive equipment may help improve a child's performance over capability. Capability refers to what physical function a child can do, generally within a specific environment and without using aids.[1,14-16] For example, a child who is unable to walk does not have the capability to ambulate and may therefore use creeping as his primary form of independent locomotion. However, while creeping may be an appropriate form of locomotion in the home, it is not an appropriate form in many community environments. Therefore, the child's performance (what he actually does in various places and situations)[1,14-16] lags behind his capability. In this case, he can locomote independently in the home but not in the community. This child's need for a locomotive form in the community could be addressed by providing him with a wheelchair. In this way, independent locomotion in the community may be attained, raising his level of performance closer to his level of capability. As an alternative, perhaps the child's performance can improve if he learns to walk using an upper extremity gait aid such as a walker. This too could improve his performance of independent locomotion in various environments, including home.[1,15,16]

A given child's motor performance may exceed his demonstrated capability, as scored on a standardized test, or his performance may lag behind his capability due to environmental barriers. Also, among children with the same diagnosis and similar capability in gross motor skills, there may be different levels of performance, depending on the environment. In a 2004 study of children with cerebral palsy, Tieman et al. proposed different reasons for discrepancies between capability and performance in various settings for a given child. Performance can differ across settings because of the impracticality of using a particular capability in some settings or because of societal expectations, such as the example above regarding the use of creeping as the primary mode of locomotion in the community. Time constraints may impact a child's performance in a particular context; the child may choose a lower level of function or a less independent function (such as being pushed in a wheelchair) because it is faster. Greater contextual demands of one environment over another, such as longer distances or uneven surfaces, will also affect, and perhaps diminish, performance.[14]

In addition to having direct therapeutic benefits that may improve a child's ability to perform some functions with increased independence, adaptive equipment can play an important role in caregiving and parenting by assisting in the daily management of the child at home. Some devices are particularly beneficial for increasing the child's independence, subsequently making caregiving easier, whereas others, such as portable seating systems and manual wheelchairs, may not increase the child's independent mobility but will decrease the physical demands on the caregiver.[4]

A 2005 study in Norway by Ostensjo et al. found that the more severe the gross motor limitations, the more a child and family needed and used assistive devices and environmental modifications. Mobility devices such as power mobility, walkers, and adapted bicycles provided benefits that most improved the child's function and independence, which in turn reduced the burden on the caregiver.[4]

Although adaptive seating was found to help decrease the amount of caregiver assistance required for feeding, parents in the study deemed many modifications that affected a child's self-care had a negative impact on caregiving, with little increased functional independence for the child. With or without assistive devices, many children need caregiver assistance for self-care ADLs such as eating, toileting, dressing, and bathing. Often, with even small improvements in self-care skills, there is a negative effect on caregiving because the activity, such as eating, takes longer for the child to do more independently. This can lead to frustration for the parent and ultimately to the parent assisting the child more or simply doing it to save time. An exception to caregivers' experiences of these negative effects with self-care devices can be toileting. Attention to good positioning for toileting increases a child's comfort. Proper positioning for toileting may not influence a child's independence in toileting, but it can benefit the child and the caregiver by improving the child's bowel and bladder function and even increasing the likelihood of timely toilet training.[4]

Often, lifts and hoists are not viewed by families as particularly helpful until the child gets older and becomes too heavy for the parent to lift. This early reliance on physically lifting a child rather than employing the use of mechanical devices is usually a consequence of time restraints on the caregiver.[4]

Although adaptive equipment should be prescribed with the goal of achieving maximum benefits with the least restriction, this ideal approach may occasionally need to be compromised. For example, some families may be unwilling to adjust the routines of all family members to meet the needs of only one member. Also, ideal goals may not be possible because of architectural barriers that prohibit using certain adaptive devices. When barriers (behavioral, architectural, or financial) exist, the therapist must analyze the short-term needs of the family and the long-term goals for the child before making a decision or recommendation. Decisions to use adaptive equipment should be made jointly by the physical therapist and the family. Also, the child's input should be considered if the child can participate in such decision making. Whenever adaptive equipment is recommended, its use must be monitored to ensure that therapeutic goals and family needs are being met.

▶ Precautions when using adaptive equipment

Can adaptive equipment be dangerous? This is a difficult question to answer, especially because most equipment has a design that is meant to be inherently free of dangers. Problems may arise from the way in which equipment is used by various caregivers. Although a particular piece of equipment may have been prescribed, fitted, and properly explained, its misuse or overuse may cause unintentional consequences and compromise the child's safety.

Misuse

Adaptive equipment is often static, and in spite of the benefits of a particular device, it may not provide a rich environment for exploration or for learning new movements and transitions from one position to another. Gross motor development in normal children requires learning through doing, moving, and feeling. Sensory input, particularly vestibular, proprioceptive, and tactile, is required to produce optimal motor output that is both effective and varied. Static positioning, which occurs when some adaptive equipment is used excessively, can retard motor development by modifying sensory input, reducing spontaneous movement activity, and limiting opportunities to move and explore.

A carefully developed plan for therapeutic use of a piece of adaptive equipment must take into consideration not only the potential benefits, but also the potential deleterious effects. Movement, by its very nature, is dynamic and requires the skillful coordination of both agonist and antagonist muscle groups to complete normal patterns of movement. Some types of adaptive equipment are static, tending to fix a child into one pattern, albeit therapeutic, while denying the opportunity to experience the competing or antagonist pattern. For example, a device for side-lying provides an opportunity for the child to play while placed in a neutral, midline orientation. Although a neutral, midline orientation may be an appropriate goal, it is important to note that an asymmetric orientation is not inherently bad or undesirable. An asymmetric orientation is a normal precursor to weight shifting, lateral flexion, and intra-axial rotation and should not be completely excluded from the child's positioning by overreliance on the side-lying device. The therapist is responsible for teaching balanced movement patterns and positions. The person responsible for positioning a child must be aware of the benefits of various positions and must avoid constant and unchanging positioning habits that might interfere with the child's development of balanced movement and postures.

Inappropriate use of equipment that places the child in static postures can also lead to other complications, such as joint contractures or skin breakdown, either of which may eventually require surgical repair. Anyone who has responsibility for the child must understand the therapeutic goals of using equipment and monitor its use to maximize the benefits and minimize the deleterious effects.

Poor Planning

A child's age and developmental level are first considerations when planning for equipment needs. However, poor planning for growth and change can lead to equipment that fails to meet the child's needs for the short and/or long term. With the increasing difficulty in receiving reimbursement for expensive equipment for the child with a physical disability, the therapist must anticipate and plan carefully for the child's physical growth, developmental changes, and acquisition of new skills. The inexperienced therapist may overlook the changing needs of the child. A child who requires positioning in sitting during the early years may be given an expensive chair that will provide positioning in sitting and optimal use of the upper extremities for fine motor skills. However, in spite of the initial advantages of the chair, it may be inappropriate for future mobility and socialization needs. Predicting the child's needs in the areas of growth and development, education, and recreational alternatives (e.g., wheelchair sports) is a monumental task, but one in which physical therapists must often participate at the request of insurers and local and state funding agencies.

Therapists must learn how various agencies and providers prefer to reconcile future needs and reimbursement patterns with the child's current needs. Some providers prefer to pay initially for less-expensive devices that must be replaced more frequently, even though a costlier device might be more cost-effective in the long term. Other providers prefer an initial, larger expenditure for a device that will last for 3 to 5 years. These considerations must be contemplated carefully. The consequences of miscalculations in these decisions may be a child poorly accommodated in an ill-fitting device that does not meet the current needs or that will meet the needs for only a short time. In such instances, the therapist must then explore difficult alternatives, such as borrowing or adapting old equipment, until the patient is eligible for new equipment. The growth potential of various pieces of equipment is discussed later in this chapter. Clearly, in addition to a child's current age and developmental level, growth and developmental change are critical aspects to consider when selecting adaptive equipment.

Equipment Use Compared with Facilitation of Function

The use of equipment instead of facilitating the development of independent skills is a concern when recommending adaptive equipment. As already discussed, positioning devices may not allow for balanced development because of their static nature. Unfortunately, some therapists and parents have the idea that, with so many equipment options, equipment is equivalent to therapy. The child is thus "plugged" into many types of equipment throughout the day, moving from high chair to car seat to side-lyer to stander. With the child nearly continuously in containers, the equipment becomes a substitute for handling or positioning of the child by the parent or physical therapist. This occurrence can be a detriment to parent–child relationships as well as a barrier to continued skill acquisition by the child. Equipment is not a substitute for treatment. Equipment may restrict the learning of active postural transitions and movement for exploration, two major aspects of normal motor development. In some cases, a child who uses no adaptive equipment may fare better through verbal instructions, feedback, and handling than the child who is extensively equipped. This suggestion does not advocate denial of needed equipment to maximize therapeutic input and function; rather, it recognizes that, just as appropriate equipment can be useful for satisfying the overall needs of a child, overuse or misuse of equipment can be detrimental.

Safety Issues

Ensuring the safe and correct use of the equipment is a top priority. Caregivers and the child, when age appropriate, must be taught the correct methods of donning, doffing, and using equipment. Strategies such as color coding and numbering straps, to make sure they are fastened to the proper endpoint in the proper sequence, help avoid mistakes in donning the device. This is particularly helpful when caregivers include a number of people in addition to the parents, such as grandparents, babysitters, day care staff, teachers, and teachers' aides.

Another safety issue relates specifically to mobility equipment. Equipment that gives a non-locomotive child the ability to locomote requires attention to the environment in which the equipment is used as well as attention to the child's cognitive and judgment abilities. If the equipment makes it possible for the child to maneuver in a previously unusable area of the home, is the area adequately childproofed? When using a motorized wheelchair instead of a manual wheelchair, does the child exhibit sufficient judgment to use the motorized chair safely within his environment, in terms of both his own safety and the safety of others?

All adaptive equipment used with children should be inspected frequently to ensure the integrity of the equipment for continued, safe utilization. Needed repairs should be addressed with preemptive action to avoid the likelihood of sudden breakage or equipment breakdown that could cause injury or abrupt loss of function.

To further avoid unsafe circumstances and injury, equipment should always be used for the intended purpose and in the intended manner for which it was manufactured. Although some guidelines for safe usage of equipment may seem to the novice therapist to be matters of common sense and common knowledge, it is the responsibility of the therapist not to make this assumption. Rather, precautions and safe usage are critical aspects of instructing the family, the child, when age-appropriate, and other caregivers and supervising adults in correct and safe use of assistive technology.

When having equipment custom-made, the inclusion of appropriate safety components is imperative. Whether the equipment is custom-made or commercially available, specific safety features of the equipment, such as seat belts, locks, and brakes, should always be employed during equipment use and should not be disabled or disconnected.

Psychosocial Issues

Carefully selected and fitted adaptive equipment can offer many opportunities and increase a child's independence, but equipment can also be psychosocially disadvantageous. Equipment, especially extensive equipment, often has a way of drawing attention to a child's disabilities and therefore the child's differences. Children tend to be honest, sometimes brutally so. Adaptive equipment, or anything else that separates a child from peers, can be emotionally and socially challenging for the child with a disability.

In addition to socially and psychologically separating a child from others, adaptive equipment can physically separate a child. A child strapped into plastic, vinyl, wood, and metal often seems to be the recipient of fewer hugs and physical affection. This may be simply because of the physical barriers caused by the equipment, but it may also be the result of adults and children who feel intimidated by the equipment and are fearful of disturbing something if they get too close to the child.

On the positive side, equipment that increases a child's mobility and functional independence such as power mobility and integrated wheelchair standers[12] has been shown to lead to better success with all types of mobility and to enhance a child's cognitive, perceptual motor, and psychosocial development.[11–13,17,18]

▶ Determining a child's equipment needs

The primary therapist who provides routine, continuing care for a child should have established continually evolving short- and long-term goals for the child. Eventually, it may become clear to the therapist that adaptive equipment is needed to achieve some functional goals. Sometimes, because of the size or nature of the facility at which the child is treated or because the physical therapist lacks experience working with and recommending equipment, a referral to an outside agency, clinic, or therapist may be helpful to determine needs and equipment to meet those needs. Whether the child is referred to a children's hospital, a wheelchair clinic in a medical center, or directly to an equipment vendor's establishment, the provision of appropriate apparatus depends mainly on detailed and accurate information about both the child and the child's environment.[19] If possible, the primary therapist should be present during the evaluation for equipment to give an accurate assessment of the child's needs. In lieu of the physical therapist's presence, a detailed report with an assessment of the child's needs and recommendations for equipment should be included in the referral.

An initial assessment of the child may include a thorough mat assessment, a movement assessment, an interview of the child (when developmentally appropriate) and parents, an environmental review, and an assessment of the child in relation to a specific piece of equipment.[19] Because of time restrictions, the assessment may concentrate on one specific type of equipment or functional need (e.g., sitting), and additional assessments may be required for other equipment needs. Once the proper equipment has been ordered and received, the primary therapist should examine the child with the equipment to ensure that the apparatus suits the child, and that it meets the identified goals. Also the child, if developmentally able, and the caregivers helping the child use the equipment must be instructed in its correct use.

Evaluation and Assessment of the Child

The parameters to be considered when evaluating a child's need for adaptive equipment are similar to those of most other evaluations. The goal of such an evaluation, however, is to direct the therapist to the most appropriate equipment options available. A number of assistive technology assessment tools (AT) have been developed.[15,20–25] Depending on the AT, the child, family, home, school, and other natural environments are assessed, along with the child's current medical status and medical history. Many of these AT are available on the internet. A therapist may want to consult some of the existing tools and use them in part or totality as guidelines. Although every child is unique, using an AT can strengthen the clinical decision-making process. The following specific items summarize what should be considered in the evaluation and assessment of the child.

Range of Motion

Range of motion (ROM) is important in selecting most equipment because accommodation of the patient in most apparatus will depend on adequate ROM and joint mobility. The device being considered will dictate the motions and ranges necessary for success.

Critical ranges of motion to be addressed when using various adaptive devices include adequate head and neck rotation to bring head to midline, trunk rotation to achieve trunk symmetry, a minimum of 90 degrees hip and knee flexion for functional sitting, and plantigrade feet (neutral dorsiflexion/plantarflexion) for standing and for using footrests or the floor when sitting. If the child has knee or hip flexion contractures, care must be taken to ensure that a particular device will accommodate the contracture while still preserving good functional alignment. For example, a prone, supine, or vertical stander (covered later in this chapter) will not facilitate adequate weight-bearing alignment if a contracture(s) is too extreme. In some cases, surgical correction of hip and knee flexion contractures may need to be considered before ordering a stander for long-term use.

Muscle Tone, Motor Control, and Strength

Muscle tone, control, and strength deserve careful consideration when selecting equipment. The degree of strength and motor control needed for functional use of the device must be determined. For example, use of a manually controlled wheelchair requires strength, motor control, and coordination of the upper extremities. If the child does not have adequate upper extremity function, or if the child is functioning asymmetrically, a standard manually controlled wheelchair is an inappropriate choice for independent function. A motorized device that does not require the strength and motor control needed for a manually controlled chair may be more useful for the child. A motorized chair also has options for control that do not require any upper extremity function. A specific, detailed assessment by an experienced technician can help the therapist identify alternative methods for optimal management of the equipment. In choosing a motorized device, the strength and motor control of the upper extremities or alternative body parts to control the device are only two considerations. One must also evaluate cognitive, sensorimotor, and coping abilities, as discussed later in this chapter.

A child's muscle tone is a particularly important factor in equipment decisions for children with sensorimotor impairments such as children with a diagnosis of cerebral palsy. Positioning devices such as standers, side-lyers, and adaptive seats and chairs often have a modifying effect on muscle tone in these children. For example, the child's orientation to gravity may have a significant bearing on muscle tone when the child tries to assume an upright position. This influence may indicate that a prone stander is a better choice than a vertical stander or supine stander for that particular child. The therapist must assess patterns of movement with regard to decreased or increased muscle tone, tone dominance, and dyskinesias (uncontrolled, involuntary, extraneous movements). Does the child exhibit hypotonus or hypertonus and to what degree? Are the dyskinesias of mild, moderate, or severe magnitude? Does the patient have cortical control, manifested by a voluntary ability to initiate a pattern of movement? Does the child's body exhibit attempts to compensate, whether volitional or not, for uncomfortable positioning and/or movement?

Examples of the effects of tone on the appropriateness of a piece of equipment for a particular child follow. A child positioned in a prone stander with too much forward tilt from the vertical position may show increased abnormal extensor tone in a compensatory attempt to achieve a more upright position against the force of gravity. In contrast, another child in a prone stander may demonstrate increased flexor tone, influenced by a tonic labyrinthine reflex in the prone position. In a child with extensor hypertonia, increased scapular retraction and hyperextension of the neck may occur secondary to positioning the child in supine, reclined sitting, or in a supine stander. These patterns will interfere with optimal upper extremity function. Another child with extensor hypertonus may attempt to counteract the body's pull into extreme extension when sitting, by protracting the shoulder girdle, posteriorly tilting the pelvis, and holding the head forward. Any position the child exhibits must be assessed for the contributing causes, including compensations.

Reflexes

A change of position with respect to gravity will also affect a child whose motor patterns are influenced by developmental reflexes. The prone or supine position may increase or decrease the impact of the tonic labyrinthine reflex on the child's posture or movement. Side-lying may facilitate the asymmetric tonic lumbar reflex. Because inadvertent facilitation of primitive or pathologic reactions may create a block in the normal developmental pattern, each piece of equipment should be evaluated for its effect on reflexes. For example, some devices for mobility, such as tricycles and bicycles, may aggravate a persistent asymmetric tonic neck reflex. As the child pushes the pedal with the right foot, the head is turned toward the right side to enhance the effectiveness of the push. The child reverses this pattern when pushing with the left foot. Only in unusual circumstances would a therapist choose to use a technique that encourages using obligatory primitive reflexes. The use of devices to restrict or inhibit the influence of primitive reflexes is more common, thus providing an opportunity for the development of more normal and symmetric patterns of movement.

Sensation

Children with myelomeningocele, or other pathologies with compromised sensation, offer tremendous challenges to the therapist attempting to develop a program involving the use of adaptive equipment. Priorities for the child with myelomeningocele include providing safe, pressure-tolerant seating and upright positioning. The therapist must have a thorough knowledge of the patient's sensation to achieve these goals. The patient and family should be consulted with regard to sensation, as they usually have a keen awareness of the sensory loss, as well as potential danger zones. This situation is especially true for the older child. Particular attention must be paid to the skin over the spinal cord lesion and to bony prominences, including the ischial tuberosities, greater trochanters, sacrum, femoral and tibial condyles, tibial tuberosities, fibular heads, and malleoli. These bony prominences must also be monitored in a child with intact sensation but limited ability to reposition because of poor motor control, weakness, or severe spasticity.

Cognitive, Sensorimotor, and Social/Emotional Skills

Many physical therapists are not trained specifically to assess cognition, some sensorimotor skills, or social/emotional development; as a result, these areas are often ignored. This is a serious omission with the pediatric patient, whose prognosis for function with adaptive equipment often depends less on physical abilities and more on cognitive function, psychosocial skills, and sensorimotor abilities, including perception, motor planning, and reaction time. Neurosensory development and stimulation are integral to the development of motor skills as well as cognitive skills in the typically developing infant.[26] Although IQ is not considered to be a good determinant of ability to use power mobility, for example, other cognitive skills are key, including judgment, problem-solving abilities, and the ability to understand cause and effect, direction, and spatial relationships.[13,17] Motivation, intelligence, and normal perception often overcome even severe physical impairments. The opposite is also true. Limitations in cognition, perception, or social/emotional skills may result in function that is lower than would be predicted by physical findings alone. To develop realistic goals for a child, the physical therapist must know the whole child and must integrate information obtained from the teacher, social worker, occupational therapist, and psychologist into the therapeutic plan.

Functional Skills

Assessing functional skills requires integration of all available information, in an attempt to determine why a child behaves in a certain manner. The physical therapist must discover what functions the child is able to perform and how, what functions he or she is unable to perform and why, and why the child does not do more. For example, some children tend to bunny hop rather than creep. It is important to know if this tendency to bunny hop is merely a developed habit without any physical foundation or is secondary to a strong symmetric tonic neck reflex, muscle weakness in the extensors of the hips and/or knees, or both. Determining appropriate physical therapy interventions is based on this type of analysis and understanding.

A similar thought process should be used when deciding whether or not the child needs equipment. For example, if a 2-year-old child is not rolling or exploring the environment, is a device aimed at the goal of assisted mobility an appropriate acquisition? The therapist must first assess why the child does not move and explore. Does the child have a cognitive disability that limits the natural curiosity to explore the environment? Is the child afraid of moving because of visual, hearing, or other sensory impairments? Does the child exhibit a strong asymmetric tonic neck reflex that acts as a physical limitation to rolling? Is abnormal muscle tone in certain body segments a barrier to movement? Has the child been placed in devices at home that limit the opportunity to develop independent mobility? Once a determination has been made as to why a child has delayed motor skills and decreased mobility, realistic recommendations for equipment can be offered. Only when working with a child who is severely limited in his or her mobility, without reasonable short- or long-term expectations of gaining device-unaided mobility, would it be appropriate to opt immediately for adaptive equipment for remediation of the problem(s).

The child with profound cognitive deficits may not use equipment that is provided because he or she lacks the motivation to explore his or her environment. For the child with visual or hearing impairments to learn to manipulate his or her environment, methods for exploration of that environment need to be improved by first addressing the specific sensory impairment. If a child lacks experience in exploring the environment owing to lack of opportunity, the therapist must offer as much freedom of movement and equipment-free mobility as is possible and educate the family about the importance of providing the child with opportunities to move. Although equipment may eventually play a role in each of these situations, adaptive equipment should not be the first type of treatment used. Adaptive equipment should supplement and complement function with the least amount of restriction of the child.

The child who is physically limited may show great improvement in cognitive ability, social interaction, and independence when mobility is improved.[11–13] When adaptive equipment or devices are used judiciously, the improvement in mobility should occur without increases in abnormal reflexes or patterns of movement in children with sensorimotor impairments.

Evaluation of a child's ROM, muscle tone, motor control, strength, reflexes, sensation, perception, cognition, social/emotional skills, and function abilities is an integral component of the assessment of the child. Only when these parameters are considered and it is understood why a child has particular motor behaviors, can goals and appropriate intervention strategies be planned for the child, including recommending appropriate adaptive equipment.

Assessment of the Family, Home, and School

After the child has been assessed, goals have been established, and appropriate equipment has been identified, at least in theory, the therapist should evaluate the family, home, and school environments. The home environment, opportunities in the home, and parental expectations have been shown to influence the development of a child, including motor development.[27-30] It stands to reason that the development of a child with disabilities is also influenced by these factors. Moreover, acquiring, learning to use, and following-through with adaptive equipment for a child will be highly influenced by the child's home and other natural environments and the family. Overall physical therapy goals for the child using adaptive equipment must be compatible with the goals of the caregivers at home and school. This is essential for enabling a child to participate well in both domains.[2] Because adaptive equipment is often used not only in both home and school settings but in several other settings as well, problems sometimes arise from conflicting needs and disparities in caregiver thinking in the differing environments. These conflicts over adaptive aids may arise in particular for the child who is institutionalized because the collaboration of several different caregivers on a rotating staff is needed.

Useful information can be obtained by asking the family members about their expectations for the apparatus being considered. This opportunity for family members to express their opinions promotes a dialogue between family and therapist, allowing the therapist to determine whether the family goals are realistic or if compromises are necessary. Objective data about the family and home include the following categories and questions:

1. *Physical layout of the home*
   - Is the dwelling a house or an apartment?
   - How many steps are found in the home?
   - Is there easy access to the home from the outdoors (i.e., no stairs, availability of an elevator, etc.)?
   - How large are the rooms?
   - Are the structure and size of the home adequate for equipment to be used in the home, particularly mobility equipment?
   - Is there space for equipment use and storage?
   - How wide are the doorways and hallways?
   - Are the floors carpeted?
   - Are bathrooms, tubs, and toilets accessible?

2. *Community factors.* The therapist should determine whether the family lives in an urban, suburban, or rural community to assess the availability of and options for transportation and socialization within the community. The availability of privately owned vehicles and/or public transportation is important when the therapist is considering the type of mobility equipment to be purchased. Issues such as the weight of mobility equipment, its versatility on various surfaces, and its ease of transport are important considerations.

3. *Socioeconomic factors.* The cost of equipment may have a serious impact on the final decision regarding adaptive equipment for the child with a disability. When making a decision about buying adaptive equipment, the therapist, often in conjunction with a social worker, must examine insurance coverage, other third-party payment systems, funding agencies within the community, and potential rental options. Before equipment is ever ordered, it is essential that the availability and source of funding is determined. Size of the family, daily routine, and the time available to spend with the child with special needs, as well as potential options for others to help the family, must be considered. Compliance with the suggested use of adaptive equipment may ultimately be the main issue to be considered in the decision to obtain the equipment. If there is little realistic expectation that the child will benefit from having the equipment or that the equipment will be used by the family, there may be little justification for its purchase.

4. *Other cultural factors.* In addition to socioeconomic factors, other cultural factors must be considered and respected.[31] Increasingly, physical therapists and other health care professionals find themselves working with patients and clients with cultures different from their own. It is imperative that physical therapists become not only culturally sensitive but also culturally competent. Some cultural issues that need to be addressed when obtaining equipment for children include the following:

   - Who makes the decisions in the family?
   - Are there cultural sensitivities regarding receiving financial aid to purchase equipment?
   - Does the equipment being considered violate any religious beliefs of the family?
   - If there are language barriers, do the family and child understand the need for the equipment and the process for acquiring the equipment?
   - Will language differences interfere with teaching the family and the child proper use of the equipment, and can these problems be overcome?
   - Is the home structure amenable to safe and easy use of the equipment being considered?
   - Are there cultural beliefs that preclude the use of certain equipment? For example, in some cultures, an infant is never placed on the floor.[32-35] Therefore, a positioning device used on the floor may be

unacceptable to the family. Another example is that technology such as electricity or computers is not used in some cultures. These beliefs may affect the use of power wheelchairs, home-suctioning equipment, and some communications aids.[36,37]

All of these questions obviously apply to obtaining equipment for any child. However, they are worth special mention in regard to a child whose culture differs considerably from the dominant culture of the community. It is the therapist's responsibility to learn enough about a child's culture to effectively and competently provide interventions, including recommendations of adaptive equipment.

When assessing a child's need for equipment, the physical therapist must consider the school setting in which the child may spend a large portion of the day. It is important to determine whether the child is enrolled in a special school for children with disabilities or mainstreamed into a regular school and/or classroom. In a special school, teachers and staff are usually very open to suggestions and are well equipped to handle any devices being considered. It is often these teachers who initiate the purchase or procurement of the equipment and they are eager to learn and work with the child.

Whether in a special school or regular community school, a child and family may encounter some barriers to acquiring and using adaptive equipment. If the therapist is able to anticipate some of these potential issues, conflict between the family and the school staff may be avoided, and the process will proceed more smoothly and more likely to the satisfaction of all involved. Of course, the primary goal is to address the child's needs sufficiently and to optimize the child's functional performance in all of his environments.

A 2004 review of the literature by Copley and Ziviani described some of the foreseeable sticking points regarding the use of assistive technology in school environments, including the following[8]:

1. Failure to do a multidisciplinary assessment; failure to do an assessment in the child's natural environment; or failure to reassess the child and the equipment over time
2. Failure to include the child and family in the decision-making process and the choice of equipment
3. Lack of adequate planning for use of adaptive equipment in the child's school environment, including lack of realistic goals, failure to include the specific equipment in the Individualized Educational Plan (IEP), or failure to specifically define the link between adaptive equipment and achievement of educational goals
4. Inadequate education of school staff about the equipment, the needs of the child, or the specific goals for using the equipment
5. High cost of adaptive equipment; high cost of maintaining equipment, including repairs, updating technology, replacement, and changes necessitated by the child's growth
6. Lack of funding and funding sources

7. Length of time to receive equipment once it is ordered and lengthy repair time, both of which may leave child without needed equipment
8. Lack of timely onsite support for troubleshooting equipment problems
9. General time constraints, including time to train staff, time to learn how to use the equipment, time to obtain the equipment, and time troubleshooting
10. Insufficient formal training and educational experiences about adaptive equipment for physical and occupational therapists
11. Teacher resistance to and/or rejection of adaptive technology, particularly high-tech devices for communication
12. Incompatibility of hardware and software; lack of available software to more directly meet a child's specific needs
13. Device-specific problems, including lack of portability, slow operation, or space requirements for storage
14. Storage of equipment so that it is difficult to access
15. Sharing equipment among children so device is not readily available for a given child

Suggestions for overcoming many of these barriers are also reported by Copley and Ziviani. Readers are encouraged to consult this excellent review, although it is somewhat dated, and other more recent literature for practical ways to prevent and address these common problems.[8]

When the child is mainstreamed into a regular school, teachers and staff may be reluctant to accept adaptive equipment because of their limited experience with special apparatus. This reluctance may be related to the health and developmental needs of the child, but also to concerns about time, space, liability, and acceptability of these devices in a classroom of mostly nondisabled children. A thoughtful compromise is often necessary to meet the physical, educational, emotional, and social needs of the child with a disability.

The Individual with Disabilities Education Improvement Act (IDEA, 2004), Part B, provides for assistive technology and assistive technology services deemed necessary for a child to access an education. The IEP should include the specific device and its features, the educational goals for use of the device, and the specific assistive technology services needed for a child to achieve the goals of the IEP, as well as definitive outcome criteria to measure the child's progress. Any equipment that is included in the IEP must be paid for by the school, unless parents choose to purchase the device.[6,38] The IDEA laws are more completely presented in Chapter 21.

Examples of equipment that might be recommended for use in the classroom to address physical impairments and disabilities include the following:

1. Special chairs, seating devices, or adaptations to the regular desk chair
2. Wheelchair lapboards
3. Wheelchair or desk easels

4. Standing frames, standing tables, and prone standers
5. Integrated wheelchair standing devices
6. Wedges for seating in chairs
7. Wedges or bolsters for positioning on the floor when same-age cohorts are on the floor, such as in a reading circle

The physical therapist can be a valuable resource person for teachers and other staff by making suggestions and helping procure equipment that can enhance a child's educational experience. Often, a piece of adaptive equipment can make the difference between a child feeling fully included in, rather than excluded from, classroom work and activities.[12]

 Equipment selection

When the child's evaluation is completed and goals are established, the types of equipment available, or alternatively, the practicality of making equipment, are determined. Equipment can be purchased, rented, borrowed, or in some cases, where only simple adaptations are needed, fabricated by the child's family or others who have the skill and are familiar with the child.

Purchasing Equipment

Many companies make devices and equipment that are identical in concept. Criteria that must be considered in choosing a specific device include the following:

1. *Dimensions of the apparatus.* The device should not only be adequate when purchased, but should also, if feasible, allow for some future growth of the child. Some pieces of equipment have a built-in system for extending or enlarging the device. The therapist must determine which company makes the particular size best suited for a given child.
2. *Availability of optional adaptations.* Are there parts that help improve the fit and specificity of the device? Are these options cost-effective, easily adjusted, and durable?
3. *Reputation of the manufacturer.* Is the product covered by a guarantee? Has the company previously provided support when problems with equipment have arisen? Is service readily available, and is equipment for trial use available? Will a company representative instruct the therapist and other appropriate staff in optimal use of the device?
4. *Promptness of delivery.* Is the product kept in stock by most local vendors or medical supply houses? Is there a backlog of orders that will delay the equipment's delivery? Is the product custom-made?
5. *Cost.* Is the price reasonable or will less-expensive alternatives provide the same benefits?
6. *Aesthetics.* Is the device cosmetically acceptable to the child and family or might it be rejected on this basis?
7. *Weight, size, and manageability.* Is the device easy to use, and can it be stored? Can it be transported if necessary? Does it fold or disassemble in some way that makes storage and transport easier?

Brochures or catalogs available from the manufacturer or vendor will provide much of this information. Most vendors of adaptive equipment also have websites with continually updated descriptions of equipment and information about new equipment and pricing. Local vendors with extensive experience with the equipment can help in answering many questions. Physical therapists in local hospitals or in the community can recommend vendors or specific salespeople. The therapist should not feel obligated to order from any vendor or person in particular. Although one salesperson might be knowledgeable about wheelchairs, another person may have more experience with positioning devices or ADL equipment.

Paying for Equipment

The cost of adaptive equipment and other aids for accomplishing ADLs can be an obstacle to a child's achievement of maximum functional potential. Limited living space and storage in most homes underscores the obvious impracticality of a child getting every promising piece of equipment available. Also, some assistive devices may have a limited period of usefulness for a particular child owing to growth or the child's making progress or, in some cases, regressing. However, the greatest limiter to acquiring adaptive equipment in most cases is probably the cost.[39]

Funds available to pay for health care for children, with or without special needs, as well as eligibility requirements to access those funds, vary greatly among the states. Likewise, the ability of a family to get health care or purchase equipment for a child may depend on whether they have private or public insurance. It is known that raising children with special needs and complex medical conditions requiring lifetime medical care is more costly than raising children without chronic pathologies, impairments, or disabilities.[40,41] However, according to 2005–2006 data, the high costs of raising children with special health care needs are mitigated if the family has a primary care medical home, which has a strong care coordination component. Families with this type of service coordination were significantly less likely to incur out-of-pocket expenses with either private or public insurance, and out-of-pocket expenses incurred tended to be 32% and 15% less, respectively, compared with families that did not have a medical home type of care coordination.[40] Mitchell and Gaskin studied access to health care for children with special needs who receive Medicaid, comparing fee-for-service plans with the managed care option. Children in managed care programs had fewer unmet health care needs and were more likely to have consistent care by a primary care physician than the fee-for-service cohort.[42]

When one considers lifetime health care costs for families of children with special needs, it is easy to see how adaptive equipment, some very costly, can be difficult to obtain, maintain, and replace with growth and change in the child. Many children with congenital pathologies and impairments require new equipment frequently, over many years in a lifetime, in the presence of other exorbitant and rising medical expenses.

The physical and occupational therapist should work in concert with the child and family, the physician and other health care professionals, the medical home care coordinator (often his primary physician), an assistive technology professional (ATP), and teachers. The process of equipment procurement must include prioritizing equipment needs, and sometimes opting for a less-expensive or less complex device, or even sacrificing some adaptations to enable the family to acquire another device to meet a second functional need.

While renting, borrowing, trading, and fabricating some equipment may be options, in some cases purchasing equipment is the best or only option. How does a family pay for equipment? What resources are available to help parents pay for adaptive equipment?

A number of resources are available to pay for adaptive equipment but will vary depending on certain conditions and qualifications. Briefly, the following resources will purchase or help a family purchase equipment for children, some through the age of 21 years[38,43–46]:

1. Private medical insurance[44]
   - If the equipment is medically necessary
   - If prescribed by a physician
   - If the family's policy covers adaptive equipment
   - Depends on policy; some limit number of devices in a lifetime or limit frequency of replacement
2. IDEA[44]
   - Under Part B of IDEA, equipment in the child's IEP is paid for by the school district
   - Under Part C, district pays for the equipment if it is in the IFSP (Individual Family Service Plan)
   - Part C will not pay if other private or public resources are available
   - If state or federal law says parents have to contribute something in the Early Childhood Program, perhaps on a sliding fee basis, parents may pay part; however, the child cannot be denied the equipment or service if parents are unable to pay
3. Medicaid (Title XIX)[44,3]
   - For families with low income; Medicaid eligibility requirements are determined by each state; age of eligible children varies by state
   - Financial eligibility is typically based on some percentage of the federal poverty level
   - Jointly funded by the state and federal government; coverage varies by state[44]
   - A state *must* fund according to minimal federal standards, but *may* elect to fund more than the minimum
   - Equipment *must* be medically necessary

   - Federal contribution will pay for assistive technology; depending on the state, state *may* pay for durable medical equipment (DME)
   - Prior Approval (PA) for services *may* be required by the state[47]
4. Early and Periodic Screening, Diagnosis and Treatment (EPSDT) program[44]
   - Included in all state Medicaid programs, required by federal government
   - Requires states to provide for children 0 through 21 years of age
   - Physical therapy and DME services not included in the standard state Medicaid plan *may be* reviewed for Medicaid coverage under EPSDT policy[47]
   - Family must meet state's financial eligibility requirement for Medicaid
   - Covers assistive technology, but is an often overlooked resource
5. Katie Beckett Waiver/TEFRA state plan option (Tax Equity and Fiscal Responsibility Act)[47]
   - Waiver program for medical assistance for children who do not qualify for Medicaid because of parents' income
   - Waiver was enacted to support home and community care instead of institutionalization for children who need long-term, institutional-level care
   - For eligibility, only the child's income is considered
   - Policies vary among states; not available in all states★
6. Children's Health Insurance Program (CHIP) [formerly SCHIP][46]
   - Provides health coverage to children in families with incomes too high to qualify for Medicaid, but can't afford private coverage
   - Jointly funded by federal and state governments, with matching federal funds to states to provide this coverage
   - Administered by the states
7. State Assistive Technology (AT) Loan Programs
   - Loan program available in many states, via Assistive Technology Act of 2004.
   - Low interest loans and long repayment schedules
8. National AT Reuse Center[44,48,49]
   - Centers nationwide that sell safe recycled equipment
9. Community Philanthropic and Service Organizations and Clubs and National Organizations
   - Local community service organizations such as the Lions, Masons, Shriners Hospital for Children, Kiwanis Clubs, Civitan, Rotary Clubs, Knights of Columbus, and local churches, synagogues, and mosques[43,44]
   - National organizations such as Easter Seal Society, Muscular Dystrophy Association, United Way, United Cerebral Palsy Association, Juvenile Arthritis Association, and March of Dimes
10. State Assistive Technology Projects[44,50]

★At this writing, less than half of the states have TEFRA or Katie Beckett Waiver for children.[45]

The Section on Pediatrics of the American Physical Therapy Association (APTA) publishes a fact sheet that lists numerous sources that can provide a therapist with additional information about funding for adaptive equipment.[43]

Many funding sources, especially private insurances, require a physician's prescription if they pay for assistive technology.[44,51] Regardless of requirement for prescription, having one at the beginning of the process usually helps ensure a smoother process and improves the likelihood of securing funding. Sometimes in educational settings, a child's care becomes fragmented because of disagreement among health care professionals about the role of the child's physician in recommending or prescribing rehabilitation therapies and DME. This is particularly true in states that allow physical therapists to practice without referral. However, in the best interests of the child, it is imperative that all who are involved in the child's health care and education work together to optimize the child's potential. Collaboration between the child's therapists and physicians, including having a physician-written prescription for adaptive equipment, can improve coordination of care, avoid duplication of services and conflicting recommendations, and prevent unnecessary expenses.[51]

In addition to a prescription, a letter of medical necessity is often required when ordering adaptive equipment. The letter of medical necessity must be written by the certified or licensed professional who performed the assessment on the child (physician, PT, or OT). Once again, a shared effort is probably most helpful.[51] If the letter was not written by the child's physician, a prescription from the physician should accompany the letter. If funding for equipment is denied, an appeal letter should be written. Examples of letters of medical necessity for assistive technology and appeal letters can be found on the internet.[52-54]

As a child ages there may be increased need for adaptive equipment, yet funding for this equipment may decrease, particularly at the postsecondary school level.[55,56] This decreased funding is due to several factors, including health insurance policies that deny or limit reimbursement for certain services (such as adaptive equipment), age limitations on government entitlement programs for children's health care, age limitations on dependent child coverage by health insurance policies, and changes in Medicaid eligibility as the child ages, as it relates to financial assets.[56] These practices not only limit the accessibility of adaptive equipment for many older children, but they frequently make a child's transition to adulthood more difficult. One initiative by the American Academy of Pediatrics (AAP) Committee on Child Health Financing is an attempt to remediate some of the assistive technology funding problems of the older child and the young adult. The AAP issued a policy statement advocating health care benefits for children through age 26. This policy recommends that all public and private health plans provide comprehensive benefits for children across the span of life from birth through 26 years of age, including "Rehabilitative and habilitative services and devices" and "Rental, purchase, maintenance, and service of DME."[57(p189)]

Issues surrounding the funding for adaptive equipment must continue to be a topic of conversation, study, and research for physical therapists and other professionals involved in the care of children with disabilities, particularly in light of changing health care policy. As suggested by advocates for the current model of a primary care medical home, children with long-term disability and complex medical problems deserve "appropriate educational and therapeutic strategies including: . . . adaptive and assistive technology."[58(p1111)]

Renting or Borrowing Equipment

Some types of equipment for short-term use can be rented. However, if particular customized features are needed in a device, the likelihood of finding the precise, appropriate apparatus is decreased. Often, concessions can be made regarding some equipment options, if renting the equipment proves to be highly cost-effective. Compromising correct fit and safety for the sake of cost-effectiveness should not be an option.

Some communities have what is commonly referred to as an equipment closet or equipment lending library. These closets, usually run by not-for-profit organizations or agencies, are repositories for used equipment in good repair that are no longer in use. This equipment is made available for other children and parents to borrow for the period of time needed, often until the child outgrows the equipment.

Also, in today's internet-connected world, it is not unusual, through social media, personal websites, or support groups, for parents to make contact with other parents who have adaptive equipment that is no longer being used. These parents with unused devices are often willing to sell or give away useful equipment or trade for another piece of equipment. However, the same exceptions and cautions mentioned regarding renting equipment also apply to borrowing or buying used equipment from equipment closets or other individuals.

Fabricating Equipment

An abundance of commercially available equipment today offers therapists, families, and children numerous options. Not only is there a wide variety of types of equipment that help a child function in multiple environments, but considerable competition exists among manufacturers and vendors regarding proprietary variations in similar types of equipment. Consequently, the need to make equipment instead of purchasing commercially available equipment has declined considerably. Nonetheless, fabricating instead of purchasing a simple piece of equipment is sometimes a practical choice, especially when limited financial resources may be better spent purchasing highly complex equipment.

The decision to make equipment is based on many variables that must be considered carefully, including who will build the equipment, the cost of building the device, who will pay for the equipment, and liability issues. Asking some carefully framed questions may help the therapist make a decision about whether or not to advocate homemade adaptive equipment.

1. Will the physical therapist be building the equipment, or be serving as a consultant to other builders? Other people who might build equipment for children include commercial woodworkers, woodworking hobbyists, volunteer organizations with appropriately skilled members, and the child's parents.

2. Is making the equipment cost-effective? Items that must be accounted for include tools, space needs, building materials, time for planning and designing, and time for measuring and building. In making a decision, the advantages of customized homemade equipment must be weighed against the expense of designing, planning, and building the apparatus. Will adapting a commercially available device be a better compromise?

3. Will parents pay out-of-pocket, or will insurance companies pay for the cost of homemade equipment?

4. Who will pay for potentially costly errors if the equipment is fitted incorrectly or is inappropriate when completed?

5. Who assumes liability for the correct and safe use and performance of equipment made by a therapist, hobbyist, or volunteer? This is an important consideration in today's society wherein manufacturers are liable for the safe use of their products. If a child is injured or otherwise harmed using noncommercial equipment, the person who made the equipment may be legally and financially responsible.

Materials commonly used for homemade equipment include wood, ABS Plastic, Ethefoam, PVC Pipe, and tri-wall (triple wall) cardboard. Tri-wall consists of triple-thickness corrugated cardboard that is lightweight, firm, and inexpensive. Tri-wall is fast and easy to use, although its use requires an electric saw, glue gun, and hand tools, such as a hammer, screwdriver, and utility knife. Although it is not waterproof, tri-wall can be treated with acrylic latex paint or fabric for sealing and preservation. Tri-wall is less durable than wood, which makes it most appropriate for temporary or trial pieces of equipment, or for children who are growing rapidly (Fig. 12.1). Like wood, tri-wall is a firm, solid medium and may require padding for comfort. Many therapists consider tri-wall useful for making customized chairs that must be measured precisely for the child. A bolster-type chair available commercially and a similar chair made from tri-wall are shown in Figures 12.2 and 12.3. Although selection of a design and measuring the child and the tri-wall are time-consuming chores, actual building with tri-wall is a fast process. Working with this material is noisy, messy, and potentially dangerous because of the tools. A separate

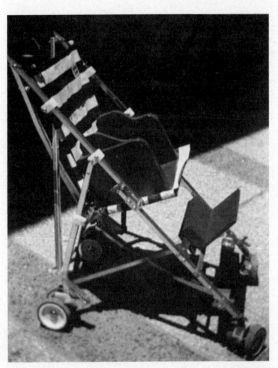

FIGURE 12.1 Umbrella-type stroller with a tri-wall insert and foot support.

workplace is recommended. As with wood, family members and volunteers can be recruited to make apparatuses from tri-wall. Special training is usually necessary, and many parents are reluctant to try because of fear of mistakes and failure. Some judicious support and praise for the family member can help overcome reluctance, and the parent

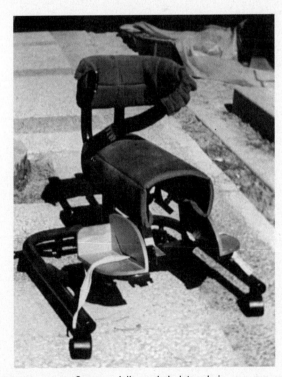

FIGURE 12.2 Commercially made bolster chair.

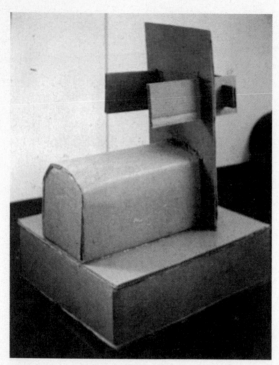

FIGURE 12.3 Tri-wall alternative to the commercially made bolster chair shown in Figure 12.2.

may become an essential part of the team that is making the adaptive equipment for the child. A seating insert made from tri-wall is shown in Figure 12.4.

In spite of the potential drawbacks, some therapists still choose to fabricate equipment themselves or have a parent do so. This may be particularly useful for the young child

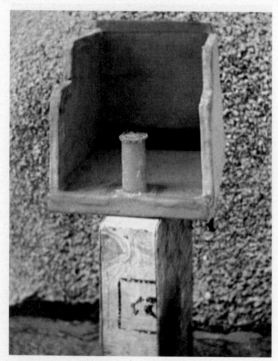

FIGURE 12.4 Tri-wall seat insert.

who is growing rapidly or for the child whose need is only temporary. In each of these situations, a simply made piece of equipment could satisfy the short-term needs of the patient. The child could use the fabricated equipment until it is outgrown, at which time another piece could be made, or if growth has slowed, a commercially available piece could be substituted. One of the main reasons for building equipment in the past was that commercially available equipment often did not satisfy the needs of a child with unique problems. However, meeting the unique needs of people to enhance function has become the primary emphasis of professionals in the rehabilitation field, including those who design and manufacture adaptive equipment. This recent emphasis has resulted in a wider variety of and improvement in commercially available devices.

▶ Equipment for positioning

General uses for equipment as adjuncts to treatment have been presented, but benefits can also accrue with proper equipment and frequent changes in position. Among those benefits are temporary inhibition of pathologic tone and movement, temporary reduction of abnormal reflexes, reduction of asymmetries, improved circulation, improved bone health, improved upper extremity functioning, prevention of soft tissue contractures and decubiti, and improved communication, cognitive and personal–social development. Some of the issues involved in providing children with equipment to support various activities as well as the sitting, standing, and side-lying positions will now be addressed.

Sitting

General Considerations

The sitting position is optimal for upper extremity function and is therefore important for the child and the adult. Maintained sitting posture is a goal achieved by most typical infants before 1 year of age, and sitting is required for many functions throughout life.

By watching children in preschool and kindergarten, it is apparent that a goal of many teachers is sitting for a reasonable amount of time for group activities. Children in the early school years younger than 7 years of age also require frequent changes in position. They prefer to play and work in the prone position, standing by a table, and in other positions that allow for easy transitional movements and change. Sitting, as a position for optimal function, occurs only after the children learn to sit for prolonged periods of time. Sitting is defined as ". . . a position in which the weight of the trunk is transferred to the support area mainly by the ischial tuberosities and surrounding tissues."[59] Proper alignment in sitting is thought to enhance overall functioning by providing an adequate and secure base of support, inhibiting abnormal tone, providing a stable base from which the upper extremities can function, and improving perception of the environment. There are also significant social benefits to being upright in sitting and being able to move.

Although a body of literature is devoted to seating for children, much of the literature reports clinical experience and empirical data rather than controlled scientific studies. The result of this lack of scientific documentation is poor standardization when evaluating and providing adaptive seating devices. Conflicts regarding the value of various positioning options could be more easily and completely resolved if a scientific basis existed for each option. Because the literature on pediatric seating is limited, the adult literature has been examined and applied to the pediatric age group.

The first consideration when selecting a chair or other seating device is the intended purpose of the chair. Chairs can be function specific. A lounge chair is uncomfortable when a person is eating a meal, yet a straight-back chair with little padding is undesirable for relaxation. Similarly, a physical therapist must consider function when recommending chairs for children with special needs.

A child's sitting ability without devices helps define the basic purpose of a chair or wheelchair. A child who is a *hands-free sitter* needs a chair to provide a comfortable and stable base of support for functional activities. The purpose of a wheelchair for this child is to provide mobility in addition to the stability. A child who depends on his upper extremities for support so as to sit independently, a *hands-dependent sitter*, needs seating that effectively stabilizes, centers, and supports his pelvis and trunk so the child can use the arms and hands for functional skills rather than supporting sitting. A child unable to self-support at all for independent sitting is considered a *propped sitter* and needs more complex seating that will provide total body support.[5]

Many therapists believe customized seating is always preferable, especially a wheelchair. In lieu of a totally customized chair, the following parameters, established for adults and modified for children, should be considered, whether choosing a conventional chair, a commercially available adaptive seat, a custom-constructed chair, or a wheelchair.

Seat

HEIGHT The height of the chair seat should allow the feet to be placed flat on the floor or a foot rest. Height should be such that with feet flat, hips are flexed to at least 90 degrees. Slightly more hip flexion is even more desirable to prevent some children from going into extensor posturing. Comfortable placement of the feet should prevent excessive pressure from the front edge of the seat on the popliteal fossae.[59,60]

DEPTH The seat should be shallow enough to provide for flexion of the knees without pressure in the popliteal area and without slouching. Slouching occurs when the child goes into a posterior pelvic tilt to allow the knees to flex over the edge of a seat that is too deep. Slouching causes sacral sitting, as the child transfers weight to the chair seat through the sacrum rather than the ischial tuberosities. Also, normal sitting posture requires anterior pelvic tilt, whereas slouching caused by too much seat depth enhances a posterior tilt of the pelvis. The seat should be deep enough to allow maximal distribution of weight.[60] If the seat is too shallow, weight is borne over a smaller area of the body, thereby increasing pressure per square inch on the posterior thighs and increasing the risk of skin breakdown. Also, a seat that is too shallow decreases the hip flexion to less than 90 degrees because the distal aspects of the thighs are not supported by the seat. This increased extension at the hips may cause the child to slide out of a chair. In a child with extensor hypertonus, increased extension of the hips may also trigger increased extensor tone throughout the body. A good rule of thumb for determining seat depth for children is to have one finger width between the edge of the seat and the popliteal space. Keep in mind that as the child grows, the length of the femur will increase and the space between the edge of the seat and the popliteal fossae will naturally increase.

PADDING Padding helps to limit pressure on the 6-mm^2 surface of each ischial tuberosity that normally bears most of the weight in sitting, which allows for increased sitting tolerance.[61,62] However, surfaces that are too soft increase the difficulty with which postural changes are made during sitting, and this lack of postural change can lead to back strain and potential skin breakdown. Akerblom judged movement while sitting to be the most important requirement of a comfortable chair.[61] He designed a chair that allowed for various conditions (i.e., the trunk away from the back support, sitting with lumbar support, or reclining back with both lumbar and thoracic support). These options reduce muscle strain and increase tolerance.[61]

Backrest

Trunk musculature and spinal ligaments must be considered when sitting to avoid back discomfort. The anterior and posterior longitudinal ligaments of the trunk provide their best support with the back in neutral position. Increasing the normal lordosis may stretch the anterior longitudinal ligament, whereas exaggerated kyphosis will stretch the posterior longitudinal ligament and may cause posterior protrusion of degenerating intervertebral discs. These changes produce low back pain and may cause difficulty in achieving adequate thoracic and lumbar extension needed to rise from sitting. The chair backrest should accommodate adequate movement while in the chair, to help offset muscular fatigue and for pressure relief. However, the backrest should also provide adequate support of the trunk to prevent muscular fatigue. Support for the weight of the trunk reduces the muscular work of sitting. The height of the backrest must be appropriate for the individual child. The child who needs extensive head, neck, and trunk support needs a tall backrest that extends above the head. Such a child may also benefit from a reclining backrest, which can provide periodic relief for muscles to combat fatigue.[63] The height of the backrest need not extend above the shoulder in many clients. Freedom to change position and improved mobility are available when limiting the height of the backrest to shoulder level.[64] In fact, for patients with excellent trunk stability and balance, the top of a wheelchair backrest is often just below the inferior angles of the scapulae. This shorter backrest allows great mobility of the upper trunk, use of the upper extremities, and general freedom of movement while in a wheelchair. These shorter backrests are usually seen on wheelchairs used by very active young people and wheelchair athletes.[65] Other considerations for wheelchair seating will be discussed later in this chapter. Finally, support for the lumbar curve and allowance for the posterior protruding sacrum and buttocks need to be taken into account in effective seating.

Seat to Backrest angle

The angle formed between the seat and the backrest of a chair is arguably most comfortable between 95 and 110 degrees. However, this angle may cause the person to slide forward, particularly those with increased extensor tone in the hips and back musculature. Using a wedged cushion, with the greatest height in the front, may help counteract this problem. Bergan suggests that chairs will provide a child with the best sensory feedback when the child's spatial orientation is that of sitting with a slight inclination backward.[66] The word *dump* in wheelchair seating refers to the number of inches closer to the ground the back of the wheelchair seat is, compared with the front of the wheelchair seat, thereby providing a slightly backward spatial orientation as described by Bergan. Wheelchair dump for adults is usually 1 inch, but for children, a 2-inch dump is more appropriate. Dump can be accomplished or enhanced in any chair by using a wedged cushion as described above, or the dump can be built into the chair[63] by decreasing, to less than 90 degrees, the angle between the seat and the backrest.

Orthopedic and biomechanical needs of all children must be considered when planning seating. While most therapists use an empirical or trial-and-error approach in determining a good seating position for a particular child, most agree that a stable pelvis serves as the keystone for seating, especially for children with neurodevelopmental disorders. Once the pelvis is aligned properly, the trunk, head, and extremities have a more stable base. This often means that fewer assistive devices and wheelchair options are necessary for optimal function.

The specific approaches to, options for, and adaptations of seating are too numerous to review here and are constantly evolving. However, providing seated weight bearing on the ischial tuberosities, maintaining a slight lumbar lordosis, positioning the hips and knees in at least 90 degrees of flexion, and maintaining plantigrade feet are principles that are fairly consistently applied to seating most children with impairments and disabilities. Variations of these basic concepts may be applied, based on a child's diagnosis and his individual clinical presentation.

Armrests

Armrests should be positioned to bear approximately 50% of the weight of the child's arms. Armrests are also used to move from a sitting to a standing position and vice versa, to do transfers, and to do sitting push-ups for regular and frequent pressure relief for the buttocks. Armrests that are too low or too high decrease the mechanical advantage of the flexed elbow when the individual performs sitting push-ups and transfers.

Seating Considerations for Specific Diagnoses and Impairments

The criteria and limits described for seating are applicable to all types of seating systems and for all diagnoses and impairments. The emphasis may change with the diagnosis and impairments, but the concepts are constant.

Appropriate seating for the child with cerebral palsy and similar neuromuscular disorders must consider the effects of various seating or wheelchair components on muscle tone, abnormal reflex activity, and function. Increase in extensor tone in the lower extremities, with increased hip adduction and internal rotation, thought to accompany the sling effect of most standard wheelchair seats and backrests is a common problem associated with wheelchair seating of a child with cerebral palsy. A solid seat and solid backrest can reduce this sling effect.

Hip flexion slightly greater than 90 degrees is advocated by many physical therapists when seating the child with cerebral palsy. The increased hip flexion resulting from the increased dump of the seat tends to break up strong extensor patterns due to hypertonia. The reduction in extensor tone reduces the likelihood of a compensatory posterior pelvic tilt that may result in increased dorsal kyphosis, scapular protraction, and hyperextension of the neck. Avoiding these postures by good hip positioning facilitates more normal upper extremity function and flexor–extensor balance of the cervical muscles. This change may produce positive consequences for swallowing, breathing, and stability and motor control of the neck and trunk. Hip flexion greater than 90 degrees may also decrease the probability of the child's lower extremities thrusting into an extension pattern and keep the child from sliding out of the chair.

In addition to altering the hip angle, the chair itself may be tilted anteriorly or posteriorly, relative to the floor, as described previously, until the desired results of positioning are achieved. Issues of concern with these adjustments, whether through chair dump or tilt, include pelvic alignment for stability while sitting and the effects on tone of the various angles of the hip and of the seat itself. Nwaobi and colleagues, using electromyograms, found that orientation of the body and head in relation to gravity plays an important role in controlling extensor activity in children with extensor hypertonus.[67] Perception and hand function will also be altered as differing angles and positions are used. Therefore, an individualized approach examining the effects of each change in position is necessary to determine optimal seating arrangements for children.

Once it appears that the various angles of hips, seat, and chair have been established and pelvic stability has been achieved in the child with cerebral palsy, the therapist must consider the trunk, head and neck, and the lower extremities. Ninety degrees of knee flexion and good weight bearing on the feet should be encouraged to enhance stability. Too much weight bearing on the plantar surface can result in a primitive extensor thrust pattern in children with neuromotor impairments that will significantly reduce stability. Alignment of the trunk should encourage maximal symmetry, yet provide for movement and active postural adjustment. A headrest or support should be used only if needed to improve positioning or to protect the child when transported. The ultimate goal of the sitting position should be to align the child without restricting the movements and postural adjustments available to the child. Reassessment of the seating device is necessary when the patient's postural tone improves and new skills are acquired.

The seating concerns are different for children with progressive or nonprogressive weakness, paresis, or paralysis, as seen in muscular dystrophy, spinal muscular atrophy, myelomeningocele, or traumatic spinal cord injury. The height of armrests, type of footrests, dump, tilt, and recline are important factors for successful transfers, mechanically efficient wheelchair push-ups for pressure relief, sit-to-stand, and stand-to-sit. The ability to recline a chair or wheelchair is particularly helpful for children with extreme or progressive weakness because it is easier to achieve periodic rest in a recumbent position. This is true both for the relief of general fatigue as well as changing and sometimes limiting the gravitational influence on various muscles. Also, as strength declines in progressive disorders, muscle imbalance in the trunk may lead to an asymmetrical sitting posture, which can be alleviated by strategically placed pads for positioning, appropriate height armrests, and lapboards or tabletops to provide and encourage postural symmetry when seated. A child with myelomeningocele or traumatic spinal cord injury may benefit from seating cushions and the ability to perform pressure relief measures due to inherent sensory deficits.

There are potential negative effects of using seating devices across disability groups. These effects include reduced joint motion secondary to static positioning, disruption of skin integrity as a result of prolonged use of a seating device, limited ability to change position thus risking skin breakdown in a child with impaired sensation, and reduced independent functional mobility resulting from overuse of seating devices.

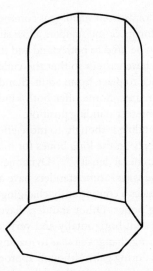

FIGURE 12.5 Corner chair. The angled sides aid in protraction of the shoulder girdle, inhibiting extensor hypertonia.

Seating Devices that Facilitate/Accommodate Specific Postures

Various specialized chairs are available commercially or can be constructed for particular seating problems. Chairs that incorporate the basic principles of seating as discussed in this chapter can have special adaptations that facilitate or accommodate a specific posture.

Two examples of specialized chairs that are available are the corner chair and the bolster chair. The corner chair (Fig. 12.5) is a chair that has lateral supports for the upper trunk. These supports position the child in shoulder girdle protraction, a strategy that tends to decrease extensor spasticity in children with tone problems such as cerebral palsy. Bolster chairs are chairs with a bolster-type seat (see Figs. 12.2 and 12.3). These chairs also aid in inhibiting excessive extensor tone in children with cerebral palsy by flexing and abducting the hips.

Many other specialized chairs and seating aids can be found by perusing equipment company catalogs and websites. Products are continually evolving, and often a commercial device is available to meet a child's specific seating needs.

Standing

The upright standing posture is the foundation for many functional activities in addition to bipedal locomotion. Standing and bearing weight on the lower extremities also can promote circulation, bone mineral density, respiratory endurance, gastrointestinal function, integumentary health, improved/maintained lower extremity ROM, modulation of spasticity, upper extremity function, vertical access (vertical reach), and social interaction with others.[12,68-70] For a child with limited options and opportunities for moving, appropriate adaptive equipment for standing provides another alternative for positioning throughout the day to help reduce or prevent skeletal deformities.[12]

Equipment for assisted standing is commercially available in a variety of forms. Some standers allow sit-to-stand movement, some can be used to both stand and to locomote, and some standers have casters so that the child can be moved easily from place to place by an adult. Standing devices can be static or dynamic. Some offer both kinds of loading in the erect or semierect standing position.

Dynamic standing is thought to more effectively increase the loading effects on the long bones for maintaining or increasing bone mineral density.[68–70] Dynamic standing can be achieved several ways. Some standers have a vibrating footplate that produces a continuously changing stimulus to the weight-bearing bones. Other standers have separate footplates that can shift horizontally and vertically to simulate the weight-bearing changes similar to loading and unloading the extremities during gait. Although appropriate body support is maintained, some standers allow body sway during standing, creating a dynamic weight-bearing environment. Mobile standers create a vibration type of dynamic input as the stander moves over various surfaces and thresholds.

Prone Standers

Prone standers are used frequently for children who require, but cannot achieve, the position of hands-free upright standing or its approximation. The child is placed in prone on the device. The trunk, buttocks, and lower extremities are all supported. The angle of the board is then increased toward a vertical position, depending on the child's tolerance and the therapist's goals. When the board is at its maximal angle, usually slightly less than 90 degrees to the floor, weight bearing is optimal through the lower extremities and feet. A knee-standing position can also be used. A prone stander is shown in Figure 12.6. The patient benefits from the physiologic changes associated with weight bearing, the freedom to use hands while upright, and the social and perceptual opportunities

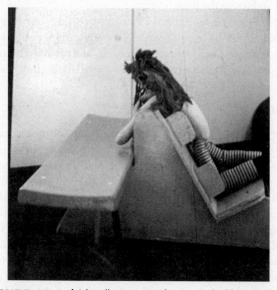

FIGURE 12.6 A tri-wall prone stander covered with enamel paint is used for kneeling.

afforded by an upright position. As the angle of the prone stander decreases to less than upright, the benefits of lower extremity weight bearing are diminished because more weight is borne increasingly by the anterior structures of the trunk.

In addition to providing weight bearing in the lower extremities, a prone stander can be used to facilitate upper extremity functional skills. A child can experience and practice upper extremity weight bearing functions if his prone stander is approximately 45 degrees or less above the horizontal to enable activities requiring upper extremity weight shifting, unilateral weight bearing, and reaching as well as bilateral upper extremity weight bearing. As the angle of tilt of the stander increases, his upper extremities are gradually freed for mobility functions, with completely hands-free standing available to the child in an upright position. Opportunities to experience hands-free standing are important for optimizing upper extremity use in socially appropriate contexts.

Use of a prone stander can also facilitate control and strength of the muscles of the neck and trunk. The demands on these muscles from body weight and gravitational forces will vary significantly with different angles of the stander. For example, as the patient approaches an upright position, the effort required of the cervical extensors for head righting will decrease. The therapist must assess the quality of movement shown by the child in the prone stander. The function of the head, neck, scapulae, and upper extremities should be included in this assessment, as should trunk alignment and positioning of the lower extremities. Hyperextension of the neck, exaggerated retraction of the scapulae with the upper extremities in the high-guard position, and poor symmetry and midline position of the trunk secondary to muscle imbalance are all common secondary postural problems when a child is placed in a prone stander.

The therapist must bear in mind the proper lower extremity alignment for weight bearing when considering the use of a prone stander for a particular child. Correct weight bearing for normal standing requires dynamic pressure through the heels, with the center of gravity passing slightly posterior to the ankle joint; this position is not feasible in a prone stander. Therefore, the use of the prone stander must be evaluated carefully. The prone stander is useful if the physiologic benefits of weight bearing are the major goal or if it is being used to accommodate hands-free standing. If the prone stander is considered for preambulation skills and conditioning, its use may be inappropriate and counterproductive.

When the prone stander is introduced into a child's program, the entire treatment regimen should be reevaluated. Although the child may appear to adapt well to the prone stander for 1 hour each day, its overuse may cause undesirable changes, particularly in children with hypertonicity. Increased abnormal extensor tone is an example of a change sometimes seen with prolonged use of a prone stander. The increased tone may affect the previously adequate positioning for sitting and may decrease function at home and school. This negative effect might require adjustments in the amount of time spent in the prone stander, or it may require a different approach to positioning in the stander or a different kind of stander.

Providing the opportunity for a child to interact with peers in play or school situations is an important benefit of using a prone stander. Being able to work at a table or play at an elevated sandbox with peers has important social and emotional benefits. Prone standers usually have casters so the child can be moved by an adult to different places for different activities while still standing. This is especially helpful in a classroom setting. A prone stander may be incorporated into a multi-position stander.

Supine Standers

A supine stander is an alternative to the prone stander and may better meet the needs of children with a goal of achieving an upright position. Similar to a standard tilt table, a supine stander allows weight bearing through the trunk and lower extremities, with the degree of weight bearing proportional to the angle of the supporting surface. The child is secured around the trunk, hips, and knees, with these areas as close to erect standing alignment as possible. With those criteria achieved, the supine stander is angled toward a 90-degree upright position. Unlike the prone stander, the supine stander does not provide for weight bearing for the upper extremities, and lower extremity weight bearing occurs through the heels rather than the forefeet. This makes the supine stander a better option when working toward weight-bearing alignment for ambulation. The supine stander also affords the child the numerous physiologic benefits of upright weight bearing provided by the prone stander and allows the child to perceive and interact with the environment from an upright posture. Variations of the supine stander are shown in Figures 12.7 and 12.8.

As with all adaptive devices, the supine stander must include a careful assessment of the child for compensations, some of which may be pathologic. Commonly noted deviations with use of a supine stander include thoracic kyphosis with forward protrusion of the head, hyperextension of the cervical spine, and asymmetry secondary to imbalanced muscle control. If tolerance for an upright position is limited and the child is reclined, increased evidence of asymmetric tonic neck reflex and the Moro reflex may be seen. These abnormal reflexes may occur in a supine or semi-reclined position for any child with poorly integrated developmental reflex activity, and the child will fix into gravity (progravity). Because normal development requires the acquisition of antigravity control, the increased reflex activity in a supine or semi-supine position may be counterproductive. Upper extremity function for the child in a supine stander usually requires a special table or easel, thus restricting the child's participation in group activities. The supine stander has become increasingly popular in recent years. As with other pieces of adaptive equipment, periodic evaluation is necessary to determine the long-term benefits and hazards associated with the supine stander with a given child. A supine stander may be incorporated into a multi-position stander.

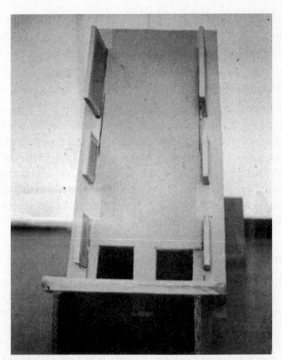

FIGURE 12.7 Supine stander made of tri-wall.

Standers with Sit-to-Stand Option

Children can be transferred from a wheelchair to a seated position in some standers, and the stander, equipped with power, can raise the child to a standing position. This

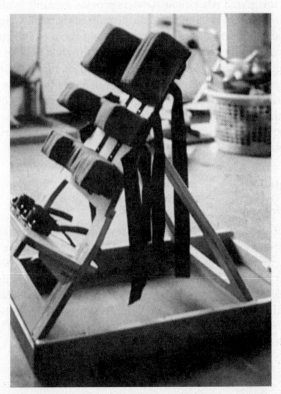

FIGURE 12.8 A Supine stander made of wood. It is padded for comfort and was designed and built entirely by parents.

device increases the ease of a child attaining a standing position, with or without assistance, and decreases the potential risks to the child during difficult transfers into a stander.

Standing Tables

Traditional standing tables are also available and although stationary, they may be all that is needed for a particular child's standing program. Standing tables have a built-in work surface and are therefore not compatible with use at other surfaces such as countertops, tables, or school chalkboards/dry erase boards. Another disadvantage of standing tables is that they usually require an adult to get the child into the device and standing.

Integrated Wheelchair Standing Devices

A wheelchair standing device is a standing device integrated into the child's personal wheelchair. It can be manually or power controlled, and it can be part of a manual or power wheelchair base. The advantage of the wheelchair stander is that the child can stand without having to be transferred to another device.[12] The child may stand more frequently and randomly, may be more independent in achieving the standing position, can accomplish functional reach at different heights, and has increased vertical reach, in addition to the other benefits of erect standing. Also, the risks involved with transfers to a standing device are eliminated, and the child and family have one less piece of equipment to deal with.[12]

Integrated wheelchair standers provide dynamic loading of the lower extremities and the benefits of dynamic weight-bearing during the rise to standing and stand-to-sit activities. Dynamic loading also occurs with the child in different standing/semi-standing positions, due to changing skeletal alignment and varying amounts of weight bearing in diverse positions. A child can move in the environment while standing in the wheelchair stander, thereby gaining increased functional opportunities and dynamic loading through the vibration effects by moving across different surfaces and thresholds.[12]

Side-lying

Side-lyers

Side-lyers are particularly useful for young children or large children with low developmental function who require an alternative to sitting, lying in bed, or lying on the floor. Side-lyers can be elaborately constructed or can be very simple devices with pillows, straps, and other commonly available items. A typical fabricated side-lyer is shown in Figure 12.9. When using a side-lyer, the objective is to place the child in a side-lying position according to the following criteria:

1. The trunk should be as symmetric as possible.
2. The head should be supported, in neutral alignment with the trunk.
3. Weight-bearing limbs (upper and lower extremity touching the surface) should be slightly flexed.

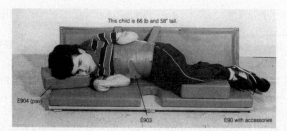

FIGURE 12.9 A commercially available side-lyer.

4. Non–weight-bearing limbs should be free to move. This position encourages play in midline, dissociation between the limbs, and symmetric and neutral head and trunk alignment. It is also a position that is neutral regarding most abnormal reflex activity. Straps are commonly used to support the trunk, the pelvis, and, occasionally, the weight-bearing lower extremity. Pillows or pommels usually support the thigh in a neutral position for hip abduction/adduction and internal/external rotation. The device should accommodate the child on either side unless circumstances prevent the child from freely lying on each side. Frequent reassessment is required to prevent compensations while using or after being removed from the side-lyer.

5. Areas of potential problems include neck hyperextension from pushing against the head support and flexion/retraction of the shoulder on the non–weight-bearing side. These problems may occur with a child who exhibits extensor hypertonicity. When using a side-lyer, the therapist must be careful when aligning the child with chronic hyperextension of the neck or with a tracheostomy. Improper positioning in either of these cases could cause airway obstruction and compromise the child's ventilation.

Although the side-lyer provides easy manipulation of toys and objects because one hand is stabilized against the surface in good midline alignment, the position is not optimal for perceptual development because the child must play with objects in a horizontal plane when the environmental backdrop is vertical. That is, toys are rotated 90 degrees with respect to the usual, functional visual field. This ironic occurrence is not a contraindication to using a side-lyer unless the child has obvious or suspected difficulties with perception or cognition. Most children compensate easily for the problem, especially when sides are alternated, and enjoy these changes of position.

Overall Considerations for Positioning

Although not a complete list of positioning devices, examples have been provided to illustrate the issues to be considered in choosing and using equipment for positioning, the benefits of various positioning devices, and some of the possible negative consequences. Negative consequences can be minimized by periodic reassessment of the child and education of the family and staff. When caregivers are aware of the potential negative effects of the equipment, they are more likely to anticipate and recognize early signs of those effects.

Physical therapists who work with children and adaptive equipment will be required to suggest the frequency and duration of use and endurance. Unfortunately, a uniform answer rarely exists. Endurance depends on variables that change daily. Rather than suggesting specific lengths of time for use, the therapist may choose to let the warning signs of fatigue guide the usage. Those warning signs include difficulty maintaining the desired posture, increased asymmetry, complaints of discomfort, facial expressions signifying discomfort or displeasure, and verbal requests to be moved. The therapist can recommend using a device until any one of those warning signs is apparent or a maximum time limit has been reached. Depending on the child and the type of equipment, 20 to 30 minutes is a recommended maximum for a child who can make few, if any, postural adjustments. For a child who is able to make postural adjustments while in the equipment, varying the distribution of weight bearing, for example, 1 hour at a time is probably a maximum. It may be worthwhile to encourage attempts to increase endurance gradually over the course of several weeks or months, realizing that minor variations in tolerance will occur daily. Because daily variations in activity level are normal for everyone, we should acknowledge these variations in the child with physical disabilities.

Prolonged positioning in any one posture is contraindicated. In addition to fatigue, negative effects of prolonged positioning include pressure ulcers, joint stiffness, and decreased passive and active range caused by hypertonus and/or immobilization.

▶ Mobility equipment

In addition to providing assistance with positioning, adaptive equipment can supplement a child's existing manner of independent locomotion or offer mobility to children who otherwise have no means of locomotion. Some devices, such as a scooter board, pre-wheelchair device, and other devices used on the floor, are appropriate only within the home or classroom. Other devices such as wheelchairs make it possible for the child to be mobile within the community.

Scooter Boards

A scooter board is a flat, padded board with casters (Fig. 12.10). While prone on the board, a child propels by using hands on the floor. Scooter boards are especially helpful for the toddler or young child who has no prone locomotion and is limited in floor play and exploration. Sometimes a scooter board is incorporated into a prone stander, such that the child can be mobile on the floor and then elevated in the stander without changing equipment.

Prewheelchair Device

These devices allow children 18 months to 5 years of age to play on the floor at peer level. Sometimes referred to as

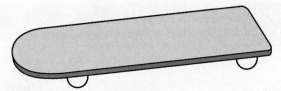

FIGURE 12.10 The scooter board is a wheeled mobility device that allows the child to locomote on the floor with his or her peers.

carts, these are hand-propelled devices on which a child assumes a long-sit position and propels the cart by moving the large wheels with the upper extremities, similar to propelling a manual wheelchair. Several commercial designs are available (Fig. 12.11). Sometimes this type of device is used for a toddler-aged child who will inevitably get a manual wheelchair and will learn how to self-propel in a wheeled device using the hands.

Wheelchairs

Providing a wheelchair for a patient requires an understanding and application of all of the criteria previously discussed about proper alignment and positioning in sitting. It is also beneficial to know about the options available when purchasing a wheelchair and the compromises involved when selecting certain options.

Before continuing, it is worth stating that the wheelchair industry is in constant flux. This is why a well-informed and capable vendor or manufacturer's representative and a certified ATP are important to the rehabilitation team. The representative can provide information about changes and innovations in DME and discuss the comparative adaptability, durability, cost, and features of wheelchairs and other equipment supplied by competing manufacturers. It may be easiest to discuss options by looking at a typical order form for a pediatric chair (see Display 12.1). These forms are traditionally completed by the vendor, patient, patient's family, and physical therapist working together to meet the patient's needs.

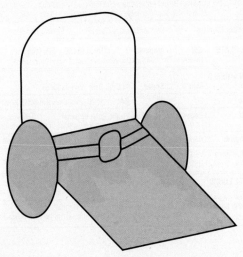

FIGURE 12.11 The pre-wheelchair device allows the child to be mobile on the floor and teaches the use of the upper extremities for propelling the wheelchair.

DISPLAY

12.1   A Sample Order Form for a Pediatric Wheelchair

Effective July 5, 1993

ORDER FORM

Date: _____ P.O.#: _____
Buyer: _____ Customer#: _____

Bill To:
Name _____
Mailing Address _____
City _____ State _____ Zip _____
Phone (___) _____

☐ **Drop Ship/Ship To:**
Name _____
Street Address _____
City _____ State _____ Zip _____
Phone (___) _____ Marked For _____

QUICKIE 2   ☐ *Adult*   ☐ *Kids*

COLOR
☐ *Blue*   ☐ *Black*   ☐ *Red*   ☐ *Midnight Purple*   ☐ *Silver*
☐ *Sky White*   ☐ *Teal*   ☐ *Hot Pink*   ☐ *Ultra Yellow*   ☐ *Lavender*
☐ *Blue Sapphire* ☐ *Blk Diamond*   ☐ *Candy Red*

FRAME DIMENSIONS
Frame Width
☐ *11″* *   ☐ *12″*   ☐ *13″*   ☐ *14″*   ☐ *15″*   (Seat Width: 1/2″ Narrower)
☐ *16″*   ☐ *17″*   ☐ *18″*   ☐ *19″*   ☐ *20″*   (*11″ Wide by Upholstery)

Sling Depth
☐ *10″*   ☐ *11″*   ☐ *12″*   ☐ 13″
☐ 14″   ☐ 15″   ☐ *16″*   ☐ 17″[1]   ☐ 18″[1]

Cushion   ☐ *2″*   ☐ *3″*   ☐ *4″*
☐ Solid Seat[3]   ☐ Omit Cushion   ☐ Omit Seat Sling

BACKREST   (Push Handles Std.)   ☐ *Low* (8 1/2″–12″)[17]   ☐ *Med* (12″–15 1/2″)[17]   ☐ *Tall* (15 1/2″–19″)[17]
Backrest Options   ☐ 8° Bend (Med & Tall)[17]   ☐ Omit Push Handles[17]   ☐ Depth Adjustable[18,11]
☐ Omit Depth Adj Solid Back & Hardware   ☐ Omit Depth Adj Solid Back Include Hardware
☐ Swing-Away Adj Stroller Handles (Avail w/ Depth Adj Back Only)   ☐ Solid Back[3,17]
☐ Backrest Cushion[17]   ☐ Adj Upholstery (Avail w/ 14″–20″ Frame Widths and Med or Tall Back Heights)[17]
☐ Omit Back Upholstery[17]   ☐ Omit Back Post & Upholstery[17]

FRAME SPECIFICATIONS
Frame Length   ☐ Kids   ☐ *Reg*   ☐ Long   ☐ Hemi[5]   ☐ Long Hemi (17″–18″ Deep)[5]

Hanger Type ☐ *60°*   ☐ *70°*   ☐ *90°*   ☐ 70° V[19]   ☐ Hemi (60°)   ☐ Omit Hangers
☐ Articulating-Adult (15″–20″ Widths)[2]
☐ Articulating-Kids (11″–16″ Widths; Std w/ 2″ footrest Ext Tubes and Adj Flip-Up Footplates)[2]
☐ Impact Guards—Plastic   ☐ Impact Guards—Neoprene

Footplates   ☐ *Composite*[9]   ☐ Plastic Cover   ☐ Reverse   ☐ High Mount[6]
☐ Foam[4]   ☐ Angle Adj[9]   ☐ Angle Adj High Mount[9]   ☐ Omit Footplate
☐ 90° Adj Flip-Up[4,8]   ☐ 90°/90° Footboard[4,7]   ☐ Extended[9]
☐ Heel Loops   ☐ Omit Leg Strap

Footrest Ext Tubes[20]   ☐ *Short* (14″–16 1/2″; N/A w/Articulating Legrest)   ☐ *Med* (16 1/2″–19″)   ☐ *Long* (19″–21 1/2″)
☐ Omit Ext Tubes

CASTERS   ☐ *8″ Pneumatic*   ☐ 8″ Polyurethane   ☐ 5″ Low-Profile Polyurethane
☐ 6″ Pneumatic   ☐ 6″ Polyurethane   ☐ Aluminum Caster Rim

Caster Options   ☐ 3/4″ Longer Fork Stem Bolt   ☐ 1 1/2″ Longer Fork Stem Bolt
☐ Caster Pin Locks   ☐ Omit Caster Wheels   ☐ Quick-Release Caster Stems[21]

ARMRESTS   ☐ Padded Swing-Away[17]   ☐ Omit Armrests
☐ Adult—Height Adjustable w/Std Pad (10″)   ☐ Adult—Height Adjustable w/Full-Length Pad (14″)
☐ Kids—Height Adjustable w/Std Pad (10″)   ☐ Kids—Height Adjustable w/Full-Length Pad (14″)

Stroller Handles   ☐ Stroller Handles (Reg)[10,17]   ☐ Stroller Handles (Tall)[10,17]

AXLE PLATE   ☐ *Std*   ☐ Amputee[11]   ☐ Quad Release Axle Nuts
☐ One-Arm Drive (Attach One-Arm Drive Supplemental Order Form)

REAR WHEELS
Rim   ☐ Mag[12]   ☐ *Spoke*   ☐ Omit Rear Wheels/Axles
Size   ☐ 20″   ☐ 22″   ☐ *24″*   ☐ 26″ (3/4″ Stem Bolt Std w/26″ Wheels)
Tire   ☐ *Pneumatic*   ☐ Full-Profile Polyurethane[12]   ☐ Airless Insert[12]
☐ Low-Profile Polyurethane[13]   ☐ Kevlar[13]   ☐ High-Pressure Clincher (24″, 26″ Only)[18]
Handrim   ☐ *Aluminum*   ☐ Plastic Coated   ☐ Long Tabs   ☐ Omit Handrims
Projections   ☐ Vertical[14]   20″/22″ _____   24″/26″ _____
☐ Oblique   ☐ 6   ☐ 8   ☐ 10   ☐ 12

WHEEL LOCKS   ☐ *High-Push*   ☐ Low   ☐ Omit
☐ High-Pull   ☐ Do Not Mount

Wheel Lock Options   ☐ 6″ Ext Handles   ☐ 9″ Ext Handles
☐ Grade Aids (N/A w/ Polyurethane High-Pressure Clincher Tires or Kids Length Frames)

ACCESSORIES
☐ Anti-Tip Tubes
☐ Armrest Pouch (Hgt Adj)
☐ Caddy
☐ Crutch Holder
☐ Front-End Stabilizer
☐ Leg Strap
☐ Leg Strap-Double
☐ Spoke Guards
☐ Transfer Board
☐ Tool Kit

Backpack & Seat Pouch
(Specify Color)
☐ Adult _____
☐ Kids _____
☐ Seat Pouch _____

Clothing
(Specify Color and Size)
☐ Long Sleeve Shirt _____
☐ Sweatshirt _____
☐ Golf Shirt _____
☐ T-Shirt _____
☐ Jacket _____
☐ Barrel Bag _____
☐ Hat _____
☐ Eyeglass Holders _____

Lifting Straps
☐ Q2 Low[10,17]
☐ Q2 Medium[10,17]
☐ Q2 Tall[10,17]

Positioning Bolts
☐ Long Velcro® Style (67″)
☐ Short Velcro® Style (57″)
☐ Long Buckle (64″)
☐ Short Buckle (54″)

Side Guards
☐ Fabric Kids
☐ Fabric Regular
☐ Plastic Kids[15]
☐ Plastic Reg[15]

Touch-Up Paint
☐ Color: _____

Wheelchair Tray Table
☐ Extra Small 10″–12″
☐ Small 13″–14″
☐ Medium 15″–17″
☐ Large 18″–20″

Special Instructions _____
_____
_____
_____
_____
_____

Items in *Bold Italic* Print are Standard
1. Available only on long frame.
2. N/A w/high-push wheel locks.
3. 8° bend not available: 11″–15″ wide, 10″–15″ deep only.
4. Not available with heel loops: single leg strap standard.
5. Hemi hangers only.
6. Only available on 60° hangers and hemi hangers.
7. Available only with 11″–16″ frame widths.
8. Available only with 11″–16″ frame widths and 90° hangers.
9. Available on 14″–20″ widths.
10. Omit push handles.
11. Not available with swing-away armrest; height adj. available at swing-away price.
12. Not available on 26″ wheels.
13. Only available on 24″ wheels.
14. Not available with low-profile polyurethane tires.
15. Not available with height adjustable armrests.
16. Not available with mag wheels.
17. Not available with depth adjustable back.
18. Standard with 20″ solid back height and stroller handles.
19. Available with 16″–20″ frame widths and composite footplates only.
20. Not available with 90° hangers or articulating legrest-kids.
21. Not available with caster pin locks; not available with 3/4″, or 1 1/2″ lock stem bolt.

Specifications Subject to Change without Notice

The first decision when matching a child with a wheelchair for mobility is determining whether the child needs dependent or independent mobility.[71] Exclusively dependent wheelchair mobility should be reserved for children who, for some reason, cannot attain independent mobility with a wheelchair—either manually propelled or powered. Dependent mobility may be the goal for children unable to operate a manual or powered wheelchair because of insufficient upper extremity function, limited fine motor control, lack of judgment, insufficient cognitive skills, or profound and multiple physical impairments and disabilities. Some children may have to be dependent in mobility because of environmental or societal barriers such as lack of funds for a power wheelchair, lack of means to transport a power chair, or inaccessibility of the home. Wheelchairs for dependent mobility of children include strollers, transport or travel chairs, manual wheelchairs, and reclining and tilt in space wheelchairs.[71] Since the goal of enhancing a child's independent function is paramount, feasible options for achieving some degree of independent mobility should be explored prior to deciding upon dependent mobility.

If a child can attain independent wheeled mobility with an appropriate wheelchair, will reaching this goal be most likely attained by a manual or powered wheelchair? Reasons for opting for a powered chair include: (1) severe upper extremity weakness, (2) paresis, paralysis, or dyskinesias that preclude manual wheelchair propulsion, (3) inadequate upper extremity control, (4) extreme fatigue, (5) respiratory compromise, (6) function in more challenging environments such as outdoors or in the community, (7) high metabolic costs of propelling a manual wheelchair, and (8) concerns about secondary impairments from overuse injuries acquired from long-term manual propulsion of a wheelchair.[11,13,17,18,72–76] Well-meaning health care professionals may suggest that selecting a powered wheelchair will lead to the child gaining weight or losing muscle strength owing to lack of exercise. This is not a good rationale for choosing a manual chair. As stated above, the choice of a primary mobility device should be determined to provide optimal independence. A child who uses powered mobility should get exercise to prevent disuse weakness and weight gain, but his ability to be mobile in the community should not be connected to his exercise habits.[13]

Wheelchair design is the first consideration in choosing a manual wheelchair. For independent mobility, two basic options exist in a manually driven wheelchair: a rigid frame and a cross-braced (X-frame) folding wheelchair. Most people are familiar with a cross-braced folding wheelchair and often choose this type as it appears easier to transport in cars and store in the home. Although the rigid-frame chair does not fold, the wheels are removable and the back folds forward, leaving a small box-type structure. The rigid-frame chair offers increased stability and ease of rolling, and it is always the chair of choice for sports and recreation. In many instances, once the child adjusts, families find the rigid chair to be as manageable as the traditional folding chair. A disadvantage of the rigid-frame wheelchair is its limited

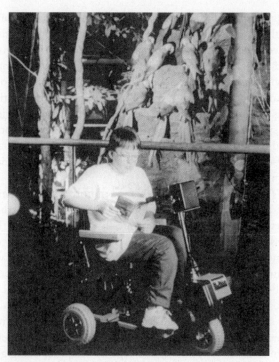

FIGURE 12.12 A three-wheeled scooter.

adjustability for growth; as a result, it is sometimes overlooked for the pediatric population. If properly fitted, the rigid-frame chair can provide years of use.[†]

For children who are not independently mobile with a manual wheelchair because of any of the previously described impairments or disabilities, a motorized device may be considered. A vendor and certified ATP should be consulted regarding alternatives, which include powered wheelchairs, three- or four-wheeled scooters, and segways. A scooter (Fig. 12.12) is much less expensive than a standard motorized wheelchair (approximately $1500 to $3500 compared with $4,000 to $12,000).[‡] It can be disassembled into components that are lighter and easier to load into a car or public transport vehicle and is relatively simple to learn to operate and maintain. Also, scooters are often preferred by a child and parents because scooters may be more readily accepted by peers. Any seating system, from a simple standard molded plastic seat to the most elaborate custom-made wheelchair seating system, can be adapted to the scooter. It must be noted that the patient must have bilateral hand use and some degree of reach to hold the scooter's handlebars, push the accelerator, and steer. Also, the child needs at least fair sitting balance.

Traditional power wheelchairs are extremely heavy, do not disassemble easily into component parts, and generally

[†]Modified rigid wheelchairs have now been devised that combine rigidity but allow for some growth. Additional information can be obtained from an informed vendor.

[‡]Prices vary dramatically, based on the seating and positioning options required and the need for additional electronic options.

require a van for transport and ramps or a stair-free entrance to the home. Additionally, they are usually quite sophisticated electronically, which may mean frequent fine-tuning and adjusting. However, they can usually accommodate environmental control systems and augmentative communication technology, can allow for changes in position (e.g., reclining, tilting), and can be operated using a variety of switches or other types of controls. Traditional motorized wheelchairs require more of a trial-and-error approach to perfectly fit and train the patient, and maintenance may be more involved.

The Segway® is a relatively new motorized device being used by some people with disabilities. This personal transporter is a two-wheeled, dynamically stabilized device that runs on large format batteries.[77] Although not originally designed for persons with disabilities, teens, young adults, veterans who are disabled, and others have found the Segway® to be a transporter that provides safe access into small indoor spaces and outdoors, even on rugged terrain.[77-81] Also, for some, such as college students, it is a safe and efficient means to get around campus without automatically being seen as disabled. The original Segway® requires being able to stand on the device, but new accessories are being developed, including seats.[82] The scooter or Segway® may be preferred for an older marginal ambulator who requires a device for long distances. A traditional motorized wheelchair is usually reserved for the individual who requires a more extensive mobility system for full-time use. Specialists in power wheelchairs should be consulted if a traditional power wheelchair system is being considered.

Power Mobility for Young Children

The use of power mobility was formerly reserved for older children under the mistaken impression that a child needed to be older to have sufficient cognitive development to learn to control a power wheelchair. However, a 2001 study by Botos et al. found children with an IQ of less than 55 could be trained to use a power wheelchair.[17] As a result of the Botos study and others, the current notion is that readiness to use a power chair depends on cognitive abilities other than IQ, such as understanding the concepts of cause and effect, direction, spatial relationships, and problem solving.[13,17,72,83-85] These cognitive abilities begin developing quite early in a child's first year of life, and independent mobility is a powerful positive factor for a child's psychosocial and cognitive development.[13,17,72,73,84-88]

Children as young as 11 months of age have demonstrated the ability to control a power wheelchair.[13,89] Other studies have revealed that children aged 14 months,[72] 20 months,[11] and 36 months[86] can learn to use power wheelchairs. Huang and Galloway report on a modified powered riding toy as an inexpensive and novel means of introducing power mobility to a very young child. These low-tech commercial toys are readily available and can be an excellent learning environment for children under 3 years of age to experience independent mobility.[87] The integrated development of locomotion, cognition, and perceptual-motor abilities in infancy and toddlerhood and studies of very young children with impairments support the consideration of power mobility for very young children as a means of achieving independent locomotion.

Suggestions for Wheelchair Fitting and Options

Once a wheelchair style has been selected, whether manual or power, the size, fit, and options must be determined. The physical therapist should consider the following criteria for wheelchairs, as well as the principles of good seating discussed earlier in this chapter:

1. Seat width should allow for growth and should be able to accommodate outerwear for cold winter climates. Most vendors consider 1 inch on each side to be appropriate. Too much room makes it very difficult to propel a manual wheelchair effectively, especially when armrests are used. In most pediatric models, chairs can be ordered in 1-inch increments to custom-fit any child. In an X-frame wheelchair, growth in width is provided by replacing the cross braces and upholstery of the wheelchair. No growth adjustment is available in a rigid-frame wheelchair. Almost all children are provided with a solid seat, used with a cushion, to avoid the slinging effect of upholstery. Cushions of various types of foam or gel as well as air-filled are available. Cushions are used not only to protect skin from breakdown, particularly over bony prominences, but also to change the patient's placement and alignment within the chair. Increasing the cushion height lowers the functional height of the wheelchair backrest and armrests, lowers the foot plates relative to the patient, and changes the patient's effective arm length and access to the wheels. This technique is often used to extend the use of a chair for several months for a patient who is growing tall but who has not outgrown the width of the chair. It is important, when measuring a chair, to remember to account for changes relating to cushion use (Fig. 12.13).

2. Seat depth should permit comfortable knee flexion without popliteal pressure. A solid seat back with hardware placed between the uprights often allows for several inches of growth in a child. The insert is placed forward of the uprights and is moved back as the child grows. However, the most energy-efficient alignment of a patient for manual propulsion places the greater trochanter over the axis of the back wheels and only 40% of the combined weight of the wheelchair and occupant on the front casters.[75,76,90] It is, therefore, unwise to use cushions behind the child to temporarily decrease the seat depth or use inserts to accommodate an excessive increase in seat depth. Axle plate adjustments that adjust both horizontally and vertically are available, but the extent of modification depends on many factors, including the frame size of the chair. Other recommendations for wheelchair seat depth were discussed previously in this chapter under general seating principles.

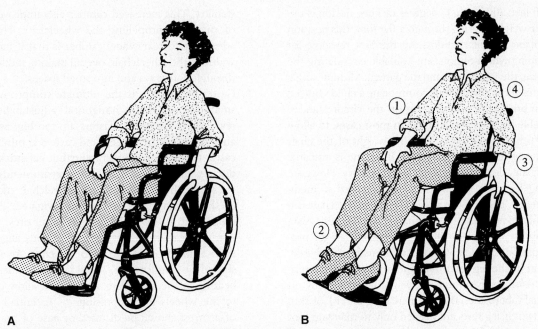

A   **B**

FIGURE 12.13 (A) Patient is accommodated without cushion. **(B)** Use of a cushion will change: (*1*) position of arm on armrest; (*2*) relative leg length; (*3*) relative arm length in relation to the wheel; and (*4*) the amount of back support (decreased).

3. As stated previously, wheelchair dump can be accomplished by a wedged cushion, with the cushion thicker in the front than at the back—where the seat meets the wheelchair back. Another way of increasing dump is to tilt the seat and backrest unit of the chair slightly backward in relation to the wheelbase and floor. This change allows gravity to push the child back into the chair to avoid sliding forward. This approach involves a tilt system in wheelchairs, both manual- and power-driven, which maintains the seat-to-back relationship but changes the angle of the seat-back unit relative to the ground.[63] Tilt systems, whether operated manually or powered, allow a child to have frequent changes in body position, while maintaining optimal postural alignment. Tilt in a wheelchair provides gravity-assisted positioning and has been shown to be effective for addressing a variety of issues that can compromise the child's comfort, health, and well-being, including problems associated with physiology, alignment, biomechanics, transfers, and deformity prevention.[63] When using a tilt system, particular attention must be paid to avoiding pressure in the popliteal spaces.[59] A reclining wheelchair does not maintain the seat-to-back angle as a tilt system does, but the reclining chair is an option for children who need to change positions frequently and/or need to rest in a near recumbent position. For children who need frequent rest periods, the reclining chair allows rest wherever the child happens to be and also reduces the risks of frequent transfers into and out of the wheelchair. A power reclining chair makes it possible for a child to achieve a rest position independently and therefore more timely throughout the day.

4. If it does not compromise good positioning or alignment, a sling wheelchair backrest can improve mobility, increase sitting tolerance, and decrease the weight of the wheelchair by eliminating heavy inserts and hardware. The preferred backrest height for maximum independent propulsion of a manual wheelchair is below the scapulae, for optimum freedom of movement, as discussed previously. However, some children require additional support provided by a higher backrest and even a head support, and these chairs should be equipped with a solid back. A dilemma arises when a head support is needed only during transport, such as bus transportation to school. Automobile safety standards require head restraints during transit.[91] Children are often more functional without a head support and need a headrest for transportation only (i.e., the patient who has fair head control when in a static position but who experiences fatigue or becomes compromised with excessive movement). It is difficult to mount a headrest on a sling-type backrest. Therefore, a need for a removable headrest usually implies changing to a solid wheelchair backrest. In certain instances, this combination may be a barrier to a child's customary independent and energy-efficient mobility. This problem can be resolved by having the child transfer into a federally approved car seat or wheelchair when being transported, thus negating the need for a headrest mounted on the child's primary wheelchair itself.

5. Selection and placement of wheelchair footplates and leg rests are dictated by a child's impairments and size and the size of the wheelchair frame and caster wheels. Individual footplates are available for each foot or one single plate

for both feet. Although 90 degrees of knee flexion is optimal for weight bearing through a flat foot, this position may not be feasible. Vendors are the best resource for determining which options are available considering the frame size, the wheel size, and the patient. Multiple-angle foot plates allow change to accommodate a child's braced and non-braced foot, depending on the circumstances. Removable leg rests are desirable in most cases, to allow ease of transfer and to decrease the weight of the chair when disassembling for transport. If recline is available in the chair, elevating leg rests are necessary. However, elevating leg rests should only be requested if medically needed, because the added weight to the chair can make maneuverability of the chair more difficult. Also, elevating the legs when sitting in a wheelchair for prolonged periods should not occur unless medically advised. Elevation of the leg rests shifts the body weight posteriorly, increasing the amount of weight borne directly on the ischial tuberosities, thereby increasing the risk of skin breakdown. If leg rests are needed only to maintain foot placement on the footplates, an alternative is a single calf strap with one footplate or heel loops at the back of each footplate. Velcro-fastening straps around a child's feet at the ankles can also be used to keep the feet on the footrests, but should not be used if the child can transfer independently. If straps closing over the child's foot are used, their placement should be at the ankle rather than across the ball of the foot and toes, since toe straps can elicit increased spasticity in those with lower extremity spasticity.

6. Wheel size is critical to achieve the most energy-efficient propulsion. Ideally, the elbow should be in 100 to 120 degrees of extension when the child grasps the push-rim at its highest point.[75,92,93] This optimal elbow angle is a product not only of wheel diameter but also of seat height, including the height of the appropriate wheelchair cushion, armrest position, and placement of the rear axle. Pneumatic tires give a smoother ride (adding some shock absorbency) but require considerable maintenance for consistent and proper inflation pressure. Underinflated tires increase the effort of manual propulsion. For small children, the child's weight may not justify the need for pneumatic tires considering the extra maintenance required, but in older, heavier children, riding on rough terrain is clearly better on pneumatic tires.

7. Stability of a manual wheelchair depends on the height of the person's center of mass (affected by individual's height and height of wheelchair seat), placement of the rear wheel axle relative to the center of gravity, and the width of the base, that is, the distance between the two rear wheels at the floor. Improved lateral stability can be achieved by increasing rear wheel camber. Wheel camber refers to the vertical orientation of the wheels. By angling the wheels inward at the top, the distance between the wheels at the floor becomes greater, thereby enlarging the base of support and increasing lateral stability. This increased camber also improves the ease of manually propelling the wheelchair. The one disadvantage to rear wheel camber is that it increases the width of the wheelchair, overall making it difficult to go through doorways and into small spaces.[71]

8. Caster wheel size is the ultimate compromise. In the small-framed chair, horizontal adjustability of the rear axle is lost if the casters are too big, as the clearance between the wheels and casters is minimal. Small caster tires add maneuverability but get stuck in cracks, ditches, and the like. The author recommends the smallest caster that will still allow wheelchair management on the terrain that is most often navigated. The options range from 2- to 8-inch diameter caster tires.[65]

9. Armrests can improve symmetrical body alignment and deter a child from falling out of the chair. Armrest height should be comfortable, should allow reduced weight-bearing in the shoulders, and should allow easy access to the wheels for propulsion.[75,93] Essentially, the type of armrest should be dictated by ease of management. Many experienced wheelchair users prefer to be without armrests; however, bus drivers, parents, and other care-givers often rely on them as an aid in transferring the chair into and out of vehicles. Removable armrests can provide the benefits of armrests when needed but can be removed for ease of some types of transfers and for moving the wheelchair into close proximity to a table or desk.

10. Wheel locks (brakes) should be positioned for easiest management and can be operated either by pushing or pulling, depending on the patient's preference and abilities. Many companies also offer high- or low-mount options for brakes.

11. A seat belt is essential on a child's wheelchair. The belt should originate at the angle of the seat and backrest on both sides, closing over the child low on the pelvis. It should not come around the child from the middle of the backrest of the wheelchair.

12. Anti-tippers are also a must on a child's wheelchair, especially for the young child and novice wheelchair user.

13. Lap desks or trays are particularly helpful for children, especially the school-aged child. The lap desk, if used, must be carefully fitted to the chair so as not to increase the overall width of the chair. Lap desks of clear Lucite or a similar material are preferable to opaque lapboards. The see-through lapboard helps facilitate positive body image by allowing the child to see the lower extremities and the lower trunk. Likewise, the ability of others to see the whole child through the lapboard tends to have a positive impact on the child's interactions with others.

14. Manual wheelchairs for young and/or small children who are independent in wheeled mobility can be outfitted with an extended push handle that allows a parent or other caregiver to push the child, when needed, in a wheelchair that is close to the ground. They can also be equipped with attendant-operated brakes and wheel locks for added safety.

15. Lightweight and ultralight manual wheelchairs are preferable for children, unless the child's weight makes propulsion of a lighter-weight wheelchair difficult. The weight of the wheelchair during use is affected by its construction, the weight of accessories and options, and the child's weight, and will impact the child's energy demands. Weight is also a factor when lifting the wheelchair into a vehicle for transport. A case study of two children with spina bifida with myelomeningocele, by Meiser and McEwen in 2007, found that children and parents preferred the ultralight rigid frame chair over the lightweight folding frame wheelchair.[94]

Children with special needs such as a deformity that must be accommodated in the wheelchair will benefit from a wheelchair custom-molded to the child's shape in one of several ways. One method uses a fluid foam-like product. The child sits on, or back against, a container filled with this fluid material allowing it to form around the deformity and solidify after several minutes. Once hardened, the foam is padded as necessary and covered (Fig. 12.14).

Once a wheelchair prescription is complete, the child's therapist and certified ATP should be satisfied that the decisions are best for a given child. Any misgivings should be discussed with more experienced therapists, another vendor,

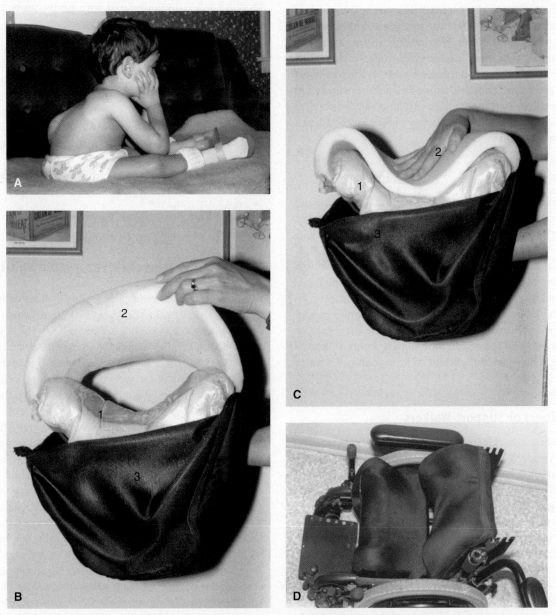

FIGURE 12.14 (A) Child with myelomeningocele with gibbus on back may require a custom-fitted wheelchair back. **(B)** (*1*) Solidified foam that conforms to child's back during fitting; (*2*) soft foam for added protection from pressure; (*3*) wheelchair back upholstery. **(C)** (*1*) Solidified foam, (2) soft foam, (3) wheelchair back upholstery. **(D)** Finished wheelchair with custom-conformed back.

or a manufacturer's representative. Therapists should always remember that equipment is expensive and, more importantly, will affect the quality of the child's life for the next 3 to 5 years.

Tricycles

Tricycles are a fun and functional way for some small children to locomote. Specially adapted tricycles are available commercially, or a standard tricycle can be modified. Modifications may include vertically turned handgrips (to inhibit flexor hypertonia of the trunk and facilitate antigravity trunk extension in children with tone disorders), abduction pommels, back supports, and foot straps. Foot straps are usually applied at the angle of the foot and lower leg, rather than across the toes, similar to ankle straps on wheelchair footplates. This placement prevents a stimulus to the ball of the foot that might cause uncontrolled plantar flexion and increase abnormal extensor tone in the lower extremities and trunk. Tricycles, although sometimes awkward to transport, are appropriate for use within the community and can be an important adjunct to a child's independence and peer interaction.

Bicycles

Bicycles for older children provide functional mobility and recreation. Adapted bicycles are available commercially, and many can be further modified. Typical seating adaptations include seatbelts and backrests, pedal and brake modifications, and wheel modifications that include a third or fourth wheel. Also, the method for propelling the bike can be modified, including hand cycling. For some children, adapted bicycles offer longer-distance mobility, energy conservation, and exercise opportunities. Because a bicycle is a mode of transportation and recreation for children without disabilities, using a bike can help a child to fit in with peers more readily.

Gait Trainers or Support Walkers

Gait trainers, also referred to as support walkers, are devices for children who need more support when walking than is supplied by traditional handheld and maneuvered walkers. Children using these devices typically need partial body weight support, trunk support, and forearm support to walk.[68] Gait trainers may be used on a long-term basis to provide a means of independent ambulation, or they may be a step in the continuum of developing independent ambulation with less support such as a wheeled walker or forearm crutches.[68,95] In a 2011 nationwide survey of clinicians, Low et al. found many clinicians using support walkers with children, and one-third to one-half of the children progress to ambulation with a handheld walker.[68,95] Several gait trainers are available commercially.[96-98]

Support walkers are not only a means of independent ambulation for some children, but are beneficial in other ways: they make possible upright position for social interaction and upper extremity function and offer many benefits of lower extremity weight bearing (discussed earlier in this chapter). The weight-bearing benefits are considered noteworthy because the weight bearing is dynamic and comes from intermittent loading, a strategy that has been found to improve cortical bone mineral density.[69,70,99]

Other Mobility Aids

A variety of other mobility aids may be used, depending on the child's impairments and degree of involvement. Mobility aids commonly used with adults can be used with children and include the following:

1. Forearm (Lofstrand), platform, or axillary crutches
2. Canes (J-cane, T-cane, quad-cane)
3. Walkers (wheeled, reverse wheeled, platform, walkers with up-turned handgrips)
4. General lower extremity orthoses (supramalleolar orthosis [SMO], ankle-foot orthosis [AFO], KAFO, HKAFO)
5. Specialized orthotic devices (parapodiums, reciprocating gait orthosis)
6. Manual or power lifts to transfer nonambulatory children[100]
7. Wheelchair lifts[100]
8. Sport wheelchairs and all-terrain wheelchairs

▶ Transporting children with disabilities

Age-appropriate restraints and seating a child, with or without special needs, in the back seat significantly reduces serious injury in automobile accidents.[101,102] The AAP recommends that all children under the age of 13 years ride in the rear seat. As of 2011, the AAP recommends that children be placed in rear-facing car seats until age 2 years or until they reach the maximum height and weight for that particular car seat and then they graduate to a forward-facing car seat until height and/or weight reach the manufacturer's limit. The AAP further recommends that a belt-positioning booster seat should be used when any child has outgrown a forward-facing car seat and should be used until the child is 8 years of age, has reached approximately 4 feet 9 inches in height, according to the manufacturer's instructions. The child who has not yet reached the suggested height at age 8 should continue to use the booster until reaching the height requirement. The AAP maintains a current list of approved car seats along with recommendations for selecting an appropriate car seat and the correct and safe usage of car seats.[102] Children who need to lie flat during transport because of impairments or disabilities should be in a crash-tested car bed.[102]

In the United States, vehicle safety restraints for the transport of all infants and young children are required in all 50 states. In spite of this requirement, nonuse of vehicle restraints for young children with disabilities remains a problem. A 2007 study by Korn et al. in Israel found frequent misuse and nonuse of child safety restraints in family vehicles with children who had complex special needs, both physical and behavioral. Reasons for incorrect or misuse of restraints included the high cost of equipment, child's refusal to use equipment, child's crying, lack of parental knowledge about the importance, appropriateness, and technical modifications of restraints for children with special needs, and a lack of availability of appropriate restraints.[103] This study emphasizes the need for education of parents and the need for manufacture of approved restraints designed to accommodate children's complex physical impairments. Although a study by O'Neil et al. in 2009 found a higher percentage of use of restraints compared with the Israeli study, frequent errors in use and misuse of restraints still occurred, in nearly 73% of study cases.[104] Demographic and cultural differences between the two study populations may account for the difference in nonuse. Nonetheless, the degree of misuse in both studies indicates a need for education of the public and the continued development of vehicle safety restraint systems for children with medical, physical, and behavioral special needs.

Parents may ask a physical therapist, familiar with their child's impairments and needs, for advice or suggestions regarding appropriate and safe car seats. A physical therapist with special training in car safety restraint systems and their application to children with impairments is best able to advise parents. The AAP guidelines for safety restraints for children with special health care needs, first published in 1999 and reaffirmed in 2006, include a standard car safety seat that meets federal motor vehicle safety standards if possible; using rolled towels to give lateral support in the safety seat if needed, without interfering with the seat's harness system; not modifying the car safety seat restraints; turning off air bags if child must ride in front seat; moving seat back as far as possible if child must ride in front seat; securing all medical equipment under the child's seat or on the floor; and having an adult ride in the back seat with medically fragile child.[104] Simple modifications, such as adding an abduction pommel, a small seat wedge, or lateral supports to a standard car seat, can be made, as long as the integrity of the seat and safety are not compromised by the adaptation.

Although an appropriately appointed standard child safety seat should be used if it meets the child's safety needs, for children with complex involvement a medical car safety seat is needed. These seats tend to be more expensive than standard safety seats but should be used when the standard safety seat cannot adequately provide for the child's safety.[104] A number of vehicle safety restraints for children with special health care needs are currently available, including the Britax Traveller Plus EL, Special Tomato MPS Car Seat, Roosevelt Car Seat, Snug Seat Pilot Special Needs Booster, Hippo (Spica Cast) Car Seat, Recaro Monza Reha Adaptive

Car Seat, Columbia Medical Spirit Adjustable Positioning System (APS) Car Seat.[105] The physical therapist should check with adaptive equipment vendors regarding seats that could meet specific needs for a child with a disability.

A child being transported in a wheelchair should have a head support,[91] and the wheelchair should be secured with a four-point tie-down device. Lap desks and other equipment attached to the wheelchair should be removed and secured separately. Another option is to transfer the child from a wheelchair to a certified transit wheelchair.[106,107] However, these chairs are frequently not available for a given child.

If a child is able to transfer from a wheelchair to a safety equipped bus seat, that should be done. For a child sitting in a school bus seat equipped with seat belts, safety vests are available that can be worn by the child and secured to a specially installed tether mount in the bus, providing adequate upper body restraint with the bus seat belt providing lower body restraint.[106,108] Federally developed safety guidelines for school buses that transport children with special needs are available on the National Highway Traffic Safety Administration website.[109,110]

Medical equipment, such as a ventilator, is often transported with the child. Any medical equipment, including unoccupied wheelchairs, also needs to be secured within the vehicle for the safety of all occupants, whether in private or public transportation.[106,111]

▶ Equipment for infants and toddlers

When considering the needs of the infant and the toddler and the availability of devices, one must remember that these younger children are often undiagnosed, or may have a developmental delay that may not result in long-term disability. Children who are developing typically who require long periods of hospitalization for cardiac, pulmonary, gastrointestinal, and other disorders may benefit from types of apparatus that enhance motor development.

Standard high chairs and strollers can be used with many infants and toddlers with disabilities. Specially designed adaptive high chairs and strollers are also available. However, they should be used sparingly for the child with sensorimotor impairments so as not to discourage or impede the child's development of functional skills. Seating equipment for feeding may offer a stable, symmetrical position that allows for optimal oral motor function, head righting and control, and freedom of movement of the upper extremities. A good feeding posture for all infants includes being semi-upright or sitting upright and in slight trunk and neck flexion, to avoid hyperextension of the trunk and neck to aid in swallowing.

Concepts of seating and positioning already discussed in this chapter should be applied to strollers and high chairs. For example, the toddler who is able to sit in a high chair or stroller should have adequate hip flexion (90 degrees) and support to facilitate trunk symmetry and midline use of the hands. The original umbrella or sling-style strollers encourage adduction and internal rotation of the hips and posterior tilt of the pelvis, which are not components of good postural alignment for sitting and are not suitable for many infants and toddlers with disabilities. Some contemporary strollers called umbrella strollers have a solid seat and back, which does not create the same kind of postural deviations as the original.

Physical therapy interventions for the infant and toddler should concentrate on encouraging normal development of controlled motor patterns, and assistive devices *should not* predominate. The therapist working with the young child should recommend the parents facilitate movement and avoid static positioning when the child is left alone to play. As these children grow older, some may no longer have a disability, but others will develop additional manifestations, and a diagnosis may become more evident. Children in the latter group are likely to have continued treatment and equipment needs, and should be evaluated when appropriate, as previously outlined.

Hospitalized Children

Normal motor development is an integrated process that requires sensory input and freedom to respond to that input through general motor output, exploration, and play. Normal patterns of movement develop when agonist and antagonist muscles learn balanced and synergistic cooperation. Because equipment may disrupt or interfere with this process by limiting or restricting sensory input as well as movement, using equipment for infants and toddlers is almost always discouraged.

Movement in hospitalized children is often restricted by monitors, telemetry devices, and therapeutic medical equipment. It would be counterproductive to the child's motor development to add apparatus to these medically necessary devices. The objective for the hospitalized child is often to provide optimal freedom of movement within the limits imposed by medical interventions and equipment. Physical therapy for hospitalized children should encourage increased activity, if safe, and should facilitate movement patterns that, because of the external limitations, are difficult for the child to initiate. As the child's medical status improves, or when the child returns home, equipment use should still be limited, except when indicated to promote physical control or safety.

Ventilator-dependent children represent a small but growing population with major equipment needs. With increasing frequency, the physical therapist is asked to assist in the discharge planning and management of ventilator-dependent children. Technologic advances have prolonged life expectancy for many children with chronic illnesses, including, for example, those with myelomeningocele with symptomatic Arnold-Chiari malformation. Portable ventilators and third-party funding have aided in transforming

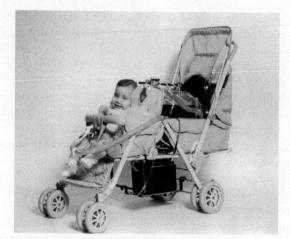

FIGURE 12.15 A commercially available double stroller.

these once chronically hospitalized children into active members of the community. They often return home, attend local schools, and participate in recreational and social activities in the community. Such participation requires a transport system for essential life-support equipment, which may include a portable ventilator and battery, humidifier, oxygen source, airway suction unit with catheters and hoses, a bag valve mask (manual resuscitator), a bag of supplies, and other items.

An innovative approach must be taken with this population to address developmental, orthopedic, and respiratory needs. It is essential to find a vendor interested in working with the family by being able to tailor the needed apparatus to the child's unique requirements. Much trial-and-error effort may be expended to resolve the problems presented by the weight of the ventilators, unusual balance points, difficult maneuverability, and the child's need to be in close proximity to these devices. The two systems shown in Figures 12.15 and 12.16 were designed to meet the specific needs of both child and family. Figure 12.15 shows a commercially available double stroller reinforced to house the ventilator in the rear seat with the battery suspended between the seats. The child can recline or sit upright using an age-appropriate and cost-effective mobility device that is aesthetically pleasing and manageable. Figure 12.16 shows a portable ventilator adapted for a Snug Seat with the battery on the front footplate and the ventilator positioned behind the seat. The child is positioned high enough to allow easy access to the equipment underneath and to accommodate caregivers who may perform suctioning and other procedures. The Snug Seat tilts 45 degrees in space and allows for easy adjustments for postural changes or growth. As the child grows and independent mobility becomes likely, manual or motorized wheelchairs can be adapted for the child's use.§

---

§A very special thank you to the DME Shoppe and Joe Thieme (Naperville, IL) for creating these units and many more similar devices.

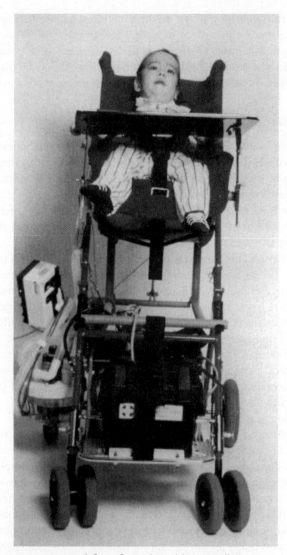

FIGURE 12.16 A Snug Seat adapted for a ventilator.

Infants and Toddlers without Physical Impairments

Let us consider the equipment used frequently for babies and toddlers without physical impairments, including infant swings, jumpers, baby walkers, and exercise saucers. It is common practice for families to purchase these devices despite little knowledge about their advantages or disadvantages.

Swings are probably the most benign device of the four just mentioned. There is little evidence to indicate that swings are unsafe during the first year of life, as long as they are used with supervision. Swings provide vestibular stimulation through linear movement. Vestibular stimulation is important for development of normal balance and postural responses, especially during the first 2 years of life. The regular rhythm of the swinging action can also be calming to an infant. Although swings are pleasant and convenient for the child and family, they should be used sparingly to avoid limiting the child's opportunities to move and explore the environment. Also, the increasing incidence of positional plagiocephaly in infants has a relationship to pressure on the posterior skull. Nonessential containment of children in devices that place sustained pressure on the skull, such as swings and infant carriers, should be limited.

Jumpers are devices suspended from doorways by large cables, springs, and clamps. Some freestanding jumpers are now available and are suspended from a stand or support. The jumper enables the child to bounce up and down by extending the lower extremities and pushing against the floor. Although the child may enjoy the vestibular stimulation provided during such an activity, caution must be exercised. The child must be supervised constantly to prevent falling, banging against the doorframe or supporting structure, or becoming entrapped in the cables or springs when reaching out for a toy. Even restricted use of the jumper may lead to the patterns of exaggerated extensor activity with components of strong internal rotation of the hips and plantar flexion of the ankles. As a result, some children may develop a tendency to toe-walk. Also, the repetitive high impact loading on the child's lower extremities may be injurious to cartilage and growth plates of the immature skeleton. In addition to these potential hazards, the jumper, like other devices, impedes development of normal motor skills by eliminating the opportunity to make transitions from one pattern to another and by restricting free movement and learning new sequences of movement. For reasons of safety and to reduce the potential of abnormal movement patterns, physical therapists generally discourage the use of these jumpers by all children.

Walkers have been used for children with ambulation difficulty by parents under the mistaken impression that these devices aid walking skills. Not only are baby walkers potentially dangerous, but they do not facilitate the development of normal walking and may actually impede motor development.[112] Ridenour studied the effects of frequent and regular use of a baby walker on bipedal locomotion in human infants. She found that walkers modified the mechanics of infant locomotion in several ways. Infants who used walkers were able to commit numerous mechanical errors while still succeeding in bipedal locomotion.[113] Patterns of locomotion with an infant walker are neither normal nor advantageous. Children who use these walkers have poor weight-bearing alignment and hold their trunk and lower extremities in considerable flexion. They also have frequent asymmetry due to leaning and commonly toe-walk. Additionally, a 1986 study by Crouchman found prone locomotion delayed in many normal babies who spent excessive time in infant walkers[114]; Garrett et al. reported similar findings in 2002.[112] Infants who spend a large portion of their days in containers of various types are probably not experiencing adequate age-appropriate neurosensory stimulation[26] or "tummy time" and are not developing a variety of options for moving. The exercise saucers, in lieu of baby walkers, put the child in a similar disadvantageous posture, depending on the relative heights of the child and saucer seat, and using exercise saucers invites similar bad habits. They are, however, safer for the child because they are not on wheels.

These observations suggest that walkers and exercise saucers may have an adverse effect on motor development, although the adverse effects may be of short duration once walker use is discontinued.[99,112–115] Further study is needed to confirm findings relative to infant walker and exercise saucer use and the development of motor skills, particularly ambulation, but most physical therapists discourage the use of walkers by all infants, and strongly discourage their use in infants with documented or suspected neurologic deficits or other physical impairments. Therapists discourage the use of baby walkers because of their inherent dangers as well as because their use may promote postures and motor behaviors that can interfere with or delay the development of typical motor skills. Exercise saucers, if used, should be used only for short periods, and the parent is advised to make sure the child's size and abilities are appropriate for the saucer.

Baby jumpers, walkers, and exercise saucers have been implicated in thousands of injuries and numerous fatalities. In 1993, more than 23,000 baby walker–related injuries, mostly to children between the ages of 5 and 15 months, were seen in hospital emergency rooms according to the U.S. Consumer Product Safety Commission.[92,116] A 2006 study by Shields and Smith revealed 197,200 baby walker–related injuries among children under 15 months of age in the United States for the years 1990–2001.[117] In 1994, a stationary activity center (exercise saucer), similar in design to the original walker but without wheels, was developed. Since that time, the number of walker-related injuries and deaths has decreased dramatically, but the use of secondhand walkers manufactured prior to that time continues, with resultant injuries.[117]

Although the incidence of injury associated with nursery products has declined in the United States over the past 20 years, injuries continue to occur. During the period 2001–2011, injuries to children under the age of 5 years associated with the use of baby walkers, jumpers, and exercisers totaled more than 43,000.[118] The number of injuries is most likely higher when one considers those injuries that are never reported or are treated in clinics or at home rather than hospital emergency rooms. During the period of 1989 through 1993, 11 walker-related deaths occurred.[92,116] From 2001 through 2009, there were 13 deaths associated with walkers, jumpers, and exercise saucers used by children under 5 years.[118] Most injuries from baby walkers have been the result of the walker tipping over, falls down stairs, walker collapse because of poor structural design, and finger entrapment. Injuries have included abrasions, lacerations, fractures, burns, poisonings, severe head trauma, and death.[92]

▶ Activities of daily living

Although not strongly emphasized in this chapter, ADLs should be mentioned briefly. ADLs are not major concerns for infants or toddlers with impairments, but they grow

increasingly important as these children grow older and become more capable of caring for themselves. Because families can usually manage the ADL needs of a young child, the issue of ADLs as a therapeutic goal may be overlooked or not considered as the child grows older.

Toileting and Bathing

Equipment for ADLs, particularly for toileting and bathing, should be assessed according to guidelines similar to those used for other pieces of apparatus as previously described. Attention to good toileting positioning increases a child's comfort. Lack of appropriate positioning and equipment can be a barrier to healthy bowel and bladder function and may also lead to delays in toilet training.[4]

Criteria for good seating apply to seating a child on a toilet. Toilets may be modified by adding abduction pommels, vertical handgrips (to keep the child symmetric and decrease flexor hypertonia), corner-style backrests, and footrests. Essential to good positioning on the toilet is for the child's hips and knees to be flexed to 90 degrees with feet flat on the floor, footrests, or a stool. This position helps limit extensor spasticity in those children affected by hypertonia and also helps all children relax their abdominal muscles and feel secure. If the child feels secure, confident, and relaxed, toileting may proceed more rapidly and easily.

Although achieving good positioning for toileting may be as simple as using a footstool with some children, many children need more support and therefore more complex seating arrangements. Various toileting aids and equipment are available, ranging from a bedside commode to wheelchair adaptations to make transfer to a toilet easier. Consult equipment catalogs and websites and confer with equipment vendors for devices appropriate for a particular client.

When choosing a bathtub seat, general principles of good seating should be considered, and ease of management in the tub and safety of the child are the major objectives. Although many bathtub seats exist, completely satisfactory seats for both practical use and safety are difficult to find for all children, but even more so when the child becomes older and heavier. Vendors should provide sample bathtub seats for both inspection and mock usage trials. The family must decide which tub seat provides the safest and most suitable solution depending on the particular environmental barriers of the home and the physical needs of the child.

Feeding

Keeping a growing child nourished in the face of physical impairments can be very challenging for parents and a source of great frustration for child and parent alike. As with bathing and toileting, good positioning is the first rule of order for feeding a child, whether for independent self-feeding or assisted feeding. Applying basic principles of good seating as discussed earlier, whether in a standard high chair, a regular kitchen or dining chair, or with the help of an adaptive seating device, can (1) make it possible for a child to be an independent feeder, (2) improve the caregiver's ability to feed the child, and (3) limit the need for other extensive feeding aids. Feeding aids can be found in rehabilitation catalogs and websites.

Playing

Toys are the tools of children's work, which is to play. Playing with toys enhances a child's sensorimotor, cognitive, psychosocial, and motor development. Often children with impairments will need help with positioning for play. Play positions should vary and be developmentally appropriate, and the support for positioning can be from an adult or from simple equipment.

Children with certain impairments may be unable to play with many commercially available toys. With a bit of creativity, many toys can be adapted for children, perhaps by changing the switching mechanism on a toy or adapting a toy so a child can grasp it more easily. In addition to adapting toys, consideration of a child's developmental level and abilities is important when selecting toys. Parents and therapists should not overlook toys made especially for children with special needs; these can be found on the internet or in special needs catalogs. Also, with the growing emphasis on universal design, more toys found in traditional toy stores, both today and in the future, may be age- and ability-appropriate for children with various impairments. Therapists can help parents find the best toys for their children. After all, providing children with suitable toys and objects for play is an important aspect of nurturing children and helping them learn in all domains of development.

▶ Access technologies

Access technologies are described as "Technologies that translate the intentions of the user with profound physical impairments into functional interactions such as communication or environmental control."[119(p204)] A specific access solution consists of the technology, a user and user interface, a task, and an environment or access site that typically changes throughout the user's day. Historically, the user interface for available access technologies has been a mechanical switch activated by changes in displacement, tilt, force, or air pressure and are controlled by a specific physical movement of the user. These mechanical switches are reliable, available, and relatively simple to operate. However, a user must have a minimum of one consistent movement to control a mechanical switch, and the switch is usually mounted such that its position precludes using different body parts to control it, making its use less than ideal for persons who have mental or physical fatigue.[119]

A 2008 literature review of access technologies identified a number of emerging technologies for persons with severe and multiple impairments, including infrared sensing;

surface electromyography; oculography, using eye movement or point of gaze to move a computer cursor; computer vision, a system that controls cursor movements by using a camera to track a specified facial feature of the user; electrodermal activity; and electroencephalography, electrocorticography, and intracortical recordings, three types of brain–computer interface. Voice-activated switches and speech recognition–based technologies also continue to evolve.[119]

Modification of the environments in which a person uses adaptive equipment (e.g., ramps, lifts, grab bars) can optimize a person's interaction with the environment.[4,120] Combined assistive technology and environmental interventions are sometimes referred to as AT-EI.[120]

Communication Systems

Communication systems are a subgroup of access technologies. Although most of this chapter has focused on adaptive equipment relative to positioning, mobility, and ADL needs (i.e., the physical needs of the child), it is important that we give brief consideration to communication devices. These devices may be equipment used by a child who is deaf or hearing impaired or has primary speech deficits, partial sight, blindness, or motor impairments.

As physical therapists, we must be generally familiar with communication equipment for two reasons. First, our interaction with children in the therapeutic environment necessarily requires our ability to communicate with them. This brief synopsis is intended to broadly familiarize the reader with various types of communication devices that may be encountered. A second reason for physical therapists to have an understanding of adaptive communication systems is that many of these strategies require controlled movement as the user interface. Knowing about these systems can help the physical therapist address movement issues to facilitate the child's successful use of a communication strategy. The physical therapist at times may work closely with a speech and language pathologist in developing appropriate motor control for a communication system.

Children with hearing impairment may need hearing aids, amplified telephones, or classroom amplification systems. They also use some of the gestural communication systems described in the next section, such as American Sign Language, which do not require adaptive technology.

Devices that use visual or vibratory cues to alert a hearing-impaired person to a telephone, doorbell, smoke alarm, alarm clock, or automobile horn are important aids for both function and safety. Using the telephone to communicate with persons who are non-hearing or hearing can be accomplished with a telecommunication device for the deaf (TDD) or video-relay technology via telephonic or internet connection.[5,6]

Persons with visual impairment use magnification devices, recorded books and newspapers, computerized reading systems that scan printed materials and produce synthesized speech or electronic Braille output, and braillers. Braillers have evolved from mechanical devices to computerized and computer-like devices that allow editing, read material back to the individual, and display in words and/or Braille.[5,6]

Augmentative communication strategies are classified as gestural, gestural assisted, or neuro-assisted.[121]

Gestural Strategies

Gestural strategies are unaided strategies, requiring no instrumentation, and therefore no adaptive equipment. Movement, generally of the face and upper extremities, is used to transmit messages visually. Smiling, nodding, shaking of the head, and other head and eye movements and hand gestures are typically used gestural communication strategies.

Additionally, several gestural communication systems may be used. These include American Sign Language (ASL), American Indian Hand Talk (Amer-Ind), finger spelling, eye-blink encoding, and gestural Morse code.[5,121–124]

Gestural Assisted Strategies

These aided communication strategies require adaptive equipment in the form of a communication board or display of a symbol system that is activated by gesture or movement. Users of this type of strategy use gestures to select components on the display to transmit their messages.[6,121,122]

Gestures may be direct movement of the head, upper extremity, or eyes. If head movements are used, a head pointer is required. Indirect use of movement occurs when the display is controlled by an electronic switching device activated by muscle contractions and includes the use of microcomputers. Movements used to activate mechanical switches include finger, head, foot, and eyebrow movements. Switches may be controlled by joysticks, pushbuttons (such as keyboards), pads, squeeze bulbs, and blowing or sucking on the end of a tube (sip and puff switches). Infrared sensing devices can be used with movement to select visual symbols, such as an infrared transmission module mounted on a head stick or eyeglasses.[119]

Gestural-assisted communication aids may simply be visual symbol sets such as photographs, drawings, the alphabet, and printed words on a display. This classification of communication strategies also includes several specific systems of symbols such as Picsyms, Sigsymbols, Blissymbols, and Rebuses.[6,121,122] Computerized communication boards known as voice output communication aids (VOCA) use gestural interfaces to directly select words, pictures, or symbols, employing switches activated by touch, joystick manipulation, a head pointer, eye gaze, or other available gestures. The output can be synthesized speech or digital speech.[5,6]

Gestural-assisted communication devices are available commercially. However, they are generally most effective for function when they are customized for a specific child. Computer software is now available to custom-create picture boards.[6]

Neuro-assisted Strategies

These aided communication strategies also use a display, but unlike the gestural assisted strategies that rely on gestural manipulation of a switching mechanism, this display is activated by bioelectrical or physiologic signals from the body. This type of device is most needed in the child with motor impairments so severe that the child is unable to control body movements adequately for gesturing. The same displays are used as in the gestural assisted systems, but the switches are controlled by surface electrodes on the scalp (electroencephalogram) or a selected muscle (electromyogram).[121] The evolving technologies of electrocorticography and intracortical recordings, both with brain–computer interfaces where electrodes are implanted in the brain, are neural-assisted technologies. Electrodermal technology uses skin electrodes to detect changes in skin conductivity through the autonomic nervous system.[119]

Environmental Controls

A person with a disability needs to function in a variety of environments. Therefore, the ability to perform specific functions in everyday life must be considered relative to context. Sometimes, a particular environment renders a person unable to effectively interact with and control the environment, making function more difficult or perhaps impossible. A person's inability to function within a particular context because of architectural or attitudinal barriers within a society has been termed a handicap by the WHO.[125] Environmental contexts in which a child must function vary, depending on the individual child and the age, interests, and family culture. Broadly, children need to function in the home, at play, and at school, and the older teenager may need to function in a work environment.

Environmental control systems are another subgroup of access technologies. Assistive technology appropriate to one environment can sometimes be modified to function in another environment. Alternatively, the environment can be modified to optimize a person's interaction with the environment with devices such as ramps, lifts, and grab bars.[4,120] Changing the environment may require architectural and/or landscaping adaptations and use of environmental access technologies. Eliminating functional architectural and landscaping barriers is beyond the scope of this chapter. However, an introduction to environmental control technologies is both fundamental and appropriate.

Depending on the age, a child needs a reasonable ability to control the home and play environment. The ability to control room lighting, television and radio, kitchen appliances, toys, ambient temperature, doors, windows, and window shades can greatly increase a child's independence and self-confidence. Controls can be separate for each device or integrated into an environmental control unit, a single device with switches to control multiple functions within the environment such as lights, kitchen appliances, and window drapes and shades.[5]

Controls can be low-tech, mid-tech, or high-tech. Environmental controls can have a variety of user interfaces, including movement of a hand, finger, or mouth stick to directly select a switch; electronic scanning, which allows the individual to select among choices; and coded access, which uses a code-activated signal to trigger switches.[5] Although the access technologies described above, including the emerging brain–computer interfaces, have been used mostly as communication access technologies, they have potential as means to control the environment as well.[119]

▶ Universal design

Universal design is a concept that refers to the development of products and environments that are universally usable, that is, usable by all people with or without disabilities. This idea is based on an understanding that all people can find certain types of equipment and environmental design to be helpful in daily life.[5,6] Ramps, elevators, automatic doors, recorded books, and talking computer software are examples of putting the concept of universal design into practice in today's society. As this concept continues to grow and be embraced by more people, the benefits for persons who have impairments and disabilities will also expand, improving access to better interactions with others and to more environments.

Tablet Computers, iPads, Androids, and Similar Devices

The growing industry of high-technology equipment such as tablet computers, iPads, Androids, smartphones, and e-readers exemplifies how universal design has been embraced in today's culture. These devices are developed and produced to increase the ease of, speed of, and access to communication, knowledge, and entertainment for people of all abilities. Children with impairments and disabilities are using these high-tech devices with increasing frequency, mostly for communication and entertainment. Some of these devices can be used, however, for environmental control, and they are extremely helpful in the classroom. These devices are portable, readily available, relatively inexpensive, and adaptable to a child's individual needs and abilities. Also, use of these ordinary high-tech devices emphasizes the similarities among children with and without disabilities. For a child, using devices that are used by peers rather than using medical devices can be empowering and motivating.

SUMMARY

The purchase, building, and use of adaptive equipment can be complex and time-consuming aspects of pediatric physical therapy. These processes are further complicated by the lack of strong evidence to help with appropriate and objective choice of equipment. The available options are so numerous and ever changing that even the most experienced physical therapist is unlikely to feel that all equipment has been considered before making a choice. The safest and most realistic approach to the selection of adaptive devices for children lies in a theoretic construct based on: (1) careful evaluation of the child, (2) assessment of the environments in which the child functions, and (3) assessment of the family and other caregivers. The goals and abilities of the child must be agreed upon before therapeutic needs can be met with various types of equipment. When this information is known, the therapist can develop a therapeutic program that includes safe and effective use of equipment without unwanted negative effects. When the child's needs and goals are considered, the specific details of the numerous devices available become less intimidating and confusing. Frequent reevaluation by the therapist will ensure that the child receives continuing benefits from adaptive equipment. Input from teachers, aides, parents, and the child will provide valuable feedback regarding the child's use of the equipment. The scheme suggested in this chapter provides the therapist with a framework for documenting the needs of the child, selecting or making appropriate equipment, evaluating the effects of the equipment, and reassessing the child's status periodically.

Anyone procuring or fabricating equipment on a regular basis should keep records on the various devices, manufacturers, and vendors used. Records should indicate ease of fit, wear of the device (how well it holds up over time), acceptance or criticism from patients and families, and the efficiency of customer service, including the elapsed time from placement of an order to delivery of equipment. Records are a useful resource for future recommendations and orders. In addition, the records may provide the basis for quantitative data regarding effectiveness of and deficiencies in various adaptive devices. Perhaps the compilation of these data can serve to help the profession evolve from an art to a science in the matter of adaptive equipment.

Keeping abreast of new developments and trends in the field of adaptive equipment is essential to optimize function in the children whom physical therapists evaluate and treat. The professional literature and the internet are two of the best resources to help therapists generate ideas for using adaptive aids and equipment and to stay informed.

REFERENCES

1. World Health Organization. Towards a common language for functioning, disability and health ICF. http://www.who.int/classifications/icf/training/icfbeginnersguide.pdf. Accessed December 16, 2012.
2. Murchland S, Parkyn H. Promoting participation in schoolwork: assistive technology use by children with physical disabilities. *Assist Technol*. 2011;23:93–105.
3. Desch LW, Gaebler-Spira D. Prescribing assistive-technology systems: focus on children with impaired communication. *Pediatrics*. 2008;121:1271–1280.
4. Ostensjo S, Carlberg EB, Vollestad NK. The use and impact of assistive devices and other environmental modifications on everyday

activities and care in young children with cerebral palsy. *Disabil Rehabil.* 2005;27(14):849–861.

5. Peterson JM, Hittie MM. *Inclusive Teaching: The Journey Towards Effective Schools for All Learners.* 2nd ed. Upper Saddle River, NJ: Pearson Education Inc; 2010.

6. Dell AG, Newton DA, Petroff JG. *Assistive Technology in the Classroom: Enhancing the School Experiences of Students with Disabilities.* 2nd ed. Boston, MA: Pearson Education Inc; 2012.

7. George Mason University. Assistive technology initiative. Equity and diversity services. http://ati.gmu.edu/what_ati.cfm. Accessed July 11, 2013.

8. Copley J, Ziviani J. Barriers to the use of assistive technology for children with multiple disbilities. *Occup Ther Inter.* 2004;11(4):229–243.

9. Angelo DH. Impact of augmentative and alternative communication devices on families. *Augmentative Alt Commn.* 2000;16:37–47.

10. Carpe A, Harder K, Tam C, et al. Perceptions of writing and communication aid use among children with a physical disability. *Assist Technol.* 2010;22:87–98.

11. Jones MA, McEwen IR, Hansen L. Use of power mobility for a young child with spinal muscular atrophy. *Phys Ther.* 2003;83:253–262.

12. Arva J, Paleg G, Lange M, et al. RESNA position on the application of wheelchair standing devices. *Assist Technol.* 2009;21:161–168.

13. Rosen L, Arva J, Furumasu J, et al. RESNA position on the application of power wheelchairs for pediatric users. *Assist Technol.* 2009;21:218–226.

14. Tieman BL, Palisano RJ, Gracely EJ, et al. Gross motor capability and performance of mobility in children with cerebral palsy: a comparison across home, school, and outdoors/community settings. *Phys Ther.* 2004;84(5):419–429.

15. Kerfeld CI, Dudgeon BJ, Engel JM, et al. Development of items that assess physical function in children who use wheelchairs. *Pediatr Phys Ther.* 2013;25:158–166.

16. Mieres AC, Lam J. Commentary on development of items that assess physical function in children who use wheelchairs. *Pediatr Phys Ther.* 2013;25:167.

17. Bottos M, Bolcati C, Sciuto L, et al. Powered wheelchairs and independence in young children with tetraplegia. *Dev Med Child Neurol.* 2001;43(11):769–777.

18. Butler C, Okamoto GA, McKay TM. Powered mobility for very young disabled children. *Dev Med Child Neurol.* 1983;25:472–474.

19. Isaacson M. Best practices by occupational and physical therapists performing seating and mobility evaluations. *Assistive Technol.* 2011;23:13–21.

20. Wisconsin Assistive Technology Initiative. AT assessment forms. http://www.wati.org/?pageLoad=content/supports/free/index.php. Accessed July 26, 2013.

21. Georgia Project for Assistive Technology. AT consideration checklist. http://www.gpat.org/Georgia-Project-for-Assistive-Technology. Accessed Oct 6, 2013.

22. University of Kentucky Assistive Technology (UKAT) project. UKAT toolkit. http://edsrc.coe.uky.edu/www/ukatii/. Accessed July 26, 2013.

23. Patient reported outcomes measurement information system (PROMIS). Dynamic tools to measure health outcomes from the patient perspective. http://www.nihpromis.org. Accessed April 11, 2012.

24. Cella D, Yount S, Roghrock N, et al. The patient-reported outcomes measurement information system (PROMIS): progress of an NIH roadmap cooperative group during its first two years. *Med Care.* 2007;45(5)(suppl 1):S3–S11.

25. Wheelchair seating and assessment guide. New York. 2009. https://www.emedny.org/providermanuals/DME/PDFS/Wheelchair%20evaluation%20template%203-09.pdf. Accessed October 6, 2013.

26. Marshall J. Infant neurosensory development: considerations for infant child care. *Early Childhood Educ J.* 2011;39:175–181.

27. Rodrigues LP, Saraiva L, Gabbard C. Development and construct validation of an inventory for assessing the home environment for motor development. *Res Q Exer Sport.* 2005;76(2):140–148.

28. Abbott AL, Bartlett DJ, Kneale Fanning JE, et al. Infant motor development and aspects of the home environment. *Pediatr Phys Ther.* 2000;12:62–67.

29. Venetsanou F, Kambas A. Factors affecting preschoolers' motor development. *Early Childhood Educ J.* 2010;37:319–327.

30. Bartlett DJ, Fanning JK, Miller L, et al. Development of the daily activities of infants scale: a measure supporting early motor development. *Dev Med Child Neurol.* 2008;50(8):613–617.

31. Kelly Y, Sacker A, Schoon I, et al. Ethnic differences in achievement of developmental milestones by 9 months of age: the millennium cohort study. *Dev Med Child Neurol.* 2006;48(10):825–830.

32. Mayson TA, Harris SR, Bachman CL. Gross motor development of Asian and European children on four motor assessments: a literature review. *Pediatr Phys Ther.* 2007;19:148–153.

33. National Science Foundation. http://www.nsf.gov/discoveries/disc_summ.jsp?cntn_id=103153. Accessed April 27, 2013.

34. Tripathi R, Joshua AM, Kotian MS, et al. Normal motor development of Indian children on Peabody developmental motor scales- 2 (PDMS-2). *Pediatr Phys Ther.* 2008;20:167–172.

35. Countries and their Cultures. http://www.everyculture.com/index.html. Accessed April27, 2013.

36. Banks MJ, Benchot RJ. Unique aspects of nursing care for Amish children. *MCN Am J Matern Child Nurs.* 2001;26(4):192–196.

37. Weyer SM, Hustey VR, Rathbun L, et al. A look into the Amish culture: what should we learn? *J Transcult Nurs.* 2003;14(2):139–145.

38. American Physical Therapy Association Section on Pediatrics. Fact sheet: assistive technology and the individualized education program. 2007. www.pediatricapta.org. Accessed June 1, 2013.

39. Judge SL. Accessing and funding assistive technology for young children with disabilities. *Early Childhood Educ J.* 2000;28(2):125–131.

40. Porterfield SL, DeRigne L. Medical home and out-of-pocket medical costs for children with special health care needs. *Pediatrics.* 2011;128:892–900.

41. Shattuck PT, Parish SL. Financial burden in families of children with special health care needs: variability among states. *Pediatrics.* 2008;122:13–18.

42. Mitchell JM, Gaskin DJ. Do children receiving supplemental security income who are enrolled in Medicaid fare better under a fee-for-service or comprehensive capitation model? *Pediatrics.* 2004;114:196–204.

43. American Physical Therapy Association Section on Pediatrics. Fact sheet: resources on reimbursement for pediatric physical therapy services and durable medical equipment. 2007. www.pediatricapta.org. Accessed June 1, 2013.

44. The Early Childhood Technical Assistance Center. Assistive technology funding sources. http://ectacenter.org/topics/atech/funding.asp. Accessed July 28, 2013.

45. Catalyst center. The TEFRA Medicaid and state plan option and Katie Beckett waiver for children: making it possible to care for children with significant disabilities at home. http://hdwg.org/catalyst/tefraindicator. Accessed July 28, 2013.

46. Children's Health Insurance Program. State and federal funding for CHIP. http://www.medicaid.gov/CHIP/CHIP-Program-Information.html. Accessed July 28, 2013.

47. Reimbursement Committee of the Section on Pediatrics, APTA. Fact sheet: what providers of pediatric physical therapy services should know about Medicaid. 2009. www.pediatricapta.org. Accessed October 17, 2012.

48. Pass It On Center–The National AT Reuse Center. http://www.passitoncenter.org/Home.aspx. Accessed July 28, 2013.

49. Pass It On Center–The National AT Reuse Center. Reuse locations. http://passitoncenter.org/locations/search.aspx. Accessed July 28, 2013.

50. AbleData. State assistive technology projects resource center. http://www.abledata.com/abledata.cfm?pageid=113573&top=16050&ksectionid=19326. Accessed July 28, 2013.

51. Sneed RC, May WL, Stencel C. Policy versus practice: comparison of prescribing therapy and durable medical equipment in medical and educational settings. *Pediatrics.* 2004;114:e612–e625.

52. Rifton. Components of a letter of medical necessity. http://www.rifton.com/adaptive-mobility-blog/letter-of-medical-necessity-tram-transfer-mobility-device/. Accessed June 12, 2013.

53. Rifton. Sample letter of medical necessity for a medical feeding chair. http://www.rifton.com/adaptive-mobility-blog/sample-ot-letter-medical-necessity-rifton-feeding-chair/. Accessed June 12, 2013.

54. National Assistive Technology Technical Assistance Partnership. What should be in a letter of medical necessity? http://www.resnaprojects.org/nattap/goals/other/healthcare/mednec.html. Accessed June 12, 2013.

55. Johnson KL, Dudgeon B, Kuehn C, et al. Assistive technology use among adolescents and young adults with spina bifida. *Am J Public Health.* 2007;97:330–336.

56. Reiss J, Gibson R. Health care transition: destinations unknown. *Pediatrics.* 2002;110:1307–1314.

57. Committee On Child Health Financing. Scope of health care benefits for children from birth through age 26. *Pediatrics.* 2012;129(1):185–189.

58. Cooley WC. Providing a primary care medical home for children and youth with cerebral palsy. *Pediatrics.* 2004;114;1106–1113.

59. Marks A. On making chairs more comfortable—how to fit the seat to the sitter. *Fine Woodworking.* 1981;31:11.

60. Keegan J. Alterations in the lumbar curve related to posture and sitting. *J Bone Joint Surg.* 1973;35A:7.

61. Akerblom B. *Chairs and sitting.* Paper presented at: the Symposium on Human Factors in Equipment Design; 1954; Sweden.

62. Knutsson B, Lindh K, Telhag H. Sitting: an electromyographic and mechanical study. *Acta Orthop Scand.* 1966;37:415–426.

63. Dicianno BE, Arva J, Lieberman JM, et al. RESNA position on the application of tilt, recline, and elevating legrests for wheelchairs. *Assist Technol.* 2009;21:13–22.

64. Keegan J. Evaluation and improvement of seats. *Industr Med Surg.* 1962;31:137–148.

65. Batavia M. *The Wheelchair Evaluation: A Clinician's Guide.* 2nd ed. Sudbury, MA: Jones and Bartlett Publishers; 2010.

66. Bergan A. *Positioning the Client with Central Nervous System Deficits: the Wheelchair and Other Adapted Equipment.* 2nd ed. New York, NY: Valhalla Press; 1985.

67. Nwaobi O, Brubaker C, Cusick B, et al. Electromyographic investigation of extensor activity in cerebral palsy children in different seating positions. *Dev Med Child Neurol.* 1983;25:175–183.

68. Low SA, Westcott McCoy S, Beling J, et al. Pediatric physical therapists' use of support walkers for children with disabilities: a nationwide survey. *Pediatr Phys Ther.* 2011;23:381–389.

69. Damcott M, Blochlinger S, Foulds R. Effects of passive versus dynamic loading interventions on bone health in children who are nonambulatory. *Pediatr Phys Ther.* 2013;25:248–255.

70. Paleg GS, Smith BA, Glickman LB. Systemic review and evidence-based clinical recommendations for dosing of pediatric supported standing programs. *Pediatr Phys Ther.* 2013;25:232–247.

71. Olson DA, DeRuyter F. *Clinician's Guide to Assistive Technology.* St. Louis, MO: Mosby; 2002.

72. Jones MA, McEwen IR, Neas BR. Effects of power wheelchairs on the development and function of young children with severe motor impairments. *Pediatr Phys Ther.* 2012;24:131–140.

73. Guerette P, Furumasu J, Tefft D. The positive effects of early powered mobility on children's psychosocial and play skills. *Assist Technol.* 2013;25(1):39–48.

74. DiGiovine C, Rosen L, Berner T, et al. RESNA position on the application of ultralight manual wheelchairs. 2012. http://resna.org/resources/position- papers/UltraLightweightManualWheelchairs.pdf. Accessed Jul 13, 2013.

75. Boninger ML, Baldwin M, Cooper RA, et al. Manual wheelchair pushrim biomechanics and axle position. *Arch Phys Med Rehabil.* 2000;81(5):608–613.

76. Lin J, Shinohara M. The effects of wheelchair configuration on propulsion efficiency. RESNA Annual Conference; 2013. Available at: http://www.RESNA.org. Accessed Aug 6, 2013.

77. Segway. Segway technology and advanced development. http://www.segway.com/about-segway/segway-technology.php. Accessed July 12, 2013.

78. Weiss TC. Segway-a legal personal assistive device? http://www.disabled-world.com/assistivedevices/mobility/segway.php. Accessed July 12, 2013.

79. Sawatzky B, Denison I, Langrish S, et al. The Segway personal transporter as an alternative mobility device for people with disabilities: a pilot study. *Arch Phys Med Rehabil.* 2007;88:1423–1428.

80. Sawatzky B, Denison I, Tawashy A. The Segway for people with disabilities: meeting clients' mobility goals. *Am J Phys Med Rehabil.* 2009;88(6):484–490.

81. Wagstaff BL. Make way for segways: mobility disabilities, segways, and public accommodations. *George Mason Law Rev.* 2013;20(2):247–359. Available at: http://www.georgemasonlawreview.org/doc/Wagstaff_Website.pdf. Accessed July 12, 2013.

82. Segway seat: the glideseat. http://www.glideseat.com/. Accessed July 12, 2013.

83. Furumasu J, Guerette P, Tefft D. Relevance of the pediatric powered wheelchair screening test for children with cerebral palsy. *Dev Med Child Neurol.* 2004;46(7):468–474.

84. Tefft D, Guerette P, Furumasu J. Cognitive predictors of young children's readiness for powered mobility. *Dev Med Child Neurol.* 1999;41:665–670.

85. O'Shea R, Boyniewicz K. Commentary on effects of power wheelchairs on the development and function of young children with severe motor impairments. *Pediatr Phys Ther.* 2012;24:140.

86. Ragonesi CB, Chen X, Agrawal S, et al. Power mobility and socialization in preschool: follow-up case study of a child with cerebral palsy. *Pediatr Phys Ther.* 2011;23:399–406.

87. Huang H, Galloway JC. Modified ride-on toy cars for early power mobility: a technical report. *Pediatr Phys Ther.* 2012;24:149–154.

88. Campos D, Goncalves VG, Guerreiro MM, et al. Comparison of motor and cognitive performance in infants during the first year of life. *Pediatr Phys Ther.* 2012;24:193–198.

89. Ragonesi CB, Galloway JC. Short-term, early intensive power mobility training: case report of an infant at risk for cerebral palsy. *Pediatr Phys Ther.* 2012;24:141–148.

90. Ambrosio F, Boninger ML, Koontz AM, et al. *A model-based criterion for assessing appropriateness of wheelchair setup.* Paper presented at: RESNA 27th International Annual Conference; 2004; Orlando, Florida. Available at: http://www.RESNA.org. Accessed Aug 6, 2013.

91. U.S Government Printing Office. Standard No. 202a; Head restraints; mandatory applicability begins on September 1 2009. http://www.gpo.gov/fdsys/granule/CFR-2010-title49-vol6/CFR-2010-title49-vol6-sec571-202a/content-detail.html. Accessed July 20, 2013.

92. Brubaker C. Ergonomic considerations. *J Rehabil R D [Clin Suppl].* 1990;27:37–48.

93. Rehabilitation Engineering and Assistive Technology Society of North America. RESNA position on the Application of Ultralight Manual Wheelchairs. 2012. http://resna.org/resources/position-papers/UltraLightweightManualWheelchairs.pdf. Accessed March 20, 2013.

94. Meiser MJ, McEwen IR. Lightweight and ultralight wheelchairs: propulsion and preferences of two young children with spina bifida. *Pediatr Phys Ther.* 2007;19(3):245–253.

95. LoveLace-Chandler V, Early D. Commentary on "Pediatric physical therapists' use of support walkers for children with disabilities: a nationwide survey." *Pediatr Phys Ther.* 2011;23:390.

96. Mulholland Positioning Systems Inc. http://mulhollandinc.com/category/gait_trainers/. Accessed February 19, 2013.

97. Rifton. Rifton pacer gait trainers. www.Rifton.com/Pacer. Accessed February 19, 2013.

98. Flaghouse Giant Leaps Special Needs Products. www.flaghouse.com. Accessed October 3, 2012.

99. Pin T, Eldridge B, Galea MP. A review of the effects of sleep position, play position, and equipment use on motor development in infants. *Dev Med Child Neurol.* 2007;49(11):858–867.

100. Vander Loop L. How to safely move your child: lift system options. http://cpfamilynetwork.org/blogs/how-to-safely-move-your-child-lift-system-options. Accessed January 8, 2013.

101. Berg MD, Cook L, Corneli HM, et al. Effect of seating position and restraint use on injuries to children in motor vehicle crashes. *Pediatrics*. 2000;105:831–835.

102. Car seats: information for families for 2013. http://www.healthychildren.org/English/safety-prevention/on-the-go/pages/Car-Safety-Seats-Information-for-Families.aspx. Accessed April 3, 2013.

103. Korn T, Katx-Laurer M, Meyer S, et al. How children with special needs travel with their parents: observed versus reported use of vehicle restraints. *Pediatrics*. 2007;119(3):e637–e642.

104. O'Neil J, Yonkman J, Talty J, et al. Transporting children with special health care needs: comparing recommendations and practice. *Pediatrics*. 2009;124(2):596–603.

105. Carseats and seatbelt guards. http://www.especialneeds.com/pediatrics- seating-mobility-carseats-seatbelt-guards.html. Accessed January 8, 2013.

106. Committee on Injury and Poison Prevention. School bus transportation of children with special health care needs. *Pediatrics*. 2001;108(2):516–518.

107. RESNA. RESNA's position on wheelchairs used as seats in motor vehicles. Available at: http://resna.org/resources/position- papers/RESNAPositiononWheelchairsUsedasSeatsinMotorVehicles.pdf. Accessed July 2, 2013.

108. eSpecial needs. Britax Traveller Plus EL http://www.especialneeds.com/special-needs-carseat-britax-standard-traveller-plus.html. Accessed July 20, 2013.

109. National Highway Traffic Safety Administration. Summary of vehicle occupant protection laws Ninth Edition. 2011. http://nhtsa.gov. Accessed May 2, 2013.

110. National Highway Traffic Safety Administration. Transporting students with special needs for school bus drivers. http://nhtsa.gov. Accessed May 2, 2013.

111. Bull M, Agran P, Laraque D, et al. Transporting children with special health care needs. *Pediatrics*. 1999;104(4, pt 1):988–992.

112. Garrett M, McElroy AM, Staines A. Locomotor milestones and babywalkers: cross sectional study. *Br Med J*. 2002;324:1494.

113. Ridenour M. Infant walkers: developmental tool or inherent danger? *Percept Mot Skills*. 1982;55:1201–1202.

114. Crouchman M. The effects of babywalkers on early locomotor development. *Dev Med Child Neurol*. 1986;28:757–761.

115. Kauffman I, Ridenour M. Influence of an infant walker on onset and quality of walking pattern of locomotion: an electromyographic investigation. *Percept Mot Skills*. 1977;45:1323–1329.

116. Consumer Product Safety Commission. Baby walkers: advance notice of proposed rulemaking. *Fed Reg*. 1994;59:39306–39311.

117. Shields BJ, Smith GA. Success in the prevention of infant walker-related injuries: an analysis of national data, 1990–2001. *Pediatrics*. 2006;117:452–459.

118. Consumer product safety commission. Nursery products: injury statistics. http://www.cpsc.gov/en/Research--Statistics/Toys-and-Childrens-Products/Nursery- Products/. Accessed May 4, 2013.

119. Tai K, Blain S, Chau T. A review of emerging access technologies for individuals with severe motor impairments. *Assist Technol*. 2008;20(4):204–219.

120. Hammel J. Technology and the environment: supportive resource or barrier for people with developmental disabilities? *Nurs Clin N Am*. 2003;38:331–349.

121. Silverman F. *Communication for the Speechless*. 3rd ed. Needham Heights, MA: Allyn & Bacon; 1995.

122. Musslewhite CR, Ruscello DM. Transparency of three communication symbol systems. *J Speech Hearing Res*. 1984;27:436–443. Available at: http://www.asha.org/. Accessed January 11, 2012.

123. O'Brien M. Hand talk—preserving a language legacy. http://www.nsf.gov/. Accessed January 11, 2013.

124. National Federation of the Blind. Communication methods. 2013. http://nfb.org/deaf-blind-resources. Accessed January 11, 2013.

125. Barbotte E, Guillemin F, Chau N, et al. Prevalence of impairments, disabilities, handicaps and quality of life in the general population: a review of recent literature. *Bul World Health Org*. 2001;79:1047–1055.

Musculoskeletal Disorders

Orthopedic Management

Michael DiIenno

Musculoskeletal Development
Musculoskeletal Examination
History
Postural Screen
Range of Motion
Strength
Lower Extremity Alignment (Rotational and Angular)
Classification of Errors of Morphologic Development
Congenital Limb Deficiencies
Nonsurgical and Surgical Management of Congenital
Limb Deficiencies
Prosthetic Training
Prenatal Deformations
Congenital Muscular Torticollis
Congenital Metatarsus Adductus and Clubfoot Deformity

Developmental Dysplasia of the Hip
Arthrogryposis Multiplex Congenita
Postnatal Deformations
Rotational Deformities
Dysplasias
Osteogenesis Imperfecta
Joint Hypermobility Syndromes
Pathologic Processes
Legg–Calvé–Perthes Disease
Slipped Capital Femoral Epiphysis
Tibia Vara (Blount Disease)
Limb Length Discrepancy
Scoliosis (Idiopathic)
Summary

T he term *orthopedics* in pediatric physical therapy is often used to refer to a specific group of pediatric diagnoses. Within the profession of physical therapy, orthopedics refers to a subspecialty of practice. As the profession has increased its focus on specialization and board certification, pediatric orthopedics has begun to emerge as a subspecialty within a specialty. Many medical professions have a tendency to compartmentalize their profession and the patients they see by body systems, such as children with orthopedic disabilities or children with neurologic disabilities. This practice lends itself to specialization or the development of clinical expertise in a well-defined area. However, this practice also may fragment the care of patients and even the thinking of the professionals involved.

The various systems of the body are intertwined, and normal or atypical influences on one system almost always have an impact on other body systems. This is especially true of a young child whose musculoskeletal system is immature and susceptible to external and internal influences. The action of muscles working within a normal neurologic system is necessary for the development of joints and the shape and contour of a child's bones. When the neurologic or muscular systems are altered or impaired, many times secondary skeletal impairments develop.

This chapter discusses the growth and development of a child's musculoskeletal system and pediatric musculoskeletal assessment, introduces a classification system based on morphogenesis, and provides an overview of pediatric orthopedic diagnoses commonly encountered by pediatric physical therapists. This chapter contains the term *orthopedic* in the title and focuses on specific orthopedic diagnoses. However, the effects of normal and atypical forces on an immature musculoskeletal system and the secondary impairments that may develop, as well as the discussion of the components of a pediatric musculoskeletal assessment, can be applied to many children seen in pediatric physical therapy. For example, most children with a primary diagnosis of neurologic origin present with impairments of their musculoskeletal system that may impact their overall function.

▶ Musculoskeletal development

The formation of the musculoskeletal system occurs during the embryonic period (second to eighth week postconception). The limb buds arise from mesenchymal cells and appear during the fourth week, with the upper limb developing 2 days ahead of the lower limb. Mesenchymal cells begin to differentiate into cartilage within 4 to 5 days of the formation of the limb bud. The formation of a cartilaginous skeleton occurs rapidly and is completed during the first fetal month (3 months from conception). The cartilaginous template then begins to be replaced by bone with the appearance of primary ossification centers in the diaphysis of the long bones. Secondary ossification centers appear near the end of fetal development and remain until puberty, when skeletal growth is complete.[1,2]

Joint formation begins as the cartilaginous template is being formed. An area of flattened undifferentiated cells forms between two areas of cartilage. The flattened area transforms into three layers, and the peripheral layers maintain contact with the cartilage and eventually become the joint capsule. The middle layer cavitates and forms the joint cavity. The original cartilage at the interface of the joint capsule remains and becomes the articular cartilage.[1,2]

The extremities are susceptible to major morphologic abnormalities during the embryonic period when the limb buds are developing. For example, exposure of the embryo to pharmacologic agents while the limb buds are forming may result in congenital limb deficiencies. During the fetal period, structures increase in size and cartilage begins to be replaced by bone formation; however, minimal bone remodeling occurs. During this time, the fetus is more susceptible to minor morphologic abnormalities that are the result of position constraints and abnormal mechanical forces.[2] For example, torticollis or clubfeet may result from position constraints late in the pregnancy. Postnatally, much bone remodeling occurs at a rapid rate of 50% annually in the infant and toddler and gradually slows to the adult rate of 5% annually.

Bone grows in length through the continuation of the process of endochondral ossification begun during the fetal period. Endochondral ossification is often referred to as epiphyseal growth because longitudinal growth occurs at the epiphyseal plate. Increases in the diameter of bone or bone thickness occur through appositional growth or the laying down of new bone on top of old bone. These two types of bone growth respond differently to mechanical loading and the forces associated with weight bearing and muscle pull. Appositional bone growth is stimulated by increased compressive forces. Increased weight bearing results in increased thickness and density of the shaft of the tibia.[3,4] However, decreased weight bearing, as seen with immobilization, results in atrophy of the bone.[3]

The response of epiphyseal growth to mechanical forces is dependent on the direction, magnitude, and timing of the force. Intermittent compressive forces applied parallel to the direction of growth cause longitudinal bone growth; however, constant compressive forces of excessive or high magnitude retard bone growth.[5] A compressive force may be applied unevenly across the physis, resulting in slowing of growth on one side only. The uneven growth produces an angulation of the physis and changes the direction of growth.[3] Mechanical loads or forces that are applied perpendicular to the longitudinal growth of the bone result in a change of direction or deflection of bone growth. New growth is deflected and results in displacement of the epiphysis if the load is maintained. A torsional stress to the physis deflects columns of cartilage around the circumference of the physis in either a clockwise or counterclockwise direction. New bone then grows away from the physis in a spiral pattern resulting in a torsional deformity.

In summary, the growth and development of the musculoskeletal system is dependent on the normal interplay of multiple factors, including hormones, nutrition, and mechanical forces.[5,6] The immature musculoskeletal system is vulnerable to abnormal mechanical forces and pressures; alterations in the timing, direction, or magnitude of forces may have a deleterious effect on the growing and developing musculoskeletal system. Congenital deformities and secondary musculoskeletal impairments that are seen in children with neurologic diagnoses are examples of the vulnerability of the immature musculoskeletal system to abnormal extrinsic forces. However, the immaturity of a child's musculoskeletal system can also be an advantage and is often used as the rationale for many treatment interventions that will be discussed throughout this chapter.

▶ Musculoskeletal examination

A thorough musculoskeletal examination should be part of a comprehensive evaluation of a child seen by a physical therapist. Depending on the history or diagnosis, certain aspects of the musculoskeletal examination should be performed while other aspects may be omitted. However, for those children with a diagnosis that includes multiple joint or system involvement, a complete musculoskeletal examination should be performed beginning as a postural screen with a more in-depth examination dependent on the findings of the initial screening. The examination should be completed in a timely and organized manner in the order outlined in the following sections. The order may be altered depending on the comfort and interaction of the child.

History

A thorough history should be obtained from the parents and the child if the child is able to convey the information to the examiner. The history should include information regarding onset of the presenting complaint, whether pain is present, what aggravates or alleviates the pain, any changes in alignment, activity or participation noted, and a comparison with normal routines. While talking with the parents, the physical therapist should be observing the child's posture, play, spontaneous movements, and activities with relevance to the child's posture, noted asymmetries, and difficulty with age-appropriate skills. For older children, questions regarding sexual maturation including Tanner staging for males and females as well as age at onset of menstruation should be considered to provide information related to bone age and development.[7]

Postural Screen

During the postural screen, the therapist examines skeletal alignment in a variety of positions, including anterior, posterior, and lateral views, depending on the age of the child. This process should include head, spinal, and lower extremity alignment, limb length, and upper extremity position. The therapist looks for typical upright head, cervical lordosis, thoracic kyphosis, lumbar lordosis, pectis excavatum or carinatum, and anterior or posterior pelvic tilt relative to the age of the child from a lateral view. From the posterior view, the physical therapist visually notes symmetry of shoulder, scapulae, pelvic height, and lateral rib asymmetries, such as a rib hump, that would indicate a rotational deformity of the spine. An anterior view can help identify asymmetries in nipple height, lateral rib position, and pelvic height.

Lower extremity alignment should also be screened from a sagittal view as well as an anterior and posterior view. The therapist looks at symmetry of pelvic height; rotational variations of the lower extremities, such as the knees or feet pointing in or out; and a valgus or varus position of the knees, forefoot, or hindfoot. From a sagittal view, the physical therapist assesses pelvic position and alignment of the hip, knee, and ankle.

Limb length should be reviewed in both a weight-bearing and non–weight-bearing position using the accepted bony landmarks of the anterior superior iliac spine and the medial malleolus. The posterior superior iliac spine may also be included to determine the presence of innominate bone up or down slip. The postural screen will direct the physical therapist to where to focus the next portion of a more in-depth musculoskeletal assessment.

Range of Motion

Although the goniometric techniques used to measure active or passive joint range of motion (ROM) in children and adults are similar, several factors must be kept in mind when assessing ROM in children. Age-related differences exist in ROM values between adults and infants and young children. For example, a full-term newborn will exhibit flexion contractures of the hips and knees secondary to intrauterine positioning.

Before any goniometric measurement is taken, attention must be given so that the child is relaxed and remains calm. Movements should be slow so as to limit anxiety and to avoid eliciting a stretch reflex in children with increased muscle tone. Slow movements should also be used if pain is present or suspected and for those children who may have more brittle bones or recent fractures.

Reliability studies of goniometry in children should guide physical therapists in their use of goniometric measures to document ROM. Several researchers have investigated the reliability of goniometric measurement of the hip, knee, and ankle of children with cerebral palsy. High intrarater reliability was present in those studies, but interrater reliability was variable from moderate to high throughout the studies.[8,9,10,11] Improved reliability is observed with strict measurement protocols and when the same therapist assesses changes in ROM over time.

Muscle length tests should also be included in the overall joint motion assessment. Specific tests and their procedures do not differ from standard procedures used with the adult population. Hip flexor muscle length is assessed using the Thomas test or the prone hip extension test. Hamstring length is usually assessed in adults using the straight leg raise test; however, the popliteal angle (PA) measurement is commonly used in pediatrics (Fig. 13.1). The PA measurement can be used in the presence of a knee flexion contracture; therefore, it is useful for children who present with involvement of multiple joints.[12] Ankle dorsiflexion should be measured with the knee flexed and extended to determine soleus and gastrocnemius contributions to limitations. Care should be taken to maintain subtalar joint neutral during the measurement to minimize midfoot dorsiflexion contributing to an overestimated hindfoot measurement.

Overall joint mobility should be measured using techniques such as the Beighton Score to determine the presence of generalized joint hypermobility.[12a]

Strength

An accurate assessment of strength requires careful consideration in the pediatric population but yields important information regarding deficits and changes over time. A variety of methods to assess strength are available, and their use may depend on the age and ability of the child. For infants and children younger than 3 or 4 years, assessment of strength is most often accomplished through observation of movement and function. Compensatory movement, poor dynamic alignment, or asymmetric movement between sides may be indicative of muscle weakness. A child must be able to follow the directions of the testing procedure to ensure accurate results using either manual muscle testing (MMT) or dynamometry.[13] Strength may also be reliably measured using isokinetic machines with some positioning modification to accommodate for small size or the use of pediatric extremity attachments as seen in the Biodex System 4.[14,15]

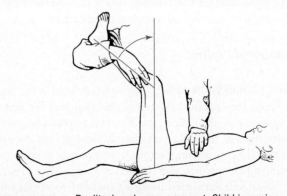

FIGURE 13.1 Popliteal angle measurement. Child is supine, hip is flexed to –90 degrees, and the knee is slowly extended until resistance is felt. The angle between the anterior aspect of the lower leg and a vertical line corresponding to the thigh is recorded as a measure of hamstring contracture.

MMT has the same inherent weaknesses with the pediatric population as with adults. The grades of "good" and "normal" are very subjective and do not account for any changes that may occur in a child over time, secondary to maturation. Handheld dynamometry has been found to be a reliable and sensitive method of assessing strength in various populations of children.[16–18] Gajdosik determined that handheld dynamometry could be used reliably with typical developing children between the ages of 2 and 5 years as long as they could follow the directions and understand the command to push as well as agree to participate in the process.[19] Normative and percentile values for isokinetic knee extension and flexion strength have been published by multiple authors for children aged 6 to 13 years.[20,21] Along with functional performance, these strength measures provide additional objective data to consider when determining a child's readiness to return to recreational or competitive sports.

Lower Extremity Alignment (Rotational and Angular)

Normal skeletal development includes rotational or torsional and alignment changes of bones and joints. These normal developmental processes may be altered secondary to abnormal muscle pull or weight-bearing forces. Consequently, impairments that impact function often result from the combination of abnormal forces on a developing skeletal system. The bones remain susceptible to deforming forces until growth is complete; therefore, the impairments may increase in severity over time.

Staheli et al. have developed a rotational profile to assess lower extremity alignment and assist in determining which component of the lower extremity contributes to the rotational variation. The rotational profile consists of six measurements: (1) foot progression angle (FPA), (2) medial rotation of the hip, (3) lateral rotation of the hip; (4) thigh–foot angle (TFA), (5) angle of the transmalleolar axis, and (6) configuration of the foot. Normal values have been established for the first five measurements and can be used to determine whether the variation falls within the wide range of normal or whether intervention is indicated.[22]

Rotational Profile

FOOT PROGRESSION ANGLE The FPA is defined as the angle between the longitudinal axis of the foot and the line of progression of the child's gait. The FPA provides an overall summation of the child's rotation during gait, but does not identify the contributing factors. A positive sign denotes out-toeing and a negative sign denotes in-toeing. The FPA can be objectively measured using a variety of footprint measures, including ink or chalk on the feet or more expensive commercially available gait mats. Many times in the clinic, the FPA is assessed subjectively to give the clinician an overall view of the child's rotation during gait. The procedures listed in the following sections assist the clinician with identifying the contributing factors to the overall rotational profile of the child (Fig. 13.2A).

HIP ROTATION Medial and lateral hip rotation in prone are assessed to determine femoral torsion. The child is in prone with hips in neutral and knees flexed to 90 degrees, and medial and lateral hip rotation measurements are then taken goniometrically. Soft tissue limitations may influence the final measure of hip rotation as well as the degree of femoral torsion. Normal medial hip rotation is less than 60 to 65 degrees (Fig. 13.2B, C).

The literature also describes a second test of femoral torsion referred to as Ryder test. The child sits or lies in prone with knees flexed to 90 degrees over the edge of a table. The greater trochanter is palpated while rotating the leg. When the greater trochanter is palpated most laterally, which should correspond to the femoral neck being parallel to the examining table, the angle of hip rotation (typically medial) is measured goniometrically. The measure of medial hip rotation should correspond to the degree of femoral anteversion, although data compared to computed tomography (CT) suggest that the test may underestimate the measurement by up to 20 degrees.[8,23]

THIGH–FOOT ANGLE The child is in the prone position with the hips extended, the knee flexed to 90 degrees, and the foot in a natural resting position; do not attempt to align the foot. The angle formed from the bisection of the axis of the thigh and the axis of the foot is measured. This TFA is used to determine rotational variation of the tibia and the hindfoot. If the foot is in an out-toeing position, the value is positive; if the foot is in an in-toeing position, the value is negative (Fig. 13.2D).

TRANSMALLEOLAR AXIS The child is positioned in prone, as previously described. A line perpendicular to the axis between the lateral and medial malleoli is drawn. The angle formed between the perpendicular line and the axis of the thigh is measured. This angle assesses the contribution of the distal tibia to the rotational profile (Fig. 13.2E).

The contribution of the foot must also be included when assessing rotational variations. Identifying the alignment of the hindfoot and forefoot in subtalar joint neutral will determine if hindfoot or forefoot varus or valgus deviations, hindfoot equinus with midtarsal hypermobility, or metatarsus adductus is contributing to the FPA.

Angular Alignment

If the initial postural screening revealed suspected lower extremity alignment deviations, such as a varus or valgus posture, an objective angular measurement should be performed. Expected values for genu varus and valgus will differ depending on the age of the child. Genu varum is measured with the child in supine with legs extended and

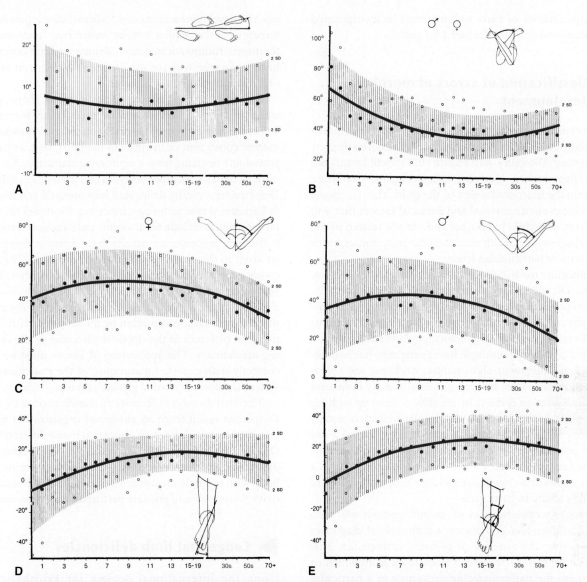

FIGURE 13.2 The five measurements in Staheli's rotational profile plotted as the mean values plus or minus 2 standard deviations (SDs) for each of the age groups. The dark line indicates the mean values as they change with age, and the shaded areas indicate the normal ranges. **(A)** Foot progression angle (FPA). **(B)** Lateral rotation of the hip in males and females. **(C)** Medial rotation of the hip in females and males (separate). **(D)** Thigh–foot angle (TFA). **(E)** Angle of the transmalleolar axis.

the patella facing upward and the medial malleoli touching. The distance between the femoral condyles is measured. Genu valgus is measured in the same position but with the knees touching. The distance between the malleoli is measured.[24] The contribution of angular variations must be delineated from rotational variations.

Additional areas that may be included in the musculoskeletal assessment include assessment of muscle tone, sensation testing, and developmental skill level. An assessment of muscle tone may reveal hypertonicity or hypotonicity of specific muscle groups and an imbalance of muscle forces around specific joints. These unbalanced muscle forces may produce impairments over time that cause pain or interfere with the child's functional abilities.

Sensation testing is performed with children just as with adults and incorporates the same rationale for inclusion of testing. Sensory testing is indicated when nerve involvement is suspected, such as with fractures or after an amputation or application of an external fixator.

Assessment of a child's developmental level is indicated if the orthopedic condition is suspected of delaying or interfering with development as seen with dysplasias and torticollis. For the ambulatory child, this includes an assessment of gait. Gait assessment is similar to assessing an adult and can be performed through systematic clinical observation or with more objective measures, ranging from video analysis to an instrumented gait laboratory. The age of the child must be considered when assessing gait, and knowledge of the characteristics of early walking must be incorporated into the assessment (see Chapter 5 for gait).

 ## Classification of errors of morphologic development

The terminology adopted by the World Health Organization's (WHO) International Classification of Functioning, Disability, and Health (ICF)[25] will be utilized in this chapter when discussing various diagnoses and their impact on the functional ability of the child. The ICF model also includes environmental and personal factors that will differ from one child to another and are not related to the child's diagnosis or health condition but may impact his or her activity or participation levels.

To illustrate the ICF model, a child with osteogenesis imperfecta (OI) will be used as an example. For a child with OI, the pathophysiology is the abnormality in the connective tissue at the cellular level. One of the impairments that results is fragile bones susceptible to deforming forces and fracture. The child may sustain multiple lower extremity fractures resulting in misalignment, short stature, weakness, and a slow labored gait. The slow labored gait is an activity limitation that may lead to an inability of the child to keep up with his or her peers during play or at school. Participation restrictions may include not permitting the child to attend a day care of peers or to play outside at recess owing to a fear of increased risk of fractures. Environmental factors such as a teacher's fears or a crowded recess area have contributed to the child's ability to participate.

Spranger's classification of morphogenesis will also be used to introduce and discuss a multitude of diagnoses that fall under the category of pediatric orthopedics. This classification system provides a framework from which to understand the pathophysiology resulting in a particular diagnosis, the impairments that may develop as the child grows, the impact of the impairments on the child's activities and participation levels, and how physical therapy may have an impact. With an understanding of the pathophysiology, the reader will be able to identify impairments that may be present or may develop and the impact of physical therapy on preventing or limiting the impairments, with the ultimate goal of minimizing the activity limitations and participation restrictions for the child.

Spranger's classification of disorders of morphogenesis consists of four divisions: malformations, disruptions, deformations, and dysplasias.[26] Malformations are morphologic defects of an organ or body part from an intrinsically abnormal developmental process. Because the abnormality is intrinsic from the moment of conception, the organ or body part never had the potential to develop normally. Examples of malformations include longitudinal limb deficiencies, cleft lip and palate, and septal defects of the heart.

Disruptions are morphologic defects of an organ or body part resulting from the extrinsic breakdown of an originally normal developmental process. Normal development is interrupted at the cellular level by an external factor such as a teratogen, trauma, or infection. Transverse limb deficiencies historically seen with the use of thalidomide are an example of a disruption.

Deformations are abnormalities in form, shape, or position of a body part caused by mechanical forces. The deforming forces may be extrinsic to the fetus, such as intrauterine constraint, or intrinsic to the fetus, such as fetal hypomobility resulting from a neuromuscular defect. Examples of deformations include torticollis and metatarsus adductus. Deformations can be delineated into prenatal and postnatal deformities versus pathologic processes. Examples of postnatal deformities include tibial varum and rotational variations. Pathologic processes are usually deformities as the result of an insult to the physis or other area of the bone. These processes include the diagnoses of Legg–Calvé–Perthes disease, slipped capital femoral epiphysis, and limb length discrepancies resulting from insults or abnormal forces to the growth plate. Deformations can often be ameliorated with the application of forces in the opposite direction of the deforming mechanism. The application of forces must be timed correctly with expected maturation of the musculoskeletal system to allow for normal growth and remodeling to occur.

The final division in Spranger's classification is dysplasia. Dysplasias result from an abnormal organization of cells into tissues, which leads to abnormal tissue differentiation. OI and Ehlers Danlos Syndrome (EDS) are examples of dysplasias. Dysplasias usually involve whole systems of the body with multiple impairments present that will lead to activity limitations and possibly participation restrictions.

Congenital limb deficiencies

Using the International Society for Prosthetics and Orthotics (ISPO) classification system, congenital limb deficiencies are described as either longitudinal or transverse (Fig. 13.3A, B).[27] Longitudinal limb deficiencies are described as reduction or absence of an element or elements within the long axis of the limb. There may be normal skeletal elements distal to the affected bone or bones.[27] A longitudinal limb deficiency is an example of a malformation in which a morphologic defect of an organ or larger region of the body occurs when normal organogenesis is interrupted. Any combination of skeletal limb involvement is possible, but certain distinct entities are more commonly seen than others. For this chapter, congenital longitudinal deficiency of the radius will be used as an example of upper extremity involvement and proximal femoral focal deficiency (PFFD) as an example of a lower extremity longitudinal limb deficiency. Both are examples of congenital malformations and are more frequent in their incidence; they are also examples of children with limb deficiencies typically seen by therapists.

Longitudinal deficiency of the radius, often commonly referred to as radial clubhand, occurs in 1 per 100,000 live

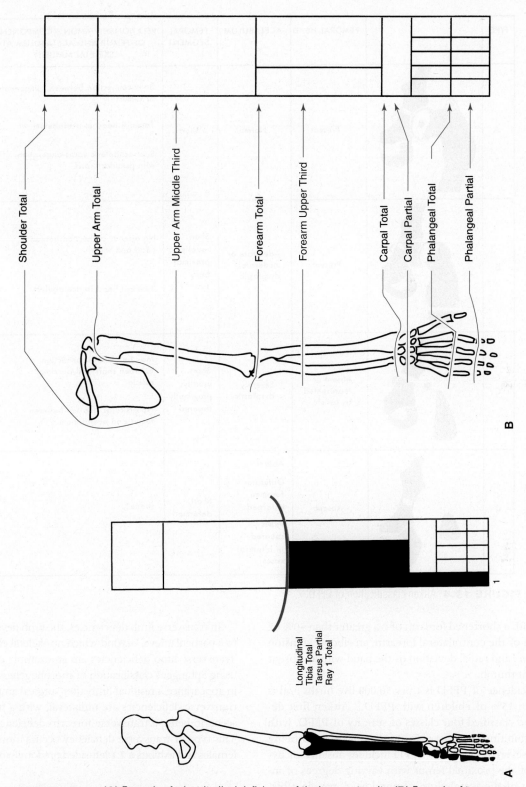

FIGURE 13.3 **(A)** Example of a longitudinal deficiency of the lower extremity. **(B)** Example of transverse deficiencies at various levels of the upper extremity.

births, with bilateral involvement present in 50% of the children. Radial deficiencies can be defined as the failure of formation of parts of deficiencies on the radial side of the upper extremity, including the radius, carpals, metacarpals, and phalanges of the first ray and thenar musculature.[28,29]

Heikel classified radial deficiencies into four types, ranging in severity from type I (consisting of delayed appearance of the distal radial physis) to type IV (involving complete absence of the radius).[30] Type IV is the most common presentation.[24] Clinically, children with type IV radial deficiency

TYPE		FEMORAL HEAD	ACETABULUM	FEMORAL SEGMENT	RELATIONSHIP AMONG COMPONENTS OF FEMUR AND ACETABULUM AT SKELETAL MATURITY
A	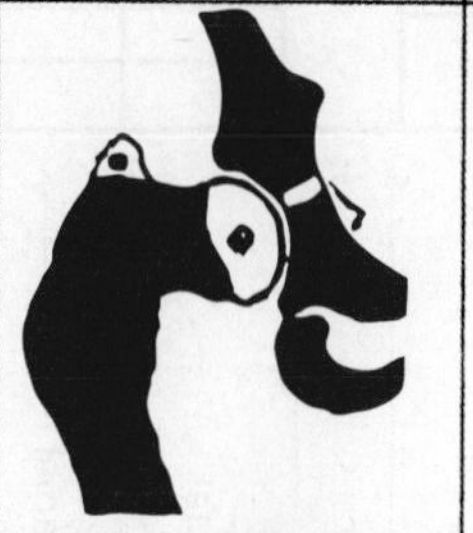	Present	Normal	Short	Bony connection between components of femur Femoral head in acetabulum Subtrochanteric varus angulation, often with pseudarthrosis
B	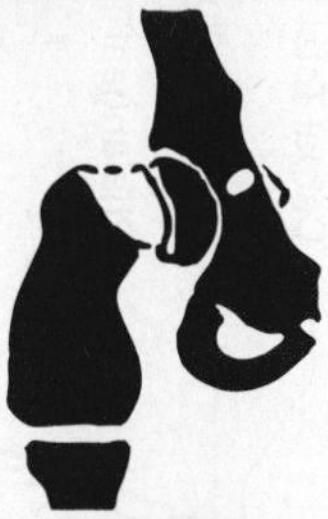	Present	Adequate or moderately dysplastic	Short, usually proximal bony tuft	No osseous connection between head and shaft Femoral head in acetabulum
C	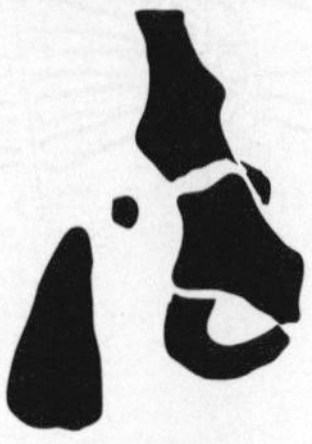	Absent or represented by ossicle	Severely dysplastic	Short, usually proximally tapered	May be osseous connection between shaft and proximal ossicle No articular relation between femur and acetabulum
D	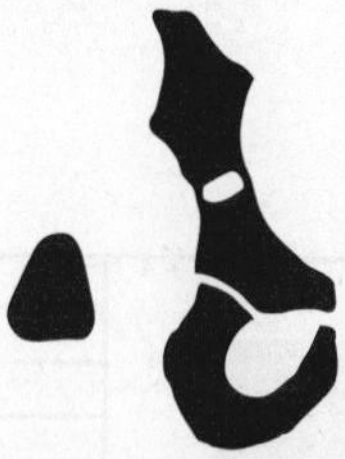	Absent	Absent Obturator foramen enlarged Pelvis squared in bilateral cases	Short, deformed	(none)

FIGURE 13.4 Aitken classification of PFFD.

present with a shortened forearm of no greater than 50% of the length of the contralateral forearm, an elbow extension contracture, and radial deviation of the hand with an absent or deficient thumb.

The incidence of PFFD is 1 per 50,000 live births and is bilateral in 15% of children with PFFD.[31] Aitken first described and classified four classes of severity of PFFD, with class A exhibiting the least involvement and class D being the most severe (Fig. 13.4).[32] PFFD includes absence or hypoplasia of the proximal femur with varying degrees of involvement of the acetabulum, femoral head, patella, tibia, fibula, cruciate ligaments, and the foot. Clinically, infants with PFFD present with an abnormally short thigh held in hip flexion, abduction, and external rotation (Fig. 13.5). Hip and knee flexion contractures are often present along with anteroposterior instability of the knee and a significant leg length difference, with the foot of the involved leg often at the height of the opposite knee.

In transverse limb deficiencies, the limb develops normally to a particular level beyond which no skeletal elements exist.[27] Transverse limb deficiencies are an example of a disruption using Spranger's classification of morphogenesis and resemble in appearance a residual limb after surgical amputation. Most transverse deficiencies are unilateral, with a frequently seen scenario being a transverse forearm deficiency (Fig. 13.6).[28] This type of transverse deficiency occurs more frequently in females and exhibits a 2:1 left-sided predominance.[33]

Nonsurgical and Surgical Management of Congenital Limb Deficiencies

Children with longitudinal limb deficiencies often require multiple surgical procedures to obtain maximal function of the involved limb. Surgical procedures may include tendon transfers, realignment or repositioning of the hand and/or fingers, and osteotomies for the upper extremity, and most

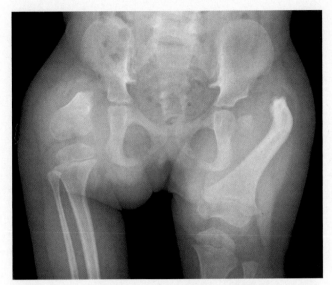

FIGURE 13.5 Radiograph of a child with bilateral PFFD with asymmetric involvement of each femur, tibia, and fibula.

commonly include a combination of amputation, fusion, limb lengthening, and osteotomies for lower extremity limb deficiencies. Surgical correction is rarely required for children with transverse limb deficiencies.

Upper Extremity: Longitudinal Radial Deficiency

Shortly after birth, the child's hand should be serially splinted or casted to stretch the shortened soft tissues and

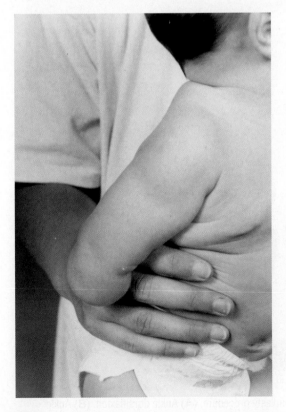

FIGURE 13.6 Child with congenital transverse below-elbow limb deficiency.

realign the hand as centrally as possible over the distal fore-arm. At the same time, therapy goals should also focus on increasing elbow ROM, especially elbow flexion. Stretching of the soft tissues is necessary before any surgical procedures. Between 6 months and 1 year of age, centralization of the hand by an orthopedic surgeon is often performed. The goal of centralization is a stable wrist centered on the distal ulna while maintaining functional wrist motion.[34]

Postoperatively, the child's hand is splinted in the newly aligned position on the distal ulna. Compliance with wearing of the splint is crucial for long-term success of the surgical centralization. The splint should be worn throughout the day and night during the healing phase. After the initial healing phase is complete, a splint should be worn at night until skeletal maturity is achieved. By skeletal maturity, the ulna has undergone epiphyseal adaptation to accommodate the centralized carpus to ensure stability of the wrist position, and use of a night splint is no longer necessary.[34]

Centralization of the hand is contraindicated in older children or adolescents who have adapted to their hand position, when severe deformity of the hand is also present that would limit hand function and when elbow flexion is less than 90 degrees. Adequate elbow flexion is needed prior to surgery so that when the hand is realigned, the child is still able to bring his or her hand to the mouth.

Lower Extremity: PFFD

Surgical intervention for children with PFFD is varied, must be individualized, and can include any combination of amputation, reconstruction, fusion, or limb-lengthening procedures. Surgery addresses the issues of the unstable hip joint and the inequality of limb lengths, the two issues that interfere with the child's overall functional abilities. Many children require multiple surgical procedures; thought must be given early to develop a long-term surgical plan for family education and to condense surgeries into one procedure when possible. Surgery is generally not recommended for children with bilateral PFFD, because their limb length is equal or near equal and they are able to ambulate with or without extension prostheses.[24,35,36]

Surgical options can be divided into those that involve amputation and reconstruction for eventual prosthetic fitting and those that involve limb-lengthening techniques. Three typical surgical scenarios include: foot amputation with proximal reconstruction, rotationplasty, and limb lengthening. Following foot amputation with proximal reconstruction, the child's limb resembles and functions as an above-knee amputation. Using an extension prosthesis on an existing residual limb is a nonsurgical approach to treatment that has been associated with greater patient satisfaction over amputation-type procedures.[37] A rotationplasty, or the turnabout procedure, is a surgical technique that allows the child to function similarly to a child with a below-knee amputation. This complex procedure involves significant limb reconstruction, including 180-degree re-alignment of the lower leg. As a result, the child's ankle then functions as a knee joint, with ankle plantar flexion acting as knee extension and ankle dorsiflexion acting as knee flexion (Fig. 13.7).[24,38] Limb lengthening may be indicated when more than 60% of predicted femoral length is present[35,39] or the discrepancy in femoral length is predicted to be less than 15 cm. An in-depth description of limb-lengthening procedures is provided later in this chapter under section Limb Length Discrepancies.

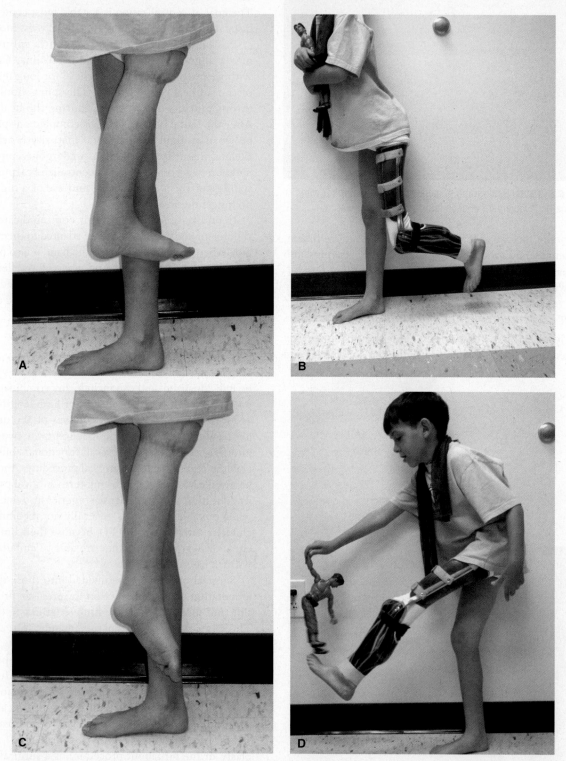

FIGURE 13.7 An 11-year-old boy who underwent a rotationplasty procedure. **(A)** Ankle dorsiflexion. **(B)** Ankle dorsiflexion produces prosthetic knee flexion. **(C)** Ankle plantar flexion. **(D)** Ankle plantar flexion produces prosthetic knee extension.

Prior to surgical intervention, physical therapy should be initiated in early infancy to improve ROM at the involved hip, promote developmental activities (including symmetry of skills and weight bearing at the age-appropriate times), and assist with the development of age-appropriate balance skills.

Postoperatively, acute physical therapy interventions will depend on the procedure and will involve improving or maintaining ROM, strength, and balance in preparation for prosthetic training. ROM and stretching activities of the ankle (now the functioning knee) following a rotationplasty are essential to ensure proper prosthesis movement and functional lower extremity alignment. Maximum plantar flexion range is needed to promote knee extension in the prosthesis. Sitting and other activities involving knee flexion will require close to 20 degrees of ankle dorsiflexion. Strengthening of these muscle groups is also important; ankle plantar flexion and dorsiflexion strength provides stability in stance and powers the prosthesis during gait. Recent literature has reported good long-term functional and quality-of-life outcomes but with persistent gait deviations following rotationplasty procedures.[40]

Prosthetic Training

Physical therapy intervention should begin before the fitting of the initial prosthesis. During infancy, physical therapy may be initiated on a weekly basis or a consultative basis, depending on the needs of the child and the family. Infants with a longitudinal limb deficiency have contractures or ROM limitations that must be addressed before surgery or prosthetic fitting. The infant with a radial deficiency requires stretching of the soft tissues, including passive exercises and splinting before surgery. The infant with PFFD requires ROM exercises to increase hip extension and adduction motions before surgery or prosthetic fitting. Infants with transverse limb deficiencies rarely exhibit contractures.

Infants with congenital limb deficiencies should also be monitored for their developmental skills. Symmetry of skills is emphasized as well as weight-bearing skills through both the upper and the lower extremities. Early weight-bearing skills promote proximal joint stability that may be needed later to use a prosthesis. Children with an upper extremity transverse limb deficiency are usually fitted with a prosthesis by 6 months of age when they begin simple two-handed activities. Children with lower extremity limb deficiencies are generally fitted with a prosthesis between 8 and 10 months, when they begin weight-bearing skills.

When an infant or child first receives a prosthesis, the fit, alignment, and overall function are assessed. The child and family must be shown the proper donning and doffing techniques, instructed in a wearing schedule, and shown how to check the skin for redness or possible breakdown. The initial goal is for the infant or toddler to accept wearing the prosthesis and gradually increase the wearing time throughout the day. The prosthesis is usually removed for naps and should be removed when going to sleep for the night.

Upper Extremity Prosthetic Training

An infant's first prosthesis has a terminal device that is soft and cosmetically appealing but nonfunctional (Fig. 13.8). A more functional terminal device is added when the child begins to engage in bimanual play. Functional terminal devices are either voluntary opening or voluntary closing. Voluntary-opening terminal devices open as the child reaches forward with the arm, whereas voluntary-closing devices mimic reaching and grasping and close as the child reaches forward to grasp an object.

The initial goals for an infant or young toddler are to wear the prosthesis, become adjusted to the weight of the prosthesis, and begin to use the prosthesis for propping in prone or sitting and bimanual skills. By the age of 15 to 18 months of age, training on the use of an active terminal device should begin (Fig. 13.9). The child is taught to open the terminal device, grasp an object, and then release the object.[41] If the child has an above-elbow prosthesis, the elbow is locked when the child is initially learning to control the terminal device so that the child only learns one movement at a time. The child with an above-elbow limb deficiency activates the terminal device through scapular movements and a cable connected to the terminal device.

Some clinicians and parents may opt to have a young toddler fitted with an externally powered myoelectric device. Initially, the child is fitted with a myoelectric hand that opens when one electrode is activated through forearm muscle contraction. By 3 to 4 years of age, the child's myoelectric hand can be converted to two electrodes so that both opening and closing of the hand are controlled by the child.[42]

As the child progresses, the use of the terminal device should include manipulation of small objects and using the prosthesis as the helper hand to hold paper for writing or coloring, holding the handlebars of a tricycle, feeding, and dressing. Expectations need to be reasonable, because the child will use the uninvolved hand as the dominant hand. By school age, the child should be independent with self-care activities including dressing, toileting, and eating. Activities should always focus on independence with age-appropriate skills. By the time the child is in high school, he or she may want to participate in various activities, including sports, driving, and social events. Various terminal device options are available to promote participation in numerous sports and to facilitate driving and control of the steering wheel, and cosmetic terminal devices are available for social times when cosmesis may be more important than function. The child, teenager, and young adult should always be a part of the discussion for therapy goals and prosthetic options.

Lower Extremity Prosthetic Training

An infant or toddler younger than 2 years of age may be fitted with a prosthesis without a knee joint. The goals for initial prosthetic training are toleration of the prosthesis and to begin standing weight-bearing activities. The prosthesis will interfere with the child's method of floor mobility and will

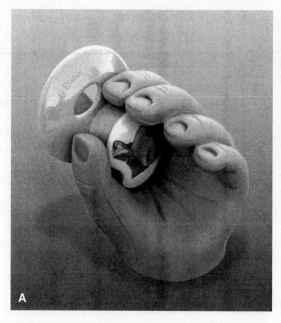

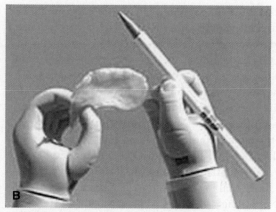

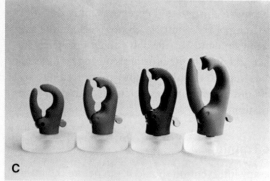

FIGURE 13.8 Terminal device options: **(A)** Passive Infant Alpha Hand (TRS, Boulder, CO). **(B)** L'il E-Z Hand promotes grasping when thumb is moved (TRS, Boulder, CO). **(C)** ADEPT voluntary closing hand (TRS, Boulder, CO).

require an adjustment period by the child. Initial standing activities should include transitions in and out of standing at a support, weight-shift activities in preparation for gait and balance reactions, and protective skills. Gait training may be

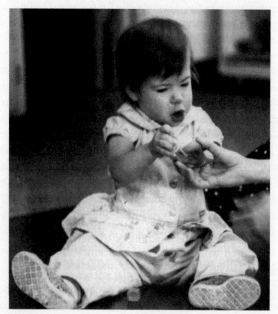

FIGURE 13.9 Child is wearing a left below-elbow prosthesis with an ADEPT voluntary closing hook. Therapist assisting child to operate the terminal device.

initiated with an assistive device; the assistive device is often discarded voluntarily by the child when it is no longer necessary. During the early preschool years, a prosthesis with a knee should be introduced to the child. Various prosthetic knee options are available that provide additional stability during the early years.

Several clinics now use articulated prosthetic knees for toddlers in their initial prosthesis. The prosthetic knee allows more typical movements seen in toddlers such as crawling, squatting, and kneeling and promotes a more normal gait pattern (Fig. 13.10).[43,44] Previously, it was difficult to fit an articulating knee in the small shank of a toddler's prosthesis, but advances in prosthetic design have enabled prosthetists to overcome this challenge.

Growth is an issue with children and lower extremity prostheses. Young infants and toddlers can outgrow their prosthesis every 6 months. For this reason, many prosthetists will fit a child with a prosthesis that accommodates some growth, stage the introduction of components, and utilize components that can be replaced as the child grows. For toddlers, spacers can be added to increase the length of the prosthesis and prolong the fit and use of the prosthesis. However, children will typically need to have their prosthesis replaced every 9 to 12 months because of growth and durability issues.

Some older children may require a second prosthesis or additional distal components for specific activities such as sports or water activities.

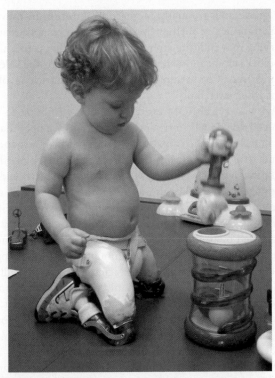

FIGURE 13.10 Toddler wearing bilateral transfemoral prosthesis with knee joint to promote age-appropriate ambulation skills and play activities on the floor.

▶ Prenatal deformations

A deformation is an abnormal form, shape, or position of a part of the body caused by mechanical forces. Deformations are normal responses of the tissue to abnormal mechanical forces that may be extrinsic or intrinsic to the fetus. Intrauterine constraint is an example of an extrinsic force, whereas fetal hypomobility secondary to a nervous system impairment such as myelomeningocele is an example of an intrinsic force. If the deforming force is removed, normal development or maturation of the body part would be expected to occur.

This chapter discusses congenital muscular torticollis (CMT) as an example of an extrinsic deformation and clubfeet as an example of either an extrinsic or intrinsic deformation. Both of these diagnoses may also have other causative factors; abnormal mechanical forces are only one of the possible contributing factors. Developmental dysplasia of the hip (DDH) is an example of a deformation that probably begins prenatally, continues to progress if the deforming forces are not altered, and may not be recognized until much later in postnatal life. Lastly, this section discusses arthrogryposis as an example of an intrinsic deformation that begins very early in fetal development and consequently results in significant deformations at birth and throughout later life.

Congenital Muscular Torticollis

The term torticollis comes from the Latin for twisted neck. CMT is a common form involving a unilateral shortening

TABLE 13.1	Head and neck features of CMT	
Left SCM Torticollis		**Right SCM Torticollis**
Left	Cervical lateral flexion	Right
Right	Cervical rotation	Left
Left	Frontal flattening	Right
Right	Occipital flattening	Left
Left	Jaw retraction	Right
Right	Pseudo-facial droop	Left

of the sternocleidomastoid (SCM) muscle. The infant with CMT presents with ipsilateral head and neck lateral flexion toward the shortened SCM, with contralateral head and neck rotation away from the shortened SCM. Facial asymmetry and plagiocephaly (flattening of the skull) often develop secondary to the persistent asymmetric positioning of the head. Table 13.1 summarizes the typical clinical presentation found in the head, neck, and face with CMT on each side. While the SCM may be the primary muscle involved, secondary shortening of other cervical muscles such as scalenes, levator scapulae, or upper trapezius occurs (Fig. 13.11).

CMT is usually noted in the first 2 to 3 weeks after birth, with a reported incidence of 0.4% to 1.9%.[45] The etiology of CMT is uncertain. A mass or fibrotic tumor is often observed or is palpable within the belly of the SCM muscle and appears within the first few weeks after birth and then gradually disappears. The exact cause of the fibrotic tumor within the SCM muscle is not known. Researchers

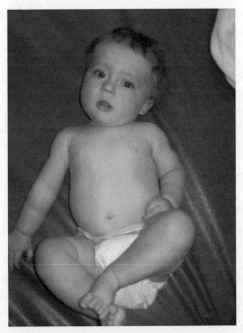

FIGURE 13.11 Infant with left congenital muscular torticollis. Note the facial asymmetry in the region of his mandible. (Used with permission from Taylor JL, Norton ES. Developmental muscular torticollis: outcomes in young children treated by physical therapy. *Pediatr Phys Ther.* 1997;9(4):173–178).

have hypothesized that occlusion of blood vessels with resultant anoxic injury to the SCM muscle may produce the fibrotic changes observed within the muscle. Intrauterine malposition and birth trauma have been hypothesized as causative factors.[46] Infants with CMT have a higher incidence of breech presentations[47] and associated congenital musculoskeletal diagnoses, such as hip dysplasia and foot deformities.[47,48]

Several authors propose that fibrosis of the SCM muscle is present in all children with CMT and ranges on a continuum of no palpable mass to a firm palpable mass.[47,48] Consequently, CMT is often classified into three clinical groups: (1) sternocleidomastoid tumor (SMT), when a definitive mass or tumor is palpable within the SCM muscle, (2) muscular torticollis (MT), when contracture of the SCM muscle is present but no palpable mass is present, and (3) positional torticollis (POST), when both contracture of the SCM muscle and a palpable mass are absent.[49,50]

The "Back to Sleep" program, initiated by the American Academy of Pediatrics in 1992 to reduce the incidence of sudden infant death syndrome (SIDS), recommended sleeping in supine for infants.[51] Since the inception of this program, SIDS rates have declined more than 50%, but the incidence of plagiocephaly and POST has increased dramatically.[52–54] The torticollis associated with positional plagiocephaly develops as a secondary impairment from the plagiocephaly. This is the direct opposite of what is seen with CMT, where the plagiocephaly develops secondary to the persistent asymmetric positioning of the head. Ultimately, the treatment for POST would follow an approach very similar to that for other forms of CMT.

A full systems review and a developmental screen are vital during the initial examination to rule out nonmuscular causes of torticollis. Almost 20% of cases of torticollis involve a more serious underlying condition, so it is important to consider an expanded differential diagnosis.[55] Physician specialist collaboration and diagnostic imaging may be necessary to rule out atlantoaxial rotary instability, hemivertibrae, cervical subluxation, posterior fossa tumors, Chiari malformations, ocular and vestibular abnormalities, and Grisel syndrome related to recurrent nasopharyngeal infection.

Conservative Management

Conservative management of CMT is generally recommended for infants 12 months and younger. Conservative management with direct physical therapist intervention includes prolonged passive stretching of the SCM muscle, active exercises to improve cervical ROM with subsequent strengthening exercises, and symmetric developmental activities to correct the infant's head, neck, and upper extremity position. Consistent caregiver education and a home exercise program (HEP) are essential to success. Passive SCM stretching can be achieved through positioning and handling techniques.[47,48] Stretching should be gentle and

low grade and gradually increase in duration to prevent microtrauma and further fibrosis.[50,56] Pain responses such as crying may indicate stretching intensity that is too high. Shoulder stabilization should be considered for the side of the involved SCM to address other cervical muscle involvement when stretching.

Active cervical ROM exercise including rotation to the involved side may be introduced in children younger than 3 to 4 months old who can visually track objects or respond to stimuli to attend to the involved side. For children older than 4 months, active cervical ROM and strengthening should be introduced via equilibrium and righting reactions[47,48] and developmental play promoting upper extremity weight bearing, weight shifting, and reaching. Intensity may be progressed by gradually increasing active head movement against gravity and duration or amount of unilateral upper extremity weight bearing during facilitation of play. Midline position for head and trunk should be emphasized as the child progresses from supported sitting to independent sitting and standing. Neutral shoulder girdle alignment should also be promoted with progression from supported to independent prone, quadruped, and reaching activities.

A heavy emphasis should be placed on caregiver education during each session with time provided for observation of HEP activities. "Tummy time" is the term used to encourage play in a prone position to facilitate active cervical movement and developmental play. Positional and stretching recommendations are important to address and incorporate into daily activities such as diaper changes, feeding, naps, play and use of equipment such as car seats, infant swings, and feeding chairs. For example, caregivers who bottlefeed should be encouraged to bottlefeed on the side that promotes rotation to the involved side, or gentle prolonged stretching may be better achieved while an infant is asleep during a nap.

Cheng reported that the most important predictors of successful response to manual stretching are the clinical group, neck rotation deficit, and age at initial presentation.[49] The POST type, neck rotation deficits of less than 15 degrees, and presentation less than 1 month old were associated with increased success of stretching protocols. Several other studies have demonstrated the success of conservative management during the first year.[47,48,56] None of these studies included a control group to assist with determining the extent of time and maturation on the resolution of the CMT. A treatment strategy algorithm based on age and cervical ROM was developed by Van Vlimmeren and colleagues based on the evidence currently available in the literature.[50]

Orthotic Devices

Plagiocephaly resulting from positioning should be treated in early infancy with a cranial orthosis aimed at correcting the cranial–facial asymmetry. There are a few band and helmet devices available commercially and through local vendors and certified orthotists, such as the Symmetry Through

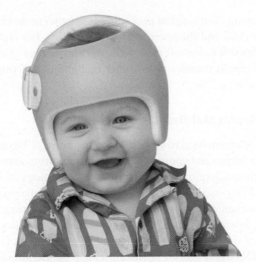

FIGURE 13.12 Infant wearing a STARband cranial orthosis to correct plagiocephaly. (Photo courtesy of Orthomerica Products© Inc; 2013)

Active Remolding (STARband®) orthosis, the Dynamic Orthotic Cranioplasty system (DOC band®), and other custom-molded helmets (Fig. 13.12). The cranial remolding devices apply pressure to the anterior and posterior prominences of the cranium, but allow growth in the flattened areas. A cranial orthosis is generally recommended between 3 and 4 months and not for children older than 12 months of age. The band or helmet is initially worn for 23 to 24 hours per day and then only while sleeping once symmetry is achieved.

It is difficult to draw conclusions for the use of helmets or cranial remolding orthoses to correct plagiocephaly as the population is not always defined and the studies often do not differentiate between plagiocephaly resulting from CMT or positional plagiocephaly.[57,58] Variability is evident in the length of the time for helmet versus no helmet intervention and outcome measurements and scores. There is agreement that helmets achieve cranial remolding more quickly compared with conservative interventions without a helmet, although long-term benefit may not outweigh the excessive cost associated with the devices.

A cervical orthosis may be beneficial for infants and young children with torticollis that is not responding to conservative treatment. The goal for an orthotic device is to help maintain cervical ROM or limit the ability to tilt toward the involved side. The TOT collar (tubular orthosis for torticollis) is a soft tubular collar with rigid struts of varying lengths that are positioned to elongate targeted muscles and limit motion in the opposite direction. The TOT collar is recommended for infants at least 4 months old who have a consistent head tilt of 5 degrees or greater for more than 80% of the day and perform all movements with a head tilt. Appropriate candidates for use of the TOT collar must also exhibit a minimum of 10 degrees of lateral neck flexion toward the noninvolved side or demonstrate the ability to laterally flex the head away from the involved side.[59]

Fabricated or modified foam soft collars may be used for infants that are unable to fit in a TOT collar. Cervical orthotic devices should be used only when the child is awake and supervised.

Persistent facial asymmetry, intermittent head tilt with fatigue or illness, and functional asymmetry resembling hemiplegia but with a normal neurologic examination have been observed in children with full resolution, indicating the complexity of this disorder as well as possible long-lasting implications.[47]

Surgical Management

Surgical treatment is indicated for infants with CMT that does not respond after 6 months of conservative treatment, who present with a residual head tilt, and who exhibit deficits of passive rotation and lateral flexion of the neck greater than 15 degrees and have a tight band or tumor.[49] The need for surgical intervention can also be predicted on the basis of classification of CMT, neck rotation deficit, and age at initial presentation. Cheng and colleagues followed 821 infants with CMT classified as SMT, MT, and postural torticollis (PT). Surgery was needed for 8% of the infants in the SMT group, 3% in the MT, and none in the PT group. Infants with greater than 15 degrees of neck rotation deficit and older ages at presentation were more likely to need surgery.[49]

Surgical intervention usually involves release of the muscle distally at one or both of the heads, depending on the severity; excision of a portion of the muscle may also be indicated.[24] Postoperatively, physical therapy is indicated for achieving and maintaining cervical ROM and for strengthening of musculature to maintain newly achieved alignment of the head.

ROM that fails to improve, worsening cranial asymmetry, and children older than 9 months at the time of presentation are all cause for concern during treatment programs. If left untreated, CMT may lead to increased facial and cranial asymmetries secondary to abnormal growth of soft tissues, including the SCM muscle and surrounding fascia and vessels. The development of a cervical scoliosis with compensatory thoracic curvature as well as ocular and vestibular impairments have been reported in cases of unresolved CMT.[24,46]

Congenital Metatarsus Adductus and Clubfoot Deformity

Metatarsus adductus is characterized by adduction of the forefoot in relation to the midfoot and hindfoot. The lateral border of the foot is convex with the curve beginning at the base of the fifth metatarsal resulting in the classic bean shape.[60] Metatarsus adductus is an example of a deformation caused by intrauterine positioning and is associated with other positional deformations, such as CMT and dysplasia of the hip.[61]

Metatarsus adductus is classified as mild Grade I with clinical correction of the foot beyond the lateral border, moderate Grade II with correction of the foot to a straight lateral border, or severe Grade III that does not correct to midline.[62] Severe metatarsus adductus may also be referred to as metatarsus varus and may include medial subluxation of the tarsometatarsal joint.[24]

Grades I and II metatarsus adductus resolve spontaneously without treatment by 4 to 6 months of age and account for about 95% of cases.[63–65] Infants with moderate or severe metatarsus adductus should be treated with serial casting until a flexible forefoot with proper alignment is achieved.[63] The height of the serial cast may need to extend above the knee to control any tibial rotation.

Clubfoot, or congenital talipes equinovarus, is a complex deformity involving ankle plantar flexion, hindfoot varus, and forefoot adduction and pronation. The incidence is 1 per 1000 live births, but the etiology is unclear.[60] Intrauterine positioning may be a causative factor in milder forms or when a primary neuromuscular impairment, such as myelomeningocele or arthrogryposis, is present. In the latter cases, decreased or absent fetal movement secondary to the primary neuromuscular impairment could lead to prolonged abnormal fetal positioning and the resultant clubfoot deformity at birth.

In the severe forms of congenital talipes equinovarus, pathologic deformities in the anatomy and alignment of the bony and cartilaginous structures of the foot are present. The muscles are also hypoplastic, giving an overall smaller appearance to both the foot and the lower leg on the involved side. The etiology may be a defect in the mesenchymal cells forming the template for the cartilaginous model of the hindfoot structures, indicating a dysplasia rather than a deformation.[24] More recently, the genetic and chromosomal abnormality links to idiopathic clubfoot are being uncovered.[66,67]

The goal of treatment for congenital clubfoot is to restore alignment and correct the deformity as much as possible and to provide a mobile foot for normal function and weight bearing. Initial treatment is begun shortly after birth. The Ponseti treatment method has demonstrated great success in reducing or eliminating the need for extensive corrective surgery.[68] It consists of serial casting with manipulation to correct the forefoot adduction and pronation and hindfoot varus along with percutaneous Achilles tenotomy to correct equinus. The cast extends above the knee to address medial tibial torsion that usually accompanies the foot deformity. Long-term post-correction brace use for up to 4 years is necessary to maintain correction.[68] Casting should continue until the foot achieves approximately 70 degrees of hyper abduction followed by 3 additional weeks to allow the Achilles tendon to heal. Children treated with the Ponseti method demonstrate minimally delayed achievement of gross motor milestones including ambulation.[69]

Surgical correction is usually performed before 6 months of age to limit the extent of secondary deformities from developing. The surgical procedure is dependent on the age of the child and the severity of the deformity, but typically includes soft tissue releases of the tight structures or an anterior tibialis transfer to promote realignment of the foot and ankle.

Developmental Dysplasia of the Hip

DDH is a term used to cover a broad spectrum of hip anomalies in infants and young children that result from abnormal growth and development of the joint. The etiology of DDH most likely includes multiple factors, such as malposition and mechanical factors in utero such as a small intrauterine space, hormone-induced ligamentous laxity, genetics, and cultural or environmental factors. The greatest risk factors for DDH are a breech position, female gender, first-born child, and a positive family history for DDH. The incidence of DDH is very variable and is dependent on environmental factors, age of diagnosis, and inclusion criteria for the diagnosis of DDH.[24] However, the incidence of DDH increases in infants with other congenital deformations, such as torticollis or metatarsus adductus.[61,70]

During early fetal development, the acetabulum is very deep, and the femoral head is spherical. Consequently, the femoral head is well covered by the acetabulum, and the hip is a stable joint. With fetal growth and development, the acetabulum increases in diameter and becomes shallower, providing less coverage for the femoral head. The shallow acetabulum, less rounded femoral head, and increased femoral anteversion values present normally in infants at birth result in a very unstable hip. In the immediate postnatal period, the depth of the acetabulum increases relative to diameter, producing a more stable ball-and-socket joint. The increased movement available to the newborn creates modeling forces that deepen the acetabulum as growth occurs. The most significant acetabular growth occurs during the first 18 months, and minimal acetabular growth occurs after 3 years of age.[2]

Any interference with the normal growth and development of the hip joint may result in DDH. Interference can include abnormal forces resulting from positioning and confined space in utero, positioning that restricts normal kicking movements postnatally, and abnormal or absent muscle pull in utero and postnatally. The timing of these factors impacts the severity of the joint changes. DDH, which results from malpositioning late in the last trimester, shows less anatomic changes and responds quickly to intervention compared with an infant whose hip development was affected early in fetal life. DDH in a newborn can be classified as subluxatable, dislocatable, subluxed, or dislocated (see Table 13.2).

Assessment

Newborn screening for DDH includes the Ortolani test and the Barlow maneuvers (Fig. 13.13A, B). Both of these tests are more reliable before 2 months of age and when the

TABLE 13.2	Classification of Newborn Infant's Hips
Classification	**Criteria**
Normal	No instability of hip joint
Subluxatable	Femoral head within the acetabulum but can be partially displaced out from under the acetabulum
Dislocatable	Femoral head within the acetabulum but can be fully dislocated using the Barlow maneuver
Subluxed	Femoral head rests partially out of the acetabulum but can be reduced
Dislocated	Femoral head is completely out of the acetabulum

infant is calm and not crying to facilitate soft tissue relaxation. As the infant grows, the unstable hip either remains in the acetabulum through normal development or remains outside the acetabulum and is prevented from relocating.

Therefore, the Ortolani and Barlow maneuvers are much less reliable for infants older than 2 to 3 months of age.[24,63] Additional signs that may be noted in the newborn period include asymmetry of thigh or gluteal folds, limitation of hip abduction ROM or asymmetric hip abduction ROM, and apparent unequal femoral lengths, referred to as Galeazzi sign. These signs become strong indicators of DDH in the older infant when the Ortolani or Barlow maneuvers are no longer reliable. In older children who are ambulatory, DDH is usually diagnosed by an abnormal gait pattern. Children with unilateral DDH exhibit a positive Trendelenburg sign, and children with bilateral DDH walk with a waddle.[24,63]

When DDH is suspected from your assessment, the infant is referred for an ultrasound or radiography, depending on his or her age. Ultrasound is used for young infants when ossification of the femoral head is minimal and would not be detected on radiography. Any time an infant

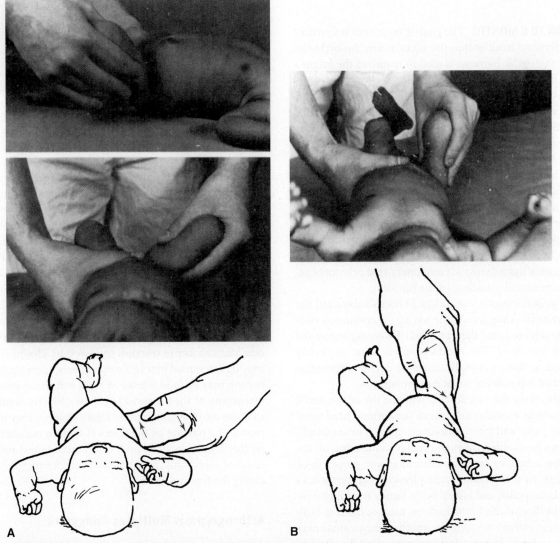

FIGURE 13.13 (A) The Ortolani maneuver. From a flexed and adducted position, the hip is abducted; the examiner feels a clunk as the femoral head moves into the socket. The examiner's other hand stabilizes the infant's pelvis. **(B)** The Barlow test. The examiner holds the infant's hip in flexion and slight abduction. The infant's hip is adducted while applying pressure in a posterior direction. Dislocation of the femoral head with pressure indicates an unstable hip.

is referred for physical therapy, regardless of diagnosis, hip stability should be assessed. If risk factors are present, such as breech presentation or other congenital deformities, and your assessment is normal, the infant may still benefit from a referral for an ultrasound to confirm that DDH is not present.

Management

The aim of treatment is to return the femoral head to its normal relationship within the acetabulum and to maintain this relationship until the abnormal changes reverse.[70] The earlier the treatment is initiated, the less abnormal changes are present in the structures of the hip joint and the less time is needed for the structures to return to their normal relationship. Treatment regimens will vary slightly between facilities and preference of the physician, but the same general concepts are followed in the management of infants and children with DDH.

NEWBORN TO 6 MONTHS The goal of treatment is to maintain the femoral head within the acetabulum. An orthosis, typically the Pavlik harness, is used to maintain the infant's hips in a flexed and abducted position.

The Pavlik harness consists of a shoulder harness with two anterior and two posterior straps, stirrups for the legs, and booties to secure the feet (Fig.13.14). In the Pavlik harness, the infant's hips are flexed 90 to 100 degrees, which locates the femoral head in the acetabulum. With the infant in supine, the hips are allowed to fall into abduction; they are not forced into abduction. The abducted position stretches the hip adductor muscles and allows the femoral head to slide over the posterior rim into the acetabulum. The anterior and posterior straps permit active hip flexion and abduction, but limit hip extension and adduction. Therefore, the Pavlik harness has a dynamic component that promotes active movement and modeling of the hip joint.

The Pavlik harness is worn 23 to 24 hours a day until the hip is stable; full-time use of the harness is continued after stability is achieved, and then a period of weaning out of the harness is instituted. The child's progress must be closely monitored to detect complications or decide alternative treatments if hip stability is not developing.

Complications that can develop with the use of the Pavlik harness include avascular necrosis of the femoral head, femoral nerve palsy, and inferior dislocation.[24,71] These complications can be avoided through regular monitoring of the child's hips, parent or caregiver education, and proper fit of the harness. At many centers, the physical therapist works with the orthopedist and instructs the family in proper donning and doffing of the Pavlik harness. In an outpatient facility, an infant you are treating for another impairment may be wearing a Pavlik harness. It is imperative that the physical therapist be knowledgeable in the fitting of the Pavlik harness and recognize signs of ill-fit when he or she is working with these infants.

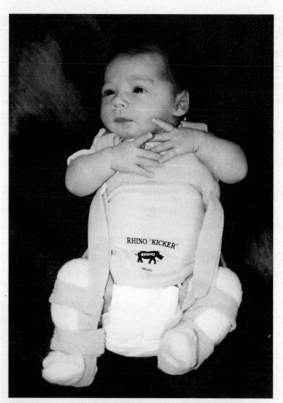

FIGURE 13.14 The Pavlik harness maintains the infant's hips in flexion and allows active movement of the hips into abduction. (Photo courtesy of RhinoPediatric Orthopedic Design, Inc.)

SIX TO 12 MONTHS After 6 months of age, it may become more difficult to relocate the femoral head in the acetabulum. Traction for a period of time may be attempted to relocate the hip and then institute wearing of the Pavlik harness. If the child is ambulatory, an abduction orthosis may be more practical than a Pavlik harness. Closed reduction under anesthesia may be required with the application of a hip spica cast to maintain the hip in the located position.[24]

AFTER 12 MONTHS Rarely will the child's hip be able to be relocated without surgical intervention. Conservative methods, such as home traction followed by closed reduction, may be attempted before a surgical procedure. Surgical correction may include release of tight soft tissue structures or osteotomy of the proximal femur to allow the femoral head to move into the acetabulum. Older children may require removal of a portion of the femoral shaft to reduce the forces on the femoral head when it is relocated in the acetabulum, femoral osteotomy, or acetabular osteotomy to aid in relocating the femoral head.[24,63]

Arthrogryposis Multiplex Congenita

Arthrogryposis multiplex congenita (AMC), also referred to as multiple congenital contracture (MCC), is a nonprogressive disorder characterized by multiple joint contractures and muscle weakness or imbalance. The reported incidence of AMC varies from 1 in 3000 to 1 in 4000 live births.[72,73] The disorder is related to a paucity of movement early in fetal development, leading to multiple contractures at birth. The exact etiology is unknown, but is probably multifactorial with genetic mutation causes currently being uncovered. AMC is associated with multiple neurogenic or myopathic disorders that exhibit a defect in the motor unit, including the anterior horn cells, roots, peripheral nerve, motor end plates, or muscle, resulting in weakness and decreased fetal movement early in development. Fetal immobility results in multiple joint contractures, fibrosis of muscles, and fibrosis of the periarticular structures.[73,74]

There is much variability among infants with AMC; however, common clinical features are generally present. These features include: (1) featureless extremities that are often cylindric in shape with absent skin creases, (2) rigid joints with significant contractures, (3) dislocation of joints, especially the hips, (4) atrophy and even absence of muscle groups, and (5) intact sensation, although deep tendon reflexes (DTRs) may be diminished or absent.[73] The infant's contractures are usually symmetric and typically include shoulder internal rotation, elbow flexion or extension, wrist flexion with ulnar deviation, hip flexion with either internal rotation or a frog-legged posture, knee flexion or extension, and equinovarus deformities of the feet (Fig. 13.15).[24]

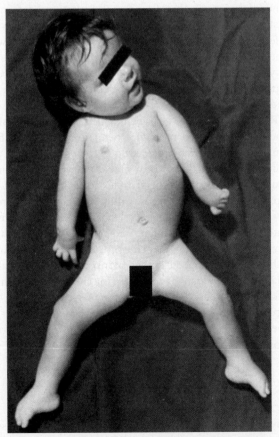

FIGURE 13.15 Arthrogryposis multiplex congenita in an infant. The shoulders are internally rotated and adducted, and the elbows and wrists are extended. The hips are flexed, externally rotated, and abducted, and the feet demonstrate talipes equinocavus.

Management

Intervention requires multiple disciplines working toward the same goal and timeline. The goal of intervention is to achieve the maximum functional level for each child. Treatment techniques include passive stretching through positioning, casting and splinting, strengthening activities, developmental skills, surgical procedures, and the use of adapted or rehabilitation equipment. The family is crucial in planning the long-term goals for the child and assisting with the carryover of activities.

INFANCY Positioning and passive stretching exercises should begin shortly after birth. Serial casting begins in the first few months for foot deformities (see Clubfoot section), knee flexion contractures, and wrist flexion contractures. Caution must be used to stretch only to the end range and maintain the stretch with a cast or a splint. Forceful aggressive stretching of a rigid joint can result in damage to the joint capsule and surrounding soft tissues.[24] Any gains in ROM must be maintained with a splint or positioning device, or the contracture will recur.

Usually between 6 and 12 months of age, residual contractures at the feet and knees are surgically corrected.[63] Surgical correction involves release of the tight joint capsule and soft tissues. Surgical correction is maintained by splinting, strengthening exercises, and active functional movement. For example, a child who had a bilateral release of posterior structures of the ankle to correct an equinovarus deformity should have a splint fabricated to maintain the ROM as well as begin a standing program with the use of a standing device or ambulation aid.

The goals of intervention for the child's upper extremities must be well planned. For optimum function and independence with self-care skills, the child should have the ability to flex and extend the elbows. If this is not possible, treatment should aim to ensure that one elbow is able to flex for feeding activities and that the other elbow is able to extend for reaching and toileting activities.

During this age range, the child should develop some mobility skills. Rolling is often difficult secondary to the lower extremity contractures. Some children may learn to scoot on the floor on their belly or their back initially. Most children can learn to sit but have difficulty achieving the sitting position independently. From sitting, floor mobility should be encouraged. Creeping on hands and knees is often difficult, and children often learn to scoot on their bottom. Pulling to stand may be limited by contractures of the lower extremity. Surgical techniques should be timed to prepare the child to stand when the child is developmentally ready. Preambulation activities should begin before 1 year of age.

12 MONTHS THROUGH PRESCHOOL The goal of treatment during this age range is to develop the maximum level of independence with mobility and self-care skills. Ambulation is possible for many children with AMC and should be considered a viable goal until proven otherwise. Upper extremity skills focus on feeding and dressing activities. Maintenance of acquired ROM is crucial, as are continued gains in ROM. Strengthening exercises through age-appropriate activities, as well as specific mobility training, are incorporated into the program.

SCHOOL AGE   The school-age time period often highlights the functional impairments that may exist for a child with AMC. The child's ambulation speed may be slow compared with his or her peers, and fine motor difficulty may interfere with writing speed and clarity. Adaptive and rehabilitation equipment may be necessary to assist the child with functioning independently in the school setting and maintaining social interaction with his or her peers.

 Postnatal deformations

Deformations can also occur postnatally secondary to the immaturity of the musculoskeletal system of a growing and developing child. The effect of growth on the musculoskeletal system can be used to correct prenatal deformities, such as seen in the treatment rationale for CMT or metatarsus adductus. However, the effect of growth can also produce additional deformities postnatally if a force is abnormal or unopposed.

Rotational Deformities

The variation of a child's rotational profile that occurs with normal growth and development produces many questions for parents and subsequent visits to an orthopedist or a physical therapist. The child with a rotational variation presents with either an in-toed or out-toed gait. Clarification on what is a true normal rotational variation, when the rotation becomes a deformity, and appropriate assessment and intervention are necessary to answer parents' questions, recognize true problems, and possibly impact those problems. The causative factors of the in-toeing or out-toeing must be evaluated and the rotational components measured using Staheli's rotational profile outlined earlier in the chapter. Staheli's rotational profile includes FPA as an overall measure, hip rotation ROM to assess femoral torsion, TFA to assess tibial torsion and the hindfoot, angle of the TMA (transmalleolar axis) to assess the distal tibia, and the configuration of the foot. The measurements can then be compared with the normative values to determine whether the child falls within the range of normal for his or her age and which component or components of the lower extremity are contributing to the in-toed or out-toed gait pattern (see Fig. 13.2).

FPA shows the greatest variability in infancy before leveling off to a mean of 10 degrees with a range of −3 to 20 degrees in childhood. Hip rotation ROM is divided into medial and lateral rotation of the hip and is a clinical measure to assess femoral torsion. The sum of medial and lateral hip

rotation is approximately 100 degrees and slightly more in infants.[75] Lateral rotation of the hip is greater than medial rotation in infants secondary to tightness of soft tissues from intrauterine positioning. Femoral anteversion is present in infancy, but is not as noticeable because of the infant's position of lateral rotation. Femoral anteversion is usually noticeable in young children, but continues to decrease from infancy throughout childhood. Persistent femoral anteversion may be classified as a rotational deformity when the following values exist: mild if medial rotation is 70 to 80 degrees and lateral rotation is 10 to 20 degrees, moderate if medial rotation is 80 to 90 degrees and lateral rotation is 0 to 10 degrees, and severe if medial rotation is greater than 90 degrees and no lateral rotation is present.[22,75] The TFA increases from a negative angle in infancy to a positive angle throughout childhood. The angle of the TMA also increases from infancy through childhood. The tibia is medially rotated in infancy secondary to intrauterine positioning. De-rotation of the tibia toward the normal lateral tibial torsion values in adulthood occurs normally through growth and development.

Infants and young children exhibit greater femoral anteversion and medial tibial torsion that gradually decrease through normal growth and development. An in-toeing gait is most common during the second year after the child begins to walk. If the measured values fall outside the two standard deviation values for normal, a rotational deformity exists. Intervention is necessary only if the deformity interferes with function or has the potential to interfere with function or development.[75] However, if a rotational deformity is cosmetically unappealing for the child, adolescent, or parent, intervention may also be considered although not medically necessary.[75]

Previously, treatment has included exercise, bracing, shoe modifications, and orthopedic correction. Shoe modifications are ineffective in correcting in-toeing problems, and devices such as the Denis Browne bar or twister cables may actually cause secondary deformities at the knee as well.[24,64] Hip, knee, ankle foot orthoses (HKAFO) and knee, ankle foot orthoses (KAFO) constructed of newer light polymer material shell and multiplane movement joints may have clinical benefits, but evidence is not more than anecdotal at this time. Orthopedic surgery consisting of a femoral or tibial osteotomy may be indicated for children who exhibit deformities greater than 3 standard deviations from the normal values (i.e., femoral anteversion greater than 50 degrees) and when the deformity interferes with function or is a cosmetic concern.

 Dysplasias

A dysplasia is an abnormal organization of cells into tissue that leads to abnormal tissue differentiation.[6,26] Children born with a dysplasia exhibit widespread involvement because the abnormal tissue differentiation is present wherever the tissue is present.

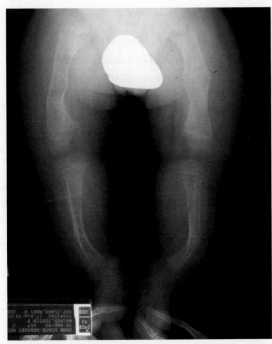

FIGURE 13.16 Radiograph of a 13-month-old child with type III OI. Note the poor bone density, previous fracture sites, bowing of the bones, and the length of the femurs in relation to the tibias.

Osteogenesis Imperfecta

OI is a congenital disorder of type I collagen synthesis that affects all connective tissues in the body. The reported incidence is dependent upon criteria used for OI and ranges from 1 in 15,000 to 1 in 100,000.[76,77] The musculoskeletal involvement is diffuse and includes osteoporosis with excessive fractures even at birth, bowing of long bones, spinal deformities, muscle weakness, and ligamentous laxity.[76–79] In addition to the musculoskeletal involvement, other clinical features of children with OI may include blue sclera in the eyes, dentinogenesis imperfecta, hearing loss, growth deficiency, cardiopulmonary abnormalities, easy bruising, excessive sweating, and loose or dislocated joints[76,77] (Fig. 13.16).

In 1979, Sillence first described OI Types I through IV based on genetic, clinical, and radiographic findings without regard for molecular involvement.[76,80] Recently, the genetic complexity of OI is becoming more transparent with approximately 2000 different type I collagen mutations identified.[80] The International Skeletal Dysplasia Society has recommended utilizing Sillence typing to classify the severity of OI or phenotypic presentation. In addition, these classifications should not include direct molecular reference to eliminate typing that only reflects newly discovered genetic variants that have little distinguishing features in the clinic.[81] Table 13.3 outlines the specific characteristics for OI Types I through VIII.

Binder et al.[79] developed a classification system based on body size and limb proportions and their expected functional outcomes (Table 13.4). Consequently, physical therapy interventions can then be aimed at potential musculoskeletal deformities that presently interfere with the child's expected functional abilities or at preventing those deformities from developing.

TABLE 13.3	Classification of OI			
Type[a]	Severity	Inheritance	Characteristics	Mobility Status
I	Mildest form of OI	Autosomal dominant	Blue sclera, dentinogenesis imperfecta, fewer bone fractures and progressive deformity, mild short stature or normal height	Ambulatory—may use an orthotic device
II	Lethal in perinatal period	Autosomal dominant	Severe bone fragility with multiple rib and long bone fractures at birth. Bones are "crumpled"; ribs may be beaded	Not applicable
III	Severe form	Autosomal dominant or recessive	Blue or normal sclera, dentinogenesis imperfecta, variable bone fragility but often severe, progressive skeletal deformity, scoliosis, very short stature	Variable; may be ambulatory with assistive device and orthotic devices, may use wheelchair for all or partial mobility
IV	Moderate	Autosomal dominant	Gray or normal sclera, dentinogenesis imperfecta, moderate fragility of bones, scoliosis, moderate short stature	Often independent at home and community, with or without assistive device
V	Moderate	Autosomal dominant	Normal sclera and teeth, frequent dislocation of radial head and calcification of forearm interosseous membrane, moderate-to-severe bone fragility, mild-to-moderate short stature	Ambulatory
VI	Moderate	Autosomal recessive	Normal sclera and teeth, vertebral compression fractures often seen, more fractures than seen in type IV but at birth, scoliosis, moderately short stature	May be ambulatory or use wheelchair
VII	Moderate	Autosomal recessive	White sclera, normal teeth, moderate bone fragility with fractures at birth, very short humeri and femurs with coax vara, mild short stature	May be ambulatory or use wheelchair
VIII	Severe to lethal in perinatal period	Autosomal recessive	Severe growth deficiency and bone demineralization	Variable to not applicable

[a]Types I to IV are based on Sillence classification system. Types V to VIII are expanded types clinically distinguishable by bone histology or recessive inheritance.

13.4 Functional Classification for OI and Focus of Rehabilitation

Type	Physical Characteristics	Functional Expectations	Focus of Rehabilitation Interventions
A	Most severely involved group Large head relative to body, very short stature, bowing of long bones with joint contractures and weakness May have severe scoliosis and/or vertebral compression fractures	Dependent for ADLs except for feeding May use manual wheelchair; more likely to use power wheelchair	Positioning, including molded seating systems, therapeutic water activities Soft tissue mobilization to increase shoulder and MCP joint ROM and soft tissue mobilization techniques to alleviate back pain
B	Severe short stature, high incidence of femoral bowing, scoliosis, hip flexion contractures Strength generally at least 3/5	Stand and/or ambulate with assistive devices and braces Partial independence with ADLs Contractures of hips and shoulders and limited forearm supination interfere with function	Posture and active ROM exercises aimed at limiting contractures Strengthening with emphasis on abdominals, hip extensors and abductors, and quadriceps Endurance through swimming and biking, developmental activities through normal sequence Many children will not crawl but scoot in sitting
C	Less growth deficiency, poor LE alignment including hip abduction and external rotation contractures Joint laxity with LE valgus and pronation of the feet Strength of 3/5 or greater, poor endurance	Community ambulation with or without orthotic devices Independent with ADLs	Strengthening exercises with weights *proximal* on limb Conditioning exercise to improve endurance and long-distance ambulation May use orthotic devices for alignment, but all orthotic devices should be articulated

ADLs, activities of daily living; LE, lower extremity; MCP, metacarpophalangeal; ROM, range of motion.

From Binder H, Conway A, Gerber LH. Rehabilitation approaches to children with osteogenesis imperfecta: a ten-year experience. *Arch Phys Med Rehabil.* 1993;74:386–390.

Management

PHARMACOLOGIC Several pharmacologic and vitamin supplements have been studied in an attempt to decrease the fragility of the bones of children with OI. Agents such as calcitonin, fluoride, hormones, and vitamins C and D have all been shown to be ineffective in preventing fractures.[82] Calcium and vitamin D may be ineffective alone but can support greater efficacy in conjunction with bisphosphonate drug therapies.[80]

Medications from the bisphosphonate family such as pamidronate, alendronate, and zoledronic acid have been administered to children and adults with OI to improve their bone density. Bisphosphonates act to inhibit osteoclast activity and have been used in postmenopausal women to decrease osteoporosis. Bisphosphonates can be administered orally or intravenously at cyclic periods. Intravenous (IV) administration has been found to be effective in improving bone density, especially vertebral body; decreasing fracture rate; decreasing back pain; improving sense of well-being; and improving grip strength, mobility, self-care skills, and ambulation.[83–86] Maximum bone density benefits are realized with pamidronate in the first 2 to 4 years of treatment, but maintenance therapy is suggested until bone growth is finished.[80] Oral administration may not be as effective as IV administration. However, significant evidence supports that oral administration of bisphosphonates is effective in improving bone density.[84,87,88] Moderate-to-strong evidence suggests oral bisphosphonate efficacy in reducing the fracture rate, improving the functional status of some subjects, and improving quality of life in children with OI types I, III,

and IV.[82,84,87] Future study regarding bisphosphonates should include further analysis of how long the child should receive the medications, whether the results are reversed if the medication is stopped, and which groups should receive which medications. Other novel approaches currently under investigation include the efficacy of gene therapy to silence allele mutations, bone marrow transplant, and selective mesenchymal stem cell transplant to treat OI.

ORTHOPEDIC Fractures are managed with a soft splint or fiberglass cast for immobilization. The period of immobilization is kept short to minimize the bone demineralization that normally occurs with inactivity. Frequent fractures can lead to further demineralization, refractures, and bony deformity, specifically bowing of the long bones. Muscle pull on long bones can also cause significant anterior bowing of the long bones of the lower extremity. Osteotomy, flexible intramedullary nails, and telescoping intramedullary rod fixation may be used to correct bowing deformities or stabilize fractures.[76,80] Surgical corrections facilitate orthotic use and standing programs as well as provide support to the bones to decrease the fracture rate.

Rehabilitation

Several practitioners from the Children's Hospital Medical Center, Washington, DC, and the National Institutes of Health have developed and revised a rehabilitation protocol for children with OI.[78,79,89] Much of this information is now published in a book with clear explanations of exercises from early infancy through gaining independence for adolescents.[90] In view of wide variability among children with OI, the protocol is meant to serve as a guideline and must be individualized for each child and family. The goals for the child with severe OI are to: (1) prevent deformities of the head, spine, and extremities, (2) avert cardiorespiratory compromise by avoiding constant positioning in supine, and (3) maximize the child's ability to move actively.[78] These goals are based on the theory that muscle strengthening and weight-bearing programs for upper and lower extremities promote active earlier use of the extremities and may lead to increased bone mineralization and less severe musculoskeletal deformities.[78,89]

Instruction in handling of an infant with OI is crucial for all parents and caregivers. The infant should be held with the head and trunk fully supported. For infants with severe OI, caregivers may be more comfortable holding the child on a pillow. Careful positioning of an infant with OI should begin in the first few days after birth with instruction from a knowledgeable physical therapist. Positioning aims to align the infant's head, trunk, and extremities and to protect the infant from hitting hard surfaces with activity. Emphasis is on midline orientation of the head and position changes to prevent the development of a laterally tilted head and misshapen skull. Active movement is encouraged as beginning strengthening exercises. Careful handling activities can be performed in straight frontal or sagittal plane movements. Rotary movements should be avoided to prevent rotational fractures.

Strengthening activities progress from active movement to playing with lightweight toys and rattles. Active movement can be further encouraged in water either at bath time or in a swim program with the parent present. Standard active-assistive and resistive exercises can be incorporated as the child becomes a little older. Emphasis is also placed on the development of head control and head righting in a variety of positions because children with OI often have a very large head. Developmental activities such as prone skills and rolling are encouraged. Independent sitting is encouraged when developmentally appropriate, as is some type of floor mobility. Those children who do not have the ability to develop independent sitting skills should be fitted for a custom-molded seat to promote head and trunk alignment and afford the child the opportunity to play in an upright position. Throughout the developmental progression, increasing or maintaining ROM and strength, especially of the pelvic girdle, is incorporated into activities.

Children should be fitted with orthoses when they have developed independent sitting skills and balance and are beginning to pull to stand. Those children who cannot sit independently but have developed head control should be fitted for a standing frame. Recent standing equipment design advances may eliminate the need for custom-molded frames. The orthoses recommended in the protocol are containment or clamshell HKAFOs.[78,90] Clamshell orthoses are similar to standard HKAFOs except that a contoured anterior shell is present to support the thigh and lower leg. Gait training begins with an assistive device and may or may not progress to independent ambulation without an assistive device. With ambulation and upright positioning, attention must be directed to the pelvic girdle. Hip flexion contractures often develop, and children with OI typically require ongoing strengthening of their hip extensors and abductors.[90]

Children who do not develop independent functional ambulation should be fitted with a manual or power wheelchair as appropriate. Positioning remains key with any seating system, and attention is given to head and trunk alignment.

In a 10-year follow-up report, Binder and colleagues emphasized the need for rehabilitation to focus on the child's functional needs.[79] These key rehabilitation strategies are outlined in Table 13.4. Binder et al. reported progress with functional skills in all groups of children with OI, ranging from improved head control to community ambulation. Progress appears related to severity of the disease, but should be expected for all children with OI if the goals address functional needs. Factors that impair independence include joint contractures and muscle weakness for those children with severe forms of OI, and endurance capabilities for children with less severe forms of OI.

Recent studies show that children with OI can participate in physical therapist–supervised exercise programs and demonstrate improved aerobic and muscle performance with decreased fatigue.[91] Detraining observed following the completion of these programs emphasizes the need for ongoing therapist developed and safely monitored exercise programs as part of a weekly routine. The use of whole body vibration (WBV) systems has been incorporated into training programs to improve muscle strength and power in healthy and motor-impaired adults, demonstrating results beyond that of training without WBV.[92,93] WBV has shown promising results in improving mobility and function and decreasing support devices needed for children with OI.[93] Current equipment costs make treatment outside of the clinical or research setting prohibitive, but further technological or home gaming system development will likely change this.

Joint Hypermobility Syndromes

EDS is another disorder of collagen synthesis, primarily type V, with an incidence of 1:10,000.[94,95] It is a clinically and genetically heterogenous group of connective tissue disorders characterized by joint hypermobility, skin hyperextensibility, and tissue fragility.[94–96] Formerly divided into 14 distinct variations, there are now 7 accepted general classification types of EDS.[95] (Table 13.5) However, the Classic and Hypermobility type account for 90% of all cases and involve mostly orthopedic complaints.[96]

In 1967, Kirk first described a similar condition known as benign joint hypermobility syndrome (BJHS), which is also characterized by generalized joint laxity with musculoskeletal complaints. It is called "benign" owing to the absence of a specific genetic, musculoskeletal or rheumatic disorder.[97] Examination and treatment approaches to EDS and BJHS are indistinguishable.

TABLE 13.5	EDS Classifications	
Current Classification	**Prior Classification**	**Clinical Presentation**
Classic	EDS I and EDS II	Joint hypermobility Skin hyperextensibility Atrophic scars Smooth velvety texture
Hypermobile	EDS III	Joint hypermobility Mild skin hyperextensibility +/– smooth velvety texture
Vascular	EDS IV	Thin skin Easily bruised Pinched nose Appearance of premature aging Rupture of medium and large arteries within uterus and bowel
Kyphoscoliotic	EDS VI	Joint hypermobility Progressive scoliosis Scleral fragility with rupture Tissue fragility Aortic dilation Mitral valve prolapse (MVP)
Arthrochalasia	EDS VII A EDS VII B	Severe joint hypermobility Joint subluxations Congenital hip dislocation Skin hyperextensibility Tissue fragility
Dermatosparaxis	EDS VII C	Severe skin fragility Decreased skin elasticity Easily bruised Hernias Premature rupture of fetal membranes
Unclassified	EDS V EDS VIII EDS X, EDS XI EDS IX EDS, Progeroid form	Classic features Classic features and periodontic disease Mild classic features, MVP (mitral valve prolapse), joint instability Classic features, occipital horns, premature aging

TABLE 13.6	Beighton Criteria for Joint Hypermobility	
Major Criteria	A Beighton score of 4/9 or more (either current or historic) Joint Pain for more than 3 mo in four or more joints	
Minor Criteria	A Beighton score of 1, 2, or 3/9 (0, 1, 2, or 3 if aged 50+) Joint pain (>3 mo) in one to three joints or back pain (>3 mo), spondylosis, spondylolysis/spondylolisthesis. Dislocation/subluxation in more than one joint, or in one joint on more than one occasion. Soft tissue inflammation >3 lesions (e.g., epicondylitis, tenosynovitis, bursitis). Marfan-like symptoms (tall, slim, span/height ratio >1.03, upper: lower segment ratio <0.89, arachnodactyly (positive Steinberg thumb/ Walker wrist signs). Abnormal skin: striae, hyperextensibility, thin skin, papyraceous scarring Eye signs: drooping eyelids, nearsighted or anti-mongoloid eye slant Varicose veins or hernia or uterine/rectal prolapse	
Beighton Score	1, 2 – Passive 5th MCP extension >90 degrees (Right and Left) 3, 4 – Passive thumb apposition to forearm (Right and Left) 5, 6 – Elbow hyperextension >10 degrees (Right and Left) 7, 8 – Knee hyperextension >10 degrees (Right and Left) 9 – Standing trunk flexion with knees extended, palms flat on floor	
Positive Diagnosis criteria	2 major criteria 1 major and 1 minor criteria 4 minor criteria	

Examination

Examination procedures for patients with EDS and BJHS should include a hypermobility scale and lower extremity rotational profile. Multiple hypermobility scales exist but the Beighton Score is frequently used in clinical settings. The Beighton Score is a component of the full Beighton Criteria used to diagnose hypermobility syndromes[98] (Table 13.6). Other areas of specific concern include the shoulders, ankles, and feet. Complaints of hypermobility are often accompanied by diffuse muscle and joint pain and general fatigue along with hand pain and fatigue with prolonged handwriting.

Management

Intervention focus and strategies will depend on the patient's age and severity of joint involvement. Most programs should include a combination of the following four areas: targeted therapeutic exercise, self-care and home management, functional training for recreation, school, or work, and orthoses or adaptive equipment.[12a]

Therapeutic Exercise

Therapeutic exercise programs should include a combination of strengthening, neuromuscular education, neuromuscular stabilization, and stretching usually of the hindfoot only. Glenohumeral joint and scapular stabilization and strengthening are important to combat recurrent subluxations. This reduction in subluxations also improves proximal stability to facilitate functional use of the hand and arm without recurrent pain. However, this level of achievement may be difficult for younger children, and goals for improvement may be delayed until a child can follow more complex instruction. Foot and ankle strengthening will promote stability and preserve foot function. Full hindfoot ROM should be achieved, as Achilles tightness usually develops due to midfoot breakdown. Abdominal and trunk strengthening for overall proximal and lumbar stabilization is frequently necessary as low back pain is a common complaint. Wrist and hand work should focus on small intrinsic muscle strengthening without joint hyperextension to facilitate hand use in fine motor tasks especially for school and work.

Self-Care

Patients require education regarding the need for joint stability and protection. End-range positions such as leaning on hyperextended elbows and standing for long periods with hips and knees hyperextended for comfort should be avoided.[12a] It is also common for patients with hypermobility to demonstrate joint "tricks" such as contortion or shoulder popping. However, these movements can result in microtrauma, further exacerbating pain symptoms. Gym class limitations include: allowance for rest periods, no somersaults, push-ups, arm hanging activities, timed exercises, or unsupervised stretching that often occurs in large classes. Aside from these, activity modification rather than elimination should be considered.

Functional Training

Patients with EDS and BJHS are at increased risk for ligamentous and repetitive use injuries because muscles perform constant double duty as joint stabilizers and movers.[99] Training will vary with the age of the child, but can include recreational or organized play, school or work activity. Patients require assessment of specific functional tasks with recommendations for modification, optimization of good body mechanics, and exercise prescription for injury prevention.

Orthoses and Adaptive Equipment

Primary equipment and device needs are related to the hands, ankles, and feet. These children benefit from wider grip pens and pencils or regular ones with grip-widening foam attached to them. Some children benefit from early use of computer or laptop use for note taking. More widespread academic use of electronic tablets may provide even more hand symptom relief.

The foot and ankle should be protected as early as possible to prevent structural deformity associated with excessive pronation. A biomechanical foot exam should be performed with the foot in subtalar joint neutral to ensure that the hindfoot mobility is accurately measured before an orthotic or orthosis is prescribed. A bracing device should provide the maximum support with the minimal amount of anatomical control possible to facilitate maximal muscle activity and bone development. Children with EDS and BJHS do well with custom and semi-customized shoe orthotics and University of California Biomechanics Lab (UCBL)–type orthoses for mild-to-moderate foot hypermobility and light weight supramalleolar orthoses in severe cases.

▶ Pathologic processes

Pathologic processes are a broad category of conditions that are abnormal and may impact the developing and growing musculoskeletal system of a child. These processes are varied in their origin and may include vascular, infectious, metabolic, mechanical, traumatic, or structural causes.

Legg–Calvé–Perthes Disease

Legg–Calvé–Perthes disease is a self-limiting disease of the hip initiated by avascular necrosis of the femoral head. The precise cause of the avascular necrosis that disrupts blood flow to the capital femoral epiphysis is not known. Microtrauma, transient synovitis, infection, insulin-like growth factor I pathway abnormalities, congenital or developmental vascular irregularities, and thrombotic vascular insults have all been theorized as producing the avascular necrosis, but recent evidence is strongly suggestive of vascular abnormalities and dysfunction.[100,101] The disease typically occurs between 3 and 13 years of age, with boys affected three to five times more frequently than girls. However, Legg–Calvé–Perthes disease is most commonly seen in boys between 4 and 10 years of age who are active yet small for their age. Bilateral presentation is seen in 10% to 20% of children with the disease.[24]

Legg–Calvé–Perthes disease progresses through four clearly defined stages: (1) initial, (2) fragmentation, (3) reossification, and (4) healed.[102] During the initial phase, a portion or all of the femoral head becomes necrotic and bone growth ceases. The necrotic bone is resorbed and fragmented; at this time revascularization of the femoral head is initiated. During this second stage, the femoral head often becomes deformed, and the acetabulum becomes flattened in response to the deformity of the femoral head. With revascularization, the femoral head begins to reossify. As the femoral head grows, remodeling of both the femoral head and the acetabulum occurs.[100,102] The stage of the disease at the time of diagnosis, sex of the child, and age at onset impact the final outcome and congruency of the hip joint.

There are several classification systems aimed at assisting with predicting outcomes of children with Legg–Calvé–Perthes disease. Herring et al. developed a classification system based on involvement of the lateral aspect of the femoral head. They found this lateral pillar classification to demonstrate good-to-excellent reliability among users.[102] The original A, B, C classification progressing from least to most lateral pillar deterioration is the most widely used. Modifications to include a fourth B/C border category have not demonstrated the same reproducibility.[103]

Clinically, children with Legg–Calvé–Perthes disease present with a limp and pain referred to the groin, thigh, or knee.[24,104] If the condition is undetected, hip ROM limitations may develop with restrictions in hip internal rotation and abduction, a hip flexion contracture may be present, and a Trendelenburg-type gait is frequently observed.[104] Muscle spasm of the hip adductors and iliopsoas may also be noted. Children who present to a physical therapist with the preceding symptoms and unknown etiology should be referred to a pediatric orthopedist.

Management

The goals of treatment are to relieve the symptoms of pain and muscle spasm, prevent or minimize femoral head deformity, contain the femoral head in the acetabulum while bone remodeling occurs, and restore ROM. Treatment for relief of pain includes anti-inflammatory medications, traction, and partial weight bearing with the use of crutches. Minimizing deformity and containment of the femoral head may be achieved by using traction, orthotic devices such as a Petrie cast, Scottish-Rite orthosis, or A-Frame orthosis (Figs. 13.17 to 13.19), or surgical procedures such as a femoral or innominate osteotomy.

If an orthotic device is used as the method of femoral head containment, it may be required for a prolonged period of time, up to 1 to 2 years. While wearing the orthosis

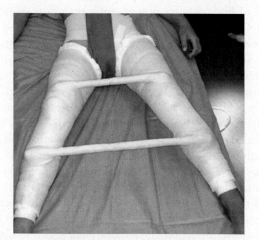

FIGURE 13.17 Petrie cast.

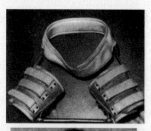

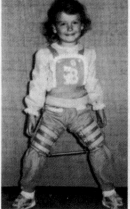

FIGURE 13.18 Scottish-Rite orthosis. The abduction bar contains a swivel joint that allows reciprocal motion of the legs.

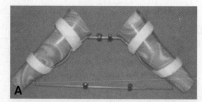

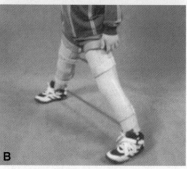

FIGURE 13.19 A-Frame Orthosis. Custom-molded in: **(A)** approximately 30 degrees of bilateral hip abduction and **(B)** slight knee flexion. (Rich MM, Schoenecker PL. Management of Legg–Calvé–Perthes disease using an A-frame orthosis and hip range of motion: a 25-year experience. *J Pediatr Orthop.* 2013;33:112–119).

and after healing, physical therapy is often warranted to address ROM limitations and strength deficits. After removal of the orthotic device, children may continue to walk with a Trendelenburg-type gait because of weakness of their hip extensors and hip abductors. Physical therapy after surgical intervention focuses on gait training and restoration of hip ROM and strength. Knee and ankle strength and ROM should also be continually addressed due to long-term immobility.

Although multiple treatment methods exist for Legg–Calvé–Perthes disease, decision making and outcomes are more correlated with certain factors such as age at onset, total amount of femoral head involvement, Herring lateral pillar classification, and the disease stage at the time of diagnosis. Children under 6 years do well regardless of treatment protocol, and surgery may not be necessary.[104–106] Children who are under 8 years of age at the time of onset and have minimal involvement of the lateral aspect of their femoral head have very favorable outcomes regardless of the type of treatment received.[105,106] However, children who are over the age of 8 years at the time of onset and have moderate involvement of the lateral aspect of the femoral head have improved outcomes with surgical intervention.[105] Children who have complete collapse of the lateral aspect of their femoral head, more total femoral head involvement, or in later stages of the disease at diagnosis typically have poor outcomes.[104–106]

Recent literature suggests a specific protocol that demonstrated excellent outcomes over a 25-year period.[107] This protocol included an adductor tenotomy as needed to achieve 35 to 40 degrees of hip abduction, Petrie casting for 6 weeks, followed by donning of a custom A-Frame orthosis for 20 out of 24 hours per day for up to 3 years, and a hip ROM HEP performed twice a day. Good spherical hip congruency was developed with an overall rate of 93% of 240 hips studied having congruency. This included 78% of the more involved B and C Herring Classification hips as well. During the bracing period, children were permitted to ambulate while wearing the brace, and they maintained a normal school schedule, thereby demonstrating minimal limitations to daily living participation.

Slipped Capital Femoral Epiphysis

Slipped capital femoral epiphysis (SCFE) is typically described as occurring when the femoral head slips, or is displaced, from its normal alignment with the femoral neck. However, it is actually caused by displacement of the femoral neck usually anteriorly and superiorly.[108] Weakness of and excessive stresses on the growth plate are thought to contribute to the displacement of the femoral head. Increased shear forces may be caused by obesity and structural problems such as femoral retroversion and physeal obliquity.[108,109] Testosterone in boys and hormonal imbalances in boys and girls, and growth spurts may contribute to growth plate weakness or instability.[108,109] SCFE is the most common hip problem of adolescence but the incidence of SCFE varies according to age, sex, and race. The incidence is higher in males and the African American population, and is often associated with the onset of puberty.[108,109] Bilateral occurrence has been reported in at least 50% of young adolescents.[108–110]

SCFE is classified by weight-bearing ability, duration of symptoms, and radiographic findings. Patients with stable SCFE (which represents greater than 90% of cases) are able to bear weight with or without support, but patients with unstable SCFE cannot.[108] Acute SCFE is defined as a sudden onset of painful symptoms of less than 3 weeks' duration, whereas chronic SCFE is characterized by a gradual onset of symptoms for greater than 3 weeks. The third type is acute-on-chronic SCFE with a history of mild pain for greater than 3 weeks and a recent sudden exacerbation of symptoms.[109] Classification according to the severity of the displacement of the femoral head is defined as follows:

(a) Grade I, displacement of the femoral head up to one-third of the width of the femoral neck;
(b) Grade II, greater than one-third but less than one-half displacement;
(c) Grade III, displacement greater than one-half (Fig. 13.20).[24,108]

Clinical presentation of young adolescents with SCFE includes pain in the groin, medial thigh, or knee; limping; external rotation of the leg; and limited hip ROM, especially flexion, abduction, and internal rotation.[64,108] External rotation is noted with attempts to flex the affected hip. With an acute onset, pain is often severe, and the adolescent is unable to bear weight on the affected lower extremity. History may include a traumatic or gradual onset. If an undiagnosed young adolescent presents to physical therapy with the preceding symptoms, the therapist should consider immediate referral to a pediatric orthopedist for further workup.

Management

The goals of treatment include growth plate stabilization to prevent further displacement and prevention of complications, including avascular necrosis, chondrolysis, and early osteoarthritis.[24,108,109] Physeal stabilization is achieved through surgical pin fixation in situ.[110,111] This may also include prophylactic fixation of an uninvolved hip, especially in younger children.[108,110] Additional arthroscopic

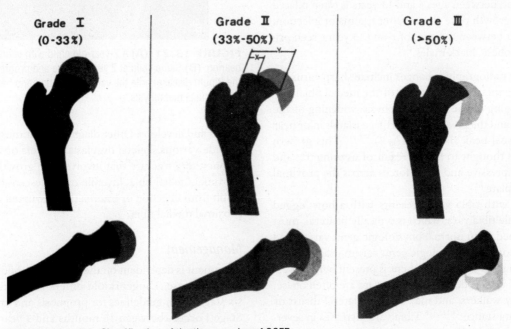

FIGURE 13.20 Classification of the three grades of SCFE.

osteochondroplasty may be utilized to treat femoral acetabular impingement, which occurs in every hip with SCFE.[111] More significant procedures such as osteotomies are required for advanced and complicated cases. Nonsurgical treatment, including bed rest, traction, and casting, is not successful; long-term outcomes may include limited hip ROM, pain, and surgical procedures necessitated by early osteoarthritis.

Physical therapy includes gait training with an assistive device postoperatively; usually, a non–weight-bearing status is recommended during the acute recovery period, but often increases within 4 to 6 weeks. Bilateral strength and ROM throughout the lower extremities should be maintained through open chain exercises and stretching, respectively, during the non–weight-bearing phase. Care should be taken to maintain full knee and ankle ROM, which can decrease from minor amounts of lower extremity immobility and previous surgery. In view of the association with obesity, strengthening of the abdominal and trunk musculature is important preparatory work prior to return to bilateral weight-bearing activities and gait training post acutely. After weight-bearing advances, interventions should focus on increasing lower extremity strength to restore proper gait patterns and functional activity. Strengthening progress may be slow and complicated by excess weight or by a premorbidly decreased activity level.

Tibia Vara (Blount Disease)

Tibia vara, or Blount disease, is a growth disorder of the medial aspect of the proximal tibia, including the epiphysis, physis, and metaphysis.[24,112] Tibia vara is classified as three types, related to the age of onset:

1. Infantile, less than 3 years of age is the most common;
2. Adolescent, between ages 6 and 13 years is often related to partial growth plate closure after trauma or infection;
3. Late onset between the ages of 6 and 15 years, seen primarily in obese, black males.[113]

Diagnostic radiographic changes include sharp varus angulation in the metaphysis, beaking of the medial tibial metaphysis, wedging of the medial epiphysis, widening of the growth plate, and the presence of cartilage islands in or near the metaphyseal beak (Fig. 13.21A–B).[114,115] This growth disturbance is thought to be the result of asymmetric and excessive compressive and shear forces across the proximal tibial growth plate.[24]

The child with tibia vara presents with a bow-legged stance. Infantile tibia vara, which is typically bilateral, must be distinguished from normal physiologic genu varum and medial tibial torsion. Physiologic genu varum gradually decreases until a genu valgus alignment is present between 2.5 and 3 years of age. Toddlers with tibia vara are often obese, are often early walkers, and may exhibit a lateral thrust of the knee during stance.[24,115,116] Tibia vara increases in severity, whereas physiologic genu varum decreases as the child

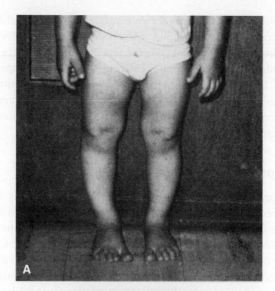

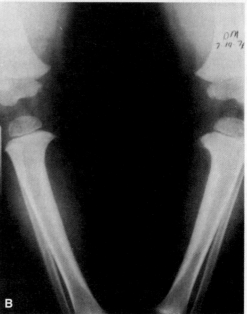

FIGURE 13.21 (A) A 2-year-old child with varus on weight bearing. **(B)** Same child at 2 years of age and progression of the Blount disease; note the varus angulation and beaking of the medial tibial metaphysis.

grows and develops. Other diagnoses that must be ruled out include various skeletal dysplasias, rickets or vitamin D deficiency, or a fracture that involved the growth plate of the proximal medial tibia. Juvenile or adolescent tibia vara may result from infection or trauma that disrupted growth of the proximal medial tibia.

Management

Treatment is dependent on the age of the child and the stage of the disease. Langenskiöld differentiated tibia vara into six stages with guidelines for prognosis and intervention.[114] Stage I occurs between 18 months and 3 years of age, and is characterized by beaking of the medial metaphysis and delay in growth of the medial epiphysis of the tibia. The stages progress in severity until stage VI. Stage VI is seen between 10 and 13 years of age and is characterized by fusion of the medial aspect of the physis while growth continues laterally.[24,114]

Treatment options include orthotic devices or surgical procedures. Orthotic intervention is recommended for children under 2 to 3 years of age, with radiographic findings consistent with stage I or II.[115,117] Of this group, children with smaller angular deformity and unilateral disease often respond better to bracing.[117] An HKAFO or KAFO used in full knee extension is recommended primarily while the child is weight bearing.[115,117] Proper fit and valgus correction adjustment should be assessed every 2 to 4 months. Physical therapy intervention may include family instruction in orthosis donning, doffing, wearing schedule, as well as skin inspection during brace use. Gait training with or without an assistive device may be warranted.

After the age of 4 years, surgical options produce better outcomes than orthotic devices.[112,115,116] Despite disease severity, stage, and age of presentation, there are ultimately two tibial osteotomy surgical categories[116]: tibial osteotomy with full angular correction using internal or external fixation; or tibial osteotomy with gradual angular correction using a multiaxial correction (MAC) monolateral external fixator device, or a circular device such as a Taylor Spatial or Ilizarov frame (see Fig 13.22).[112,116] Gradual corrections are performed by the patient actually being responsible to turn the screws on external fixation devices at a set daily rate to correct angular deformities. Recently, MAC devices have demonstrated comparable outcomes to circular frame devices but with easier application and improved patient ROM and decreased interference with general mobility.[112] Guided growth procedures such as lateral hemiepiphysiodesis, stapling, or tension band plate ("8-plate") placement are not indicated for correction of angular deformity related to Blount disease.[118]

Physical therapy intervention includes lower extremity strengthening, knee and ankle ROM, and gait training. Loss of knee flexion, terminal extension, and ankle dorsiflexion ROM can slow progress with functional activities during gradual correction procedures if consistent stretching is not performed in an HEP. Infection is one of the most common complications.[112] Patients and families will need education in skin and pin care when external fixator devices are used to prevent pin site infections as well as tissue mobility. ROM and strengthening interventions may be complicated for the obese patient who presents with limited premorbid joint mobility and muscle strength.

Limb Length Discrepancy

A limb length discrepancy may be caused by shortening or overgrowth of one or more bones of the leg. Inequality of leg lengths may result from congenital conditions such as limb deficiencies or hemihypertrophy, infections or fractures

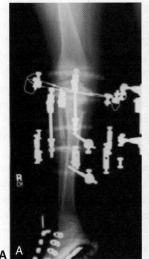
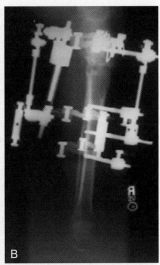
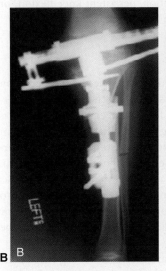
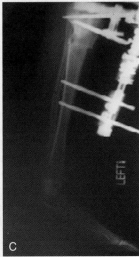

FIGURE 13.22 **(A)**. Ilizarov placement on right lower extremity **(B)** Left tibia with MAC device.
(Used with permission from Clarke SE, McCarthy JJ, Davidson RS. Treatment of Blount disease: a comparison between the multiaxial correction system and other external fixators. *J Pediatr Orthop.* 2009;29:103–109).

that injure the physis, neuromuscular disorders, tumors, or trauma that results in overgrowth and disease processes. Injuries to the physes are often asymmetric and result in angular deformities in addition to the shortening of the affected limb. Leg length differences range from 1 to 10 cm or greater.

Measurements must be taken when a leg length difference is suspected. Functional measurements can be taken by placing blocks of known height under the shorter leg until bilateral pelvic landmarks are level, assuming there is no pelvic deformity. Clinical measurement may be taken with the patient supine by measuring from the anterior superior iliac spine to the medial malleolus. Reliability of this measurement is affected by soft tissue asymmetries, excess fat tissue, and identification of bony landmarks.[119] More precise measurements are needed to predict the leg length discrepancy that will be present at maturity, evaluate treatment options, and predict the timing of surgical intervention if necessary. To assist with prediction of future growth and treatment options, the orthopedist uses radiographic methods to obtain accurate measurements and determine bone age, and uses growth charts or mathematical prediction models to estimate future skeletal growth of the child.[120] Leg length is generally assessed using plain film, computed radiography, or CT scanogram.[119]

Significant leg length discrepancies greater than 2 cm are a cosmetic as well as functional issue. Gait is less efficient and awkward, and postural compensations of the leg, pelvis, and spine often develop. Postural compensations may not lead to a structural deformity, but they may cause discomfort in adulthood. Functional compensatory mechanisms include toe walking or foot and ankle supination on the short side or vaulting, circumduction, persistent knee flexion, or foot and ankle pronation on the longer side.[120]

Management

Treatment is dependent on the age of the child, expectation of remaining limb growth, severity of the leg length difference, and preference of the family and child. Intervention is usually not indicated for leg length differences of less than 2 cm.[24] A lift inside the shoe or a custom-fabricated external heel-sole lift may be used for differences of 1 to 2 cm. Surgical treatment options are suggested for discrepancies of greater than 2 to 2.5 cm.[120] These procedures fall into one of two categories: shortening of the longer limb or lengthening of the shorter limb, but the approaches may be combined.

Shortening procedures are indicated for leg length discrepancies of 2 to 5 cm.[24,64,120] Limb shortening is commonly achieved through epiphysiodesis on the longer limb. Permanent physeal ablation methods include percutaneous drilling or curettage through the growth plate. Or "temporary" methods can be performed by staple or tension band ("8 plate") fixation in the metaphysis and epiphysis across both the medial and lateral sides of the growth plates of the distal femur and/or the proximal tibia. The medial-lateral "8 plate" approach has not been shown as effective as medial or lateral use for angular conditions. Percutaneous transphyseal screw implantation is a newer technique that is becoming a standard approach.[120] Most physicians opt for lengthening the shorter limb when the discrepancy is greater than 5 cm.

If the adolescent has reached skeletal maturity, then epiphysiodesis is not an option. In these cases, shortening of the longer limb is accomplished through osteotomy involving removal of a portion of the bone to equalize leg lengths. The maximum for removal in the femur is 5 to 6 cm, and 2 to 4 cm is the maximum for the tibia. The disadvantages of shortening by osteotomy are the reduction in overall height of the individual, body proportions may be cosmetically unappealing, the amount of equalization is limited, and the uninvolved leg has undergone surgery, which can impact muscle performance and efficiency.

Limb-lengthening techniques are directed at the involved leg and allow for equalization of discrepancies greater than 5 cm.[24] Limb-lengthening techniques are based on the concept of distraction osteogenesis, which means that new bone is formed as two segments of bone are slowly moved apart. Despite the surgical technique or apparatus used, the procedures are most successful when based on the Ilizarov biologic principles and the Law of Tension Stress.[121] These principles are named for the physician who proposed them and include minimizing bone disturbance, delaying distraction, rate and frequency of distraction, and the number and site of osteotomies.

A corticotomy minimizes bone disturbance by only cutting the cortex of bone while keeping the periosteum and nutrient artery within the medullary cavity intact. Delaying distraction 5 to 10 days depending on the age of the child allows the osteogenesis process to sufficiently initiate before the segments are pulled apart. The rate of distraction is about 1 mm/day, but the process should be broken down into a frequency of 0.25-mm increases every 6 hours to boost the osteogenesis process. The patient or family performs the distraction by turning bolts or knobs at set intervals throughout the day. Corticotomies can be performed in the metaphyseal or diaphyseal region, but tend to do better with less complications when done in the metaphyseal region. And while two simultaneous corticotomy sites in the same tibia can produce satisfactory results, this is not recommended in the femur.

The original Wagner technique, once popular in the United States, did not follow a majority of these principles and had high rates of complication.[121] A complete diaphyseal osteotomy was performed with a monolateral frame external fixator placed. Distraction was immediately initiated at a rate of 1.5 to 2.0 mm/day performed at one interval. After full distraction was achieved, an iliac crest bone autograft was implanted and plated to support the bone gap, and the external fixator was removed. After the graft was incorporated into the bone, the plates were removed. The entire process involved three operative procedures and could not be used to correct angular or rotational deformities.

Ilizarov introduced a circular frame external fixator with telescoping rods to employ his biologic principles during a metaphyseal lengthening procedure (Fig. 13.23).[121] But the Ilizarov principles are successfully applied with the use of newer devices previously discussed with Blount disease. The Taylor Spatial Frame (TSF) is another circular frame with telescoping rods, while the Limb Reconstruction System (Orthofix®) and the Multiaxial Correction System (Biomet®) devices are monolateral frames used successfully for limb-lengthening procedures. After the desired length is achieved, the external fixator device is kept in place for approximately 1 month for every 1 cm of distraction until the bone consolidation phase is complete.[121] All of these systems are used to correct angular and rotational components of limb leg

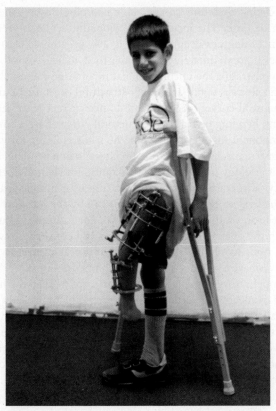

FIGURE 13.23 A 9-year-old boy with a diagnosis of PFFD who is presently undergoing an Ilizarov lengthening. The lengthening will provide a longer level arm when wearing his prosthesis and bring the height of his knees closer together.

discrepancies as well. The pins can be removed in an outpatient procedure. The disadvantages of the Ilizarov and TSF are the multiple pin sites and bulkiness of the apparatus. The overall length of time required to achieve the desired length and keep the fixator in place are disadvantages of all external systems.

The Intramedullary Skeletal Kinetic Distractor (Orthofix®) is an internally implanted device utilized for limb lengthening. The patient controls the lengthening process through rotational movements of the lower leg. These systems eliminate the spatial problems and extended duration of external frames. Dror Paley introduced the lengthening on nail (LON) procedure, which combines traditional external fixators with an intramedullary nail to decrease the overall duration of external fixator placement and bone healing time.[122] This procedure has been shown to result in a higher incidence of treatable hindfoot equinus likely due to accelerated lengthening.[122]

Limb-lengthening procedures bring their own set of problems to the child, family, and professionals involved in the care of the child. Families must be able to make multiple appointments over a period of time, perform daily pin care, and carry out exercise programs. Problems that may be encountered during the course of a lengthening procedure include infection at the pin sites, joint stiffness, subluxation or

dislocation (especially of the proximal tibia), nonunion, and fractures. ROM limitations occur secondary to shortening of the soft tissues and the rate of soft tissue growth compared with that of bone.

Physical Therapy

Physical therapy intensity varies with the five phases of the process: latency, distraction, consolidation, fixator removal and healing, and the rehabilitation phase. Immediately after surgery during the latency or delayed distraction period, the physical therapist is involved for gait-training activities and promoting early weight bearing, which further facilitates bone growth for most children who have undergone a lengthening procedure. Instruction in pin care must also begin immediately postoperatively to prevent infection. Pins can also be wrapped with gauze to provide soft tissue compression, which reduces pain resulting from tissue movement or microtearing around pin sites. Stretching can be initiated to minimize ROM limitations.

During the distraction phase, physical therapy should be frequent and focused on ROM and stretching along with corresponding strengthening activity. Decreased knee and ankle joint ROM are common and should be addressed consistently. Splinting can be utilized during this phase, especially for the ankle. Hip ROM may become limited to a lesser extent. It is important for the therapist to acknowledge that maintaining the same ROM measurement over the duration of the distraction phase actually represents increased muscle and soft tissue length, and this should be considered successful ROM intervention progress. Therapists should be considerate of fixator pin placement, especially in the thigh and around the knee. Typical lateral pin placement, especially distal on the femur, will contribute to soft tissue impalement of the tensor fascia lata and iliotibial band complex, thereby limiting achievable knee ROM. As a result, ROM losses may occur during the distraction phase. But aggressive intervention is still necessary during the lengthening process. Strengthening can safely include modalities such as electric stimulation and aquatic therapy. Limited motion and muscle atrophy may also contribute to muscle adhesion. Tissue mobilization should be used to facilitate soft tissue movement and improved joint motion.

During the consolidation phase, strengthening and tissue mobilization activities should be continued while previously achieved ROM should be at least maintained. This phase should include formal program supervision or weekly monitoring by the therapist. However, insurance restrictions may require the use of a comprehensive HEP rather than supervised therapy sessions. A cast is placed following fixator removal to protect the new bone during continued healing. During this phase, an HEP is sufficient to promote continued allowable stretching and strengthening of nonimmobilized joints.

The rehabilitation phase may last up to 1 year. During this phase, aggressive stretching is advanced to achieve as much functional ROM as possible. Flex casting and dynamic splinting are often utilized as a stretching adjunct to address knee flexion or extension and ankle plantar flexion contractures. ROM status often regresses, so the therapist should remain steadfast and utilize soft tissue mobilization techniques to maintain progress. Strengthening activities are progressed as muscles and soft tissue is further lengthened. Functional activities and gait normalization can be implemented as bone healing progresses and muscle strength and ROM increase. Postural reactions and balance training should be addressed as the body accommodates to the new limb length, limits of stability, base of support, and center of gravity.

Scoliosis (Idiopathic)

Scoliosis is a lateral curvature of the spine greater than 10 degrees. Idiopathic denotes that the scoliosis is of unknown origin—the most common form of scoliosis. Idiopathic scoliosis can be further delineated by age of onset: infantile occurs in children from birth to 3 years of age, juvenile occurs between the ages of 3 and 10 years, and adolescent develops after 10 years of age.[123] This section of the chapter focuses on adolescent idiopathic scoliosis (AIS). However, the pediatric therapist should be mindful that not all scoliosis is

idiopathic; therefore, congenital or neurologic causes should be ruled out. The incidence of idiopathic scoliosis greater than 10 degrees is approximately 2%, greater than 20 degrees is approximately 1%, greater than 40 degrees is 0.4%, demonstrating the uncommon nature of large curves.[124,125]

Scoliosis is defined as either structural or nonstructural. Structural curves are fixed and do not correct with lateral trunk bending or traction. Structural curves have a rotary component that is visible when the trunk is flexed forward. Nonstructural curves correct on lateral trunk bending, and their etiology is often a pelvic obliquity, limb length discrepancy, or medical factors such as a tumor or muscle spasm. Structural scoliosis is further identified by the location and direction of the apex of the curve. For example, a curve with the apex in the thoracic region and convexity toward the right would be labeled as a right thoracic curve. Most curves have a primary curve and a compensatory curve. The compensatory curve is the body's attempt to keep the head and trunk aligned vertically. In the preceding example of the right thoracic curve, there may be smaller compensatory curves in the cervical or lumbar regions with their convexity toward the left (Fig. 13.24A). More than 90% of AIS is right thoracic or left lumbar, and an atypical presentation should be cause for further investigation.[123]

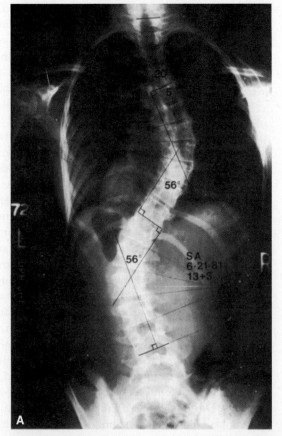

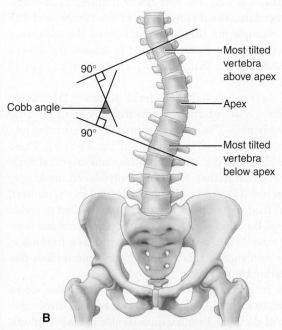

FIGURE 13.24 **(A)** Right thoracic, left lumbar scoliosis. **(B)** The degree of curvature is measured using the Cobb method. The end vertebrae, or the vertebrae that tilt toward the concavity the most, are identified. Lines are drawn extending the end plate of the top and bottom vertebrae for each curve. Perpendicular lines to the end plate lines are then drawn. The degree of curvature is defined as the angle of intersection of the end plate and perpendicular lines.

Multiple structural changes occur with scoliosis and their severity is related to the severity of the curve.[24] Changes occur in the growing spine in response to compression and distraction forces that are altered in the presence of a curvature. The vertebrae become wedge shaped, higher on the convex side and compressed on the concave side, and muscles on the concave side become shortened. The vertebral body rotates toward the convex side so that the spinous process is rotated toward the concave side. Because the ribs are attached to the thoracic vertebrae, the vertebrae may rotate. The rotation of the ribs produces a posterior rib hump, which is noted on the forward-bend test (Fig. 13.25). Thoracic scoliosis can also decrease normal kyphosis, further exemplifying the three-dimensional nature of the disorder.

Screening

School-based screenings for scoliosis are mandated in many states but have been a source of controversy with recent conflicting recommendations from two major health policy groups.[123] Screening should be targeted at girls aged 10 and again at 12 years and for boys at 13 or 14 years. A screening should include anterior and posterior views of the trunk with the shirt removed and a forward-bend Adams test (Fig. 13.25).[123] On the anterior and posterior views, the examiner looks for asymmetries in shoulder, nipple, scapular, or pelvic heights; asymmetric inguinal or gluteal folds; and curvature of the spine. The adolescent is then asked to bend over, keeping the knees extended, and allowing the arms to dangle toward the floor. During the forward-bend test, the examiner looks for asymmetries in the contour of the back (classic rib hump), indicating the rotary component of the curvature.

When scoliosis is detected, the adolescent should be referred to an orthopedist. Accurate measurement of the curve is performed through a variety of methods. A common method of measurement is a radiograph and the Cobb angle (Fig. 13.24A–B). To limit radiographic exposure, other measurement methods include Moiré topography and the Integrated Shape Imaging System 2 (ISIS2).[126] Moiré topography is a photogrammetric technique that visually depicts shadow patterns that identify asymmetries. ISIS2 utilizes computer images in the transverse, frontal, and sagittal planes to develop contours of the adolescent's trunk.[126] The goal of measurement is to determine a baseline and monitor progression of the curve.

Management of Scoliosis

Treatment intervention is based on the sex, age, and skeletal maturity of the adolescent and the severity of the curvature.[123,127] Prepubertal children are almost certain to exhibit progression of their curvature, especially when initially presenting with a curve of greater than 20 degrees. Females with a bone age of 15 years and males with a bone age of 17 years with curves less than 30 degrees generally do not

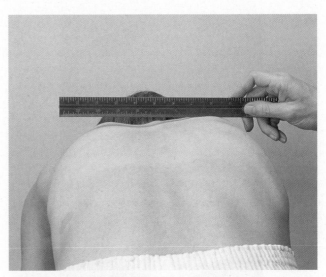

FIGURE 13.25 Forward-bend test. Rib hump is visible on bending forward.

require treatment.[123] Curves less than 25 degrees can be observed on a regular basis to monitor progression of the curve. Curves between 25 and 40 degrees should be treated with nonsurgical methods. Adolescents with curves greater than 40 degrees are candidates for surgical intervention.[123,127]

NONOPERATIVE MANAGEMENT The goal of nonoperative intervention is to maintain the curvature during growth, not to correct the curvature although improved alignment can occur.[127] Nonoperative intervention methods have included exercise, electrical stimulation, and orthoses. Evidence supporting the beneficial effects of therapeutic exercise or electric stimulation in reducing or altering the progression of a curvature is inconsistent and lacking supportive controlled studies.[123] Exercise is still indicated to maintain strength of muscles when an orthosis is used.

Orthosis management has been used in the treatment of scoliosis for many years. A recently published randomized controlled trial was stopped early owing to the efficacy of bracing.[128] Most orthotic devices operate on the principle of three-point pressure against the apex of the curve and may also incorporate a traction component. The cervicothoracic lumbosacral Milwaukee brace was one of the first orthoses developed for scoliosis. It incorporates a custom-molded trunk shell with metal uprights attached to a collar that supports the chin and occiput. Although it is effective, it is no longer a brace of choice on account of significant cosmetic concerns and patient preference.

Much slimmer and lighter-weight thoracic–lumbar–sacral orthoses (TLSO) (Fig. 13.26) that eliminate the chin and occiput component of the Milwaukee brace are the gold standard for most curves. The Boston Brace or similar variations are the most common TLSOs used in North America.[128] The pelvic stabilization and lateral pressure pads are present in a TLSO. Adolescents are generally instructed to wear the orthosis until skeletal maturity or unless the curve continues

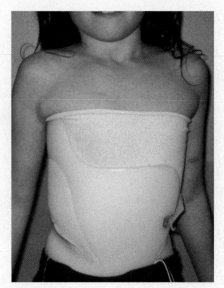

FIGURE 13.26 Boston brace (thoracic–lumbar–sacral orthosis [TLSO]).
(Sponseller PD. Bracing for adolescent idiopathic scoliosis in practice today. *J Pediatr Orthop.* 2011;31:S53–S60).

to progress and surgery is indicated. Recommended wear time is at least 18 hours. Published controlled data demonstrate the positive correlation between success rate and increased average wear time.[128]

Instruction in donning and doffing the orthosis, developing a wearing schedule, skin care, and an exercise program to maintain ROM and strength while wearing the orthosis are provided by a physical therapist. Exercise should be focused on maintaining flexibility and muscle strength of the trunk. Hip flexion contractures can develop with use of the orthosis; routine stretching of the hip flexors should be instituted when orthosis wearing is initiated. Muscle strength must be maintained while wearing the orthosis to prepare the trunk muscles for when the orthosis is discontinued. Exercise should include strengthening for abdominals, gluteal muscles such as squats and lunges, and paraspinal musculature through traditional core and lumbar stabilization programs.

OPERATIVE MANAGEMENT Surgical intervention is warranted if the curve is greater than 40 degrees, the curve is progressing with conservative management, or there is decompensation of the spine or thoracic cavity.[123,127] The goal of surgery is to obtain as much correction as possible and to stabilize the spine and maintain the correction over time. The Lenke Classification, which considers the curve type, relationship between lumbar and sacral alignment, and the sagittal curve profile, was developed to guide operative treatment decisions for orthopedic surgeons.[127]

Two main surgical approaches exist: the anterior and the posterior approach. The anterior approach goes through the chest cavity and has been associated with increased morbidity due to decreased pulmonary function.[127] The posterior approach is becoming the option of choice for AIS. This

option has been further facilitated by the development and progression of pedicle screw technology. Pedicle screws provide solid fixation through a majority of the vertebrae. The screws are then connected by rods allowing deformity correction in all three planes. That is, primary curve in the frontal plane, vertebral rotation in the transverse plane, and kyphosis or lordosis restoration or stabilization in the sagittal plane. Recent approaches target surgical correction of the primary structural curve allowing flexible compensatory curves to self-correct over time.[127] This approach preserves as much natural spinal motion as possible limiting previous detrimental effects of unnecessary lumbar spine anchoring. Pedicle screws and shorter segment rod fixation have replaced a majority of hook, wire, and Harrington rod procedures with good outcomes and less complication.

Physical Therapy

Ideally, physical therapy has been involved preoperatively with ROM and trunk-strengthening exercises as well as bed mobility instruction. Instruction in deep breathing and coughing exercises should be initiated preoperatively and adhered to immediately postoperatively. The adolescent is always encouraged to begin early mobilization, including transfers and gait training, to expedite healing and recovery. Balance, vestibular, and field of vision changes should be considered during gait training as the head position and height may be immediately altered and elevated following spinal straightening. Time frames for early mobilization and ambulation depend on the surgical technique, surgeon's preference, and whether or not a supportive orthosis is needed, but in some cases can begin as early as postoperative day one. Physical therapy is one of the important interventions for the adolescent with AIS, regardless of whether conservative or surgical care has been employed.

SUMMARY

The growth and development and disorders of a child's musculoskeletal system were discussed in this chapter. The immature musculoskeletal system of a child is susceptible to abnormal forces and stresses. Physical therapists must be alert to those forces and the consequences they may have on the developing musculoskeletal system. Many orthopedic diagnoses that were discussed in this chapter are the result of the effect of abnormal forces on the developing child and morphologic defects occurring during fetal development. However, the examination and intervention principles that were discussed and the assessment procedures that were outlined can be applied to any child seen by a physical therapist, not just those children with a diagnosis of orthopedic origin. Identifying the underlying causes, estimating the risk of further deformity or disease progression, and developing an evidence-based plan of care based on your complete assessment is the challenging but very rewarding aspect of pediatric physical therapy.

REFERENCES

1. Crelin ES. Development of the musculoskeletal system. *Clin Symp*. 1981;33:2–36.
2. Walker JM. Musculoskeletal development: a review. *Phys Ther*. 1991;71:878–889.
3. Arkin AM, Katz JF. The effects of pressure on epiphyseal growth. *J Bone Joint Surg Am*. 1956;38:1056–1076.
4. Storey E. Growth and remodeling of bone and bones. *Dent Clin North Am*. 1975;19:443–454.
5. LeVeau BF, Bernhardt DB. Developmental biomechanics: effect of forces on the growth, development and maintenance of the human body. *Phys Ther*. 1984;64:1874–1882.
6. Dunne KB, Clarren SK. The origin of prenatal and postnatal deformities. *Pediatr Clin North Am*. 1986;33:1277–1297.
7. Puberty and the Tanner Stages. www.childgrowthfoundation.org/CMS/FILES/Puberty_and_the_Tanner_Stages.pdf. Accessed November 10 2013.
8. Stuberg WA, Metcalf WK. Reliability of quantitative muscle testing in healthy children and in children with Duchenne muscular dystrophy using a hand-held dynamometer. *Phys Ther*. 1988;68:977–982.
9. Allington N, Leroy N, Doneux C. Ankle joint range of motion measurements in spastic cerebral palsy children: intraobserver and interobserver reliability and reproducibility of goniometry and visual estimation. *J Pediatr Orthop Part B*. 2002;11:236–239.
10. McWhirk LB, Glanzman AM. Within-session inter-rater reliability of goniometric measures in patients with spastic cerebreal palsy. *Pediatr Phys Ther*. 2006;18:4:262–265.
11. Glanzman AM, Swenson AE, Kim H. Intrarater range of motion reliability in cerebral palsy: a comparison of methods. *Pediatr Phys Ther*. 2008;20:4:369–372.
12. Bleck EE. *Orthopedic Management in Cerebral Palsy*. Philadelphia, PA: JB Lippincott; 1987.
12a. Russek LN. Examination and treatment of a patient with hypermobility syndrome. *Phys Ther*. 2000;80(4):386–398.
13. Kendall FP, McCreary EK. *Muscles: Testing and Function*. Baltimore, MD: Williams & Wilkins; 1993.
14. Merlini L, Dell'Accio D, Granata C. Reliability of dynamic strength knee muscle testing in children. *J Sports Phys Ther*. 1995;22:73–76.
15. Tsiros MD, Grimshaw PN, Shield AJ, et al. The Biodex isokinetic dynamometer for knee strength assessment in children: advantages and limitations. *Work*. 2011;39(2):161–167.
16. Effgen SK, Brown DA. Long-term stability of hand-held dynamometric measurements in children who have myelomeningocele. *Phys Ther*. 1992;72:458–465.
17. Hinderer K, Gutierrez T. Myometry measurements of children using isometric and eccentric methods of muscle testing (Abstract). *Phys Ther*. 1988;68:817.
18. Stuberg WA, Koehler A, Wichita M, et al. Comparison of femoral torsion assessment using goniometry and computerized tomography. *Pediatr Phys*. 1989;1:115–118.
19. Gajdosik CG. Ability of very young children to produce reliable isometric force measurements. *Pediatr Phys Ther*. 2005;17(4):251–257.
20. Holm I, Fredriksen P, Fosdahl M, et al. A normative sample of isotonic and isokinetic muscle strength measurements in children 7 to 12 years of age. *Acta Paediatrica*. 2008;97(5):602–607.
21. Wiggin M, Wilkinson K, Habetz S, et al. Percentile values of isokinetic peak torque in children six through thirteen years old. *Pediatr Phys Ther*. 2006;18(1):3–18.
22. Staheli LT, Corbett M, Wyss C, et al. Lower-extremity rotational problems in children. *J Bone Joint Surg*. 1985;67A:39–47.
23. Cusick BD, Stuberg WA. Assessment of lower-extremity alignment in the transverse plane: implications for management of children with neuromotor dysfunction. *Phys Ther*. 1992;72:3–15.
24. Tachdjian MO. *Pediatric Orthopedics*. 2nd ed. Philadelphia, PA: WB Saunders Co.; 1990.
25. World Health Organization. *International Classification of Functioning, Disability, and Health*. Geneva, Switzerland: World Health Organization; 2001.
26. Spranger J, Benirschke JG, Hall W, et al. Errors of morphogenesis: concepts and terms. *J Pediatr*. 1982;100:160–165.
27. Day HJB. The ISO/ISPO classification of congenital limb deficiency. *Prosth Orthot Int*. 1991;15:67–69.
28. Wright PE, Jobe MT. Congenital anomalies of the hand. In: Canlae ST, Beaty JH, eds. *Operative Pediatric Orthopedics*. Philadelphia, PA: Mosby–Year Book; 1991:253–330.
29. Swanson AB, Barsky AJ, Entin MA. Classification of limb malformations on the basis of embryological failures. *Surg Clin North Am*. 1968;48:1169–1179.
30. Heikel HVA. Aplasia and hypoplasia of the radius. *Acta Orthop Scand (Suppl)*. 1959;39:1.
31. Morrissy RT, Giavedoni BJ, Coulter-O'Berry C. The limb-deficient child. In: Lovell WW, Winter RB, eds. *Pediatric Orthopedics*. 5th ed. Philadelphia, PA: Lippincott Williams & Wilkins; 2001:1217–1272.
32. Aitken GT. Proximal femoral focal deficiency: definition, classification and management. In: *Proximal Femoral Focal Deficiency: A Congenital Anomaly*. Washington, DC: National Academy of Sciences; 1969:1–22.
33. Shurr DG, Cook TM. *Prosthetics and Orthotics*. East Norwalk, CT: Appleton & Lange; 1990:183–193.
34. Bayne LG, Klug MS. Long-term review of the surgical treatment of radial deficiencies. *J Hand Surg Am*. 1987;12:169–179.
35. Herzenberg JE. Congenital limb deficiency and limb length discrepancy. In: Canale ST, Beaty JH, eds. *Operative Pediatric Orthopedics*. Philadelphia, PA: Mosby–Year Book; 1991:187–252.
36. Kruger LM. Lower-limb deficiencies: surgical management. In: Bowker JH, Michael JW, eds. *Atlas of Limb Prosthetics: Surgical, Prosthetic, and Rehabilitation Principles*. Philadelphia, PA: Mosby–Year Book; 1981:795–834.
37. Kant P, Koh SH, Neumann V, et al. Treatment of longitudinal deficiency affecting the femur: comparing patient mobility and satisfaction outcomes of Syme amputation against extension prosthesis. *J Pediatr Orthop*. 2003;23:236–242.
38. Krajbich JL. Rotationplasty in the management of proximal femoral focal deficiency. In: Herring JA, Birch JG, eds. *The Child with a Limb Deficiency*. Rosemont, IL: American Academy of Orthopedic Surgeons; 1998:87.
39. Gillespie R. Principles of amputation surgery in children with longitudinal limb deficiencies of the femur. *Clin Orthop Rel Res*. 1990;256:29–38.
40. Ackman J, Altiok H, Flanagan A, et al. Long-term follow-up of Van Nes rotationplasty in patients with congenital proximal focal femoral deficiency. *Bone Joint J*. 2013;95-B:192–198.
41. Gover AM, McIvor J. Upper limb deficiencies in infants and young children. *Infants Young Child*. 1992;5:58–72.
42. Cummings DR. Pediatric prosthetics, current trends and future possibilities. *Phys Med Rehabil Clin N Am*. 2003;11:653–679.
43. Wilk B, Karol L, Halliday S, et al. Transition to an articulating knee prosthesis in pediatric amputees. *J Prosthet Orthot*. 1999;11:69–74.
44. Coulter-O'Berry C. Physical therapy considerations in pediatric acquired and congenital lower limb amputees. In: Smith DG, Michael JW, Bowker JH, eds. *Atlas of Amputations & Limb Deficiencies: Surgical, Prosthetic and Rehabilitation Principles*. 3rd ed. Rosemont, IL: American Academy of Orthopedic Surgeons; 2004:831.
45. Suzuki S, Yamamura T, Fujita A. Aetiological relationship between congenital torticollis and obstetrical paralysis. *Int Orthop*. 1984;8:175–181.
46. Bredenkamp JK, Hoover LA, Berke GS, et al. Congenital muscular torticollis. *Arch Otolaryngol Head Neck Surg*. 1990;116:212–216.
47. Binder H, Eng GD, Gaiser JF, et al. Congenital muscular torticollis: results of conservative management with long-term follow-up in 85 cases. *Arch Phys Med Rehabil*. 1987;68:222–225.
48. Emery C. The determinants of treatment duration for congenital muscular torticollis. *Phys Ther*. 1994;74:921–929.

49. Cheng JCY, Wong MWN, Tang SP, et al. Clinical determinants of the outcome of manual stretching in the treatment of congenital muscular torticollis in infants. *J Bone Joint Surg.* 2001;83A(5):679–687.

50. Van Vlimmeren LA, Helders PJM, Van Adrichem LNA, et al. Torticollis and plagiocephaly in infancy: therapeutic strategies. *Pediatr Rehabil.* 2006;9(1):40–46.

51. American Academy of Pediatrics. Changing concepts of sudden infant death syndrome: implications for infant sleeping environment and sleep position. *Pediatrics.* 2000;105:650–656.

52. Kane AA, Mitchell LE, Craven KP, et al. Observations on a recent increase in plagiocephaly without synostosis. *Pediatrics.* 1996;97:877–885.

53. Persing J, James H, Swanson J, et al. Prevention and management of positional skull deformities in infants. *Pediatrics.* 2003;112:199–202.

54. De Chalain TM, Park S. Torticollis associated with positional plagiocephaly: a growing epidemic. *J Craniofac Surg.* 2005;16(3):411–418.

55. Ballock RT, Song KM. The prevalence of nonmuscular causes of torticollis in children. *J Pediatr Orthop.* 1996;16(4):500–504.

56. Taylor JL, Norton ES. Developmental muscular torticollis: outcomes in young children treated by physical therapy. *Pediatr Phys Ther.* 1997;9(4):173–178.

57. Vles JSH, Colla C, Weber JW, et al. Helmet versus nonhelmet treatment in nonsynostotic positional posterior plagiocephaly. *J Craniofac Surg.* 2000;11(6):572–574.

58. Lipira AB, Gordon S, Darvann TA, et al. Helmet versus active repositioning for plagiocephaly: a three-dimensional analysis. *Pediatrics.* 2010;126:e936–e945.

59. Jacques C, Karmel-Ross K. The use of splinting in conservative and post-operative treatment of congenital muscular torticollis. *Phys Occup Ther Pediatr.* 1997;17:81–90.

60. Hensinger RN, Jones ET. Developmental orthopedics: the lower limb. *Dev Med Child Neurol.* 1982;24:95–116.

61. Dunn PM. Congenital postural deformities. *Br Med Bull.* 1976;32:71–76.

62. Furdon SA, Donlon CR. Examination of the newborn foot: positional and structural abnormalities. *Advances in Neonatal Care.* 2002;2(5):248–258.

63. Beaty JH. Congenital anomalies of the lower and upper extremities. In: Canale ST, Beaty JH, eds. *Operative Pediatric Orthopedics.* Philadelphia, PA: Mosby–Year Book; 1991:73–186.

64. Staheli LT. *Fundamentals of Pediatric Orthopedics.* Philadelphia, PA: Lippincott-Raven; 1992.

65. Hart ES, Grottkau BE, Rebello GN, et al. The newborn foot: diagnosis and management of common conditions. *Orthop Nurs.* 2005;24(5):313–321.

66. Weymouth KS, Blanton SH, Bamshad MJ, et al. Variants in genes that encode muscle contractile proteins influence risk of isolated clubfoot. *Am J Med Genet Part A.* 2011;155:2170–2179.

67. Alvarado DM, Aferol H, McCall K, et al. Familial isolated clubfoot is associated with recurrent chromosome 17q23.1q23. 2 microduplications containing TBX4. *Am J of Hum Genet.* 2010;87(1):154–160.

68. Morcuende JA, Dolan LA, Dietz FR, et al. Radical reduction in the rate of extensive corrective surgery for clubfoot using the Ponseti method. *Pediatrics.* 2004;113:376–380.

69. Sala DA, Chu A, Lehman WB, et al. Achievement of gross motor milestones in children with idiopathic clubfoot treated with the Ponseti method. *J Pediatr Orthop.* 2013;33(1):55–58.

70. Hensinger RN. Congenital dislocation of the hip, treatment in infancy to walking age. *Orthop Clin North Am.* 1987;18:597–616.

71. Mubarak MD, Garfin S, Vance R, et al. Pitfalls in the use of the Pavlik harness for treatment of congenital dysplasia, subluxation, and dislocation of the hip. *J Bone Joint Surg Am.* 1981;63:1239–1247.

72. Darin N, Kimber E, Kroksmark A, et al. Multiple congenital contractures: birth prevalence, etiology, and outcome. *J Pediatr.* 2002;140:61–67.

73. Thompson GH, Bilenker RM. Comprehensive management of arthrogryposis multiplex congenita. *Clin Orthop Rel Res.* 1985;194:6–14.

74. Banker BQ. Neuropathic aspects of arthrogryposis multiplex congenita. *Clin Orthop Rel Res.* 1985;194:30–43.

75. Staheli LT. Torsional deformity. *Pediatr Clin North Am.* 1986;33(6):1373–1383.

76. Forlino A, Cabral WA, Barnes AM, et al. New perspectives on osteogenesis imperfecta. *Nat Rev Endocrinol.* 2011;7(9):540–557.

77. Basel D, Steiner RD. Osteogenesis imperfecta: recent findings shed new light on this once well-understood condition. *Genet Med.* 2009;11(6):375–385.

78. Binder H, Hawks L, Graybill G, et al. Osteogenesis imperfecta: rehabilitation approach with infants and young children. *Adv Pediatr.* 1984;65:537–541.

79. Binder H, Conway A, Gerber LH. Rehabilitation approaches to children with osteogenesis imperfecta: a ten-year experience. *Arch Phys Med Rehabil.* 1993;74:386–390.

80. Amor MB, Rauch F, Monti E, et al. Osteogenesis imperfecta. *Ped Endocrinol Rev.* 2013;10(S2):397–405.

81. Cundy T. Recent advances in osteogenesis imperfecta. *Calcif Tissue Int.* 2012;90:439–449.

82. Seikaly MG, Kopanati S, Salhab N, et al. Impact of alendronate on quality of life in children with osteogenesis imperfecta. *J Pediatr Orthop.* 2005;25(6):786–791.

83. Plotkin H, Rauch FH, Bishop NJ, et al. Pamidronate treatment of severe osteogenesis imperfecta in children under 3 years of age. *J Clin Endocrinol Metab.* 2000;85:1846–1850.

84. Castillo H, Samson-Fang L. Effects of bisphosphonates in children with osteogenesis imperfecta: an AACPDM systematic review. *Dev Med Child Neurol.* 2008;51:17–29.

85. Vourimies I, Toiviainen-Salo S, Hero M, et al. Zoledronic acid treatment in children with osteogenesis imperfecta. *Horm Res Paediatr.* 2011;75:346–353.

86. Land C, Rauch F, Montpetit K, et al. Effect of intravenous pamidronate therapy on functional abilities and level of amulation in children with osteogenesis imperfecta. *J Pediatr.* 2006;148:456–460.

87. Ward LM, Rauch F, Whyte MP, et al. Alendronate for the treatment of pediatric osteogenesis imperfecta: a randomized placebo-controlled study. *J Clin Endocrinol Metab.* 2011;96:355–364.

88. Sakkers R, Kok D, Englebert RH, et al. Skeletal effects and functional outcome with olpadronate in children with osteogenesis imperfecta: a 2 year randomized, placebo-controlled study. *Lancet.* 2004;363:1427–1431.

89. Gerber LH, Binder H, Weintrob J, et al. Rehabilitation of children and infants with osteogenesis imperfecta. *Clin Orthop Rel Res.* 1990;251:254–262.

90. Cintas HL, Gerber LH. *Children with Osteogenesis Imperfecta: Strategies to Enhance Performance.* Gaithersburg, MD: Osteogenesis Imperfecta Foundation Inc; 2005.

91. Van Brussel M, Takken T, Uiterwaal CSPM, et al. Physical training in osteogenesis imperfecta. *J Pediatr.* 2008;152:111–116.

92. Osawa Y, Oguma Y, Ishii N. The effects of whole-body vibration on muscle strength and power: a meta-analysis. *J Musculoskelet Neuronal Interact.* 2013;13(3):342–352.

93. Semler O, Fricke O, Vezyroglou K, et al. Results of a prospective pilot trial on mobility after whole body vibration in children and adolescents with osteogenesis imperfecta. *Clin Rehab.* 2008;22:387–394.

94. Mitchell AL, Schwarze U, Jennings JF, et al. Molecular mechanisms of classical ehlers-danlos syndrome. *Hum Mutat.* 2009;30:995–1002.

95. Childs SG. Musculoskeletal manifestations of ehlers-danlos syndrome. *Orthop Nursing.* 2010;29(2):133–139.

96. Voermans NC, van Alfen N, Pillen S, et al. Neuromuscular involvement in various types of ehlers-danlos syndrome. *Ann Neurol.* 2009;65:687–697.

97. Kirk JA, Ansell BM, Bywaters EG. The hypermobility syndrome. Musculoskeletal complaints associated with generalized joint hypermobility. *Ann Rheum Dis.* 1967;26:419–425.

98. Grahame R. The revised (Beighton 1998) criteria for the diagnosis of benign joint hypermobility syndrome (BJHS). *J Rheumatol.* 2000;27:1777–1779.

99. Wolf JM, Cameron KL, Owens BD. Impact of joint laxity and hypermobility on the musculoskeletal system. *J Am Acad Orthop Surg.* 2011;19:463–471.

100. Kim HKW. Legg-Calve-Perthes disease: etiology, pathogenesis and biology. *J Pediatr Orthop.* 2011;31(2 suppl):S141–S146.

101. Perry DC, Green DJ, Bruce CE, et al. Abnormalities of vascular structure and funtion in children with perthese disease. *Pediatrics.* 2012;130:e126–e131.

102. Kim HKW, Herring JA. Pathophysiology, classifications, and natural history of perthes disease. *Orthop Clin N Am.* 2011;42:285–295.

103. Rajan R, Chandrasenan J, Price K, et al. Legg-Calve-Perthes disease: intraobserver and intraobserver reliability of the modified herring lateral pillar classification. *J Pediatr Orthop.* 2013;33:120–123.

104. Nguyen NT, Klein G, Dogbey G, et al. Operative versus nonoperative treatments for legg-calve-perthes disease: a meta-analysis. *J Pediatr Orthop.* 2012;32:697–705.

105. Herring JA, Kim HT, Browne R. Legg-Calve-Perthes disease. Part II: prospective multicenter study of the effect of treatment on outcome. *J Bone Joint Surg.* 2004;86A(10):2121–2134.

106. Terjesen T, Wiig O, Svenningsen S. The natural history of perthes' disease: risk factors in 212 patients followed for 5 years. *Acta Orthop.* 2010;81(6):708–714.

107. Rich MM, Schoenecker PL. Management of legg-calve-perthes disease using an A-frame orthosis and hip range of motion: a 25 year experience. *J Pediatr Orthop.* 2013;33:112–119.

108. Gholve PA, Cameron DB, Millis MB. Slipped capital femoral epiphysis update. *Curr Opin Pediatr.* 2009;21:39–45.

109. Loder RT, Aronsson DD, Dobbs MB, et al. Slipped capital femoral epiphysis. *Instr Course Lect.* 2001;50:555–570.

110. Riad J, Bajelidze G, Gabos PS. Bilatateral slipped capital femoral epiphysis: predictive factors for contralateral slip. *J Pediatr Orthop.* 2007;27:411–414.

111. Millis MB, Novais EN. In situ fixation for slipped capital femoral epiphysis: perspectives in 2011. *J Bone Joint Surg Am.* 2011;93(suppl 2):46–51.

112. Clarke SE, McCarthy JJ, Davidson RS. Treatment of blount disease: a comparison between the multaxial correction system and other external fixators. *J Pediatr Orthop.* 2009;29(2):103–109.

113. Langenskiold A. Tibia vara: a critical review. *Clin Orthop Relat Res.* 1989;246:195–207.

114. Langenskiöld A. Tibia vara: osteochondrosis deformans tibiae: a survey of 23 cases. *Acta Chir Scand.* 1952;103:1–8.

115. Zionts LE, Shean CJ. Brace treatment of early infantile tibia vara. *J Pediatr Orthop.* 1998;18(1):102–109.

116. Gilbody J, Thomas G, Ho K. Acute versus gradual corretion of idiopathic tibia vara in children: a systematic review. *J Pediatr Orthop.* 2009;29:110–114.

117. Richards BS, Katz DE, Sims JB. Effectiveness of brace treatment in early infantile Blount's disease. *J Pediat Orthop.* 1998;18(3):374–380.

118. Wiemann JM, Tryon C, Szalay EA. Physeal stapling versus 8-plate hemiephiphysiodesis for guided correction of angular deformity about the knee. *J Pediatr Orthop.* 2009;29:481–485.

119. Sabharwal S, Kumar A. Methods for assessing leg length discrepancy. *Clin Orthop Relat Res.* 2008;466:2910–2922.

120. Friend L, Widmann RF. Advances in management of limb length discrepancy and lower limb deformity. *Curr Opin Pediatr.* 2008;20:46–51.

121. Birch JG, Samchukov ML. Use of the Ilizarov method to correct lower limb deformities in children and adolescents. *J Am Acad Orthop Surg.* 2004;12:144–154.

122. Sun XT, Easwar TR, Manesh S, et al. Complications and outcome of tibial lengthening using the Ilizarov method with and without a supplementary intramedullary nail: a case-matched comparative study. *J Bone Joint Surg (Br).* 2011;93-B:782–787.

123. Hresko MT. Idiopathic scoliosis in adolescents. *N Engl J Med.* 2013;368:834–841.

124. Yawn BP, Yawn RA, Hodge D, et al. A population-based study of school scoliosis screening. *JAMA.* 1999;282:1427–1432.

125. Rogala EJ, Drummond DS, Gurr J. Scoliosis: incidence and natural history, a prospective epidemiological study. *J Bone Joint Surg Am.* 1978;60:173–177.

126. Berryman F, Pynsent P, Fairbank J, et al. A new system for measuring three-dimensional back shape in scoliosis. *Eur Spine J.* 2008;17(5):663–672.

127. Hoashi JS, Cahill PJ, Bennett JT, et al. Adolescent scoliosis: classification and treatment. *Neurosurg Clin N Am.* 2013;24:173–183.

128. Weinstein SL, Dolan LA, Wright JG, et al. Effects of bracing in adolescents with idiopathic scoliosis. *N Engl J Med.* 2013;369:1512–1521.

Sports Injuries in Children and Adolescents

Elliot M. Greenberg and Eric T. Greenberg

Introduction

Anatomic and Physiologic Differences of the Skeletally Immature Athlete
Bone Composition
Muscular Properties

Examination Principles
History
Physical Examination

Upper Extremity
Examination and Treatment Principles
The Pediatric Throwing Athlete
Elbow Injuries
Other Shoulder Pathologies
Other Elbow Injuries
Forearm, Wrist, and Hand Injuries

Pelvis, Hip, and Thigh Injuries
Examination Principles
Specific Injuries to the Pelvis, Hip, and Thigh

Knee Injuries
Examination Principles
Ligamentous Injuries
Intra-articular Injuries
Overuse injuries

Lower Leg Injuries
Shin Splints

Ankle Injuries
Ankle Sprains
Ankle Fractures
Ankle Impingement

Foot injuries
Overuse Injuries
Traumatic Injuries
Bony Abnormalities
Forefoot Injuries

Spine Injuries
General Examination
Spondylolysis and Spondylolisthesis
Other Spine Pathologies
General Treatment Principles

Sports-related Concussion
Pathophysiology
Signs and Symptoms
Risk Factors
Diagnosis and Assessment
Management and Return to Play
Special Considerations
Prevention

The Female Athlete
Special Considerations
Female Athlete Triad

Summary

▶ Introduction

It is currently estimated that nearly 38 million children and adolescents participate in youth sports each year in the United States.[1] The participation in sports allows children to learn about teamwork, competitiveness, and sportsmanship. At the same time, it helps develop physical fitness, promote improved self-esteem, lay a foundation of a healthy active lifestyle, and, most importantly, allow them to have fun. Participation in any sport carries inherent risk of injury, and with the increased popularity of youth sports has come a concomitant rise in youth sports injuries. Each year, more than 3.5 million children require medical treatment for sports-related injuries.[1] Pediatric and adolescent athletes differ from adult athletes in several ways and require

a specialized treatment approach. The goal of this chapter is to familiarize the reader with the physiologic differences between children and adults, describe specific injury patterns commonly seen among youth athletes, outline rehabilitation for these injuries, and identify strategies to promote injury prevention within this population.

▶ Anatomic and physiologic differences of the skeletally immature athlete

Bone Composition

The anatomic or physiologic differences between children and adult bone growth and development lead to altered patterns of injuries. The presence of epiphyseal growth plates

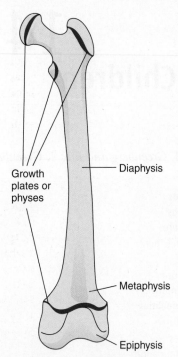

FIGURE. 14.1 Schematic of pediatric bone.

or physes is unique to the skeletally immature patient, and injuries to the physis are common due to its inherent vulnerability (see Fig.14.1).[2] Physeal fractures are usually caused by falls, but can also occur as a result of overuse. These fractures are commonly classified using the Salter–Harris scheme, which describes five distinct types of fractures. A visual schematic and detailed written description are outlined in Figure 14.2 and Display 14.1.

Physeal fractures result in a risk of premature physeal closure, creating a shorter limb or angular limb deformity as the patient progresses toward skeletal maturity. Type I and II fractures typically carry a lower risk of growth disturbance; however, close monitoring by an orthopedic physician over time is typically recommended for all physeal fractures.

The presence of secondary growth centers, known as the apophysis, is also unique to the skeletally immature patient. An apophysis is a prominence containing growth cartilage that is located on the bones and serves as an attachment site for muscle tendons.[3] Apophyseal injuries occur owing to the large traction forces applied by muscles to the bone complex. In the skeletally immature child, the bone interface is

the weaker link of the musculoskeletal complex and therefore more prone to injury. An apophysitis results from the cumulative effects of repeated microtrauma to these growth centers, resulting in chronic irritation and inflammation at the bone–cartilage interface.[3] Decreased muscle-tendon flexibility, which commonly occurs during the adolescent growth spurt, has been associated with an increased risk of developing an apophysitis injury.[4] If the tensile force is large enough, it may create an avulsion fracture in which the entire apophysis is separated from the underlying bone.

Physiologic differences also give pediatric patients an advantage in bone healing when compared with adults. The bones of children are more highly vascularized, which allows for improved availability of healing factors after injury. Furthermore, the periosteum of bone in children is thicker and stronger than adults, which makes it less likely to be fully disrupted during injury. Both of these factors will lead to improved rates of bone healing after fracture.

Juvenile osteochondritis dissecans (OCD) is a lesion of the subchondral bone that often results in articular cartilage softening, fibrillation, and fragmentation, which may result in loose bodies within the joint. Juveniles with OCD lesions have been shown to have improved healing potentials than those who have reached skeletal maturity.[5] The pathogenesis of OCD is not fully understood; however, many agree that repetitive stress to the subchondral bone results in cumulative microtrauma in a region with poor blood supply, resulting in damage.[6,7] This hypothesis of pathology is supported by study findings that note increased incidences of juvenile OCD lesions in highly active populations.[5] Males are more affected than females, and the knee is the most commonly affected joint.[8] Treatment of OCD will depend on the lesion severity, location, and degree of skeletal maturity. Conservative treatment will typically consist of a period of prolonged rest or immobilization, followed by rehabilitation and gradual return to sports over a 3-to-6-month period. Surgical treatment is usually recommended

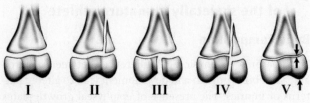

FIGURE. 14.2 Salter–Harris classification of fractures.

for unstable lesions and those that fail conservative treatment.[5] Additionally, adolescent patients nearing skeletal maturity have decreased healing capacity, and early operative treatment is usually advocated to maintain the integrity of the joint.[8] A variety of surgical techniques have been developed in an attempt to replace the articular cartilage defect. Drilling, abrasion arthroplasty, and microfracture procedures attempt to recruit pluripotential cells from marrow elements. The recruited cells will eventually differentiate in fibrocartilage that restores the articular surface, but is weaker than the hyaline cartilage typically found in the joint. Rehabilitation principles specific to the affected joint will be covered in detail later in this chapter.

Muscular Properties

At one point in time, it was suggested that owing to the lack of circulating androgens, prepubescent children would be unable to demonstrate increases in muscular strength in response to a resistance training program. However, recent reports have evidenced that children can demonstrate strength gains with proper training programs. The physiologic mechanism of strength gains in children is different than that of adults. It appears that the strength gains observed in prepubescent children are more related to improving neuromuscular control, such as increased motor unit activation and/or coordination, rather than true muscular hypertrophy.[9] In summary, the scientific literature supports the safety and efficacy of strength training in children, as long as they are properly supervised by adults.

Muscular flexibility has been shown to decrease during the adolescent growth spurt and may result in an increased potential for injury.[4] A regular static stretching program is effective at producing gains in muscle flexibility. It has been advocated that a generalized flexibility program be incorporated before or after athletic activity in order to reduce the injury potential in this high-risk group.[10]

▶ Examination principles

The examination of the pediatric or adolescent athlete will entail history taking, systems review, palpation, muscle performance testing, range of motion (ROM), flexibility, and special testing. Although these are common parts to most orthopedic evaluations, the child athlete examination differs from that of a typical adult examination. Pediatric-specific injuries require selection of alternative tests and measures, while differences in emotional maturity will also influence the examination.

History

The history-taking process is very important and serves many functions. Details regarding the mechanism of injury and acute response to injury can give the examiner many clues regarding the nature of injury (overuse versus trauma), the tissue involved, and help with initiating treatment planning. In addition, the history-taking process can serve as a period to help the child relax and become more familiar with the treating therapist. This may help decrease patient anxiety and provide for a more effective physical examination. During historical questioning, the pediatric or adolescent patient will typically forget or gloss over details that may be important for the examiner. Utilizing very specific questioning, with age-specific terminology, is usually helpful in ascertaining a complete history. When available, the parent's recollection of injury specifics should also be inquired.

Determination of the athlete's sports-specific history is also important in order to judge possible contributing factors of overtraining and to initiate goal planning for treatment outcomes. The clinician should address what sports they participate in, positions played, level of mastery (recreational or elite), whether they are currently in-season, volume of practice, how long they have participated in a certain sport, whether they play year round, and if they are currently participating in any other outside training regimens.

Physical Examination

A complete review of all physical examination procedures is beyond the scope of this textbook. The practitioner should be familiar with standardized examination procedures such as ROM, flexibility assessment, manual muscle testing (MMT), and commonly used injury-specific special tests. This section will focus on examination elements specific to the pediatric sports population. Special tests that are specific to pediatric injuries will be covered during the discussion of that injury; however, for detailed descriptions of these tests, the reader is referred to special test-specific texts.

Generalized ligamentous laxity is a condition in which most of the synovial joints of an individual tend to have more than normal ROM.[11] This condition is commonly encountered in the pediatric population and decreases with increasing age. There tends to be a familial predisposition, and females are more commonly affected.[11] Determination of ligamentous laxity is important as it may affect clinical decision making and play a role in injury pathogenesis in certain conditions such as patellofemoral pain, patella dislocations, and shoulder instability. The Beighton–Horan ligament laxity scale is the most frequently utilized assessment scale. The index includes examination of fifth-finger extension, opposition of the thumb to forearm, and trunk and hip flexion. One point is given on the basis of performance of these tasks, with a total of 9 points possible. The composite score gives an understanding of the level of laxity present, with a score of 5 to 9 typically utilized to indicate a high degree of laxity.[11] Refer to Display 14.2 for a detailed description of each test.

Muscle performance testing for the athletic population requires more detail than that elicited by MMT or dynamometry alone. Functional movement testing, such as the single-leg squat or lateral step-down test, gives the examiner much needed information regarding how the neuromusculoskeletal system performs as a unit. In the lower extremity, the biomechanical contributions of femoral internal rotation (IR), femoral adduction, tibial IR, and foot pronation lead to a position of dynamic knee valgus that has been linked to knee injuries, such as anterior cruciate ligament (ACL) tears and patellofemoral dysfunction.[12],[13] During functional testing, the clinician is observing to determine whether the patient can maintain proper trunk, pelvic, and lower extremity positioning during the movement (Fig. 14.3) The subject should be able to maintain steady balance with an upright trunk. In the frontal plane, the knee should be kept in alignment with the second metatarsal (i.e., no dynamic valgus). In the sagittal plane, forward projection of the knee in front of the toes should be limited. Specific descriptive classification schemes have been developed and have demonstrated adequate reliability.[14] However, it is the author's experience that written description of the compensatory strategies is often adequate and may even prove more useful in terms of repeat testing to evaluate specific improvement. The clinician should also seek information regarding pain associated with movement and whether any mechanical symptoms are present.

In athletes with injuries that involve low levels of pain, more aggressive functional testing may be necessary in

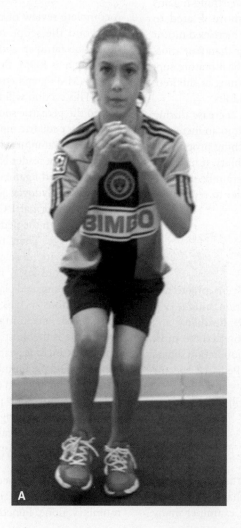
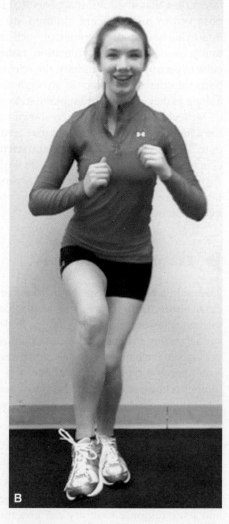

FIGURE. 14.3 Functional assessment of single-leg squat.
(A) Good lower extremity alignment and neuromuscular control with a single-leg squat. **(B)** Poor lower extremity control with femoral adduction, femoral internal rotation, knee dynamic valgus, and foot pronation.

order to stress their system adequately to identify impairments. These athletes are typically suffering from overuse syndromes and report the onset of pain after performing activity for several minutes or more. The Drop Vertical Jump is one clinical test that allows for the identification of pathologic lower extremity alignment during a more sports-specific task.[15] For this test, the patient stands on top of a box approximately 12 inches in height and is instructed to jump directly down off the box and then immediately perform a maximal vertical jump raising both arms overhead. The clinician evaluates for the degree of knee valgus, lack of pelvic or trunk control, and overall quality of movement (Fig. 14.4). This test has been shown to be predictive for identifying female athletes at risk for ACL injury and may also provide a tool for the identification of more subtle biomechanical faults that may contribute to overuse injuries.[15]

Running athletes represent a specialized group of patients and require detailed analysis of running mechanics. Although there is no agreed-upon "perfect" style of running, studies have identified biomechanical factors that may predispose a runner to certain injuries. Running analysis is most easily performed on a treadmill. The athlete should be viewed from the front, back, and side. From the side, the clinician should note the athlete's cadence (steps per minute), trunk position, degree of knee flexion at loading, stride length, foot strike pattern (forefoot versus rearfoot), and the distance of the foot at ground contact in relation to the body's center of mass (Fig. 14.5). Posteriorly, the clinician

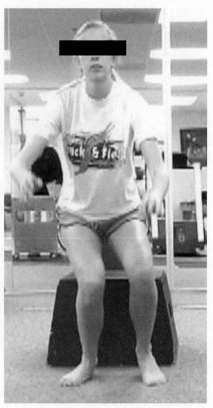

FIGURE. 14.4 Drop vertical jump. Poor neuromuscular control, asymmetrical weight acceptance, and right dynamic valgus collapse throughout lower kinetic chain.

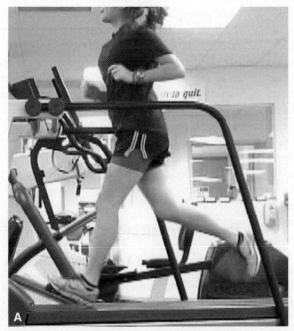
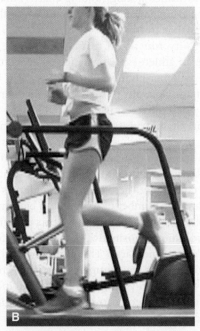

FIGURE. 14.5 Running assessment lateral view. (A) Rearfoot strike pattern, over striding and contacting anterior to base of support with knee extended; leaning forward from the hip. **(B)** Forefoot strike pattern contacting closer to base of support and greater knee flexion angle; upright posture.

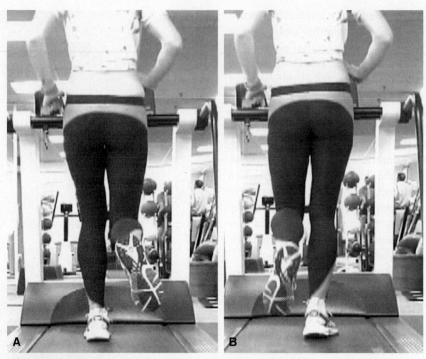

FIGURE. 14.6 Running assessment posterior view. **(A)** Maintenance of level pelvis during left midstance with good lower extremity alignment. **(B)** Contralateral left pelvic drop, excessive toe out, and poor lower extremity alignment during right midstance.

should look to identify abnormal trunk lean, pelvic instability during stance phase, presence of dynamic knee valgus, position of the foot at ground contact (degree of supination and relationship to body midline), and the amount and timing of foot pronation that occurs during stance (Fig. 14.6). Abnormalities identified during running analysis may lead to more detailed examination of strength, ROM, or flexibility and will help guide treatment.

Upper extremity functional testing allows the clinician to analyze an athlete's performance on specific tasks and determine whether biomechanical flaws exist. Upper extremity testing is generally less defined in the literature. One commonly described test is the Closed Kinetic Chain Upper Extremity Stability Test.[16] In the test, two lines are placed on the ground 36 inches apart. The patient assumes a push-up position with one hand on each piece of tape. The athlete will have 15 seconds to reach across their body and touch the tape under the opposite shoulder, as many times as they can. The number of touches can be compared with normative data for similar age and sports participants; however, the volume of normative data available for the pediatric population is not large. The clinician can also utilize this test to look for any compensatory patterns that may indicate weakness in the kinetic chain. The inability to maintain a neutral spine posture while in the push-up position could be related to core weakness. Scapular winging or asymmetries in shoulder positioning are also commonly seen compensatory patterns. Sport-specific functional testing such as throwing for a baseball player can also

be included as part of the examination. Owing to the high speeds involved with this motion, video assessment utilizing slow motion replay or motion analysis software may be necessary and useful.

The assessment of the entire kinetic chain is required for almost every injury treated by a sports physical therapist. Most sports activities involve the transfer of energy from the lower extremities, through the trunk to some other distal segment such as the hand to throw or the foot to kick a ball. Deficits in kinetic chain function have been linked to a wide array of overuse and traumatic injuries in the upper extremity, lower extremity, and trunk. The comprehensive evaluation should include assessment of single-limb balance, core stability, and hip muscle function even if the patient presents with a seemingly unrelated injury, especially if the injury is of the overuse etiology. Incomplete rehabilitation of any kinetic chain deficits may predispose this patient to repeat injury or suboptimal outcomes.

▶ Upper extremity

Examination and Treatment Principles

Generally, the examination of an athlete's shoulder should begin with a detailed postural examination. In particular, the examiner should note resting scapular position, degree of thoracic kyphosis, and general muscular bulk or appearance. An excessive thoracic kyphosis is typically associated with a position of scapular protraction and downward rotation. These factors have been linked to decreased shoulder mobility, increased likelihood of shoulder pathology, and impaired muscle activation.[17] When assessing muscular bulk, the clinician may be able to identify areas of muscle atrophy, which may prompt further investigation during specific muscle performance testing. It is important to note that it is not uncommon for the athlete's dominant shoulder to be slightly depressed relative to the contralateral limb. As discussed earlier, the patient should be screened for generalized ligamentous laxity, and pathology-specific special tests should be utilized to rule in or out specific diagnoses. These tests are outlined in Addendum B.

Scapular dysfunction is a common clinical problem in many athletes, and normal scapular motion and stability are crucial for optimal function of the shoulder.[18] The clinician should observe the patient from behind while the patient actively elevates and lowers both shoulders. The scapulae should be observed, judging for an abnormal degree of motion or altered pattern of mobility. Several visual observation methods of determining scapular dyskinesis have been described and shown to be reliable in distinguishing normal from abnormal motion.[19-21] If scapular dyskinesia is present, the surrounding anatomic structures should be evaluated in order to determine the cause. This should include assessment of thoracic spine mobility and flexibility of the pec minor, lattissimus dorsi, and teres major. In addition, isolated muscle performance testing of scapular stabilizing muscles (serratus anterior, middle and lower trapezius) and rotator cuff function should be performed.

Examination of shoulder ROM is also a key concept that must be assessed. It has been shown that overhead athletes, particularly pitchers, are likely to develop unique shoulder ROM characteristics. When measured in 90 degrees of abduction, the throwing athlete will typically demonstrate limited IR with an excessive degree of external rotation (ER) when compared with the nonthrowing shoulder. This unique ROM profile is considered normal and reflective of tissue adaptive changes that have occurred owing to the stress of throwing. However, if there is a relative difference of greater than 20 degrees of loss of IR between sides, the patient is then considered to have developed a pathologic condition, thought to contribute to shoulder injury, known as glenohumeral internal rotation deficit (GIRD). GIRD has been linked to deficits in posterior shoulder tissue length, as well as alterations in bony alignment. The clinician should attempt to identify posterior tissue tightness that may contribute to this pathology through examination of cross-body adduction, spinal level reached behind the back, and degree of posterior glenohumeral capsular laxity.[17] Additionally, the concept of total rotational motion (TRM) is important. The total arc of IR + ER should be within 5 degrees of the nonthrowing shoulder. Any differences greater than 5 degrees should once again prompt further evaluation of anatomic structures to identify the cause of asymmetry.

Examination of the elbow, wrist, and hand should include general ROM, strength assessment, and careful palpation of the involved structures. Injury-specific special testing can help confirm suspected diagnosis and should be conducted toward the end of the physical examination out of respect for the provocative nature of these procedures.

The clinician should be aware that many upper extremity pathologies, both traumatic and overuse, may involve dysfunction at remote anatomic locations that would alter body function and contribute to the athlete's symptoms. This concept is commonly referred to as regional interdependence.[22] For example, the mechanics of throwing involves a transfer of energy from the lower body and trunk to the upper extremity. Owing to the integrated nature of this activity, an inclusive evaluation should also address any limitations in the entire kinetic chain that may alter biomechanics and contribute to injury. Balance, core stability, hip/leg strength, and ROM may all need to be evaluated and addressed in a comprehensive treatment plan.

As with all other areas of physical therapy management, the findings on the initial evaluation will guide treatment decisions. It is important that the athlete be instructed and continually monitored to ensure that they are performing their exercises with proper form. One common mistake is allowing the athlete to perform upper extremity exercises in a position of scapular protraction, which would reinforce pathologic mechanics. Visual demonstration, tactile cuing, and mirror feedback are all excellent measures to help ensure proper form.

Scapular stabilizing muscles function in an endurance role to provide proper alignment of the scapula for optimal glenohumeral function. Therapists should keep this physiologic role of the muscles in mind while developing rehabilitation programs and implement a scapular stabilization program that emphasizes longer hold times and repetitions, as opposed to high-load exercises. If deficits in posterior tissue tightness are identified during examination, the clinician should implement exercises targeted at the restricted tissue. As demonstrated in Figure 14.7, the sleeper stretch, towel IR stretch behind the back, and cross-body adduction are all effective means of increasing posterior soft tissue flexibility. If posterior capsular tightness is limited, glenohumeral joint mobilizations should be implemented.

The shoulder is required to be utilized overhead for many of the demands of sports. With this in mind, the clinician should progress an athlete's rehabilitation from less provocative positions below 90 degrees of elevation to more sports-specific activities involving overhead activity. Similarly, the exercise program should also be adapted to meet the muscular demands of the imposed stresses of the athlete's sport. For example, the rotator cuff is responsible for deceleration of the shoulder after ball release in throwing. The rehabilitation program should include exercises that focus on eccentric control from similar positions. Working with the athlete to develop working knowledge of the biomechanical

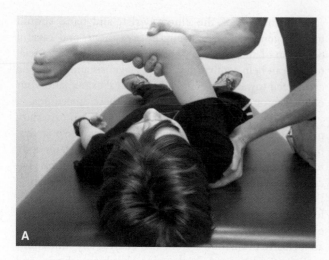

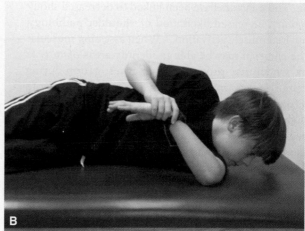

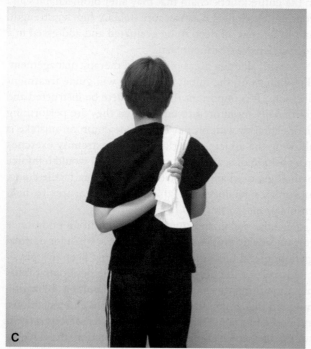

FIGURE. 14.7 Methods of stretching posterior shoulder soft tissues. (A) Shoulder horizontal adduction with scapular blocking, **(B)** sleeper stretch, and **(C)** towel internal rotation stretch.

demands of their sport or position is important during the late phases of shoulder rehabilitation.

As the throwing athlete regains function, a return-to-throwing program can be initiated. Typically, these programs vary by position, consist of many phases, and progress over several weeks. Typically, they include warm-up, throwing at progressively longer distances, and significant rest periods between bouts of throwing in a given session. The reader is referred to Axe et al.[23] for a detailed description of a return-to-throwing program.

The Pediatric Throwing Athlete

Baseball is one of the most popular sports among children and adolescents in the United States. Although baseball is

inherently a very safe sport, the biomechanical stress placed across the throwing arm and the repetitive nature of throwing predisposes these athletes to specific patterns of injury. The following sections will summarize the most frequently encountered diagnoses in the pediatric thrower. It should be noted that although this section is directed toward throwing athletes, other overhead athletes that participate in activities such as tennis, volleyball, or swimming are also likely to present with these diagnoses.

Little League Shoulder

Little league shoulder is an overuse injury caused by rotational torque and stress across the proximal humeral physis, leading to a type of Salter I fracture.[3,7] Plain films may show a widening of the proximal humeral physis, but may not be definitive. Clinically, the patient will complain of throwing- or activity-related shoulder pain. The pain may resolve after rest, but quickly return upon resuming activity. The patient will typically have tenderness to palpation over the physis. The initial treatment for little league shoulder is rest from throwing for 6 to 12 weeks.[24] Physical therapy treatment may begin during this period of relative rest. Rehabilitation should be structured along the continuum, as previously discussed, with the latter phases of rehabilitation including plyometric exercises and return-to-throwing simulation. Review and education of proper pitching mechanics, suggested pitch types, appropriate rest intervals, and pitching volume limits should be reviewed as these have been identified as risk factors for shoulder injury in youth throwing athletes.[7] The latest recommendations for pitch count, pitch type progression, and rest intervals are summarized in Tables 14.1 through Table 14.3.

TABLE 14.1	Pitch Count Recommendations for Youth Pitchers[a]
Age (yr)	**Maximum Pitches Per Day**
7–8	50
9–10	75
11–12	85
13–16	95
17–18	105

[a]2012 Little League Pitch Count Limits and Mandatory Rest Rules

Source: Stop Sports Injuries. www.stopsportsinjuries.org/blog/entryid/96/warnings-signs-for-youth-sports-burnout.aspx

Prevention and Emergency Management of Youth Baseball and Softball Injuries. American Orthopaedic Society for Sports Medicine; 2005.

Little League Baseball. www.littleleague.org/ Assets/ old_assets/media/pitchcount_faq_08.pdf

American Sports Medicine Institute. www.asmi.org

TABLE 14.2	Recommended Rest Periods for Youth Pitchers[a]	
Number of Pitches Thrown		**Mandatory Days of Rest Between Pitching**
Ages 14 and under	**Ages 15–18**	**Days**
1–20	1–30	0
21–35	31–45	1
36–50	46–60	2
51–65	61–75	3
66 and over	76 and over	4

[a]2012 Little League Pitch Count Limits and Mandatory Rest Rules

Source:http://www.stopsportsinjuries.org/blog/entryid/96/warnings-signs-for-youth-sports-burnout.aspx

Prevention and Emergency Management of Youth Baseball and Softball Injuries. American Orthopaedic Society for Sports Medicine; 2005.

Little League Baseball. www.littleleague.org/ Assets/ old_assets/media/pitchcount_faq_08.pdf

American Sports Medicine Institute. www.asmi.org

TABLE 14.3	Recommended Pitch Type Progression for Youth Pitchers
Type of Pitch	**Age (yr)**
Fastball	8 ± 2
Slider	16 ± 2
Changeup	10 ± 3
Forkball	16 ± 2
Curveball	14 ± 2
Knuckleball	15 ± 3
Screwball	17 ± 2

Source: Stop Sports Injuries. www.stopsportsinjuries.org/blog/entryid/96/warnings-signs-for-youth-sports-burnout.aspx

Prevention and Emergency Management of Youth Baseball and Softball Injuries. American Orthopaedic Society for Sports Medicine; 2005.

Little League Baseball. www.littleleague.org/ Assets/ old_assets/media/pitchcount_faq_08.pdf

American Sports Medicine Institute. www.asmi.org

Superior Labrum Anterior-to-posterior Lesions

Superior labrum anterior-to-posterior (SLAP) lesions occur in adolescents as a result of trauma and overuse. Traumatic injuries are typically related to a fall onto an outstretched arm or a traction injury. Throwing athletes are particularly vulnerable to overuse SLAP lesions because of the high stresses that repetitive overhead throwing place on the shoulder. Several theories regarding the pathophysiology of SLAP lesions in throwers have been proposed and include (1) a traction injury from the pull of the biceps tendon on the labrum during the deceleration phase of throwing, (2) contracture of the posterior shoulder capsule resulting in a posterosuperior migration of the humeral head, and (3) "peel back" mechanism where the biceps tendon imparts torsional forces to the posterosuperior labrum in the late cocking phase of throwing.[25] SLAP lesions can result in laxity of the shoulder since the structural integrity of the shoulder is impaired. Typically a patient will complain of vague shoulder pain with overhead or cross-body activities. Complaints of popping, clicking, or catching are also common. Numerous physical examination tests for detecting SLAP lesions have been described and include O'brien's active compression test, anterior slide test, resisted supination ER test, and crank test. Clinical diagnosis of SLAP lesions is challenging as most studies have shown that these tests demonstrate a high degree of sensitivity, but lack specificity.[25]

Initial treatment of SLAP lesions typically consists of a period of rest followed by rehabilitation. The rehabilitation program will typically focus on restoring normal scapular mechanics, strengthening of scapular stabilizers and rotator cuff musculature, dynamic stabilization, and proprioceptive awareness. GIRD is typically present with SLAP lesions and should be addressed accordingly. If the athlete is unable to resume their previous level of activity after a proper course of conservative treatment, surgical intervention is then indicated as SLAP lesion likely will cause ongoing limitations. There are several surgical techniques described, ranging from simple debridement to labral reattachment.[25] Postoperative rehabilitation will vary depending upon the extent of injury and procedure performed. However, the overriding principle that will apply to all SLAP rehabilitation programs is protection of the healing tissue. ROM will be slowly progressed after an initial period of immobilization, and comprehensive rehabilitation activities will progress in a graded fashion.

Elbow Injuries

Injuries to the elbow, especially amongst pitchers, appear to be on the rise. A recent review of pediatric sports elbow injuries noted that 50% to 70% of adolescent baseball players develop elbow pain yearly, with overuse being implicated as the major causative factor.[26] Poor pitching mechanics and pitching too often with inadequate rest have been implicated as major risk factors for pediatric elbow injuries.[7] Excessive pitching might not occur during a single game, but is often the summation of pitches thrown during practice, while at home, or while playing on multiple teams in the same season. The mechanics of the throwing motion place a significant degree of stress across the elbow. During late cocking and early acceleration phases of the throwing motion, valgus tension stresses are placed across the medial elbow, while the lateral aspect of the elbow receives compressive forces. During deceleration, shearing forces occur across the elbow as the forearm fully pronates and the elbow extends. Medial elbow injuries commonly encountered in the pediatric thrower include little league elbow, medial epicondyle apophysitis, and medial epicondyle avulsion fractures. Lateral elbow injuries include Panner's disease and OCD of the capitellum.

Little League Elbow

Little league elbow is a traction injury to the medial epicondylar physis due to valgus distraction forces during the late cocking and early acceleration phases of throwing. Players typically complain of medial elbow pain during throwing activities. In hindsight, players or coaches may note a period of decreasing throwing velocity or accuracy prior to symptom onset. In highly irritable elbows, the pain may be present during normal activities such as writing or lifting objects. Radiographs may reveal a widening of the apophysis or an avulsion fracture in more severe cases. Comparison views of the contralateral limb are usually recommended because of a variation in the size of normal growth centers between individuals.[3] Treatment consists of rest from throwing and activity modification until pain free, which may take 3 to 6 weeks. Rehabilitation focuses on scapular and rotator cuff strengthening and endurance, addressing any limitations in shoulder ROM, localized pain-free wrist and forearm

muscle strengthening, strengthening of abdominal and hip musculature, and optimizing throwing mechanics. An interval return-to-throwing program can be initiated after the resolution of all impairments. The athlete should be closely monitored during this period for any return of symptoms, and the program should be adjusted accordingly.

The influence of pitch type on injury is a topic of significant debate. Recent studies have more highly correlated the volume of pitching and poor biomechanics with an increased risk of elbow injuries rather than the type of pitch thrown.[7] The therapist must emphasize the importance of early instruction in proper pitching mechanics and volumes to the athlete, parents, and coaches. The fastball should be the foundation for all young pitchers, and the mechanics of this pitch should be mastered early in a pitcher's career.[27] The increased volume of practice and breakdown of mechanics that occurs with attempting to learn breaking pitches may place the athlete at a higher risk of overuse injuries, such as little league elbow. The changeup is recommended as a safe secondary pitch that can be added only after fastball mechanics are mastered. The curveball can then be added in the later phases of the athlete's baseball participation (Table 14.3).

Medial Epicondyle Apophysitis

Apophysitis may develop at the medial epicondyle as a result of repetitive tensile forces subjected to attachment of the medial elbow musculature. Symptoms generally consist of pain with activity, pain with resisted muscle testing, and pain with palpation. In the case of medial epicondyle apophysitis, clinical exam is similar to that of little league elbow, and imaging studies may be required for differential diagnosis. Treatment is consistent with previous outlined programs of activity modification and progressive resolution of impairments noted on evaluation.

Medial Epicondyle Avulsion Fracture

An acute valgus stress to the medial epicondyle may result in an avulsion fracture.[28] This injury is most often seen in baseball pitchers and gymnasts. Nonoperative management for minimally displaced fractures consists of a period of immobilization followed by rehabilitation. Recently, some reports favor operative management for these injuries owing to an increased understanding of the detrimental effects medial elbow instability may have on high-demand sports.[28]

Elbow Ulnar Collateral Ligament Injury

Ulnar collateral ligament (UCL) tears have been an injury of high-level skeletally mature throwing athletes.[28] However, recent reports indicate that UCL tears and surgical reconstruction are being seen with increasing frequency in youth athletes.[29] Evidence regarding this alarming trend incriminates cumulative trauma due to overuse in the throwing arm of youth pitchers. High pitching volumes, pitching with arm fatigue, and poor pitching mechanics appear to place the athlete at the most risk of developing UCL injury.[7,30] The patient will complain of medial elbow pain typically noted during or immediately following a bout of throwing. A prolonged trial of rest may resolve symptoms initially; however, pain will return immediately upon resuming high-velocity throwing. Surgical reconstruction, commonly known as "Tommy John" surgery, is considered only after a failure of at least 6 months of conservative care.[28] Surgical procedures are similar to those used in adults and target return to throwing roughly 6 months postoperatively. Outcomes studies are limited in children, but similar success rates have been noted in adults and high school–age athletes.[31]

Panner's Disease

Panner's disease occurs generally in younger children aged 4 to 8 years and is a self-limiting avascular necrosis of the developing ossific nucleus of the capitellum.[28] It is associated with degeneration and necrosis of the capitellum, followed by regeneration and recalcification. It is a self-limiting disorder of nontraumatic origin. Treatment consists of rest with avoidance of valgus stress and splinting for pain relief. Outcomes are typically good with resumption of full activity common after treatment.

Osteochondritis Dissecans

OCD of the capitellum typically affects the young adolescent athlete involved in high-demand, repetitive overhead, or weight-bearing activities.[6] OCD is most common in 12- to 17-year-olds involved in baseball, gymnastics, racquet sports, football, or weightlifting.[6] The pathogenesis of OCD is not fully understood; however, it likely results from cumulative injury from repetitive microtrauma in a region with tenuous blood supply.[6,7] During the late cocking and early acceleration phases of baseball throwing, the lateral radiocapitellar joint undergoes significant compressive forces, and repeated exposures may lead to subchondral bone fatigue fracture. The athlete typically complains of localized lateral elbow pain and has swelling, decreased ROM, and tenderness to palpation over the radiocapitellar joint upon physical examination.

Conservative treatment involves complete elbow rest from offending forces for up to 6 months. Rehabilitation may begin with gentle ROM and strengthening exercises when the patient is asymptomatic. Repeat imaging studies and clinical examination will help determine readiness to progress back to sports.[6] A gradual return to full activity may occur after 6 to 12 months.[28]

Several operative techniques exist for OCD lesions that fail to respond to conservative measures. Loose fragment removal with microfracture or drilling of the lesion are the most commonly seen procedures.[6,28] For microfracture procedures, postoperative rehabilitation typically begins after 6 weeks of immobilization or protected use. Return to sports may begin as early as 3 to 6 months, but may be delayed depending upon the achievement of necessary strength, ROM, and muscular endurance goals.

Other Shoulder Pathologies

Multidirectional Instability

Chronic multidirectional instability (MDI) of the shoulder in the young athlete can be caused by an acute traumatic dislocation or by an underlying capsular laxity. MDI is typically associated with generalized ligamentous laxity, and bilateral involvement is common. Presenting symptoms usually consist of bilateral shoulder pain with a loose or unstable feeling during activities such as overhead lifting, swimming, tennis, and throwing. The patient may also note shoulder subluxation during normal activities of daily living such as rolling over in bed or lifting a backpack.

Clinical examination reveals increased glenohumeral translation during passive mobility testing, with a positive sulcus sign and increased anterior–posterior glide during the load and shift test. Associated injuries such as impingement syndrome or labrum tears should be investigated. Imaging is usually not indicated for MDI, except to rule out other possible diagnoses.[3] Patients with MDI often present with scapular dyskinesis and weakness in the scapular stabilizing and rotator cuff muscles. Physical therapy is the preferred initial management strategy for MDI.[32] Patient education regarding avoiding provocative positions and subsequent dislocations is a key component to successful rehabilitation. Exercises should focus on normalizing scapular mechanics, regaining rotator cuff strength, and dynamic shoulder stabilization activities. These exercises should be performed in both open- and closed-chain positions in order to maximize active control of the humeral head in the glenoid. The patient should begin these activities with the arm in low-stress positions and limited weight bearing, while the therapist ensures that the scapula is in a desired position. Progression should include higher-demand overhead positions and increased body weight in the closed chain while incorporating exercise principles to maximize local muscular endurance. Return-to-sport training should include exercises that replicate the forces the shoulder must endure during sporting activity. For example, throwing athletes would benefit from open-chain plyometric activities, while a wrestler's program should include more aggressive closed-chain upper extremity, weight-bearing activities.

Traumatic Shoulder Dislocation

Acute traumatic shoulder dislocations occur most commonly in the anterior direction, with male athletes involved in contact sports most at risk. The typical mechanism of injury is a fall onto the arm while the shoulder is in an abducted and externally rotated position. Closed reduction is usually performed and radiographs used to rule out associated fracture and confirm relocation. Neurovascular examination should be performed before and after relocation, as secondary injury to vascular or neural structures can occur. A high risk of associated injuries is seen including Hill–Sachs lesion, glenoid rim fracture, anterior inferior glenoid labrum tear or avulsion (Bankart lesion), and capsular avulsion fracture. Advanced imaging with magnetic resonance imaging (MRI), magnetic resonance angiography (MRA), or computed tomography (CT) scan may be indicated if these injuries are suspected. Identifying associated pathologies and directing proper initial treatment is important as young athletes have been noted to be at high risk for recurrent dislocations, with some studies reporting rates as high as 90%.[33]

Nonoperative management includes rest or sling immobilization for 1 to 3 weeks. Rehabilitation should focus initially on pain management, gentle ROM, and muscle activation. The provocative position of 90 degrees abduction and ER should be avoided until late phases of rehabilitation. Treatment will progress on the basis of symptoms and stability. Principles of progression and return-to-sport training are similar to those discussed with MDI.

Because secondary injuries and recurrent instability are common after first-time dislocation, several open and arthroscopic procedures may be customized to the patient's specific intra-articular pathology. Postoperative treatment will vary depending upon the specific procedure performed; however, most protocols share a period of immobilization lasting 4 to 6 weeks. Rehabilitation will progress focusing on restoring ROM, strength, normalizing scapular movement, and dynamic stabilization of the shoulder. Aggressive ROM techniques are contraindicated as they may violate the stabilization procedure performed and lead to recurrent instability. The patient progresses slowly to more stressful overhead and 90/90 positions over the course of rehabilitation, using principles already discussed. Return to contact sports typically occurs after 6 months.

Acromioclavicular Joint Separations

Acromioclavicular (AC) joint separations also occur in this population and are often caused by a fall onto the shoulder. These injuries are generally treated nonoperatively with good results.[34] The AC joint may not return to its normal configuration after injury, and a noticeable "bump" may result. This abnormality is cosmetic and will not affect function. Occasionally, this bump may be painful with direct irritation from equipment, such as football shoulder pads. A simple donut pad can be fabricated to relieve pressure. Rehabilitation is fairly uncomplicated and should focus on regaining lost shoulder mobility and pain-free strengthening.

Clavicle Fractures

Clavicle fractures usually occur as a result of a fall onto the shoulder. Most clavicle fractures in children remain nondisplaced or minimally displaced on account of the thick periosteum in a child and can be treated nonoperatively.[35] The treatment of displaced clavicle fractures remains controversial; however, recent literature reports indicate that surgeons

are favoring surgical fixation for completely displaced, comminuted, or open-type fractures.[35,36] Nonsurgical treatment consists of 2 to 4 weeks of immobilization in a shoulder sling or a figure-of-eight brace, followed by ROM and strengthening exercises. Rehabilitation is usually minimal and return to sports activity is usual around 6 to 8 weeks. Following surgical management, the patient is immobilized in a sling for 3 weeks, after which they may begin progressive ROM and strengthening exercises. Return to sports is allowed at 12 weeks if there are clinical and radiographic evidence of healing.[36]

Other Elbow Injuries

Pediatric athletic elbow injuries include traumatic fractures and dislocations, as well as overuse injuries already discussed. Traumatic injuries usually occur as a result of falling and are common in sports such as gymnastics, snowboarding, and football. An elbow fracture or dislocation may represent a medical emergency in view of the possibility of associated neural or vascular compromise. Commonly encountered injuries will be summarized in the following section.

Supracondylar Elbow Fractures

Supracondylar fractures commonly occur in children and carry a risk of secondary neurovascular damage. This damage can lead to long-term functional deficits in the upper extremity and, therefore, prompt treatment is required.[37] Treatment is based upon the severity of fracture displacement and identification of any associated injuries. Nonsurgical immobilization is typically recommended for nondisplaced fractures, while most other injury patterns require surgical fixation.[37] Elbow stiffness and loss of elbow extension is a large concern after the initial management of supracondylar fractures and may take up to 1 year for elbow ROM to approach normal. Patients with more severe injuries, surgically managed fractures, and younger age have the most difficulty regaining motion.[38] The therapist should initiate progressive elbow ROM and upper extremity strengthening exercises when cleared by the surgeon. Methods such as dynamic splinting or serial casting may be necessary to regain motion in difficult cases.

Lateral Condyle Fractures

Lateral condyle fractures occur less commonly than supracondylar humeral fractures but have a similar mechanism of injury. Stable, minimally displaced fractures have been treated successfully with cast immobilization; however, surgical fixation is required for most displaced injuries.[39] The healing of lateral condyle fractures is slower than supracondylar fractures, and longer immobilization time may be required. As with supracondylar fractures, elbow stiffness is a serious concern after initial management, and physical therapy treatment will be similar.

Monteggia Fracture

Monteggia fracture dislocations describe a radial head dislocation with concomitant ulnar fracture. This rare injury accounts for fewer than 1% of pediatric elbow fractures.[40] Complications of Monteggia fractures can include posterior interosseus nerve palsy, radial nerve palsy, and ulnar deformity. There is no agreed-upon optimal management strategy for Monteggia fractures with regard to surgical versus nonsurgical treatment. Conservative management with closed reduction and immobilization has shown good results; however, open reduction internal fixation (ORIF) may be indicated if anatomic reduction cannot be achieved.[40] Rehabilitation time frames are based upon the method of treatment and healing and will be directed by the surgeon.

Forearm, Wrist, and Hand Injuries

Forearm fractures occur as a result of a fall and can occur in the distal, proximal, or midshaft of the radius or ulna. In children, forearm shaft fractures are usually treated with closed reduction and cast immobilization. Indications for surgery include open fractures, unstable fractures, fractures that have failed closed reduction, and sometimes in the management of older adolescents.[41]

Distal Forearm Fractures

Distal forearm fractures occur most commonly in the distal radius owing to bony architecture at the articulation with the wrist. Fractures of the distal radius metaphysis rarely require surgery and are treated with cast immobilization for 4 to 6 weeks.[42] Most injuries of the distal radius physis are of the Salter–Harris type II classification, and nonsurgical treatment is usually successful. Injury to the physis can cause growth arrest with resulting angular deformity, and close monitoring by the physician is required. Torus or Buckle fractures occur at the diaphyseal–metaphyseal junction with impaction of trabecular bone on the dorsal aspect of the radius creating a characteristic bulge on radiographs.[43] Similar to other injuries in the forearm, conservative management is the preferred treatment method.

Gymnast Wrist

Wrist pain is a common complaint among gymnasts, and "gymnast wrist" refers to an overuse injury caused by mechanical overload to the distal radius.[44] The wrist is subjected to large amounts of static and dynamic stress in gymnastics owing to the regular use of the upper extremity to support body weight during activities such as tumbling. Symptoms include pain over the distal radius with wrist extension, especially with weight-bearing positions. Early detection is important in order to prevent physeal injury or premature physeal closure with resulting wrist deformity.[44] Typically, activity modification with restriction of painful activities is required for a period of at least 4 weeks. If pain occurs with normal activities of daily living, bracing may help with pain resolution. Rehabilitation should focus on addressing local and systemic deficits that may impart increased stress across the wrist. The gymnast should be counseled regarding progressive return to weight-bearing activities and in variation of training to reduce the risk of recurrent injury.

Scaphoid Fractures

Scaphoid fractures are the most commonly encountered carpal bone fracture, but account for only 0.45% of all pediatric upper extremity fractures.[45] The most common mechanism of injury is a fall onto an outstretched hand. Although rare, accurate diagnosis and treatment of scaphoid fractures is important in view of the likelihood of nonunion or avascular necrosis with improper treatment.[46] The patient with a scaphoid fracture will typically complain of lateral wrist pain, which is increased with radial deviation and wrist extension. Point tenderness is typical with palpation of the scaphoid in the anatomic snuff box, located between the abductor pollicis longus and brevis tendons. Treatment typically consists of cast immobilization in a thumb spica cast for 6 weeks, followed by rehabilitation. If the fracture is unstable or if nonunion develops, surgical fixation may be indicated.[47] Scaphoid fractures are sometimes difficult to diagnose as the fracture may not be evident on initial radiographs. Owing to the severe consequences of misdiagnosis, a suspected scaphoid fracture is typically immobilized for 2 weeks followed by repeat examination.[46]

Fracture of the Hook of the Hamate

Hook of the hamate fractures can occur during sports like baseball, golf, or hockey. The typical mechanism of injury is a mistimed swing that contacts a solid object, translating excessive forces through the hamate.[47] Acute tenderness will exist over the hook of the hamate, and pain will typically be experienced when gripping a racquet or club. Conservative treatment consists of cast immobilization for 6 weeks; however, surgical excision of the fracture fragment may be necessary.[47]

Boxer's Fracture

A boxer's fracture involves the neck of the fifth metacarpal and typically occurs as a result of a closed fist striking an immovable object. Owing to the effect of muscular attachments, there is a resulting volar angulation of the head of the fifth metacarpal.[48] Treatment will typically consist of closed reduction with cast immobilization for 3 to 6 weeks.

Finger Fractures

Finger fractures and tendon injuries to the fingers also occur during sports participation. In general, the majority of finger fractures in pediatric patients can be treated by closed means with excellent outcomes expected.[49] Mallet finger is an injury in which the extensor digitorum tendon is avulsed from the distal phalynx, causing an inability to extend the distal interphalangeal (DIP) joint of the finger. This typically occurs owing to an unexpected flexion force such as jamming a finger on a ball or with sliding into a base. Jersey finger is an avulsion of the flexor digitorum profundus (FDP) from the distal phalynx. This injury most commonly occurs in the ring finger, and may result from the forceful contraction of the FDP when the finger gets caught in another player's jersey. Treatment for these mallet or jersey finger injuries typically consists of splint immobilization.

▶ Pelvis, hip, and thigh injuries

Examination Principles

Pelvis, hip, and thigh injuries in youth athletes can be a result of isolated traumatic events, overuse, and idiopathic origins. The pelvis is composed of a series of bones, including the ischium, ilium, pubic bone, sacrum and femur, and their articulations. These bones serve as attachment sites for a number of muscles and ligaments. Knowledge of this anatomy is paramount in the understanding and diagnosing of injury. With complaints of hip, pelvis, thigh, or knee pain, careful examination must be performed to rule out pathologic disease processes and other orthopedic and nonorthopedic conditions (Display 14.3).

A detailed history is important in the diagnosis and treatment of injuries to the hip and pelvis. Mechanism of injury, location and description of pain, and aggravating activities will assist in ensuring proper diagnosis and direction of examination. Inspection of diffuse or localized swelling and bruising will help identify locations of trauma. Careful palpation, with attention to localized swelling, pain, and tenderness, is crucial and should include bony landmarks, sites of muscle attachments, and surrounding soft tissues. Active and passive ROM testing of the hip in all planes will help identify any limitations when compared with the contralateral limb. Selective tissue muscle tension testing and tests of muscle performance will help discern involvement of contractile tissues and their ability to function properly. It is important to screen the surrounding joints, including the lower thoracic spine, lumbar spine, and knee to rule out potential distant contribution of hip pain.

Specific Injuries to the Pelvis, Hip, and Thigh

Pelvic Apophysitis

During periods of rapid growth, the immature skeleton of the pediatric athlete is at risk for overuse injuries. Bone growth exceeds the ability of muscle tissue to sufficiently lengthen and stretch, thus increasing tensile forces across pelvic apophyses, the weakest point in the muscle-tendon unit of a growing athlete.[50] Repetitive pulling of the muscle along the apophysis will cause microtrauma and progressive weakness and inflammation at the cartilaginous muscular attachment. With progression of the injury, there is a slight widening of the apophysis and may place the athlete at greater risk of avulsion injury.

The most common sites for pelvic apophysitis are the anterior inferior iliac spine (AIIS), anterior superior iliac spine (ASIS), and ischial tuberosity. The lesser trochanter, iliac crest, and greater trochanter are also possible, but less frequently encountered locations for apophysitis.[3] The site of the apophysitis is dependent upon the skeletal age and maturity of the athlete as the apophysis will fuse during certain age ranges and will no longer cause pathology (see Table 14.4). The type of activity performed may predispose athletes to apophysitis in particular locations. For example, soccer players often experience AIIS aphophysitis from ballistic rectus femoris contractions performed with repetitive kicking.

DISPLAY 14.3 Differential Diagnoses of Hip Pain

Causes of Hip Pain in Athletes

Apophyseal injury/fracture

Stress fracture

Slipped capital femoral epiphysis, septic/inflammatory arthritis, Legg–Calve–Perthes disease

Femoral acetabular impingement, acetabular labral tears, loose body

Snapping hip syndrome, tendonitis or bursitis

Muscle strain

Traumatic hip dislocation

Osteitis pubis, osteomyelitis, sport hernia

Nerve entrapments

Lumbar radiculopathy

TABLE 14.4 Hip Apophysitis Locations

Apophysitis Site	Muscle Attachments	Age of Ossification
ASIS	Sartorius, tensor fascia lata	14–16
AIIS	Rectus femoris	14–16
Ischial tuberosity	Hamstring group	21–25
Iliac crest	Tensor fascia lata, deep abdominal muscles	16–18
Greater trochanter	Gluteus maximus and medius, hip external rotator group	14–16
Lesser trochanter	Iliopsoas	14–16

Well-localized, dull pain with activity at the involved location is the common complaint with apophysitis. Pain often worsens with increased activity and decreases with rest. Progression to pain with daily activities such as walking and stair negotiation, with or without a limp, may occur without adequate rest. Examination will find tenderness at the apophysis with possible inflammation. Tensioning the muscle attachment at the apophysis will reproduce the athlete's symptoms. This can be done either by stretching or forcefully contracting the muscle of interest. Owing to rapid growth, generalized bilateral muscle inflexibility is often noted along with limited ROM on the involved side. Distinction between avulsion fractures can be appreciated upon physical exam and diagnostic imaging, as radiographs in the presence of apophysitis are generally normal.

Treatment of a pelvic apophysitis begins with rest, activity modification, and management of pain and inflammation. Weight bearing is permitted as long as it is pain free and the athlete demonstrates a nonantalgic gait. In some cases with significant pain, a short course of protected weight bearing with crutches may be needed. Once pain is controlled, the focus of treatment shifts to improving muscle flexibility and ROM. Muscle strengthening to the surrounding lumbopelvic musculature and lower extremity is also of paramount importance to restore pelvic balance and lower extremity control. Return to sport should be in a progressive manner, depending on symptoms and quality of movement and may take up to 6 weeks for full, unrestricted participation.[51]

Pelvic Avulsion Fractures

Avulsion fractures may occur with the progression of an unmanaged apophysitis in the pelvis and are found at similar locations. They most commonly occur in adolescent athletes from 14 to 25 years old, as a result of an acute injury with a distinct mechanism of injury. Strong and violent contraction of a muscle against its apophyseal attachment site, especially during the eccentric phase of a sporting activity where higher forces are generated, contributes to failure and subsequent avulsion.[52]

The athlete will often recall the isolated event and time of injury and will report feeling or hearing a "pop." Symptoms include tenderness and swelling over the site of the avulsion. Weight bearing is usually painful and results in an antalgic gait. Associated bruising is also characteristic of avulsion fractures. As occurred during the injury, pain is elicited upon a strong muscle contraction of the associated muscle group. Radiographs can confirm diagnosis in the suspicion of avulsion in most cases. Some smaller avulsions not seen on plain films may be diagnosed with CT scan. MRI is also available for soft tissue injuries and partial avulsions, but should be used when other more serious concerns exist.[3,53]

Treatment of pelvic avulsion fractures depends on the degree of widening and displacement of the apophysis. Injuries with less than 2-cm displacement will respond to a conservative course of management. The athlete is placed on relative rest from activity for the first 3 weeks and may include a short course of protected weight bearing. Once pain has subsided and time has been allotted to allow for bony healing, regaining full pain-free motion is of next concern. A short course of muscle strengthening is initiated, and once restored, a progressive return to sports-specific activities may begin 6 to 8 weeks following injury, barring no other complications.[52]

Surgical ORIF of the avulsion has been more effective than conservative care when there is evidence of greater than 2-cm or complete displacement of the fragment or with involvement of the ischial tuberosity.[52]

Snapping Hip Syndrome

Snapping hip syndrome is characterized by audible and/or palpable "popping" of the hip caused by tendons moving over bony prominences. It is usually accompanied by pain, and is consistently replicated with certain movements of the hip. Snapping hip syndrome is classified as external and internal. "Intra-articular" snapping hip is no longer considered appropriate nomenclature owing to the improved accuracy, description, and diagnosis of intra-articular hip pathology.[54] Snapping hip is often seen in performing artists, distance runners, and hurdlers.

The friction of the iliotibial (IT) band and/or anterior aspect of the gluteus maximus passing over the greater trochanter causes external snapping hip syndrome. A thickened portion of the IT band, located posterior to the greater trochanter, will pass over the anterior portion of the trochanter with hip flexion. When the hip is extended, the IT band will return to its posterior position, contributing to repetitive snapping and clicking.[54] Between the IT band and the greater trochanter lies the greater trochanteric bursa that may become inflamed with repetitive snapping, resulting in trochanteric bursitis. Tendinopathy, degeneration, and tears of the gluteus medius tendon are also likely to develop owing to the mechanical irritation at its bony attachment.[54]

External snapping hip syndrome may present in athletes in two different ways. True snapping hip syndrome is characterized by lateral hip pain and tenderness around the greater trochanter, and occurs with repetitive hip flexion and extension. The snapping is located along the greater trochanter with standing from a chair, stair climbing, and athletic activities. An athlete may also report snapping with a description of the "hip dislocating." The sensation is often repeatable with pelvic tilting activities and not usually painful. This snapping does not usually contribute to altered athletic participation or performance.[54] Dynamic ultrasound will help identify and confirm the snapping phenomenon.[50]

Treatment of external hip snapping is usually conservative and varies depending upon the level of irritability. When snapping is not painful, soft tissue techniques and stretching to the IT band, tensor fascia lata, and gluteus maximus will aid in decreasing friction and improve function. Activity modification and pain control are of primary importance in the symptomatic external snapping hip. As the level of irritability in the tissue decreases, stretching and soft tissue techniques can be progressed. In both cases, the normalization of trunk control, stability, and balance is necessary for full recovery. With a failed course of conservative management, surgical release is indicated and effective.[55]

Internal snapping hip occurs commonly in dancers and other performing artists. The snapping phenomenon occurs as the iliopsoas tendon chronically subluxes from lateral to medial while the hip is brought from a flexed, abducted, externally rotated position into extension with IR.[56] Internal snapping hip may be present but asymptomatic in approximately 10% of the population.[54]

An athlete with complaints of symptomatic internal snapping hip describes a deep, often painful and audible clunking sensation in the anterior groin. Symptoms are easily reproduced with repeated flexion and extension, or moving from a position of hip flexion, abduction, and ER to a position of hip extension and IR.[57] Though less likely, symptoms may also be reported as posterior achiness to the buttocks and sacroiliac (SI) region, owing to the origin of the iliopsoas tendon on the lumbar spine. Examination elicits the snapping upon anterior hip palpation when performing incriminating motions. When the snapping occurs, the athlete will likely become apprehensive owing to replication of pain. Direct pressure over the iliopsoas tendon may decrease the snapping phenomenon and aid in the diagnosis of internal snapping hip. Dynamic ultrasound and bursography of the iliopsoas tendon may identify the snapping phenomenon and any associated pathologic changes of the iliopsoas tendon and its bursa.[58] Although MR arthrogram cannot detect the dynamic snapping phenomenon, it may be useful in detection of intra-articular hip injury. This may be important as nearly half of those with complaints of internal snapping hip syndrome have an associated intra-articular pathology.[59] Treatment of internal snapping hip syndrome is similar in scope to external snapping hip syndrome. Activity modification and pain control is the primary goal to reduce irritability. Physical modalities, medication, and injection may be necessary. Stretching and soft tissue mobilization to the iliopsoas or anterior hip structures is utilized to normalize mobility. Exercises should be directed at improving trunk control, stability, and lower extremity positioning.[54] Again, in the failure of conservative measures, positive responses have been associated with surgical release and muscle lengthening interventions.[60]

Femoral Stress Fracture

Stress fractures to the femoral neck are frequently associated with physically active athletes and long-distance runners. Abnormal compression stress along the medial aspect of the femoral neck and excessive tensioning along the lateral side represent the two varieties of fractures. Microtrauma during repetitive stress from successive foot strikes in long-distance runners is usually the mechanism for this type of stress fracture. Factors such as poor training regimens, bone composition, vascular supply, and anatomic alignment have been linked with femoral neck stress fractures. Female athletes have up to four times higher risk of bone stress injury than their male counterparts.[61] Females with menstrual abnormalities such as amenorrhea, delayed menarche, eating disorders, and osteoporosis are at even greater risk.[62,63]

Athletes with femoral stress fractures will present with thigh, knee, or groin pain that increases with weight-bearing activities. Symptoms are often decreased or relieved following inactivity and rest. Compensatory gait strategies are often used to decrease weight acceptance on the involved limb. Tenderness along the proximal femur and groin are consistent findings, along with limitations in hip ROM, especially hip flexion and medial rotation. Plain radiographs may not initially detect stress fractures for the first 2 weeks, though follow-up films may demonstrate sclerosis or evidence of fracture. MRI is more sensitive for early diagnosis.

Treatment of suspected femoral stress fracture with protected weight bearing and crutches should occur immediately, regardless of radiographic evidence. A compression-side fracture is treated conservatively with protective weight bearing. A slow and progressive course of care is expected and should be monitored with frequent repeat imaging. Tension-side fractures are at higher risk of displacement and require surgical intervention and fixation. In the event that treatment is not initiated early, complications of nonunion, avascular necrosis of the femoral head, early-onset arthritis, and deformity are likely. Nutritional and psychological consultation is also recommended with suspicions of disordered eating.[64] Only after the athlete is pain free, demonstrates evidence of radiographic bony healing, and maintains a satisfactory clinical exam should a gradual running progression or sport-specific activities be initiated. This process will usually take several months.

Femoral Acetabular Impingement And Labral Tears

Femoral acetabular impingement (FAI) is a diagnosis that has been recognized recently as a source of hip pain and sequelae of hip pathology in the young athlete. FAI is the abutment and approximation of the femoral head or neck with the acetabular rim. This pathology is more likely found in males and has been linked to hip osteoarthritis, slipped capital femoral epiphysis, and femoral neck fracture.[65] FAI can be a result of a cam lesion, pincer lesion, or a combination of the two. Cam lesions are a result of an abnormally shaped femoral head repeatedly impinging upon an acetabulum that cannot accommodate this altered bone morphology. More commonly found in the young athletic male, resultant increased shearing forces might result in labral and chondral lesions to the anterior superior acetabulum.[66] Pincer lesions occur with excessive coverage of the acetabular rim, resulting in abutment of the femoral head and neck when the hip is flexed. This is most commonly found in the more mature athletic woman and will eventually lead to pathology along the anterior labrum and/or posteroinferior acetabulum. The hip labrum functions more like the meniscus in the knee, and with injury will result in decreased shock absorption, joint lubrication, pressure distribution, and hip joint stability.

Patients with FAI complain of deep hip and groin achiness, pain, and associated clicking that is reproduced with isolated or combined movements of hip flexion, adduction, and IR. The athlete will often describe the location of pain by making a "C" with their hand ("C sign"), placing the thumb posteriorly and the remaining fingers anteriorly, surrounding the lateral aspect of the hip. The athlete may complain of pain with prolonged weight bearing, cutting and pivoting, impact activities, and sustained positions of hip flexion, such as sitting. As the condition progresses, the pain will become more constant and debilitating, affecting more of the surrounding tissues including labrum, joint surfaces, and surrounding musculature. Clinical exam will often reveal a limitation in ROM to IR, especially with the hip flexed and adducted, and positive provocative tests for hip impingement. Reproduction of the athlete's pain with combined hip flexion and IR is considered positive for anterior hip impingement. Posteroinferior hip impingement is tested with a reproduction of pain with hip extension and ER.[67] Although these provocative tests have also been thought to be suggestive of labral hip tears, specific labral stress tests do exist. The anterior labrum is stressed by moving the hip from a position of flexion, ER, and abduction into extension, IR, and adduction. Moving the hip from flexion, adduction, and IR into extension, abduction, and ER is diagnostic for posterior labral tears.[68] Although plain radiographs will be able to detect bony abnormalities and adaptive changes, MRI is more commonly used in the detection of FAI.[69,70] When labral tear or chondral damage is suspected, MR arthrogram is the diagnostic test of choice, with the sensitivity and specificity of 90% and 91%, respectively.[71,72]

Conservative treatment is attempted in the treatment of FAI and labral tears, though it is usually not effective for long-term pain relief. Treatment includes a period of rest, activity modification, pain and inflammation control modalities, and trunk motor control and strengthening exercises.[73] Attempts are made at regaining ROM with joint mobilization and stretching activities; however, because of the mechanical nature of the pain, surgical measures are more effective in regaining function in the highly active, athletic populations. Surgical intervention involves either open or arthroscopic reshaping of the associated lesion and can occur simultaneously with labral debridement, direct repair, osteotomy, and/or chondroplasty. Physical therapy following surgical interventions is dependent upon the performed procedure. In more simple arthroscopic procedures, such as labral debridement, the athlete may be permitted to weight-bear as tolerated immediately. Initially, focus is placed on pain control, inflammation control, and gait normalization. Progression to exercises and interventions aimed at ROM

restoration, muscle functioning, and faulty movement patterns are performed in the subacute phases. Exercises that strain the anterior hip musculature, such as straight leg raises, sit-ups, and lunges, should be avoided early in the rehabilitation process to decrease the likelihood of hip flexor tendinopathy.[74] Gradual and slow return to sport should be initiated once the athlete no longer has significant impairment, asymmetry, or pain with provocative testing upon clinical exam.

Muscle Strains

Muscle strains are not commonly seen in young athletes; instead, these athletes tend to incur more apophyseal avulsion injuries. However, in the older adolescent whose apophyses are beginning to ossify, muscle strains should be considered as a possible differential diagnosis. Muscle strains can occur in the same locations as apophyseal injuries. Most common muscle strains to the hip and thigh include adductor, hip flexor, and hamstring strains. Strains are commonly a result of extreme lengthening or forceful eccentric muscle contractions to the involved muscle group, contributing to overload and microtearing.[75] These injuries are often seen in high-velocity sports, including track, football, and soccer, and activities requiring large arcs of motion, such as dancing or kicking. Injuries can occur within the muscle belly or at the musculotendinous junction. Location of the injury has a relationship with expected healing times. For instance, distal strains within the hamstring muscles tend to follow a shorter, more predictable course of recovery than injuries to the proximal tendon.[75] Classification of muscle strains helps determine severity of injury and is based upon pain, weakness, and loss of motion. Muscle strains are graded as grade 1 (minimal muscle damage), 2 (moderate amounts of microtears), or 3 (complete muscle rupture). This classification will assist in injury prognosis and management.

Athletes with acute muscle strains will present with reports of a sudden onset of pain that can be attributed to a specific activity or event. They may report feeling a pull or a "pop" in the location of the involved muscle-tendon unit. Pain will be present within the muscle or along the musculotendinous junction and usually limits the athlete from continuing sport participation. Bruising and diffuse swelling over the injured muscle may be present in the more acute and subacute phases. An antalgic gait may also be present in attempts to unload the involved extremity. Physical examination and palpation of the muscle tissue may identify muscle spasm and a palpable defect within the muscle belly. Stressing the tissue with active contraction and extreme lengthening will help confirm the diagnosis. ROM and strength limitations occur commonly from muscle strains. MRI can assist in the diagnosis and help define the extent of the muscle strain, but is usually reserved for more severe injury.[75,76] Plain radiographs are usually not indicated, but may be helpful in differentiating between avulsion injury and true muscle strain. Additional sources of pain must be considered in the suspicion of muscle strains of the thigh, hip, and pelvic musculature. For example, adverse neural tension along the sciatic tract, due to adhesions and scarring from reoccurring hamstring injuries, can contribute to posterior thigh pain and replicate symptoms of a true hamstring strain. Combined injuries to multiple muscle groups, such as the hamstrings and adductors, are possible due to their close proximity and related functions.[75] Contusions to the iliac crest or greater trochanter, called "hip pointers," are caused by a direct blow and are common in adolescents approaching skeletal maturity. Therefore, a complete and thorough evaluation is needed to determine the true nature of the athlete's complaints.

There is a high rate of muscle strain recurrence in the athletic population. Recurrence is thought to result from persistent weakness in the injured muscle, reduced extensibility of the muscle-tendon unit due to residual scar tissue, and adaptive changes in the biomechanics and motor patterns of sporting movements following the original injury.[75] The primary objective for the treatment of muscle strains is to return the athlete to the previous level of functioning while decreasing the likelihood of reinjury.

In the more severe, grade 3 complete ruptures, surgical repair or reattachment is warranted. However, most grade 1 and 2 hamstring strains will respond to conservative care. Initial treatment of acute muscle strains should follow a similar course. The principle of PRICE (protection, rest, ice, compression, and elevation) should be used to assist in pain control and tissue healing. Protection of the injured muscle is paramount at this time. Muscle stretching to the injured tissue should be avoided to allow for muscle regeneration and decrease the likelihood of scarring. Instead, pain-free ROM activities are encouraged to the associated joint segments. Pain should be avoided and may require the use of crutches or alteration of gait (shorter strides with hamstring strain) until the athlete can ambulate pain free and normally. Therapeutic exercises may be initiated to the lumbar-pelvic, hip, and knee musculature, while avoiding isolated contraction of the injured muscle or other painful activity. As the athlete progresses, attention to normalization of ROM and muscle strength should be of concern. Neuromuscular control, balance, and trunk stability activities also become a focus. Eccentric muscle training should also be encouraged to enhance neuromuscular control and protection during muscle lengthening activities.[75] Sports-specific progression can be initiated once the athlete has a satisfactory physical exam without pain during muscle stretching, normal strength based upon symmetry to the contralateral limb, and proper control with functional activities.

Corticosteroid injection has been utilized in the adult population for the management of muscle strains without any long-term side effects. This treatment is used mostly in professional athletes, but should not be a treatment option for the adolescent population.[77]

Traumatic Hip Dislocation

Traumatic hip dislocation is a high-velocity, high-impact injury during sports such as football, skiing, and motocross. The majority of hip dislocations occur in the posterior direction as a result of a high-energy, posteriorly directed force into a flexed knee. Associated fractures may occur in combination with a dislocation owing to abutment of the femoral head against the posterior acetabular wall. With this injury, the athlete will have intense pain with the limb in a position of flexion, adduction, and IR. Weight bearing and limb motion are unlikely due to the severity of pain. Hip dislocation is an emergent situation and warrants immediate medical attention. On-field joint reduction is not often performed owing to the proximity and potential damage to neurovascular structures. Instead, splinting and prompt transport to a medical facility is recommended to allow reduction within a few hours of injury. Standard radiographs will reveal the dislocated hip, and should coincide with MRI and/or CT scan to assess the potential of associated injury. After relocation and repeat radiographs, the athlete is treated with non–weight bearing for 6 weeks. Following that time, repeat imaging studies are performed in view of the risk of the development of avascular necrosis or chondrolysis. With an uncomplicated course of recovery including normalization of hip mobility and strength, return to athletics can begin at 12 weeks following satisfactory physical exam.[77]

Slipped Capital Femoral Epiphysis

Slipped capital femoral epiphysis (SCFE) is one of the most prevalent hip disorders seen during adolescence. SCFE occurs with increased mechanical shearing forces across the physis of the femoral head, resulting in posterior slippage of the proximal epiphysis, and is rarely associated with distinct traumatic event. SCFE is more prevalent in boys, especially those with an increased body mass index (BMI) and recent rapid growth. In females, the greatest incidence occurs around 9 years of age, while in males the peak incidence is at 11 years. Early onset of SCFE usually manifests with an associated endocrine disorder.[78] Despite a keen understanding of the risk factors and symptoms of SCFE, the diagnosis is still frequently overlooked or delayed. Early diagnosis of SCFE helps decrease the likelihood of subsequent hip pathology, including chondrolysis, femoral head avascular necrosis, and osteoarthritis.[79]

SCFE should be considered a differential diagnosis for any adolescent who presents with a significant limp. Pain may be described as insidious and gradual in onset to the groin, thigh, or medial knee that increases with physical activity. However, a more diffuse hip or thigh ache or complete absence of pain may coincide with an adolescent with SCFE. In acute cases, the limb of interest may assume a resting position of extension, adduction, and ER. In more chronic slips, the limb will likely fall into hip ER with painful and limited combined flexion and IR. Radiographic or clinical evaluation of the contralateral limb may also be indicated as the incidence of bilateral involvement has been reported to range from 20% to 80%.[80]

Treatment of SCFE is surgical with open fixation of the slipped epiphysis immediately following diagnosis. More stable slips tend to fare better postoperatively, with less deformity and comorbidity. Following fixation, the athlete is treated with protected weight bearing on crutches for 6 to 8 weeks. Physical therapy is initiated with the goals of maximizing ROM, muscle strength and endurance, balance, and proprioception. Most athletes are permitted a progressive return to sports once they are pain free and demonstrate symmetrical limb strength and function. However, some literature advocates restricting a return to contact sports until the physis has fully fused. More severe cases of SCFE with associated loss of motion, stiffness, and pain may require salvage procedures such as arthrodesis or osteotomy and will have difficulty returning to higher-level sport participation.[81]

Legg–Calve–Perthes Disease

Legg–Calve–Perthes disease (LCPD), or Perthes, is the eponym given to idiopathic osteonecrosis of the capital femoral epiphysis of the femoral head, usually presenting among males 4 to 8 years old. However, bilateral diagnoses are more commonly seen in girls and account for 8% to 24% of all cases.[79] The lack of blood flow and subsequent necrosis to the femoral head promotes a cascade of events resulting in impaired growth and development of the hip joint. Early onset, early diagnosis, and early intervention are favorable to allow more time for bone growth and remodeling.

Children with LCPD present with an insidious onset of a limp usually without any associated pain. However, with exercise, mild pain may be reported to the hip, groin, thigh, and/or knee. Limitations in hip IR and abduction mobility are classically associated with LCPD. Complete blood workup and radiographs are helpful in determining the presence of infection and existence and/or degree of disease progression.

The primary goals of LCPD management include maintenance of hip mobility, decreased pain with weight bearing, and containment of the femoral epiphysis within the acetabulum. The treatment remains highly controversial. However, in children with severe disease, surgical intervention appears preferable compared with nonoperative treatment, because surgery improves the shape and sphericity of the femoral head, providing greater acetabular coverage.[79] The two most common surgical methods for containment include the femoral varus osteotomy and the Salter innominate osteotomy. Once the femoral head demonstrates signs of healing, the athlete is more than likely able to return to impact activities and sports, though the level of participation may be limited.

▶ Knee injuries

Examinaton Principles

As with most other body-specific examination procedures, a detailed history gives the examiner good insight into the injury and guides the differential diagnosis. The mechanism of injury, via traumatic or insidious onset, and resultant forces transferred to the joint during injury offer clues to what knee structure may be involved. The degree and timeline of any edema should also be determined, with more acute swelling indicating injury to a highly vascularized structure. With insidious onset, symptom response to activity should be explored in detail. A child may require more specific questioning regarding pain with activity than an adult, as children typically do not offer many details with open-ended questions. The painful area should be identified, and in cases where the patient cannot verbalize the extent of pain, it is sometimes helpful to have them point to the most painful area with one finger. The parents and patient should be questioned regarding any prior orthopedic injuries or predisposing factors such as W-sitting as a child, which may impact current functioning.

Physical examination should include special tests to rule in or out specific pathologies, ROM, and muscle testing. As discussed earlier in this chapter, functional testing of the lower extremity to identify poor limb control and impairments in balance or functional strength is important. Gait assessment also provides valuable information. It might be helpful to view gait pattern without patients being aware, as they may not walk "naturally" while you are watching. Another helpful technique is to distract them by asking them to count backward or tell a story while walking. Gait abnormalities such as trunk shifting, pelvic motion, decreased weight bearing, excessive femoral IR, knee valgus, and abnormal foot movements should all be noted and guide further examination.

Ligamentous Injuries

ACL Injuries

ACL injuries are among the most severe and frequent activity-related injuries sustained by children participating in sports.[4] In the skeletally immature child, failure of the ACL complex can occur at different sites. Intrasubstance tears may occur, but failure may also present as an avulsion fracture at the insertion site of the ACL into the tibial spine. Tibial spine avulsion fractures are rarely seen after skeletal maturity. Some propose that a higher degree of cartilage within the area of the tibial spine, with the bone–tendon interface being weaker than the ligament itself, leads to failure of the bone rather than ligament.[82] This injury with the loss of continuity of the ACL results in an unstable knee complex. The mechanism of injury is similar to that of ACL tears, with failure typically during a deceleration or pivoting maneuvers with the knee undergoing valgus, hyperextension, or rotational forces.[83] The patient will typically present with a large and rapidly developing joint effusion (hemarthrosis), decreased knee ROM, and decreased ability to bear weight. Owing to the resultant loss of integrity of the ACL complex, joint laxity with increased anterior translation of the tibia on the femur may exist, which can be assessed utilizing a Lachman or anterior drawer test. Radiographs or MRI may be necessary to classify the injury and determine the extent of any secondary damage.[83]

Treatment is based upon the degree of fragmentation or displacement. Minimally displaced fractures can be treated nonoperatively with cast immobilization for 6 to 8 weeks.[82,83] Several options exist for arthroscopic or open surgical fixation and vary depending upon injury specifics and surgeon preference. Rehabilitation goals are to restore knee ROM, strength, balance, coordination, and dynamic knee stability in preparation for return to sports.

Intrasubstance ACL tears are encountered with increasing frequency in the skeletally immature population.[84] ACL injury typically occurs during sports or activities that involve running, cutting, jumping, or pivoting maneuvers. Sports that carry a high risk of ACL injury include soccer, basketball, volleyball, and football. The youngster with an ACL tear will have a similar history and physical examination findings of their adult counterparts. They will typically describe a "giving way" sensation of the knee and possibly hearing a "pop" at injury. Hemarthrosis, decreased knee ROM, and increased laxity with Lachman or anterior drawer testing are also typical. Specialized devices, such as a KT-1000™ arthrometer, may help quantify the degree of translation between the tibia and femur. Children tend to have more available joint translation than adults, and comparison with the uninjured side is necessary for accurate assessment.

The natural sequelae of the ACL-deficient knee in the young athlete typically include recurrent knee instability, cumulative intra-articular damage (meniscus tears or osteochondral defects), and decreased activity levels.[82,85] Owing to the ACL's proximity to the physes of the distal femur and proximal tibia, there is a risk of damage when typical adult ACL reconstruction surgical techniques are performed. Damage to the physis could lead to limb-length discrepancy or angular deformity as skeletal growth continues. Pediatric-specific ACL reconstruction techniques minimize this risk and are successful at restoring a stable knee complex. With the development of these innovative techniques, surgeons are more likely to favor operative reconstruction over conservative management.[86–88]

Early postoperative rehabilitation should focus on effusion management, maintaining full knee extension, regaining flexion ROM, and restoration of quadriceps activation. Progression of rehabilitation incorporates open- and closed-chain lower extremity strengthening. Initially, open-chain knee extension should stay within the safe limits of 90 degrees to 40 degrees of knee flexion to protect the ACL graft from excessive strain, but can be progressed to

full range after 8 to 10 weeks. Neuromuscular electrical stimulation (NMES) has been shown to improve quadriceps strength return after surgery[89]; however, some pediatric patients may not tolerate this modality well, and use should be on a case-by-case basis. Integrated lower extremity activities using balance exercises, perturbation training, and proprioceptive exercises should be incorporated. Additionally, core stabilization and hip strengthening should be included as part of an inclusive rehabilitation program.

Progression to jogging and bilateral jumping activities typically begin around 3 to 4 months postoperatively. Single-leg plyometrics, agility activities, and general conditioning should be progressed after this period, with return to sports participation ranging from 6 to 12 months postoperatively.[82,90] A fusion of time-based criterion and functional performance testing has been advocated to determine the athlete's readiness for high-level training and return-to-sports integration.[91] Typical requirements are 90% limb symmetry index in quadriceps strength testing and 90% symmetry with a battery of single-leg hop tests.[82,90,92]

ACL Injury Prevention

Female adolescent athletes are the highest risk population for a noncontact ACL injury, with injury rates ranging from two to nine times higher than male counterparts.[91,93,94] Similarly, trends have demonstrated that the risk of ACL injury for any adolescent athlete, regardless of gender, steadily increases from the age of 10 through adolescence.[95] Altered lower extremity movement patterns such as dynamic knee valgus, femoral IR, and limited hip/knee flexion during jumping and cutting motions have been shown to increase stress on the ACL and increase the likelihood of rupture.[12,93] Deficits in strength or neuromuscular control in the growing adolescent, especially females, predispose to these pathologic patterns and a higher risk of injury. This recognition has led to the devlopment of injury prevention programs designed to retrain the athlete by improving dynamic limb control. Efficacy of these injury prevention programs have been studied and proven successful for athletes involved in many high-risk sports.[94,96,97] There are several well-designed ACL injury prevention programs readily available, such as Sportsmetrics™ or Prevent injury Enhance Performance (PEP).

Medial Collateral Ligament Injuries

Medial collateral ligament (MCL) injuries usually occur from a valgus stress to the knee. The mechanism of injury commonly reported is another athlete falling onto the lateral aspect of the patient's knee as occurs frequently in sports like football, soccer, and basketball. The athlete will typically present with a small effusion and tenderness localized to the medial knee, along the MCL.[98] In the young patient with open physes, the possibility of avulsion of the MCL at its tibial attachment should be suspected. As a general rule, avulsion injuries should be suspected in the younger, more skeletally immature patient, while older adolescents have a higher probability of soft tissue MCL injury.[98] Clinical examination will help discern between these two injuries, but imaging will likely be necessary. The patient with an MCL injury will have tenderness to palpation along the ligament, while the patient with avulsion injury will be more tender near the distal attachment on the tibia. Special tests, such as the Valgus Stress Test at 30 degrees and 0 degrees flexion, will also help determine the degree of laxity, structures involved, and severity of injury. MCL injuries are graded 1, 2, and 3 depending upon the degree of laxity present, end feel, and degree of fiber disruption. This classification system is commonly utilized to grade most ligamentous sprains throughout the body and is detailed in Display 14.4.

MCL injuries typically respond well to conservative management.[99] A hinged knee brace may be utilized early after injury for protection against valgus forces. Early rehabilitation is advocated with focus on ROM, early and pain-free weight bearing, strengthening, balance, and dynamic stability activities. Grade 1 and 2 injuries typically do not require extended rehabilitation with an average return-to-sport time of 1 to 3 weeks and 4 to 6 weeks, respectively.[100] Grade 3 injuries are more complex and may require 9 to 12 weeks of rehabilitation.[101]

Posterior Cruciate Ligament Injuries

The posterior cruciate ligament (PCL) serves as the primary restraint to posterior translation of the tibia on the femur. This ligament is typically injured from a direct blow to the anterior aspect of the knee such as falling onto a flexed knee during activity or the knee contacting the dashboard in a car accident. Isolated injuries to the PCL are not common. The patient with a torn PCL will demonstrate posterior laxity on physical examination. Special tests, such as the posterior drawer or sag sign, will help identify instability; the dial test is helpful for determining isolated PCL or multiligament involvement.[102]

Most PCL injuries are treated conservatively. Avoidance of activity is necessary, and a brief period of immobilization may be recommended. Initial rehabilitation focuses on resolving impairments related to the acute injury such as pain, effusion, and gait abnormality. ROM exercises into the extremes of flexion cause increased stress across the PCL and should

be avoided until several weeks after injury as this motion may delay healing. Similarly, open-chain hamstring exercises are contraindicated as they may also stress the PCL complex.[102] A heavy emphasis is placed upon quadriceps strengthening and dynamic stabilization or proprioceptive training. Rehabilitation can range anywhere from 2 to 6 months. As with ACL rehabilitation, functional performance measures, such as quadriceps strength and functional hop tests, should be used to determine readiness for sports participation.

Lateral Collateral Ligament Injuries

Lateral collateral ligament (LCL) injuries are rarely seen in the pediatric athlete. An injury to the LCL is usually in conjunction with injury to the entire posterolateral corner (PLC) of the knee and results from a high-energy blow to the medial aspect of an extended knee.[98] Once again, the ligament is not the weakest link in the pediatric athlete, and bony avulsion of the LCL from the fibula can mimic the laxity associated with an LCL injury. Surgery may be necessary to fixate a displaced fracture of this nature.

Intra-articular Injuries

Meniscus Injury

Most meniscal injuries in children younger than age 10 occur in the setting of a congenital malformation known as a discoid meniscus.[103,104] The discoid meniscus is shaped like a disc, instead of the normal semilunar shape, and is more likely to develop tears. Discoid menisci occur most commonly in the lateral meniscus. The overall prevalence of discoid menisci in the United States has been reported to be between 3% and 5%, with male and female occurrence rates being similar.[104,105] Younger, preschool-aged children with a discoid meniscus may be asymptomatic and only complain of a snapping sensation in the knee. Symptomatic snapping with pain will usually be present in older, elementary-aged children. This pain may be accompanied by intermittent effusion, joint line tenderness, positive McMurray test, and gait abnormalities. The entire meniscus may also be unstable, in which a palpable prominence along the joint line may be seen with knee flexion and extension.

Treatment of the asymptomatic discoid meniscus usually consists of observation only. Although the likelihood of developing meniscal tears is higher, currently it is unclear whether surgical intervention in this population would lessen this risk.[103] Surgical intervention is recommended for the symptomatic discoid meniscus. Arthroscopic reshaping of the meniscus is typically performed using a procedure called saucerization.[104] Any associated meniscus tears are treated with partial meniscectomy or repair. Stabilization procedures are performed for unstable discoid variants. Rehabilitation programs and expected time for full recovery will vary depending upon the procedure performed. A period of limited weight bearing or ROM restrictions may be required and will be directed by the treating surgeon.

DISPLAY 14.4	Ligament Sprain Grading Scale
Grade	**Description**
1	Pain with stress testing without associated joint laxity
2	Pain with stress testing with increased joint excursion; presence of distinct end point
3	Complete ligament disruption with excessive excursion; no distinct end point

Traumatic meniscal tears, absent a congenital meniscus malformation, usually occur in older children or adolescents as a result of a twisting injury in sports. The meniscus of the developing child is more vascular than that of adults and has thus been noted to have better capacity for healing.[103] Clinical diagnosis is sometimes challenging with physical examination and special tests yielding somewhat limited diagnostic reliability.[106] The most consistent findings during meniscus tear physical examination include history of a twisting injury, joint effusion, and joint line tenderness. Other special tests such as McMurray test, Apley compression or distraction, Thessaly or Ege's test may also aid in diagnosis. The patient may complain of the knee becoming "stuck" or "catching" if a fragment of meniscus is blocking motion between the tibia and the femur. An MRI is often obtained to assist in diagnosis; however, it should be noted that the MRI is less accurate in diagnosing meniscus tears in children compared with adults.[103]

Treatment of meniscus tears will vary depending upon the location of the tear within the meniscus, tear orientation, and degree of displacement of the torn fragment. As mentioned earlier, certain characteristics of the meniscus of the skeletally immature patient allow for more healing potential than adults, and thus most tears in children are managed using repair rather than meniscectomy. Postoperatively, a patient will typically be treated with non- or partial weight bearing for 4 to 6 weeks with use of hinged knee brace. Knee flexion ROM is also typically limited from 0 degrees to 90 degrees for the first 4 to 6 weeks, with progressive flexion permitted beyond that point. Rehabilitation should continue with addressing deficits in strength, coordination, and limb control. Return to sports usually occurs around 3 to 4 months postoperatively.

Osteochondritis Dissecans in the Knee

As discussed earlier, OCD is a condition in which damage to the subchondral bone causes secondary damage to the overlying articular cartilage. The knee is the most commonly involved joint, with the lateral aspect of the medial femoral condyle being the most commonly affected site within the knee.[8] Patients with OCD typically complain of activity-related anterior knee pain. Differential diagnosis should include patellofemoral pain, chondromalacia patella, and plica syndrome, as these may all have similar symptoms. With the knee in varying degrees of flexion, the examiner may note a distinct area of point tenderness at the medial femoral condyle where the lesion is located. Wilson's sign is a special test that has been described, but may have limited diagnostic value.[107] If the lesion has progressed to being unstable, mechanical symptoms are more likely to be noted such as crepitus, knee effusion, and an abnormal gait.[108] Plain radiographs are typically part of the initial diagnostic workup of a patient suspected to have an OCD lesion. If positive, MRI or other advanced imaging will typically be utilized to gain more information and improve decision making for treatment.[109]

Treatment will vary depending upon the extent of the lesion. Nonsurgical treatment is advocated for the stable lesion. In the classic treatment protocol, the patient is non–weight bearing with the knee immobilized in a brace for a period of 6 weeks.[108] Recently, some authors have advocated that immobilization and weight-bearing restrictions are not necessary. In these cases, the patient may bear full weight, but should avoid any sports or impact activity for a period of 6 to 8 weeks.[109] In either scenario, adherence is typically an issue and considerable education regarding the long-term risks associated with improper treatment of OCD may be necessary. After this period of immobilization or activity modification, rehabilitation is initiated and focuses on deficits in strength, ROM, and other kinetic chain deficits that impact lower extremity control. Return to running, jumping, and sports can usually begin around 3 months, with a progressive introduction of activity, while continuing to monitor for return of symptoms. When initiating plyometric training, proper lower extremity alignment and impact absorption during jump landing should be emphasized.

Surgical management is typically recommended for unstable lesions or those that do not heal with conservative measures. Several surgical treatment options exist and include antegrade or retrograde drilling procedures, fragment removal, internal fixation, microfracture, autologous chondrocyte implantation, or osteochondral autograft or allograft transplantation.[108,109] Rehabilitation protocols will vary depending upon the procedure performed; however, typical protocols will require an early period of immobilization and weight-bearing restrictions. Rehabilitation is similar in scope to most other postoperative knee procedures addressing local deficits about the knee as well any other noted kinetic chain deficits. Return to sports will typically not occur until 6 to 9 months postoperatively.

Acute Patella Dislocations and Osteochondral Fractures

Most acute dislocations of the patella are caused by planting or twisting maneuvers, which usually occur while rapidly changing directions during sports. The patient will note the knee "giving way" and can occasionally recall seeing the patella located on lateral aspect of the knee. Relocation is usually accomplished by simply straightening the involved leg. The knee will be swollen, generally tender, and ROM will typically be limited owing to guarding. Lateral displacement of the patella may evoke an apprehension sign. Radiographs or MRI will be necessary to rule out the possibility of osteochondral fractures. If no osteochondral damage is noted, acute patella dislocations are usually treated conservatively with immobilization in extension for 4 weeks, followed by progressive ROM and rehabilitation. If a patient continues to experience recurrent patella dislocations, surgical intervention may be indicated. Medial patellofemoral ligament (MPFL) reconstruction is one procedure that is often seen and has been associated with good functional outcomes.[110] Weight bearing is protected early with the knee locked in extension. Early ROM and quadriceps activation are emphasized. Comprehensive rehabilitation after MPFL reconstruction overlaps considerably with the principles discussed after ACL reconstruction with return to sports around 6 to 12 months.

Osteochondral fractures typically occur with an acute lateral patella dislocation, and are most frequently located in the medial patella facet and/or lateral femoral condyle. During relocation of the patella, the medial patella surface shears across the lateral femoral condyle/trochlea, damaging the articular surface.[111] Although the frequency of this injury is difficult to quantify, some reports have found occurrence with patella dislocations to be as high as 25% to 75%.[111] The presentation of the patient with an osteochondral fracture will be similar to that of an acute patella dislocation; however, there may be palpable crepitus during movement or a mechanical, bony block to motion, due to a loose body. Plain films may not always detect the lesion, and MRI is typically the image of choice.[111] Surgical treatment is indicated in most cases of displaced osteochondral fractures with arthroscopic fixation or removal of the fragment. A resurfacing procedure, such as microfracture, is performed when the fragment is removed.[111] The microfracture procedure stimulates bone marrow, which causes bleeding, and a resulting fibrin clot forms that eventually differentiates into fibrocartilage to repair the defect.[112] To protect the healing tissue, most surgeons recommend a period of protected weight bearing and ROM restrictions postoperatively on the basis of lesion location and procedure performed. Rehabilitation will be similar to other knee disorders previously discussed. The projected time frame for return to sports is 4 to 6 months.[111]

Overuse Injuries

Anterior knee pain is a common complaint among skeletally immature athletes and can stem from a variety of causes, many of them related to overuse. Commonly encountered diagnoses that cause anterior knee pain are patellofemoral pain syndrome (PFPS), Osgood–Schlatter disease (OSD), Sinding–Larsen–Johansson disease (SLJ), inflamed synovial plica, and patella tendinopathy.

Patellofemoral Pain Syndrome

PFPS is a broad diagnosis that refers to pain in the patellofemoral joint and the surrounding structures. PFPS is the most common cause of all knee overuse injuries.[3] Biomechanical alterations in lower extremity function result in abnormal stress across the patellofemoral joint and tissue overload, which results in anterior knee pain. The interaction among several intrinsic and extrinsic factors is thought

to be responsible for causing PFPS. Structural abnormalities such as femoral anteversion, femoral trochlea dysplasia, and bipartite patella may contribute to the development of PFPS. Flexibility limitations in the quadriceps, hamstrings, hip flexors, IT band, and gastrocsoleus complex, as well as strength/neuromuscular control deficits in the gluteus medius, gluteus maximus, and quadriceps have all been implicated as factors related to PFPS.[113] Extrinsic factors related to PFPS include training errors such as inadequate rest, rapid progression of training volume, and improper shoe wear.

The patient will usually complain of a dull ache from underneath or around the patella that increases with activities such as squatting, ascending/descending stairs, running, or prolonged sitting. As mentioned above, proximal and distal factors may contribute to the development of PFPS, and thus a comprehensive physical examination is required. Special attention should be paid to examination of gluteus medius and gluteus maximus strength and the resulting coordination during closed-chain limb control, as there is a mounting body of evidence that these deficits play a large role in the development of PFPS.[113–115] Distal factors such as excessive foot pronation and limited ankle dorsiflexion may also contribute to the pathomechanics involved in PFPS and should be assessed accordingly.[116] Limb control can be assessed utilizing the Eccentric Step Down test, which may help identify limb control deficits. Locally, patella alignment and mobility should be assessed looking for evidence of either restricted or excessive patella mobility and abnormal tilting. The articulating surface of the patella should be palpated as it will usually be painful in PFPS. Pain with compression of the patellofemoral joint should also be noted (grind test). Radiographs are not necessary for diagnosing PFPS, but they may be helpful in ruling out any other possible diagnosis or related issues.[3]

Treatment must first focus on removing the offending forces during everyday activities. Relative rest from painful activities during sports should be advocated, and complete rest may be necessary in severe cases. All exercises in physical therapy should be closely monitored and should remain pain free. Correction of biomechanical problems should be the primary goal of all interventions. Close supervision and feedback are required during functional exercises to ensure proper lower extremity alignment. The multifactorial nature of PFPS dictates a diverse and extensive treatment plan. Strength training, flexibility, balance, core strengthening, neuromuscular control exercises, and orthotic intervention have all been shown to be helpful in treating PFPS.[113,117] Adjunct treatments such as patellofemoral taping or bracing may be effective for pain relief and may be used to enhance the patient's ability to participate in corrective exercises. If a patient fails to respond to conservative treatment and symptoms continue to limit function, surgical treatment could be considered. Lateral release and patellar realignment procedures for the correction of PFPS have been described. Rehabilitation from these procedures is usually extensive, and a prolonged absence from sports is required.

Apophysitis

OSD and SLJ are common overuse injuries that will cause anterior knee pain. Both are caused by traction forces from muscle contraction leading to increased stress across the apophysis. These repetitive forces lead to cumulative microtrauma, inflammation, and pain.[3] OSD represents injury at the tibial tubercle, while SLJ represents an apophysitis at the inferior pole of the patella. Symptoms typically present between the ages of 9 and 15 years in children who participate in activities that involve excessive running and jumping. The symptoms include achy pain in the anterior knee that is aggravated by activity or with direct pressure, such as kneeling. Tenderness to palpation will exist at the location of apophysitis (tibial tubercle or inferior pole of patella) and will help with differential diagnosis. Contractile testing of the involved muscle attachments will also produce pain. Radiographs are helpful at ruling out any other possible diagnoses such as avulsion fractures.

OSD and SLJ are self-limiting processes with symptoms resolving at skeletal maturity. Acute management consists of rest from aggravating activities, ice, and possibly non-steroidal anti-inflammatory drugs (NSAIDs). Treatment should focus on normalizing lower extremity flexibility, especially to the quadriceps and hamstring muscle groups. Strengthening of the quadriceps, hip abductors, and external rotators may help improve lower extremity alignment and efficiency during functional activities, and should be employed. Exercises should not provoke symptoms.

Patellar Tendinopathy

Older adolescents with fused growth plates are more likely to develop a tendinopathy with overuse, as opposed to an apophysitis. Patellar tendinopathy or "jumpers knee" is commonly seen in adolescents who play basketball, volleyball, and running. This is a mechanical overuse syndrome due to the cumulative effects of repetitive microtrauma within the patellar tendon.[3] Patients report anterior knee pain aggravated by activity. Contractile testing of the quadriceps will be painful, and tenderness to palpation along the patella tendon is common.

Treatment consists of relative rest refraining from any painful activities, improving flexibility, strength training, and improving dynamic control of lower extremity. Eccentric strengthening is an effective treatment for patellar tendinopathy, and should be incorporated into a comprehensive rehabilitation plan.[118,119] Lack of flexibility in quadriceps and hamstrings has been implicated as a risk factor for lower extremity overuse syndromes; therefore, a long-term flexibility program should be advocated for injury prevention.[120]

Plica Syndrome

Plicae are bands of tissue in the synovial lining of the knee that arise from remnants of embryologic knee development.[121] Although plica can be found at multiple locations, the medial plica is most commonly symptomatic. A medial plica should be considered a normal variant in anatomy, as its presence does not always cause symptoms. A plica can become symptomatic when it rubs across the medial femoral condyle with movement, causing inflammation and subsequent anteromedial knee pain. The patient will occasionally complain of "pseudo" locking episodes or snapping sensation with flexion/extension of the knee, making diagnosis difficult.[122] Palpation of a symptomatic plica is important for clinical examination, but can be difficult. The plica is usually felt as a painful, taut band, running from the medial patella to the medial femoral condyle and orientated perpendicular to the patella. Treatment is similar to that discussed for PFPS involving activity modification, inflammation control, flexibility restoration, pain-free strengthening, and emphasis on dynamic limb control. If conservative measures fail, arthroscopic excision may be recommended.

▶ Lower leg injuries

The lower leg refers to the area of the tibia, fibula, and all the surrounding tissues. The term "shin splints" is a generic term to describe pain to the lower leg. However, the lower leg pain can be due to various injuries to the lower leg tissues. The lower leg is susceptible to both traumatic and overuse-type injuries in athletes. Common differential diagnoses of lower leg pain include medial tibial stress syndrome, tibia and/or fibula stress fracture, chronic exertional compartment syndrome, acute compartment syndrome, muscle strains and tendinopathy, and traumatic tibia and/or fibula fracture.

Shin Splints

Medial Tibial Stress Syndrome

Medial tibial stress syndrome (MTSS) is the most common cause of pain to the lower leg. It is characterized by pain and inflammation along the anteromedial plane of the distal to central one-third of the tibia with running and jumping activities. Although not fully understood, MTSS was initially thought to be due to overuse of the posterior tibialis and/or soleus muscles contributing to subsequent periosteal reaction along the medial border of the tibia. High, repetitive loads and rapid foot pronation will contribute to microtears at the soft tissue and periosteal attachments. However, Moen recently suggested that MTSS is caused by bony overload, resulting in an osteopenic cortex and bone marrow edema, and not periostitis.[123] Contributing factors to MTSS include decreased hip internal rotation ROM, excessive plantarflexion ROM, excessive midfoot mobility, poor shock attenuation, rapid changes in exercise intensity, weakness or imbalance about the lower leg, and high BMI.[123,124]

An athlete with MTSS complains of pain and tenderness to the distal to central one-third of the lower leg along the posteromedial border of the tibia. Initially, the athlete may report pain with the start of the run that decreases as the run continues. However, as symptoms worsen, pain will continue throughout the duration of the run and may carry over into other activities. Physical exam may demonstrate weakness and imbalances about the lower leg muscles, namely the posterior tibialis and flexor hallicus longus. Biomechanical deformities to the lower kinetic chain that contribute to excessive compensatory foot pronation are also likely. Diagnostic imaging will help discern MTSS from tibial stress fracture. Initially, plain radiographs will be normal. Bone scans may confirm the diagnosis of MTSS by showing diffuse longitudinal area of uptake, as opposed to a focal, transverse line that is indicative of a stress fracture. MRI remains the most sensitive and specific test for diagnosing and discerning between an MTSS and stress fracture.

Treatment for MTSS begins with a period of active rest from painful activities such as running and jumping. Low-impact activities such as swimming, cycling, and other modes of cardiovascular training are recommended to maintain fitness levels and decrease the effects of deconditioning. Pain control modalities including ice, compressive taping/wrapping techniques, and NSAID may be helpful in alleviation of symptoms. A rehabilitation program should consist of flexibility and strength training of the lower leg musculature, with a special focus on the gastrocsoleus complex. Treatment should also restore balance and dynamic control of the lower kinetic chain and trunk. A thorough functional evaluation should also be performed to identify any contributory factors present during sport-specific movements. Shoes with adequate foot support and/or orthotic intervention may be helpful during the initial phases of treatment to control excessive foot pronation. With proper management, it may take 6 to 8 weeks before returning to running and impact activities. Return to running is performed with a progressive running program. Running distance, frequency, and intensity should not be increased simultaneously or more than 10% each week and should take into consideration patient fitness level, pain response, and goals.

Tibial Stress Fracture

Tibial stress fractures are common with activities that include repetitive loading to the lower leg, including running, basketball, gymnastics, and dance. Stress fractures are osseous fractures caused by repetitive bony overload and the inability to meet the demands of the levels of force. Contributing factors for tibial stress fracture are improper training regimens, poor bone health, high BMI, abnormally high or low medial longitudinal arch heights, and excessive foot pronation.[125] Owing to the high incidence in distance runners, certain characteristics of running mechanics have been studied and linked to tibial stress fracture. These include high vertical loading rates, heel striking at ground contact, increased step length, decreased cadence, and high tibial accelerations.[126–128]

Tibial stress fractures will cause localized, acute, and sharp pain on the tibial surface. This can occur anywhere along the length of the tibia, but is usually along the central to upper one-third of the anterior cortex. Focal tenderness and pain is reported along the site of the fracture and may be associated with a palpable thickening. Pain will usually not be present at the start of activity, but will gradually worsen as activity continues and may eventually occur at rest. Diagnosis may be confirmed with diagnostic imaging. Initially, plain radiographs may be normal, but will demonstrate periosteal healing or callus formation identifying an area of bony healing. Bone scan is not specific, but will demonstrate a focal uptake along the anterior tibia. MRI is more specific and can better assist in the diagnosis and determine the severity of the tibial stress fracture.

Initial treatment for tibial stress fractures is relative rest and activity limitation to allow for bony healing. Pain-free weight bearing, muscle activation, and flexibility activities can be initiated. In cases where weight bearing is painful, a walking boot or restriction of weight bearing may be warranted. Once there are signs of radiographic healing, progressive weight bearing and a more advanced strengthening and flexibility program can be implemented. As strength is normalizing, sport-specific training can begin with an emphasis on quality of movement and progressive return. Running gait retraining with the goals of limiting vertical and torsional loading has also been effective in the management of tibial stress fractures.[126,128] When the athlete fails to improve and continued limitation persists, or with a long history or bone health compromise, a more thorough medical workup may be warranted. This includes blood testing and nutritional consult.

Compartment Syndrome

The lower leg is comprised of four compartments: anterior, lateral, superficial posterior, and deep posterior. Each compartment comprises muscle, vascular, and nervous tissues, all encapsulated by a facial membrane.

Acute compartment syndrome is an emergent condition that results from acute trauma to the lower leg. An increase in intracompartmental pressure is caused by soft tissue swelling and contributes to localized pain, parasthesia, and weakness. In suspicion of acute compartment syndrome, immediate attention is required. Fasciotomy is performed to relieve the compartment pressure and prevent permanent tissue damage.

Chronic exertional compartment syndrome (CECS) or exercise-induced compartment syndrome is not an emergent situation but can be functionally disabling to athletes and commonly seen in long-distance runners. Pain results from muscle ischemia, which occurs with exercise, due to significantly elevated intracompartmental pressures. During exercise, increased muscle contractions can lead to increased blood flow and volume within the affected lower leg compartment. Normally, the surrounding fascia will adapt and expand to meet the demands of the increased muscle volume. However, in CECS, the containing fascia is unable to expand, thereby constricting blood flow and resulting in ischemia. Complaints of pain and tightness result, with or without neurovascular compromise. The location and presentation of symptoms will vary depending on the affected compartment. The anterior and lateral compartments are the most commonly affected; however, any of the four compartments of the lower leg can be involved.

An athlete with CECS will commonly report aching pain, tightness, and/or squeezing sensations about the lower leg in the distribution of the affected compartment. Commonly, the athlete will first report tightness or cramping, but may progress to altered sensation and motor weakness. Symptoms are usually predictable, exacerbated by a given exercise intensity and time, and relieved shortly after cessation of activity. Diagnosis of the syndrome is confirmed with intracompartmental pressure testing. Conservative treatment of activity modification, soft tissue mobilization and massage, muscle stretching and strengthening, and orthotic prescription has not been very successful in the management of CECS.[129] However, research is emerging regarding success in altering the running mechanics and technique for the treatment of CECS of the anterior compartment.[130] In the event that conservative treatment fails, surgical fasciotomy of the involved compartments is recommended, and often allows the athlete to return to full activity within 8 to 12 weeks.[124]

▶ Ankle injuries

The ankle is the most common site for athletic injuries, accounting for 20% to 30% of all musculoskeletal injuries.[131] The ankle joint comprises the three main joint articulations. The talocrural joint is the bony articulation between the distal tibia and fibula and the proximal surface of the talus, and is responsible for nearly all of ankle plantarflexion and dorsiflexion. The subtalar joint comprises the talocalcaneal and talocalcaneonavicular joints. Inversion and eversion occur predominately at the subtalar joint. It is important to note that despite the dominance of one motion occurring at a given joint, mobility occurs simultaneously in all three planes of motion owing to joint axis orientation. Therefore, triplanar movement about the ankle is often described as "supination"—or combined plantarflexion, inversion, and adduction—and "pronation," or combined dorsiflexion, eversion, and abduction.

More common differential diagnoses for ankle pain are lateral ankle sprain, syndesmosis sprain, distal physeal fracture, peroneal longus subluxation, osteochondral fracture of the talar dome, Maisonneuve fracture or combination of a distal syndesmosis tear and a proximal fibular fracture, and sinus tarsi impingement.

Ankle Sprains

Stability to the lateral ankle is due primarily to the lateral ligament complex consisting of the anterior talofibular ligament (ATFL), calcaneofibular ligament (CFL), and posterior talofibular ligament (PFL). All three ligaments aid in the restriction of excessive ankle inversion, with the ATFL also resisting anterior translation of the talus. The medial ankle ligaments are comprised of the thicker and stronger deltoid ligament, and are responsible for restraining ankle eversion, pronation, and anterior displacement of the talus. The tibia and fibula are connected distally by the anterior and posterior distal tibiofibular ligaments and the distal interosseous ligament. Together, they comprise the distal portion of the interosseous membrane that traverses the entire lengths of the shafts and contributes to lower leg stability and force transmission.

Eighty-five percent of all ankle pathology is due to acute ankle sprains, and most often involve injury to the lateral ligaments. Mechanism of injury is usually excessive inversion and plantarflexion. Deltoid sprains are also known as eversion sprains due to their mechanism of injury. Syndesmotic sprains, commonly named "high ankle sprains," usually occur in conjunction with medial ankle sprains and are caused by forced eversion and ER of the ankle causing a widening of the distal tibiofibular joint. Injuries to the medial ankle or along the tibiofibular syndesmosis are less common on account of their inherent strength.[132]

In examining an ankle injury, careful inspection of foot position at the time of injury, location of tenderness, and mobility testing aid in the recognition of the injured ligaments. The athlete will often report a distinct injury with a sudden pain or "pop." With more severe sprains, pain will not allow continued participation in athletic activity. The athlete will initially present with pain, swelling, and ecchymosis throughout the ankle and into the foot and toes. It should be noted that because of gravity, swelling and bruising may not always correspond to the site of injury. Weight bearing may also be limited and painful.

Physical exam should include careful palpation along the ankle ligaments to help discern the ligaments involved. ROM will be limited especially in motions that stress the involved ligament. Isolated ligamentous stress testing may also be beneficial in the diagnosis of ankle instability. Lateral ligamentous stress testing includes the anterior drawer and talar tilt tests. The anterior drawer test assesses the stability of the ATFL. The talar tilt test assesses the integrity of the CFL. The Kleiger test, or forced foot eversion and ER, and squeeze test stress the medial ankle's deltoid ligament and syndesmosis ligaments, respectively. All tests should be performed bilaterally to compare the amount of excursion, provocation of pain, and appreciation of a distinct end point to the uninjured ankle. In the acute stage, the ankle is often too swollen and painful to perform the tests with accuracy. Resistive muscle testing performed in midrange is usually pain free, except in the cases of an associated injury to a musculotendinous unit, such as concomitant peroneal tendon strain with a lateral ankle injury.

Like any acute injury, treatment of ankle sprains initially follows the principles of PRICE: protection, rest, ice, compression, and elevation of the involved extremity (Table 14.5). A few days of rest and immobilization may be necessary to allow for pain and swelling to subside; however, early joint mobility and weight bearing has been shown to be more favorable for functional return in comparison with prolonged immobilization.[133]

The severity of ligament disruption will affect the treatment plan design. Grade 1 ankle sprains may respond more quickly than grade 2 or 3 sprains. Owing to the higher chances of the recurrence of ankle sprain following previous injury,[133] a rehabilitation program is recommended for all ankle sprains to assist in the restoration of mobility, proprioception, and muscle performance. ROM activities can begin in the acute phases of injury, starting with ankle dorsiflexion and plantarflexion. Progression to frontal plane inversion and eversion may be initiated in pain-free, limited ranges and monitored by pain response to facilitate tissue remodeling and ligamentous healing. Straight-plane weight-bearing activities should follow a similar progression, with eventually challenging the athlete in multiplanar and unilateral activities on various surfaces. Careful attention to muscle activation, recruitment, and timing should be paramount owing to the associated increase in muscle latency following lateral ankle sprains.[134] In the case of continued ankle instability and impaired function following a rehabilitative course, especially in grade 3 injuries where there is complete ligamentous disruption, surgical reconstruction of ankle stabilizers may be warranted and yields favorable results.

Ankle Fractures

When evaluating the pediatric ankle following acute injury, it is important to discern between ligamentous sprain and growth plate injury due to the inherent weakness of the physis. Ankle fractures in sports occur with deceleration or rotational forces about a fixed foot. In children under 12 years with an immature skeletal system, a physeal fracture of the distal fibula is highly probable with a lateral ankle injury.[135] Nondisplaced Salter–Harris type I is the most common fracture of the distal fibular physes. Pain on palpation is over the physeal growth plate, which is located about one finger width above the distal portion of the lateral malleolus (Fig. 14.8). Management is with cast immobilization for 3 weeks followed by a rehabilitation program similar to that of a lateral ankle sprain. Plain radiographs are able to assist in the diagnosis of ankle fracture. The Ottawa ankle rules have been shown to be sensitive in detecting fractures to the foot in children over 5 years of age and should be utilized in the clinical decision process and diagnosis of traumatic ankle injuries in children[136,137] (Display 14.5).

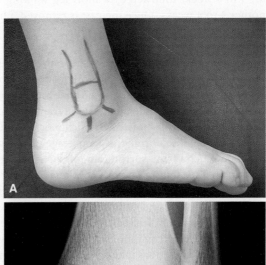
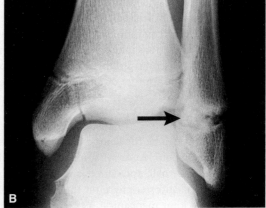

FIGURE. 14.8 **(A)** Location of distal fibular physis and lateral ankle ligaments **(B)** distal fibular physis location (arrow) with and an associated Salter-Harris II fracture of distal tibia.

TABLE 14.5	PRICE Principles for Acute Injury Management
Principle	**Management Options**
Protection	Splinting, bracing, walking boot, taping procedures
Rest	Activity modification, altered weight bearing, cross-training
Ice	Localized ice bath, cold pack, ice massage
Compression	Ace wrap, open basket weave tape application, felt padding, compressive sleeve
Elevation	Elevate injured area above level of heart to promote lymph drainage

DISPLAY 14.5	Ottawa Ankle Rules

An ankle X-ray series is required only if there is any pain in malleolar zone and any of these findings:
1. Bone tenderness at posterior edge or tip of lateral malleolus
2. Bone tenderness at posterior edge or tip of medial malleolus
3. Inability to bear weight both immediately and in emergency room

Triplane fractures and Tillaux fractures occur as the athlete approaches skeletal maturity, usually around 15 and 17 years in girls and boys, respectively. Both fractures result from partially closed growth plates. The growth plate will first fuse centrally, followed by medial and lateral closures, leaving the lateral portion vulnerable for injury. A triplane fracture occurs in three planes: coronal, sagittal, and transverse. A Tillaux fracture is a Salter–Harris type III fracture of the unfused anterolateral segment of the distal tibial epiphysis caused by avulsion of the epiphyseal segment by the ATFL.[135] Forceful ER of the foot is the common mechanism of injury. Both fractures are managed with a long leg non–weight-bearing cast for 3 to 4 weeks followed by a short leg walking cast for another 3 to 4 weeks. Once the cast is removed, physical therapy can be initiated to regain normal strength and mobility to the entire lower extremity.

Osteochondral fractures of the talar dome can result from an ankle sprain if the talus abuts the medial or lateral malleolus during the injury. Injury to the bone and overlying cartilage can produce a free-floating, painful fragment in the joint space and may limit motion. Osteochondral fractures are difficult to diagnose during the acute stage of an ankle sprain, when much of the surrounding tissue is inflamed. Persistent pain after the sprain with continued edema and intermittent clicking or locking may suggest an osteochondral fracture.[135] Casting and orthotic interventions are the treatments of less severe lesions in the younger athletes, to provide a controlled environment for chondral healing. However, more severe lesions may require surgical intervention with either arthroscopic drilling, loose body removal, pinning, or cartilaginous transfer or grafting.

Ankle Impingement

Ankle impingement can be the source of anterior, anterolateral, or posterior pain. Anterior impingement is often seen in football, basketball, and dance, and is often caused by the formation of an osteophyte on the distal tibia due to abnormal ankle joint mechanics. As the ankle is forced into maximal dorsiflexion, the osteophyte contacts the talus and causes pain. Anterolateral ankle impingement is often an area of chronic pain, which persists after an ankle sprain. Possible causes are impingement of the tibiofibular ligament, impingement of the synovium, or osteochondral fracture.[135] Pain is reported in the area between the fibula and the lateral talus, within the sinus tarsi, or near the ATFL. Treatment includes rest, NSAIDs, bracing, joint mobilization, and possible arthroscopic debridement.

Posterior impingement is described as pain in the posterior ankle when the foot is plantarflexed, and is commonly experienced by ballet dancers or athletes who repetitively point their foot. The pain is caused by a bony protrusion such as an os trigonum, a small, round bone behind the ankle joint. An os trigonum is found in about 5% to 15% of normal, asymptomatic ankles near the posterior talus.

When the os trigonum fails to fuse with the talus, it can impinge on the soft tissue during forced, end-range plantarflexion.[135] Management consists of rest, NSAIDs, and surgical excision of the bony ossicle.

Foot injuries

Overuse Injuries

Sever's Disease

The cause of foot and heel pain in the young athlete will vary depending on skeletal maturity. Achilles tendonitis and plantar fasciitis are observed more frequently in the skeletally mature athlete. However, in the skeletally immature athlete, atraumatic pain along the posterior calcaneus is likely due to Sever's disease. Sever's disease is a traction apophysitis of the calcaneus at the site of the attachment of the Achilles tendon, plantar fascia, and intrinsic muscles of the foot. This occurs during periods of rapid skeletal growth in athletes 9 to 12 years old.[138] Pain is reported along the heel, and will increase during sports such as soccer, gymnastics, and basketball with repetitive running and jumping. Pain is usually bilateral; however, it can also occur unilaterally, and can occur in conjunction with Achilles tendonitis.

A young athlete with Sever's disease will complain of sharp or dull pain along the calcaneal apophysis. A patient history of any rapid recent changes in activity levels, training errors, changes in shoe wear, and rapid skeletal growth will be consistent with Sever's disease. Gently squeezing the lateral borders of the calcaneus will often replicate painful symptoms. Musculoskeletal evaluation will often find muscle length restrictions to triceps surae muscle complex, excessive foot pronation, and possible swelling. In more severe cases, weight bearing and walking will also be asymmetric and painful.[3]

Treatment of Sever's disease begins with pain control modalities, including activity modification, ice, and NSAIDs. This condition is benign and self-limiting without any long-term consequences. Therefore, continuation with normal athletic activities should be permitted if tolerated. However, the presence of gait and running asymmetries, pain at rest, and persistent debilitating pain following sport should exclude an athlete's participation in the painful activity owing to the risk of further injury. Interventions are aimed at the restoration of flexibility and length to impaired musculature, and strengthening to calf and foot musculature. The incorporation of a gel heel lift in the athlete's shoe may also be appropriate to unload the Achilles tendon and cushion the heel. In the presence of an excessively dropped medial longitudinal arch, temporary use of orthotics may assist in unloading the Achilles tendon and the apophysis. The condition usually resolves within a few weeks or months with proper treatment. In persistent cases, casting and immobilization may be needed.

Iselin's Disease

Iselin's disease, similarly to Sever's disease, is a traction apophysitis to the proximal fifth metatarsal. This condition is seen in children 10 to 12 years old. Traction to the insertion site of the peroneus brevis muscle on the proximal aspect of the fifth metatarsal and lateral aspect of the foot will contribute to inflammation, irritation, and pain in adolescents who participate in sports with repetitive running and jumping.[3]

Upon examination, the athlete may present with localized swelling and tenderness along the proximal physis of the fifth metatarsal. Upon weight bearing, pain may increase. Resistive testing into eversion thus tensioning the peroneus brevis will replicate symptoms, along with end-range plantarflexion, dorsiflexion, and inversion.

Treatment of Iselin's disease is similar to that of Sever's disease. A short period of activity modification and pain control modalities are the initial treatment options of choice. Treatment should also include ankle flexibility to the evertors and plantarflexors, general ankle strengthening, and proprioceptive activities. In the more mild cases, the athlete can return to unrestricted activity within 3 to 6 weeks. However, in those instances where the athlete is not responding and pain is limiting functional activity, a short period of immobilization may be warranted, increasing recovery time.[3]

Tendonitis and Plantar Fasciitis

The diagnosis of a tendonitis, though not as common in the young, skeletally immature athlete, can contribute to pain and disability. Achilles tendonitis is typically reported as pain along the Achilles tendon just proximal to the superior margin of the calcaneus, often seen in ballet dancers, runners, basketball players, and other field athletes. Causative factors include rapid increases in training duration and intensity, rapid skeletal growth, and excessive foot pronation.[139] Examination should include palpation along the entire length of the tendon, starting proximally and continuing inferiorly to the heel pad, noting the area of maximal tenderness. Swelling, decreased dorsiflexion ROM, and pain with resisted plantarflexion are common findings. Single-leg heel raise and hopping reproduces pain at the Achilles tendon.

Interventions should begin with rest, ice, NSAIDs, gentle stretching of gastrocnemius and soleus muscles, and changes in footwear. A temporary heel lift or orthotic may aid in tendon unloading and should be discontinued gradually as pain subsides. As symptoms become less acute, strengthening of the plantarflexors is initiated in non–weight-bearing positions and progresses to weight-bearing postures. In treating the more chronic Achilles tendinopathy, eccentric weight-bearing exercises to the plantarflexors have been shown to be effective.[140] Balance exercise, proprioception, and entire lower extremity and core strengthening are also recommended to control excessive compensatory foot pronation. Impact activities are added slowly with a graduated return to running and sport-specific training.

Other regions of the foot and ankle are susceptible to tendonitis. Treatment of tendonitis follows a similar course, including activity modification, pain control, normalization of mobility, and strengthening. Activity can be gradually increased in a progressive manner, once symptoms have resolved, on the basis of quality of movement and soreness. Posterior tibialis tendonitis can be seen in running athletes, skaters, and gymnasts. Pain is localized to the posterior aspect of the medial malleolus. Flexor hallicus longus tendonitis is commonly seen in athletes who repetitively point their toes such as dancers working "on pointe," gymnasts, and runners. Pain can be reported on the plantar aspect of the foot and/or along the posterior aspect of the medial malleolus. Peroneal tendonitis is seen in skaters, dancers, and running athletes. Pain is typically located posterior to the lateral malleolus.

Traumatic Injuries

Lisfranc (MidFoot) Injury

The tarsometatarsal joint complex is more commonly known as the Lisfranc joint. This joint aids in the intrinsic, osseus stability of the foot. The middle three metatarsal bases and the cuneiforms form the transverse arch of the foot. Injuries to this joint complex include ligamentous sprains and/or fracture dislocations, with the ligament extending from the base of the second metatarsal to the medial cuneiform being most commonly injured. Although commonly associated with high-energy motor vehicle accidents, Lisfranc injuries are also seen in sports owing to a low-energy axial load on a plantarflexed foot with the knee anchored on the ground. This is often seen in football while a player is lying prone on the ground and another player falls on the athlete's heel. Lisfranc injuries can often occur owing to excessive abduction stress to the midfoot, where the forefoot is abducted around a fixed hindfoot. This mechanism is commonly associated with sports that require the use of a foot stirrup, such as equestrian and windsurfing.[141]

A Lisfranc injury can be difficult to identify because of the often subtle instability. More severe injuries, such as a fracture dislocation, present with noticeable foot deformity. An athlete with a Lisfranc injury often complains of pain to the dorsum of the foot following a specific mechanism of injury. Forefoot edema and bruising along the plantar arch are paramount findings of a Lisfranc injury. Weight bearing is painful and increases when asked to stand on their tiptoes.[142] Physical exam reveals tenderness upon palpation along the tarsometatarsal joints and gapping between the hallux and second toe when compared with the contralateral limb. Mobility testing will replicate pain upon abduction and pronation of the forefoot, while maintaining a fixed hindfoot. Mobility of the first and second metatarsals in all planes, along with their association with one another, should be assessed noting any pain and/or joint subluxation. It is important to discern between a stable, ligamentous sprain and complete rupture that will contribute to a gross midfoot instability.[141] Radiographs with the athlete standing that stresses the tarsometatarsal joints are helpful in diagnosis, as non–weight-bearing films may not capture a slight instability and appear normal.[143]

Stable Lisfranc injuries are managed conservatively. The athlete is immobilized with a CAM walking boot for 6 to 10 weeks, and allowed to weight-bear according to pain tolerance. Physical therapy is recommended to aid in restoration of normal gait, balance, mobility, and strength. A full-length insert is often helpful during the transition from the CAM boot to a supportive shoe. Complete recovery will take about 4 months, though some injuries may not permit an athlete to return to the prior level of sports participation. Unstable Lisfranc injuries, even subtle ones, are treated surgically.[141]

Bony Abnormalities

Tarsal Coalition

Tarsal coalition is a congenital malformation where two or more of the tarsal bones fail to differentiate, resulting in a cartilaginous, fibrous, or bony union. This often occurs bilaterally, involving the calcaneonavicular and talocalcaneal articulations. Symptoms restricting mid- and hindfoot mobility begin to appear during the second or third decade of life, as the coalition attempts to ossify. Fractures within the coalition will result in pain following fusion of the associated joints.

An athlete presenting with tarsal coalition typically complains of an insidious onset of foot or ankle pain. Pain is often exacerbated with sports requiring cutting, pivoting, changing direction, and running on uneven surfaces. Recurrent and chronic ankle sprains are also reported owing to the lack of available foot mobility, thus stressing the surrounding tissues. Physical exam often reveals a fixed, hyperpronated foot type. Limited accessory joint mobility to the midfoot and/or hindfoot is a paramount finding with tarsal coalition. A suspicion of tarsal coalition can be most accurately confirmed with CT imaging.

Treatment for tarsal coalition is directed at controlling foot motion to decrease stresses about the fusing joints. Orthotics are recommended to help support the foot and control excessive mobility. Strengthening for the intrinsic and extrinsic foot musculature is helpful for dynamic support of the foot and ankle complex, as are ankle joint flexibility activities, to decrease compensatory subtalar joint mobility. Advanced pain may respond more favorably to aggressive immobilization in a cast. If conservative treatment fails, referral for surgery prior to joint ossification is recommended and is successful in resolving pain and restoring mobility.

Accessory Navicular

Accessory navicular is the congenital formation of a small ossicle adjacent to the navicular bone or within the tibialis posterior tendon. Also known as an os navicular secundum, this condition is not always asymptomatic upon diagnosis. However, when problematic, an athlete will present with localized pain and inflammation along the navicular tuberosity and medial arch. High-impact sports and activities are often painful, especially when wearing tight-fitting shoes or cleats. Pain is often replicated with resistive foot inversion owing to one of the attachment sites of the tibialias posterior muscle. Both plain radiographs and CT scans will help confirm the diagnosis.

Conservative and surgical treatment options are available for an accessory navicular. Activity modification, NSAIDs, and orthotic interventions that control excessive midfoot motion are the primary nonsurgical options. However, a period of more aggressive immobilization within a CAM boot or cast may be necessary in more painful cases. Padding along the navicular tuberosity within the shoe will also assist in pain control by alleviating direct pressure along the bony prominence. Surgical excision of the ossicle is recommended when pain continues to limit activity following attempts at conservative management.

Forefoot Injuries

Forefoot Fractures

Metatarsal fractures in children are usually a result of direct trauma, with the fifth metatarsal being most frequently injured.[144] Metatarsal stress fractures are rare in children, but may be seen in dancers and runners owing to repetitive loading.[145] Sites of fracture include the physes, located distally in metatarsals 2 to 5, metatarsal shafts, and fifth metatarsal styloid. Localized pain, tenderness, and swelling over the fracture site are reported, and can include deformity when the fracture is displaced. Plain radiographs of the foot will assist in the diagnosis of acute fractures. The Ottawa foot rules are sensitive in detecting fractures to the foot in children over 5 years of age and should be utilized in the clinical decision process and diagnosis of traumatic foot injuries in children[136,137] (Display 14.6).

Nondisplaced fractures are treated conservatively with immobilization and closed reduction in a short leg walking cast, CAM boot, or postop walking shoe for 4 to 6 weeks. Management of displaced fractures may require surgery. Once there is evidence of bony healing, physical therapy

---

DISPLAY 14.6 **Ottawa Foot Rules**

A foot X-ray series is required only if there is any pain in midfoot zone and any of these findings:

1. Bone tenderness at the base of the fifth metatarsal
2. Bone tenderness at the navicular
3. Inability to bear weight both immediately and in emergency room

may assist to normalize gait, improve balance, and manage the adverse effects of prolonged immobilization.

In addition to shaft and physeal fractures, a fracture of the proximal diaphysis of the fifth metatarsal is called a Jones fracture. Owing to a decreased blood supply to this area, there is a greater risk of nonunion and refracture.[146] Athletes closer to skeletal maturity, ranging from 15 to 21 years of age, are most affected. This injury, often seen in basketball players and track athletes, is caused by hyper-inversion of the foot or by high-impact loading along the fifth metatarsal. Symptoms are tenderness to palpation over the proximal shaft of the fifth metatarsal, localized swelling, and decreased ability to bear weight. Management of Jones fractures in athletes has been much debated and will vary depending on the stability of the fracture, the healing process, and the athlete's functional goals. Conservative management is typically longer than management for basic fractures. The athlete is placed in a non–weight-bearing cast for 6 weeks, followed by another 6 weeks in a weight-bearing cast, brace, or orthotic. With nonunion or in high-level athletes, surgical ORIF with various techniques may be indicated.[146,147] Return to sport should be permitted once the athlete demonstrates radiographic healing of the fracture site and has progressed through a comprehensive physical therapy program.

Turf Toe

Turf toe is a hyperextension injury to the first metatarsophalangeal (MTP) joint, resulting in damage to the plantar capsuloligamentous structures. Mechanism of injury is a forceful, hyperextension of the great toe, especially while playing on hard, artificial surfaces as in soccer, basketball, and football. This is a ligamentous sprain, and severity is classified with grades 1 through 3, as previously described. A patient will present with pain along the plantar surface of the toe along with possible bruising and swelling. Pain is replicated with active or passive great toe extension.

Treatment is initiated with PRICE modalities and will progress on the basis of severity of the injury. Minor sprains can often be taped, allowing the athlete to continue with sports participation with or without a period of rest. More severe grade 3 injuries will often be treated with a few days of crutches and a steel spring plate shoe insert to limit and protect great toe hyperextension. Early mobility of the first MTP joint is recommended owing to the high incidence of long-term mobility loss (hallux rigidus). An athlete may return to play within 6 weeks once there is full, pain-free extension to the great toe.

▶ Spine injuries

Low back pain is a frequent complaint in young athletes. Characteristics of the developing spine predispose these athletes to patterns of injuries that are different than those in adults. While disc-related pathology is commonly seen in adults, it is relatively rare in the youth athlete. Similarly, children are more likely to present with pathology-related repetitive stress injury to the pars interarticularis (spondylolysis), and the presence of growth centers makes them vulnerable to developing apophyseal injuries.[148] Young athletes who present with low back pain are more likely to have structural injuries, and therefore full investigation, including imaging studies, will likely be necessary.[148,149]

General Examination

Examination begins with a thorough history via open-ended questions to ascertain whether there was a traumatic onset, specific mechanism of injury, previous injuries, and symptom behavior. The clinician should also question athletes regarding the sports-specific history including sports in which they participate, level of participation, volume of practice, how long they have participated in a certain sport, whether they play year round and outside training regimens. Symptomatic onset, duration, response to certain activities, and training/sports participation history will help the clinician differentiate between possible diagnoses and improve clinical decision making for treatment.

Posture should be assessed from the front, behind, and to the side. The clinician should note postural abnormalities that may contribute to altered biomechanical forces during function. These may include scoliosis, rounded shoulders, excessive thoracic kyphosis, hyperlordotic lumbar spine, or anterior pelvic tilt. ROM should also be assessed in all planes of movement (flexion, extension, lateral flexion, and rotation), and the clinician should note not only the range of available motion, but also the quality of the movement and symptomatic response during or after each movement. It is important to assess lower extremity and upper extremity flexibility, as decreased mobility in these structures may predispose the athlete to increased stress across the spine during activity. The clinician should be sure to assess hip and shoulder ROM, flexibility of the hip flexors, quadriceps, hamstrings, and adductors.

Palpation should identify areas of localized tenderness in the spine or SI joints, as well as areas of tenderness or muscle spasm in adjacent soft tissue. Segmental mobility of thoracic and lumbar vertebrae should be assessed, looking for areas of hyper- or hypomobility. Special tests should be utilized to help rule in or exclude certain pathologies that may exist in lumbar spine, SI joints, or hips.

Spondylolysis and Spondylolisthesis

Spondylolysis

Spondylolysis is a fracture in the pars interarticularis of the lumbar spine, with the L5 segment most commonly involved.[150] Spondylolysis is a common injury for young athletes, with one study indicating that 47% of young athletes with complaints of back pain had spondylolysis.[148] Spondylolysis is often referred to as a stress fracture, and is typically caused by repetitive stress within an area of spine during hyperextension and rotational stresses. Certain athletes, such as gymnasts, figure skaters, and dancers, are more prone to developing spondylolysis, as the demands of their sport predispose them to these typical injury patterns. The mean age for spondylolysis is 15 to 16 years. Diagnostic imaging is typically used to determine accurate diagnosis. Radiographs are performed first and may visualize the fracture through the pars interarticularis, which is referred to as a "scotty dog fracture."[151] However, radiography has shown poor sensitivity in detecting spondylytic injuries, and further diagnostic imaging is usually recommended.[152] Single photon emission computed tomography (SPECT) is a very sensitive but nonspecific imaging procedure that will show increased uptake in areas where there is increased bone metabolism, such as a stress reaction or fracture.[152] CT scan provides good visualization of osseous anatomy and can be used in cases where SPECT is positive in order to provide an accurate diagnosis. CT scan is the most accurate imaging modality for detecting spondylolysis; however, its drawbacks include high exposure to radiation and decreased ability to detect early stress reactions when no fracture line is present. Recently, MRI has become an attractive alternative to CT scan owing to the lack of radiation exposure and its ability to assess osseous edema at the pars, along with visualization of soft tissues.[152] The diagnostic utility of MRI in identifying spondylolysis varies in the literature, and most continue to refer to CT scan as the gold standard.[152,153] Nonetheless, MRI may provide valuable information during the diagnostic process without ionizing radiation exposure, and clinicians may find it used with increasing frequency.

Spondylolisthesis

Spondylolisthesis describes an anterior slippage of one vertebral body on another. This commonly occurs at the L5–S1 level, and is often graded on a I to IV scale representing the amount of anterior displacement relative to vertebral body width (see Display 14.7). Grades I and II spondylolisthesis respond well to conservative management, and sports participation has not been shown to increase the degree of slippage.[154] Sports participation is more controversial in grade III or IV spondylolisthesis.

Clinical examination findings guide treatment of the patient, and the general examination principles discussed earlier will apply. Additionally, it should be noted that most patients with spondylolysis or spondylolisthesis will typically demonstrate pain with spinal extension and combined extension rotation movements. Their pain is often aggravated by activity, especially those that place the spine in an extended position. A "step-off" sign of adjacent spinous processes may be palpated if spondylolisthesis is present.

The mainstay of treatment of spondylolysis and spondylolisthesis revolves around reducing the offending forces so the athlete can become pain free. The patient may utilize a custom-molded TLSO (Thoracolumbar sacral orthosis) or soft corset-type brace to aid pain relief via partial immobilization, protection from spinal extension, or hyperlordotic posturing. Bracing is controversial, but some studies have demonstrated improved rates of bone healing with bracing in early treatment.[155,156] As discussed earlier, the therapist should examine the spine to identify areas of hyper- or hypomobility that may focus the stress of movement to an isolated area. Owing to the effect of tight lower extremity musculature on lumbopelvic motion, close examination of flexibility is also required. In addition, the clinician should examine functional movements required by the patient's sport activity and determine whether any dysfunctional movement would correlate with pathologic stress in the spine. Core muscle strengthening and endurance training are necessary during rehabilitation, and these principles will be discussed later in this chapter.

Other Spine Pathologies

Posterior Element Overuse Syndrome

Posterior element overuse syndrome refers to a constellation of conditions involving muscle tendons, ligaments, facet joints, and joint capsules that creates pain in the lower back.[150] Symptoms may be similar to spondylolysis, and imaging is important in differential diagnosis. Treatment will usually consist of rest, activity modification, and rehabilitation to address flexibility, strength, and motor control deficits. A trial of bracing may be helpful for pain relief.

Apophysitis

Apophysitis is another common cause of pain in the spine of the young athlete. Clinically, it is marked by mechanical pain that is irritated with repeated motions of the spine and improves with rest. In the spine, the apophysis is a ring at the vertebral end plates and is not palpable. Apophysitis can also occur at the iliac crest. If this occurs, patients will typically be tender to palpation along this region and may have pain with resisted contraction of the oblique muscles.

Stingers

Injuries to the cervical spine can occur from sports participation. A "stinger" or "burner" is a traction injury of the brachial plexus that usually involves the C-5 and C-6 nerve roots, and occurs most commonly in collision athletes.[157] The athlete will often complain of stinging or burning pain with parasthesias in the affected upper extremity. Muscular

DISPLAY 14.7	Spondylolisthesis Grading System
Grade I	0%–25% vertebral body width
Grade II	25%–50% vertebral body width
Grade III	50%–75% vertebral body width
Grade IV	75%–100% vertebral body width

weakness in shoulder abduction, ER, and flexion may be present. The symptoms usually resolve quickly and allow the athlete to return to play without significant loss of playing time. If symptoms persist for more than 24 hours, further diagnostic workup including imaging studies is recommended. In more severe injuries, treatment consists of supportive rest in a sling and pain relief modalities until the symptoms resolve. After resolution of symptoms, rehabilitation for lost strength is required. The decision to return to sports is based upon normal imaging studies and satisfactory clinical strength examination. The role of electromyographic testing is usually minimal as it is not a valid tool for stinger diagnosis or an indicator of recovery for return to play decision making.[157]

General Treatment Principles

Many injuries to the spine share common rehabilitation principles. The functional requirements of the spine are somewhat paradoxical. The spine requires a high degree of mobility for the performance of functional tasks, while there is a concurrent need for stability. When treating the spine, the therapist must remember these requirements while treating deficits that may inhibit function in either realm.

Regional interdependence is evident in spine rehabilitation, and deficits in upper extremity or lower extremity flexibility, strength, or neuromuscular control may contribute to an athlete's back pain. Similarly, any areas of hypomobility in the vertebral segments above or below the injury should be examined to ensure adequate contribution of movement throughout the spine as a unit.

Core stabilization is an essential component of spine rehabilitation in the young athlete. An inclusive exercise program should be developed to target important core stabilizing muscles, such as the multifidus, transverses abdominus, erector spinae, internal/external obliques, and gluteus muscles. The therapist and athlete must incorporate the concepts of core stabilization training into functional activities that replicate the sport demands on the patient. Willardson has advocated that development of core muscle endurance, not necessarily strength, be the primary goal of rehabilitation.[158] Lumbar stabilizing muscles are composed mainly of type 1 muscle fibers and only relatively low loads are needed to improve their performance.[159] Thus, the clinician should incorporate exercises with longer periods of "hold" or higher repetition of movement, as opposed to heavy-weight, low-repetition training. Finally, as many sports activities occur in standing or involve single-limb support, balance training should be incorporated as part of an inclusive rehabilitation program.

Guidelines for resuming activity after spinal injury are not easy to generalize owing to the highly variable nature of athletic activities. Generally, resumption of activity should occur in a graded fashion, beginning with less stressful and pain-free activities. Activities can be gradually progressed

monitoring for response to increasing sport demands. Owing to the prolonged nature of many spinal injuries, the athlete may require increased time to return to baseline level of fitness prior to being ready to resume full sports participation.

▶ Sports-related concussion

Between 1.7 and 3.8 million sports-related concussion injuries occur in the United States each year, accounting for 5% to 9% of all sports injuries.[160,161] Approximately 50% of all concussions go unreported and undiagnosed.[161] Concussion in sports is a growing problem that affects athletes at all ages, and numbers are likely to increase with heightened awareness. Concussion injuries in youth athletes between the ages of 5 and 19 are rising and comprise 30% of all sports-related concussions. Though more common in contact sports, such as football, rugby, soccer, and hockey, all athletes are potentially at risk of a concussive event.

Pathophysiology

The American Medical Society for Sports Medicine (AMSSM) defines concussion, also termed mild traumatic brain injury (mTBI), as a "traumatically induced transient disturbance of brain function, caused by a complex pathophysiological process."[161] They are a less severe form of brain injury and are generally self-limited in duration and symptom resolution. Concussions are caused by a direct blow either to the head, face, neck, or elsewhere on the body, resulting in excessive linear and rotational forces transmitted to the brain. "Coup" injuries define the injuries when a stationary skull is hit by a moving object at high velocity (head being struck by a baseball). Conversely, "countercoup" injuries result from the sudden deceleration of the skull moving at a high velocity (head contacting the ground/floor or goalpost).

When the brain sustains a concussion, microscopic axonal injury occurs in conjunction with a complex cascade of ionic, metabolic, and pathophysiologic events.[161] In order to regain ionic balance and normal brain metabolism, the brain requires increased energy. However, damage to mitochondria and a decrease in cerebral brain flow contribute to a shortage of energy, and results in decreased overall brain function.[161] If, during this time of decreased function prior to full recovery, there is a second injury, the brain is at even greater risk for cellular metabolic changes and significant cognitive defects. This finding is more pronounced in youth where the immature brain is still developing, thereby placing this population at a greater risk of repeat concussion prior to complete symptom recovery.[161]

Signs and Symptoms

Signs and symptoms of concussion often vary with the individual (Table 14.6). Headache is the most common sign of

TABLE 14.6 Concussion Signs and Symptoms		
Physical	**Cognitive**	**Emotional**
Headache	Mentally "foggy"	Irritable
Fatigue, nausea, vomiting	Got "bell rung"	Sadness
Dizziness, balance disturbance	Feeling run down	More emotional
Visual problems	Difficulty concentrating	Nervousness
Sensitivity to light, noise	Impaired memory	
Numbness, tingling	Confusion	
Drowsiness	Slowed responses	
Sleep disturbances	Loss of consciousness	

concussion, followed by dizziness.[161] Loss of consciousness occurs in 10% of concussions, but is not a reliable predictor of severity. Most symptoms are not specific to concussion and may mimic other conditions, including but not limited to cardiac compromise, acute gastroenteritis, attention deficit disorder, and depression. Therefore, it is helpful to determine whether the symptoms were present prior to the concussion injury to allow for more accurate determination of symptom resolution. In 80% to 90% of concussions, symptoms resolve within 7 days following injury.[161] Despite the resolution of subjective concussive symptoms, complete cognitive impairment may still exist with further neuropsychological testing.

Risk Factors

History of previous concussion puts an athlete at a two to five times greater risk of sustaining another concussion.[161] The more concussions sustained, the greater the severity of the concussion, and duration of symptoms are all predictors of prolonged recovery. In sports with similar rules, females are at greater risk of concussion than their male counterparts. The type of sport and position is also correlated with an increased risk. For example, athletes who are in frequent high-velocity-contact situations, such as football quarterbacks, running backs, wide receivers, and defensive backs, are at greater risk of injury than other position players such as linemen. History of migraine headaches, learning disabilities, attention deficit disorders, and mood disorders may be associated with increased cognitive dysfunction and a prolonged recovery following a concussion, and could potentially complicate diagnosis and management.[161]

Physiologic differences exist between the adult and the youth brain. When dealing with the immature brain, it is important to understand their inherent increased risk of sustaining a concussion in combination with a catastrophic injury and associated prolonged recovery times. For instance, one study reported that athletes 13 to 16 years of age take longer to return to their baseline levels of

symptoms and normal neurocognitive function compared with athletes 18 to 22 years old.[160]

Diagnosis and Assessment

A health care provider specially trained and knowledgeable in recognition and evaluation of concussions is best qualified to make the clinical diagnosis. Concussions are graded retrospectively following symptoms resolution. Therefore, grading a concussion at the time of injury is considered unreliable and is no longer performed. Diagnosis should include thorough neurologic, balance, and cognitive assessments. A graded checklist should serve as an objective assessment tool for assessing the symptoms associated with a concussion, while also tracking the severity, longevity, and changes over serial reevaluations. Other assessment tools include baseline symptom scoring, balance testing, sideline evaluation tools, and computerized neurophysiologic (NP) testing. Some commonly used sideline measures include symptom scores, Maddocks Questions, Standardized Assessment of Concussion (SAC), and the Balance Error Scoring System (BESS).[161] It is important to understand that certain tests are more appropriate at different times during the recovery time period. Balance testing is typically normal after 3 days, making it a useful test for sideline management of an athlete, and less useful for later follow-up. Baseline testing prior to sports participation may aid in the identification of high-risk individuals and allow for comparison purposes following injury. This approach is somewhat controversial as the role of preinjury baseline testing remains unclear and has yet to be validated.[161] However, baseline testing may be most beneficial in those with prior history of concussion, confounding medical conditions, and high-risk sports. Testing should be performed routinely with attempts to control certain variables, including the athlete's age, fatigue level, mood, and testing environment, among other factors.

Neurophysiologic Testing

NP testing in athletes began in the 1980s, and its role has increased in recent years with the availability of computers. NP tests are objective measures of brain behavior, and are more sensitive than clinical exam for subtle cognitive impairment. However, NP testing should be an adjunct to clinical assessment and as one component of a comprehensive concussion management plan, and not in isolation. NP testing will evaluate several domains of cognitive function such as memory, cognitive processing speed, and reaction time.[161,162] There are two commonly utilized testing: paper and pencil and computerized. Owing to the ease of administration and cost-effectiveness, there has been a shift toward the use of computerized testing.

NP testing has been shown to have moderate sensitivity in the detection of post-concussive cognitive deficits,[163] and is still recommended and used in high-risk athletes with and without prior concussion. NP tests aid in the return-to-sport decision-making process, especially for athletes who deny symptoms with the desire to return to activity sooner than otherwise likely. However, the validity of the tool has yet to be determined as it shows cognitive deficits longer than athletes are symptomatic, and should be a monitoring tool in the event of a concussion.[161]

Management and Return to Play

The first step in the management of concussion will usually occur at the time of injury. The level of consciousness should be assessed. In an unresponsive athlete, assessment of airway, breathing, and heart function is of primary concern. Once established, physical evaluation of the cervical spine and other more serious injuries should be performed. In the event of even remote suspicion of cervical spine injury, the athlete should be immobilized and transferred to the emergency department for advanced imaging and care. Other reasons for immediate emergency transport include deteriorating mental status, focal neurologic findings, and worsening of symptoms. Only when serious cognitive and emergent medical situations are excluded can secondary concussion examination including symptoms, cognition, and balance be initiated.

If sideline testing appears normal and concussion is not suspected, the athlete is permitted to resume playing. Serial evaluations should be performed during and following the event to ensure the decision was correct. When concussion is suspected, the athlete should not return to play on that day. The athlete should be monitored incrementally over a period of time, recognizing deterioration of mental status, cognition, and/or consciousness. It was previously recommended to frequently wake up the concussed athlete throughout the night to ensure consciousness. However, this is no longer recommended as sleep is important in allowing the brain to rest and recover.[161] Because of the theoretical risk of bleeding, aspirin and NSAIDs are generally avoided. Other medications that mask symptoms should also be avoided.

Athletes with concussion should have a medical follow-up by a physician. The primary treatment includes physical and cognitive rest. Activities and environments that exacerbate symptoms should be avoided and moderated. Dim, quiet environments assist in moderating headache and symptoms of phonophobia and photophobia. Youth athletes will require accommodations in school, including a reduced workload and extended time to take tests. In most cases, the athlete should be permitted to miss school or only attend part of the day.

Return-to-play progression should be individualized, gradual, and progressive. The process should begin once the athlete is free of symptoms at rest and demonstrates a normal neurologic exam when compared with baseline measures, including balance and cognitive function. Only then should the athlete begin a medically supervised stepwise return (Display 14.8). The progression may take a few

DISPLAY 14.8	Activity Progression Following Concussion

Stepwise Return-to-play Protocol

Activity Level	Examples
No activity/rest	Dim environments, school accommodations, no television or radio
Light aerobic activity	Stationary bike, elliptical trainer, brisk walking
Sport-specific exercise	Shoot baskets, swinging a bat, running, submaximal resistance training
Noncontact training drills	Practice drills, complex sports movements
Full contact drills/practice	Incorporate live play and/or contact drills in practice
Return to play	Scrimmages followed by games

days to a few weeks to complete depending on the severity of concussion and individualized response to physical demands. If the athlete develops symptoms at any point during the progression, the aggravating activity should be stopped, symptoms allowed to subside, and eventually resume the previous phase of the progression. A licensed health care provider specifically trained in the management of concussions should be consulted for medical clearance prior to unrestricted activity.

Special Considerations

Second Impact Syndrome

A young athlete who returns to play while experiencing symptoms is at risk for persistent symptoms, more severe concussion, cerebral swelling, and second impact syndrome (SIS). SIS is the loss of autoregulation of the brain's blood supply leading to vascular enlargement, increase in intracranial pressure, brain herniation, and subsequent coma and/or death.[161] SIS is not fully understood; however, it is seen typically in those under the age of 18. Therefore, management of concussion in the youth athlete should be done carefully with the assurance that symptoms have resolved and all brain function has returned to baseline prior to permitting the athlete to return to play.

Postconcussion Syndrome

Postconcussion syndrome is defined as the signs and symptoms of a concussion that persist for longer than the expected time frame, such as weeks or months. Symptoms are similar to those initially following concussion, but are often more vague and nonspecific, making the diagnosis complicated. Factors associated with an increased likelihood of postconcussion syndrome are not fully clear; however, compared with other forms of concussion, sports-related concussions are less likely to result in the condition.

Rest is the paramount treatment for postconcussion syndrome. As time progresses and symptoms continue, other multifactorial treatment options may be explored. These include cognitive therapy, integrated neurorehabilitation programs, supervised progressive exercise programs, and sleep disturbance programs. A physical therapist's role may involve overseeing the progressive exercise program, including having the athlete exercise until the onset of symptoms, followed by exercising at 80% of that symptom threshold every other day. Retesting of the threshold should be performed on a regular basis with progression being a slow and steady process, symptom permitting.

Prevention

Education and awareness are the hallmarks of concussion prevention. Modification and enforcement of rules in place to reduce the risk of concussion should be strictly followed. Fair play and respect for opposing players and coaches have been shown to decrease the likelihood of concussion in sports such as hockey.[161] Coaches, parents, educators, and referees should be educated on the signs and symptoms of a concussion to allow for better detection and injury assessment. They can also assist in the safety of the youth athlete by teaching correct sport-specific techniques, emphasizing body control and proper movements, education on appropriate athletic behaviors, and limiting the number of contact exposures in practice.

Proper protective equipment should be worn at all times during competition, and athletes should be monitored for correct size and fit. This includes helmets, shoulder pads, and mouthpieces. Despite the lack of data to suggest that the use of these pieces of equipment can minimize the risk of concussion and mTBI, they have been found to be an effective means of limiting scalp lacerations, skull fractures, intracranial bleeds, and dental injuries.[161]

Strengthening of neck musculature has been studied to determine its effectiveness on concussion prevalence. Some believed that increased strength of neck musculature could enable an athlete to better attenuate the acceleration forces associated with a forceful blow to the head. However, because of the unpredictable nature of a sports concussion, no association between neck muscle strength and concussion has been identified.[161]

▶ The female athlete

Special Considerations

As a female athlete progresses through sexual maturity, physiologic and anatomic changes occur, which leave her vulnerable to injury. Earlier in this chapter, we noted that female adolescent athletes are two to nine times more likely to suffer a noncontact ACL tear than their male counterparts.[91]

In addition, female athletes are more likely to suffer other knee pathologies such as patellofemoral syndrome or patella dislocations. A wider pelvis, increased femoral anteversion, increased ligamentous laxity, increased knee valgus postioning, and altered neuromuscular firing patterns have all been implicated as factors related to the increased incidence of knee injuries in females. Measurements of dynamic knee valgus during a jumping task have been shown to be predictive of knee injuries.[12] Neuromuscular retraining programs that focus on reducing dynamic knee valgus, improving knee flexion during landing, and lessening ground impact forces have been effective at reducing this injury risk.[94] The clinician should focus on identifying any female athletes exhibiting the noted biomechanically risky movement patterns and provide instruction and training to help lessen the possibility of injury.

Female Athlete Triad

The female athlete triad refers to a constellation of three clinical entities: menstrual dysfunction, low energy availability from diminished caloric intake (with or without an eating disorder), and decreased bone mineral density.[164] Prevelance rates for individual factors involved in the triad vary widely in the athletic population, but studies have shown that 23% to 70% of female athletes can be affected.[164] There is generally a higher rate of presence in sports that require weight classes and those that emphasize aesthetics such as ballet and gymnastics. It is important to note that a female athlete need not demonstrate all three factors of the triad in order to suffer negative health sequelae.

Menstrual dysfunction in the athlete includes a wide spectrum of disorders, but amenorrhea is the most commonly discussed. Amennorrhea, defined as the absence of menses for 3 months or more, can be subcategorized into primary or secondary types. Primary refers to a delay in the age of onset of menarche, while secondary refers to a loss of menses after menarche inception. Delayed or altered menarche can lead to decreased bone density associated with the female athlete triad. Normally, the greatest accumulation of bone mass occurs during the adolescent years, but compromised bone development during this period can have severe consequences. In the short term, low bone density places the athlete at an increased risk for stress fractures, while long-term consequences can include suboptimal peak bone mass acquisition and higher risk of premature osteoporosis.[164]

Energy availability refers to the amount of dietary intake required in order to support the needs of an athlete's caloric expenditure. Low energy availability may result from a diagnosed eating disorder such as anorexia nervosa, bulimia nervosa, or eating disorder not otherwise specified (EDNOS).[164] However, low energy availability can also occur without a diagnosed disorder in cases where the caloric deficit is a result of poor dietary choices or lack of nutritional knowledge. The adverse effects of disordered eating can include

TABLE	
14.7 Female Athlete Triad	

Signs and Symptoms of Female Athlete Triad	Signs and Symptoms of Disordered Eating
Weight loss	Continued dieting in spite of weight loss
Absent or irregular periods	Preoccupation with food, weight, and/or exercise
Fatigue and decreased ability to concentrate	Frequent trips to the bathroom during and after meals
Stress fractures with or without significant injury	Use of laxatives
Longer healing times	Always wearing baggy clothing
Muscle injuries	Brittle hair or nails
	Cold hands and feet
	Dental cavities and eroding tooth enamel due to frequent vomiting
	Heart irregularities and chest pain
	Low heart rate and blood pressure

cardiac dysfunction, gastrointestinal problems, hair loss, decreased sports performance, and decreased concentration.

Treatment of the female athlete triad involves a multidisciplinary team approach consisting of a physician, nutritionist, psychiatrist, team coach, and the athlete's family. A physical therapist or athletic trainer may become part of the treatment team for resolving impairments to help the athlete make a return to sports. The primary goals of treatment are to restore normal menstrual cycle, enhance bone mineral density, and improve psychological health related to body image and sports performance.

Prevention of the female athlete triad should be of paramount importance. Early recognition of the female athlete triad allows for early intervention and limits the resulting damage. Screening for symptoms during regular sports preparticipation physicals is an excellent opportunity for early recognition and should be encouraged. Furthermore, the education of coaches, players, and families in recognizing the signs and risk factors may lead to increased reporting of issues and early treatment (Table 14.7).

SUMMARY

Developing good exercise habits earlier in life establishes healthier lifestyles throughout adulthood. There has been a dramatic increase in youth recreational and competitive sports participation over recent years. The choices are endless for most children, with gymnastics, dancing, swimming, field sports, running, skateboarding, rock climbing, riding a bike, and jumping rope all acting as modes of physical activity. Sports can provide children with psychological, social, and physical benefits; however, it can also heighten the inherent risk of sustaining an injury. Increased exposures, improper training methods, and early sports specialization have all been attributed to athletic injuries in the youth.

Proper prevention strategies and education of parents, coaches, and health care providers will allow children and adolescents to participate in sports and recreational activities in a safer and more enjoyable fashion.

Youth athletes will participate in sports similar to their adult counterparts, but anatomic, physiologic, and psychological differences exist between adults and children. Despite the similar nature of the sporting events, it is important to understand that skeletally immature athletes are vulnerable to sustain different kinds of musculoskeletal injuries. The physical therapist working with these children must take these differences into account during rehabilitation of the youth athlete. Awareness of the special needs of the youth athlete will allow a health care provider to diagnose and administer appropriate medical care, increasing the likelihood of a safe return to full and unrestricted sports participation following injury.

REFERENCES

1. Mickalide A, Hansen L. *Coaching Our Kids to Fewer Injuries: A Report on Youth Sports Safety.* Washington, DC: Safe Kids World Wide; 2012.
2. Musgrave DS, Mendelson SA. Pediatric orthopedic trauma: principles in management. *Crit Care Med.* 2002;30(11)(suppl):S431–S443.
3. Hoang QB, Mortazavi M. Pediatric overuse injuries in sports. *Adv Pediatr.* 2012;59(1):359–383.
4. Caine D, Maffulli N, Caine C. Epidemiology of injury in child and adolescent sports: injury rates, risk factors, and prevention. *Clin Sports Med.* 2008;27(1):19–50, vii.
5. Wall E, Von Stein D. Juvenile osteochondritis dissecans. *Orthop Clin North Am.* 2003;34(3):341–353.
6. Baker CL 3rd, Romeo AA, Baker CL, Jr. Osteochondritis dissecans of the capitellum. *Am J Sports Med.* 2010;38(9):1917–1928.
7. Ray TR. Youth baseball injuries: recognition, treatment, and prevention. *Curr Sports Med Rep.* 2010;9(5):294–298.
8. Kocher MS, Tucker R, Ganley TJ, et al. Management of osteochondritis dissecans of the knee: current concepts review. *Am J Sports Med.* 2006;34(7):1181–1191.
9. Ozmun JC, Mikesky AE, Surburg PR. Neuromuscular adaptations following prepubescent strength training. *Med Sci Sports Exerc.* 1994;26(4):510–514.
10. Carter CW, Micheli LJ. Training the child athlete for prevention, health promotion, and performance: how much is enough, how much is too much? *Clin Sports Med.* 2011;30(4):679–690.
11. Boyle KL, Witt P, Riegger-Krugh C. Intrarater and Interrater reliability of the Beighton and Horan joint mobility index. *J Athl Train.* 2003;38(4):281–285.
12. Hewett TE, Myer GD, Ford KR, et al. Biomechanical measures of neuromuscular control and valgus loading of the knee predict anterior cruciate ligament injury risk in female athletes: a prospective study. *Am J Sports Med.* 2005;33(4):492–501.
13. Powers CM. The influence of altered lower-extremity kinematics on patellofemoral joint dysfunction: a theoretical perspective. *J Orthop Sports Phys Ther.* 2003;33(11):639–646.
14. Chmielewski TL, Hodges MJ, Horodyski M, et al. Investigation of clinician agreement in evaluating movement quality during unilateral lower extremity functional tasks: a comparison of 2 rating methods. *J Orthop Sports Phys Ther.* 2007;37(3):122–129.
15. Myer GD, Ford KR, Khoury J, et al. Development and validation of a clinic-based prediction tool to identify female athletes at high risk for anterior cruciate ligament injury. *Am J Sports Med.* 2010;38(10):2025–2033.
16. Roush JR, Kitamura J, Waits MC. Reference values for the Closed Kinetic Chain Upper Extremity Stability Test (CKCUEST) for collegiate baseball players. *N Am J Sports Phys Ther.* 2007;2(3):159–163.

17. McClure P, Greenberg E, Kareha S. Evaluation and management of scapular dysfunction. *Sports Med Arthrosc.* 2012;20(1):39–48.

18. Ludewig PM, Reynolds JF. The association of scapular kinematics and glenohumeral joint pathologies. *J Orthop Sports Phys Ther.* 2009;39(2):90–104.

19. Kibler WB, Uhl TL, Maddux JW, et al. Qualitative clinical evaluation of scapular dysfunction: a reliability study. *J Shoulder Elbow Surg.* 2002;11(6):550–556.

20. McClure P, Tate AR, Kareha S, et al. A clinical method for identifying scapular dyskinesis. part 1: reliability. *J Athl Train.* 2009;44(2):160–164.

21. Uhl TL, Kibler WB, Gecewich B, et al. Evaluation of clinical assessment methods for scapular dyskinesis. *Arthroscopy.* 2009;25(11):1240–1248.

22. Wainner RS, Whitman JM, Cleland JA, et al. Regional interdependence: a musculoskeletal examination model whose time has come. *J Orthop Sports Phys Ther.* 2007;37(11):658–660.

23. Axe M, Hurd W, Snyder-Mackler L. Data-based interval throwing programs for baseball players. *Sports Health.* 2009;1(2):145–153.

24. Wasserlauf BL, Paletta GA Jr. Shoulder disorders in the skeletally immature throwing athlete. *Orthop Clin North Am.* 2003;34(3):427–437.

25. Knesek M, Skendzel JG, Dines JS, et al. Diagnosis and management of superior Labral Anterior Posterior tears in throwing athletes. *Am J Sports Med.* 2012.

26. Greiwe RM, Saifi C, Ahmad CS. Pediatric sports elbow injuries. *Clin Sports Med.* 2010;29(4):677–703.

27. Fortenbaugh D, Fleisig GS, Andrews JR. Baseball pitching biomechanics in relation to injury risk and performance. *Sports Health.* 2009;1(4):314–320.

28. Kramer DE. Elbow pain and injury in young athletes. *J Pediatr Orthop.* 2010;30(2):S7–S12.

29. Fleisig GS, Weber A, Hassell N, et al. Prevention of elbow injuries in youth baseball pitchers. *Curr Sports Med Rep.* 2009;8(5):250–254.

30. Fleisig GS, Andrews JR. Prevention of elbow injuries in youth baseball pitchers. *Sports Health.* 2012;4(5):419–424.

31. Petty DH, Andrews JR, Fleisig GS, et al. Ulnar collateral ligament reconstruction in high school baseball players: clinical results and injury risk factors. *Am J Sports Med.* 2004;32(5):1158–1164.

32. Guerrero P, Busconi B, Deangelis N, et al. Congenital instability of the shoulder joint: assessment and treatment options. *J Orthop Sports Phys Ther.* 2009;39(2):124–134.

33. Dumont GD, Russell RD, Robertson WJ. Anterior shoulder instability: a review of pathoanatomy, diagnosis and treatment. *Curr Rev Musculoskelet Med.* 2011;4(4):200–207.

34. Shah RR, Kinder J, Peelman J, et al. Pediatric clavicle and acromioclavicular injuries. *J Ped Orthop.* 2010;30:S69–S72 10.1097/BPO.1090b1013 e3181ba1099e1094.

35. Caird MS. Clavicle shaft fractures: are children little adults? *J Pediatr Orthop.* 2012;32(suppl 1):S1–S4.

36. Pandya NK, Namdari S, Hosalkar HS. Displaced clavicle fractures in adolescents: facts, controversies, and current trends. *J Am Acad Orthop Surg.* 2012;20(8):498–505.

37. Howard A, Mulpuri K, Abel MF, et al. The treatment of pediatric supracondylar humerus fractures. *J Am Acad Orthop Surg.* 2012;20(5):320–327.

38. Spencer HT, Wong M, Fong YJ, et al. Prospective longitudinal evaluation of elbow motion following pediatric supracondylar humeral fractures. *J Bone Joint Surg Am.* 2010;92(4):904–910.

39. Song KS, Waters PM. Lateral condylar humerus fractures: which ones should we fix? *J Pediatr Orthop.* 2012;32(suppl 1):S5–S9.

40. Leonidou A, Pagkalos J, Lepetsos P, et al. Pediatric monteggia fractures: a single-center study of the management of 40 patients. *J Pediatr Orthop.* 2012;32(4):352–356.

41. Weiss JM, Mencio GA. Forearm shaft fractures: does fixation improve outcomes? *J Pediatr Orthop.* 2012;32(suppl 1):S22–S24.

42. Stutz C, Mencio GA. Fractures of the distal radius and ulna: metaphyseal and physeal injuries. *J Ped Orthop.* 2010;30:S85–S89. 10.1097/BPO.1090b1013e3181c1099c1017a.

43. van Bosse HJ, Patel RJ, Thacker M, et al. Minimalistic approach to treating wrist torus fractures. *J Pediatr Orthop.* 2005;25(4):495–500.

44. DiFiori JP, Caine DJ, Malina RM. Wrist pain, distal radial physeal injury, and ulnar variance in the young gymnast. *Am J Sports Med.* 2006;34(5):840–849.

45. Elhassan BT, Shin AY. Scaphoid fracture in children. *Hand Clin.* 2006;22(1):31–41.

46. Evenski AJ, Adamczyk MJ, Steiner RP, et al. Clinically suspected scaphoid fractures in children. *J Pediatr Orthop.* 2009;29(4):352–355.

47. Prosser R, Herbert T. The management of carpal fractures and dislocations. *J Hand Ther.* 1996;9(2):139–147.

48. Haughton D, Jordan D, Malahias M, et al. Principles of hand fracture management. *Open Orthop J.* 2012;6:43–53.

49. Cornwall R. Pediatric finger fractures: which ones turn ugly? *J Pediatr Orthop.* 2012;32(suppl 1):S25–S31.

50. Patel DR, Lyne ED. Overuse injuries of the hip, pelvis and thigh. In: Patel DR, Greydanus DE, Baker RJ, eds. *Pediatric Practice Sports Medicine.* New York, NY: The McGraw-Hill Companies; 2009.

51. Soprano JV, Fuchs SM. Common overuse injuries in the pediatric and adolescent athlete. *Clin Pediatr Emergency Med.* 2007;8(1):7–14.

52. Porr J, Lucaciu C, Birkett S. Avulsion fractures of the pelvis—a qualitative systematic review of the literature. *J Can Chiropr Assoc.* 2011;55(4):247–255.

53. Anderson K, Strickland SM, Warren R. Hip and groin injuries in athletes. *Am J Sports Med.* 2001;29(4):521–533.

54. Ilizaliturri VM Jr, Camacho-Galindo J, Evia Ramirez AN, et al. Soft tissue pathology around the hip. *Clin Sports Med.* 2011;30(2):391–415.

55. Provencher MT, Hofmeister EP, Muldoon MP. The surgical treatment of external coxa saltans (the snapping hip) by Z-plasty of the iliotibial band. *Am J Sports Med.* 2004;32(2):470–476.

56. Byrd JWT. Snapping hip. *Oper Tech Sports Med.* 2005;13(1):46–54.

57. Allen WC, Cope R. Coxa saltans: the snapping hip revisited. *J Am Acad Orthop Surg.* 1995;3(5):303–308.

58. Cardinal E, Buckwalter KA, Capello WN, et al. US of the snapping iliopsoas tendon. *Radiology.* 1996;198(2):521–522.

59. Byrd JWT. Evaluation and management of the snapping Iliopsoas tendon. *Tech Orthopaedic.* 2005;20(1):45–51.

60. Taylor GR, Clarke NM. Surgical release of the 'snapping iliopsoas tendon'. *J Bone Joint Surg Br.* 1995;77(6):881–883.

61. Brunet ME, Cook SD, Brinker MR, et al. A survey of running injuries in 1505 competitive and recreational runners. *J Sports Med Phys Fitness.* 1990;30(3):307–315.

62. Lassus J, Tulikoura I, Konttinen YT, et al. Bone stress injuries of the lower extremity: a review. *Acta Orthop Scand.* 2002;73(3):359–368.

63. Bennell K, Matheson G, Meeuwisse W, et al. Risk factors for stress fractures. *Sports Med.* 1999;28(2):91–122.

64. Goolsby MA, Barrack MT, Nattiv A. A displaced femoral neck stress fracture in an amenorrheic adolescent female runner. *Sports Health.* 2012;4(4):352–356.

65. Fraitzl CR, Kafer W, Nelitz M, et al. Radiological evidence of femoroacetabular impingement in mild slipped capital femoral epiphysis: a mean follow-up of 14. 4 years after pinning in situ. *J Bone Joint Surg Br.* 2007;89(12):1592–1596.

66. Imam S, Khanduja V. Current concepts in the diagnosis and management of femoroacetabular impingement. *Int Orthop.* 2011;35(10):1427–1435.

67. Philippon MJ, Stubbs AJ, Schenker ML, et al. Arthroscopic management of femoroacetabular impingement: osteoplasty technique and literature review. *Am J Sports Med.* 2007;35(9):1571–1580.

68. Huffman GR, Safran M. Tears of the acetabular labrum in athletes: diagnosis and treatment. *Sports Med Arthroscopy Rev.* 2002;10(2):141–150.

69. Crawford JR, Villar RN. Current concepts in the management of femoroacetabular impingement. *J Bone Joint Surg Br.* 2005;87(11):1459–1462.

70. Ito K, Minka MA II, Leunig M, et al. Femoroacetabular impingement and the cam-effect. A MRI-based quantitative anatomical study of the femoral head-neck offset. *J Bone Joint Surg Br.* 2001;83(2):171–176.

71. Ferguson TA, Matta J. Anterior femoroacetabular impingement: a clinical presentation. *Sports Med Arthroscopy Rev.* 2002;10(2):134–140.

72. Czerny C, Hofmann S, Neuhold A, et al. Lesions of the acetabular labrum: accuracy of MR imaging and MR arthrography in detection and staging. *Radiology.* 1996;200(1):225–230.

73. Samora JB, Ng VY, Ellis TJ. Femoroacetabular impingement: a common cause of hip pain in young adults. *Clin J Sport Med.* 2011;21(1):51–56.

74. Groh MM, Herrera J. A comprehensive review of hip labral tears. *Curr Rev Musculoskelet Med.* 2009;2(2):105–117.

75. Heiderscheit BC, Sherry MA, Silder A, et al. Hamstring strain injuries: recommendations for diagnosis, rehabilitation, and injury prevention. *J Orthop Sports Phys Ther.* 2010;40(2):67–81.

76. Koulouris G, Connell DA, Brukner P, Schneider-Kolsky M. Magnetic resonance imaging parameters for assessing risk of recurrent hamstring injuries in elite athletes. *Am J Sports Med.* 2007;35(9):1500–1506.

77. Cline S. Acute Injuries of the hip, pelvis and thigh. In: Patel DR, Greydanus DE, Baker RJ, eds. *Pediatric Practice Sports Medicine.* New York, NY: The McGraw-Hill Companies; 2009.

78. Wells D, King JD, Roe TF, et al. Review of slipped capital femoral epiphysis associated with endocrine disease. *J Pediatr Orthop.* 1993;13(5):610–614.

79. Kocher MS, Tucker R. Pediatric athlete hip disorders. *Clin Sports Med.* 2006;25(2):241–253, viii.

80. Riad J, Bajelidze G, Gabos PG. Bilateral slipped capital femoral epiphysis: predictive factors for contralateral slip. *J Pediatr Orthop.* 2007;27(4):411–414.

81. Uglow MG, Clarke NM. The management of slipped capital femoral epiphysis. *J Bone Joint Surg Br.* 2004;86(5):631–635.

82. Hinton RY, Sharma KM. Anterior cruciate ligament injuries. In: Micheli LJ, Kocher MS, eds. *The Pediatric and Adolescent Knee.* Philadelphia, PA: Saunders Elsevier; 2006.

83. Anderson CN, Anderson AF. Tibial eminence fractures. *Clin Sports Med.* 2011;30(4):727–742.

84. Moksnes H, Engebretsen L, Risberg MA. Management of anterior cruciate ligament injuries in skeletally immature individuals. *J Orthop Sports Phys Ther.* 2012;42(3):172–183.

85. Lawrence JT, Argawal N, Ganley TJ. Degeneration of the knee joint in skeletally immature patients with a diagnosis of an anterior cruciate ligament tear: is there harm in delay of treatment? *Am J Sports Med.* 2011;39(12):2582–2587.

86. Wojtys EM, Brower AM. Anterior cruciate ligament injuries in the prepubescent and adolescent athlete: clinical and research considerations. *J Athl Train.* 2010;45(5):509–512.

87. Milewski MD, Beck NA, Lawrence JT, et al. Anterior cruciate ligament reconstruction in the young athlete: a treatment algorithm for the skeletally immature. *Clin Sports Med.* 2011;30(4):801–810.

88. Vavken P, Murray MM. Treating anterior cruciate ligament tears in skeletally immature patients. *Arthroscopy.* 2011;27(5):704–716.

89. Kim KM, Croy T, Hertel J, et al. Effects of neuromuscular electrical stimulation after anterior cruciate ligament reconstruction on quadriceps strength, function, and patient-oriented outcomes: a systematic review. *J Orthop Sports Phys Ther.* 2010;40(7):383–391.

90. Greenberg EM, Albaugh J, Ganley TJ, et al. Rehabilitation considerations for all epiphyseal acl reconstruction. *Int J Sports Phys Ther.* 2012;7(2):185–196.

91. Logerstedt DS, Snyder-Mackler L, Ritter RC, et al. Knee stability and movement coordination impairments: knee ligament sprain. *J Orthop Sports Phys Ther.* 2010;40(4):A1–A37.

92. Noyes FR, Barber SD, Mangine RE. Abnormal lower limb symmetry determined by function hop tests after anterior cruciate ligament rupture. *Am J Sports Med.* 1991;19(5):513–518.

93. Myer GD, Chu DA, Brent JL, et al. Trunk and hip control neuromuscular training for the prevention of knee joint injury. *Clin Sports Med.* 2008;27(3):425–448, ix.

94. Hewett TE, Ford KR, Myer GD. Anterior cruciate ligament injuries in female athletes: part 2, a meta-analysis of neuromuscular interventions aimed at injury prevention. *Am J Sports Med.* 2006;34(3):490–498.

95. DiStefano LJ, Blackburn JT, Marshall SW, et al. Effects of an age-specific anterior cruciate ligament injury prevention program on lower extremity biomechanics in children. *Am J Sports Med.* 2011;39(5):949–957.

96. Mandelbaum BR, Silvers HJ, Watanabe DS, et al. Effectiveness of a neuromuscular and proprioceptive training program in preventing anterior cruciate ligament injuries in female athletes: 2-year follow-up. *Am J Sports Med.* 2005;33(7):1003–1010.

97. Hewett TE, Myer GD, Ford KR, et al. The 2012 ABJS Nicolas Andry Award: the sequence of prevention: a systematic approach to prevent anterior cruciate ligament injury. *Clin Orthop Relat Res.* 2012;470(10):2930–2940.

98. Shea KG, Apel PJ, Pfeiffer R. Injury of the medial collateral ligament, posterior cruciate ligament, and posterolateral complex in skeletally immature patients. In: Micheli LJ, Kocher MS, eds. *The Pediatric and Adolescent Knee.* Philadelphia, PA: Saunders Elsevier; 2006.

99. Miyamoto RG, Bosco JA, Sherman OH. Treatment of medial collateral ligament injuries. *J Am Acad Orthop Surg.* 2009;17(3):152–161.

100. Derscheid GL, Garrick JG. Medial collateral ligament injuries in football. Nonoperative management of grade I and grade II sprains. *Am J Sports Med.* 1981;9(6):365–368.

101. Indelicato PA, Hermansdorfer J, Huegel M. Nonoperative management of complete tears of the medial collateral ligament of the knee in intercollegiate football players. *Clin Orthop Relat Res.* 1990(256):174–177.

102. McAllister DR, Petrigliano FA. Diagnosis and treatment of posterior cruciate ligament injuries. *Curr Sports Med Rep.* 2007;6(5):293–299.

103. Kramer DE, Micheli LJ. Meniscal tears and discoid meniscus in children: diagnosis and treatment. *J Am Acad Orthop Surg.* 2009;17(11):698–707.

104. Stanitski CL. Discoid meniscus. In: Micheli LJ, Kocher MS, eds. *The Pediatric and Adolescent Knee.* Philadelphia, PA: Saunders Elsevier; 2006.

105. Jordan MR. Lateral meniscal variants: evaluation and treatment. *J Am Acad Orthop Surg.* 1996;4(4):191–200.

106. Konan S, Rayan F, Haddad FS. Do physical diagnostic tests accurately detect meniscal tears? *Knee Surg Sports Traumatol Arthrosc.* 2009;17(7):806–811.

107. Conrad JM, Stanitski CL. Osteochondritis dissecans: Wilson's sign revisited. *Am J Sports Med.* 2003;31(5):777–778.

108. Ganley TJ, Flynn JM. Osteochondritis dissecans of the knee. In: Micheli LJ, Kocher MS, eds. *The Pediatric and Adolescent Knee.* Philadelphia, PA: Saunders Elsevier; 2006.

109. Pascual-Garrido C, Moran CJ, Green DW, et al. Osteochondritis dissecans of the knee in children and adolescents. *Curr Opin Pediatr.* 2013;25(1):46–51.

110. Buckens CF, Saris DB. Reconstruction of the medial patellofemoral ligament for treatment of patellofemoral instability: a systematic review. *Am J Sports Med.* 2010;38(1):181–188.

111. Kramer DE, Pace JL. Acute traumatic and sports-related osteochondral injury of the pediatric knee. *Orthop Clin North Am.* 2012;43(2):227–236, vi.

112. Lewis PB, McCarty LP 3rd, Kang RW, et al. Basic science and treatment options for articular cartilage injuries. *J Orthop Sports Phys Ther.* 2006;36(10):717–727.

113. Davis IS, Powers CM. Patellofemoral pain syndrome: proximal, distal, and local factors, an international retreat, April 30-May 2, 2009, Fells Point, Baltimore, MD. *J Orthop Sports Phys Ther.* 2010;40(3):A1–A16.

114. Robinson RL, Nee RJ. Analysis of hip strength in females seeking physical therapy treatment for unilateral patellofemoral pain syndrome. *J Orthop Sports Phys Ther.* 2007;37(5):232–238.

115. Dierks TA, Manal KT, Hamill J, et al. Proximal and distal influences on hip and knee kinematics in runners with patellofemoral pain during a prolonged run. *J Orthop Sports Phys Ther.* 2008;38(8):448–456.

116. Barton CJ, Bonanno D, Levinger P, et al. Foot and ankle characteristics in patellofemoral pain syndrome: a case control and reliability study. *J Orthop Sports Phys Ther.* 2010;40(5):286–296.

117. Bolgla LA, Boling MC. An update for the conservative management of patellofemoral pain syndrome: a systematic review of the literature from 2000 to 2010. *Int J Sports Phys Ther.* Jun 2011;6(2):112–125.

118. Peers KH, Lysens RJ. Patellar tendinopathy in athletes: current diagnostic and therapeutic recommendations. *Sports Med.* 2005;35(1):71–87.

119. Larsson ME, Kall I, Nilsson-Helander K. Treatment of patellar tendinopathy—a systematic review of randomized controlled trials. *Knee Surg Sports Traumatol Arthrosc.* 2012;20(8):1632–1646.

120. Witvrouw E, Bellemans J, Lysens R, et al. Intrinsic risk factors for the development of patellar tendinitis in an athletic population. A two-year prospective study. *Am J Sports Med.* 2001;29(2):190–195.

121. Bellary SS, Lynch G, Housman B, et al. Medial plica syndrome: a review of the literature. *Clin Anat.* 2012;25(4):423–428.

122. De Carlo M, Armstrong B. Rehabilitation of the knee following sports injury. *Clin Sports Med.* 2010;29(1):81–106, table of contents.

123. Moen MH, Bongers T, Bakker EW, et al. Risk factors and prognostic indicators for medial tibial stress syndrome. *Scand J Med Sci Sports.* 2012;22(1):34–39.

124. Patel DR, Lyne ED. Overuse injuries of the leg, ankle, and foot. In: Patel DR, Greydanus DE, Baker RJ, eds. *Pediatric Practice Sports Medicine.* New York, NY: The McGraw-Hill Company; 2009.

125. Beck BR. Tibial stress injuries. An aetiological review for the purposes of guiding management. *Sports Med.* 1998;26(4):265–279.

126. Crowell HP, Davis IS. Gait retraining to reduce lower extremity loading in runners. *Clin Biomech (Bristol, Avon).* 2011;26(1):78–83.

127. Lieberman DE, Venkadesan M, Werbel WA, et al. Foot strike patterns and collision forces in habitually barefoot versus shod runners. *Nature.* 2010;463(7280):531–535.

128. Heiderscheit BC, Chumanov ES, Michalski MP, et al. Effects of step rate manipulation on joint mechanics during running. *Med Sci Sports Exerc.* 2011;43(2):296–302.

129. Diebal AR, Gregory R, Alitz C, et al. Effects of forefoot running on chronic exertional compartment syndrome: a case series. *Int J Sports Phys Ther.* 2011;6(4):312–321.

130. Diebal AR, Gregory R, Alitz C, et al. Forefoot running improves pain and disability associated with chronic exertional compartment syndrome. *Am J Sports Med.* 2012;40(5):1060–1067.

131. Sharma P, Maffulli N. Tendon injury and tendinopathy: healing and repair. *J Bone Joint Surg Am.* 2005;87(1):187–202.

132. McCollum GA, van den Bekerom MP, Kerkhoffs GM, et al. Syndesmosis and deltoid ligament injuries in the athlete. *Knee Surg Sports Traumatol Arthrosc.* 2013;21(6):1328–1337.

133. Tiemstra JD. Update on acute ankle sprains. *Am Fam Physician.* 2012;85(12):1170–1176.

134. Knight AC, Weimar WH. Effects of previous lateral ankle sprain and taping on the latency of the peroneus longus. *Sports Biomech.* 2012;11(1):48–56.

135. Chambers HG. Ankle and foot disorders in skeletally immature athletes. *Orthop Clin North Am.* 2003;34(3):445–459.

136. Runyon MS. Can we safely apply the Ottawa ankle rules to children? *Acad Emerg Med.* 2009;16(4):352–354.

137. Plint AC, Bulloch B, Osmond MH, et al. Validation of the Ottawa ankle rules in children with ankle injuries. *Acad Emerg Med.* 1999;6(10):1005–1009.

138. Pontell D, Hallivis R, Dollard MD. Sports injuries in the pediatric and adolescent foot and ankle: common overuse and acute presentations. *Clin Podiatr Med Surg.* 2006;23(1):209–231, x.

139. Rowe V, Hemmings S, Barton C, et al. Conservative management of midportion Achilles tendinopathy: a mixed methods study, integrating systematic review and clinical reasoning. *Sports Med.* 2012;42(11):941–967.

140. Alfredson H, Cook J. A treatment algorithm for managing Achilles tendinopathy: new treatment options. *Br J Sports Med.* 2007;41(4):211–216.

141. Watson TS, Shurnas PS, Denker J. Treatment of Lisfranc joint injury: current concepts. *J Am Acad Orthop Surg.* 2010;18(12):718–728.

142. Mantas JP, Burks RT. Lisfranc injuries in the athlete. *Clin Sports Med.* 1994;13(4):719–730.

143. Nunley JA, Vertullo CJ. Classification, investigation, and management of midfoot sprains: lisfranc injuries in the athlete. *Am J Sports Med.* 2002;30(6):871–878.

144. Zwitser EW, Breederveld RS. Fractures of the fifth metatarsal; diagnosis and treatment. *Injury.* 2010;41(6):555–562.

145. Niemeyer P, Weinberg A, Schmitt H, et al. Stress fractures in the juvenile skeletal system. *Int J Sports Med.* 2006;27(3):242–249.

146. Hunt KJ, Anderson RB. Treatment of Jones fracture nonunions and refractures in the elite athlete: outcomes of intramedullary screw fixation with bone grafting. *Am J Sports Med.* 2011;39(9):1948–1954.

147. Murawski CD, Kennedy JG. Percutaneous internal fixation of proximal fifth metatarsal jones fractures (Zones II and III) with Charlotte Carolina screw and bone marrow aspirate concentrate: an outcome study in athletes. *Am J Sports Med.* 2011;39(6):1295–1301.

148. Micheli LJ, Wood R. Back pain in young athletes. Significant differences from adults in causes and patterns. *Arch Pediatr Adolesc Med.* 1995;149(1):15–18.

149. Rodriguez DP, Poussaint TY. Imaging of back pain in children. *AJNR Am J Neuroradiol.* 2010;31(5):787–802.

150. Purcell L, Micheli L. Low back pain in young athletes. *Sports Health.* 2009;1(3):212–222.

151. Leone A, Cianfoni A, Cerase A, et al. Lumbar spondylolysis: a review. *Skeletal Radiol.* 2011;40(6):683–700.

152. Kim HJ, Green DW. Spondylolysis in the adolescent athlete. *Curr Opin Pediatr.* 2011;23(1):68–72.

153. Yamaguchi K Jr, Skaggs D, Acevedo D, et al. Spondylolysis is frequently missed by MRI in adolescents with back pain. *J Child Orthop.* 2012;6(3):237–240.

154. Muschik M, Hahnel H, Robinson PN, et al. Competitive sports and the progression of spondylolisthesis. *J Pediatr Orthop.* 1996;16(3):364–369.

155. Sairyo K, Sakai T, Yasui N, et al. Conservative treatment for pediatric lumbar spondylolysis to achieve bone healing using a hard brace: what type and how long?: Clinical article. *J Neurosurg Spine.* 2012;16(6):610–614.

156. Sys J, Michielsen J, Bracke P, et al. Nonoperative treatment of active spondylolysis in elite athletes with normal X-ray findings: literature review and results of conservative treatment. *Eur Spine J.* 2001;10(6):498–504.

157. Weinberg J, Rokito S, Silber JS. Etiology, treatment, and prevention of athletic "stingers". *Clin Sports Med.* 2003;22(3):493–500, viii.

158. Willardson JM. Core stability training: applications to sports conditioning programs. *J Strength Cond Res.* 2007;21(3):979–985.

159. Arokoski JP, Valta T, Airaksinen O, et al. Back and abdominal muscle function during stabilization exercises. *Arch Phys Med Rehabil.* 2001;82(8):1089–1098.

160. Zuckerman SL, Lee YM, Odom MJ, et al. Recovery from sports-related concussion: days to return to neurocognitive baseline in adolescents versus young adults. *Surg Neurol Int.* 2012;3:130.

161. Harmon KG, Drezner JA, Gammons M, et al. American medical society for sports medicine position statement: concussion in sport. *Br J Sports Med.* 2013;47(1):15–26.

162. Ellemberg D, Henry LC, Macciocchi SN, et al. Advances in sport concussion assessment: from behavioral to brain imaging measures. *J Neurotrauma.* 2009;26(12):2365–2382.

163. Fazio VC, Lovell MR, Pardini JE, et al. The relation between post concussion symptoms and neurocognitive performance in concussed athletes. *NeuroRehabilitation.* 2007;22(3):207–216.

164. Nazem TG, Ackerman KE. The female athlete triad. *Sports Health.* 2012;4(4):302–311.

Juvenile Idiopathic Arthritis

Susan E. Klepper

Criteria for Diagnosis and Classification of JIA
Incidence and Prevalence of JIA
Etiology and Pathogenesis
Pathology
General Goals of Management in JIA
    Pharmacologic Therapies
Prognosis and Outcomes
Physical Therapy Examination and Evaluation
    Examination of Activities and Participation
    Examination of Body Structures and Functions

Evaluation, Diagnosis, Prognosis, and Plan of Care
Intervention
    Coordination, Communication, and Documentation
    Procedural Interventions
    Issues Related to School Participation
    Patient and Family Education and Support
Summary
Case Study

J uvenile idiopathic arthritis (JIA) is the most common of the rheumatic diseases of childhood. It is characterized by joint inflammation, but can impact multiple body systems, causing impairments, activity limitations, and participation restrictions in a growing child.

The purpose of this chapter is to describe the role of the physical therapist in the management of children and adolescents with JIA. The first section describes the criteria for diagnosis and classification of JIA, prevalence and incidence, etiology, pathology, and pharmacologic management. The second section provides a framework, based on the *Guide to Physical Therapist Practice* and the World Health Organization's (WHO) International Classification of Functioning, Disability, and Health (ICF) model, for physical therapist examination, evaluation, and plan of care (POC). Standardized assessments and outcome measures developed for JIA are discussed. The third section describes interventions to address common problems in JIA. Evidence for the efficacy of interventions, where available, is presented. Issues related to home, school, and community participation are discussed. A case study illustrates the physical therapist's management of an older child with JIA.

Other pediatric rheumatic conditions that may result in arthritis include connective tissue diseases like scleroderma, juvenile dermatomyositis, systemic lupus erythematosus, and various forms of vasculitis. Rheumatologists also manage noninflammatory disorders in children such as benign

hypermobility, localized and diffuse chronic pain syndromes, and heritable disorders of connective tissue. The principles that guide physical therapist management for the child with chronic arthritis are applicable to these other diagnoses.

▶ Criteria for diagnosis and classification of JIA

Table 15.1 compares three systems historically used to diagnose and classify childhood arthritis, including the American College of Rheumatology (ACR) criteria for juvenile rheumatoid arthritis (JRA), the European League Against Rheumatism (EULAR) criteria for juvenile chronic arthritis (JCA), and the International League of Associations for Rheumatology (ILAR) criteria for JIA. The term JIA and the ILAR classification system are now universally accepted and used in this chapter.

JIA is defined as definite arthritis of unknown etiology beginning before age 16 years and lasting for at least 6 weeks. The ILAR system includes seven distinct disease onset types plus an eighth type, "undifferentiated," which includes signs and symptoms that do not fit into one disease type or overlap more than one type.[1] Table 15.2 lists the classification criteria and exclusion criteria based on signs and symptoms during the first 6 months of disease, frequencies, onset age, and sex distribution for each JIA type.[2] In the

<table>
<tr><td colspan="2">TABLE
15.1 Comparison of Classification Systems of Childhood Arthritis</td></tr>
</table>

Characteristic	ACR (JRA)	EULAR (JCA)	ILAR (JIA)
Basis of classification	Clinical (onset and course)	Clinical (onset only) and serologic (RF)	Clinical (onset and course) and serologic (RF)

Onset types	Three
	sJRA
	polyJRA
	pauciJRA
		Six
		Systemic JCA (sJCA)
		Polyarticular JCA (polyJCA) JRA
		Pauciarticular JCA (pauciJCA)
		JPsA
		JAS
			Seven
			sJIA
			Polyarticular RF negative (RF-negative polyJIA)
			Polyarticular RF positive (RF-positive polyJIA)
			oligoJIA
			  Persistent
			  Extended
			Psoriatic arthritis (JPsA)
			ERA
			Undifferentiated

ACR, American College of Rheumatology; EULAR, European League Against Rheumatism; ILAR, International League of Associates for Rheumatology; RF, rheumatoid factor.

absence of a specific laboratory test for JIA, the diagnosis is based on clinical presentation that may change over time. The ultimate goal of classification criteria is for each disease type to be as homogeneous as possible and mutually exclusive of the other categories.

Systemic onset JIA (sJIA) can begin at any age, with an equal male-to-female ratio and represents approximately 4% to 17% of all children with JIA. The diagnostic hallmark is a fever that spikes to 39°C once or twice a day, typically during the afternoon or evening, with a rapid return to normal or slightly below normal, for at least 2 weeks. A migratory, salmon-colored rash on the trunk or limbs accompanies the rash. Children may be quite ill while febrile, but feel well during other times. Other systemic signs that may precede onset of arthritis by months or even years include pleuritis, pericarditis, myocarditis, generalized lymphadenopathy, and enlargement of the liver or spleen. Laboratory tests for rheumatoid factor (RF) and antinuclear antibodies (ANAs)

<table>
<tr><td colspan="2">TABLE
15.2 Classification Criteria, Frequency, Onset Age, and Sex Ratio for the ILAR Categories of JIA[11]</td></tr>
</table>

JIA Disease Type	Diagnostic Criteria	Frequency*	Onset Age	Sex Ratio
Systemic Arthritis	Arthritis in ≥ one joints with or preceded by fever for ≥ 2 weeks that is documented to be daily for ≥ 3 days, and accompanied by one or more of the following: 1. Evanescent erythematous rash 2. Generalized lymphadenopathy 3. Enlarged liver or spleen 4. Serositis Exclusions†: a,b,c,d	4%–17%	<16 years	F=M
Oligoarthritis	Arthritis in one to four joints during the first 6 months of disease; two categories are recognized: 1. Persistent: affecting no more than four joints throughout disease course 2. Extended: Affecting more than a total of four joints after the first six months of disease Exclusions†: a,b,c,d,e	27%–56%	Peak: 2–4 years	F>M (3:1)
Polyarthritis (RF positive)	Arthritis affecting five or more joints during the first 6 months of disease; IgM RF detected in two or more tests at least 3 months apart during the first 6 months of disease Exclusions: a,b,c,e	2%–7%	Late childhood to early adolescence	F>M 2:1
Polyarthritis (RF negative)	Arthritis affecting five or more joints during the first 6 months of disease; test for RF is negative. Exclusions: a,b,c,d,e	11%–28%	Early peak: 2–4 years Later peak: 6–12 years	F>M 2:1
Psoriatic arthritis	Arthritis and psoriasis t arthritis plus at least two of the following: 1. Dactylitis 2. Nail pitting or onycholysis abnormalities 3. Psoriasis in a first-degree relative Exclusions: b,c,d,e	2%–11%	Early peak: 2–4 years Later peak: 9–11 years	F>M

JIA Disease Type	Diagnostic Criteria	Frequency*	Onset Age	Sex Ratio
ERA	Arthritis and enthesitis, *or* arthritis or enthesitis plus at least two of the following: 1. Presence or history of sacroiliac joint tenderness and/or inflammatory lumbosacral pain 2. Presence of HLA-B27 antigen 3. Onset of arthritis in a male older than 6 years 4. Acute anterior uveitis 5. History of AS, ERA, sacroiliitis with inflammatory bowel disease, Reiter's syndrome, or acute anterior uveitis in a first-degree relative Exclusions: a,d,e	3%–11%	Late childhood or adolescence	M: 2 to 1
Undifferentiated	Arthritis that does not fulfill criteria in one of the above categories or fulfills criteria in more than one category	11%–21%		

*Reported frequencies are based on percentage of all JIA disease types as reported in Ravelli A, Martini A., 2007[2]
†Exclusion criteria reflect the principle of the ILAR classification that all JIA categories are mutually exclusive.
a. Psoriasis or a history of psoriasis in the patient or first-degree relative
b. Arthritis in an HLA-B27 positive male beginning after the 6th birthday
c. AS, ERA, sacroiliitis with inflammatory bowel disease, Reiter's syndrome, or acute anterior uveitis, or a history of one of these disorders in a first-degree relative
d. Presence of IgM RF on at least two occasions at least 3 months apart
e. Presence of systemic JIA in the patient

are both negative. Objective arthritis may be present initially or may not appear for weeks. The most common differential diagnoses for sJIA include systemic infection, malignancies, rheumatic fever, connective tissue disease, inflammatory bowel disease, and other autoimmune inflammatory conditions.

Disease course is variable. Systemic symptoms may subside after several months to a few years or may occur in repeated episodes or persistent systemic disease. Some children recover completely with arthritis in a few joints, while others follow a progressive course, with persistent arthritis in an increasing number of joints.[3] A small percentage (5% to 8%) develop a serious complication, macrophage activation syndrome (MAS), characterized by a sudden combination of fever and systemic and neurological symptoms that can be life-threatening. Early recognition and treatment of the syndrome are essential to prevent or minimize the effects of this multisystem involvement.

Polyarticular onset JIA (polyJIA) is defined as arthritis in five or more joints during the first 6 months of disease. Figure 15.1 shows the hands of a child with polyJIA. Onset is usually insidious with a progressive increase in the number of joints involved. Systemic symptoms are generally mild and include a low-grade fever, slight-to-moderate enlargement of the spleen and liver, and lymphadenopathy. Clinically evident pericarditis or pleuritis is infrequent. The ILAR classification recognizes two types of polyJIA, RF positive and RF negative. Children with RF-positive polyJIA meet the above criteria plus test positive for the RF on at least two occasions at least 3 months apart. This type occurs in 2% to 7% of all children with JIA and affects mostly adolescent girls. Disease course is similar to that seen in adults with RF-positive rheumatoid arthritis (RA), with early onset symmetric, aggressive, and erosive polyarthritis in the small joints of the hands and feet, the potential for classic boutonnière and swan neck deformities, cervical spine, and temporalmandibular joint arthritis.[4–6] Knees and ankles

may be involved in association with arthritis in the feet. Rheumatoid nodules are found on the forearm and elbow.

RF-negative polyJIA is defined as arthritis in five or more joints in the first 6 months of disease and the absence of IgM RF. It accounts for 11% to 28% of all children with JIA and affects more girls than boys. There appear to be two peak onset periods, 2 to 4 years of age and 6 to 12 years.[2] Current research suggests there may be three subsets of this disease type. The first is similar to early onset oligoarticular JIA with

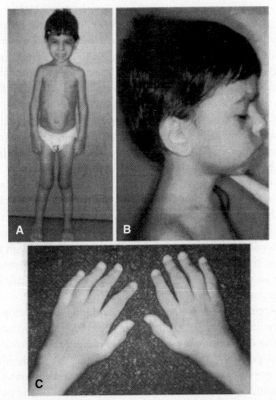

FIGURE 15.1 (A) General appearance, **(B)** Temporomandibular joint, and **(C)** Hands of a child with polyarticular onset JIA.

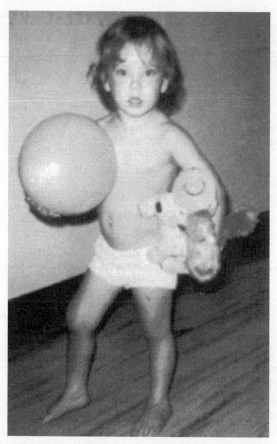

FIGURE 15.2 A child with asymmetric arthritis resulting in a LLD.

asymmetric arthritis but with a rapid increase in the number of joints involved. The second form is similar to RF-negative adult RA, with onset at school age, obvious synovitis of large and small joints, and variable outcome. The third form includes a dry synovitis with stiffness, and tendency for flexion contractures and a potential joint destruction.[2]

Oligoarticular onset JIA (oligoJIA) is defined as arthritis in four or fewer joints in the first 6 months of disease and represents the largest group (27% to 56%) of children with JIA.[2] Arthritis is typically asymmetric and affects primarily the lower extremities, with the knees most commonly involved, followed by the ankles and elbows. Figure 15.2 shows a child with asymmetric arthritis resulting in a leg length discrepancy (LLD). The hips are rarely involved, and the small joints of the hands and feet are usually spared, although this is not true in all children. The disease may initially present in one joint, frequently a knee, and the physician must rule out infection or trauma as the cause.

Approximately 30% of children with oligoJIA develop iridocyclitis, an insidious and often asymptomatic inflammation of the eyes that leads to functional blindness if untreated. ANA-positive patients are at the highest risk for developing eye disease, most within 5 to 7 years after the onset of arthritis. Some children with RF-negative polyJIA and psoriatic arthritis (PsA) may also develop iridocyclitis, especially if they are ANA positive.[2] Children must be screened periodically by an ophthalmologist using a slit-lamp examination.

Screening frequency is determined by the expected risk for eye disease and may range from every 3 to 4 months to once a year.[2,7]

The ILAR criteria recognize two separate groups of children with oligoJIA, persistent and extended. Persistent oligoJIA is defined in a child who continues to have four or fewer joints involved after the first 6 months of disease. Medical and functional outcomes for these children are typically very good; however, they remain at risk for eye disease. Extended oligoJIA is defined as arthritis affecting more than four joints after the first 6 months of disease, although fewer total joints are involved than in polyJIA. The presence of ankle, wrist, or hand arthritis, symmetric arthritis, arthritis in two to four joints, and the presence of an elevated ANA titer or erythrocyte sedimentation rate may be predictors of extended oligoJIA.[8]

The remaining disease types were previously grouped under the category of juvenile spondyloarthropathy or spondyloarthritis (JSpA). Although the prototype for SpA in adults is ankylosing spondylitis (AS), children initially present with less back pain and more hip and peripheral arthritis along with enthesitis.[9,10] The ILAR criteria recognize three disease types within JSpA, enthesitis-related arthritis (ERA) and PsA, each with a frequency of 2% to 11% of all children with JIA, and undifferentiated arthritis, a category that includes children who meet criteria for no individual disease type or meet criteria for more than one type. This group represents 11% to 21% of all children with JIA.[10]

The term *enthesitis* describes inflammation of the entheses, the attachment sites of tendons, ligaments, or joint capsules to bone. Figure 15.3 shows the most common sites of tenderness associated with enthesitis in the knees, ankles, and feet. Inclusion and exclusion criteria for ERA are shown in Table 15.2. A diagnosis of ERA requires arthritis and enthesitis *or* arthritis or enthesitis plus two of the following: presence or history of sacroiliac joint tenderness and/or inflammatory low back pain; presence of the HLA-B27 antigen; onset of arthritis in a male over the age of 6 years; acute anterior uveitis; history in a first-degree relative of AS, ERA, sacroiliitis with inflammatory bowel, Reiter's syndrome, or acute anterior uveitis.[11] Ten percent to 20% of children eventually diagnosed with AS show disease symptoms before 16 years of age and may be regarded as having "juvenile-onset AS."[12] Children who meet the criteria for juvenile AS before the age of 16 years would be diagnosed as having AS.[10] Although the ERA criteria do not address two accepted features of SpA in adults, reactive arthritis and irritable bowel disease (IBD), a child with IBD who otherwise meets the criteria for ERA would not be excluded from this diagnosis.[13]

Juvenile psoriatic arthritis (JPsA) is defined in a child, younger than 16 years, with arthritis and psoriasis or the presence of arthritis and two of the following: dactylitis, nail pitting or onycholysis, and family history of psoriasis in a first-degree relative. Dactylitis represents the combined effects of arthritis and tenosynovitis and is characterized by swelling of one or more digits that extend beyond the joint margins (Fig. 15.4). Children who are RF positive or have signs of another form of JIA are excluded from this

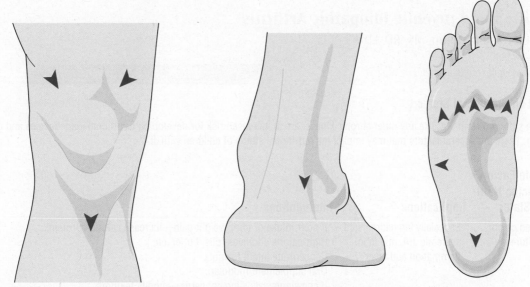

FIGURE 15.3 The most common sites of tenderness associated with enthesitis in the knees, ankles, and feet.

category. Arthritis may precede psoriasis by several years, and the disease at onset may appear more similar to asymmetric oligoJIA than adult PsA.

Incidence and prevalence of JIA

The reported prevalence and incidence rates for JIA vary widely on account of differences in study design. Prevalence in North America and Europe varied from 132 per 100,000 for population-based studies to 12 per 100,000 for clinic-based studies.[14] Reports of worldwide prevalence varied from 0.07 to 4.01 cases per 1000.[15] The most recent estimate by the National Arthritis Data Workgroup published from the 2005 United

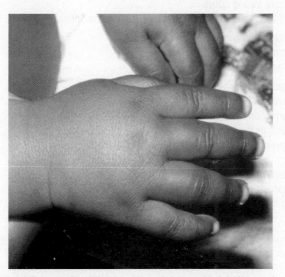

FIGURE 15.4 Dactylitis represents the combined effects of arthritis and tenosynovitis and is characterized by swelling of one or more digits that extends beyond the joint margins. (Courtesy of Thomas D. Thacher, MD.)

States census indicated that there are 294,000 children with some form of childhood arthritis.[16,17] Worldwide incidence rates for all childhood arthritis range from 0.008 to 0.226 cases per 1000 children at risk.[15] Studies representing North America and white European populations estimated between 2 and 20 new cases per 100,000 children at risk per year.[18]

Clinic-based studies found the prevalence of JIA by racial group in North America to be 32 per 100,000 for Caucasians, 40 per 100,000 for North American Indians (NAI), 26 per 100,000 for African American, and 26 per 100,000 for "others."[14,19] No differences were found in the percentage of patients with systemic JRA (sJRA) among racial groups. The proportion with oligoJIA was higher than that for polyJIA among Caucasian patients.

Gender distribution and onset age vary by disease type. Boys and girls are equally affected in sJIA; however, girls outnumber boys in oligoJIA (3:1) and polyJIA (2.8:1). Boys are more represented in juvenile AS while more females are represented in JPsA. Peak age at onset also varies by disease type. One study of 300 children with JRA reported peak age at onset was between 1 and 3 years in the total group and for girls with pauci- or polyJRA.[20] Two peak onset periods were seen in boys; one at 2 years of age for boys with polyJRA and another between 8 and 10 years for boys later diagnosed with SpA. For JPsA, there was one peak period in the preschool years, mainly in girls, with a second peak during mid- to late childhood. Onset for juvenile AS usually occurs in late childhood or adolescence.

Etiology and pathogenesis

The exact etiology and pathogenesis of JIA is not fully understood; however, there is agreement that these diseases are immune system disorders resulting in inflammation in joints and other body tissues. Disease onset appears to occur in a genetically predisposed host who encounters an external

Nutrition and Juvenile Idiopathic Arthritis

Megan Johnston Mullin, MS, RD, LDN
Clinical Dietitian,
Children's Hospital of Philadelphia

Impact on Nutritional Status

Children suffering from JIA, like any other chronic illness, are at increased risk for developing nutritional inadequacies and growth faltering. There are several factors that may impact the nutritional status of children with JIA.

Possible Factors Influencing Nutritional Status	Implications	Interventions
Increased caloric expenditure	Especially in children with systemic JIA, due to inflammation and fever	If poor intake or poor weight gain—increase calories/protein: High-calorie additives (oils, butter, etc.) Concentrate infant formula Oral supplement/modulars If chewing/swallowing concerns—modify textures Consider multiple vitamin and mineral supplements or supplementation of individual nutrients as needed. Avoid food struggles or battles: Educate parents about: what are the appropriate feeding roles of parent and child, how to provide meals and snacks at consistent times and in a relaxed and loving environment. Consider tube feedings.
Limited motion/ physical activity	Causing an inability to consume adequate calories, muscle wasting, or weight gain	If poor weight gain or poor oral intake, follow guidelines for increasing calorie intake (above). If excessive weight gain or risk for obesity: Encourage increase in physical activity. Limit intake of high-calorie/fat foods. Limit juices, sugar-added beverages. Encourage fruits, vegetables, whole grains, lean meats, low-fat dairy products.
Anorexia	Caused by chronic pain and/or due to medication	Attempt to control pain and minimize side effects of medications. Maximize calorie intake (see above). Other strategies for improving intake: Encourage small, frequent meals. Avoid hot meals that have strong odors. Use colorful foods and foods with appetizing aromas to increase appeal.
Food fads and quackery	Fasting, experimental, or elimination diets may cause nutrient deficiencies	Identify potential nutrient deficiencies. Educate patient and family on rich food sources. Vitamin/mineral supplement as needed.
Drug interactions (Commonly used medications: Salicylates (Aspirin), Tolmetin, Naproxen, Ibuprofen, Methotrexate, Corticosteroid)	Possible gastrointestinal side effects: Decreased absorption of vitamin C and folate, increased or decreased appetite, weight loss or gain, glucose intolerance	Attempt to minimize gastrointestinal side effects of medications. Identify nutrient deficiencies. Educate patient and family on rich food sources. Provide supplementation as needed. Follow guidelines for promoting weight gain or loss (see above). If glucose intolerance: Consistent eating pattern/meal schedule. Limit juices/avoid sugar-added beverages. Plan healthy, balanced meals to avoid excess carbohydrate content.

SUGGESTED READINGS

Behrman RE, Nelson WE, Vaughn VC. Nelson textbook of pediatrics. 13th Edition. In: *Immunology, Allergy, And Related Diseases: Juvenile Rheumatoid Arthritis*. Philadelphia, PA: WB Saunders Company; 1987:515–523.

Ekvall SW. Pediatric nutrition in chronic diseases and developmental disorders-prevention, assessment, and treatment. In: Lovell D, Henderson C, eds. *Juvenile Rheumatoid Arthritis*. New York, NY: Oxford University Press; 1993:263–267.

Lea F. Modern nutrition in health and disease 8th edition. In Bollet AJ, ed. Nutrition and Diet in Rheumatic Disease. Vol 2. Chicago, IL: Waverly Company;1994:1362–1372.

stimulus that may be a viral or bacterial infection. While some parents report disease onset in their child following physical trauma, it is unclear whether the trauma is the cause or simply brings attention to the disease. Different etiologic factors may be responsible for each onset type, or a single pathogen may cause distinct clinical patterns as it interacts with the specific characteristics and vulnerabilities of the child.

The presence of altered immunity, abnormal immune regulation, and production of pro-inflammatory cytokines may help explain the onset and persistence of inflammation in JIA. T-cell abnormalities and the pathology of inflamed synovium in affected joints suggest that there is a cell-mediated pathogenesis. Humoral abnormalities are evident from the presence of multiple autoantibodies, immune complexes, and complement activation. The evidence for genetic predisposition to many of these conditions is increasing, but is not completely understood. One study of over 3000 children with arthritis found there was concordance between siblings with JRA for age at onset, clinical manifestations, and disease course.[21] Although many suspected genetic characteristics are within the major histocompatibility complex (MHC) region of chromosome 6, the pathogenesis may involve the interactions of multiple genes. Correlation between HLA specificities and various types of JIA may have risk and protective effects that are age-related for each onset type and some course types.[22]

▶ Pathology

Figure 15.5 illustrates changes caused by inflammation within and surrounding a synovial joint. The cardinal signs of joint inflammation include swelling, end-range stress pain, and stiffness. Changes within the joint include villous hypertrophy, hyperplasia of the vascular endothelium, and intra-articular (IA) effusion, with swelling and distension of the joint capsule. The joint may appear enlarged because of bony overgrowth caused by increased blood flow to the inflamed tissues. Distension of the joint capsule from increased synovial fluid, stretching of periarticular tissues, and protective muscle spasm results in pain and stiffness. The presence and duration of morning stiffness is often an indicator of disease activity.

Synovial cells multiply, forming a massive overgrowth called a pannus that spreads over the articular cartilage, causing it to soften and weaken. Degradative enzymes released from the cartilage matrix into the synovial fluid further disrupt the normal cartilage fiber network. IA adhesions and osteophytes occur later. Articular surfaces become irregular, and joint congruency, alignment, and stability are compromised as erosions occur in articular cartilage and subchondral bone. Fibrosis of periarticular tendons and ligaments results in joint contractures. Subluxation may occur at the wrist and small joints of the hands and feet. Posterior subluxation of the tibia on the femur may occur in the presence of long-standing knee flexion contractures. Muscle imbalance, quadriceps weakness, and impaired mobility of the patella contribute to joint stiffness and instability.

Early radiographic changes include soft tissue swelling and widening of the joint space due to effusions, juxta-articular bone loss, and periosteal new bone, especially in the phalanges, metacarpals, and metatarsals. In persistent disease, radiographs may show joint space narrowing,

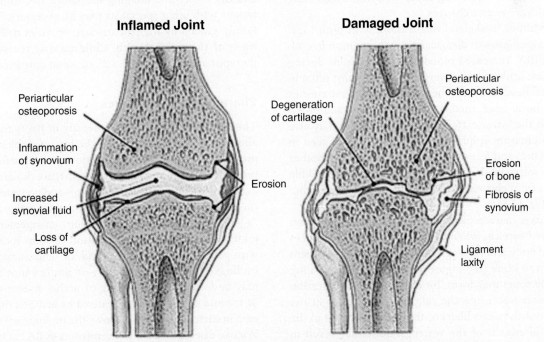

FIGURE 15.5 Changes caused by the inflammatory process within and surrounding synovial joints.

marginal erosions, and osteophytes due to thinning and loss of articular cartilage. Fibrous or bony ankylosis may occur with severe or persistent inflammation. Pathologic changes in the apophyseal and sacroiliac joints in children with juvenile ankylosing spondylitis (JAS) include endochondral and capsular ossification. In early stages of the disease, the surface of the sacroiliac joints shows little change; subchondral inflammation results in granulation tissue with few inflammatory cells and no pannus formation. A balance of erosive synovitis and capsular or ligamentous ossification often occurs in synovial joints, although the ossification process usually dominates in joints of low mobility.

The negative effects of JIA on bone health are well known and include low volumetric bone mineral density (vBMD) and decreased bone strength compared with healthy children.[23,24] Burnham et al. found significantly lower muscle cross-sectional area (mCSA) and bone strength in patients with polyJIA and SpA, aged 5 to 22 years, compared with healthy controls. Trabecular vBMD was significantly lower in these two groups as well as those with sJIA. Low bone strength was also seen in children with normal mCSA. Severe persistent arthritis was a significant predictor of these deficits and also increases the risk of fracture and failure to achieve optimal peak bone mass in adolescence and young adulthood. Other risk factors for poor bone development in JIA include delayed pubertal maturation, malnutrition, muscle atrophy and weakness, inadequate weight-bearing physical activity (PA), and long-term use of systemic corticosteroids.[25] Periarticular muscles may atrophy as a result of reflex inhibition from swelling and pain, disuse, and protein-energy malnutrition.[26] Soft tissue shortens when joints are held in flexed positions to accommodate swelling and reduce pain, contributing to joint instability and compliance during loading under motion and increasing the risk for degenerative changes.

Abnormalities in skeletal maturation, with both local and generalized growth disturbances, are common in children with JRA. Increased blood flow to the joint during active disease leads to bony overgrowth, seen most often in the humeral head and radial head of the upper extremities and the femoral head, medial femoral condyle, and proximal tibia in the lower extremities. Active disease may also result in premature epiphyseal closure, as may be seen in the small hands and feet of children with poly-JIA. Another example is micrognathia, or undergrowth of the mandible that results from chronic arthritis of the temporomandibular joints (Fig. 15.6).

Enthesitis is characterized by a nonspecific inflammation and localized osteitis, whereby granulation tissue replaces the normal bony and cartilaginous attachment of ligament and tendon to bone (see Figure 15.3). During the healing phase, bony spurs may form, for example, at the insertion of the plantar fascia into the calcaneus. Enthesitis at the attachment of the outer fibers of the annulus fibrosis to the anterolateral aspects of the vertebral body may result in syndesmophyte.

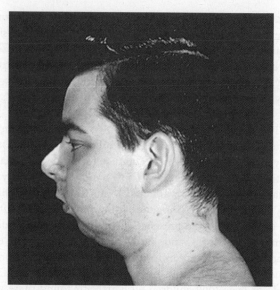

FIGURE 15.6 Micrognathia, or undergrowth of the mandible, that results from chronic arthritis of the temporomandibular joints.

▶ General goals of management in JIA

The overall goals of management in JIA are to: (1) suppress inflammation using the most effective drug therapy with the least adverse effects, (2) preserve joint structure and function, (3) promote independence and competence in daily activities, and (4) provide education and support to the child and family. The child's care is often managed at a tertiary center by a multidisciplinary team that includes a pediatric rheumatologist, rheumatology nurse, occupational therapist (OT), physical therapist, social worker or psychologist, and laboratory and imaging specialists. Occasional consultations with other specialists may be necessary. The child's family, guided by the pediatrician, provides daily management of the child's health. Children may receive physical therapist and OT at home, school, or an outpatient clinic.

Pharmacologic Therapies

The goal of pharmacologic therapy in JIA is to eliminate all signs of active disease with the least possible toxicity, to preserve joint structure and function, prevent deformity, and promote age-appropriate activities. Inactive disease is defined as having no joint with active arthritis and no systemic symptoms attributable to JIA. The ACR defines active arthritis as "a joint with swelling not due to bony enlargement, or if no joint swelling is present, limitation of joint motion along with pain on motion (POM) and/or tenderness." Isolated findings of POM, tenderness, or limited motion (LOM) may be found in the absence of active disease as a result of trauma or joint damage caused by arthritis now considered inactive. Display 15.1 shows the preliminary criteria for inactive disease and clinical remission in JIA.[27] Display 15.2 shows the ACR core set of outcome measures that has been

15.1 Preliminary Criteria for Inactive Disease and Clinical Remission in JIA* Inactive Disease

1. No joints with active arthritis*
2. No fever, rash, serositis, splenomegaly, or generalized lymphadenopathy due to JIA
3. No active uveitis
4. Normal erythrocyte sedimentation rate (ESR) or CRP (C-Reactive Protein)
5. Physician's global assessment of disease shows no disease activity based on activity

Clinical Remission

1. Clinical remission on medications: criteria for inactive disease must be met for a minimum of 6 consecutive months while the patient is on medications
2. Clinical remission off medications: criteria for inactive disease must be met for a minimum of 12 consecutive months while patient is off all antiarthritis medications

*As defined by the ACR, a joint with swelling not due to bony enlargement or if no swelling, limited motion with pain or motion and/or tenderness.[27]

validated and used in clinical trials for JIA.[28] Additional measures include the parent's global assessment of the child's pain and arthritis using separate 100-mm visual analogue scales (VAS) and a child's assessment of discomfort using the facial affective scale.[4] The definition of improvement with intervention is based on the ACR Pedi 30 response that requires at least 30% improvement from baseline in at least 3/6 variables, with no more than one of the variables worsening by more than 30%. The ACR Pedi 50 and 70 responses require 50% and 70% improvement, respectively, in 3/6 variables and no more than a 30% worsening in ≤ one variable. A disease flare is defined as worsening in any two of the six CRVs (Core Response Variables) by greater than or equal to 40% without concomitant improvement in more than one of the other CRVs by less than or equal to 30%.[26]

Therapy is targeted to the child's disease characteristics and course.[4,29,30] For children with severe persistent disease who are at risk for significant disability, early and aggressive treatment with a combination of drugs may be used. The 2011 ACR guidelines for pharmacotherapy

15.2 Core Set of Outcome Measures in JIA[27]

- Physician global assessment of disease activity on a 10-cm VAS anchored by the words "remission" and "very severe" (MD Global)
- Parent or patient global assessment of overall well-being on a 10-cm VAS anchored by the words "very well" and "very poor" (Parent/Patient Global)
- Functional ability
- Number of joints with limited range of motion (JC-ROM)
- Number of joints with active arthritis (NJAA)
- Erythrocyte sedimentation rate (ESR)

in JIA are defined by treatment group, current drug treatment, disease activity, and features of poor prognosis.[31] A summary of the guidelines is available at: http://www.rheumatology.org/Practice/Clinical/Guidelines/Juvenile_Idiopathic_Arthritis_(Members__Only)/.

Nonsteroidal anti-inflammatory drugs (NSAIDs) are the most frequently used first-line therapy to control inflammation and may be used as monotherapy in children with oligoJIA. Several NSAIDs approved for use in JIA, including naproxen, ibuprofen, meloxicam, and indomethacin, are available in liquid formulations, making it easier to administer to young children. NSAIDs reduce fever and inflammation and have an analgesic effect, but do not alter disease course. Eight weeks of therapy is considered necessary to determine the effectiveness of an NSAID. NSAIDs are generally well tolerated, although some children may experience adverse effects including stomach pain and headache. Routine monitoring for possible toxicities is necessary for all children.

IA glucocorticoid injections are used to induce disease remission in children who have one or two joints with persistent arthritis that has not responded to a trial of NSAIDs. In some children with oligoJIA, this may be the first line of therapy. Sherry et al. reported children who received IA steroid injections of lower extremity joints within the first 2 months of disease onset showed significantly lower incidence of LLD, a major cause of gait abnormalities in JIA.[32] Brostrom et al. also found decreased pain and improved gait parameters following lower limb IA steroid injections in 18 children with polyJIA.[33] The effects of IA steroid injections are often immediate and long lasting. Zulian et al. reported that 70% of patients showed no recurrence of arthritis in injected joints at a 1-year follow-up exam; 40% still had no symptoms after 2 years.[34] Triamcinolone hexacetonide is the medication preferred by many rheumatologists.[35] A joint may be injected up to three times in 1 year if disease signs and symptoms return.

Systemic absorption of the steroid from multiple injections performed in a single session may result in a cushingoid appearance; however, this is usually temporary. Other potential problems, including steroid leakage and subcutaneous atrophy, can be reduced by following scrupulous administration techniques. Therapists should consult with the treating physician regarding weight-bearing precautions after lower extremity IA injection.

Most children with severe polyJIA will require a disease-modifying antirheumatic drug (DMARD) or a biologic agent to achieve adequate disease control. Methotrexate (MTX), the most frequently prescribed DMARD in JIA has been used for over 25 years with demonstrated safety and efficacy. It is usually administered in a single oral dose of 10 to 15 mg/m² each week, although doses up to 30 mg/m² may be used in children with refractory disease. A subcutaneous injection may be useful for children who experience GI upset with the oral dose. MTX has been shown in controlled trails to slow the progression of arthritis and is more effective than either a placebo or other DMARD.[36-38] In one study, 86% of children with polyJIA achieved an ACR Pedi 70 response after 2 years of treatment with MTX compared with another DMARD. Because it may take several weeks for MTX to reach a therapeutic effect, children with severe arthritis may require short-term treatment with corticosteroids to provide immediate disease control. When taken with folic acid, MTX is well tolerated and safe in children with JIA. General precautions include avoiding the use of live vaccines while taking MTX. Patients should abstain from alcohol and women of childbearing age should be counseled to avoid pregnancy because of the potential damage to the fetus in the early stages of gestation. Liver toxicity due to MTX has not been reported in children with JIA and pulmonary toxicity is rare. Blood counts and liver enzymes are monitored every 4 to 6 weeks; if a child shows transient elevation of liver enzymes, MTX may be discontinued until lab values return to normal.[4] Research to determine the best time to stop treatment with MTX once a child achieves clinical remission is ongoing to balance the risk of relapse with the potential for adverse effects of long-term use.[38] Another DMARD, sulfasalazine, has been shown to be more effective than a placebo in suppressing disease activity in some children with oligoJIA, but the risk of toxicity is high. Blood counts and transaminase levels are monitored before and frequently during therapy.[4]

Children who do not respond to MTX alone may be treated with one of the biologic agents that target specific components of the inflammatory cascade, alone or in combination with MTX. The most frequently used agents target tumor necrosis factor-alpha (TNF- α), a cytokine responsible for many adverse effects of inflammation. The most frequently used anti-TNF-α is etanercept (ETN) administered by injection. Safety and efficacy data from an 8-year study of 318 children with JIA on continuous ETN therapy alone or in combination with MTX found no serious adverse effects from the therapy. The most common serious adverse event beyond 4 years of ETN therapy was disease flare.[39] Several studies support additional benefits of ETN therapy, including improved physical growth and quality of life (QOL) in children with JIA.[40-42] Other anti-TNF-α biologic therapies used in inflammatory arthritis include infliximab (Remicade) and adalimumab (Humira). Adalimumab, administered by subcutaneous injection, was FDA-approved in 2008 for use in JIA after a multicenter, randomized study of 190 children with active polyJIA showed an ACR Pedi 50 and 70 response in 86% and 77%, respectively, of children after 100 weeks of treatment.[43] Although not currently FDA-approved for use in JIA, intravenous infliximab is often used "off-label" by rheumatologists because of their personal experience in using the medication and data showing its efficacy.[4] Two biologic agents that target different components of the immune system have shown significant reductions in disease activity in children with JIA who do not respond to ETN. These include Abatacept for severe polyJIA, and both anakinra and tocilizumab for

sJIA. Biologic therapies are costly, oral administration is not available, and long-term studies of potential adverse effects are lacking. Because these agents inhibit the immune system, there is increased risk for infection and response to vaccination. Before starting any biologic therapy, a child should be up-to-date on vaccinations and avoid all live vaccination while on these medications; treatment is temporarily discontinued in the event of infection or exposure to varicella. Despite these limitations, biologic therapies have had a dramatic and positive impact on the lives of children with JIA.

Systemic glucocorticoids are reserved for children with severe sJIA. They have potent anti-inflammatory effects, but do not alter disease course or duration. Long-term use is associated with serious adverse effects, including Cushing syndrome, generalized growth deficits, osteoporosis and fracture, diabetes mellitus, obesity, steroid myopathy, and increased susceptibility to infection. Low-dose or alternate-day oral steroids or periodic intravenous pulsed steroid therapy may be used in severe polyJIA unresponsive to other treatments. Topical glucocorticoids are used to manage acute iritis and chronic uveitis.

▶ Prognosis and outcomes

Reports of prognosis and functional outcomes in JIA are inconsistent and at times conflicting because of differences in study design and the period of time examined. Most studies report that children with persistent oligoJIA have the best prognosis for disease outcome, although they remain at high risk for eye disease and require regular examinations by an ophthalmologist. In contrast, children with polyJIA often experience persistent disease, achieve clinical remission at lower rates, and have a lower probability of remission within 10 years.[44] Of this group, children with RF-positive polyJIA have the worst prognosis for clinical remission. A 2002 study of 392 patients reported that the probabilities of remission 10 years after disease onset by disease type were oligoJIA (47%), sJIA (37%), RF-negative polyJIA (23%), and RF-positive polyJIA (6%).[45] A more recent study of 437 patients with JIA followed for up to 4 years found very few (6%) episodes of clinical remission off medications that were sustained for more than 5 years.[46] Predictors of poor outcome include the presence of a positive RF, symmetrical disease, severe or extended arthritis at disease onset, early signs of wrist or hip disease, and persistence of active disease.[44,47,48] Children not in remission by age 16 years have a high probability of active disease into their adult years.

Reports of functional outcomes in JIA over the past decade are also inconsistent, although most studies conclude that children with persistent oligoJIA have the least physical limitations, while those with RF-positive polyJIA experience significant activity limitations that can have a negative impact on their QOL.[49] A study of young adults with a history of JRA reported that 40% had no physical limitation while 33% with poly- and sJIA had moderate-to-severe disability. Compared with national statistics for the same age group, fewer females with JRA completed postsecondary education, and unemployment rates in young adults with JRA were higher.[50] A large multicenter study conducted in 32 countries found that the strongest predictors of poor health-related quality of life (HRQOL) were high scores for physical disability and pain.[51] Their findings were supported by a subsequent study by Amine et al.[49]

In contrast to these reports, several studies suggest that long-term functional outcomes in this population, including educational and occupational status, as well as self- or parent-reported HRQOL have improved in recent years and are similar to same-age healthy controls.[2,52–54] Reports on the effect of disease type and duration on functional outcomes have been inconsistent, with some studies finding no significant impact of disease type, severity, or duration on educational or occupational status, while others indicate lower HRQOL in patients with extended oligoJIA and polyJIA.[55,56]

Most of these studies have been cross-sectional, assessing functional outcome at one point in time. The only longitudinal study examined physical function in 227 children with JIA from 1987 to 2002 using a parent-completed measure of disability validated for JIA. Each patient was followed for at least 1 year, and one parent completed the questionnaire at least twice during that time. Although degree of disability varied widely between and within patients during the study period, after a median follow-up period of 3.4 years, 75% had no disability, while only 3% had severe disability, suggesting that most children with JIA have a somewhat good long-term prognosis for functional abilities. Baseline predictors of poor long-term functional outcome included age less than 7 years at disease onset, tender joint count (JC) >8, limited JC > 10, and an initial level of disability in either the mild-to-moderate or severe category. The authors suggest that children who fit this clinical profile might need more aggressive treatment to prevent disease progression and physical disability.[57]

The reported prognosis for ERA among studies is also inconsistent.[10] One study found the presence of HLA-B27, evidence of arthritis rather than arthralgia, and disease onset after 5 years of age predicted definite or possible SpA.[58] Two other studies reported a poorer outcome in SpA than either oligJIA or RF-negative polyJIA, and a similar outcome to RF-positive polyJIA.[59,60] Predictors of poor outcome included genetic risk factors for AS and ankle or hip arthritis in the first 6 months of disease.[59] Disease onset younger than 16 years is associated with more severe hip disease, unlike adults who demonstrate more severe spinal disease. The presence of HLA-B27 appears to be associated with older age at disease onset and an extended disease course within the first 3 years in boys.[61] Frequency of enthesitis increases during the disease course, and children must be monitored for subtle losses in joint motion and tissue extensibility in the thorax and lumbar spine.[62]

▶ Physical therapy examination and evaluation

Display 15.3 shows the components of the physical therapy assessment. A top-down approach, beginning with the child's activities and participation, allows the therapist to focus the physical examination on areas that most impact the child's participation in home, school, and community settings. The therapist must be alert to changes in joint mobility and integrity or loss of muscle bulk and strength that signal a disease flare or joint damage. The child's age, cognitive and emotional development must also be considered as well as the amount of support and resources available to the family.

Examination of Activities and Participation

The impact of JIA on a child's daily activities and participation depends on disease type, course, and severity. Lower extremity arthritis may cause difficulty in transitions from the floor to standing, community, and school ambulation, stair ascent/descent, and recreational activities. Children with disease onset at a young age may demonstrate subtle motor deficits, including impaired balance, coordination, agility, and speed.[63] Chronic arthritis, pain, and stiffness in the cervical spine and upper limbs may cause problems with

---

DISPLAY 15.3 Components of the Physical Therapist Examination in JIA

- Clinical observation
- Medical history
- Examination of the child's activities and participation in typical life settings (home, school, community) through standardized questionnaires, informal interview, or observation of child performing activities
- Examination of the child's gross motor skills for daily activities, play, and sports
- Systems review
  - Integumentary system
    - Examine skin for presence of rash, nodules
    - Examine nails for pitting, onycholysis
  - Musculoskeletal system
    - Joint status and integrity
    - Joint range of motion
    - Soft tissue extensibility
    - Muscle bulk
    - Muscle strength and endurance
    - Postural alignment
  - Cardiopulmonary system
    - Resting and exercise heart rate
    - Aerobic capacity or performance on field test
  - Multiple systems
    - Pain
    - Gait pattern and parameters
    - Postural control

basic activities of daily living (ADLs), handwriting, carrying books, and other instrumental ADLs.

The child's personality and drive to be independent, as well as the expectations of caregivers and friends impact the child's functional performance and adaptation to a chronic disease. Frequent disruptions to the child's school day as a result of visits to the nurse for medications or rest periods, and lateness and absence due to illness or medical appointments can negatively impact the child's education. Participation in physical education (PE) and sports may be limited or inconsistent owing to disease flares. Obtaining services to address these problems within the school setting can be difficult.[64]

Table 15.3 lists standardized measures used in JIA. Self- or parent- as proxy report questionnaires, including the Childhood Health Assessment Questionnaire (CHAQ), Pediatric Outcomes Data Collection Instrument (PODCI), and the Activities Scale for Kids (ASK) measure the child's capability (what he or she *was able to do*) during a defined period of time (e.g., previous 1 to 2 weeks). The ASK also measures the child's performance (what he or she *actually did* during the defined time period). Only one measure, the Juvenile Arthritis Functional Assessment Scale (JAFAS), assesses the child's functional capacity or what he or she actually does under standardized conditions.

The CHAQ is the most frequently used measure of disability in JIA and has been translated and validated in more than 40 languages.[65,66] The original CHAQ, shown in Display 15.4, targets children aged 1 to 19 years and includes 30 activities organized into eight categories. A child aged 9 years or older, or a parent as proxy for a younger child, may serve as the respondent who scores each statement based on how much difficulty (0 = no difficulty, 1 = some difficulty, 2 = much difficulty, 3 = unable to do) the child had in performing the task during the previous week. An item is scored as "not applicable" if the child is too young to perform the task. The highest scored item in each section dictates the score for that category; if the respondent reports needing an assistive device or assistance from another person to perform any task in that category, the minimum score for the category is 2. The global disability index (DI), calculated as the average of the eight category scores, has a range of 0–3, with higher scores indicating greater disability. Some studies employ a range of DI scores to categorize levels of disability: 0 = no disability, 0–0.5 = mild, 0.6–1.5 = moderate, and >1.5 = severe.[65] Dempster et al. found that a minimum decrease of 0.13 in the DI significantly correlated with a parent's assessment of clinical improvement in the child's functional abilities, while a minimum increase of 0.75 correlated with parents' assessment of decline in function.[67]

Pain intensity during the previous week is rated on a 15-cm VAS, anchored on the left side with a happy face and the words "no pain" and on the right side with a sad face and the words "worst pain." The discomfort index ranges from 0 to 3, with higher scores indicating greater pain. A second VAS is used to report overall health status, with higher scores indicating poorer health.

An important limitation of the CHAQ is its focus on disability rather than the entire spectrum of a child's physical function. With 0 as the best possible score, the CHAQ DI suffers from a ceiling effect whereby scores are often clustered at the lower end of the scale, making it less sensitive to subtle indicators of the child's true functional capability.

TABLE 15.3 Standardized Assessment Instruments in JIA

Level of ICF	Instrument	Outcome Measured	Reference
A&P, I	CHAQ	BADLs and IADLs, pain, overall health status	Singh et al., 1994[65,67,68]
A&P	ASK	BADLs, IADLs, play, transfers	Young et al.*
A&P, I	PODCI	BADLs and IADLs, pain, overall health status	American Academy of Orthopedic Surgeons (AAOS)§
A	JAFAS	BADLs, IADLs (observed performance of activities under standardized conditions)	Lovell et al., 1989[69]
A&P, I	JAQQ	BADLs, IADLs, pain, HRQOL	Duffy et al., 1997[70]
A&P, I	PedsQL	BADLs, IADLs, pain, HRQOL	Varni et al., 2002[71]
QOL	QOML scale	Overall and HRQOL	Gong et al.[72]
I	GROMS	Joint ROM	Epps et al., 2002[79]
I	pEPM-ROM	Joint ROM	Len et al., 1999[80]
I	JC-LOM	Joint ROM loss	Klepper et al., 1992[83]
I	JC-Swelling	Joint effusions	
I	JC-POM	Joint stress pain	
I	JC-T	Joint tenderness	

ICF, World Health Organization International Classification of Functioning, Disability, and Health; A, activity; P, participation; I, impairment; CHAQ, Childhood Arthritis Health Questionnaire; ASK, Activities Scale for Kids; PODCI, Pediatric Outcomes Data Collection Instruments; JAFAS, Juvenile Arthritis Functional Assessment Scale; JAQQ, Juvenile Arthritis Quality of Life Questionnaire; PedsQL, Pediatric Quality of Life Questionnaire; QOML, Quality of My Life Questionnaire; GROMS, Global Range of Motion Scale; pEPM-ROM, Pediatric Escola Paulista de Medicina Range of Motion Scale; JC-LOM, Joint Count-Limitation of Motion; JC-POM, Joint Count-Pain on Motion; JC-T, Joint Count-Tenderness; BADLs, basic activities of daily living; IADLs, instrumental activities of daily living; HRQOL, health-related quality of life.
*Available at: http://www.activitiesscaleforkids.com/
§Available at: http://www.aaos.org/research/outcomes/outcomes_peds.asp

DISPLAY 15.4   Health Assessment Questionnaire*

In this section, we are interested in learning how your child's illness affects his or her ability to function in daily life. Please feel free to add any comments on the back of this page. In the following questions, please check the one response that best describes your child's usual activities (averaged over an entire day) *over the past week*. If your child has difficulty in doing a certain activity or is unable to do it because he or she is too young but NOT because he or she is *restricted by arthritis*, please mark it as "Not Applicable." *Only note those difficulties or limitations that are due to arthritis.*

	Without Any Difficulty	With Some Difficulty	With Much Difficulty	Unable To Do	Not Applicable
Dressing and Grooming					
Is your child able to:					
• Dress, including tying shoelaces and doing buttons?	_____	_____	_____	_____	_____
• Shampoo his or her hair?	_____	_____	_____	_____	_____
• Remove socks?	_____	_____	_____	_____	_____
• Cut fingernails/toenails?	_____	_____	_____	_____	_____
Arising					
Is your child able to:					
• Stand up from a low chair or floor?	_____	_____	_____	_____	_____
• Get in and out of bed or stand up in crib?	_____	_____	_____	_____	_____
Eating					
Is your child able to:					
• Cut his or her own meat?	_____	_____	_____	_____	_____
• Lift a cup or glass to mouth?	_____	_____	_____	_____	_____
• Open a new cereal box?	_____	_____	_____	_____	_____
Walking					
Is your child able to:					
• Walk outdoors on flat ground?	_____	_____	_____	_____	_____
• Climb up five steps?	_____	_____	_____	_____	_____

*Please check any *aids* or *devices* that your child usually uses for any of the above activities:

Devices used for dressing (button hook,

_____ Cane   _____ zipper pull, long-handled shoe horn, etc.)

_____ Walker   _____ Built-up pencil or special utensils

_____ Crutches   _____ Special or built-up chair

_____ Wheelchair   _____ Other (specify: _____)

*Please check any categories for which your child usually needs help from another person *because of arthritis*

_____ Dressing and grooming   _____ Eating

_____ Arising   _____ Walking

	Without Any Difficulty	With Some Difficulty	With Much Difficulty	Unable To Do	Not Applicable
Hygiene					
Is your child able to:					
• Wash and dry entire body?	_____	_____	_____	_____	_____
• Take a tub bath (get in and out of tub)?	_____	_____	_____	_____	_____
• Get on and off the toilet or potty chair?	_____	_____	_____	_____	_____
• Brush teeth?	_____	_____	_____	_____	_____
• Comb/brush hair?	_____	_____	_____	_____	_____
Reach					
Is your child able to:					
• Reach and get down a heavy object, such as a large game or books, from just above his or her head?	_____	_____	_____	_____	_____
• Bend down to pick up clothing or a piece of paper from the floor?	_____	_____	_____	_____	_____
• Pull on a sweater over his or her head?	_____	_____	_____	_____	_____
• Turn neck to look back over shoulder?	_____	_____	_____	_____	_____

(continued)

Grip

Is your child able to:

- Write or scribble with a pen or pencil?   _____   _____   _____   _____   _____
- Open car doors?   _____   _____   _____   _____   _____
- Open jars that have been previously opened?   _____   _____   _____   _____   _____
- Turn faucets on and off?   _____   _____   _____   _____   _____
- Push open a door when he or she has to turn a doorknob?   _____   _____   _____   _____   _____

Activities

Is your child able to:

- Run errands and shop?   _____   _____   _____   _____   _____
- Get in and out of car or toy car or school bus?   _____   _____   _____   _____   _____
- Ride bike or tricycle?   _____   _____   _____   _____   _____
- Do household chores (e.g., wash dishes, take out trash, vacuum, do yard work, make bed, clean room)?   _____   _____   _____   _____   _____
- Run and play?   _____   _____   _____   _____   _____

*Please check any *aids* or *devices* that your child usually uses for any of the above activities:

_____ Raised toilet seat   _____ Bathtub bar

_____ Bathtub seat   _____ Long-handled appliances for reach

_____ Jar opener (for jars previously opened)   _____ Long-handled appliances in bathroom

*Please check any categories for which your child usually needs help from another person *because of arthritis*

_____ Hygiene   _____ Gripping and opening things

_____ Reaching   _____ Errands and chores

Pain

We are also interested in learning whether or not your child has been affected by pain because of his or her illness.

- How much pain do you think your child has had because of his or her illness *in the past week*? Place a mark on the line below to indicate the severity of the pain.

No Pain   Very Severe Pain

_____

0   100

Health Status

1. Considering all the ways that arthritis affects your child, rate how your child is doing on the following scale by placing a mark on the line.

_____

0   100

Very Well   Very Poorly

2. Is your child stiff in the morning?   _____ Yes   _____ No
   If YES, about how long does the stiffness usually last (in the past week)?   Hours/Minutes _____

*Adapted from Singh G, Athreya B, Fries JF, et al. Measurement of health status in children with juvenile rheumatoid arthritis. *Arthritis Rheum.* 1994;37:1761–1769.

Two revised versions of the CHAQ, the VAS$_{CHAQ-38}$ and the Cat$_{CHAQ-38}$ have been proposed by Lam et al. to address these problems.[68] Each contains eight additional items targeting more physically challenging tasks, eliminates the separate domains and the questions about aids or assistance, and calculates the DI as the simple mean of scores on all 38 items. Both versions provide the following instructions to the responder: "This section will ask you how well you were able to do activities on your own in the last week, compared with most other kids your age." In the VAS$_{CHAQ-38}$, the child responds by placing a mark on a 10-cm VAS anchored on the left end by the statement "Much worse than most other kids my age" and on the right side by "Much better than most other kids my age." The Cat$_{CHAQ-38}$ retains the original 0–3 scoring system of the CHAQ. Display 15.5 shows the additional eight items included in the revised versions.

The JAFAS is the only measure of physical capacity designed for children with arthritis.[69] The child is observed

---

DISPLAY

15.5 **Eight Additional Items Included in the CAT$_{CHAQ38}$ and the VAS$_{CHAQ38}$[68]**

1. I think I could have done climbing activities by myself.
2. I think I could have played team sports with others in my class.
3. I think I could have played some sports by myself.
4. I think I could have played team sports in competitive leagues.
5. I think I could have kept my balance while playing rough games.
6. I think I could have done activities I usually enjoy for a long time without getting tired.
7. I think I could have run a race.
8. I think I could have worked carefully with my hands.

---

and timed performing 10 common daily tasks (buttoning a shirt or blouse, putting on a shirt over the head, pulling on socks, cutting food with a knife and fork, getting in and out of bed, rising to stand from sitting on the floor, picking up an object from the floor, walking 50 feet, and walking up a flight of steps). The child's time to complete each task is compared with a criterion standard based on a healthy control group. Items are scored 0 if the time is equal to or less than the criterion, 1 if the time is more than the criterion, and 2 if the child is unable to complete the task. Administration and score takes 10 minute and requires minimal training and equipment. The scale and directions for administering the test are provided in the original paper.[69]

Several measures have been developed to assess health status and QOL in children with arthritis. Three of the most frequently used are the Juvenile Arthritis Quality of Life Questionnaire (JAQQ),[70] Pediatric Quality of Life Inventory (PedsQL) Rheumatology Module 3.0,[71] and Quality of My Life (QOML) Questionnaire.[72] The QOML questionnaire consists of two separate VAS that measure overall QOL and HRQOL in children and adolescents. The QOL scale asks, "Overall, my life is," and the HRQOL scale asks, "Considering my health, my life is." The respondent (child or parent as proxy) records their response to each question on the 100-mm VAS for each question stem; scoring ranges from 0 ("the worst") to 100 ("the best"). Patients and parents also complete a 5-point ordinal measure of change in QOL (much worse, somewhat worse, the same, somewhat better, much better) since the last visit. A study by Gong et al. reported the minimal clinically important difference (MCID) that indicates improvement was 7 mm for the overall QOL and 11 mm for the HRQOL scale. The MCID that indicated deterioration was −33 mm for QOL and −38 mm for HRQOL.[72]

Two norm-referenced assessments that may be useful in JIA include the Peabody Developmental Motor Scales–2 (PDMS-2) and the Bruininks-Oseretsky Test of Motor Proficiency-2 (BOT-2). The School Function Assessment (SFA)[73] and the informal school checklist shown in Appendix A can provide information on the child's function in school.

Examination of Body Structures and Functions

Joint Motion and Integrity

Figure 15.7 shows one format used for recording findings of a joint examination, including swelling or joint effusion, joint tenderness, stress pain, and limitation of motion.[74] The signs of active joint inflammation are swelling, tenderness, or stress pain. Limited joint motion alone does not indicate active disease, but may be the result of long-standing disease. Joint effusions are detected by demonstrating fluctuation of synovial fluid from one area of the joint to another (Fig. 15.8). In examining the fingers and toes, one should place the sensor fingers proximal to the base of the middle phalanx and dorsal to the collateral ligaments to detect movement of the synovial fluid. Small effusions in the knee joint can be detected by eliciting a bulge sign. This is done by stroking in an upward direction along the medial aspect of the joint to empty the synovial pouch, followed by stroking upward or downward on the lateral side of the joint while using the other hand to detect a bulge of fluid as the pouch refills. The joint is scored as normal if there is not a clear indication of effusion.

Firm pressure applied directly over the joint line may elicit joint *tenderness*. In active disease, tenderness felt by pressure over the joint line should be greater than that elicited by pressure on the bone adjacent to the joint. The amount of pressure applied to detect joint tenderness is about 20% less than that needed to cause pain when squeezing the triceps or lower calf muscles. To assess *stress pain*, the therapist moves the limb to the end of the available range and applies slight overpressure.

An examination of joint motion provides valuable baseline information about joint integrity and function. Asking the child to perform a series of functional movements directs the physical therapist's attention to problem areas. In very young children, active motion can be elicited by playing games like "Simon Says." If screening suggests pain or limited motion, standard goniometric measurement should be used. Checking accessory joint motions may help determine the cause of impaired joint dysfunction. Limited motion, pain, and crepitus suggest joint damage. Radiographs will show joint damage in long-standing arthritis; however, ultrasound is more sensitive in identifying subclinical disease.[75] Magnetic resonance imaging (MRI) is more sensitive than either a clinical exam or the core outcome variables to detect hip damage in JIA.[76]

Common patterns of joint impairments and subsequent activity restrictions in JIA are shown in Table 15.4. Although there is a bias toward arthritis in large joints, the small joints of the hands and feet are frequently involved in polyJIA. Hip arthritis occurs in 30% to 50% of children, primarily in those with an sJIA and polyJIA and often predicts greater disability.[48,77] Pain associated with hip disease is typically referred to the groin, buttocks, medial thigh, or knee. The child may exhibit a gluteus medius limp when walking due to pain or weakness. Hip flexion contractures occur subsequent to active joint inflammation as the child holds the joint in flexion to relieve pressure and pain. Hip contractures may also occur secondary to knee arthritis or an LLD.

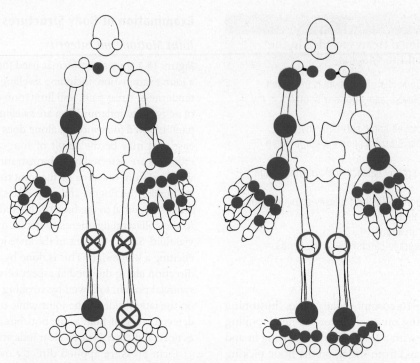

FIGURE 15.7 Example of the visual format used to record active joint count in a child with polyarticular disease. The left figure shows joints with an effusion (*solid circle*) or soft tissue swelling (*X*). The right figure shows joints with stress pain or tenderness (*solid circle*). (From Wright V, Smith E. Physical therapy management of the child and adolescent with arthritis. In: Walker J, Helewa A, eds. *Physical Therapy in Arthritis*. Philadelphia, PA: W. B. Saunders; 1996:211–244, with permission.)

The knee is the joint most often involved in oligoJIA, but knee arthritis is common in all disease types. Limited joint mobility, spasm of the hamstrings, and shortening of the tensor fascia latae (TFL) and iliotibial band (ITB) contribute to loss of knee extension and changes in postural alignment and gait. Chronic synovitis causes overgrowth of the femoral condyle, resulting in a valgus deformity of the knee. Shortening of the TFL and ITB exacerbate this impairment.

Ankle and foot arthritis occur in all JIA types, often resulting in limited dorsiflexion (DF) and subtalar motion. Although calcaneal eversion and forefoot pronation are common, many children exhibit a cavus forefoot and loss of subtalar eversion. Foot problems in polyJIA are underappreciated and have a significant impact on gait. Impairments include hallux valgus, hallux rigidus, hammer toes, and overlapping toes. Metatarsalgia and subluxation of the metatarsophalangeal (MTP) joints cause pain during stance and ambulation.

Arthritis in the shoulder girdle results in pain, restricted motion, and altered biomechanics in shoulder rotation, flexion, and abduction. Elbow flexion contractures are common, occur early in the disease course, and are often accompanied by limited forearm supination. Wrist arthritis is also seen in polyJIA with long-standing disease; the

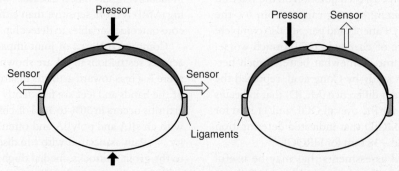

FIGURE 15.8 Two ways of detecting joint effusions. (From Smythe H, Helewa A. Assessment of joint disease. In: Walker J, Helewa A, eds. *Physical Therapy in Arthritis*. Philadelphia, PA: W. B. Saunders; 1996:129–148, with permission from H. Smythe, MD, FRC[C].)

TABLE

15.4   Common Patterns of Joint and Soft Tissue Impairments in JIA

Cervical Spine
- Most common in PoJIA and SoJIA
- Loss of extension, rotation
- Loss of normal lordosis
- May develop torticollis if asymmetric
- Chronic inflammation may lead to joint space narrowing with nerve root irritation
- Fusion of zygapophyseal joints—often occurs first in C-2–C-3 but may progress to other levels
- Dysplasia of vertebral bodies
- Instability of C-1–C-2 articulation may occur, but less common than in adult RA

Temporomandibular Joints
- Most common in PoJIA; less common in oligoJIA
- Restriction in opening mouth; pain on chewing
- Greater functional loss if cervical spine extension is limited
- Mandibular asymmetry if unilateral involvement
- Undergrowth of the mandible (micrognathia)
- Malocclusion of the teeth
- May require orthodontic treatment

Shoulder Complex
- Most common in PoJIA
- Limited glenohumeral ABD and MR noted first; limited shoulder flexion
- Shortening of pectorals and scapular abductors
- Overgrowth of humeral head with irregular shape
- Shallow glenoid fossa with increased risk of subluxation
- Functional loss increases if elbow and wrist arthritis is present

Thoracolumbar Spine
- Most common in ERA; sacroiliac arthritis common in JAS
- Motion may be limited by spasm of spinal extensors or short hip flexors
- Scoliosis secondary to long-standing LLD
- Kyphosis in association with neck and shoulder arthritis
- Excessive lumbar lordosis secondary to hip flexion contracture
- Long-term systemic steroid therapy contributes to osteoporosis, wedging vertebral bodies, small compression fractures

Hip
- Occurs in PoJIA and SoJIA; primary cause of disability
- Loss of extension, MR, and ABD
- Weakness of gluteus medius and deep hip LR; may cause Trendelenburg gait deviation
- Flexion contracture may be masked by increased lumbar lordosis
- May have marked pain on weight bearing; pain may be referred to groin, buttocks, medial thigh, knee
- Femoral head overgrowth
- Osteoporosis
- Limited weight bearing in young child contributes to poorly developed hip joint with shallow acetabulum and trochanteric growth abnormalities
- Lateral subluxation of femoral head, aggravated by short hip adductors
- Potential for protrusio acetabuli and AVN in persistent severe disease
- Potential for repair of articular cartilage with fibrocartilage during disease remission with improved weight bearing and mobility

Elbow
- Occurs in all types
- Involved early in disease course
- Loss of extension, forearm supination
- Overgrowth of radial head restricts ROM
- Proximal radioulnar joint involved
- Ulnar nerve entrapment possible

Wrist
- Occurs in all types; occurs early in disease course
- Accelerated carpal maturation
- Undergrowth of ulna; ulna may migrate dorsally
- Radial and intercarpal fusion
- Rapid loss of extension; shortening of wrist flexors; volar subluxation
- Wrist rests in flexion and ulnar deviation
- In older onset or RF-positive PoJIA, wrist may deviate radially
- Distal radioulnar disease causes loss of forearm pronation and supination
- Flexor tenosynovitis

Hand
- Involvement later in PoJIA and SoJIA than oligoJIA; small joints of hand least commonly affected in JAS
- Premature epiphyseal fusion and growth abnormalities
- MCP and CMC subluxation
- Flexor tenosynovitis
- Loss of MCP flexion, terminal extension
- PIP contractures more common than DIP
- Marked decrease in grip strength
- Boutonniere less common than swan neck deformities

Knee
- Most common joint involved early in all disease types
- Rapid weakness and atrophy of quadriceps, loss of patellar mobility
- Flexion contracture; may cause secondary hip flexion contracture
- Loss of hip flexion
- Overgrowth of distal femur contributes to LLD in unilateral disease
- Knee valgus aggravated by short hamstrings, TFL, and ITB
- Posterior tibial subluxation secondary to prolonged arthritis or aggressive stretching of shortened hamstrings
- Risk of femoral fracture associated with osteoporosis

Ankle and Foot
- Occurs in all disease types
- Altered growth causes bony changes in the tarsals, with potential for fusion
- Growth abnormalities due to early closure of epiphyses
- Early loss of ankle inversion, eversion; later loss of D-FL, Pl-FL, especially if standing and walking are limited
- Excessive hindfoot valgus or varus
- Excessive forefoot pronation or supination
- Loss of extension at MTP joints, with subsequent loss of push-off at terminal stance
- MTP subluxation
- Hallux valgus; hammertoes
- Overlapping of IPs
- Enthesitis at heel or knee is common in ERA

ABD, abduction; AVN, avascular necrosis; CMC, carpometacarpal; D-FL, dorsiflexion; DIP, distal interphalangeal; ERA, enthesitis-related arthritis; IP, interphalangeal; ITB, iliotibial band; JAS, juvenile ankylosing spondylitis; LR, lateral rotation; MCP, metacarpophalangeal; MR, medial rotation; MTP, metatarsal phalangeal; oligoJIA, Oligoarticular onset JIA; PIP, proximal interphalangeal; Pl-FL, plantar flexion; polyJIA, polyarticular onset JIA; RF-positive, rheumatoid factor positive; ROM, range of motion; sJIA, systemic onset JIA; TFL, tensor fascia latae.

Data in this table are summarized from Cassidy JT, Petty RE, eds. *Textbook of Pediatric Rheumatology*. 4th ed. Philadelphia, PA: W. B. Saunders; 2001. This listing is not inclusive, nor do all of the characteristics listed occur in every child with arthritis.

severity and pattern of deformity varies based on age and skeletal maturation. In disease onset at a young age, wrist subluxation and undergrowth of the ulna result in ulnar deviation. In those 12 years or older at disease onset, a pattern of radial deviation is more common. Persistent arthritis in the joints of the hands and tenosynovitis result in pain and limited motion in the carpometacarpal (CMC), metacarpophalangeal (MCP), and proximal interphalangeal (PIP) joints.

Joint motion can be recorded in standard chart format or on the stick figure shown in Figure 15.7. Specific goniometric measurements should be used for initial and follow-up physical therapist examinations. Therapists should be familiar with several standardized scales used in clinical studies to measure joint motion, although these are rarely used in clinical settings. The Articular Severity Index (ASS) scores global LOM for each joint, averaged for right and left sides, includes using an ordinal scale (0 = no LOM; 1 = 1% to 25% LOM; 2 = 26% to 50% LOM; 3 = 51% to 75% LOM; 4 = 75% to 100% LOM) to record joint motion.[78] The Global Range of Motion Score (GROMS) includes all joints and provides a single score for global joint motion in children with arthritis.[79] A reduced 10-joint GROMS includes only those joints weighted by experts as essential for function and most often involved in JIA. The Pediatric Escola Paulista de Medicina Range of Motion (PEPM-ROM) scale includes 10 joint movements judged to be most often involved in children with arthritis and most important for essential functions.[80]

Muscle Structure and Function

Impairments in muscle structure and function are documented in children and adolescents with JIA. In the acute stage, muscles supporting affected joints show protective spasm and may be hyperreactive to stretch, although their ability to support the joint is diminished. Periarticular muscle atrophy and weakness are more evident in subacute and chronic disease. Factors contributing to these impairments include the production of pro-inflammatory cytokines, alterations in anabolic hormones, abnormal protein metabolism, high resting energy metabolism, and pain-induced inhibition of motor unit activity.[14,45,46] Early onset and persistent disease impair muscle development near inflamed joints but also in distant areas that may persist even after clinical remission.[47–50,81–90]

Common patterns of weakness include hip extension and abduction, knee extension, ankle plantar and DF, shoulder abduction and flexion, elbow flexion and extension, wrist extension, and grip. Weak ankle musculature negatively impacts gait in JIA.[33,81,83] Brostrom et al., using a custom-built isokinetic dynamometer to measure ankle strength, found that girls with JIA had 40% less plantar flexion (PF) and 50% less DF strength compared with age- and sex-matched healthy controls.[33] The ratio of PF to DF strength was similar in both groups, suggesting the disease affects both muscle groups equally. Children with JIA also perform poorly on standardized measures of trunk flexor strength compared with age, sex, and size-matched healthy controls and age- and sex-based norms.[83]

Two recent studies examined anaerobic capacity in JIA. van Brussel et al. reported 94% of their sample (N = 62, ages 7 to 16 years) had significantly lower mean and peak anaerobic capacity (65% and 67%, respectively) compared with predicted values.[84] Deficits were larger in girls and were found in children in clinical remission off meds as well as those with active disease. The largest impairments were in children with RF-positive polyJIA. Children with oligoJIA did not differ significantly from predicted values. Lelieveld et al. confirmed these findings in older adolescents. Strong negative correlations between anaerobic capacity, physical function, and overall well-being suggest that higher muscle fitness contributes to feeling better and being able to perform daily activities with less difficulty.[85]

Muscle bulk, strength, and endurance should be assessed at the initial and follow-up visits. Measures of limb circumference (calf and thigh) document any asymmetries in muscle bulk and changes over time. Manual muscle tests (MMTs) can be used to measure isometric strength in older children, but reliability is questionable for grades above 3 (fair). Handheld or isokinetic dynamometers provide more objective and reliable measures of strength in children with arthritis.[88–90] Figure 15.9 shows a modified blood pressure cuff used as an alternative to a commercial handheld dynamometer. The rolled cuff is placed distally as far as possible on the limb without crossing a painful joint. The tester applies pressure to the cuff with a flat hand. The patient pushes against the cuff, while the tester increases pressure

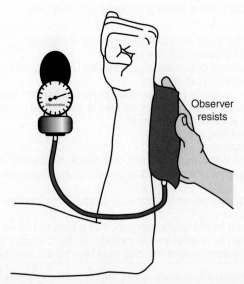

FIGURE 15.9 Use of modified blood pressure cuff to measure isometric triceps strength. (From Walker J, Helewa A, eds. *Physical Therapy in Arthritis.* Philadelphia, PA: W. B. Saunders; 1996: 129–148, with permission from H. Smythe, MD, FRC[C].)

gradually for 5 seconds. Grip strength can also be measured by having the child squeeze the cuff.[74]

Measures of dynamic strength in functional muscle group provide information about the child's daily activities. Special attention is given to the antigravity muscles and those known to be weak in children with arthritis. In very young children, strength is estimated by observing age-appropriate motor skills. In older children, strength can be assessed using free weights to determine the repetition maximum (RM) for a muscle group. A 6 to 10 RM (maximum weight the child can lift through the available ROM, using proper form, for 6 to 10 repetitions) is a sufficient measure of strength to establish a baseline, determine a training protocol, and evaluate progress.[91] Isometric testing performed at multiple joint angles provides an estimate of dynamic strength and may indicate weakness at specific points within the ROM. Muscle endurance is measured by having the child perform as many repetitions as possible, lifting a specified percentage, usually 60% to 80%, of the 6 or 10 RM. Tests of strength and endurance are performed on different days to avoid fatigue. A warm-up light activity precedes testing.

Aerobic Capacity and Performance

A large body of evidence shows that aerobic fitness is lower in children with JIA than in healthy peers (Display 15.6).[84–87,92–94] In a recent study, van Brussel et al. measured peak oxygen uptake (VO_{2peak}) during a progressively graded exercise test on a cycle ergometer.[84] VO_{2peak} was significantly reduced (75% of predicted values for healthy controls) in 95% of their sample of 62 children with JIA, aged 6.7 to 15.9 years. Lelieveld et al. confirmed their findings in a sample of adolescents with JIA, aged 16 to 18 years.[85] These studies support an earlier meta-analysis that indicated mean VO_{2peak}/kg body mass was 22% lower in children with JIA compared with age- and sex-matched healthy controls and reference values.[92] In one of the studies reviewed, Giannini and Protas also reported children with JIA had a lower peak workload and peak heart rate (HR_{peak}) during exercise and shorter exercise time than matched controls.[93] Heart rate during submaximal exercise was also higher in children with

JIA, suggesting that they work at a higher percentage of their peak exercise capacity than healthy children. This may partly explain the fatigue frequently reported by children with JIA.

Performance-related field tests have also been used to estimate aerobic fitness in children with chronic arthritis. Klepper et al.[83] reported that children with polyJIA scored significantly lower on the 9-Minute Walk–Run Test than healthy matched controls. Unlike the controls, many children with JIA were unable to maintain a steady running pace. Test scores did not correlate significantly with active JC or articular severity score (ASS), suggesting performance may have been limited by other impairments, including low aerobic and muscular fitness, low motivation, or inexperience in distance or timed run tests.

The cause of impaired aerobic fitness is most likely multifactorial. Physiologic factors related to the disease process, including pain, mild anemia, and poor mechanical efficiency that results from muscle atrophy, weakness, and joint stiffness, can impact the child's willingness and ability to be active. These impairments particularly impact children who develop JIA at a very young age and those with persistent active disease. However, there is also evidence that hypoactivity, whether secondary to disease symptoms or a sedentary lifestyle, contributes to poor fitness. Several studies of school-age children found that neither active JC nor the ASS were significantly correlated with aerobic fitness.[83,89,93] However, studies using the JIA classification system and the PRINTO criteria for disease activity and remission report differences in aerobic fitness based on sex and disease type, although not on disease activity. The largest deficits in VO_{2peak} were found in girls and children with RF-positive polyJIA, while no impairment was found in children with oligoJIA.[84,85] Significant deficits were seen in children whose disease was in clinical remission off medications as well as those with active disease. It appears that aerobic fitness in JIA does not improve without direct intervention despite improvement in disease status.

Aerobic fitness should be assessed prior to the child's participation in a physical conditioning program. Test results can guide intervention and help to monitor the child's response to overall management of the disease. Recent work by Takken et al. reported a significant and strong correlation ($r = 0.95$, $p < .001$) between peak workload (W_{peak}) and VO_{2peak} in children with JIA during a progressive exercise test on a cycle ergometer.[95] This suggests that VO_{2peak} can be predicted from W_{peak}, weight, and gender using the equation:

$$VO_{2peak} \text{ (L/min)} = (0.008 \times W_{peak} \text{ [Watts]}) + (0.005 \times \text{weight [kg]}) + (-0.138 \times \text{gender [1=male, 2 = female]}) + 0.588$$

Alternately, simple inexpensive field tests like the 1-mile or 9MRW provide an indication of the child's aerobic performance compared with published age- and sex-based health fitness criteria. The 6-minute walk test (6MWT) is another performance-related test developed to assess aerobic fitness in adults with severe cardiopulmonary disease, but increasingly used to assess functional walking capacity

DISPLAY 15.6	Comparison of Physiologic and Performance Variables in Children with and without Arthritis
Variable	**Children with Arthritis Compared with Healthy Children**
Peak VO_2	↓
Peak heart rate (HR_{peak})	↓
Submaximal HR	↑
Peak workload	↓
Peak anaerobic power	↓
Performance-based fitness	↓
Muscle strength and bulk	↓

in healthy children as well as those with limited mobility or chronic health disorders. In this test, the child is told to walk continuously back and forth along a straight path to cover as much distance as possible in 6 minutes. Standard guidelines for test administration have been published by the American Thoracic Society (ATS).[96] Reference values or prediction equations for the 6MW distance (6MWD) in healthy children living in the United States have been published.[97] Lelieveld et al. found a low correlation between 6MWD and VO_{2peak} in children with JIA, indicating that the test is not a good surrogate measure of VO_{2peak} in this population.[98] However, another study reported that children with JIA worked at 80% to 85% of their peak VO_2 and HR during the test, indicating it is an intensive submaximal exercise test in children with JIA.[99] Post-walk HR can be used to determine exercise intensity for an aerobic training program.

Pain

Acute pain occurs in active arthritis and during some routine medical procedures. Chronic pain is common despite improvement in medical control of the disease.[100] Anthony and Schanberg found that a high percentage of children with JIA reported pain during clinic visits, many rating pain intensity in the higher range of the measurement scale.[101] Data on 462 children from the Cincinnati Juvenile Arthritis Databank indicated that 60% of children reported pain at disease onset, 50% had pain at 1-year follow-up, and 40% reported pain 5 years later.[102] Pain is especially common in polyJIA and significantly impacts daily activities. Schanberg et al. studied 41 children who completed daily diaries over a 2-month period to assess disease symptoms and function.[103] More than 60% reported having pain, described as "sharp," "aching," "burning," and "uncomfortable," on most days; 31% rated their pain as severe. Symptoms were significantly associated with decreased participation in school and social activities. Pain is often associated with sleep disturbance, fatigue, and lower QOL.[104]

The source of chronic pain in JIA is multifactorial. Children with JIA appear to have a lower pain threshold and tolerance compared with healthy peers. One cause may be prolonged activation of peripheral and central nociceptive systems, resulting in changes in pain processing and increased sensitivity to noxious stimuli.[105–107] Other factors that may contribute to a child's rating of pain include family pain histories, fluctuations in mood, stressful events, coping mechanisms, and overall health status.

Pain assessment should be comprehensive and ongoing, and include a pain history, self-report for children over the age of 4 years, parent report, and behavioral observations. In very young children, the therapist should be alert for pain behaviors validated in JIA, including bracing, guarding, rubbing, rigidity, and flexing.[108] Display 15.7 lists self-report instruments that are useful in young children, including the Oucher, Wong-Baker Faces Pain Rating Scale, and the Poker Chip Tool.[109–111] The child can also indicate pain distribution

DISPLAY 15.7	Pediatric Pain Assessment Instruments Useful in Children with JIA
Instrument (References)	**Description**
Oucher Scale[109]	• Ages 3–12 years • Measures pain intensity • Includes six faces and a scale from 0 to 100, from happy to very sad, scored as 0–5
Faces RatingScale[110]	• Suitable for children aged 3 years and older • Scale includes six faces from happy to very sad, scored as 0–5; record face number child chooses • Child chooses face that best represents current feeling • Measures pain intensity and affect
Poker Chip Tool[111]	• Four red chips each representing a "piece of hurt" • Measures intensity from 1 piece to 4 pieces of hurt • Used for 3- to 4-year-olds • Correlates with Oucher

and intensity on a body map using different colors to represent levels of pain intensity (Fig. 15.10). Children at least 5 years old can report pain intensity on a numeric scale, a word graphic rating scale, or a VAS. The Varni/Thompson Pediatric Pain Questionnaire (PPQ) is a comprehensive pain

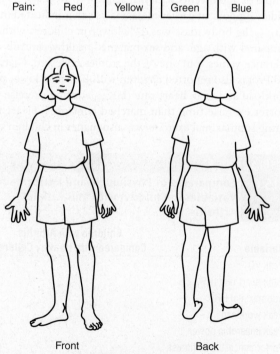

Pain: | Red | Yellow | Green | Blue |

Front   Back

FIGURE 15.10 Example of a body outline figure and rating scale used to assess pain intensity and location in children.

assessment with both child and parent reports; however, because of its length, it is used primarily in research.[112]

Growth and Postural Alignment

Height, weight, body composition, and posture should be included in the initial and follow-up physical therapy assessment to monitor the effects of the disease on growth and skeletal alignment. Potential problems include a forward head posture, kyphosis, excessive lumbar lordosis, scoliosis, lower limb flexion contractures, genu valgus, and ankle and foot deformities. Torticollis may occur in children with asymmetric cervical spine arthritis.

Leg length differences may cause pelvic obliquity and the appearance of a scoliosis in standing. Leg length should be examined in supine, measuring from the anterior superior iliac spine (ASIS) to the medial malleolus. The length of the femur and tibia should be measured separately if the child has a hip or knee flexion contracture. When differences are found, recheck spinal alignment after placing small lifts of known thickness under the shorter leg to level the pelvis. Mobility of the lumbar spine should be examined in children with ERA using the modified Schober test (Fig. 15.11). With the child standing, with feet together and pointing forward, draw a line between the two dimples of Venus to mark the lumbosacral junction. Place a mark on the spine 5 cm below and 10 cm above this line and measure the distance between the two marks. The increase in distance between the marks from baseline to a position of maximum forward flexion is used as an indicator of spinal mobility. An increase of less than 6 cm is considered abnormal. Assessment of sitting posture is also important to determine potential causes of muscle pain and fatigue during functional activities. Habitually sitting in a "slumped" posture characterized by a posterior pelvic tilt, thoracic kyphosis, and forward head position contributes over time to shortening of the anterior chest muscles and over-lengthening of scapular stabilizers, resulting in limited and/or painful shoulder motion during reaching and other upper limb activities.

Gait

Gait deviations in children with JIA are not uncommon.[82,113–115] Their gait pattern is often described as "cautious." Compared with healthy controls, children with JIA demonstrate decreased gait speed, cadence, and shorter step and stride length. Kinematic deficits include increased anterior pelvic tilt throughout the gait cycle, decreased peak hip extension at terminal stance, hip abduction during stance, peak knee extension at the end of single limb support, increased ankle DF throughout the gait cycle, decreased PF at initial contact, push-off, and throughout the swing phase. Data on ground reaction force during gait in JIA indicate lower heel-strike and push-off force.[115]

Positive changes in gait kinematics and muscle function following IA steroid injections in children with JIA support the belief that pain, stiffness, muscle weakness, and impaired joint mobility contribute to their gait deviations.[33,114] Hartmann et al. speculated that limited hip extension and ankle PF at the end of stance may contribute to shortened step length in children with JIA and recommend intervention aimed at reducing these impairments and improving joint mobility.[115] Foot pain and deformities from long-standing arthritis also negatively impact gait pattern and activities. Dekker et al. found strong associations between foot-related impairments (active disease, limited joint motion, and pain), activity limitations, and participation restrictions in 31 of 34 children with JIA.[116] The mean age of the sample was 12.4 ± 3.7, 76% had polyJIA, and median disease duration was 1.5 years. Using the Juvenile Arthritis Foot Disability Index (JAFI), 88% of participants reported some foot problems, 82% reported activity limitations, and 62% reported some restrictions in school and social participation related to foot impairments. These findings reinforce the need for standard screening for foot-related impairments in JIA.[117]

Observational gait assessment using a standardized recording form can provide useful information. The child should be observed walking with and without shoes, although walking barefoot is often painful for some children. The gait symmetry, step and stride length, and alignment of the lower limb at heel strike, mid-stance, terminal stance, and swing are noted. Data from an instrumented gait mat provide a permanent record of the child's gait pattern. A low-cost alternative is footprint analysis using craft paper and painting the soles of the child's feet.[118] Velocity and cadence can be calculated by timing the walk. A video of the child's gait provides a permanent record and is useful to monitor change. A full assessment should include walking on level surfaces, inclines, stairs, and curbs, and while running. Use of any assistive devices for mobility should be noted.

▶ Evaluation, diagnosis, prognosis, and plan of care

The ICF provides a framework to help the physical therapist synthesize findings from the examination and medical history, identify priority problems, formulate hypotheses about the causes of those problems, and develop treatment goals

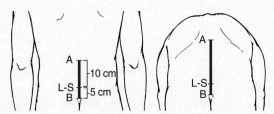

FIGURE 15.11 The modified Schober test of lumbar spine mobility. (Modified from Oatis CA. *Kinesiology: The Mechanics and Pathomechanics of Human Movement.* Baltimore, MD: Lippincott Williams & Wilkins; 2004.)

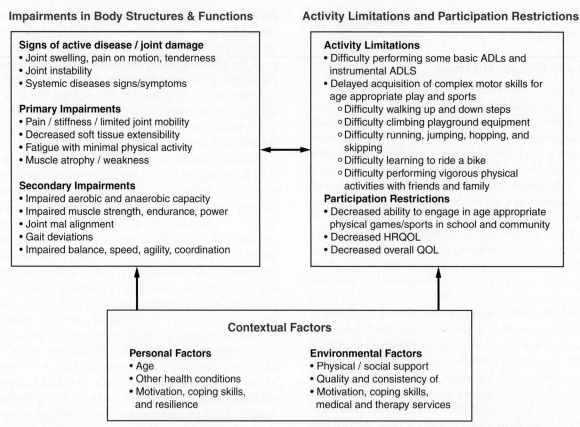

Impairments in Body Structures & Functions

Signs of active disease / joint damage
• Joint swelling, pain on motion, tenderness
• Joint instability
• Systemic diseases signs/symptoms

Primary Impairments
• Pain / stiffness / limited joint mobility
• Decreased soft tissue extensibility
• Fatigue with minimal physical activity
• Muscle atrophy / weakness

Secondary Impairments
• Impaired aerobic and anaerobic capacity
• Impaired muscle strength, endurance, power
• Joint mal alignment
• Gait deviations
• Impaired balance, speed, agility, coordination

Activity Limitations and Participation Restrictions

Activity Limitations
• Difficulty performing some basic ADLs and instrumental ADLS
• Delayed acquisition of complex motor skills for age appropriate play and sports
  ◦ Difficulty walking up and down steps
  ◦ Difficulty climbing playground equipment
  ◦ Difficulty running, jumping, hopping, and skipping
  ◦ Difficulty learning to ride a bike
  ◦ Difficulty performing vigorous physical activities with friends and family

Participation Restrictions
• Decreased ability to engage in age appropriate physical games/sports in school and community
• Decreased HRQOL
• Decreased overall QOL

Contextual Factors

Personal Factors
• Age
• Other health conditions
• Motivation, coping skills, and resilience

Environmental Factors
• Physical / social support
• Quality and consistency of
• Motivation, coping skills, medical and therapy services

FIGURE 15.12 The therapist synthesizes the examination findings and information from the medical history and interview with the parent and child, analyzes the data, and formulates hypotheses regarding the relationship between disease status, impairments, and activity limitations. BADLs, basic activities of daily living; HRQOL, health-related quality of life; IADLs, instrumental activities of daily living; QOL, quality of life.

(Fig. 15.12). Disease type and course, current and anticipated problems, as well as personal and environmental factors are considered. Because few studies provide strong evidence for the effectiveness of any particular interventions, the physical therapist must often draw from literature in other areas to determine the best interventions.

 Intervention

Display 15.8 lists overall goals of intervention in JIA. Treatment must be appropriate for the child's age, cognitive, and psychosocial development. Physical activities and exercise must be graded on the basis of disease activity and severity. Developmentally based play can be useful to encourage young children to be active; however, joints with active disease or limited motion require direct attention.

Coordination, Communication, and Documentation

Coordination of services and communication among individuals providing care for the child can be challenging. Often children with JIA receive disease-specific care from a pediatric rheumatology team in a tertiary clinic that may be several hours from the child's home. The clinic physical therapist may perform the initial evaluation and develop a POC with the child and family. Children with well-controlled disease who have no serious physical impairments often receive a home exercise program (HEP), with suggestions for managing disease symptoms and participating in age-appropriate activities. Those who require ongoing or periodic physical therapist may receive services in their home, a local clinic, or school. Working with the family, the community or school therapist can obtain information from the rheumatology team about the child's diagnosis, disease status, medications, and precautions. The clinic nurse is often in the best position to facilitate communication among health care providers. Periodic physical therapist progress reports help the rheumatology team monitor the child's response to medical therapies, physical function, and adherence to exercise recommendations. Therapists can find forms to guide an initial history and physical examination and to document follow-up in the book "Occupational and Physical Therapy for Children with Rheumatic Diseases: a clinical handbook" by Kuchta and Davidson. (Display 15.9)

15.8   General Goals of Physical Therapist Intervention

Reduce impairments in body structures and functions
- Maintain/improve joint range of motion
- Maintain/improve muscle bulk, strength, and endurance
- Maintain/improve health-related fitness
  - Reduce fatigue, improve stamina for physical activity
  - Reduce postural deviations/improve postural alignment

Maintain/improve child's activities and participation in the home, school, and community
- Basic and instrumental ADLs
- Functional mobility
- Gross motor skills for age-appropriate play, recreational activities, and sports
- Provide information and support to the child and caregivers
- Provide information on the effects of arthritis on the body systems
- Explain the benefits of daily exercise and provide clear instructions and illustration
- Provide information to help the child manage pain and stiffness
- Consult with school personnel to ensure child's full participation
- Assist child and family to set achievable and meaningful goals
- Encourage child and caregivers to actively participate in medical and therapy regimen

Procedural Interventions

Pain Management and Comfort Measures

The first line of intervention to manage pain in JIA is adequate disease control using one or more of the systemic medications preciously discussed. IA steroid injections are effective in reducing inflammation, pain, and swelling in individual joints. Children with chronic pain despite adequate disease control may benefit from non-pharmacologic treatments that provide temporary relief, give the child and parent some control over disease symptoms, and potentially increase adherence to exercise recommendations. A warm bath or shower can reduce morning stiffness. Exercising in a warm pool relieves pain and improves mobility. However, superficial or deep heat applied directly over inflamed joints is contraindicated because locally applied heat increases IA temperatures and may increase activity of cartilage-degrading enzymes.[119,120] In contrast, locally applied cold decreases IA temperature and is used to reduce joint pain and muscle spasm.[121] Cold along with rest, ice, compression, and elevation (RICE) applied immediately after an injury reduces inflammation, swelling, and pain. Placing a dry or damp warm towel between the cold source and skin allows the cold to penetrate slowly without stinging.

Balanced rest and exercise are necessary to manage pain and maintain joint mobility and function. Studies suggest children with JIA have decreased pain after participating in water- or land-based exercise programs.[122,123] Restorative sleep is also essential for adequate pain management as

15.9   Resources for Children with Arthritis, Their Families, and Arthritis Health Professionals

Organizations
Arthritis Foundation (AF)
  1330 West Peachtree Street
  Atlanta, GA 30309
  1-800-238-7800
  www.arthritis.org

Juvenile Arthritis (JA) Alliance
This virtual community of parents, volunteers, health professionals, and anyone affected by JA is connected through the AF website and provides resources and opportunities for members to connect and share with others. An annual national conference brings together families and health professionals for education and recreation.
http://www.arthritis.org/juvenile-arthritis.php

American College of Rheumatology/Association of Rheumatology Health Professionals
The Association of Rheumatology Health Professionals (ARHP) is a multidisciplinary section of the ACR that provides education and resources to all health professionals caring for individuals with rheumatic diseases. Educational products and programs include the slide collection, online rehabilitation case studies, and training programs. The Annual Scientific Meeting brings together international researchers, clinicians, and educators with the purpose of sharing the latest research and clinical information related to the care of children and adults with rheumatic disease. The Pediatric Rheumatology Symposium (PRSYM) occurs every 3 years and is dedicated exclusively to the needs of pediatric rheumatology clinicians and researchers.
www.rheumatology.org

(continued)

15.9   Resources for Children with Arthritis, Their Families, and Arthritis Health Professionals *(continued)*

Camps
Several state AF chapters sponsor summer residential camps for children with arthritis or other rheumatic diseases. Contact your local AF chapter for information.

Arthritis Foundation Exercise Programs and Videos
Arthritis Foundation Exercise Program (land-based)
Aquatic Exercise Program—warm water exercise program
Take Control with Exercise—Thera-Band Combo
Tai Chi (DVD)

Water Exercise Programs for Children
The National AF, in conjunction with the national office of the YMCA, developed a recreational aquatic program for children with JA. Contact the local AF chapter for information.

Range-of-Motion Exercise Program for Young Children
This video uses a story to engage young children in ROM exercises to maintain joint and soft tissue flexibility.
Carmen D.
Scottish Rite Hospital for Children
2222 Welborn
Dallas, TX 75219

Publications for Parents and Children

Raising a Child With Arthritis: A Parent's Guide
Arthritis Foundation, 2008

Kids Get Arthritis Too Newsletter
Arthritis Foundation periodic publication

Your Child with Arthritis—A Family Guide for Caregiving
Authors: Tucker Lori B., DeNardo Bethany A., Stebulis Judith A., Schaller Jane G. Baltimore: John's Hopkins University Press, 1996

It's Not Just Growing Pains
Author: Thomas J. A. Lehman, MD: Oxford University Press, 2004

The Official Patient's Sourcebook on Juvenile Rheumatoid Arthritis
A Revised and Updated Directory for the Internet Age
Editors: James N. Parker, MD
Philip M. Parker, PhD
ICON Health Publications, 2002
ICON Group International, Inc.
4370 La Jolla Village Drive, 4th Floor
San Diego, CA 02122

Publications for Clinicians
Kutcha G, Davidson I. Occupational and Physical Therapy for Children with Rheumatic Diseases: a clinical handbook. New York: Radcliffe Publishing 2008
http://www.radcliffehealth.com/shop/occupational-and-physical-therapy-children-rheumatic-diseases-clinical-handbook.

---

poor sleep and fatigue negatively impact daytime function.[104,124] Simple measures to improve sleep and reduce morning stiffness include performing active ROM exercises before bed, using a sleeping bag to maintain body warmth during the night, and wearing resting splints to support joints in a functional position. Stretch gloves provide gentle compression and may relieve wrist and hand stiffness and pain. A cervical pillow helps reduce neck pain. One study found that children who received a massage by a parent before bed reported less pain and stress than control subjects.[125]

Cognitive-behavioral techniques, such as progressive muscle relaxation (PMR), meditative breathing, hypnosis, guided imagery, electromyographic (EMG) biofeedback, and modification in pain behaviors, may help the child manage pain. Reductions in self-rated pain intensity and expression of pain behaviors have been reported in children who participate in pain management programs that included PMR, EMG biofeedback, meditative breathing, and guided imagery.[126,127] Distraction and imaginative play are useful in young children. Children with severe pain may require a multidisciplinary pain program.

Surgery and Postoperative Physical Therapy

Well-timed selective surgical procedures can relieve pain and restore joint health and function in young children when conservative measures have failed. Older children with joint damage may require reconstructive surgery to relieve pain and restore function. The decision to perform surgery is made by an interdisciplinary team on the basis of an analysis of the risks and benefits. The physical therapist is involved in the preoperative assessment and planning, as well as the postoperative rehabilitation.

Soft tissue releases (STRs) are performed to manage joint contractures that are unresponsive to conservative measures. Reduced IA pressure and increased joint mobility improve joint nutrition and healing of the articular cartilage by fibrocartilage. The most common procedures include adductor and psoas tenotomies to reduce hip flexion contracture, ITB fasciotomy, hamstring lengthening, and posterior capsulotomy to relieve knee flexion contracture. Postoperative care is aimed at preserving muscle length and joint motion through splinting and ROM exercise. After STR at the hip, the joint is positioned in an abduction and extension splint; following STR for knee flexion contractures, the joint is positioned in extension. However, immobilization is kept to a minimum to avoid further loss of motion, and ROM exercises begin within the first 48 hours unless there are problems with wound healing. Gait training begins as soon as possible. Strengthening exercises can begin when soft tissue inflammation resolves. To maintain ROM following discharge, the child must lie prone for periods during the day and avoid prolonged sitting. The use of splints may be discontinued after about 8 weeks, but the child must continue physical therapy for several months to achieve optimal results.

Supracondylar osteotomy may be performed in conjunction with STRs for a severe flexion contracture at the knee or when there is a valgus deformity and evidence of joint damage. An arthrotomy is usually done at the same time if there is a poorly formed or overgrown patella that is fixed to the femoral condyle, limiting joint motion.[128] Postoperatively, the leg is immobilized in a cylindrical cast with immediate weight bearing. The cast is removed when there is evidence of adequate bone union.

Synovectomy is rarely performed in JIA because of the risk for postoperative pain and spasm and poor long-term results. However, the procedure may be done in combination with STRs to treat hip flexion contractures. It may also be done arthroscopically for acute synovitis of the knee, when effusion and overgrowth of inflamed synovium stimulate the adjacent epiphysis, resulting in lengthening of the limb.[128] Tenosynovectomy may be indicated in a child with severe hand arthritis to prevent tendon rupture or reduce nerve entrapment from synovial proliferation.

Arthrodesis may be considered when a child has disabling pain and a high risk for natural joint ankylosis, for example, in advanced arthritis of the wrist, interphalangeal joints, ankle or subtalar joints. Postoperative care includes immobilization in a cast, exercise, and positioning of adjacent joints to maintain mobility. After lower limb surgery, the child is allowed to stand and walk with crutches or walker. Immobilization continues until there is radiographic evidence of successful fusion. Epiphysiodesis, or temporary surgical arrest of the growth plate, may be useful in some children with bony overgrowth leading to LLD.[129]

Children with irreversible joint damage may be candidates for total joint arthroplasty (TJA). Several factors are considered in the decision to perform TJA in a child with JIA, including the child's age, skeletal maturity, physical status, upper limb function, and the potential ability of the child and family to complete the lengthy and intensive postoperative rehabilitation. Ideally, surgery is delayed until the epiphyses have fused or there is little chance of further growth of the limb, although TJA may be necessary in younger children who have severe joint damage, disabling pain, and loss of function.[130] Custom-designed hip prostheses that are porous are typically used to accommodate the smaller bones in children with JIA and allow for biologic fixation, because cemented prostheses are more susceptible to loosening after several years. Timing of procedures is extremely important in a child who requires multiple joint replacements. In children with severe upper limb arthritis, fusion of a damaged or painful wrist may be necessary first to allow the child to use crutches after hip or knee surgery. When hips and knees must be replaced, the hip joints are usually done first. Both hips are replaced at the same time if there is severe bilateral hip damage.[131]

Preoperative physical therapist includes a conditioning program to improve strength, ROM and general stamina, and gait training with crutches or walker. The child and parent also receive instruction in postoperative precautions to protect the implant during daily activities. Postoperative care for total hip arthroplasty (THA) is influenced by the surgical approach and type of implant used. Protected weight bearing for several weeks is required for an uncemented implant. With a posterior surgical approach, the child progresses from walking with crutches or a walker to a cane. To protect the abductor muscles after an anterior lateral approach, the child must use an assistive gait device for 6 to 8 weeks and avoid active hip abduction for 12 weeks.[132] The postoperative program includes active ROM exercises with precautions to avoid hip flexion past 90 degrees, adduction past neutral, and internal rotation. A foam abduction pillow is used for 6 weeks, alternating with a CPM (Continuous passive motion) machine and prone positioning. Submaximal isometric exercises of the hip extensors and abductors and quadriceps may be started early. The child must also practice transfers and ADLs. Elevated toilet seats and dressing aids are used to help the child maintain hip precautions. Gait training with an assistive device can begin during the first week. Active exercise in shallow water and ambulation in chest-deep water may begin as soon as wound healing is complete. Hip precautions are usually maintained for the first two to three postoperative months, although this may vary based on the surgeon. Activities that cause high-impact loading on the lower limbs should be avoided.

Total knee arthroplasty (TKA) is usually done using a cemented prosthesis, and may be accompanied by STRs to resolve a flexion contracture, release of the lateral retinaculum to prevent further valgus deformity, and resurfacing of the underside of the patella. Postoperative therapy begins with ROM exercises on day 2. A CPM machine can be used immediately, with an extension splint worn at other times. Prone positioning is also encouraged to preserve knee extension. The goal is to achieve knee ROM from full extension to 100 degrees of flexion. A program to strengthen lower extremity musculature is begun with isometric and straight leg–raising exercises. Aquatic exercise and stationary cycling, using a range limiter on the pedal to control the amount of knee flexion, may also be used. Full weight bearing, using a knee immobilizer, is begun on the second postoperative day. Ambulation without assistive devices is allowed when the child demonstrates at least 90° of knee flexion and adequate lower extremity strength and endurance. Parvizi et al. studied long-term clinical outcome of TKA in 13 children (25 knees) with JIA using the Knee Society Score (KSS) that measures pain and function; each scale has a maximum of 100 points, with higher scores indicating less pain and improved function.[130] The KSS for pain improved from 27.6 preoperatively to 88.3 at the last follow-up period, 10.7 years after surgery. Scores for function improved from 14.8 preoperatively to 39.2 at follow-up. The overall arc of knee flexion also improved from a mean of 70 degrees to 81 degrees at follow-up.

The most common complications with THA include infection, dislocation, and biologic loosening of the components, especially with cemented THA. Improved outcomes have been reported for non-cemented procedures in children with JIA, even in those with active disease and in children as young as 12 years at the time of surgery.[133] Outcome from TJA may be complicated by several factors in children with JIA, including smaller bones, extent of osteoporosis, and presence of skeletal malalignment. Also, significant periarticular changes prior to the TJA may cause difficulty in regaining full ROM in the involved and adjacent joints. Additional procedures may be necessary to improve long-term outcomes, including STRs, soft tissue transfers, and correction of skeletal deformities.

Exercise

Daily exercise is essential to maintain joint health, remediate impairments, and achieve health-related physical fitness (HRPF). Display 15.10 illustrates the components of a physical conditioning program that is graded to accommodate disease activity. Specific exercise recommendations are reviewed below.

DISPLAY 15.10 Recommendations for Staging Physical Activity and Exercise in JIA

	Disease State		
Exercise type	**Acute disease**	**Subacute and chronic disease**	**Inactive disease/Clinical remission on/off medications**
ROM/flexibility	Daily AROM or AAROM of all active joints and adjacent joints • 1–2 reps, 1–2 times/day	Daily AROM of all active joints and adjacent joints • 1–2 reps 1×/day • Active flexibility exercise • Modified yoga poses	Daily AROM of all active joints and adjacent joints
Aerobic activity	Balance rest for active joints with low-intensity, low-impact PA to maintain physical stamina, reduce load on inflamed joints • Exercise in warm pool • Tricycle or bicycle	Increase weight-bearing PA to promote bone health and lower limb muscle strength • Walking, low-impact dance • Use joint supports, splints, orthoses as recommended	Accumulate 60 min/day of moderate-to-vigorous PA • Aerobic dance, "step" aerobics, Tai chi, biking, swimming, jumping rope*
Neuromuscular training • Minimize muscle atrophy Muscle strength • Muscle endurance • Muscle power • Neuromuscular control • Proprioception • Postural control • Coordination • Agility • Speed	One set of 1–6 repetitions of *submaximal* isometric muscle contractions performed at multiple points within the available pain-free ROM (performed several times/day) • One rep includes "ramp" up contraction for 2 s, hold for 6 s, "ramp" down for 2 s • 20s rest between reps	Dynamic exercises • Must be able to perform 8–10 reps against gravity with good form and without pain before adding resistance • Use functional movements • To ⇑ muscle endurance, perform 15–20 reps with no added resistance • Use light weights, 0.5–2.5 Kg; (bottles filled with water or sand, handheld or cuff weights, elastic bands)	Resistance Training • Determine starting weight based on a 6–10 RM or targeted number of reps • Include closed chain activities to promote bone health and improve proprioception Include coordination, speed, and agility drills to promote motor skills for safe age-appropriate physical play and sports

Range-of-Motion Exercise and Stretching

Techniques to preserve or increase joint mobility and soft tissue extensibility include ROM exercise, positioning, and splinting. All joints with arthritis and adjacent joints should be moved through the available range for three to five repetitions, preferably twice a day. Active ROM (AROM) is optimal to preserve muscle function as well as joint mobility. Active assisted ROM (AAROM) is used when the child is unable to perform AROM. Passive ROM is avoided during active disease to prevent overstretching and tissue trauma. Games that elicit functional limb and trunk movement patterns are useful in very young children.

Daily positioning in prone for at least 30 minutes allows a low-load prolonged stretch on hip and knee flexors. The child can lie prone on a bed or other firm surface with legs extended and feet hanging off the edge. A pillow placed under the abdomen keeps the pelvis level, while a small rolled towel placed under the forehead positions the cervical spine to accommodate limited neck rotation. Commercial or custom-made resting splints can support inflamed joints, maintain proper joint alignment, and apply a gentle low-load stretch on the soft tissues. Figure 15.13 shows custom-made resting splints for the hands and knees. A posterior "shell" keeps the knee extended and maintains hamstring length during the night; this may reduce stiffness and allow the child to stand more easily upon arising.

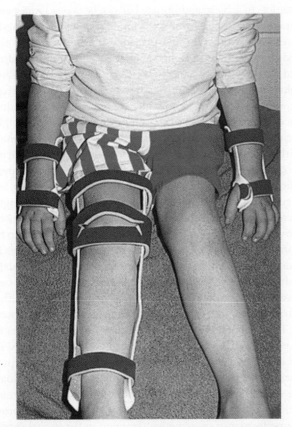

FIGURE 15.13 Custom-made resting splints for the hands and knees.

Gentle manual stretching to lengthen shortened soft tissues can begin once arthritis is under adequate control. Although there is little evidence for the effectiveness of any specific stretching regimen in JIA, research in adults indicates that holding a static stretch at the end of available ROM for 30 to 60 seconds is needed to increase muscle extensibility.[134] This may lengthen tissues prior to placing the limb in a splint. Neuromuscular stretching techniques that promote autogenic or reciprocal inhibition of shortened muscle, including contract-relax, agonist contraction, and a combination of both, are useful in treating limited joint motion. The amount of resistance applied varies according to the child's tolerance.

Stretching techniques and ROM exercises must be graded according to disease status of individual joints. It is important to gain the child's cooperation to minimize pain and reflex muscle spasm. Soaking in a warm bath prior to stretching facilitates relaxation and tissue extensibility. Aggressive passive stretching is avoided because of the risk for damage to epiphyseal areas at the tendon–bone interface. Using a long lever arm when stretching stiff hamstrings may cause posterior subluxation of the tibia. Stretching is always combined with active exercise to encourage active use of the muscles in their new resting length and to actively use the joint throughout the new ROM.

Radiologic assessment is necessary to examine available joint space and rule out ankylosis prior to instituting any program to reduce joint contractures. Conservative approaches that provide a static progressive low-load stretch include serial splints or casts and dynamic splints. Custom-made serial splints are convenient because the therapist can mold and modify the splint as needed to accommodate the child's ROM. However, because these splints can be easily removed, their effectiveness depends on the child's adherence. In contrast, serial casts require a considerable amount of time and skill to apply and cannot be modified, but also cannot be removed by the child. Protocols vary across clinics; however, typically the child wears the cast for 48 to 72 hours, after which it is removed and bivalved. During the next 1 to 2 weeks, the cast is worn for 18 to 24 hours a day, removing it only for exercise sessions. Active exercise in a warm pool helps the child move the joint in its new ROM. If the child still has limited joint mobility, a new cast is applied, and the process is repeated until full functional ROM is achieved.[135]

Commercially available dynamic splints can be ordered to fit specific joints. The tension can be controlled by the physical therapist and set to patient tolerance. Figure 15.14 shows a brace with a dial-lock knee joint that allows the physical therapist to adjust the degree of extension as the child gains motion. Most patients will tolerate a dynamic splint for 1-hour periods during the day. However, this type of splint is not generally used on a joint with acute arthritis.

Exercise to Improve Muscular Performance

The evidence supporting strength training in JIA is limited to several small nonrandomized studies. These suggest that children with medically controlled arthritis can

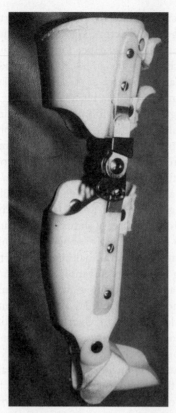

FIGURE 15.14 Example of a dial-lock knee joint.

improve muscle function through individualized progressive resistance training, with no exacerbation of disease symptoms.[136–138] Oberg et al. found increased quadriceps strength in children with JIA following a 3-month program of combined land and water exercise twice a week for 40 minutes.[136] A study by Fisher et al. published only in abstract form, reported significant improvements in quadriceps and hamstring strength and endurance, contraction speed, and performance of timed tasks following an 8-week (3×/week) program of isokinetic strength training in 19 children with JRA, aged 6 to 14 years.[137] The regimen was individualized and progressed based on the child's initial tests and response to training. Muscle function in controls who did not exercise declined during the same period.

Specialized neuromuscular training has also been shown to be effective in improving neuromuscular control. Myer et al. described such a program in a single case study of a 10-year-old girl with quiescent oligoJIA who wished to return to competitive basketball.[138] The regimen included treadmill walking to improve symmetry in lower limb muscle function, progressive core and lower limb strengthening to improve postural control and kinesthesia during jumping and landing. Resistance bands used during multidirectional movements simulated unanticipated challenges during games and practice sessions. Outcomes included improved control in single limb stance, improved lower limb symmetry during gait and landing, and improved isokinetic strength ratio between lower limb flexors and extensors.

Strengthening exercises target muscles supporting joints with arthritis, although any specific deficits identified during the assessment must be addressed. Exercise mode and total volume are graded to the child's age, disease status, condition of individual joints, and current muscle function. During active disease, the main concern is to maintain muscle bulk, strength and endurance, prevent deformities, and help the child maintain normal daily activities. Isometric exercise is used when movement is painful. Resistance can be provided manually or by a stable external object, nonelastic webbing, or heavy elastic bands placed close to and proximal to the joint. Prolonged maximal isometric contractions are avoided because this may increase the IA pressure and constrict blood flow through the exercising muscles.[139] The child can be taught to regulate intensity by first contracting the muscle maximally, then letting go slightly and holding a submaximal contraction for about 6 seconds, exhaling during the contraction, and inhaling during the relaxation phase. EMG biofeedback may help the child isolate the muscle group and learn to regulate the intensity of the contraction. Because strength gains with isometric exercise are specific to the joint angle, isometric contractions should be performed every 15 degrees to 20 degrees throughout the ROM. Five to ten repetitions daily may be sufficient to maintain muscle strength.[140]

Dynamic resistance exercise is initiated once the disease is under medical control and the child can move the limb against gravity for 8 to 10 repetitions without pain.[140] Training includes concentric and eccentric contractions and attempts to achieve appropriate balance between agonist and antagonist muscle groups. To increase dynamic strength, external resistance can be provided by the weight of the body part, light free weights, or elastic bands. Young children and those with musculoskeletal impairments should use lighter weights and perform two to three sets of 10 to 15 repetitions of each exercise to build strength and muscle endurance. Exercise intensity is based on the amount of weight the child can move through the ROM for 6 to 10 repetitions without discomfort, maintaining proper exercise form. Progression is determined by the child's performance at periodic reassessment. If elastic bands are used, lighter bands are used first, progressing to more resistive bands as strength increases, provided there is no joint pain or other signs of active disease. Resistance training twice a week appears to be sufficient for healthy prepubertal children to achieve gains in muscle strength.[91] However, children with JIA may benefit from shorter sessions three times a week, with a day or two between sessions for recovery. Training sessions begin with a warm-up of light aerobic activity and end with a cooldown.

The prescription should include diagrams of all exercises to be performed. A useful resource is the Quick-Fit for Kids (SPRI Products, Inc., Buffalo Grove, IL) that includes clear, reproducible diagrams and instructions for each exercise. Goals are established in collaboration with the child and parent, including increasing strength, reducing fatigue, and improving performance of activities. Training in functional movement patterns increases transfer of strength gains to everyday activities. Periodic reassessment of the child's activity performance provides information about the impact of training.

Aerobic Conditioning

A 2008 Cochrane review found only three published RCTs (Randomized control trial) that investigated the effects of aerobic training in JIA.[141] These studies compared land-based physical therapy with combined water and land-based exercise, aquatic training versus standard medical care, and high-intensity land-based exercise to qigong, a form of gentle relaxation program similar to Tai chi.[124,142,143] All three studies reported that there were no adverse effects from exercise, but none found significant improvement in VO_{2peak} following aerobic training. Possible reasons cited by the authors included low exercise frequency, insufficient intensity, poor adherence to center-based sessions or failure to perform home exercise. However, several non-randomized studies found significant improvements in other indicators of aerobic function, including higher distance run scores (land-based exercise), lower submaximal VO_2, increased exercise time (water, combined water, and land exercise), and decreased time to HR recovery (water). Most studies also report decreased disease signs and symptoms following training. Several review papers that provide an overview of exercise studies and recommendations for children with rheumatic diseases may be useful to clinicians in planning an exercise program for this population.[144–147] According to the literature, the recommendation for children with JIA who have impaired aerobic fitness is to train at least twice a week at an intensity of 60% to 85% of HR_{max} for 45 to 60 minutes per session for at least 6 to 12 weeks.[144] Children who cannot tolerate a 30-minute session can begin with frequent short bouts of activity, increasing duration as their endurance improves. The child can monitor exercise intensity by counting pulse rate for 6 to 10 seconds, using a portable HR monitor, or estimating the exercise intensity on a rating of perceived exertion (RPE) scale.

The specific exercise mode appears to be less important than the intensity, duration, and frequency. However, weight-bearing exercises should be encouraged to maintain or improve bone density. A 2007 review of eight randomized trials reported improved bone density in healthy children following repeated impact activities (jumping rope) performed two to three times a week for 8 to 16 weeks.[148] Sandstedt et al. recently found a similar response in a controlled trial of children with JIA, aged 8 to 21 years.[149] Subjects were randomly assigned to a physical exercise (N = 33) or control (N = 21) group. The exercise program consisted of 100 two-footed jumps with a rope, core exercises, and upper body strength training (3 sets of 10 repetitions with a load of 0.5 to 2 kg) three times a week for 12 weeks. Twenty-eight of the 33 participants completed the exercise program without difficulty with a 70% adherence rate. Bone mineral density increased significantly in the exercise group compared with the control group after 3 months. A recent study by van Brussel et al. suggested that anaerobic training (high-intensity interval training) might be as useful as aerobic exercise for children with JIA.[150] The suggested exercise set is 15 bouts (15 to 30 seconds/bout) of "all-out" cycling sprints with 1 to 2 minutes of active rest (cycling with low resistance) between bouts. A single training session could include three to five bouts with active rest periods of 5 minutes between sets. The authors caution that this type of physical training has not been studied in JIA; however, improvements in fitness and physical function have been reported in children with other chronic conditions.

Activities to improve proprioception, postural control, and coordination should be incorporated into the program. Teaching the child proper exercise form at the beginning of a training program and frequent monitoring are essential. Pain reported by the child should be carefully assessed for specific cause. Delayed-onset muscle soreness may occur early in the program but should resolve with time. Overuse injuries accompanied by joint swelling and pain should be treated with cold, elevation, and rest, and the exercise program should be modified to reduce potential injuries. Several exercise programs developed by the Arthritis Foundation (AF) for adults may be suitable for older children with JIA (Display 15.10). Some commercial exercise videos for healthy children may be useful in JIA; however, the physical therapist should review programs to determine their suitability for a child with JIA. Physical therapists can also develop an individualized exercise video for the child's use at home. We currently use two videos developed at our center to provide a general conditioning program for children with JIA.

Maintaining an Active Lifestyle: Recreation and Sports

Multiple studies report that children and adolescents with JIA engage in less vigorous PA and fewer organized sports than their healthy peers.[87,94,151–153] Significant associations between PA level and VO_{2peak}, but not with disease activity, suggest a possible cause–effect relationship that provides direction for intervention.[152,153] The Center for Disease Control and Prevention (CDCP) recommends 60 minutes of moderate-to-vigorous physical activity (MVPA) on most days of the week for all children to achieve and maintain optimal health. These recommendations apply to children with JIA, although the type and intensity of activity may need to be graded to the child's disease status and physical abilities. Low-impact activities like swimming, walking, dance, modified yoga, Tai chi, and cycling are the most appropriate choices when a child has active arthritis in weight-bearing joints. Bicycles can be adapted to lessen the stress to lower limb joints by setting seat height so the knee is at an angle of 10 degrees to 15 degrees of flexion when the child's foot is at the apex of the downstroke.[154] Exercise in a heated (88° to 92°F) pool is recommended throughout the year for children who have limited or painful mobility on land. Cooler pool temperatures (82° and 86°F) are more suitable for aerobic exercise.

Sports become more important as children reach school age. Safe and successful participation depends on the child's motor competence as well as physical stamina. Several studies report delayed motor development in young children with JIA.[64,155] The most recent, by van der Net et al. (2008), examined motor development and functional skills in preschool age (PSA) and early school-age children (ESA) with JIA, using standardized norm-referenced tests.[156] They found 45% of the PSA group, all with polyJIA, scored more than 2 standard deviations (SD) below the mean on the Bayley Scales of Infant Motor Development. Mean score for the ESA group on the Movement Assessment Battery for Children was within the normal range; however, 12% had severe delay and 20% were at risk for developmental delay. Functional skills assessed on the Pediatric Evaluation of Disability Inventory indicated that 70% of the ESA group scored greater than −2 SD on the mobility scale, suggesting that motor skill deficits become more evident as the demands for motor competence increase. Poor motor skills may limit a child's ability to participate in age-appropriate sports and contribute to a child's feelings of being less physically competent than their peers.

School-age children should be encouraged to participate in PE class. The therapist can consult with the instructor to adapt activities for the child. Somersaults and headstands should be avoided to prevent injury to the cervical spine.

Children with wrist and hand arthritis should avoid weight bearing on the hands. Children with mild-to-moderate arthritis can participate in sports without disease exacerbation; however, high-impact loading on inflamed or damaged joints should be avoided.[156] Sports with a high potential for collision, including football, hockey, and boxing, should be discouraged. Figure 15.15 illustrates a flow chart the physical therapist can use to determine whether the child's preferred sport or recreational activity is a good "fit" for his or her physical abilities and motor skills. The activity should be analyzed to determine its collision or contact potential, demands for aerobic and muscular work, ROM, and neuromuscular skill. An exercise program designed to remediate specific problems may decrease the child's risk for injury. If the child chooses to play on a sports team, coaches should be made aware of the child's diagnosis and safety considerations, and allow occasional breaks from play during practice and games. The physical therapist can develop a preseason and in-season conditioning regimen if none exists.

Self-care Activities

A primary goal for the child with JIA is to achieve independence in age-appropriate activities in all environments. The

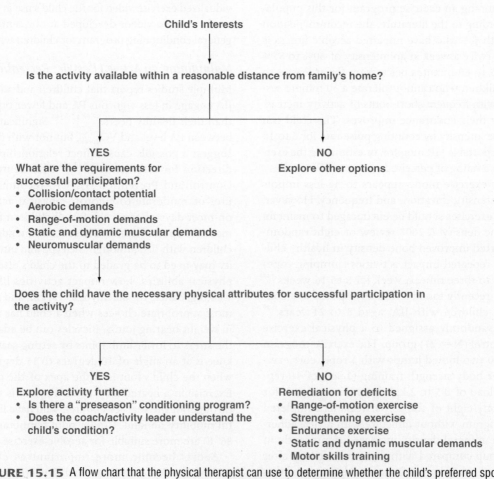

FIGURE 15.15 A flow chart that the physical therapist can use to determine whether the child's preferred sport or recreational activity is a good "fit" for his or her physical abilities and motor skills.

emphasis in young children is on basic ADLs and motor skills for play. Although these skills remain important, older children become more interested in sports and other social activities. Independence for an adolescent or young adult may revolve around the ability to drive, socialize with friends, and acquire a job.

The role of the therapist is to: (1) assess the child's functional abilities using one of the standardized assessments described previously, (2) provide education and direct training in self-care activities, mobility, and motor skills, (3) suggest appropriate assistive devices, environmental modifications, and adaptive equipment, and train the child in their use, and (4) consult with school personnel and suggest adaptations to the child's educational program. A child with minimal physical limitations may only need advice about the most efficient method of performing tasks, whereas a child with severe limitations may need instruction in the use of adaptive equipment or environmental modifications to promote independence. Dressing and hygiene aids that may be useful include Velcro closures on clothing and shoes, elastic shoelaces, a dressing stick, a buttonhook, a long-handled shoehorn, and a bath brush. Built-up handles on grooming items, eating utensils, and drawing and writing implements allow the child to be independent in these activities. The child with limited neck extension may need to use a straw to drink from a glass.

Parents and children need information on joint protection to reduce pain, muscle fatigue, and potentially deforming mechanical forces on vulnerable joints during activity. Children should use large joints to perform tasks when possible, because they tolerate stress better than the small joints. For example, the child can carry large objects on the forearms instead of grasping them with the hands, and use a backpack positioned close to the body's center of gravity or a rolling backpack to hold schoolbooks. Diagrams, demonstration, and practice of joint protection techniques may improve adherence.[157] Functional wrist and hand splints may decrease pain with grasping, gripping, or manipulative activities. Splints may also be useful in minimizing deforming mechanical forces during hand use.

Simple modifications in the home can increase a child's independence. These include replacing traditional doorknobs and faucets with levers, using a raised toilet seat, and installing safety bars in the bathtub or shower and additional handrails in stairways. The child should also have easy and safe access to the bathtub, toilet, and sink. More substantial modifications may be needed if a child uses a wheelchair within the home, including widening doorways and adding a ramp or wheelchair lift at the entrance to the house.

Functional Mobility

Continued weight bearing and walking are necessary to increase bone density, improve muscle strength, and prevent contractures for a child with JIA. Standing, cruising, and walking should be encouraged at the expected age. Young children should walk within the home and outside play area and for short distances in the community. Shoes should fit well and provide cushioning and support to the joints of the foot. High heels, platforms, and wedges are discouraged because they place added stress on the ankles and feet and increase the risk of falling. Sneakers with a flexible sole, good arch support, and deep heel cup are often a good choice for most children. A shoe with a wide, deep toe box may be needed for children with foot deformities such as hallux valgus, hammer toes, or claw toes. An off-the-shelf full-length shoe insert or metatarsal pad may alleviate pressure and pain on weight-bearing joints; however, a study by Powell et al. supports the use of custom-made foot orthoses for children with active ankle and foot arthritis.[158] They randomly assigned 40 children, aged 5 to 19 years, with arthritis in the ankle, subtalar, and/or metatarsal joints to one of three intervention groups: custom-made semirigid orthotics with shock-absorbing functional posts; prefabricated off-the-shelf show inserts made of 1/8-inch flat neoprene; or supportive athletic shoes with a medial longitudinal arch support and shock-absorbing soles worn alone. All children received new athletic shoes at the start of the study. Outcome measures at baseline and after 3 months of intervention included self-reported pain (1-cm VAS), 50-m walk time, the self-administered Foot Function Index (FFI) that measures pain, activity limitations, and disability, and the Physical Functioning Scale of the PedsQL. Assessors were blinded to group allocation. Children in the custom-made orthotics group showed significantly greater improvement in overall pain, walking speed, all subscales of the FFI, and physical functioning compared with the other two groups.

Careful assessment of the lower quarter, with emphasis on the foot and ankle, should be done to determine the orthotic prescription. Assess ROM at the ankle and subtalar and midtarsal joints, and the toes. Deformities that impact fit and comfort of shoes include hammer toes, claw toes, overlapping toes. Examination of the child's shoes and sole of the foot helps identify pressure points from weight bearing or improper alignment. Palpation of the foot can also locate problems such as tenosynovitis, enthesitis, or plantar fasciitis. The type of orthosis varies based on whether the deformities are fixed or flexible. Flexible deformities may be managed by an orthosis that holds the joint in good anatomic alignment. Fixed deformities require accommodative orthoses. For example, a patient with hallux rigidus, with loss of great toe extension, may need a metatarsal bar added to the sole of the shoe to create a mechanical means of rolling over in gait.

Few children with JIA require an assistive device for ambulation; however, when changes in gait pattern are observed, or the child refuses to walk, the cause should be determined and addressed immediately. LLD, found most often in children with oligoJIA, should be corrected within a quarter inch to prevent postural compensations, such as knee flexion of the longer limb, pelvic obliquity, or scoliosis. A child with pain or weakness in one leg can use a cane on the opposite side to unload the involved limb. A walker may be necessary for a child who has significant bilateral lower limb impairments. Platform attachments can be added for the child who also has limited upper limb motion, although this is rarely necessary.

Some children will need to use wheeled mobility for long distances in school or the community to preserve energy. Tricycles or bicycles with training wheels are good options for young children. Older children can use a lightweight sports wheelchair or powered scooter to move around their school, college campus, or community. Some children with upper extremity arthritis find it easier to maneuver the wheelchair with their feet. The child should be encouraged to get out of the wheelchair often during the day, standing and walking as tolerated to preserve muscular function and prevent contractures. Powered wheelchairs are generally reserved for children with severe disability.

Issues Related to School Participation

Frequent absences due to illness or medical appointments, or decreased attention because of pain, stiffness, and fatigue can cause problems in school performance.[159,160] The school checklist (Appendix A) can be used to identify school-based problems. The physical therapist can provide information to school personnel about the potential impact of JIA on school performance, and suggest adaptations to the educational program. Accommodations might include a second set of books for home, adapted writing tools, laptop computer for taking notes, and an easel-top desk for a child with cervical spine arthritis. Modifications in the child's schedule may be necessary, including visits to the nurse for medications or rest periods during the day and allowing the child to stand and move periodically to prevent stiffness from long periods of sitting, and using an elevator for transitions between floors.

Some schools provide these services and modifications voluntarily, but a formal evaluation by the school and development of an IEP (Individualized Education Plan) may be necessary. Children with arthritis may qualify for related services under the Individuals with Disability Act (IDEA) or under Section 504 of the Vocational Rehabilitation Act. Educational and vocational counseling is beneficial for adolescents and should begin no later than age 16 years to prepare for the transition to postsecondary education or work.[161]

Patient and Family Education and Support

The demands placed on the family when a child is ill can be overwhelming. Successful management of JIA depends to a great extent on the ability of the child and caregivers to manage the medical and therapeutic regimen. The therapist plays an important role in helping parents and the child to understand the effects of the disease and the benefits of medication, exercise, and other therapeutic procedures. Educational materials for families should be culturally appropriate and in the parent's preferred language. Materials for children should be appropriate to the child's cognitive and emotional development. Display 15.10 shows resources for children with arthritis, their families, and health professionals who care for them. HEPs should be individualized to target the child's needs and limited to no more than seven simple exercises, requiring 20 to 30 minutes. The book *Raising a Child with Arthritis: A Parent's Guide* provides illustrations and instructions for ROM and postural exercises.[162] Exercises can be incorporated into daily activities for young children. Older children should be encouraged to express their personal goals and participate in developing the exercise program. Periodic reassessment and progression of the exercise prescription provide encouraging feedback to the child and parent.

The effectiveness of treatment is highly dependent on adherence to the plan by the child and caregivers. Studies indicate that adherence to medications is higher than for exercise and is associated with lower disease activity. Moderate-to-high adherence to exercise is associated with better physical function, lower pain, and parental perception of global improvement. Parental adherence to exercise appears to be higher for younger children. Lack of time and failure to see the benefits of the prescribed activities contribute to lower adherence to exercise in older children and adolescents.[163-165] Active participation in managing the child's health care may be enhanced when both parent and child understand the effects of the disease and benefits of medication, exercise, and other therapeutic procedures.

Transition to Adult Healthcare

Effective self-management of health care needs becomes especially important in late adolescence because estimates indicate that only 30% to 60% of adolescents with JIA enter adulthood with their disease in clinical remission and many continue to report pain and activity limitations as a result of their JIA. Hilderson et al. followed 44 patients with JIA, who were older than 16 years of age, had left pediatric care, and did not participate in a structured program of transitional care (PTC). The majority of patients (56.8%) who had persistent disease and associated activity limitations were still in specialized rheumatology care, 13.6% were followed by a general practitioner, and 29.6% were no longer in medical follow-up. Of this latter group, 16.7% had disabilities and 42% reported persistent pain. The authors stress the need for interdisciplinary care programs throughout follow-up of children with JIA and structured transition from pediatric to adult health care.[166] A multicenter study by McDonagh et al. supports the use of an individualized PTC designed to reflect the developmental stages of adolescence. They found significant improvement in adolescent and parent ratings of HRQOL, arthritis-related knowledge, and satisfaction with rheumatology care. Although not statistically significant, improvements were also found for independent health behaviors (managing medications and independent medical consultations) in the 12-month assessment.[167]

Older children and adolescents who participate in setting goals and making decisions about their own health care feel a greater sense of control. A study by Stinson and colleagues described how adolescents developed effective self-management skills through a dual process that included "letting go" by adults who manage their health care and "gaining control" of managing their own illness.[168] Common subthemes expressed by participants included "knowledge and awareness about the disease, listening to and challenging care providers, communicating with the doctor, managing pain, and managing emotions."[168] Adolescents universally agreed on the need for more information and believed that web-based interventions could improve accessibility to this information. A study by Lelieveld et al. supports this belief. They found that an internet-based program directed at children with JIA, aged 8 to 12 years, who had low daily PA, was safe, feasible, and effective in improving PA levels, endurance, and adherence to PA recommendations.[169]

SUMMARY

This chapter presents information on the heterogeneous disorders included under the umbrella term JIA. These conditions are classified on the basis of signs and symptoms during the first 6 months after disease onset, although the exact diagnosis may not be clear for some time. Seven disease types are recognized: systemic, RF-negative polyarthritis, RF-positive polyarthritis, oligoarthritis-persistent, oligoarthritis-extended, ERA, and PsA. An eighth category, *undifferentiated*, includes disease signs and symptoms that do not fit into any one or fit into more than one specific disease type. Although the exact etiology of JIA is not entirely understood, great strides continue to be made. Most children with JIA do well with early diagnosis and appropriate medical treatment to manage the inflammatory process. However, some with severe and persistent disease experience significant impairments, including joint pain and swelling, limited ROM, and muscle atrophy and weakness. Secondary impairments in aerobic fitness and exercise tolerance are common and may contribute to activity limitations and participation restrictions. The long-term prognosis depends on the child's age at disease onset, disease type and course, and the quality and consistency of health care. The goal of management is for the child to lead as normal a life as possible. Physical therapists play an important role on the multidisciplinary team to help the child and family achieve this goal.

CASE STUDIES

CASE STUDY 1 **Sara** Sara is a 13-year-old girl with RF-negative polyJIA of 8 years' duration. After several years of mild disease activity, Sara presents with swelling in multiple joints, most notably both knees and the right ankle. She complains of pain and morning stiffness lasting 30 to 60 minutes and neck pain during the day. She lives with her parents, an older brother, and sister and is in the eighth grade at a local public school.

Medical History
Sara was diagnosed with polyarticular JIA at 5 years of age. Her parents stated signs of the disease, including stiffness and irritability upon awakening, "bumps" on her elbows and shins, and altered gait pattern, were evident for at least a year before the diagnosis. At her first visit to the pediatric rheumatologist, she had active disease in most extremity joints and the cervical spine. Rheumatoid nodules were found on the extensor surface of the ulna and tibial crest bilaterally. She was originally treated with naproxen; however, after 6 months, during which she continued to have active disease, MTX given orally once a week was initiated. Signs of systemic disease were not evident at this time.

During the next several years, Sara continued to have disease flares in both knees, both hips, and the right ankle that were managed by IA steroid injections. Following each injection, she reported significant pain relief and was able to return to her normal activities. At the age of 11 years, Sara's JIA was determined to be in clinical remission on medication. However, her disease flared 6 months ago, with increased joint pain, morning stiffness, and fatigue that affected her school attendance and participation in PE and sports.

Current Complaints
Sara is seen in clinic today to review her medications and HEP. She takes her MTX, but misses at least 30% of the prescribed dose of naproxen each week. She admits to poor adherence to the HEP, stating it doesn't help. According to Sara's mother, she has missed school or been late at least once a week for several months owing to disease symptoms. She does not meet the school's PE or sports requirement because of her JIA. She receives Physical therapy and Occupational therapy once a week in school and several accommodations under a 504 plan. These include lockers at either end of the school, a set of books for home, laptop computer for class notes, extra time for written exams, and excuse from PE when she is unable to participate. Sara is also not bound by the school's attendance policy.

The rheumatologist confirmed that Sara has active arthritis in both of her wrists, knees, and right ankle. Active and PROM is limited in the cervical spine, wrists, hips, right knee, and ankle; she has deformities of the toes in both feet. He added ETN once a week to Sara's medication regimen, continuing the once/weekly MTX and naproxen twice/day. IA steroid injections were scheduled for her next visit in 1 week, and she was referred to physical therapist for an evaluation and review of her HEP, and to OT for revision of her wrist splints and suggestions for adaptive equipment to improve her hand function. Sara was also referred to the child life specialist for assistance in managing her own health care needs.

Sara's Goals

Sara expressed two major concerns: (1) She would always have this disease and never be able to do the same activities as her friends; (2) She would not be able to keep up physically with the demands of high school. She stated her goals were to be like other kids, play on a sport team like basketball or soccer, and hike and ski with her family.

Physical Therapist Examination
QUESTIONS GUIDING THE EXAMINATION

1. Are there specific activity limitations that negatively impact Sara's participation and overall QOL and prevent her from achieving her current goals?
2. Are there specific impairments that contribute to these problems?

ACTIVITY AND PARTICIPATION FINDINGS

To answer the first question, several standardized assessments validated for children with JIA were used. The QOML questionnaire includes two 100-mm VAS that measure overall QOL and HRQOL; higher scores indicate better QOL.[73] Sara rated both her overall QOL and HRQOL as 40/100 mm. Using the 5-point categorical scale (much better to much worse), Sara rated her life as "much worse" than at her last clinic visit 3 months ago, indicating her JIA has a negative impact on her QOL.

Sara also completed the CAT$_{CHAQ38}$; the Disability Index (DI), calculated as the mean score for all 38 items, has a range of 0 to 3 where higher scores indicate greater disability.[69] Her DI was 1.50, suggesting moderate disability. She scored the following tasks as "unable to do" during the previous week: "play team sports with others in my class," "run a race," and "perform activities for a long time without getting tired." Pain during the previous week was scored as 60/100 mm on a VAS (higher scores indicate greater pain).

To answer the second question, several measures were performed, including a systems review, observational gait analysis, and two composites of the BOT-2, Body Coordination (Balance and Bilateral Coordination) and Strength and Agility (Running Speed and Agility and Strength). The tables below show Sara's scores on the BOT-2.

Composite Score Profile (Normative mean on Standard Score = 50, SD = 10)

Composite	Standard Score	90% CI	Compared with Normative Values	Descriptive Category
Body coordination	36	32–40	>−1 SD	Below average
Strength & agility	37	33–41	>−1 SD	Below average

Subtest Profile (Normative mean on Scale Score = 15; SD = 5)

Subtest	Scale Score	90% CI	Compared with Normative Values	Descriptive Category
Bilateral Coordination	14	12–16	−1 SD	Average
Balance	3	0–5	>−2 SD	Well below average
R & A	8	6–10	>−1 SD	Below average
Strength	8	5–11	>−SD	Below average

BODY STRUCTURES AND FUNCTION FINDINGS

1. Signs of active joint disease
   - Both wrists, knees, and ankles had effusions with loss of joint contours; swelling was also noted around the right Achilles tendon.
   - Tenderness to palpation and mild withdrawal were noted at the above joints and at the right Achilles tendon.
2. ROM: All joints showed PROM within normal limits (WNL) with these exceptions:
   - Cervical spine rotation and lateral flexion to either side: limited by 50%.
   - Right shoulder flexion: −20 degrees (0 to 160 degrees)
   - Elbow extension: −20 degrees (R), 30 degrees (L)
   - Wrist DF: (R) −25 degrees (0 to 45 degrees); (L) −15 degrees (0 to 55 degrees)
     - Resting position of R wrist/hand: ulnar deviation, MCP, and PIP flexion (alignment corrected with passive motion)
   - Pelvis in anterior tilted position; lumbar spine in excessive lordosis
   - Hip extension (modified Thomas test): −10 degrees (R) and (L).
   - Ober test: short Tensor Fascia Lata (R)
   - Knee extension, measured in prone: −10 degrees (R), −5 degrees (L)
     - Hamstring length test (supine): −45 degrees (R), −35 degrees (L)
     - Prudential Fitnessgram (PF) Sit & Reach score: 8″, below the minimum health fitness standard (HFS) of 10″ for her age and gender[180]
   - Feet and ankles
     - (R) ankle PF: 0 degrees to 30 degrees; (R) ankle DF with the knee extended: 0 degrees
     - Hindfoot eversion: 0 degrees (R) and (L); inversion WNL
     - Pes cavus (R) and (L)
3. Muscle strength
   - Gross strength (MMT): lower limb = 4/5; upper limb = 3+/5
   - Functional ankle PF muscle endurance: able to perform eight bilateral heel rises
   - Grip strength measured with a modified blood pressure cuff: 60/20 mm Hg (R) and 80/20 mm Hg (L). According to Smythe and Helewa,[74] a rise of 20 mm Hg from the baseline of 20 mm Hg is equal to approximately 5 lb (2.27 kg)

of force; Sara's grip strength, measured in pounds, was 10 lb (R) and 15 lb (L), considerably below the reported range of values for healthy, typically developing 13-year-old females: (39 to 79 lb [R], 25 to 76 lb [L]).[170]

- PF curl-up test (abdominal strength and endurance) score: 8, below the minimum HFS of 18; PF modified pull-up test (upper body strength and endurance) score: 1, below the minimum HFS of 4.[171]

4. Aerobic performance/exercise tolerance
   - 6MWD: 550 m, less than mean distance of 663±50.8 m (95% CI: 651.0 to 675.0) reported for 12- to 15-year-old females[172]
     - Post-walk HR (170 bpm) was approximately 82% of age-related HR_{max} and indicates a good effort and provides a target HR for exercise training
   - Self-rated fatigue during the previous week: 50 on a 100-mm VAS

5. Body composition: Body mass index and skinfold thickness measures WNL for her age

6. Gait pattern: Footprint analysis with video
   - Decreased walking velocity: 75 cm/sec compared with 138.8±4.7 cm/sec reported for a 12.6 y/o males and females combined[173]
   - Shortened right step length compared with left
   - Majority of weight borne on lateral side of foot throughout stance phase
   - Lack of push-off at terminal stance: decreased active ankle PF ROM and decreased hip extension

Evaluation and Diagnosis
GUIDING QUESTIONS

1. Which impairments contribute to Sara's current activity and participation problems?
2. Which impairments must be addressed to prevent or minimize secondary problems?
3. What strengths and resources does Sara have that could support her overall QOL?

Participation Restrictions	Activity Limitations	Impairments
- Frequent school absence and tardiness - Inconsistent participation in PE - Unable to participate in sports with friends or family	- Difficulty transitioning between sitting on floor and standing - Difficulty negotiating steps - Difficulty with reach, grasp, and manipulation activities - Difficulty performing activities (complex motor skills) for PE and sports	*Musculoskeletal* - Active arthritis (joint swelling and pain) - Limited joint ROM / ↓ soft tissue extensibility - Muscle weakness (hand grip, core trunk, and lower limb muscles) *Cardiopulmonary* - Impaired aerobic fitness - Impaired anaerobic fitness (speed/power) *Neuromuscular/ Multisystem* - Gait deviations: Slow walking speed, uneven step, stride length

- Lower limb and foot pain when walking
- Poor postural control (steady state on narrow base of support; anticipatory)
- Poor bilateral coordination/ movement speed

The first two columns in the table above list the priority activity and participation problems identified by Sara and her parents on the basis of information from the CHAQ, JAQQ, and interview. Column three lists the impairments believed to contribute to these problems.

- Active arthritis contributes to pain, tenderness, and limited active and passive ROM
- Limited joint motion and soft tissue shortening contribute to impaired movement patterns, fatigue, and pain during physical activities
- Muscle weakness, fatigue, and poor power contribute to gross motor deficits
- Impaired joint mobility and muscle performance contribute to gait deviations
- Impaired proprioception, coordination, and speed may contribute to poor muscular control and postural stability during challenging physical activities
- Poor adherence to prescribed medications and HEP and Sara's limited participation in her health care contribute to poor disease control and functional outcome

STRENGTHS AND RESOURCES
Although Sara's adherence to her medical and therapy regimen has been inadequate, she now appears more interested in managing her disease and improving her health status and functional capacity. Her parents are very supportive, and the school appears to be willing to accommodate her needs by making requested modifications to her educational program.

Prognosis
GUIDING QUESTIONS

1. What would improve Sara's active participation in her health care?
2. What is the best POC with regard to medications and rehabilitation?

Question 1: The rheumatology team believed that inadequate disease control and poor adherence to her therapy regimen contributed to Sara's current problems. They thought adherence would improve if Sara were more involved in her own health care. Sara stated she wanted to participate in PE and sports with her family and friends. She is also concerned about adjusting to the physical and work challenges of high school next year. The child life specialist helped her understand how she might achieve her goals if her JIA was under better control by regular use of medication and adherence to her exercise regimen.

Question 2: The team believed that Sara's arthritis and functional status would improve following IA injections, the addition of etanercept (Enbrel™), and improved adherence to the NSAID prescription and daily exercise regimen.[31] Sara agreed to a 6-month contract, listing her goals, therapy objectives, and a POC aimed at achieving these. An interim reevaluation was scheduled for 3 months. The contract included: (1) following her full medication regimen, (2) performing home ROM and strengthening exercises, and (3) participating in an aerobic conditioning program designed by the physical therapist. She also agreed to wear resting hand splints each night while sleeping. Sara and her parents agreed to a 3-month trial of direct physical therapist and occupational therapist twice a week, with goals of improving ROM and strength, and her parents signed permission for the clinic physical therapist and OT to consult with the school PE instructor to discuss activity modifications so Sara could safely participate in PE.

Expected Outcomes (Goals to be achieved in 6 months with progress toward the goals observed at the 3-month follow-up visit):

- Improved adherence to medication should result in improved disease control, reduced joint pain, improved physical function, and HRQOL.[164–166]
  - Goal: Sara will show at least a 75% improvement in adherence to her medication schedule based on a daily log, with entries verified by one parent.
  - Goal: Sara will demonstrate improved capability to perform necessary and desired activities based on a reduction of ≥ 0.13 on her self-reported CAT_{CHAQ38} DI.[67]
  - Goal: Sara's self-reported HRQOL score will show improvement based on an increase of ≥ 11 mm in her score on the QOML VAS.[72]
- Sara's gait pattern will improve following joint injections and supportive therapy
  - Goal: Sara will demonstrate increased walking speed and symmetry in step and stride length based on observational gait analysis and footprint recording.
- Available evidence suggests that Sara can improve her performance-related physical fitness through a physical conditioning regimen performed twice a week.[144,174]
  - Goal: Sara's 6MWD will increase by at least 48 meters, the minimal detectable change (MDC) reported for healthy children on the 6MWT.[97]
  - Goal: Sara will demonstrate decreased fatigue with physical activity based on self-report using a 100-mm VAS where higher values equal greater fatigue.
- Daily ROM and flexibility exercises should improve joint ROM and soft tissue extensibility, resulting in decreased stiffness and pain.
  - Goal: Sara will demonstrate improved passive joint ROM based on goniometric measurement of the shoulders, hips, knees, and ankles.
- Improved physical status should allow Sara to increase her participation in physical activities with her family and friends. Sara will record progress using a daily dairy.

- Goal: Sara will actively participate in at least 75% of all PE activities each week, with or without modifications.
- Goal: Sara will participate in at least one recreational PA with family or friends each week for at least 1 hour.

Intervention Plan

Following IA injections to the knees, right wrist, and right ankle, Sara was on non–weight bearing for 1 day. After 1 week of modified PA, she resumed all typical activities.

Coordination, Communication, and Documentation

The rheumatology team worked with Sara and her parents to determine techniques that would improve her adherence to the treatment plan. The nurse provided instruction to Sara and her parents to ensure correct administration of the weekly injections of etanercept and reasons for following the exact prescription for taking the NSAID. The physical therapist provided written and oral instructions, demonstration, and illustrations of Sara's exercises. The OT made new resting wrist/hand splints and gave Sara assistive devices to improve her ability to perform ADLs. The child life specialist helped Sara establish a schedule for taking medications and develop a daily diary to keep a record of her medications, use of splints, HEP, PE, and recreational activities. Each section of the diary included space for Sara's comments. She was encouraged to contact the team with questions about her program or symptoms. The team, with the permission of Sara and her parents, sent a copy of the physical therapist and occupational therapist evaluations to the school and requested the PE instructor to consult with the clinic physical therapist to adjust activities so that Sara could increase her participation.

Patient Education

The clinic physical therapist discussed the findings of the physical examination with Sara and her parents. She discussed the impact of arthritis on joints and muscles, the potential sources of pain and stiffness, and secondary problems, including poor exercise tolerance and impaired motor skills. She explained that Sara's current functional problems were likely related to limited joint mobility and soft tissue extensibility, pain, and poor aerobic and muscular fitness. She explained that intervention would be directed toward reducing these impairments. The therapy program would also include practice of the activities that were difficult for Sara.

Procedural Interventions

- Direct physical therapy 30 to 45 minutes twice a week and instruction in HEP.

INTERVENTIONS FOR IMPAIRED JOINT MOBILITY AND MUSCLE FUNCTION

Direct therapy: Initial instruction in maintaining control of the trunk and lumbar spine by engaging abdominal muscles during all activities

1. AAROM for shoulder flexion, abduction in scapular plane, medial and lateral rotation, with attention to scapular position, movement, and scapulohumeral rhythm
2. Prone scapular progression exercises; progress to standing scapular exercises against a wall; progress to using light

handheld weights when Sara can perform exercises without pain or compensatory movements

3. AAROM and AROM for serratus anterior; progress to exercise against resistance
4. Instruction in isometric exercise to improve neck stability
5. Stretching of shortened latissimus dorsi, lateral shoulder rotators and posterior capsule, hip flexors, hamstrings, right gastrocnemius using autogenic and reciprocal inhibition
6. Stretching of right TFL
7. Strength training for hip extensors, deep external rotators, and abductors
   - Begin with AROM to teach correct technique for each muscle group
   - Progress to graded resistance exercise using light weights or elastic bands
   - Closed kinetic chain (CKC) exercise, including graded squats, lunges, and "step" training to improve strength, endurance, and control of lower extremity musculature
8. Gait training to improve lower limb weight bearing, step and stride length

INTERVENTIONS TO ADDRESS IMPAIRED MOTOR SKILLS

1. Activities to improve proprioception, agility, and coordination once joint ROM and muscle strength improve and pain decreases
2. Gait training to increase walking velocity, using timed walks
3. Activity- or sport-specific training to ensure safe participation in physical activities and recreational sports

HOME EXERCISE PROGRAM

1. Daily AROM exercises concentrating on cervical spine, shoulders, wrists, hips, knees, and ankles using illustrations from *Raising a Child with Arthritis*
2. Daily aerobic activity (Sara's choice), gradually increasing duration to at least 30 minutes a day and intensity to at least 75% of her age-based HR_{max}

RECOMMENDATIONS/REFERRALS

1. Referral to orthotist for custom insoles to accommodate pes cavus deformity and decrease pain under MTP joints
2. Recommendation for semirigid cervical collar when riding in school bus and car, and easel top for desk to decrease neck strain when reading

Reexamination

Sara was seen by the clinic physical therapist at her 3-month follow-up rheumatology appointment. She reported receiving physical therapy twice a week at school before classes begin and OT once a week during school time. She also attends all PE classes each week and participates in approximately 50% of the activities with some modifications. The school PE instructor and physical therapist are working together to improve Sara's gross motor skills and adapt difficult activities to allow her to participate with her classmates.

FINDINGS OF REEXAMINATION

Activities and Participation

1. Sara's CAT_{CHAQ38} DI decreased from 1.50 to 1.30, exceeding the reported minimal clinically important improvement of ≥ 0.13
2. Her self-reported HRQOL improved from 40 to 70 mm, and she reported her life as somewhat better since her last clinic visit

Body Structures and Functions

1. Signs of active joint disease
   - Mild swelling noted in the right knee, no tenderness or pain on passive motion
2. ROM, flexibility, and joint alignment
   - No change in cervical spine AROM, but no c/o POM
   - (R) shoulder PROM: 0 to 170 degrees with stress pain at end range
   - Wrist DF: 0 to 60 degrees (R), 0 to 60 degrees (L)
   - Passive hip extension limitation: 5 degrees
   - Knee extension (examined prone): − 5 (R); WNL (L)
   - (R) Ankle PROM: PF = 0 to 40 degrees; DF with knee extended = 0 to 5 degrees
   - Passive calcaneal eversion increased: 0 to 5 degrees
3. Standing posture
   - Sara continued to stand with an increased anterior pelvic tilt and lumbar lordosis, although she could correct this upon request by engaging her abdominal muscles.
   - Barefoot, Sara continued to stand with most of her weight over the lateral border of her foot; when wearing her custom-made in-shoe orthoses and sneakers, her weight was borne more evenly over the plantar surface of the foot.
4. Muscle strength and flexibility
   - Grip strength: 100/20 mm Hg (20 lb) (R); 140/20 mm Hg (30 lb) (L)
   - Score on the PF reported by Sara's school physical therapist improved
     - Curl-up test: increased from 8 to 12 (HFS = 18)
     - Modified pull-up test: increased from 1 to 5 (HFS = ≥4)
     - Sit & reach test: increased from 8″ to 9″ (HFS = 10″)
5. 6MWD increased from 550 m to 610 m, exceeding the MDC of 48 m.
6. Gait velocity increased from 75 cm/sec to 110 cm/sec. Gait pattern showed improved heel contact, weight more evenly distributed over the plantar surface of the foot during midstance, improved push-off on the medial side of the forefoot and hip extension at terminal stance, and increased step length.

Outcomes

1. A review of Sara's medication and activity diary indicated improved adherence to her medication regimen and HEP program; this was supported by Sara's parents as well as decreased signs of active arthritis and improved ROM in most joints.

2. Improvements in self-reported worst pain from 60 mm to 40 mm and worst fatigue from 50 mm to 20 mm over the previous week on the VASs reflect improved disease control.

3. Improvements in PF scores, walking speed, and 6MWD suggest increased stamina, as a result of improved adherence to her exercise program.

4. Clinically meaningful improvements in her physical function and QOL lend support to her improved health status and ability to manage her condition.

Plan

On the basis of Sara's improved physical status, the clinic therapist recommended continuing with direct physical therapy in school with an emphasis on increasing aerobic fitness, strength, and gross motor proficiency. She also suggested that the school physical therapist and the PE instructor work together with Sara on specific training for basketball to allow her to participate in an intramural league at school. Reevaluation was scheduled for her next clinic appointment in 3 months.

REFERENCES

1. Prakken B, Albani S, Martini A. Juvenile idiopathic arthritis. *Lancet.* 2011;377:2138–2149.

2. Ravelli A, Martini A. Juvenile idiopathic arthritis. *Lancet.* 2007; 369:767–778.

3. Cassidy JT, Levinson JE, Bass JC, et al. A study of classification criteria for a diagnosis of juvenile rheumatoid arthritis. *Arthritis Rheum.* 1986;29:274–281.

4. Kahn P. Juvenile idiopathic arthritis—an update on pharmacotherapy. *Bul NYU Hosp Jt Dis.* 2011;69(3):264–276.

5. Weiss JA, Ilowite NT. Juvenile idiopathic arthritis. *Arthritis Rheum Dis Clin N Am.* 2007;33(3):441–470.

6. Cannizzano E, Schroeder S, Muller LM, et al. Temporomandibular joint involvement in children with juvenile idiopathic arthritis. *J Rheumatol.* 2011;38(3):510–515.

7. American Academy of Pediatrics section on rheumatology and section on ophthalmology: guidelines for ophthalmologic examinations in children with juvenile rheumatoid arthritis. *Pediatrics.* 1993;92:295–296.

8. Al-Matar MJ, Petty RE, Tucker LB, et al. The early pattern of joint involvement predicts disease prognosis in children with oligoarticular (pauciarticular) juvenile rheumatoid arthritis. *Arthritis Rheum.* 2002;46(10):2708–2715.

9. Rosenberg AM, Petty RE. A syndrome of seronegative enthesopathy and arthropathy in children. *Arthritis Rheum.* 1982;25:1041–1047.

10. Colbert RA. Classification of juvenile spondyloarthritis: enthesitis-related arthritis and beyond. *Nat Rev Rheumatol.* 2010;6(8):477–485.

11. Petty RE, Southwood TR, Manners P, et al. International league of associations for rheumatology classification of juvenile idiopathic arthritis: second revision, Edmonton, 2001. *J Rheumatol.* 2004;31:390–392.

12. Gomez KS, Raza K, Jones SD, et al. Juvenile onset ankylosing spondylitis—more girls than we thought? *J Rheumatol.* 1997;24:735–737.

13. Tse Sm, Laxar RM. Juvenile spondyloarthropathy. *Curr Opin Rheumatol.* 2003;15:374–379.

14. Oen K, Cheang M. Epidemiology of chronic arthritis in childhood. *Semin Arthritis Rheum.* 1996;26:575–591.

15. Manners PJ, Bower C. Worldwide prevalence of juvenile arthritis—why does it vary so much? *J Rheumatol.* 2002;29:1520–1530.

16. Helmick GG, Felson DT, Lawrence RC, et al. Estimates of the prevalence of arthritis and other rheumatic conditions in the United States. *Arthritis Rheum.* 2008;58:15–25.

17. Sacks JJ, Helmick CG, Luo YH, et al. Prevalence and annual ambulatory health care visits for pediatric arthritis and other rheumatologic conditions in the United States in 2001–2004. *Arthritis Rheum.* 2007;57:1439–1445.

18. Cassidy JT, Petty RE. *Textbook of Pediatric Rheumatology.* 4th ed. Philadelphia, PA: W.B. Saunders; 2001.

19. Hochberg MC, Linet MS, Sills EM. The prevalence and incidence of juvenile rheumatoid arthritis in an urban black population. *Am J Public Health.* 1983;73:1202–1203.

20. Sullivan DB, Cassidy JT, Petty RE. Pathogenic implications of age onset in juvenile rheumatoid arthritis. *Arthritis Rheum.* 1975;18:251–255.

21. Clemans LE, Albert E, Ansell BM. Sibling pairs affected by chronic arthritis of childhood: evidence for a genetic predisposition. *J Rheumatol.* 1985;12:108–113.

22. Murray KJ, Moroldo MB, Donnelly P, et al. Age-specific effects of juvenile rheumatoid arthritis-associated HLA alleles. *Arthritis Rheum.* 1999;42:1843–1853.

23. Burnham JM, Shultz J, Dubner SE, et al. Childhood onset arthritis is associated with an elevated risk of fracture: a population-based study using the General Practice Research Database. *Ann Rheum Dis.* 2006;1074–1079.

24. Burnham JM, Shultz J, Dubner SE, et al. Bone density, structures, and strength in juvenile idiopathic arthritis. *Arthritis Rheum.* 2008;58(8):2518–2527.

25. Kotaniemi A, Savolainen A, Kroger H, et al. Weight-bearing physical activity, calcium intake, systemic glucocorticoids, chronic inflammation, and body constitution as determinants of lumbar and femoral bone mineral in juvenile chronic arthritis. *Scand J Rheumatol.* 1999;28:19–26.

26. Henderson C, Lovell D. Assessment of protein-energy malnutrition in children and adolescents with juvenile rheumatoid arthritis. *Arthritis Care Res.* 1989;2(4):108–113.

27. Wallace CA, Ravelli A, Huang B, et al. Preliminary calidation of clinical remission criteria using the OMERACT filter for select categories of juvenile idiopathic arthritis. *J Rheumatol.* 2006;33(4):1789–795.

28. Gianinni EH, Ruperto N, Ravelle A, et al. Preliminary definition of improvement in juvenile arthritis. *Arthritis Rheum.* 1997; 40(70):1202–1209.

29. Kahn P, Imundo L. Juvenile rheumatoid arthritis and spondyloarthropathy syndromes. In Burg F, Ingelfinger J, Polin R, et al, eds. *Current Pediatric Therapy.* Philadelphia, PA: Saunders Elsevier; 2006.

30. Haskers PJ, Laxer RM. Medical treatment of juvenile idiopathic arthritis. *JAMA.* 2005;294(13):1671–1684.

31. Beukelman T, Patkar NM, Saag KG, et al. American College of Rheumatology recommendation for the treatment of juvenile idiopathic arthritis: initiation and safety monitoring of therapeutic agents for the treatment of arthritis and systemic features. *Arthritis Care Res.* 2001;63(4):465–482.

32. Sherry DD, Stein LD, Reed Am, et al. Prevention of leg length discrepancy in young children with pauciarticular juvenile rheumatoid arthritis by treatment with intra-articular steroids. *Arthritis Rheum.* 1999;42:2330–2334.

33. Brostrom E, Hagelberg S, Haglund-Akerlind Y. Effect of joint injections in children with juvenile idiopathic arthritis: evaluation of 3-D gait analysis. *Acta Paediatr.* 2004;93:906–910.

34. Zulian F, Martini G, Gobber D, et al. Triamcinolone acetonide and hexacetonide intra-articular treatment of symmetrical joints in juvenile idiopathic arthritis: a double-blind trial. *Rheumatol (Oxford).* 2004;43(10):1288–1291.

35. Huppertz JI, Tschammler A, Horowitz AE, et al. Intra-articular corticosteroids for chronic arthritis in children: efficacy and effects on cartilage and growth. *J Pediatr.* 1995;127(2):317–321.

36. Gianinni EH, Brewer EJ, Kuzmina N, et al. Methotrexate in resistant juvenile rheumatoid arthritis. Results of the U.S.A.–U.S.S.R. double-blind, placebo-controlled trial. The Pediatric Rheumatology Collaborative Study Group and The Cooperative Children's Study Group. *N Engl J Med.* 1992;326(16):1043–1049.

37. Gianinni EH, Cassidy JT, Brewer EJ, et al. Comparative efficacy and safety of advanced drug therapy in children with juvenile rheumatoid arthritis. *Semi Arthritis Rheum.* 1993;23(1):34–46.

38. Foell D, Frosch M, Schulze zuk Wiesch A, et al. Methotrexate treatment in juvenile idiopathic arthritis: when is the right time to stop? *Ann Rheum Dis.* 2004;63(2):206–208.

39. Lovell DJ, Reiff A, Ilowite NT, et al. Safety and efficacy of up to eight years of continuous etanercept therapy in juvenile rheumatoid arthritis. *Arthritis Rheum.* 2008;58(5):1496–1504.

40. Vojvodich PF, Hansen JB, Andersson U, et al. Etanercept treatment improves longitudinal growth in prepubertal children with juvenile idiopathic arthritis. *J Rheumatol.* 2007;34(12):2481–2485.

41. Robinson RF, Hahata MC, Hayes JR, et al. Quality of life measurements in juvenile rheumatoid arthritis patients treated with etanercept. *Clin Drug Investig.* 2003;23(8):511–518.

42. Gianinni EH, Iliowite NT, Lovell DJ, et al. Effects of long term etanercept treatement on growth in selected categories of juvenile idiopathic arthritis. *Arthritis Rheum.* 2010;62(11):3259–3264.

43. Lovell DJ, Ruperto N, Goodman S, et al. Adalimumab with or without methotrexate in juvenile rheumatoid arthritis. *N Engl J Med.* 2008;359(8):810–820.

44. Ravelli A. Toward an understanding of the long-term outcome of juvenile idiopathic arthritis. *Clin Exp Rheumatol.* 2004;22(3):271–275.

45. Oen K. Long-term outcomes and predictors of outcomes for patients with juvenile idiopathic arthritis. *Best Pract Res Clin Rheumatol.* 2002;16:347–360.

46. Wallace CA, Huang B, Bandeira M, et al. Patterns of clinical remission in select categories of juvenile idiopathic arthritis. *Arthritis Rheum.* 2005;52:3554–3562.

47. Ravelli A, Martini A. Early predictors of outcome in juvenile idiopathic arthritis. *Clin Exp Rheumatol.* 2003;21(5)(suppl 31):S89–S93.

48. Spencer CH, Berstein BH. Hip disease in juvenile rheumatoid arthritis. *Curr Opin in Rheumatol.* 2002;4:536–541.

49. Amine B, Rostom S, Benhouazza K, et al. Health related quality of life survey about children and adolescents with juvenile idiopathic arthritis. *Rheumatol Int.* 2009;29:275–279.

50. Oen K, Malleson PN, Cabral DA, et al. Disease course and outcome of juvenile rheumatoid arthritis in a multi-center cohort. *J Rheumatol.* 2002;29:1989–1999.

51. Oliveria S, Ravelli A, Pistoria A, et al. Proxy health-related quality of life of patients with juvenile idiopathic arthritis: the Pediatric Rheumatology International Trials Organization (PRINTO) multinational quality of life study. *Arthritis Rheum.* 2007;57(1):35–43.

52. Arkela-Kautiainen M, Haapassari J, Kautiainen H, et al. Favorable social functioning and health-related quality of life of patients with juvenile idiopathic arthritis in early adulthood. *Arthritis Rheum.* 2005;65(6):875–880.

53. Boiu S, Marniga E, Bader-Meunier B. Functional status in severe juvenile idiopathic arthritis in the biologic treatment era: on assessment in a French paediatric rheumatology referral centre. *Rheumatol.* 2012;51:1285–1292.

54. Halberg M, Herneff G. Improvement of functional ability in children with juvenile idiopathic arthritis by treatment with etanercept. *Rheumatol Int.* 2009;30:229–238.

55. Gerhardt CA, McGoren KD, Vannatta K, et al. Educational and occupational outcomes among young adults with juvenile idiopathic arthritis. *Arthritis Care Res.* 2008;59(10):1385–1396.

56. Ringold A, Wallace CA, Rivara FP. Health-related quality of life, physical function, fatigue, and disease activity in children with established polyarticular juvenile idiopathic arthritis. *J Rheumatol.* 2009;36:130–1336.

57. Magni-Maazemi S. A longitudinal analysis of physical functional disability over the course of juvenile idiopathic arthritis. *Ann Rheum Dis.* 2008;67:1159–1164.

58. Cabral DA, Oen KG, Petty RE. SEA syndrome revisited: a long-term follow-up of children with a syndrome of seronegative entheosopathy and arthropathy. *J Rheumatol.* 1992;19:1282–1285.

59. Selvang AM, Lien G, Sorskaar D, et al. Early disease course and predictors of disability in juvenile rheumatoid arthritis and juvenile spondyloarthropathy: a 3-year prospective study. *J Rheumatol.* 2005;32:1122–1130.

60. Flato B, Hoffman-Vold AM, Reif A, et al. Long-term outcome and prognostic factors in enthesitis-related arthritis: a case control study. *Arthritis Rheum.* 2006;54:3573–3582.

61. Lillemore B, Damgard M, Andersson-Gare B, et al. HLA B27 predicts a more extended disease with increasing age at onset in boys with juvenile idiopathic arthritis. *J Rheumatol.* 2008;35:2055–2061.

62. Burgos-Vargas R, Clark J. Axial involvement in the seronegative enthesopathy and arthropathy syndrome and its progression to ankylosing spondylitis. *J Rheumatol.* 1989;16:192–197.

63. Morrison CD, Bundy RC, Fisher AG. The contribution of motor skills and playfulness to the play performance of preschoolers. *Am J Occup Ther.* 1991;45:687–694.

64. Lineker SC, Badley EM, Dalby DM. Unmet service needs of children with rheumatic diseases and their parents in a metropolitan area. *J Rheumatol.* 1996;23:1054–1058.

65. Singh G, Athreya B, Fries J, et al. Measurement of health status in juvenile rheumatoid arthritis. *Arthritis Rheum.* 1994;37:1761–1769.

66. Ruperto N, Ravelli A, Pistorio A, Malattia C et al. Cross-cultural adaptation and psychometric evaluation of the Childhood Health Assessment Questionnaire (CHAQ) and the Child Health Questionnaire (CHQ) in 32 countries. Review of the general methodology. *Clin Exp Rheumatol.* 2001 Jul–Aug;19 (4 Suppl 23):S1–9.

67. Dempster H, Porpera M, Young N, et al. The clinical meaning of functional ourcome scores in children with juvenile arthritis. *Arthritis Rheum.* 2001;44:1768–1774.

68. Lam C, Young N, Maruahn J, et al. Revised versions of the Childhood Health Assessment Questionnaire (CHAQ) are more sensitive and suffer les from a ceiling effect. *Arthritis Care Res.* 2004;51:881–889.

69. Lovell DJ, Howe S, Shear E. Development of a disability measurement tool for juvenile rheumatoid arthritis: the Juvenile Arthritis Functional Assessment Scale. *Arthritis Rheum.* 1989;32:1390–1395.

70. Duffy CM, Arsenault HL, Duffy KN, et al. The Juvenile Arthritis Quality of Life Questionnaire—development of a new responsive index for juvenile rheumatoid arthritis and juvenile spondyloarthritides. *J Rheumatol.* 1997;24(4):738–746.

71. Varni J, Seid M, Smith Knight T, et al. The PedsQL in pediatric rheumatology: reliability, validity, and responsiveness of the Pediatric Quality of Life Inventory generic core scales and rheumatology module. *Arthritis Rheum.* 2002;46:714–725.

72. Gong GUK, Young NI, Dempster H, et al. The quality of my life questionnaire: minimal clinically important difference for pediatric patients. *J Rheumatol.* 2007;34:581–587.

73. Coster W, Deeney T, Haltiwanger J, et al. *School Function Assessment.* Boston, MA: Harcourt Brace & Co; 1998.

74. Smythe H, Helewa A. Assessment of joint disease. In Walker J, Helewa A, eds. *Physical Therapy in Arthritis.* Philadelphia, PA: WB Saunders; 1996.

75. Janow GL, Panghaal V, Frinh A, et al. Detection of active disease in juvenile idiopatic arthritis: sensitivity and specificity of the physical exam vs ultrasound. *J Rheumatol.* 2011;38(12):2671–2674.

76. Nistala K, Babar J, Johnson K, et al. Clinical assessment and core outcome variables are poor predictors of hip arthritis diagnosis by MRI in juvenile idiopathic arthritis. *Rheumatol(Oxford).* 2007;46(4):699–702.

77. Bekkering WP, ten Cate R, van Suijlekom-Smit LW, et al. The relationship between impairments in joint function and disabilities in independent function in children with systemic idiopathic arthritis. *J Rheumatol.* 2001;28:1099–1105.

78. Brewer EJ, Gianinni EH. Standard methodology for segment I, II, and III pediatric rheumatology collaborative study group studies. I. Design. *J Rheumatol.* 1982;9:109–113.

79. Epps H, Hurley M, Utley M. Development of a single score to assess global range of motion in juvenile idiopathic arthritis. *Arthritis Care Res.* 2002;47:398–402.

80. Len C, Ferraz M, Goldenberg J, et al. Pediatric Escola Paulista de Medicina range of motion scale: a reduced joint count score for general use in juvenile rheumatoid arthritis. *J Rheumatol.* 1999;26:909–913.

81. Hendrengren E, Knutson LM, Haglund-Akerlind Y, et al. Lower extremity isometric torque in children with juvenile rheumatoid arthritis. *Scand J Rheumatol.* 2001;30:69–76.

82. Lechner DE, McCarthy CF, Holden MK. Gait deviations in patients with juvenile rheumatoid arthritis. *Phys Ther.* 1987;67:1335–1341.

83. Klepper S, Darbee J, Effgen S, et al. Physical fitness levels in children with polyarticular juvenile rheumatoid arthritis. *Arthritis Care Res.* 1992;5:93–100.

84. van Brussel M, Lelieveld OT, van der Net JJ, et al. Aeroibc and anaerobic capacity in children with juvenile idiopathic arthritis. *Arthritis Care Res.* 2007;57:891–897.

85. Lelieveld OT, van Brussel M, Takken T, et al. Aerobic and anaerobic capacity in adolescents with juvenile idiopathic arthritis. *Arthritis Care Res.* 2007;57:898–904.

86. Fan J, Wessel J, Ellsworth J. The relationship between strength and function in females with juvenile rheumatoid arthritis. *J Rheumatol.* 1998;3:1399–1405.

87. Takken T, van der Net J, Helders P. Relationship between functional ability and physical fitness in juvenile rheumatoid arthritis. *Scand J Rheumatol.* 2003;32:174–178.

88. Dunn W. Grip strength of children aged 3 to 7 years using a modified sphygmomanometer: comparison of typical children and children with rheumatic disease. *Am J Occup Ther.* 1993;47:421–428.

89. Giannini MJ, Protas EJ. Comparison of peak isometric knee extensor torque in children with and without juvenile arthritis. *Arthritis Care Res.* 1993;6:82–88.

90. Wessel J, Kaup C, Fin J, et al. Isometric strength measurements in children with arthritis: reliability and relation to function. *Arthritis Care Res.* 1999;12:238–246.

91. Faigenbaum AD, Milliken LA, Laud Rl, et al. Comparison of 1 and 2 days per week of strength training in children. *Res Q Exerc Sport.* 2002;73(4):416–424.

92. Takken T, Hemel A, van der Net JJ, et al. Aerobic fitness in children with juvenile idiopathic arthritis. *J Rheumatol.* 2002;29:2643–2647.

93. Giannini MJ, Protas EJ. Aerobic capacity in juvenile rheumatoid arthritis patients and healthy children. *Arthritis Care Res.* 1992;4:131–135.

94. Hebestreit H, Muller-Scholden J, Huppertz HI. Aerobic fitness and physical activity in patients with HLA-B27 positive juvenile spondyloarthropathy that is inactive or in remission. *J Rheumatol.* 1998;25:1626–1633.

95. Helders PJ, Klepper SE, Takken T, et al. Juvenile idiopathic arthritis. In Campbell SK, Palisano RJ, Orlin MN, eds. *Physical Therapy for Children.* St. Louis, MO: Elsevier Saunders; 2012.

96. American Thoracic Society. ATS statement: guidelines for the six-minute walk test. *Am J Respir Crit Care Med.* 2002;166:111–117.

97. Klepper SE, Muir N. Reference values on the 6-minute walk test for children living in the United States. *Ped Phys Ther.* 2011;23:32–40.

98. Lelieveld OT, Takken T, van der Net JJ, et al. Validity of the 6-minute walking test in juvenile idiopathic arthritis. *Arthritis Care Res.* 2005;53:304–307.

99. Paap E, van der Net JJ, Helders PJ, et al. Physiologic response of the six-minute walk test in children with juvenile idiopathic arthritis. *Arthritis Care Res.* 2005;53:351–356.

100. Kimura Y, Walco G. Treatment of chronic pain in pediatric rheumatic disease. *Nature Clinical Practice Rheumatol.* 2007;3(4):210–218.

101. Anthony KK, Schanberg L. Pain in children with arthritis: a review of the current literature. *Arthritis Rheum (Arthritis Care Res).* 2003;49:272–279.

102. Lovell DJ, Walco GW. Pain associated with juvenile rheumatoid arthritis. *Pediatr Clin N Am.* 1989;36:1015–1027.

103. Schanberg L, Anthony KK, Gil KM, et al. Daily pain and symptoms in children with polyarticular arthritis. *Arthritis Rheum.* 2003;48:1390–1397.

104. Aviel YB, Stremler R, Bensler SM, et al. Sleep and fatigue and the relationship to pain, disease activity and quality of life in juvenile idiopathic arthritis and juvenile dematomyositis. *Rheumatol.* 2011;50:2051–2060.

105. Hogeweg JA, Kuis W, Huygen AC, et al. The pain threshold in juvenile chronic arthritis. *Br J Rheumatol.* 1995;4:61–67.

106. Thatsum M, Zachariae R, Scholer M, et al. Cold pressor pain: comparing responses of juvenile rheumatoid arthritis patients and their parents. *Scand J Rheumatol.* 1997;26:272–279.

107. Hogeweg JA, Kuis W, Oostendorp RA, et al. General and segmental reduced pain thresholds in juvenile chronic arthritis. *Pain.* 1995;62:11–17.

108. Jaworski TM, Bradley LA, Heck LW, et al. Development of an observational method for assessing pain behaviors in children with juvenile rheumatoid arthritis. *Arthritis Rheum.* 1995;38:1142–1151.

109. Beyer JE, Denyes MJ, Villarruel AM. The creation, validation, and continuing development of the Oucher: a measure of pain intensity in children. *J Pediatr Nurs.* 1992;7:335–346.

110. Wong DL, Baker CM. Pain in children: comparison of assessment scales. *Pediatr Nurs.* 1988;14:9–17.

111. Hester NO, Foster R, Kristensen K. Measurement of pain in children: generalizability and validity of the pain ladder and the poker-chip tool. In: Tyler DC, Kane EJ, eds. *Advances in Pain Research and Therapy.* New York, NY: Raven Press; 1990.

112. Varni JW, Thompson KL, Hanson V. The Varni/Thompson pediatric pain questionnaire. I. Chronic musculoskeletal pain in juvenile rheumatoid arthritis: an empirical model. *Pain.* 1987;28:27–38.

113. Frigo C, Bardare M, Corona F, et al. Gait alteration in patients with juvenile idiopathic arthritis: a computerized analysis. *J Orthopedic Rheumatol.* 1996;9:82–90.

114. Brostrom E, Haglund-Akerlind Y, Hagelberg S, et al. Gait in children with juvenile chronic arthritis. Timing and force parameters. *Scand J Rheumatol.* 2002;31:317–323.

115. Hartman M, Kreupointner F, Haefner R, et al. Effects of juvenile idiopathic arthritis on kinematics and kinetics of the lower extremities call for consequences in physical activity recommendations. *Int J Pediatr.* 2010; pii 835984. Available at: http://www.ncbi.nlm.nih.gov/pubmed/20862334. Accessed October 19, 2012.

116. Dekker M, Hoeksma AF, Dekker JHM, et al. Strong relationships between disease activity, foot-related impairments, activity limitations and participation restrictions in children with juvenile idiopathic arthritis. *Clin Exp Rheumatol.* 2012;28:905–911.

117. Hendry G, Gardner-Medwin J, Watt GF, et al. A survey of foot problems in juvenile idiopathic arthritis. *Musculoskeletal Care.* 2008;6(4):221–232.

118. Adams MA. *Clinical Gait Measurement with Pedographs.* 1st ed. Bellevue, WA: Pickle Point Press; 2005.

119. Oosterweld FG, Rasker JJ. Effects of local heat and cold treatment on intra-articular temperature of arthritis knees. *Arthritis Rheum.* 1994;37:1578–1582.

120. Wiltink A, Nijweide PJ, Oosterbon WA, et al. Effect of therapeutic ultrasound on endochondral ossification. *Ultrasound Med Biol.* 1995;21:121–127.

121. Oosterweld FG, Rasker JJ. Treating arthritis with locally applied heat and cold. *Semin Arthritis Rheum.* 1994;24(2):82–90.

122. Bacon MC, Nicholson C, Binder H, et al. Juvenile rheumatoid arthritis: aquatic exercise and lower extremity function. *Arthritis Care Res.* 1991;4:102–105.

123. Takken T, van der Net JJ, Helders PJ. Do juvenile idiopathic arthritis patients benefit from an exercise program? A pilot study. *Arthritis Care Res.* 2001;45:81–85.

124. Zamir G, Press J, Tal A, et al. Sleep fragmentation in children with juvenile rheumatoid arthritis. *J Rheumatol.* 1998;25:1191–1197.

125. Field T, Hernandez-Reif M, Seligman S, et al. Juvenile rheumatoid arthritis: benefits of massage therapy. *J Pediatr Psychol.* 1997;22:607–617.

126. Lavigne JV, Ross CK, Barry SL, et al. Evaluation of a psychological treatment package for treating pain in juvenile rheumatoid arthritis. *Arthritis Care Res.* 1992;5:101–110.

127. Walco GA, Varni JW, Ilowite NT. Cognitive-behavioral pain management in children with juvenile rheumatoid arthritis. *Pediatrics.* 1992;89:1075–1079.

128. Swann M. The surgery of juvenile chronic arthritis. *Clin Orthop Rel Res.* 1990;259:70–75.

129. Skytta ET, Savolainen HA, Kautiainen HJ, et al. Long-term results of leg length discrepancies treated with temporary epiphyseal stapling in children with juvenile chronic arthritis. *Clin Exp Rheumatol.* 2003;21:669–671.

130. Parvizi J, Lajam CM, Trousdale RT, et al. Total knee arthroplasty in young patients with juvenile rheumatoid arthritis. *J Bone Joint Surg.* 2003;85:1090–1094.

131. Emery HM, Bayer SL, Sisung CE. Rehabilitation of the child with a rheumatic disease. *Pediatr Clin North Am.* 1995;42:1263–1285.

132. Nestor BJ, Figgie MP, Wright FV, et al. Surgical management of juvenile rheumatoid arthritis. In Melvin J, Wright FV, eds. *Rheumatologic Rehabilitation: Pediatric Rheumatic Diseases.* Bethesda, MD: AOTA; 2003.

133. Odent T, Journeau P, Prier AM, et al. Cementless hip arthroplasty in juvenile idiopathic arthritis. *J Pediatri Orthop.* 2005;25(4):465–470.

134. Bandy WD, Irion JM. The effect of time of static stretch on the flexibility of the hamstring muscles. *Phys Ther.* 1994;74:845–852.

135. Melvin J, Wright FV. Procedure for serial casting of contractures form juvenile arthritis. In: Melvin J, Wright FV, eds. *Rheumatologic Rehabilitation: Pediatric Rheumatic Diseases.* Bethesda, MD: AOTA; 2003.

136. Oberg T, Karszina B, Gare A, et al. Physical training of children with juvenile chronic arthritis. *Scand J Rheumatol.* 1994;23:92–95.

137. Fisher NM, Venkatraman JT, O'Neil K. The effects of resistance exercises on muscle function in juvenile arthritis. *Arthritis Rheum.* 2001;44(suppl 9):S276.

138. Myer G, Brunner HI, Melson PG, et al. Specialized neuromuscular training to improve neuromuscular function and biomechanics in a patient with quiescent juvenile rheumatoid arthritis. *Phys Ther.* 2005;85:791–802.

139. James MJ, Cleland LG, Gaffney RD, et al. Effect of exercise on 99mTc-DTPA clearance from knees with effusions. *J Rheumatol.* 1994;21:501–504.

140. Minor MA, Westby MD. Rest and exercise. In: Robbins L, Burckhardt C, Hannan M, et al., eds. *Clinical Care in the Rheumatic Diseases.* 2nd ed. Atlanta, GA: American College of Rheumatology; 2001.

141. Takken T, van Brussel M, Engelbert RH, et al. Exercise therapy in juvenile idiopathic arthritis: a Cochrane review. *European J Phys Rehabil Med.* 2008;44:287–297.

142. Epps H, Ginnelly L, Utley M, et al. Is hydrotherapy cost-effective? A randomized controlled trial of combined hydrotherapy programmes compared with physiotherapy land techniques in children with juvenile idiopathic arthritis. *Health Technol Assess.* 2005;9:1–5.

143. Singh-Grewal D, Schneiderman-Walker J, Wright V, et al. The effects of vigorous exercise training on physical function in children with arthritis: a randomized controlled, single-blinded trial. *Arthritis Care Res.* 2007;57:1202–1210.

144. Klepper SE. Exercise in pediatric rheumatic diseases. *Curr Opin in Rheumatol.* 2008;20:619–624.

145. Gualano B, Sa Pinto AL, Perondi B, et al. Evidence for prescribing exercise as treatment in pediatric rheumatic diseases. *Autoimmun Rev.* 2010;9:569–573.

146. Long AR, Rouster-Stevens KA. The role of exercise therapy in the management of juvenile idiopathic arthritis. *Curr Opin in Rheumatol.* 2010;22:213–217.

147. Takken T. Exercise testing and training in children with juvenile idiopathic arthritis and dermatomyositis: state of the art. *Annals of the Rheum Dis.* 2006;V:25.

148. Gannoti ME, Nahorniak M, Gorton GE, et al. Can exercise influence low bone mineral density in children with juvenile rheumatoid arthritis? *Pediatr Phys Ther.* 2007;19:128–139.

149. Sandstedt E, Fasth A, Fors H, et al. Bone health in children and adolescents with juvenile idiopathic arthritis and the influence of short-term physical exercise. *Pediatr Phys Ther.* 2012;24:155–162.

150. van Brussel M, van Doren L, Timmons BW, et al. Anaerobic to Aerobic power ratio in children with juvenile idiopathic arthritis. *Arthritis Care Res.* 2009;61(6):787–793.

151. Takken T, van der Net JJ, Kuis W, et al. Physical activity and health-related physical fitness in children with juvenile idiopathic arthritis. *Annals of Rheum Dis.* 2003;62(9):885–889.

152. Lelieveld OT, Armbrust W, van Leeuwen MA, et al. Physical activity in adolescents with juvenile idiopathic arthritis. *Arthritis Care Res.* 2008;57:898–904.

153. Tarakci e, Yelden I, Mutlu EK, et al. The relationship between physical activity level, anxiety, depression, and functional ability in children and adolescents with juvenile idiopathic arthritis. *Clin Rheumatol.* 2011;30:1415–1420.

154. Scull S, Athreya B. Childhood arthritis. In: Goldberg B, ed. *Sports and Exercise for Children with Chronic Health Conditions.* Champaign, IL: Human Kinetics; 1995.

155. van der Net J, van der Torre P, Engelbert RH, et al. Motor performance and functional ability in preschool and early school aged children with juvenile idiopathic arthritis: a cross-sectional study. *Pediatr Rheumatol Online J.* 2008;16(6):2. Available at: http://www.ncbi.nlm.nih.gov/pmc/?term=2246124.

156. Kirchheimer JC, Wanivenhaus A, Engel A. Does sport negatively influence joint scores in patients with juvenile rheumatoid arthritis: an 8-year prospective study. *Rheumatol Int.* 1993;12:239–242.

157. Carmen D, Browne R. Joint protection education for children with arthritis: can handouts replace professional instruction? *Arthritis Rheum.* 1996;39:S1714.

158. Powell M, Seid M, Szer IS. Efficacy of custom foot orthotics in improving pain and functional status in children with juvenile idiopathic arthritis. *J Rheumatol.* 2005;32:943–950.

159. Whitehouse R, Shape J, Sullivan D, et al. Children with juvenile rheumatoid arthritis at school. *Clin Pediatr.* 1989;28:509–514.

160. Stoff E, Bacon M, White P. The effects of fatigue, distractibility, and absenteeism on school achievement in children with rheumatic disease. *Arthritis Care Res.* 1989;2:54–59.

161. Lovell DJ, Athreya B, Emery HM, et al. School attendance and patterns, special needs in pediatric patients with rheumatic disease. *Arthritis Care Res.* 1990;3:196–203.

162. Arthritis Foundation: Raising a Child with Arthritis. 2012. Available at: http://www.afstore.org/Products-By-Topic/Juvenile-Arthritis/RAISING-A-CHILD-WITH-ARTHRITIS.

163. Feldman DE, deCivita M, Dobkin PL, et al. Effects of adherence to treatment on short-term outcomes in children with juvenile idiopathic arthritis. *Arthritis Rheum.* 2007;57(6):905–912.

164. Feldman DE, deCivita M, Dobkin PL, et al. Perceived adherence to prescribed treatment in juvenile idiopathic arthritis over a one year period. *Arthritis Care Res.* 2007;57:226–233.

165. April KT, Feldman DE, Zunzunequi MV, et al. Association between treatment adherence and health-related quality of life in children with juvenile idiopathic arthritis: perspectives of both child and parent. *Patient Prefer Adherence.* 2008;2:121–128.

166. Hilderson D, Corstjens F, Moons P, et al. Adolescents with juvenile idiopathic arthritis: who cares after age 16? *Clin Exp Rheumatol.* 2010;28:790–797.

167. McDonagh JE, Southwood TR, Shaw KL, et al. The impact of a coordinated transitional care programme on adolescents with juvenile idiopathic arthritis. *Rheumatol(Oxford).* 2007;46:161–168.

168. Stinson JN, Toomey PC, Stevens BJ, et al. Asking the experts: exploring the self-management needs of adolescents with arthritis. *Arthritis Care Res.* 2008;59(1):65–72.

169. Lelieveld OT, Armbrust W, Geertzen JH, et al. Promoting physical activity in children with juvenile idiopathic arthritis through an internet-based program: results of a pilot randomized controlled trial. *Arthritis Care Res.* 2012;62(5):697–703.

170. Mathiewetz V, Wiemer DM, Fedman SM. Grip and pinch strength: norms for 6 to 9 year olds. *Am J Occup Ther.* 1986;40:705–711.

171. Prudential Fitnessgram: Cooper Institute; available at Human Kinetics: http://www.humankinetics.com/products/all-products/The-FitnessgramActivitygram-Test-Administration-Manual-Updated-4th-Edition

172. Geiger R, Strasak A, Treml B, et al. Six-minute walk test in children and adolescents. *J Pediatr.* 2007;150:395–399.

173. Lythgo N, Wilson C, Galea M. Basic gait and symmetry measures for primary school aged children and young adults whilst walking barefoot and with shoes. *Gait Posture.* 2009;30:502–506.

174. Tarakci E, Ipek Yeldan, PhD, PT1, S. Nilay Baydogan, MSc, PT, Seref Olgar, MD, Ozgur Kasapcopur, MD. Efficacy of a land-based home exercise programme for patients with juvenile idiopathic arthritis: a randomized, controlled, single-blind study. *J Rehabil Med.* 2012;44:962–967

School Activity and Participation Checklist

Children with arthritis or other musculoskeletal disorders may experience difficulty performing some necessary or desired activities in school. These activity limitations may negatively impact the child's participation in school programs. The list below includes many of the typical tasks performed in school. Please check any activity that is difficult for you/your child; please add any other activities that are difficult.

▶ School Attendance

_____ Getting to school on time is difficult for me because:

• I am stiff or hurt in the morning
• I'm too tired to get ready for school
• I need help getting dressed

_____ I am often absent, late, or have to leave school early often because:

• I do not feel well
• I have a doctor's appointment
• I am tired

▶ Classroom Activities

_____ I have trouble taking off/putting on my coat, hat, gloves, boots, etc.

_____ I have trouble using a pen, pencil, or crayons in school because:

• My arm or hands (fingers or wrist) hurt or □ get tired
• The pen, pencil, crayon is too small to hold

_____ I have trouble writing on the chalkboard

_____ I have trouble raising my hand to ask or answer a question

_____ I get stiff sitting in my chair for a long time

_____ My teacher(s) will not let me stand up or walk around when I'm stiff

_____ I get tired during the day and need to rest

_____ I have trouble finishing my schoolwork on time

_____ I have trouble writing fast when I take a test or class notes

_____ My school doesn't have the things that help me do things at home (splints, easel for writing, chair cushion, other)

▶ Physical Education/Recess

_____ I have trouble opening my gym locker

_____ I have trouble changing clothes for gym

_____ I have trouble taking a shower after gym class

_____ I have trouble walking to the playground as fast as the other kids

_____ I have trouble doing the same things in gym/on the playground as the other kids in my class

_____ My gym teacher is afraid to let me do the same things as the other kids

_____ My gym teacher doesn't understand that I can't do some of the things the other kids do. (List the things you have trouble doing.)

▶ Getting Around School

_____ I have trouble getting around the school (I am often late for the next activity) because:

• My classes are too far apart
• The cafeteria or gym is too far away

_____ I have trouble standing in lines for a long time, like in the cafeteria or during assemblies

_____ I have trouble carrying my books, lunch tray, or other things while walking in school

_____ I have trouble opening my milk carton, lunch box, or using a knife and fork during lunch

_____ I have trouble opening heavy doors

_____ I have trouble going up/down stairs

_____ I have trouble using the bathroom at school

_____ I have trouble during fire drills, earthquake drills, and other emergency drills

_____ I often miss field trips because I have trouble walking long distances

▶ **Other Problems**

_____ My teacher(s) don't understand the problems I have because of my condition

_____ My teacher(s) make a big deal of my condition, and it makes me feel different

_____ Other kids make fun of me or say things that make me feel bad

_____ I don't want anyone to know that I have arthritis (other condition)

_____ I have hand splints but don't want to wear them in school

_____ I sometimes forget to take my medicine because it is in the nurse's office

Please add any other school-related problems you/your child have because of their arthritis or other health condition

_____

_____

_____

Klepper S, Lopez R, Winn R, 2004

Rheumatology Transition Checklist for Teenagers

This checklist is to help you prepare to move on to adult care. You can achieve independence in matters of your health and future by actively participating in your care and planning transition to the next step: Care with an Adult Rheumatologist and Center.

	Plan to Start	Needs Practice	Can Do Independently Already	Comments and Contacts
Describe and understand your chronic condition				
Discuss concerns, any issues about transfer of care				
Participates in support group, camp, and teen programs. Interacts with teen, young adult "role models."				
Understands differences between pediatric and adult care, verbalizes expectations for moving on				
Prepares questions and speaks up at medical visit				
Participates in "Teen Visits"; partial visits without parent				
Takes medications, does exercises, treatment correctly				
Keeps "diary" information – medication, doses, provider names, phone numbers, and tracks relevant medical info				
Calls for prescription refilled, lab results, and schedules appointments; keeps contact numbers in cell phone				
Calls to report change in illness, new symptoms, concerns				
Knows insurance and has plans for continuous medical coverage after transfer				
Continues primary care visits—plans for primary care after transfer				
Understands and obtains reproductive health information and appointments				
Independent with self-care, chores, uses devices for ADLs if needed, volunteers, works part time				
Discusses how drugs, alcohol, cigarettes affect illness, pregnancy, and medication toxicities				
Contacts resources/agencies, i.e., Vocational Rehab, driving, college office for students with disabilities, financial aid, other:_____				
Discusses and plans for time to transfer care				
Chooses an adult physician—makes appointment				

Adult Rheumatologist:_____Address:_____

Phone Number: _____ FAX # _____ First Appointment Date: _____

Comment:_____

Patricia A. Rettig, MSN, RN, CRNP, The Children's Hospital of Philadelphia, revised 10/1/10

Healthcare Transition Resources

Visit the Health Care Transition Web site at:
http://hctransitions.ichp.edu/
This mailing list is a service of the Division of Policy and Program Affairs at the Institute for Child Health Policy (www.ichp.edu)

Arthritis Foundations
Atlanta, Georgia 30357-0669
(800) 283-7800
   a. Decision Making for Teenagers with Arthritis brochure
   b. JA Alliance/AF National and Regional Conferences for families and professionals

On TRAC – Taking Responsibility for Adolescent/Adult Care
British Columbia Children's Hospital
Room 2 D20 4480 Oak Street
Vancouver, B.C.
Canada 3V4
(604) 875-3472
   a. Annotated Bibliography
   b. Workshops, training, and consultation

RAP Journal for teens with JIA
Resource Handbook for Parents of Adolescent s with JIA
Janet McDonagh MD and Karen Shaw MD, Rheumatology
Institute of Child Health
Diana, Princess of Wales children's Hospital
Steelhouse Lane
Birmingham, B4 6NH UK
Tel: 0121 333 8743

Parent Training and Information Center
PACER Center, Inc.
4826 Chicago Avenue South
Minneapolis, MN 55412
(612) 827-2966
   a. Speak Up for Health – handbook for parents
   b. Living Your Own Life – handbook for teenagers written by young people and adults with chronic illnesses or disabilities

Other Medical/
Surgical Disorders

Pediatric Oncology

Victoria Gocha Marchese

Common Types of Pediatric Cancer
- Leukemia
- Central Nervous System Tumors
- Lymphoma
- Neuroblastic Tumors
- Sarcoma
- Retinoblastoma
- Wilms Tumor

Disease and Medical Intervention Factors that Influence Physical Therapy Practice
- Chemotherapy
- Radiation Therapy
- Surgery
- Bone Marrow Transplantation and Peripheral Stem Cell Transplantation

Physical Therapy Examination and Evaluation
- Systems Review
- Medical and Social History
- Tests and Measurements
- Body Function and Structure (Impairments)
- Activity (Activity Limitations)
- Participation (Participation Restrictions)

Diagnosis, Prognosis, and Plan of Care
- Physical Therapy Intervention
- Coordination, Communication, and Documentation
- Patient/Client Instruction
- Procedural Intervention

Survivorship

Each year more than 11,000 children and adolescents in the United States are diagnosed with cancer.[1] As a result of improved diagnostic testing and medical interventions, survival rates of young adults who had cancer in childhood are approaching 80%.[2] It is estimated that 328,000 survivors of childhood cancer are living in the United States, which means that approximately 1 in 570 adults 20 to 34 years of age is a survivor of childhood cancer.[3] Therefore, more young adults than ever before are now living with the short- and long-term effects of the cancer and the medical interventions used to save their lives. As the numbers of children with cancer and survivors increase, so does the need for physical therapists to learn more about early detection, treatment interventions for common types of pediatric cancer, and the short- and long-term side effects arising from the cancer and its treatment. As physical therapists, we have a responsibility to understand the continuum of care for our patients, from the first indication that a diagnosis of cancer is a possibility to appropriate types of physical therapy interventions, to educating our patients about long-term complications they may experience as they relate to the scope of physical therapy practice primarily in the areas of the musculoskeletal, neuromuscular, integumentary, and cardiopulmonary systems.

Physical therapists are in a unique position to assist patients with their cancer care and advance the body of research, considering our education and training in those functional areas most adversely impacted by the disease and its treatment. These areas include disease prevention, education, and intervention, with a focus on a variety of impairments including range of motion (ROM), strength, motor planning, balance and coordination, fatigue, assistive devices, prosthetics and orthotics, and functional mobility. The ultimate goal is to improve the patients' quality of life and ability to participate in family and community activities.

Cancer is the uncontrolled growth of cells that do not function properly. As these cells increase in number, they tend to crowd out normal healthy cells or develop into a solid mass, causing signs and symptoms of disease to appear. Typically, the cancer develops at a primary site, but it may *metastasize* or spread to other areas of the body. The term *cancer* is often used to refer to various types of cancer. In children, leukemia, brain tumors, lymphomas, Wilms tumor, neuroblastoma, retinoblastoma, rhabdomyosarcoma, osteosarcoma, and Ewing sarcoma family of tumors are the most common types.[1] In contrast, adults most frequently develop prostate, breast, lung, colon, and rectal cancer.[4]

Common types of pediatric cancer

Leukemia

Leukemia is the most prevalent type of pediatric cancer, accounting for 25% of all cancer cases in children younger than 15 years of age.[5] The disease takes its name from *leukocyte* (white blood cell) and the Greek word ending *emia,* which indicates a condition of the blood. Normal leukocytes are essential in helping the body remove foreign substances such as viruses, bacteria, and fungi. Leukemia, a malignant disorder of the blood and the blood-forming tissues of the bone marrow, is characterized by an overproduction of abnormal leukocytes. There are several different types of leukemia and they are typically classified by the type of cell that gives rise to the cancerous cells (lymphoid or myeloid) and by the speed at which the cells replicate, quickly (acute) or slowly (chronic).

The most common pediatric leukemia is acute lymphoblastic leukemia (ALL), also known as acute lymphocytic leukemia or acute lymphoid leukemia. ALL accounts for 72% of all leukemia cases in children younger than 15 years of age.[5] It is most common in children 2 and 3 years of age. ALL is considered acute because immature lymphocytes proliferate rapidly and because the disease is fatal without treatment. However, with appropriate medical intervention, survival rates for children with ALL are now approaching 94%.[6]

The second most common pediatric leukemia is acute myeloid leukemia (AML), also referred to as myelocytic, myelogenous, or nonlymphoblastic leukemia; it accounts for 15% to 20% of all leukemia cases in children younger than 15 years of age.[7] AML is the rapid proliferation of immature myeloid cells. The survival rate of children with AML is less favorable than that of children with ALL; however, recent survival rates have risen to approximately 71%.[6] In contrast to acute leukemias, chronic leukemia is less common in children, accounting for less than 5% of the cases of pediatric leukemia.[8]

Genetic factors are assumed to play a role in causing the acute leukemia. For example, children with Down syndrome, Klinefelter syndrome, and neurofibromatosis are more likely to develop leukemia than are children without these conditions.[9–12] Another possible factor in the development of acute leukemia is exposure to ionizing radiation and certain toxic chemicals.[5,7]

The signs and symptoms for leukemia are typically caused by an overproduction of a specific cell type that crowds out normal healthy cells, causing anemia, thrombocytopenia, and neutropenia and producing the identifiable side effects of leukemia such as fatigue, bruising, bleeding, infection, bone pain, fever, and enlarged lymph nodes and spleen.[5,7]

Medical intervention for children with leukemia includes multi-agent chemotherapy, which can be given for 2 to 3 years, depending on the type of leukemia and the protocol. It is typically only when ALL relapses, that is, when the cancer cells return, that children will receive a stem cell transplant. However, for children with AML, stem cell transplantation is often the first choice of treatment, if a donor is available.[6,7]

Central Nervous System Tumors

Central Nervous System (CNS) tumors are the second most commonly diagnosed pediatric cancer and the most commonly diagnosed solid tumor in children (Table 16.1).[13] These tumors account for 25% of childhood malignancies and most frequently occur in children during the first decade of life.[13] The most common types of CNS tumors found in children and adolescents are astrocytoma, primitive neuroectodermal tumors (including medulloblastoma), brainstem gliomas, ependymomas, and craniopharyngioma.[6,13] Signs and symptoms of brain tumors in children vary widely according to the size and location of the tumor. They may include headaches, seizures, drowsiness, dysphasia (impaired speech), dysphagia (difficulty with swallowing), impaired vision, behavioral changes, sudden vomiting, poor coordination, weakness, impaired balance, and paresthesia.[6,14,15]

Medical intervention for children with brain tumors depends on the type and location of the tumor and may include surgery, radiation therapy, and chemotherapy.[13] Survival rates for children with CNS tumors vary depending on the type of tumor, size, and location. Children and adolescents with a CNS cancer have an overall survival rate of 74%.[13]

Lymphoma

The third most common type of cancer in children is lymphoma, including Hodgkin disease and non-Hodgkin lymphoma (NHL). Lymphomas account for 8% of all pediatric cancers.[1] These malignancies arise in the lymphoid cells

TABLE 16.1 Common Pediatric CNS Tumors[6,13–15]				
Type of Tumor	**Histology**	**Location**	**CNS Occurrences (%)**	**Peak Age of Incidence**
Astrocytoma (juvenile pilocytic astrocytoma, anaplastic astrocytoma, glioblastoma multiforme)	Astrocytes (glial cells)	Cerebellum, cerebrum, thalamus, or hypothalamus	52	5
Medulloblastoma	Neuroepithelial	Cerebellum	20	1–10
Primitive neuroectodermal tumor (cerebral, neuroblastoma, cerebral medulloblastoma)	Neuroepithelial	Cerebrum	20	1–10
Brainstem gliomas	Glial cells	Midbrain/pons/medulla	10	5–10
Ependymoma	Ependymal	Fourth ventricle	6	<5

and have their own biologic subtypes.[16] Hodgkin disease is more common in older children and adolescents, whereas NHL is more prevalent in younger children.[1] The signs and symptoms of Hodgkin disease include painless supraclavicular or cervical adenopathy, nonproductive cough, fatigue, anorexia, slight weight loss, and pruritus.[16] NHL is typically classified into four subcategories[16]:

1. Burkitt and Burkitt-like lymphoma (small noncleaved cell lymphoma)
2. Lymphoblastic lymphoma
3. Diffuse large B-cell lymphoma
4. Anaplastic large cell lymphoma

The clinical signs and symptoms of NHL may include changes in bowel habits; nausea; vomiting; swelling of the abdomen, face, neck, or upper limbs; pain dysphagia; and dyspenia.[17] The survival rate for children and adolescents with Hodgkin disease is 91% for low-stage disease and greater than 80% for advanced disease; for those with NHL, the rate is nearly 80%.[6,17] Medical treatment of lymphoma typically includes chemotherapy and radiation therapy.[16,17]

Neuroblastic Tumors

The neuroblastic tumors include neuroblastoma, ganglioneuroblastoma, and ganglioneuroma.[18] These tumors develop from primordial neural crest cells and account for 50% of infant malignancies.[6] Two-thirds of children diagnosed with neuroblastoma are under 5 years of age.[3] Neuroblastomas commonly develop in the adrenal glands, sympathetic nervous system, ganglia of the abdomen, and sympathetic ganglia of the chest or neck.[1,18] The signs and symptoms of neuroblastoma depend largely on the location of the tumor. These include a palpable fixed hard mass in the neck or abdomen area and pain and paralysis if the tumor involves the spinal cord or peripheral nerves.[18] Surgery, chemotherapy, and radiation therapy are used to medically manage cases of neuroblastoma. The survival rate of children with neuroblastoma depends on the child's age at diagnosis, disease stage, and tumor histology.[3,18] The younger the child is at diagnosis, the greater the chances of survival. Those who are less than 1 year of age at the time of diagnosis have a survival rate of 90%. The 5-year survival rate of children 1 to 4 years of age at diagnosis of neuroblastoma is approximately 68%; for children 5 to 9 years of age at diagnosis, the survival rate is 52%, and for those children 10 to 14 years of age at diagnosis, the survival rate is 66%.[3]

Sarcoma

The word *sarcoma* means a malignant tumor arising from cells of mesenchymal origin. These cells typically mature into skeletal muscle, smooth muscle, fat, fibrous tissue, bone, and cartilage.[19] The medical intervention for sarcoma may include neoadjuvant (preoperative chemotherapy)

and adjuvant (after surgery) chemotherapy, surgery, and/or radiation therapy. The primary goal of medical treatment is to improve survival of the patient and to preserve as much function of the affected extremity as possible. Factors used to determine the type of medical intervention include the tumor's size, location, and response to presurgical chemotherapy and containment of the disease to the primary site.[20]

Osteosarcoma

Also called osteogenic sarcoma, osteosarcoma is the most common bone tumor in adolescents.[21] They occur most commonly in the long bones, primarily in the metaphyseal area of the distal femur, proximal tibia, or proximal humerus.[21] Teenagers are at the greatest risk of developing osteosarcoma; this is thought to be due to their rapid growth spurts.[21] The primary symptom of osteosarcoma is pain in the involved site with or without the presence of a palpable mass or decreased ROM.[6,21] Medical intervention for sarcoma includes neoadjuvant chemotherapy, adjuvant chemotherapy, and surgery—limb sparing (salvage), amputation, or rotationplasty (Figs. 16.1 through 16.4). Factors used to determine the form of surgery include: the tumor's size, location, and response to presurgical chemotherapy and containment of the disease to the primary site.[20] Survival rates for children with metastatic osteosarcoma (30%) are not as favorable as those for children whose disease is localized (75%).[6]

Ewing Sarcoma

Ewing sarcoma is the second most common type of bone malignancy in children and adolescents.[22] It is thought that Ewing sarcoma originates from neural crest cells; however, Ewing sarcomas are considered to be a tumor primarily of the bone or soft tissue.[22] Common sites for Ewing sarcoma are the vertebral column, pelvis, rib, and long bones such as the femur, tibia, and fibula.[22] Approximately 56% of patients who develop Ewing sarcoma are 10 to 20 years old.[22] Signs and symptoms include pain and/or swelling at the tumor

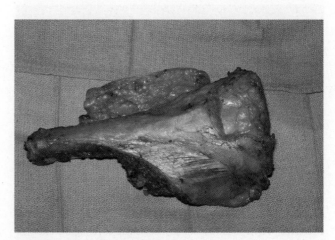

FIGURE 16.1 Excised osteosarcoma.

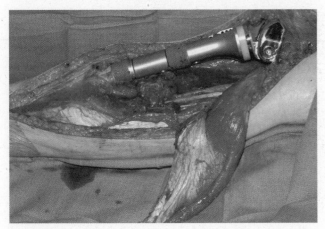

FIGURE 16.2 Internal prosthesis in place during surgery.

location.[22] Medical intervention for children with Ewing sarcoma includes surgery, chemotherapy, and radiation therapy. The prognosis for Ewing sarcoma in children varies widely, depending on the tumor location. The overall 5-year survival rate for children with localized Ewing sarcoma is approximately 70%.[1] The survival rate is lower for those patients who develop metastatic disease (15% to 30%).[1]

Rhabdomyosarcoma

The most common soft tissue sarcoma in neonates to children 14 years of age, rhabdomyosarcoma is the sixth most common cancer in children and adolescents.[1,19] The most prevalent sites for a rhabdomyosarcoma are the head and neck, followed by the urinary and reproductive organs, extremities, and trunk.[6,19] Signs and symptoms of rhabdomyosarcoma include the appearance of a mass or the disturbance in a normal body function such as a tumor in the nasopharynx that causes an obstruction and discharge.[19] Medical treatment for children with rhabdomyosarcoma includes surgical removal of the tumor, chemotherapy, and radiation therapy.[19] As was the case with the other sarcomas, the survival rate for children

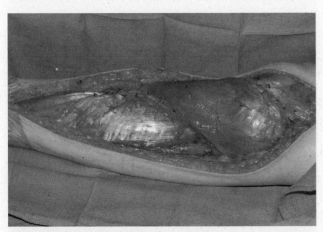

FIGURE 16.3 Gastrocnemius muscle flap covering the internal prosthesis before closing the surgical wound.

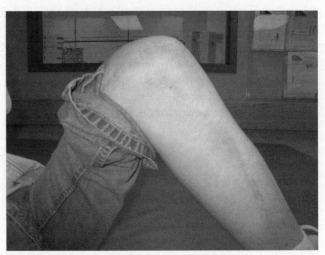

FIGURE 16.4 Surgically repaired lower extremity approximately 3 months after repair with good wound closure.

with rhabdomyosarcoma depends on the tumor size, location, and cellular composition, how successful surgical removal was, and whether the tumor is contained to one site. Children younger than 15 years at diagnosis have a 5-year survival rate of 65% in contrast to those 15 to 19 years of age, who have a 47% survival rate.[1,3]

Retinoblastoma

Retinoblastoma, a malignancy of the retina that originates from multipotent precursor cells, accounts for only 3% of the cases of cancer in children younger than 15 years of age; however, it accounts for 13% of cancers in infants.[3,6,23] The disease may be hereditary or nonhereditary; the hereditary form presents primarily in infants.[23] The nonhereditary form occurs when the gene spontaneously develops a new mutation and is more prevalent in children than in infants.[23] The median age of retinoblastoma is 2 years of age.[1] Three out of four children will have unilateral involvement, while one out of four will have bilateral involvement.[1] The two most common signs and symptoms of retinoblastoma are leukocoria (lack of the normal red reflex of the eye) and strabismus (eyes cross).[23] Medical intervention for children with retinoblastoma is very multifaceted and may include enucleation (removal of the eye), external beam radiotherapy, plaque radiotherapy, laser photocoagulation, cryotherapy, thermotherapy, and systemic chemotherapy.[23] The 5-year survival rate for infants and children with retinoblastoma now exceeds 95%.[6]

Wilms Tumor

Wilms tumor, also called nephroblastoma, is the most common malignancy of the kidney in children.[24] Children younger than 6 years of age are more likely to have Wilms tumor than are older children; it is commonly diagnosed between 3 and 4 years of age.[1,24] The primary signs and symptoms of Wilms tumor are abdominal swelling or mass, fever, anemia, and hypertension.[24] Medical intervention for Wilms tumor consists of surgical resection, chemotherapy, and radiation therapy.[24] The 5-year survival rate for children with Wilms tumor is 92%.[2]

 ## Disease and medical intervention factors that influence physical therapy practice

When a patient presents with signs and symptoms suggestive of cancer, a physician orders specific diagnostic tests. A complete blood count test is very frequently performed to evaluate the function of the bone marrow. The normal blood values listed in Table 16.2 are only a general range because these values vary slightly according to the child's gender and age.[25] The ranges listed as acceptable for participation in exercise are a guideline only. Because children with cancer often have low blood counts, it is highly recommended that the physical therapist contact the child's physician and discuss these parameters. Physical therapists at the leading children's oncology centers, with the approval of physicians, may continue to provide physical therapy services even when a child has low blood counts. For example, the physical therapist may encourage gentle active ROM exercises or a light game of toss with a patient who has a platelet count less than 20,000 μg/L or slow walking for a child with a hemoglobin concentration less than 8 g/100/mL rather than no exercise. Therefore, the standard of care must include structured activities with parameters guided by the blood count levels that were previously agreed upon.

A bone marrow aspiration or bone marrow biopsy is performed by direct insertion of a needle into the bone, typically the iliac crest bone; the sample is then examined microscopically to detect the presence of cancer cells. A lumbar puncture is performed by insertion of a needle into the lumbar vertebrae area; cerebrospinal fluid is withdrawn to determine whether the cancer involves the cerebrospinal fluid. Physical therapists must understand that a child who has undergone either a bone marrow aspiration or a lumbar puncture may experience discomfort with movement or feel sore in these areas for a few days and take this into consideration when performing the physical therapy examination and planning for that session's intervention program. For example, if a patient has difficulty transitioning from a sitting position to standing, it may not be due to lower extremity weakness but instead to discomfort in the hip or low back area, and in a few days the problem will resolve.

If a patient presents with pain or swelling in an extremity, radiography, ultrasound, computed tomography (CT), or magnetic resonance imaging (MRI) is performed. Examination of the imaging results is helpful in identifying the tumor's location, but further testing, for example, of a needle biopsy sample, is required to determine the type of tumor on the basis of the cell's morphologic characteristics. This information is important to the physical therapist because the location of the tumor may have an impact on the surrounding tissues such as causing joint contractures or change the patient's lower extremity weight-bearing status, thus limiting ambulation and functional mobility.

Before prescribing a course of medical treatment, the oncologist will determine the tumor's grade and stage by identifying the specific type of cancer on a cellular level, its exact location, and whether the cancer has spread to other areas of the body. The tumor's grade, which indicates its degree of malignancy, is determined on the basis of the microscopic appearance of the tumor cells, the tendency of the tumor to spread, and its growth rate. A system frequently used in the determination of cancer grade is that of the World Health Organization (WHO).[15] The system starts with grade I (a tumor that grows slowly and has a slightly abnormal appearance) and ends with grade IV (a tumor that reproduces most rapidly and has the undifferentiated cells).[15] Staging classifications are used to describe whether the disease is contained to the primary site, and if not, the extent of its spread. Although the exact cause of the cancer is often unknown, genetic and environmental factors have been linked to many of the common pediatric cancers. It is important for the oncologist to understand these genetic factors because they may also affect the type of intervention

TABLE 16.2	Blood Count, Symptoms, and Exercise Guidelines[26]			
	Red Blood Cells (Erythrocytes)	**Platelets (Thrombocytes)**	**Hemoglobin**	**White Blood Cells (Leukocytes)**
Function	CO_2 and O_2 transport	Clotting of blood	CO_2 and O_2 transport	Defense against infection
Normal values	Male: $4.7–5.5 \times 10^6/\mu L$ Female: $4.1–4.9 \times 10^6/\mu L$	150,000–350,000/μL	10–13 g/100 mL	4500–11,000/mm³
Name of low value	Anemia	Thrombocytopenia	Anemia	Bacterial, viral, and/or fungal infection
Symptoms of low values	Pallor Fatigue	Bruising Petechiae	Pallor Fatigue	Infection
Exercise guidelines	See Hemoglobin	No exercise: <20,000 Light exercise: 20,000–50,000 Resistive exercise: >50,000	No exercise: <8 Light exercise: 8–10 Resistive exercise: >10	No exercise: <5000 Light exercise: >5000 Resistive exercise: >5000

chosen for the patient. The physical therapist too must understand the grading and staging systems to tailor the physical therapy intervention program and plan of care around the child's specific needs. For example, if a child has a lower extremity osteosarcoma and the therapist is working on gait training and the patient is becoming short of breath with increased work of breathing, the therapist will want to know if the patient has lung metastases, and modify the session accordingly.

Pediatric cancers are typically treated with multiple modalities such as surgery, chemotherapy, radiation therapy, or stem cell transplantation. Medical intervention is based on the type of cancer and the extent of disease. There are different phases of treatment: induction, consolidation, and maintenance. During the induction phase, the patient receives high doses of chemotherapy and possibly other modalities such as radiation therapy, with the goal of achieving remission as quickly as possible (no cancer cells present). To eliminate any remaining cancer cells, patients continue to receive high doses of chemotherapy during the consolidation phase. During the maintenance phase, patients receive lower doses of chemotherapy with the goal of preventing disease relapse.

Chemotherapy

Chemotherapeutic agents are chemicals used to interfere with rapidly dividing cancer cells, thus resulting in cell death. Multi-agent chemotherapy is used to prevent resistance to one drug and allows administration of higher doses. Chemotherapy is the primary intervention for many types of cancers such as leukemia and lymphoma. It is often combined with other treatment modalities such as surgery and radiation therapy. For example, children with osteosarcoma or Ewing sarcoma often receive neoadjuvant chemotherapy for approximately 10 to 12 weeks before surgery to help shrink the tumor.[26,27] They also receive adjuvant chemotherapy to aid in elimination of any cancer cells that have spread into other areas of the body.

Chemotherapeutic agents are administered in a variety of ways, including intravenous, oral, and intramuscular routes. Most do not readily cross the blood–brain barrier; therefore, to target disease in the CNS, these agents are injected directly into the cerebrospinal fluid, typically through a catheter inserted in the lumbar area or in the brain.[28] This mode of administration, which is called intrathecal, is commonly used for administration of methotrexate.

Chemotherapeutic agents cause secondary side effects (Table 16.3).[29–41] Not all agents cause the same side effects, nor do they occur within the same period of time. For example, drugs such as vincristine are known to cause sensory/motor peripheral neuropathy, primarily affecting the hands and feet, within weeks of administration.[29,40,42–45] The earliest and most common clinical sign related to vincristine toxicity is a decreased Achilles tendon reflex, which can occur within a month of chemotherapy. The primary indication of peripheral neuropathy is foot drop, decreased ankle dorsiflexion strength and active ROM, and neuropathic pain.[35,40,46] However, the order in which the clinical presentation occurs may vary; the physical therapist may observe weakness in a patient's intrinsic muscle of the hands and feet followed by weakness of the anterior tibialis, or the patient may experience neuropathic pain without any signs of

---

TABLE

16.3 Specific Chemotherapeutic Agents and Common Side Effects Pertinent to Physical Therapy[35–49]

Chemotherapeutic Agents	Common Side Effects		Common Types of Cancer
	Short Term	**Long Term**	
Vincristine	Hypertension, motor difficulties, CNS depression, peripheral neuropathy, alopecia, constipation, anorexia, jaw pain, leg pain, weakness, paresthesia, numbness, myalgia, cramping	Peripheral neuropathy, decreased gross and fine motor skills	Leukemia, Hodgkin disease, neuroblastoma, lymphomas, Wilms tumor, and rhabdomyosarcoma
Cisplatin	Bradycardia, nausea, vomiting, bone marrow suppression, ototoxicity, peripheral neuropathy	Ototoxicity, nephrotoxicity	Osteosarcoma, Hodgkin disease and non-Hodgkin lymphoma, brain tumors
Methotrexate	Malaise, fatigue, dizziness, alopecia, photosensitivity, nausea, vomiting, diarrhea, anorexia, mucositis, glossitis, myelosuppression, arthralgia, osteopenia	Osteoporosis, bone fracture, infertility, renal toxicity, hepatotoxicity, neuropsychological-cognitive deficits	Leukemia, osteosarcoma, non-Hodgkin lymphoma
Dexamethasone	Hypertension, increased susceptibility to infection, myopathy, increased appetite, mental changes	Growth suppression, bone demineralization, osteonecrosis	Leukemia, brain tumors, and other types of malignancy
Ifosfamide	Somnolence, dizziness, polyneuropathy, alopecia, dermatitis, nausea, vomiting, anorexia, diarrhea, constipation, myelosuppression	Cardiotoxicity, nephrotoxicity	Hodgkin disease and non-Hodgkin lymphoma, acute and chronic lymphocytic leukemia, sarcoma
Doxorubicin	Alopecia, nausea, vomiting, mucositis, diarrhea, bone marrow suppression	Cardiotoxicity, myocarditis	Lymphoma, leukemia, soft tissue sarcoma, neuroblastoma, osteosarcoma

muscle weakness. As soon as the dose of the vincristine is decreased or administration of the drug is stopped, the symptoms of neurotoxicity generally decrease; however, some researchers report residual deficits of gross motor skills.[34,43] Drugs such as methotrexate cause problems such as myelosuppression within a week of their administration and long-term neuropsychological problems with memory deficits and visual-spatial and motor coordination impairments.[47–49] Myelosuppression is a process in which bone marrow activity is decreased, resulting in low production of platelets, red blood cells, and white blood cells and a corresponding increase in the risk of bleeding, fatigue, and infection.

Radiation Therapy

Radiation therapy uses ionizing radiation to disrupt the structure of the tumor cells' DNA, which limits the cells' ability to further reproduce. Radiation therapy is delivered by an external radiation beam or internal placement of radiation material near the tumor. Radiation therapy is often used alone or more frequently combined with other treatments such as surgery and chemotherapy.[50,51] Radiation therapy delivered before surgical removal of a tumor can shrink the tumor mass, thus decreasing the amount of damage to the surrounding healthy tissues.[52] Radiation is used after surgery to destroy any cells that may have spread from the primary site.[52] Total body irradiation is also combined with chemotherapy to destroy the child's bone marrow in preparation for receiving a stem cell transplant. Radiation therapy may cause numerous short- and long-term side effects (Table 16.4), which are mainly related to the area and the surrounding tissues that received the radiation.[50–57] Side effects from radiation are particularly severe in infants and children who are still growing. Their neuropsychological and musculoskeletal systems are affected.

Surgery

Surgical procedures typically performed for the pediatric patient with cancer include tumor biopsy, central line and shunt placement, and tumor resection, with or without extensive surgical reconstruction.

Tumor Biopsy

Typically, before any medical intervention takes place, a biopsy of a portion of the tumor or a bone marrow aspiration is obtained. These procedures are performed under general anesthesia, conscious sedation, or local anesthesia. Unfortunately, with some brain tumors, primarily those of the brainstem, a biopsy cannot be performed due to the high risk of damage to surrounding tissue.

Central Line and Shunt Placement

Because most children receive intravenous chemotherapy agents over an extended period of time, a surgically placed indwelling catheter that leads directly into a major blood vessel near the heart may be required. These lines are often called a central line, Broviac, or Hickman catheter. The Broviac catheter is an external catheter that leads into a major vessel such as the external or internal jugular. An internal catheter is placed into the same major vessel, but it remains under the skin and is accessed with a needle each time the child needs to receive medication or to have blood drawn. A central line being pulled out accidentally constitutes a medical emergency owing to the risk of infection and bleeding. Therefore, special precautions must be taken to keep the area around the catheter clean, dry, and protected from injury.

Surgical placement of a ventriculoperitoneal shunt is often required when a brain tumor results in increased intracranial pressure. It is important for physical therapists to know the following signs and symptoms of increased cranial pressure owing to a brain tumor or a shunt malfunction: headaches, vomiting, diplopia, disturbances of consciousness, papilledema, and changes in motor function.[14]

Surgical Resection

Most solid tumors will require surgical resection. However, some are too large to be resected, or are located where surgical resection would be risky. Examples include brainstem glioma or neuroblastoma that extends into the spinal cord. However, for malignant tumors, surgical resection is typically the optimal choice. To increase the chance that the tumor does not return or spread to other areas of the body, the surgeon will make every effort to completely resect the

TABLE 16.4	Short- and Long-term Side Effects of Radiation[50–57]	
Short Term	**Long Term**	**Implication for Physical Therapists**
Skin	Fibrosis	Pain
Redness	Pathologic fracture	Decreased ROM
Blistering	Bone growth abnormalities	Decreased strength
Hair loss	Osteonecrosis/avascular necrosis	Decreased endurance
Fibrosis	Osteoporosis	Decreased functional mobility
Fatigue	Cardiac complications	Decreased balance
Cognitive deficits	Hypertension	Decreased neuropsychological function
	Thyroid dysfunction	Motor accuracy, sensory integration, Memory, concentration
		Decreased quality of life and participation in community and family activities

tumor with a clean margin of tissue with no cancer cells. Because it is not always known whether any cells have spread beyond the primary tumor site, chemotherapy and radiation therapy may also be given to the patient.

Other Surgical Procedures

For patients with an upper or lower extremity bone or soft tissue tumor, surgical options such as amputation, rotationplasty, and limb-sparing procedures are available.[58–60] Limb-sparing procedures may include the use of a custom endoprosthetic device, allograft reconstruction, or autograft reconstruction, or combine the use of endoprostheses and bone grafts.[20] For children who have not reached skeletal maturity, the lower extremity can be reconstructed by using an expandable endoprosthesis or contralateral epiphysiodesis.[20] Use of the expandable endoprosthesis, also referred to as a repiphysis prosthesis, is the common choice.[58] After the expandable prosthesis is implanted, the surgeon can lengthen the child's leg without opening the surgical site. Use of this noninvasive procedure decreases the risk of infection and the time required for healing. The short-term limitations of the limb-sparing procedure (Table 16.5) include slow wound healing due to use of chemotherapeutic agents, infection, and poor joint ROM[61,62] (Fig. 16.5). Long-term side effects include the need for frequent surgical revisions due to loosening of the prosthesis, leg length discrepancy, fractures, infection, poor joint ROM, extensive problems requiring amputation, and local tumor recurrence.[20,58,61–63] Thus, it is important for physical therapists to plan for these types of complications and provide preventive measures if possible, such as exercises to prevent contractures and activity recommendations to decrease the wear and tear on the prosthesis, recommending biking and swimming activities versus running and contact sports.

AMPUTATION This surgical procedure results in removal of a portion of an extremity; the extent of the amount of limb removed depends on the tumor's location, type, and size. Amputation is typically performed when it is not possible to make a wide-enough excision to achieve clean margins, or when surgery is so extensive that the extremity is no longer functional.[61] After deciding that a child needs an amputation,

the surgeon makes every effort to provide the patient with a residual limb that is conducive to the functional use of a prosthetic device. The short-term complications of an amputation may include psychological distress related to a drastic change in body image, slow healing of the surgical site if the child is receiving chemotherapy, inadequate wound coverage, neuropathic pain, phantom limb sensation, and increased energy expenditure for functional activities.[61] Long-term complications include psychological distress related to a drastic change in body image; skin blisters, redness, or bruising on the residual limb due to growth or weight changes; phantom limb pain and sensation; musculoskeletal pain; and increased energy expenditure for activities of daily living.[61]

ROTATIONPLASTY This surgical procedure is sometimes performed in lieu of an amputation; however, it is still considered a form of amputation.[61] Rotationplasty is not the standard of care at many of the children's hospitals in the United States. Rotationplasty removes a femoral tumor while preserving the neurovascular bundle and the distal portion of the lower leg and foot. The lower leg is turned 180 degrees and attached to the proximal femur in such a way that the foot can serve as the functional knee joint and as a weight-bearing surface for a prosthesis. The resultant residual limb does not require multiple surgical revisions and it is longer than if a below-knee amputation had been performed.[20] This longer limb provides the patient with the chance for higher functional abilities.[64] Furthermore, patients who have undergone rotationplasty can participate in recreational activities and sports, as can patients who have had an amputation.[65,66] In the short term, the wound heals poorly; and in both the short and long term, the extremity appears odd. Researchers have studied quality of life in patients who have undergone a rotationplasty and determined that patients do not show reduction in psychosocial adaptation compared with the healthy population.[67,68]

Bone Marrow Transplantation and Peripheral Stem Cell Transplantation

Bone marrow transplantation (BMT) or peripheral blood stem cell transplantation (PSCT) is performed for children

---

TABLE 16.5 Short- and Long-term Side Effects of Limb-sparing Procedures, Amputation, and Rotationplasty

Limb-sparing Procedures		Amputation		Rotationplasty	
Short term	Long term	Short term	Long term	Short term	Long term
Slow wound healing	Multiple surgical revisions	Slow wound healing	Body image difficulties	Slow wound healing	Poor body image
Infection	Leg length discrepancy	Infection	Skin blisters	Infection	Leg length discrepancy
Poor ROM	Fractures	Inadequate wound coverage	Redness	Increased energy expenditure	Increased energy expenditure
Increased energy expenditure	Infection	Increased energy expenditure	Phantom limb pain		
	Poor joint ROM	Neuropathic pain	Muscle pain		
	Increased energy expenditure		Increased energy expenditure		
	Converted to amputation				
	Local recurrence				

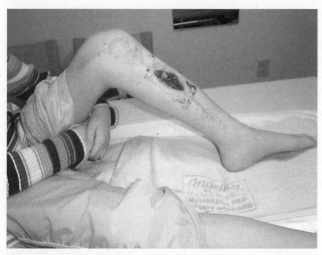

FIGURE 16.5 Patient 3 months after a limb-sparing procedure for proximal tibia osteosarcoma, presenting with wound closure problems.

with leukemia (relapsed ALL or chronic myelogenous leukemia) or other hematologic diseases (e.g., aplastic anemia, severe combined immunodeficiency [SCID], and sickle cell disease) that involve the bone marrow. The purpose is to replace the patient's bone marrow with his or her own marrow or donor bone marrow capable of producing healthy cells. Bone marrow is typically harvested by the repeated insertion of a large needle into the donor's bone (e.g., the iliac crest) and withdrawal of the marrow. The stem cells, the most immature cell that further differentiates into mature cells, are obtained by taking blood from the donor via a process called apheresis. There are three common forms of BMT or PSCT:

1. Allogeneic transplants from a histocompatible donor
2. Autologous transplants from the patient's own cells
3. Syngeneic transplants from an identical twin

The protocol being used and the policies of the institution where the transplantation takes place will determine whether the child receives a BMT or PSCT. The more common procedure currently performed is the PSCT. Some institutions are also now performing umbilical cord blood transplants.

Children who receive a BMT or a PSCT first receive combination chemotherapy to achieve a state of remission (no identifiable cancer cells in the body). The child is then admitted to the hospital for the conditioning phase. For approximately 1 week, the child receives chemotherapeutic agents (e.g., thiotepa) and total body irradiation, depending on his or her age and the treatment protocol. The goal of the conditioning phase is to provide complete bone marrow suppression. Because the child's white blood cell, red blood cell, and platelet counts drop, the child requires special care during this period to prevent infection and hemorrhaging. The child then receives an infusion of bone marrow or peripheral stem cells. For approximately 6 weeks, the child stays in an isolated room equipped with a positive pressure and an air filtration system to help prevent infection.

Engraftment, the process by which donor marrow begins to produce healthy cells, typically takes 10 to 17 days.[69] However, until the body produces its own cells, the child will require antibiotics to prevent infection and transfusions of red blood cells and platelets. Children may require red blood cell and platelet transfusions for up to 6 months and may not have adequate white blood cells to fight infection for 6 to 12 months.[69] Thus, physical therapists must be knowledgeable of the patient's blood count levels to plan for the physical therapy session.

Transplant recipients do not produce healthy bone marrow cells for a period of time. Therefore, the recipient has an increased risk of infection, bleeding, and severe fatigue. Children who receive allogeneic transplants may develop some form of graft-versus-host disease (GVHD), a process by which the transplanted marrow (graft) starts to attack the patient's (host) organs. There are two types of GVHD: acute and chronic. Acute GVHD can begin as early as the first month after the transplantation, when the engraftment process is taking place. Acute GVHD most commonly affects the skin, the gut, and the liver; the patient experiences a rash, itchy skin, skin discoloration, dry mouth, mouth ulcers, diarrhea, and weight loss. Chronic GVHD occurs months after the patient receives the transplant and affects the skin and gastrointestinal system. Specific complications may include changes in the skin pigmentation and texture; possible development of joint contractures; dry mouth and ulcer formations; difficulty in swallowing and malabsorption, which may cause the child to lose weight; chronic liver disease; and problems with the eyes such as dryness, pain, and sensitivity to light.[70] The drugs prednisone, cyclosporine, and methotrexate are commonly given to patients to prevent GVHD or to decrease the severity of the reaction.[70] Long-term complications include those that were previously listed under chemotherapy and radiation therapy. Physical therapists should evaluate and provide intervention for children with GVHD to assist in the prevention of the development of joint contractures, decreased strength, and functional mobility.

Stem cell rescue is a process by which the child's own stem cells are extracted and stored. The child is then able to receive very high doses of chemotherapeutic agents, after which he or she receives a transfusion of his or her own cells. This procedure allows patients with cancer such as medulloblastoma and neuroblastoma to receive multiple rounds of very high doses of chemotherapy.

▶ Physical therapy examination and evaluation

Systems Review

Because patients with cancer are often fatigued before the physical therapy examination begins, it is important that the therapist identify areas of concern immediately and focus the examination on those target areas. The systems review is a helpful way to guide the physical therapy examination. As soon as the therapist sees the patient, whether this occurs in the patient's hospital room, the clinic, the child's classroom, or home, he or she can identify key issues. Keeping a list of the essentials in mind helps with speed and thoroughness:

1. Musculoskeletal: obvious joint contractures or foot drop
2. Neuromuscular: signs of pain such as antalgic gait pattern, facial grimacing, guarding an area, increased or decreased muscle tone, facial paralysis, difficulty hearing when the therapist says "hello" ; neurocognitive deficits that will limit the child's ability to follow directions; or impaired balance
3. Cardiovascular and pulmonary: nasal flaring, increased work of breathing or respiratory rate
4. Integumentary: facial skin color that demonstrates possible low hemoglobin or liver function problems, for example, bruising that signals a low platelet count

Medical and Social History

Obtaining a thorough medical and social history is one of the key components of any physical therapy examination. This process helps the physical therapist select the types of questions to ask the patient, directs the specific types of tests and measurements that are chosen, and ultimately guides the plan of care. If the patient's chart is available, it is ideal to obtain the following information before meeting the patient:

1. Diagnoses
2. Disease grade and stage
3. Medical history, including patient's growth and development
4. Current medical treatment, including the types of chemotherapeutic agents the patient is receiving and other medical treatments
5. Current blood values, that is, hemoglobin concentrations, white and red blood cell counts, and platelet counts

However, physical therapists are not always fortunate enough to have the patient's medical chart available before meeting the patient. If the child or caregiver is unable to provide the therapist with the pertinent information, then it is most appropriate to call the physician or nurse.

After obtaining the required medical information, it is important for the therapist to build a rapport with the child and the family. This is when the therapist asks about the child's social history. With whom does the child live? Does he or she have any siblings? What grade has he or she completed in school? What sports or other leisure activities does the child enjoy? The therapist will use the answers to these questions as a basis for discussing areas with which the child is having difficulty at home, at school, or in the hospital. Often, it isn't until the therapist begins the examination that the child and family realize how much trouble the child is really having with a specific task such as climbing onto a school bus or that he or she is frequently tripping when walking on grass or other uneven surfaces.

Tests and Measurements

Before the therapist conducts any tests or measurements, it is important that he or she plan the session. To make sure the examination is thorough and comprehensive, the therapist can use a disablement model such as the WHO's International Classification of Functioning, Disability, and Health (body functions/structures, activity, and participation) or the model of the National Center for Medical Rehabilitation Research (pathophysiology, impairment, functional limitation, disability, and societal limitations).[71] In this chapter, the WHO model will be used as a reference. According to the WHO, the term *body function and structure* refers to the physiologic functions of body systems, including the body's psychological functions and anatomic parts, such as organs and limbs and their components. *Activity* refers to the execution of a task or action by an individual and *participation* refers to involvement in a life situation.[71] The WHO model takes into account the interactions between all three components of the model and the child's individual environmental and personal factors. Each child will require an individualized examination based on the specific diagnoses and common side effects of the medical intervention the child has received or is receiving. Table 16.6 outlines the key areas of focus in each category. For individual patients, some areas will be more applicable and will require further testing.

Body Function and Structure (Impairments)

Musculoskeletal

The musculoskeletal component of the examination is important for children with cancer because they oftentimes have problems with ROM, strength, and postural alignment. When performing the ROM examination, the therapist should give particular attention to the joints above and below any area where a surgical procedure has recently been performed. Children will often guard the area around the surgical site because of pain or fear. For example, immediately after a brain tumor resection, a child may have decreased cervical spine ROM or may tilt his or her head laterally to compensate for visual deficits. For a few days after a central line placement, a child may not want to perform full-shoulder flexion or trunk ROM because the chest area is sore. After an aggressive distal femur or proximal tibia limb-sparing procedure, a child's hip, knee, and ankle ROM may be limited. Another important factor to consider when testing a child's ROM is the type of chemotherapy the child is receiving or has received because agents such as vincristine cause a decrease in active ankle dorsiflexion ROM; over time, this decreased ROM can develop into a contracture. Therefore, the therapist will want to focus on the ankle and hand grip strength in patients receiving vincristine.

When performing the strength component of the examination, the therapist must consider the child's blood count

TABLE 16.6	Recommended Tests and Measurements			

Body Function and Structure		Activity	Participation
Musculoskeletal	**Integumentary**	**Ambulation**	**Quality of Life**
ROM	Skin	Quality of gait pattern	School
Goniometer	Temperature		Work
Functional ROM	Color	Assistance required	Play
	Texture	Forearm crutches	Sports
		Axillary crutches	Marriage
Strengthening	Wound	Walker	Travel
Manual muscle test	Healing	Wheelchair	Palliative care
Handheld goniometer	Drainage	Orthoses	Talking
Functional abilities	Smell	Prosthesis	
		Manual guidance	
Postural alignment	Scar mobility		Questionnaires
		Locomotion and developmental skills	SF-36
		Walking	PedsQL
Neuromuscular	**Cardiopulmonary**	Sit-to-stand	
Pain	Endurance	Stand-to-sit	
FLACC scale	2-, 6-, 9-minute run/walk tests	Pull to stand	
FACES scale		Creeping	
Visual analog scale	Rate of perceived exertion	Crawling	
	Physiological Cost Index	Rolling	
Type of pain	Heart rate	Stair climbing	
Neuropathic	Respiratory rate		
Nociceptive		Standardized tests	
		Peabody Developmental Motor Scales	
Muscle tone and motor control	Cervical and thoracic asymmetry	Pediatric Evaluation of Disability Inventory	
Ataxia	Nasal flaring		
Spasticity	Belly breather	Balance and coordination	
Hypotonicity	Increased work of breathing	Single-limb stance	
Clonus		Timed up and down stairs	
Paresis		Timed up and go	
		Start/stop on oral cue	
Visual exam		Tandem walking	
Vision		Walking on uneven surfaces (grass, hills)	
Tracking		Dual-task activities	
Diplopia			
Eye–hand coordination			
Sensation			
Light touch			
Sharp dull			
Two-point discrimination			
Sensory integration			

levels. For children with a low platelet count, the typical manual muscle test and dynamometry is not appropriate. However, the therapist can observe the child's functional strength abilities while performing activities such as walking, climbing stairs, and performing transitional movements such as sit-to-stand.

Neuromuscular

When examining a child's neuromuscular system (i.e., conducting tests of pain, muscle tone, balance, motor control, vision, sensation, and sensory integration), it is important for the therapist to consider the complex interplay of the neuromuscular system with all the other systems in the body, the environment, and the task. If a child with a brainstem glioma presents with increased or decreased muscle tone or stiffness in the right lower and upper extremity, the therapist must consider how this impairment affects the child's active and passive ROM, isolated muscle strength, proprioception, functional abilities, and activities of daily living, while also taking into account the child's cognitive abilities, age, family support, and motivation.

It is important that the physical therapist determine whether a child is experiencing pain, and if so, to identify the location, intensity, quality, onset/duration, and aggravating and alleviating factors. Pain is measurable in all individuals regardless of age. Depending on the patient's age and cognitive abilities, a variety of tools are available: (1) the

FLACC (Face, Legs, Activity, Cry, Consolability) scale for infants to children 5 years of age; (2) the FACES scale for patients 5 to 13 years of age; and (3) self-reporting numeric scales (0 to 10) or a visual analog scale for children older than 13 years. A child may experience nociceptive pain and/or neuropathic pain. Nociceptive pain, commonly described as aching or throbbing pain, is typically caused by bone, joint, muscle, skin, or connective tissue damage from the disease itself, from medications such as steroids, or from surgery. In contrast, neuropathic pain is typically described as burning, tingling, or piercing, and it is caused by injury to a nerve, either from surgery, chemotherapeutic agents, or radiation therapy.[72–74]

Integumentary

Examination of the integumentary system tells the therapist a great deal about a child. The color and texture of the skin alone may offer the therapist some information that will lead to further examination. For example, pallor suggests anemia; jaundice, liver dysfunction; dry and itchy skin, GVHD; cold skin, poor circulation; hot skin, infection; drainage with a foul odor, infection; blisters, poorly fitted brace; red/blistered skin, radiation burns; and ulcers, pressure sores. Physical therapists will want to examine the mobility of a scar and note any scar adhesions. Physical therapists play a critical role in the identification and management of the integumentary issues that children with cancer may experience. The physical therapist must take the time to examine the integumentary system thoroughly, document the findings, and communicate and coordinate the plan of care with the physician.

Cardiopulmonary

Children with cancer may experience cardiopulmonary complications due to the effects of chemotherapy, radiation, prolonged bed rest, generalized fatigue, or skeletal abnormalities caused by a tumor, surgery, or radiation therapy. Therefore, the physical therapist must perform a comprehensive respiratory, skeletal (rib cage), and endurance examination. A good starting point is observation of the child, which will reveal increased work of breathing, nasal flaring, respiratory rate, and skeletal asymmetries that affect the cardiorespiratory system. More detailed assessments will include using a pulse oximeter to obtain a child's resting heart rate before he or she performs an endurance examination and the therapist calculates his or her target heart rate range.

The child's age and abilities will guide the type of endurance tests the therapist chooses. For infants and toddlers, endurance testing may include observation of skin color, vital signs, and breathing patterns while the child is playing. For testing of the older child and adolescent, more structured methods are available such as a treadmill test at a variety of levels, step tests, and run/walk tests, including the 2-, 6-, and 9-minute tests.[75,76] While the child is performing the endurance tests, the therapist can monitor the child's heart and respiratory rates. Tools are available to examine the energy required to perform specific tasks. The physiologic cost index is an objective way to calculate a child's energy expenditure. The rating of perceived exertions scale is a subjective scale of how hard the child reports that he or she is working.[77–82]

Activity (Activity Limitations)

Ambulation and Locomotion

Children with cancer may experience difficulty with ambulation and locomotion as a result of the disease and treatment effects. These deficits may occur due to the effects of drugs such as vincristine that cause foot drop, weakness due to nerve root impingement, bone pain from the buildup of blast cells in the bone marrow, or structural changes from a limb-sparing or amputation procedure. The therapist will first identify the child's primary means of mobility, whether it is walking, crawling, or using a wheelchair. Second, the therapist will identify the amount of assistance or the type of assistive device required for the patient to perform the task. Third, the therapist will examine the quality of the gait pattern or other means of mobility.

Balance and Coordination

Balance and coordination deficits are common in children who have had a CNS or peripheral nervous system tumor or who have experienced side effects of chemotherapy or radiation therapy, surgical alterations of the skeletal system, or weakness from prolonged inactivity. As previously stated in the neuromuscular section, therapists must consider other systems (e.g., vision, hearing, sensation, muscle tone, and cognition) and environmental factors when examining a child's balance and coordination abilities. A few common tests (Table 16.6) include eyes open or closed, single-limb stance, timed up and down stairs, timed up and go, dual-task activities, and tandem walking.[83,84]

Participation (Participation Restrictions)

The most important component of the examination is identification of how the child's body structure/function and activity limitations are affecting the child and the family at home, work, school, or play. This can be achieved by using oral communication, observation, and structured questionnaires. Two commonly used pediatric-specific questionnaires are the PedsQL and the Short Form 36.[85,86] Often, a therapist will ask children and parents how things are going at home and the reply is "just fine"; however, it is the role of the physical therapist to focus the child and family on specific tasks such as getting in and out of bed, eating at the dinner table with the family, bathing, going to the mall with friends, going to school, climbing stairs at school, walking to class at school, and participating in sports. It is also important to discuss with the child and caregiver the child's level of involvement in activities because the child may feel isolated, lonely, and left out when he or she returns to school.[87]

 Diagnosis, prognosis, and plan of care

The physical therapy diagnosis and prognosis for pediatric cancer will vary depending on the specific type of cancer, medical intervention, and family dynamics. The following physical therapy diagnoses are common for patients with cancer: pain (neuropathic/nociceptive), fatigue, decreased ROM, decreased strength, decreased endurance, developmental delays, poor wound closure, decreased functional mobility, and decreased participation in community activities (Table 16.7). For each patient, the plan of care and goals will require individual consideration depending on the child's unique circumstances. The physical therapist's role is to assist children with cancer in the prevention of secondary complications of the cancer and medical interventions; to promote health, wellness, fitness, and normal development; to limit the degree of disability; to promote rehabilitation; and to restore function in patients with chronic and irreversible disease.[88] To fulfill this role, the physical therapist should provide physical therapy intervention for children with cancer with an equal emphasis on body structure/function impairments, activity limitations, and participation restrictions.[89] The time line for physical therapy intervention and the child and caregiver's goals will depend on the individual child and the medical diagnosis and prognosis.

Physical Therapy Intervention

The evidence to support the need for physical therapy services for children with cancer is overwhelming. Furthermore, our clinical experience has clearly demonstrated that physical therapy intervention for children with cancer is beneficial on all levels of care from body function/structure limitations to activity limitations to participation limitations. Despite the documented cases of children with cancer who have had complications with ROM, strength, endurance, decreased balance, and functional activities, the effects of a comprehensive physical therapy program for children with cancer have not been well documented in the literature. The few studies specifically related to physical therapy intervention for children with cancer have been focused primarily on children with leukemia. On the basis of the results of these studies,

TABLE 16.7   Possible Physical Therapy Diagnoses Based on Medical Diagnosis

Medical Diagnosis	Physical Therapy Diagnosis	Possible Causes
Leukemia/lymphoma	Pain	Peripheral neuropathy, bone pain from buildup of blast cells in the bone marrow, joint, and bone mainly due to osteonecrosis
	Decreased sensation	Peripheral neuropathy, nerve root compression
	Decreased strength	Peripheral neuropathy, steroids, inactivity
	Decreased ROM	Peripheral neuropathy, osteonecrosis
	Decreased endurance and fatigue	Inactivity, chemotherapy, radiation therapy, stem cell transplant
	Decreased functional mobility	Decreased strength, endurance, pain
	Decreased participation in community activities	Self-confidence, fear, other social concerns such as friendships and previously listed impairments, limited handicapped-accessible accommodations
CNS and peripheral nervous system tumor	Pain	Tumor impingement (spinal cord or peripheral nerve root impingement), peripheral neuropathy or surgical pain
	Decreased sensation	Peripheral neuropathy, CNS damage
	Decreased strength	Tumor impingement, surgical pain, fear, immobility, inactivity
	Decreased ROM	Surgical incision site, decreased motor control, abnormal muscle tone
	Decreased balance and coordination	Poor motor control, ataxia, paralysis/paresis, decreased vision, vestibular dysfunction
	Decreased functional mobility	Visual deficits, decreased strength, endurance
	Decreased participation in community activities	Previously listed impairments and limited handicapped-accessible accommodations
Bone and soft tissue tumors	Pain	Tumor impingement, surgical pain, neuropathic pain, chemotherapy, osteoporosis
	Decreased sensation	Surgical nerve damage, chemotherapy
	Decreased strength	Immobility, nerve damage, CNS metastases
	Decreased ROM	Immobility, nerve damage, scar adhesions
	Open wound	Failure of incision site to close, infection

children currently receiving medical intervention for ALL demonstrate significant improvements in lower extremity strength and ankle dorsiflexion ROM when they participate in a physical therapy program.[35,43,90] Furthermore, the literature also supports the following benefits of exercise for adults with cancer: improved hemoglobin concentrations, reduced duration of neutropenia and thrombocytopenia, reduced severity of diarrhea and pain, reduced duration of hospitalization, reduced reports of nausea, decreased emotional distress, increased lean body weight, improved physical performance, improved functional capacity, improved quality-of-life index, improved flexibility, decreased fatigue, improved concentration, and increased skeletal mass.[91–102]

Coordination, Communication, and Documentation

Because of the rapidly changing needs of children with cancer, it is important that the physical therapist take the time to appropriately coordinate, communicate, and document all aspects of the physical therapy care. Physical therapy coordination, communication, and documentation require different approaches, depending on the location of services such as inpatient, outpatient, and school-based services. Regardless of the location of services, it is oftentimes challenging to coordinate appointment times around the child's nap, a procedure that requires sedation, and other medical appointments; to identify the child's blood counts before physical therapy; and to talk with the physician or nurse if changes are observed. To maximize the physical therapy session, it is imperative that the physical therapist take responsibility in all three of these areas.

Patient/Client Instruction

A primary role of the physical therapist is to provide information, to educate, to motivate and inspire, and to instruct patients, caregivers, and siblings. Fulfillment of this role is essential in optimizing the benefits of physical therapy services. Therefore, a responsibility of the physical therapist is to empower the child and family to take an active role in improving the child's health and well-being. The physical therapist must discuss with the child and family activities that are of interest to them and offer positive encouragement for the activities the child can do.

Physical therapy interventions must be age appropriate and, most importantly, meaningful to the child and the caregiver. Physical therapy instruction for a child with cancer may consist of showing a child how to get out of bed for the first time after surgery; helping him or her learn how to properly use an assistive device, orthosis, or prosthesis; or helping him or her perform specific therapeutic exercises. The physical therapist may deliver the instructions orally or by manual guidance, visual demonstration, or written handouts. Through child, family, and therapist collaboration, ideas are generated on how the child and family can

participate in activities together, with the goal of enhancing the child's performance, functioning, and, ultimately, quality of life.

Procedural Intervention

Each intervention session between the therapist and a child with cancer is unique because of the complexity of the disease, the medical intervention, and the individual needs of the child and family. A physical therapy session may require modifications because the child has a low blood count, fever, pain, headache, vomiting, diarrhea, generalized fatigue, or drainage from a wound, or because the child has a specific request. Therefore, the physical therapist should be prepared to modify the intervention session on the basis of the child's needs at that moment, keeping in mind the short- and long-term goals of the therapy. Physical therapy interventions (Table 16.8) may include nonpharmacologic pain

TABLE 16.8 Suggested Physical Therapy Interventions		
Area of Focus	**Intervention**	**Frequency**
Pain	Modalities	As needed
	Ice, heat, massage	
	Positioning	
	Assistive device	
	Neuropathic pain	
	Compression stocking	
	Deep pressure	
	Physician-prescribed medications	
	Gabapentin, Elavil, morphine	
Strengthening	Therapeutic exercises	3–5 days a week
	Functional activities	
	Stair climbing	
	Squats	
Stretching	CPM machine	Five times a week to daily
	Splinting, bracing, orthotic	
	Manual stretching, self-stretching	
Aerobic/endurance	Walking	5 days a week
	Treadmill	
	Bike	
	Stair stepper	
	Swimming	
	Dancing	
Manual techniques	Manual guidance	As needed
	Neurodevelopmental treatment	
	Self-directed	
Motor learning principles	Knowledge of performance	As needed
	Knowledge of results	
	Blocked practice	
	Random practice	

management, therapeutic exercise, aerobic exercise, gait training, or a fitting for an assistive device, wheelchair, orthosis, or prosthesis. Most importantly, the pediatric physical therapists must be creative.

▶ Survivorship

There are an estimated 328,000 survivors of childhood cancer in the United States, 80% of whom survived for at least 5 years beyond diagnosis, largely because of significant improvements in the medical management of these cancers.[103] With this increase in life expectancy, three out of five of these childhood cancer survivors will experience adverse late effects as a result of the cancer itself or the treatment received.[104] Late effects are the complications or adverse events that occur months or years following the completion of treatment and can impact any organ system in the body. Survivors often develop mild to severe long-term impairments of the musculoskeletal (muscle weakness, osteonecrosis, osteoporosis, leg length discrepancy), neuromuscular (peripheral neuropathy, pain, poor motor control), cardiopulmonary (cardiomyopathy, pulmonary fibrosis, fatigue, decreased exercise tolerance, obesity) and integumentary systems (fibrosis, radiation dermatitis), as well as neurocognitive dysfunction (memory and processing delays).[105,106] Both the risk of developing late effects and their severity increases as the time since completion of treatment increases. Early recognition of these late effects offers the best opportunity to provide appropriate treatment, thus minimizing the impairments associated with late effects.

Long-term follow-up by a multidisciplinary team is essential in providing the care required to optimize the health and quality of life of childhood cancer survivors. Unfortunately, long-term follow-up care is often not provided or accessed by these survivors. Physicians and physical therapists should routinely monitor these survivors for identifying the onset of adverse late effects and initiating appropriate therapeutic interventions. It is critical that physical therapists obtain a detailed medical history from the patient, family, or physician regarding the diagnosis, treatments, and medications received during cancer-related care so as to more appropriately evaluate and treat any identified late effects. Reports indicate that only 72% of survivors of childhood cancer can accurately report their diagnosis and only 35% understand the severity and risk of impairments that might arise as a result of treatment.[106,107]

The Children's Oncology Group has developed guidelines that provide the physical therapist advice on appropriately screening and managing this growing population of childhood cancer survivors in an effort to provide them with consistent care and reduce the long-term health risks they face. These Guidelines, as well as "Health Links" (patient education on guideline-specific topics), are available at www.survivorshipguidelines.org.[108] Research has demonstrated the effectiveness of early intervention and education and has

demonstrated the ability of exercise and physical therapy interventions to moderate many of the late effects reported by survivors.[109–113] In summary, childhood cancer survivors and their families can benefit from physical therapy interventions as they transition from diagnosis through active treatment and to survivorship.

CASE STUDIES

CASE STUDY 1

ACUTE LYMPHOBLASTIC LEUKEMIA

History

Three-year-old Emily presented to her pediatrician with excessive bruising, accompanied by reports of wanting her parents to carry her rather than having to walk. She had no significant past medical history and was performing all age-appropriate skills until 3 weeks ago. Her white blood cell count was high. Analysis of bone marrow aspirate and cerebrospinal fluid from a lumbar puncture showed an overproduction of blast cells and CNS involvement. Emily's disease was diagnosed as ALL, and she was referred to a hospital approximately 60 minutes from her hometown to receive treatment. She was enrolled on a standard risk protocol to receive combination chemotherapy (prednisone, dexamethasone, vincristine, daunorubicin, doxorubicin, L-asparaginase, methotrexate, cyclophosphamide, and cytarabine). Chemotherapy will last approximately 2.5 years and will be administered in four main phases: induction, CNS preventive therapy, consolidation, and re-induction and maintenance therapy. Today, Emily's blood counts were mildly low (WBC 4.6 [normal range, 4.9 to 12.9/mm^3]; RBC 3.2 [normal range, 3.90 to 5.30/mm^3]; Hbg 10.0 [normal range, 11.5 to 14.0]; platelet 98,000 [normal range, 190,000 to 490,000]) (St. Jude Children's Research Hospital normal blood value ranges for a 3-year-old child).

Emily lives at home with her mother, father, and two older brothers. She enjoys playing with her dolls, riding her bike, and going to the playground. She used to attend a preschool 2 hours a day, 3 days a week, before her diagnosis. Emily's mother works out of the home and her father is an accountant. Emily's parents report that their daughter has not attended preschool in 8 weeks.

Emily was referred to the physical therapy department 3 weeks after her initial diagnosis, with the goal of increased functional mobility. Her parents were very concerned because Emily was not walking.

Physical Therapy Systems Review

Emily is bright and was very comfortable talking with the physical therapist when her father was holding her. She appeared fearful of movement. Her muscle tone appears within normal limits to mildly low. Vision, hearing, and sensation appear intact. She doesn't appear to have any pain while her father is holding her. She is mildly pale with a few healing bruises. Her respiratory rate and breathing pattern appear normal at rest.

Physical Therapy Tests and Measures

Emily presented with full active range of motion (AROM) in her neck, trunk, upper extremities, and lower extremities. Her strength was examined while she was playing with toys and was grossly 4 (0 to 5 scale). Emily tracked right/left/up/down.

She followed directions when spoken to at a normal voice level. Her sensation was within normal limits (WNL) as measured by light touch, and her muscle tone was WNL. Emily had no pain, as measured by the FLACC scale, when she was sitting and playing; however, when she was in a standing position, her FLACC pain score was 5, indicating pain in her lower extremities. Emily's skin color was mildly pale and she presented with three large bruised areas, which were healing. Emily's skin around her central line was clean and dry. Emily presented with decreased endurance, as indicated by her increased work of breathing and increased heart and respiratory rates while she performed functional tasks such as transitioning from sitting to standing and ambulating.

Emily ambulated independently for 2 feet, slowly with a short step length, and then began to cry. Emily stood independently with her hand on a bench and cruised right and left for 3 feet. Emily transitioned from sitting on a bench to standing with moderate assistance, and from standing to sitting on the floor by half-kneeling with her hand on her knees and then on the floor, with minimal assistance for balance. She crawled on her hands and knees for a distance of 4 feet independently. She would not attempt to ascend a step.

Physical Therapy Diagnosis

- Nociceptive pain caused by increased blast cell production in the bone marrow and arthralgia from high-dose methotrexate and intrathecal cytarabine
- Decreased strength from inactivity
- Decreased endurance from inactivity
- Decreased functional mobility due to pain, limited strength, and nausea
- Decreased participation in play and nonattendance at school

Physical Therapy Prognosis

Emily is expected to have a full recovery from her physical therapy diagnoses. After she receives chemotherapy for a few more weeks, she should have no more bone pain from her initial disease. Over the next 3 months, Emily will increase her strength and endurance so she can participate in family activities.

GOALS AS DETERMINED WITH EMILY AND HER FAMILY

- At 1 week, ambulate independently with a rolling walker
- At 4 weeks, ambulate independently without assistance, transition from ring sitting to standing independently, ascend and descend three steps with one hand on a rail
- At 6 weeks, ascend and descend three steps independently, jump up independently with both feet leaving the floor 1 inch
- Ongoing goals, including family independently assisting Emily with the exercise program

Plan of Care

Emily will receive physical therapy three times a week for the first 2 weeks. She is scheduled to be an inpatient for a week while she receives chemotherapy. The frequency of her physical therapy will then be decreased to two times a week for 2 weeks, and then once a week. As soon as Emily is ambulating independently and performing age-appropriate gross motor skills, she will receive physical therapy services on an as-needed basis only. The plan for physical therapy services with Emily will involve educating Emily and her family in the following areas: activities to regain function, normal development, resuming activities that are important to Emily and her family such as going to the park and riding their bikes together as a family, and future concerns such as the development of peripheral neuropathy or osteonecrosis. The physical therapist may find that Emily could benefit from a referral to occupation therapy to assist with fine motor skills or activities of daily living with a focus on age-appropriate developmental skills.

Physical Therapy Patient-related Instruction

Activity: Ankle dorsiflexion passive ROM and family instruction on signs and symptoms of peripheral neuropathy due to vincristine (foot drop, tripping, poor grip strength)—Frequency: Five times a week. Intensity: Mild stretch. Duration: Hold for 30 seconds.

Activity: Strengthening exercises—Frequency: Five times a week. Intensity: Fun, functional, strengthening activities such as squatting to pick up a toy off the ground; tossing a ball overhead, from the mid-chest region, and underhand; painting a picture while standing at the kitchen table, squatting to pick up a different color marker; and doing ankle pumps while listening to music. Duration: Throughout the day, because she will not tolerate long periods of exercise at one time; therefore, three sets of 10 repetitions are recommended.

Activity: Ambulation with a walker—Frequency: When she needs to transition from one activity to another. Intensity: Short distances to start and buildup. Duration: Throughout the day.

Activity: Aerobic exercise, tricycle riding—Frequency: 7 days a week. Intensity: Slow and controlled. Duration: 5 minutes to start and buildup to 10 minutes. She should be wearing a helmet (Fig. 16.6).

Physical Therapy Procedural Intervention

The physical therapist will help Emily perform ankle dorsiflexion stretching and review procedures for ensuring proper alignment with Emily's parents. The therapist will encourage Emily to play a game such as basketball that requires her to transition from standing to squatting to pick up the ball, walking over to the basket, and tossing the ball into the basket. This activity will assist Emily with her upper and lower extremity strength and ambulation skills. While Emily rides a tricycle, the therapist will monitor her heart rate with a pulse oximeter and visually observe her respiratory rate, skin color, and breathing pattern. During the physical therapy session, the therapist will be able to determine

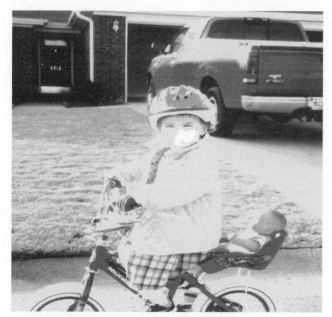

FIGURE 16.6 Emily playing outside on her bike.

Emily's improvements in ROM, strength, endurance, and functional mobility, and then make recommended suggestions to Emily and her family on how to modify her home or inpatient exercise program.

Episode of Care

Three months after Emily received the initial diagnosis of ALL, she met all her previously set goals. However, 1 month later, she developed peripheral neuropathy, as indicated by frequent tripping while she was walking and running. The physical therapy examination indicated that Emily had weak intrinsic musculature in her feet and hands and decreased active ankle dorsiflexion strength. Emily's doctors decreased her dose of vincristine to reduce the effects of the peripheral neuropathy, and the physical therapist provided Emily with bilateral solid ankle–foot orthoses to help prevent falls and to protect the alignment of her ankle structure. Emily continued to perform her ankle dorsiflexion stretching and strengthening exercises as previously recommended. Fourteen months after the diagnosis of ALL, she developed severe pain in her right foot. Emily's mother was very concerned because this was the initial symptom of ALL; however, it did not signal a return of leukemia, but was a symptom of avascular necrosis that had developed in her calcaneus. Her physician modified Emily's corticosteroid dose and recommended that she use her walker again for a few weeks. After 1 month, Emily no longer required the use of the walker to ambulate and was pain free unless she ambulated for long distances. When Emily completed her medical intervention, she no longer needed to use an ankle–foot orthosis. Emily has osteopenia due to the effects of chemotherapy with methotrexate and corticosteroids. She is now in kindergarten, riding her bike, and playing with her friends without difficulty. Emily still runs slowly and not as smoothly as her friends, but she is hopeful her running will improve.

CASE STUDY 2

OSTEOSARCOMA

History

John, a 14-year-old boy with no significant medical history, presented to his pediatrician with leg pain after a soccer injury. John's physician referred him to the physical therapy department for treatment of a left hamstring strain, three times a week for 6 weeks. After 2 weeks, the physical therapist noticed that John's condition was not improving and called the physician. The physician ordered a CT scan of John's left lower extremity; imaging results indicated a large mass. The physician then ordered a biopsy of the mass; on the basis of the results, he diagnosed John's condition as osteosarcoma of the left distal femur. John had no signs of metastatic disease. John lives in a large metropolitan city with a well-known children's hospital, where he is scheduled to begin 3 months of neoadjuvant chemotherapy (ifosfamide, carboplatin, and doxorubicin). John went to one session of physical therapy to review training on how to use forearm crutches for a non–weight-bearing left lower extremity. Previous physical therapy had consisted of training on use of axillary crutches and left knee AROM exercises. A central line was surgically placed. After 10 weeks of chemotherapy, John was reevaluated by his orthopedic surgeon and oncologist. John, his family, and the doctors agreed that John would receive a limb-sparing procedure, specifically an expandable endoprosthesis because John is still growing. After the surgical procedure, the physician requested that the physical therapist provide John with a continuous passive motion (CPM) machine in the surgical recovery room. The physician also requested that physical therapy services start on postoperative day 1 for functional mobility training, left knee ROM therapeutic exercises, and family education.

John's blood test results were WNL on postoperative day 1 (WBC 10.2 [normal range, 4.2 to 12.2/mm^3]; RBC 4.75 [normal range, 4.50 to 5.30/mm^3]; Hbg 14.2 [normal range, 12.5 to 16.5]; platelet 250,000 [normal range, 170,000 to 430,000]) (St. Jude Children's Research Hospital normal blood value ranges for a 16-year-old boy).

Social History

John lives at home with his mother and two younger brothers. He is in the eighth grade in school and enjoys playing soccer and basketball and motorcycle riding. John's mother has a full-time job outside the home, and he sees his father only once every few months.

Physical Therapy Systems Review

When the physical therapist arrived in John's hospital room, he was in bed. A Foley catheter, central venous line, and pain pump had been placed. He was receiving an analgesic through an epidural catheter in his lumbar spinal area to assist with lower extremity pain management. His mom and both brothers were present. John was alert and oriented, but reluctant to begin physical therapy.

Physical Therapy Tests and Measures

John presented with full active ROM in his neck, upper extremities, and right lower extremity. John's CPM had been set at 0 to 45 degrees of motion after his surgery the previous night, and the settings had not been changed. The therapist removed John's left leg from the CPM and performed gentle passive ROM exercises; the left hip and ankle demonstrated a full ROM and 50 degrees of left knee flexion. He had decreased trunk mobility due to the placement of his epidural catheter. His strength was 5/5 as measured by manual muscle testing in bilateral upper extremities and right lower extremity. John's strength in the left lower extremity was limited because of pain and fear of movement. With moderate assistance for support of John's left lower extremity, he flexed his left hip to 90 degrees and actively dorsiflexed his left ankle to the neutral position.

He followed directions spoken at a normal voice level. He had lost sensation to light touch in his bilateral lower extremities owing to the effects of the epidural. John reported pain in his left lower extremity as a 3 on the 0 to 10 self-report scale. His incision was covered with dressings.

John required minimal assistance to protect the epidural while transferring from a supine to a sitting position in his bed. He required maximum assistance for support of his left lower extremity to scoot to the edge of the bed. The physical therapist placed a hinged knee brace, which was locked in extension, on John's left lower extremity before John got out of bed. With the brace locked in full-knee extension, John then transferred from sitting on the edge of the bed to standing by using his forearm crutches. He required minimal assistance for balance and maximum assistance for support of his left lower extremity to maintain non–weight bearing. John ambulated 5 feet to a chair in his room and transferred from standing to sitting with maximum assistance for support of his left lower extremity.

Physical Therapy Diagnosis

- Nociceptive pain from the surgical site
- Neuropathic pain from nerve damage during surgery
- Decreased strength from change in alignment of the muscle pull
- Increased energy expenditure with functional activities such as walking
- Decreased functional mobility due to pain, limited strength and balance, and nausea from the anesthesia
- Decreased participation in school, sports, and socialization with friends

Physical Therapy Prognosis

John's strength and functional mobility are expected to improve. He may continue to lack full-knee extension secondary to the changes in the biomechanical alignment of his knee structure.

GOALS AS DETERMINED WITH JOHN AND HIS FAMILY

John will transfer from a supine position to sitting independently (the same day his epidural catheter is removed). John will transfer from a sitting to a standing position with forearm crutches and non–weight bearing on the left lower extremity,

with standby assistance (3 days). John and his mother are able to independently use the CPM and don and doff John's lower extremity brace. John will independently ambulate 50 feet with forearm crutches and non–weight bearing on left lower extremity (4 days). John will ascend and descend 12 steps with one hand on the rail and one hand on a forearm crutch, non–weight bearing on left lower extremity with contact guard assistance for safety (6 days).

Plan of Care

John will receive physical therapy daily while in the inpatient unit. After he is transferred home, he will return for outpatient physical therapy five times a week for 1 month, and then be followed up once a week to make modifications to his home exercise program.

Physical Therapy Client-related Instruction

The physical therapist will provide John and his mother with instruction on the use of his equipment, exercises, and safety.

Activity: Instruction on use of the CPM and how to increase the ROM by 10 degrees each day

Activity: Instruction on donning and doffing the lower extremity brace, which John is to wear when getting out of bed and during ambulation

Activity: Instruction on active left lower extremity ROM exercises

Activity: Transfer training

Activity: Gait training on non–weight-bearing left lower extremity

Physical Therapy Procedural Intervention

The physical therapist will provide John with manual guidance, tactile cues, and oral instruction to achieve his goals.

Episode of Care

John was discharged from the hospital on postoperative day 5. He began outpatient physical therapy 2 days after his discharge from the hospital. He reported pain as a 6 on the 0 to 10 numerical scale; therefore, the physical therapist called the pain team working with John, and the team increased his short-acting pain medication. He delayed resumption of chemotherapy until 3 weeks after surgery to allow his surgical incision time to heal. Therefore, the physical therapist had to check the computer during each session to check John's blood counts to determine the appropriate physical therapy intervention for that day. For example, if John's platelet count was less than 50,000, he would not use weights for strength training in view of the increased likelihood of hemorrhage. Instead, he would perform active ROM exercises for stretching his left knee.

After 6 weeks of outpatient physical therapy that included strengthening and stretching exercises, John achieved 100 degrees of passive left knee flexion and 92 degrees of active left knee flexion. He had a knee extension lag of approximately 20 degrees. John's full active ROM in his left knee was 20 to 92 degrees of knee flexion.

His left lower extremity strength was hip flexion/extension and abduction/adduction 5/5, hip internal rotation 4–/5, hip external rotation 4/5, knee extension 3+/5, knee flexion 4–/5, and ankle dorsiflexion/plantar flexion/inversion/eversion 5/5. John's orthopedist approved full weight bearing on his left lower extremity. Therefore, gait training and exercises to help John shift onto the left lower extremity were added to the physical therapy sessions, which continued to be focused on ROM, strength, and weight.

John used the CPM for 6 weeks at night only. When he was not performing his exercises during the day, he wore his knee brace unlocked to continue to work on increasing his knee flexion ROM. After he completed the use of the CPM, John wore his knee brace at night locked in full extension to assist him in preventing the development of a knee flexion contracture because he still did not have full active knee extension ROM.

After 1 month of physical therapy five times a week, John's sessions were decreased to once a week because he was independent in his exercise program and was showing signs of progress. He had achieved active knee flexion to 110 degrees and continued to lack 10 degrees of active knee extension to achieve full extension. He ambulated with a mild lateral trunk deviation to the left; however, with oral cues, he could ambulate with his trunk in the midline position. He could ascend and descend 12 stairs, alternating feet to step slowly with his hand on the rail for minimal support. John now wore the lower extremity brace only to sleep in at night, and he wore a small knee brace during the day to provide tactile cues and comfort to his left lower extremity.

Eight months after John's surgery, he completed his chemotherapy. John and the physical therapist noticed he had increased trunk flexion to the left. John had grown over the past 8 months. As a result, his prosthesis needed to be lengthened. After it was lengthened, John's left lower extremity was sore, and he required gentle knee ROM exercises and the use of crutches for 2 days. He then returned to his normal pre-lengthening functioning.

Twelve months after John's surgery, he came to the physical therapist once every 3 months for checkup visits. He had returned to school and was planning to swim on his high-school swim team.

REFERENCES

1. American Cancer Society. www.cancer.org. Accessed 2013.
2. Scheurer ME, Bondy ML, Gurney JG. Epidemiology of childhood cancer. In: Pizzo PA, Poplack DG, eds. *Principles and Practices of Pediatric Oncology*. 6th ed. Philadelphia, PA: Lippincott Williams & Wilkins; 2011:2–16.
3. National Cancer Institute. www.cancer.gov. Accessed 2013.
4. Jemal A, Murray T, Samuels A, et al. Cancer Statistics, 2003. *CA Cancer J Clin*. 2003;53:5–26.
5. Margolin JF, Rabin KR, Steuber CP, et al. Acute lymphoblastic leukemia. In: Pizzo PA, Poplack DG, eds. *Principles and Practices of Pediatric Oncology*. 6th ed. Philadelphia, PA: Lippincott Williams & Wilkins; 2011:518–565.
6. St. Jude Children's Research Hospital. www.stjude.org. Accessed February 2013.
7. Cooper TM, Hasle H, Smith FO. Acute myelogenous leukemia, myeloproliferative and myelodysplastic disorders. In: Pizzo PA, Poplack DG, eds. *Principles and Practices of Pediatric Oncology*. 6th ed. Philadelphia, PA: Lippincott Williams & Wilkins; 2011:566–610.
8. Altman AJ, Fu C. Chronic leukemias of childhood. In: Pizzo PA, Poplack DG, eds. *Principles and Practices of Pediatric Oncology*. 6th ed. Philadelphia, PA: Lippincott Williams & Wilkins; 2011:611–637.
9. McBride ML. Childhood cancer and environmental contaminants. *Can J Public Health*. 1998;89(suppl 1):S53–S62, S58–S68.
10. Muts-Homshma S, Muller H, Geracost J. Klinefelter's syndrome and acute non-lymphocytic leukemia. *Blut*. 1981;44:15.
11. Shearer P, Parham D, Kovnar E, et al. Neurofibromatosis type I and malignancy: review of 32 pediatric cases treated at a single institution. *Med Pediatr Oncol*. 1994;22:78–83.
12. Woods W, Roloff J, Lukens J, et al. The occurrence of leukemia in patients with Schwachman syndrome. *J Pediatr*. 1981;99:425.
13. Blaney SM, Haas-Kogan D, Pussaint TY, et al. Tumors of the central nervous system. In: Pizzo PA, Poplack DG, eds. *Principles and Practices of Pediatric Oncology*. 6th ed. Philadelphia, PA: Lippincott Williams & Wilkins; 2011:717–808.
14. Thapar K, Taylor MD, Laws ER, et al. Brain edema, increased intracranial pressure, and vascular effects of human brain tumors. In: Kaye AH, Laws ER, eds. *Brain Tumors: An Encyclopedic Approach*. London, England: Churchill Livingston; 2001:189–215.
15. American Brain Tumor Association. www.abta.org. Accessed February 2013.
16. Metzger M, Krasin MJ, Hudson MM, et al. Hodgkin lymphoma. In: Pizzo PA, Poplack DG, eds. *Principles and Practices of Pediatric Oncology*. 6th ed. Philadelphia, PA: Lippincott Williams & Wilkins; 2011:638–662.
17. Gross TG, Perkins S. Malignant non-hodgkin lymphomas in children. In: Pizzo PA, Poplack DG, eds. *Principles and Practices of Pediatric Oncology*. 6th ed. Philadelphia, PA: Lippincott Williams & Wilkins; 2011:663–682.
18. Brodeur BM, Hogarty MD, Mosse YP, et al. Neuroblastoma. In: Pizzo PA, Poplack DG, eds. *Principles and Practices of Pediatric Oncology*. 6th ed. Philadelphia, PA: Lippincott Williams & Wilkins; 2011:886–922.
19. Wexler LH, Meyer WH, Helman LJ. Rhabdomyosarcoma. In: Pizzo PA, Poplack DG, eds. *Principles and Practices of Pediatric Oncology*. 6th ed. Philadelphia, PA: Lippincott Williams & Wilkins; 2011:923–953.
20. Hosalkar HS, Dormans JP. Limb sparing for pediatric musculoskeletal tumors. *Pediatr Blood Cancer*. 2004;42:295–310.
21. Gorlick R, Bielack S, Teot L, et al. Osteosarcoma: biology, diagnosis, treatment and remaining challenges. In: Pizzo PA, Poplack DG, eds. *Principles and Practices of Pediatric Oncology*. 6th ed. Philadelphia, PA: Lippincott Williams & Wilkins; 2011:1015–1044.
22. Hawkins DS, Bolling T, Dubois S, et al. Ewings sarcoma. In: Pizzo PA, Poplack DG, eds. *Principles and Practices of Pediatric Oncology*. 6th ed. Philadelphia, PA: Lippincott Williams & Wilkins; 2011:987–1014.
23. Margolin JF, Rabin KR, Seuber CP, et al. Retinoblastoma. In: Pizzo PA, Poplack DG, eds. *Principles and Practices of Pediatric Oncology*. 6th ed. Philadelphia, PA: Lippincott Williams & Wilkins; 2011:809–837.
24. Fernandez C, Geller JI, Ehrlich PF, et al. Renal tumors. In: Pizzo PA, Poplack DG, eds. *Principles and Practices of Pediatric Oncology*. 6th ed. Philadelphia, PA: Lippincott Williams & Wilkins; 2011:861–885.
25. Ghasemi Z, Martin T. *Laboratory values in the intensive care unit*. Newsletter of the acute care/hospital clinical practice section. Alexandria, VA: American Physical Therapy Association; 1995.
26. Meyers PA, Schwartz CL, Krailo M, et al. Osteosarcoma: a randomized, prospective trial of the addition of ifosfamide and/or muramyl tripeptide to cisplatin, doxorubicin, and high-dose methotrexate. *J Clin Oncol*. 2005;23(9):2004–2011.
27. Womer RB, West DC, Krailo MD, et al. Randomized controlled trial of interval-compressed chemotherapy for the treatment of ewing sarcoma: a report from the Children's Oncology Group. *J Clin Oncol*. 2012;30(33):4148–4154.
28. Adamson PC, Bagatell R, Balis FM, et al. General principles of chemotherapy. In: Pizzo PA, Poplack DG, eds. *Principles and Practices of Pediatric Oncology*. 6th ed. Philadelphia, PA: Lippincott Williams & Wilkins; 2011:279–355.
29. Vainionpaa L, Kovala T, Tolonen U, et al. Vincristine therapy for children with acute lymphoblastic leukemia impairs conduction in the entire peripheral nerve. *Pediatr Neurol*. 1995;13:314–318.

30. Mattano LA, Sather HN, Trigg ME, et al. Osteonecrosis as a complication of treating acute lymphoblastic leukemia in children: a report from the Children's Cancer Group. *J Clin Oncol.* 2000;18(18):3262–3272.

31. Kaste SC, Jones-Wallace D, Rose SR, et al. Bone mineral decrements in survivors of childhood acute lymphoblastic leukemia: frequency of occurrence and risk factors for their development. *Leukemia.* 2001;15:728–734.

32. Galea V, Wright MJ, Barr RD. Measurement of balance in survivors of acute lymphoblastic leukemia in childhood. *Gait Posture.* 2004;19:1–10.

33. Lehtinen SS, Huuskonen UE, Harla-Saari AH, et al. Motor nervous system impairment persists in long-term survivors of childhood acute lymphoblastic leukemia. *Cancer.* 2002;94:2466–2473.

34. Wright MJ, Halton JM, Martin RF, et al. Long-term gross motor performance following treatment for acute lymphoblastic leukemia. *Med Pediatr Oncol.* 1998;31:86–90.

35. Wright MJ, Hanna SE, Halton JM, et al. Maintenance of ankle range of motion in children treated for acute lymphoblastic leukemia. *Pediatr Phys Ther.* 2003;15:146–152.

36. Lesink PG, Ciesielski KT, Hart TL, et al. Evidence for cerebellar-frontal subsystem changes in children treated with intrathecal chemotherapy for leukemia: enhanced data analysis using an effect size model. *Arch Neurol.* 1998;55:1561–1568.

37. Langer T, Martus P, Ottensmeier H, et al. CNS late-effects after ALL therapy in childhood. Part III: neuropsychological performance in long-term survivors of childhood ALL: impairments of concentration, attention, and memory. *Med Pediatr Oncol.* 2002;38:320–328.

38. Reimers TS, Ehrenfels S, Mortensen EL, et al. Cognitive deficits in long-term survivors of childhood brain tumors: identification of predictive factors. *Med Pediatr Oncol.* 2003;40:26–34.

39. Fletcher BD. Effects of pediatric cancer therapy on the musculoskeletal system. *Pediatr Radiol.* 1997;27:623–636.

40. Vainonpaa L. Clinical neurological findings of children with acute lymphoblastic leukemia at diagnosis and during treatment. *Eur Pediatr.* 1993;152:115–119.

41. Yonemoto T, Tatezaki S, Ishii T, et al. Marriage and fertility in long-term survivors of high grade osteosarcoma. *Am J Clin Oncol.* 2003;26:513–516.

42. Bradley WG, Lassman LP, Pearce GW, et al. The neuromyopathy of vincristine in man clinical, electrophysiological and pathological studies. *J Neurol Sci.* 1970;10:107–131.

43. Wright MJ, Halton JM, Barr RD. Limitation of ankle range of motion in survivors of acute lymphoblastic leukemia in childhood: a cross-sectional study. *Med Pediatr Oncol.* 1999;32:279–282.

44. Tanner KD, Reichling DB, Gear RW, et al. Altered temporal pattern of evoked afferent activity in a rat model of vincristine-induced painful peripheral neuropathy. *Neuroscience.* 2003;118:809–817.

45. Jew R, ed. *The Children's Hospital of Philadelphia Formulary 2001–2002.* Hudson, OH: Lexi-Comp Inc.

46. Gocha Marchese V, Chiarello LV, Lange BJ. Strength and functional mobility in children with acute lymphoblastic leukemia. *Med Pediatr Oncol.* 2003;40:230–232.

47. Wheeler DL, Vander Griend RA, Wronski TJ, et al. The short- and long-term effects of methotrexate on the skeleton. *Bone.* 1995;16:215–221.

48. Harten G, Stephani U, Henze G, et al. Slight impairment of psychomotor skills in children after treatment of acute lymphoblastic leukemia. *Eur J Pediatr.* 1984;142:189–197.

49. Mattano L. The skeletal remains: porosis and necrosis of bone in the marrow transplantation setting. *Pediatr Transplant.* 2003;7:71–75.

50. Krasin MJ, Rodriguez-Galindo C, Billups CA, et al. Definitive irradiation in multidisciplinary management of localized Ewings sarcoma family of tumors in pediatric patients: outcome and prognostic factors. *Int J Radiat Oncol Biol Phys.* 2004;60:830–838.

51. Oberlin O, Rey A, Anderson J, et al. Treatment of orbital rhabdomyosarcoma: survival and late effects of treatment—results of an international workshop. *J Clin Oncol.* 2001;19:197–204.

52. Davis AM, O'Sullivan B, Turcotte BR, et al. Function and health status outcomes in a randomized trial comparing preoperative and postoperative radiotherapy in extremity soft tissue sarcoma. *J Clin Oncol.* 2002;20:4472–4477.

53. Grossi M. Management and long-term complications of pediatric cancer. *Pediatr Clin N Am.* 1998;45:1637–1651.

54. Cooper JS, Fu K, Marks J, et al. Late effects of radiation therapy in the head and neck region. *Int J Radiat Oncol Biol Phys.* 1995;31:1141.

55. Jentzsch K, Ginder H, Cramer H, et al. Leg function after radiotherapy for Ewings sarcoma. *Cancer.* 1981;47:1267–1278.

56. Williams KY, Cox RS, Donaldson SS. Radiation induced height impairment in pediatric Hodgkin's disease. *Int J Radiat Oncol Biol Phys.* 1993;28:85–92.

57. Nysom K, Holm K, Michaelsen KF, et al. Bone mass after allogeneic BMT for childhood leukaemia or lymphoma. *Bone Marrow Transplant.* 2000;25:191–196.

58. Neel MD, Wilkins RM, Rao BN, et al. Early multicenter experience with a noninvasive expandable prosthesis. *Clin Orthop Rel Res.* 2003;415:72–81.

59. Rougraff BT, Simon MA, Kneisl JS, et al. Limb salvage compared with amputation for osteosarcoma of the distal end of the femur. A long-term oncological, functional, and quality-of-life study. *J Bone Joint Surg Am.* 1994;76:649–656.

60. Tunn PU, Schmidt-Peter P, Pomraenke D, et al. Osteosarcoma in children. *Clin Orthop Rel Res.* 2004;421:212–217.

61. Nagarajan R, Neglia JP, Clohisy DR, et al. Limb salvage and amputation in survivors of pediatric lower-extremity bone tumors: what are the long-term implications? *J Clin Oncol.* 2002;20:4493–4501.

62. Renard AJ, Veth RP, Scchreuder HWB, et al. Function and complications after ablative and limb-salvage therapy in lower extremity sarcoma of bone. *J Surg Oncol.* 2000;73:198–205.

63. Jeys LM, Grimer RJ, Carter SR, et al. Risk of amputation following limb salvage surgery with endoprosthetic replacement, in a consecutive series of 1261 patients. *Int Orthop.* 2003;27:160–163.

64. McClenaghan BA, Krajbich JI, Prone AM, et al. Comparative assessment of gait after limb-salvage procedure. *J Bone Joint Surg Am.* 1989;71:1178–1182.

65. Fuchs B, Sims FH. Rotationplasty about the knee: surgical technique and anatomical considerations. *Clin Anat.* 2004;17:345–353.

66. Fuchs B, Kotajarvi BR, Kaufman KR, et al. Functional outcome of patients with rotationplasty about the knee. *Clin Orthop Rel Res.* 2003;415:52–58.

67. Veenstra KM, Sprangers MAG, Van Der Eyken JW, et al. Quality of life in survivors with Van Ness-Borggreve rotationplasty after bone tumour resection. *J Surg Oncol.* 2000;73:192–197.

68. Hillman A, Hoffman C, Gosheger G, et al. Malignant tumor of the distal part of the femur or the proximal part of the tibia: endoprosthetic replacement or rotationplasty: functional outcome and quality-of-life measurements. *J Bone Joint Surg.* 1999;81:462–468.

69. Horwitz EM. Bone marrow transplantation. In: Steen G, Mirro J, eds. *Childhood Cancer: A Handbook from St. Jude Children's Research Hospital.* Cambridge, MA: Perseus Publishing; 2000:155–165.

70. Bain LJ. *A Parent's Guide to Childhood Cancer (The Children's Hospital of Philadelphia).* New York, NY: Dell Publishing; 1995:89–100.

71. World Health Organization. International Classification of Functioning, Disability, and Health. http://www.who.int/classifications/icf/en/. Accessed January, 2005.

72. Schechter NL, Berde CB, Yaster M. *Pain in Infants, Children, and Adolescents.* 2nd ed. Philadelphia, PA: Lippincott Williams & Wilkins; 2003.

73. Jensen MP, Karoly P, Braver S. The measurement of clinical pain intensity: a comparison of six methods. *Pain.* 1986;27:117–126.

74. Wong DL, Hockenberry-Eaton M, Wilson D, et al. *Wong's Essentials of Pediatric Nursing.* 6th ed. St. Louis, MO: Mosby; 2001.

75. Jackson AS, Coleman AE. Validation of distance run tests for elementary school children. *Res Q.* 1976;47:86–94.

76. Steele B. Timed walking tests of exercise capacity in chronic cardiopulmonary illness. *J Cardiopulm Rehabil.* 1996;16:25–33.

77. *Health Related Physical Fitness: Test Manual.* Reston, VA: American Alliance for Health, Physical Education, Recreation and Dance; 1980.

78. Butler P, Engelbrecht M, Major RE, et al. Physiological cost index of walking for normal children and its use as an indicator of physical handicap. *Dev Med Child Neurol.* 1984;26:607–612.

79. Nene AV. Physiological cost index of walking in able-bodied adolescents and adults. 1993;7:319–326.

80. Chin T, Sawamura S, Fujita H, et al. The efficacy of physiological cost index (PCI) measurement of a subject walking with an Intelligent Prosthesis. *Prosthet Orthot Int.* 1999;23:45–49.

81. Marchese VG, Ogle S, Womer RB, et al. An examination of outcome measures to assess functional mobility in childhood survivors of osteosarcoma. *Pediatr Blood Cancer.* 2004;42:41–45.

82. Grant S, Aitchison T, Henderson E, et al. A comparison of the reproducibility and the sensitivity to change of visual analogue scales, Borg scales, and Likert scales in normal subjects during submaximal exercise. *Chest.* 1999;116:1208–1217.

83. Habib Z, Westcott S. Assessment of anthropometric factors on balance tests in children. *Pediatr Phys Ther.* 1998;10:101–108.

84. Zaino CA, Gocha Marchese V, Westcott SL. Timed up and down stairs test: preliminary reliability and validity of a new measure of functional mobility. *Pediatr Phys Ther.* 2004;16:90–98.

85. Varni JW, Seid M, Kurtin PS. Reliability and validity of the pediatric quality of life inventory version 4.0 generic core scales in healthy and patient populations. *Med Care.* 2001;39:800–812.

86. Ware JE, Snow KK, Kosinski M, et al. *SF-36 Health Survey Manual and Interpretation Guide.* Lincoln, NE: Quality Metric Inc; 2000.

87. Eiser C, Vance YH. Implications of cancer for school attendance and behavior. *Med Pediatr Oncol.* 2002;38:317–319.

88. American Physical Therapy Associaton. Guide to physical therapist practice. Second edition. *Phys Ther.* 2001;81:9–744.

89. Marchese VG, Chiarello LA. Relationships between specific measures of body function, activity, and participation in children with acute lymphoblastic leukemia. *Rehabil Oncol.* 2004;22:5–9.

90. Marchese VG, Chiarello LA, Lange BJ. Effects of physical therapy intervention for children with acute lymphoblastic leukemia. *Pediatr Blood Cancer.* 2004;42:127–133.

91. Dimeo FC, Tilmann MHM, Bertz H, et al. Aerobic exercise in the rehabilitation of cancer patients after high dose chemotherapy and autologous peripheral stem cell transplantation. *Cancer.* 1997;79:1717–1722.

92. Dimeo FC, Stieglitz RD, Novelli-Fischer U, et al. Effects of physical activity on the fatigue and psychological status of cancer patients during chemotherapy. *Cancer.* 1999;85:2273–2277.

93. Dimeo FC, Fetscher S, Lange W, et al. Effects of aerobic exercise on the physical performance and incidence of treatment-related complication after high-dose chemotherapy. *Blood.* 1997;90:3390–3394.

94. Winningham ML, MacVicar MG, Bondoc M, et al. Effects of aerobic exercise on body weight and composition in patients with breast cancer on adjuvant chemotherapy. *Oncol Nurs Forum.* 1989;16:683–689.

95. MacVigar MG, Winningham ML, Nickel JL. Effects of aerobic interval training on cancer patients' functional capacity. *Nurs Res.* 1989;38:348–351.

96. Young-McCaughan S, Sexton D. A retrospective investigation of the relationship between aerobic exercise and quality of life in women with breast cancer. *Oncol Nurs Forum.* 1991;18:751–757.

97. Courneya KS, Keats MR, Turner AR. Physical exercise and quality of life in cancer patients following high dose chemotherapy and autologous bone marrow transplantation. *Psychooncology.* 2000;9:127–136.

98. Courneya KS, Friedenreich CM, Sela RA, et al. The group psychotherapy and home-based physical exercise (group-hope) trial in cancer survivors: physical fitness and quality of life outcomes. *Psychooncology.* 2003;12:357–374.

99. Hayes S, Davies PSW, Parker T, et al. Quality of life changes following peripheral blood stem cell transplantation and participation in a mixed-type, moderate-intensity, exercise program. *Bone Marrow Transplant.* 2004;33:553–558.

100. Hayes S, Davies PSW, Parker T, et al. Total energy expenditure and body composition changes following peripheral blood stem cell transplantation and participation in an exercise program. *Bone Marrow Transplant.* 2003;31:331–338.

101. Mock V, Burke MB, Sheehan P, et al. A nursing rehabilitation program for women with breast cancer receiving adjuvant chemotherapy. *Oncol Nurs Forum.* 1994;21:899–907.

102. Courneya KS, Friedenreich CM. Relationships between exercise during treatment and current quality of life among survivors of breast cancer. *J Psychosoc Oncol.* 1997;15:35–56.

103. The childhood cancer survivor study: an overview. The National Cancer Institute website. http://www.cancer.gov/cancertopics/coping/ccss. Accessed February 2013.

104. Children's Oncology Group. www.childrensoncologygroup.org. Accessed February 2013.

105. Marchese VG, Miller M, Niethamer L, et al. Factors affecting childhood cancer survivors' choice to attend a specific college: a pilot study. *Rehabil Oncol.* 2012;30(1):3–11.

106. Landier W, Bhatia S. Cancer survivorship: a pediatric perspective. *Oncologist.* 2008;13(11):1181–1192.

107. Armenian SH, Meadows AT, Bhatia S. Late effects of childhood cancer and its treatment. In: Pizzo PA, Poplack DG, eds. *Principles and Practice of Pediatric Oncology.* 4th ed. Philadelphia, PA: Lippincott Williams and Wilkins; 2011:1368–1387.

108. Children's Oncology Group. Long-term follow-up guidelines for survivors of childhood, adolescent, and young adult cancers. www.survivorshipguidelines.org. Accessed February 2013.

109. Ness KK, Leisenring WM, Huang S, et al. Predictors of inactive lifestyle among adult survivors of childhood cancer: a report from the childhood cancer survivor study. *Cancer.* 2009;115(9):1984–1994.

110. Ness KK, Morris EB, Nolan VG, et al. Physical performance limitations among adult survivors of childhood brain tumors. *Cancer.* 2010;116(12):3034–3044.

111. Wampler MA, Galantino ML, Huang S, et al. Physical activity among adult survivors of childhood lower-extremity sarcoma: a report from the Childhood Cancer Survivor Study. *J Cancer Surviv.* 2012;6:45–53.

112. Järvelä L, Niinikoski H, Lähteenmäki P, et al. Physical activity and fitness in adolescent and young adult long-term survivors of childhood acute lymphoblastic leukaemia. *J Cancer Surviv.* 2010;4(4):339–345.

113. Mulrooney DA, Dover DC, Li S, et al. Twenty years of follow-up among survivors of childhood and young adult myeloid leukemia: a report from the Childhood Cancer Survivor Study. *Cancer.* 2008;112(9):2071–2079.

Rehabilitation of the Child with Burns

Suzanne F. Migliore

Epidemiology

Etiology
  Child Abuse and Neglect

Prevention

Structures and Functions of the Skin

Classification of Burns
  Burn Depth
  Burn Size
  Mechanism of Injury
  Minor, Moderate, and Major Classifications

Pathophysiology
  Dimensions of Injury
  Burn Wound Healing

Scar Hypertrophy and Contraction

Burn Center

Burn Team

Initial Treatment and Medical Management

Systems Review
  Pulmonary System
  Cardiovascular System
  Renal System
  Circulatory System
  Musculoskeletal System

Nutrition

Pain Management

Burn Wound Management
  Nonsurgical Interventions
  Surgical Management
  Cultured Autografts and Dermal Substitutes

Physical Therapy Examination
  Examination/Evaluation

Interventions
  Pain Management
  Wound Care
  Splinting and Positioning
  Casting
  Range of Motion
  Massage
  Ambulation
  Exercise
  Scar Management
  Patient/Client-Related Instructions

Outcomes

Burn Camp

Summary

Case Studies

The purpose of this chapter is to provide a basic description of pediatric burn care and to discuss the therapist's role in providing interventions for a child with a thermal injury—from the acute phase through the rehabilitation phase.

Examinations and interventions for children with thermal injuries are unique. Certainly, appropriate treatment for adults with burn injuries is not necessarily applicable to children with these same injuries and vice versa. Moreover, the treatment for a 9-month-old baby may differ from that for a 3-year-old child, which, in turn, may be different from the approach used for a 10-year-old child. The information presented will be applicable for the pediatric physical therapist across the continuum of care.

The role of the therapist is broadly addressed. The specific role of the therapist is defined, in part, by the individual setting and may also be dependent on the particular facility's medical and surgical techniques and approach.

▶ Epidemiology

According to the Centers for Disease Control and Prevention (CDC), unintentional injuries ranked as the number one cause of death for children between the ages of 1 and 18 years. Injuries sustained via fire or burns were the fourth leading cause of unintentional fatal injuries.[1] In 2011, the CDC reported over 140,000 fire- or burn-related nonfatal injuries in the United States.[2] In addition, fire/burn-related injuries that were listed as violence-related/intentional injuries ranked in the top 10 causes of nonfatal injuries in children from birth through 9 years of age.[3]

The National Safe Kids organization publishes burn and scald safety information for children and their caregivers. They too track statistics regarding fire-related deaths and injuries as their program seeks to aid in prevention awareness. In 2008, 366 children under the age of 14 years died of fire or burn-related injuries. In addition, in 2010, children under the age of 14 accounted for 40% of fireworks-related injuries, with burns accounting for more than half of all fireworks-related injuries.[4]

▶ Etiology

There are numerous causes of burns. They include thermal injuries attributed to residential fires, automobile accidents, playing with matches, improper handling of firecrackers, and scalds caused by kitchen or bathroom accidents. Chemical burns occur because of contact, ingestion, inhalation, or injection of acids, alkalis, or vesicants. Electrical burns happen when there is contact with faulty electrical wiring, electrical cords, or high-voltage power lines.[5]

The mechanism of thermal injury may most closely correlate with the child's age. For example, toddlers often sustain a scald burn from pulling hot liquids off surfaces (e.g., boiling water off a stove, hot tea off a table); they also sustain unintentional scald burns from bathtub accidents, where the home's water heater temperature is set too high. Hot tap water accounts for almost 25% of all scald burns among children and correlates with more deaths and hospitalizations than any other hot liquid burns.[4] Tap water can cause a full-thickness burn in under 5 seconds at the temperature of 140° F. Hot liquids such as coffee, tea, soup, or cocoa can reach temperatures hot enough to cause a scald burn.[6]

Toddlers are also at risk for electrical burns due to putting objects into uncovered electrical outlets or by chewing on wires leading to electrical products. Flame burns from playing with matches and contact burns due to touching hot objects (iron/stove/curling irons) happen with the school-age group. As children grow and become more adventurous, the mechanism of burn injury correlates with the risks these children and adolescents take.

Male children are at higher risk of burn-related death and injuries than their female counterparts. Children under the age of 4 years and those with disabilities are at higher risk of burns. The mortality rates from burn injuries for Native Americans and African Americans are two to three times higher than that for Caucasian children.[4]

Lorch et al. in 2011 studied the etiology of burn injuries in infants brought for medical attention in the emergency department. They found that males outnumbered females (55% and 45%, respectively), and that African Americans comprise 47% of the patients seen. Most burns seen in this study occurred in the home, and most commonly in the kitchen. Scald burns were the most common (hot liquids either in the bath or in the kitchen) followed by contact burns due to touching a hot appliance such as the stove, iron, or heater.[7]

Shah et al. in 2011 studied the epidemiology and profile of pediatric burns looking at data from the national burn registry. They too found scalds to be the most common

mechanism of injury due to hot liquids, cooking oils, or bath water. As a single food item, they found hot noodles (microwaved) were responsible for a large majority of burns reviewed. They also found that gasoline burns, electrical burns, and burns due to motor vehicle accidents were more likely in children older than 10 years. Non-accidental or child abuse accounted for 6.7% of all the burns reviewed.[8]

Child Abuse and Neglect

According to the National Clearinghouse on Child Abuse and Neglect, in 2011, there were over 740,000 children confirmed to be victims of child abuse in the United States. Overall, the national child victim rate continued a downward trend.[9] The National Center for Injury Prevention and Control lists fire/burn intentional injuries among the top nine causes of nonfatal injuries for children under the age of 9 years as of 2007.[3] Shah et al. revealed that children under the age of 1 year were more likely to be burned by non-accidental causes, attributed to the demands of a newborn on new or single parents.[7]

Up to 8% of infants and children admitted to the hospital for burns are victims of abuse. Suspicion of abuse arises when the injuries are non–splash related, linear demarcations (e.g., glove/stocking distribution), or burns to the buttocks and no other portion of the body (i.e., dipped into hot water). Contact burns with symmetric shapes may also signify intentional burns (e.g., circular lines consistent with a stovetop burner). Children with inflicted burns are more likely to have burns on both hands, feet, and legs, and there may be a higher total body surface area (TBSA) involved.[10] To try to distinguish between an accidental and an intentional burn, notation should include the pattern, location, and depth of the burn. Certain burn patterns will raise suspicions including scald burns to the perineum, buttocks, and lower extremities, especially those with sharply defined lines between burned and unburned skin.[11] In the hospital setting, suspicion of abuse or neglect is investigated by an interdisciplinary team including physicians, nurses, social workers, psychologists, and physical therapists. Factors in a child's case that may indicate abuse or neglect include:

- Child is brought for treatment by an unrelated adult
- An unexplained delay of 12 or more hours in seeking treatment
- Inappropriate parental affect: Parents appear inattentive to child; lack empathy; may appear to be under the influence of alcohol or drugs
- Attribution of guilt for injury to the patient's sibling or to the patient
- An injury inconsistent with its description
- History of injury inconsistent with the developmental capacity of the patient
- History of accidental or non-accidental injury to the patient or siblings
- History of failure to thrive

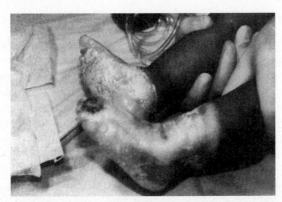

FIGURE 17.1 "Mirror image" burns to bilateral feet and lower legs, a pattern consistent with abuse via dunking in hot water.

- Historical accounts of the injury that differ with each interview
- Injury localized to genitalia, perineum, and buttocks (because of frequency with which injury occurs related to toilet training)
- "Mirror image" injury of extremities (Fig. 17.1)
- Inappropriate affect of child; child appears withdrawn with flattened affect
- Evidence of unrelated injuries, for example, scars, bruises, welts, fractures

All states have laws requiring that certain professionals, including physical therapists and occupational therapists, report suspected cases of child abuse. The physical therapist will aid in the determination of abuse by doing a thorough examination and evaluation of the burn mechanism, size, location, and depth of injury.

Prevention

Because of the high incidence and common pattern of distribution of types of burn injuries among children of various age groups, prevention efforts have been directed toward educating parents, children, and others as to how these injuries occur and how they can be prevented. The National SAFE KIDS Campaign was the first national organization dedicated to prevention of childhood injuries. It was founded in 1988 and has over 600 SAFE KIDS coalitions and chapters across the United States. Injury prevention efforts in the area of thermal injuries include distribution of smoke alarms and assistance in amending plumbing codes to include "anti-scald" technology and a maximum water heater temperature of 120° F. Other prevention tips include using the back burner of the stove and turning pot handles inward so as to avoid young children pulling down on the handles. For older children, cooking safety is imperative, including use of the microwave. Safety training by parents may include not allowing children to use the microwave until they are tall enough to reach the items, using oven mitts to remove the item, and slowly opening the container

after removing it from the microwave. For other household areas, parents should consider using a sturdy screen around a fireplace or outdoor fire pit, keeping candles away from anything that can burn, and placing matches and flammable liquids out of the reach of children.[12]

Injury prevention is commonly called the three E's: education, engineering (including environmental change), and law enforcement. Such prevention initiatives led to changes in the laws for children's sleepwear, smoke detector use, and setting water heaters to less than 120° F.[13]

Several suggestions for preventing childhood burn injuries include the following:

- Lowering water heater temperature settings to 120° F or lower
- Keeping cords to coffee pots and cups with hot liquids out of reach of young children
- Keeping young children in a safe place during food preparation and serving
- Turning pot handles toward the back of the stove and cooking on rear burners when possible
- Supervising children in the bathtub and testing bath water with a liquid crystal thermometer before placing the child in the tub
- Keeping young children in a safe place when using appliances such as a clothes iron or curling iron, and allowing these items to cool while out of the reach of children
- Discouraging the use of infant walkers
- Placing safety caps on electrical outlets
- Teaching children that matches are tools, not toys
- Teaching older children and adolescents about: (1) the dangers of high-voltage wires and (2) the dangers of and safe use of gasoline and other flammable liquids
- Teaching children about the dangers of fireworks

Additionally, other prevention efforts have focused on federal regulations mandating the use of flame-retardant fabrics and materials in such articles as children's sleepwear and mattresses to help decrease the number and severity of burns resulting from the ignition of these items. In April 1996, the Consumer Product Safety Commission relaxed the standard for children's sleepwear flammability, which became effective January 1, 1997. However, as of June 2000, all manufactured or imported sleepwear must be flame resistant or snug fitting, and a warning label must be attached to each item.[14]

Structures and functions of the skin

The skin, like the heart and lungs, is a vital organ of the body. In fact, it is the largest organ of the body, varying in thickness from 0.5 mm in the eyelids to 4 mm in the palms and soles.[15] The skin is composed of the more superficial and thinner (20 to 400 μ) layer, the epidermis, and of the deeper and thicker (440 to 2500 μ[14]) layer, the dermis. The dermis can be divided into two layers, the more superficial papillary dermis and the deeper reticular dermis. The depth classification of the burn will be determined by the structures involved. In the basal layer of the epidermis are granules of melanin that give skin its color. The dermis is vascular, and the epidermis, although avascular, has its deeper layers nourished by fluid from the dermis (Fig. 17.2). Sweat glands, hair follicles, and sebaceous glands are contained in the skin, and nails are found on the fingers and toes. Sensory nerves and sympathetic fibers to vessels, to arrector pili muscles, and to sweat glands abound in the skin.[15] The skin helps regulate body temperature, preserves body fluids, protects against infection (by serving as a barrier and also by having certain bactericidal abilities), protects against radiation, and acts as a barrier to help protect vital organs and other body structures against external objects and fluids. Because of nerve endings that sense touch, pain, and temperature, the skin aids in both protective and discriminatory sensation. The skin also assists in vitamin D production. The skin, along with its appendages, can help reveal an individual's race, age, sex, and health. Ridges in the skin on the fingertips give each person a unique set of fingerprints. The skin on the face, with fluctuations in blood flow (e.g., blushing) and with the action of the underlying muscles, can express an individual's emotions. Whenever the skin is significantly damaged or destroyed, these functions may become impaired. Because skin is an organ, when skin is damaged or destroyed, there are both local and systemic effects.[15]

▶ Classification of burns

Burns can be classified by depth of tissue involvement and by size via the percentage of TBSA and by mechanism of injury. For purposes of triage, burns are also classified as minor, moderate, or major.

Burn Depth

Burns can be classified according to the depth of skin damaged or destroyed (Fig. 17.3). Superficial burns (formerly referred to as first-degree burns) are most commonly sunburn. They will heal without scar formation or pigment changes. Deeper burns are classified as partial-thickness burns (formerly known as second-degree burns) or as full-thickness burns (previously referred to as third-degree burns). Partial-thickness burns can be either superficial or deep. Superficial partial-thickness burns involve the epidermis and the papillary dermis. Nails, hair, oil and sweat glands, and nerves are spared. They are painful, appear red, and frequently present with blisters. Superficial partial-thickness burns will heal in about 2 weeks or less without scarring.[16]

Deep partial-thickness burns injure structures deep into the reticular dermis. Structures affected include nails, hair follicles, and the function of sebaceous glands. These burns are waxy white in appearance and are pliable. Such burns may be insensitive to light touch but painful to deep pressure. If they become infected, dry out, or have impaired circulation, deep partial-thickness burns can convert to full-thickness wounds. Deep partial-thickness burns will heal spontaneously by epithelial cells from remaining dermal appendages, but the time required for healing may be 3 to 6 weeks or longer, and such burns heal with scar tissue that can hypertrophy and contract. Although deep partial-thickness burns will heal spontaneously without skin grafting, because of the prolonged healing time and frequently poor functional and cosmetic outcome, as well as other reasons listed later, many surgeons elect to excise and apply skin grafts to these wounds when possible and indicated.

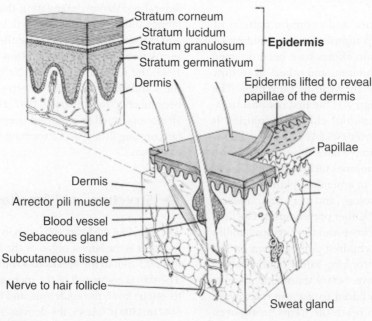

FIGURE 17.2 Structure of the skin.

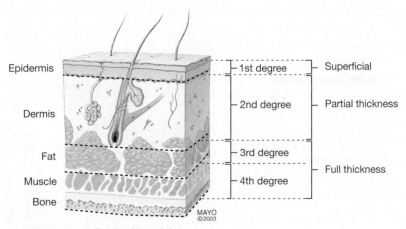

FIGURE 17.3 Depth of burn injury.

Full-thickness burns, by definition, destroy the full thickness of the skin. Such burns can appear as cherry red, white, or brown and leathery, and thrombosed veins may be visible. Hairs can be easily extracted owing to the death of hair follicles.[16] Because the nerves have been destroyed, full-thickness burns are anesthetic to touch. (This does not mean that there is no pain associated with such burns. Activation of the nerves around the periphery of the burn, exposure of the wound to air by removal of dead tissue, or manipulation of the wound can cause extreme pain.) Full-thickness burns will not heal without skin grafting. Even with skin grafting, such burns may result in scar contraction and hypertrophy. Figure 17.4 demonstrates both deep partial- and full-thickness burns to the shoulder and chest.

The actual depth of injury may not be accurately or easily determined on the first day, even by the most experienced clinician. Burn injuries frequently present with varying depths of involvement and usually are not of uniform depth; such factors as how the injury occurred, the thickness of body skin in the area of the burn, and whether or not the individual was wearing clothes have a bearing on the depth of injury. The skin of infants and young children is thinner than that of adults, so, for example, a hot liquid that would cause a superficial, partial-thickness burn in an adult may cause a deeper injury in an infant or toddler. Knowing the depth of the burn is important in determining triage, resuscitation, wound care and closure, and prognosis.

Burn Size

Burns are also classified according to size or TBSA burned. The TBSA is counted as 100%. There are three widely accepted means of determining the extent of body surface area involved. The first is the palmar method, where the palm of an individual's hand is estimated to be about 1% of the TBSA. A second method, more traditionally utilized in the triage of adults, is the "Rule of Nines." According to this rule, in an adult, the head represents 9% of the TBSA, each upper extremity counts as 9%, the trunk represents 36%, each lower extremity represents 18%, and the genitalia are assigned 1%. However, a child's head (especially that of a baby) is larger in proportion to the body than an adult's head, and a child's lower extremities are smaller in proportion to the body than an adult's lower extremities are. For example, the head of a baby who is younger than 1 year is counted as 18%, whereas each lower extremity represents 13.5%. Because of such differences, modified versions of the "Rule of Nines" are used to calculate the TBSA burned in children. The most accurate measurement across the age groups and one that has been modified for the pediatric population is the Lund and Browder chart.[16] The Lund and Browder chart assigns different percentages to body parts, according to the patient's age. Use of a body diagram and the appropriate age-matched percentage will allow for more accurate triage and initial emergency care.[17] The examination form in Figure 17.5 shows the body diagrams and surface area percentages associated with the Lund and Browder chart.

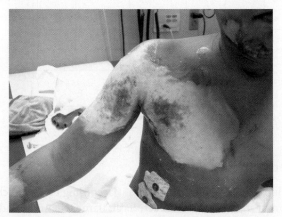

FIGURE 17.4 Deep partial- and full-thickness burns to right upper extremity and trunk. Darkened areas with no capillary refill and no pain sensation are signs of a full-thickness injury.

BURN ASSESSMENT

(PATIENT PLATE IMPRINT)

5+ Years   1-5 Years

CAUSE OF BURN: _____

DATE OF BURN: _____ TIME OF BURN: _____

WEIGHT: _____

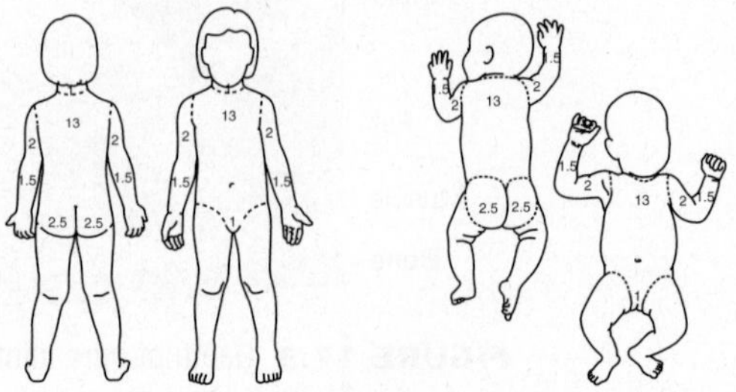

Lund & Browder Chart

Area: *For all body parts except trunk, buttocks, and genitalia, the number in the table represents only the anterior or posterior surface of the body. Need to double number if both anterior and posterior are burned.	Age/Years					% of Body Surface Area Burned: _____		
	0-1	1-4	5-9	10-15	ADULT	PARTIAL THICKNESS	FULL THICKNESS	TOTAL
*Head	9.5%	8.5%	6.5%	5%	3.5%			
*Neck	1%	1%	1%	1%	1%			
Anterior Trunk	13%	13%	13%	13%	13%			
Posterior Trunk	13%	13%	13%	13%	13%			
Right Buttock	2.5%	2.5%	2.5%	2.5%	2.5%			
Left Buttock	2.5%	2.5%	2.5%	2.5%	2.5%			
Genitalia	1%	1%	1%	1%	1%			
*Right Upper Arm	2%	2%	2%	2%	2%			
*Left Upper Arm	2%	2%	2%	2%	2%			
*Right Lower Arm	1.5%	1.5%	1.5%	1.5%	1.5%			
*Left Lower Arm	1.5%	1.5%	1.5%	1.5%	1.5%			
*Right Hand	1.25%	1.25%	1.25%	1.25%	1.25%			
*Left Hand	1.25%	1.25%	1.25%	1.25%	1.25%			
*Right Thigh	2.25%	3.25%	4.25%	4.25%	4.75%			
*Left Thigh	2.25%	3.25%	4.25%	4.25%	4.75%			
*Right Leg	2.5%	2.5%	2.75%	3%	3.5%			
*Left Leg	2.5%	2.5%	2.75%	3%	3.5%			
*Right Foot	1.75%	1.75%	1.75%	1.75%	1.75%			
*Left Foot	1.75%	1.75%	1.75%	1.75%	1.75%			
					TOTAL			

Signature: _____

Date: _____

FIGURE 17.5 Lund and Browder chart for burn size estimation.

The importance of accuracy with burn size estimation has implications for proper fluid resuscitation in the acute medical treatment and overall morbidity and mortality due to the large inflammatory and hypermetabolic response. Attention to the changing body proportion size of a growing child must be taken into account.[18]

Mechanism of Injury

A third way of classifying burns is according to the mechanism of injury: scald, contact, flash, flame, chemical, radiation, or electrical. Knowing the causative agent or method can be important in giving appropriate treatment. For example, if an individual sustains a chemical burn, knowing which chemical caused the burn is necessary in order to apply the correct antidote and in determining the need for copious water lavage, which would not necessarily be done for an electrical burn or a flame burn. Recognizing the mechanism of injury and correlating the presentation of the burn will aid in ruling out child abuse.

Minor, Moderate, and Major Classifications

Burns can be classified as minor, moderate, or major according to guidelines established by the American Burn Association (ABA) for purposes of triage. For example, a minor burn for an adult might be a partial-thickness burn involving less than 15% of the TBSA; such a patient could be treated as an outpatient. A minor burn for a child might be a partial-thickness burn involving less than 10% of the TBSA, but hospitalization might be considered for such a patient. The ABA recommends that an individual with the following injuries be referred to a burn center:

- Partial-thickness burns greater than 10% TBSA
- Burns of the face, hands, feet, genitalia, perineum, or major joints
- Full-thickness burns in any age group
- Electrical burns
- Chemical burns
- Burn injury in patients with preexisting medical disorders that could complicate management
- Burns in children at a hospital without qualified personnel or equipment
- Burn injury in patients that will require special social, emotional, or rehabilitative intervention.[19]

▶ Pathophysiology

Dimensions of Injury

Regardless of the mechanism of injury, each burn wound consists of three zones that are identified concentrically around the center portion of the injury. The most central area of the burn is the zone of coagulation; this is the area that had the most contact with the heat source. The cells in this zone have been permanently damaged. Extending outwardly is the zone of stasis. The cells in the zone of stasis have decreased blood flow and respond to resuscitation to save viable tissue. The outermost zone of burn injury is the zone of hyperemia. These cells have sustained the least damage and should recover within 10 days.[16]

Burn Wound Healing

Burn wound healing can be categorized into three phases: inflammation, proliferation, and maturation/remodeling.

Inflammatory Phase

Once an injury has occurred, the disruption of epidermal and dermal structures signals the healing process to occur.

Platelets come in contact with the injured tissue, fibrin is deposited, more platelets are trapped, and a thrombus is formed. There is also a local vasoconstriction that occurs, and in combination with the thrombus, it blocks the injured tissue from systemic circulation, thus achieving hemostasis. The major goals of the inflammatory phase are to provide for this hemostasis and breaking down and removing cellular, extracellular, and pathogen debris, which will in turn signal the repair process to start. Cytokines and growth factors attract responder cells and help regulate the repair process.[20]

Proliferative Phase

The proliferative phase, which is dominated by fibroblast activity, follows the inflammatory phase. The goals of the proliferative phase are to assist wound healing and restore skin integrity. The main processes involved in this second stage are angiogenesis, collagen synthesis, and wound contraction. Collagen is deposited at the wound site as early as 48 hours after a burn. Type I collagen is seen by days 4 to 7 after injury. Granulation tissue forms as endothelial cells migrate to the wound and will continue until the wound is completely re-epithelialized. The cells migrate from the periphery toward the center of the wound (i.e., the wound will heal from the outside toward the middle).[20] Reepithelialization is more rapid when the stratum granulosum layer of the epidermis is intact, as with superficial partial-thickness burns. The burn wound will remain in this phase until epithelialization is complete or until the wound is surgically treated (e.g., covered with a skin graft).

Maturation/Remodeling Phase

The maturation or remodeling phase is the final phase of wound healing. This final phase actually began as granulation tissue formed in the earlier proliferative phase. During the remodeling phase of burn wound healing, collagen synthesis and lysis occurs, thus creating scar tissue. During the remodeling phase, the collagen is reorganized into a more compact area. An imbalance in collagen synthesis will result in a hypertrophic or keloid-type scar (discussed later).[20]

▶ Scar hypertrophy and contraction

As previously mentioned, there are two common, though often avoidable, sequelae of deep partial-thickness and full-thickness burns: scar hypertrophy and scar contraction. Scar hypertrophy and scar contraction can impede both physical and psychological functioning. Scar hypertrophy is a raised, thick, usually hard, often knotty-appearing area of scar tissue (Fig. 17.6) that results from an imbalance of collagen synthesis and collagen lysis. A hypertrophic scar is raised, but does not exceed the original boundaries of the wound. A keloid scar is raised and extends beyond the boundaries of the original wound. Factors that may predict scar formation

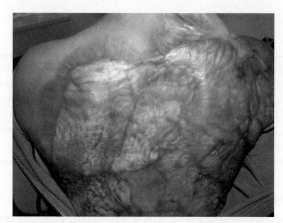

FIGURE 17.6 Hypertrophic scarring along patient's back following split-thickness skin grafts.

include depth of the wound, extended healing time, wounds in individuals with more skin pigment, and young people who tend to scar more than the elderly.[21]

Hunt[22] stated that increased tension, which promotes collagen deposition and lessens collagen lysis, may contribute to the formation of hypertrophic scars, evidenced by the appearance of hypertrophic scars in areas of motion, such as the joints (Fig. 17.7).

Chan et al. in 2012 examined the correlation of the time to skin grafting and hypertrophic scarring. They acknowledged that in addition to the age of the patient and the mechanism of the burn injury, factors that played a role in hypertrophic scar formation included race, genetic predisposition, site and depth of the burn. Other complications such as a prolonged inflammatory phase or wound colonization also increased the scarring process. They performed split thickness skin grafting in porcine models and concluded that early grafting of deep dermal burns had better histology and clinical scar outcomes. They noted that contemporary surgical practice was to delay grafting until 14 to 21 days post injury, but their study advocated for earlier grafting as the best scar outcomes were observed in skin grafts performed within 14 days of the injury.[23]

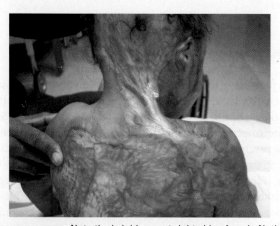

FIGURE 17.7 Note the keloid scar at right side of neck. Notice the band-like formation.

Scar contraction is the pulling or shortening of scar tissue, which can result in loss of joint motion or skin mobility. Scar contracture is a fixed shortening of the scar tissue that may be amenable only to surgery. Contraction may be attributed to myofibroblasts, cells with contractile properties, found in the healing burn wound.[21] Scar contraction not located over a joint can lead to disfigurement, especially if such contraction involves the face. Scar contraction over a joint can lead to loss of joint range of motion (ROM) or postural and gait deviations. Because of the contracting force of scar tissue, which results in loss of skin mobility, loss of joint ROM can also result from contracting scar tissue adjacent to, although not covering, a joint.[21] What is initially just loss of motion from contracting scar can, if left uncorrected, lead to a gradual shortening of joint capsules, muscles, tendons, and ligaments.

The processes of scar contraction and hypertrophy begin almost as soon as the burn wound begins healing, although initially may not be readily visible. Collagen formation begins within 24 hours of the burn injury. There is a high rate of collagen synthesis in the wound,[24] and such activity returns to a normal pace by 6 to 12 months.[25] The scar is initially red because of an increased blood supply, but it usually fades over time. When the scar is no longer actively hypertrophying and contracting, it is said to be mature. The period of scar maturation for most children is approximately 12 to 18 months. For adults, this period may be shorter. While the scar is active, particularly during the first 6 months, the processes of hypertrophy and contraction can be controlled or corrected by nonsurgical approaches, such as pressure, splinting, and ROM exercises, which will be discussed later. As scar maturation progresses, these treatments become less effective in altering scar. After the scar is mature, most nonsurgical treatments are no longer effective, and surgery, if indicated, may afford the only treatment alternative.

▶ Burn center

In 1999, the ABA published guidelines for the development and operation of burn centers, and updated the guidelines for verification for burn centers in 2006. To achieve verification as a burn center, the center has to meet rigorous standards, and participate in onsite and ongoing review by the ABA. As of 2013, there are over 60 verified burn centers in the United States.[26]

▶ Burn team

In its guidelines for burn centers, the ABA specifies which personnel should staff the burn center, as well as which specialists and personnel should be on call or available for consultation. (The criteria state that "both physical and occupational therapy should be represented in the burn center staff.") Within the ABA guidelines, each burn center establishes its own burn team. Personnel who comprise the burn team and their specific roles may vary from institution to institution or according to the individual needs of a given patient or the particular phase of healing, although there generally is a core team.[26] The pediatric burn team frequently includes a surgeon, a nurse, an occupational therapist, a physical therapist, a social worker, a respiratory therapist, a dietitian, a child life therapist, a hospital chaplain, a discharge planner, various specialists (pediatrician, pulmonologist, psychiatrist, plastic surgeon, infection control specialist, etc.), and most importantly, the child and family. Because many children do not have a traditional nuclear family, it is often necessary to determine who, in the child's view, comprises the family.

Initial treatment and medical management

The initial treatment and medical management of the pediatric burn patient depends, in part, on the depth, size, and location of the burn; the presence of other concomitant injuries, such as smoke inhalation; the age of the child; and the premorbid health of the child. The injury itself will trigger physiologic responses that, in turn, will affect treatment requirements.

Systems review

Pulmonary System

Establishing and maintaining an adequate airway and breathing are the first concerns when treating a thermally injured patient. If the patient has inhaled steam or noxious gases, intubation may be necessary because bronchospasm and upper airway edema[27] may develop, possibly resulting in airway obstruction within hours. Oxygen is administered if the patient has inhaled high levels of carbon monoxide. The endotracheal tube may be removed once edema has subsided, usually within a few days.[27] Patients with more extensive airway or lung injuries will require sustained or more involved treatment.

Cardiovascular System

The circulatory changes that occur following a burn injury have been discussed earlier. These changes are termed *burn shock*. The loss of fluid, increased capillary permeability, and vasodilation that occur all cause decreases in the circulatory volume and reduced cardiac output. Proper fluid resuscitation is key to recovering normal cardiac output. Inadequate fluid replacement can lead to poor tissue perfusion, organ dysfunction, and death.[16]

Fluid Resuscitation

Because of the inflammatory process and increased capillary permeability in patients with deep partial-thickness or full-thickness burns, fluid leaves the blood and is dispersed into the interstitial spaces. Patients with burns of less than 10% to 20% of their TBSA, depending on other considerations, may be able to compensate for this fluid shift physiologically through such measures as vasoconstriction and urine retention.[27] Patients with burns involving a greater percentage of TBSA will develop hypovolemic shock and can die if not treated. Replacement of the circulating fluid loss is termed *fluid resuscitation*. Fluids cannot be administered orally to patients with larger area burns because of ileus (obstruction of the bowel), which occurs secondary to shock. Fluids, with electrolytes similar to serum, and colloid are given intravenously. Patients with smaller burns may be able to take fluids orally. However, children, in particular, may be unwilling to drink and may therefore require intravenous fluids. In a few days, with adequate fluid replacement, the fluid in the interstitial spaces returns to the intravascular spaces, and the patient will have a diuresis, signalling successful fluid resuscitation.[27] After fluid resuscitation, the patient may still require replacement of fluids because fluid is also lost through the burn wound and because the patient may be unwilling or unable to take sufficient fluids orally.

A urinary catheter is placed in patients with large burns so as to monitor urine output during resuscitation. Patients with perineal burns may also require catheterization to keep bandages dry or to protect newly placed skin grafts during the skin graft phase.

Renal System

As a result of loss of fluid from intravascular spaces, renal vasoconstriction can occur and may cause renal failure due to decreased renal blood flow and decreased glomerular filtration. With electrical burn injuries, extensive tissue may be damaged, thus releasing myoglobin, which may occlude the kidneys, thus leading to renal failure.

Circulatory System

Full-thickness burned skin is inelastic. Because of the body's response to injury and fluid resuscitation, the patient will become edematous. This is a systemic response that also occurs in the unburned parts of the body. In the case of circumferential burns of the extremities, the combination of inelastic skin and increasing edema can cause a tourniquet effect, resulting in compromised circulation to the distal extremities. If treatment is not initiated, ischemia and tissue damage or necrosis can occur. Signs of compromise include pallor, decreased skin temperature, delayed capillary refill, numbness/tingling, and decreased chest wall excursion in the case of trunk burns. Compartment pressures of greater than 30 mm Hg also indicate the need for surgical

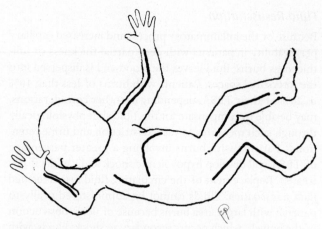

FIGURE 17.8 This diagram shows where surgical incisions (escharotomy) are performed in patients who have compromised blood flow due to circumferential full-thickness burns. The incisions are made laterally and/or medially with the patient in the true anatomic position, as shown.

intervention. The trauma surgeon will attempt to relieve the pressure by performing an escharotomy, which is a surgical incision through the burned tissue. These incisions are usually along the lateral and medial sides of the affected extremity. At the chest, longitudinal incisions are made along the anterior axillary lines and a transverse incision at the costal level.[16] Figure 17.8 shows common sites for escharotomy.

In 2009, Orgill and Piccolo released practice guidelines for burn care clinicians regarding escharotomy and decompressive therapies. Their review of the burn care literature supports the implementation of decompressive techniques following a burn injury to alleviate further tissue necrosis and preserve nerve function. If pressure is still not relieved by an escharotomy, these incisions may need to be extended, and the fascia released as well via a fasciotomy.[28]

Musculoskeletal System

Owing to the association between fire and traumatic injuries, it is not uncommon to have a burn injury and concomitant fracture. Examination of the musculoskeletal injury will often be delayed while the potential life-threatening injuries are assessed. Patients who are unresponsive or unable to report specific pain may be at risk for having fractures or other musculoskeletal injuries unnoticed upon primary or secondary surveys. The therapist may be the first clinician to discover an undiagnosed musculoskeletal injury. Children likely to have musculoskeletal injuries are those involved in an automobile accident with a resulting fire or those who jumped from a burning building. Both burns and fractures can cause soft tissue swelling, thus requiring an escharotomy in the case that circulation is compromised (see Circulatory system). Nonoperative management of fractures includes using a splint or traction. Use of a circumferential cast is discouraged because of swelling and the inability to examine

the wounds properly. Internal fixation is also beneficial as it increases the rate of fracture healing. Surgery for internal fixation should occur within 48 hours after injury; otherwise, bacterial colonization is presumed. Surgical fixation of the fracture will allow for reduction in pain at the fracture site and for physical therapy interventions.[29]

▶ Nutrition

In response to the burn injury, the patient is in a hypermetabolic state, and caloric and nutritional requirements are greatly increased. The hypermetabolic and inflammatory response caused by a burn is demonstrated by an increase in protein, proinflammatory cytokine, and catabolic hormone levels. These findings increase energy requirements, which can result in muscle wasting due to a catabolic state. If this posttraumatic response is prolonged, it can lead to multiple organ dysfunction and death. Raising of room temperatures and nutritional supplementation have been efficient in modulating the hypermetabolic responses.[30] Adequate nutrition is necessary to prevent wasting and to promote proper wound healing. The child with a burn may be unwilling to eat because of the injury and a strange environment. The severity or location of the burns may make it difficult or impossible to eat. A patient with a larger burn may find it hard to consume the volume of food necessary to obtain sufficient calories. Additionally, the patient will be prohibited from eating on days when a surgical procedure is scheduled. Because of such factors, the patient may receive a large portion of nutrition through enteral tube feedings or through peripheral vein infusions. Enteral nutrition is the preferred route of nutritional support since it offers maintenance of the gastrointestinal (GI) mucosal integrity by delivering nutrients into the GI tract. A nutritional assessment should be done upon admission following a thermal injury. This will include review of medical, nutritional, and medication histories, and laboratory data, and a patient examination. The clinician will evaluate plasma protein levels, more specifically, albumin and prealbumin. The normal range for serum albumin is 3.5 to 5 g/dL. Low levels of albumin may signify poor potential to heal. Prealbumin is a transport protein for thyroid hormone. Normal serum prealbumin levels range from 16 to 40 mg/dL, with values greater than 16 mg/dL associated with malnutrition. The half-life of prealbumin is 2 to 3 days, thus making it a good predictor of nutritional status.[31]

▶ Pain management

Burn-associated pain is one of the most relevant complaints in patients with burn injuries. Burn pain intensity can vary because of the inflammatory response and the changes in levels of inflammatory mediators. In partial-thickness burns, nerve endings are still viable and cause significant pain, while full-thickness burns are less painful owing to the damage to the nerve endings. Medical and therapeutic interventions such as dressing changes, wound cleansing, and physical therapy can cause pain. Tengvall et al. in 2010 did a retrospective study on patients' memories of pain after their burn injury. They found that patients remember pain throughout the recovery from the initial injury, to care within the hospital or burn center, and through transition to home with any new physical limitations.[32]

In 2003, Martin-Herz et al. investigated pediatric pain control practices in North American Burn Centers. Their study results were compared to a study completed in 1982, which revealed at that time that 17% of burn units recommended using no opioid analgesics and 8% did not use any analgesics during pediatric wound care.[33] The newer survey revealed significant changes in the use of opioids during pediatric burn dressing changes. Morphine appeared to be the "gold standard" for medicating the child before, during, and after a painful procedure.[34] Twenty-five percent of the responders in the survey utilized psychotropic medications in combination with opioids. Background pain control and breakthrough pain control was also best controlled by IV morphine. Only 8% of centers responding stated that they routinely utilized an anesthesia-based pain service for helping with pain management.[35]

In 2010, Bayat et al. studied analgesia and sedation for children undergoing burn wound care. They identified the different types of burn pain experienced by children. These included background pain, which was relatively constant from the time of injury through the initial healing period. Next was procedural pain, which was described as burning or stinging during wound cleansing and dressing changes, and often included significant anxiety and distress. Next was breakthrough pain, which was worsening of background pain either due to a decrease in blood levels of analgesia and may require additional medication or use of a patient-controlled analgesia (PCA) pump. The last type of pain they looked at was postsurgical pain, which was longer lasting but less severe than procedural pain.[36] Medications used for procedural analgesia or sedation should have a rapid onset, limited side effects, and allow for resumption of activities and oral intake following the procedure. Common medications might include nonsteroidal anti-inflammatory drugs (NSAIDs), opiates (morphine, oxycodone, fentanyl), benzodiazepines (for sedation and anxiety), and ketamine (for sedation and amnesia/analgesia).[36]

The services of child life specialists and music therapists can aid with the nonpharmacological approach as well as with preparing the child for the procedure. The child's pain and anxiety must be considered and treated appropriately throughout all phases of healing. Age-specific distraction techniques can be seen in Table 17.1.

Medication for pruritus should also be considered, as itching can be a source of discomfort and pain, and may limit patient tolerance for interventions. Antihistamines were the most commonly prescribed medications for pruritus.

TABLE 17.1	Non-Pharmacologic Pain Management
Age Range	Participation Motivators/Distraction Techniques
Under 2 yr	Use parents to help; rattles, bubble blowing, singing, videos
2–7 yr	Singing, looking at a book, videos, magic wand
7–11 yr	Allow them to participate as indicated; headphones for music, videos, sticker chart
11 yr and above	Give precise information regarding the intervention; music, videos, video games, reward chart

Opioids themselves can cause itching, so careful documentation of the occurrence of itching and whether or not it is related to burn wound healing or medication is important.[35]

Besides specific medications and pain management techniques, the facility and each professional should have a treatment approach that has as a goal caring for the burn patient in a way that causes the least amount of pain. Some suggestions for minimizing patients' pain are made throughout the chapter.

▶ Burn wound management

The primary goals of wound management are to provide an optimal environment for wound healing, to provide a healthy tissue bed to receive a skin graft, and to protect healing tissue or a recently placed graft. Such goals are accomplished mainly through removing dead tissue, keeping the wound clean and minimizing bacterial invasion, preventing the wound or new skin graft from drying out, and protecting newly healing tissue or recent skin graft(s) from disruptive mechanical abrasion. There are nonsurgical and surgical interventions that comprise overall burn wound management. Prior to any wound cleansing or dressing changes, the child should be premedicated.

Nonsurgical Interventions

Wound Cleansing

HYDROTHERAPY Hydrotherapy is used in some burn centers as a part of wound management. Showering, immersion, or use of a spray table can accomplish it. The purpose of hydrotherapy is to help remove the old topical antimicrobial agent, to clean the wound, to help superficially debride the wound (through the effect of the agitator), to increase circulation to promote wound healing, and to provide an environment for exercise. Agitation may be used in the presence of a highly necrotic wound (e.g., road burn). The drawbacks of hydrotherapy are that it can spread infection, it can increase the length of time required for a dressing change, it can increase cost (because of the additional personnel required to perform the procedure and clean the equipment), it can increase edema (especially if a limb is placed in a dependent position), and patients, particularly children, may find it traumatic, especially if a bathtub was the mechanism of original injury. Because of the drawbacks of hydrotherapy, some burn centers limit its use to specific wounds or to certain phases of wound healing, or use hand-held shower heads to help clean the wound.

In 2010, Davison et al. reviewed hydrotherapy in North American Burn Centers. The results of their study showed a decrease in the use of hydrotherapy from as high as 95% of the burn centers using it in 1990 to 83%. With the trend toward early excision of dead tissue and the increase in nosocomial infections, the use of immersion hydrotherapy decreased from 81% to 45%, using showering methods instead.[37]

Dressing Changes

Most burn patients will undergo bandage (also called dressing) changes from daily to every few days depending on the dressings used. Even very young children can participate in removing their dressings, which may help minimize pain and offer some sense of control and independence in a situation in which they might otherwise feel helpless. Because some of the pain experienced during a dressing change is caused by exposure of the wound to air, such exposure time should be limited. Limiting the exposure time to air will help prevent the tissue from drying out and will also limit exposure to bacteria. To minimize the time required for a dressing change, bandages should be prepared ahead of time so that they may be quickly applied. Health care professionals who wish to observe the patient's wound should be present at the time of the dressing change so that the patient is not waiting with an undressed wound for them to arrive. If the parent desires, and if appropriate, the parent's presence during the dressing change can be beneficial for both the parent and the child. In some cases, however, children may cry more in the presence of a parent because they expect the parent to "rescue" them from the dressing change.

In some burn centers, therapists are responsible for or may assist with daily wound care for both inpatients and outpatients. (It may also be the case that the therapist, before or during performance of outpatient therapy, will need to change the patient's bandage.) During a dressing change, the old bandage is removed and the wound may be superficially debrided (nonviable tissue removed). At the same time the wound is cleaned and examined, ROM is measured without the dressings in place to establish how much ROM the patient should work toward for the remainder of the therapy day.

Topical Agents

In a burn injury, the protective barrier of the skin is lost, and the burn wound becomes a host for bacteria. Topical antimicrobial agents play a vital role in helping minimize bacterial colonization of the wound, decrease vapor loss, prevent desiccation, and control pain.[38] Several topical antimicrobial agents may be employed depending on the specific wound and the organisms to be controlled.

Silver sulfadiazine (Silvadene) is the most commonly used topical agent.[5] Silvadene is a white, opaque cream that is painless upon application, has fair eschar penetration, and has a broad antibacterial spectrum.[38] Silvadene can't be used by patients with sulfa allergies.[5] Silvadene has also been shown to cause neutropenia when applied on large surface area burns.[38] Mafenide acetate (Sulfamylon) is another topical agent available in liquid or cream form, is painful upon application, has excellent eschar penetration, and has a broad antibacterial spectrum. Mafenide acetate is utilized on burns of the external ear to reduce suppurative chondritis.[38] Sulfamylon can be used on partial-thickness burns that are resistant to Silvadene and to increase eschar penetration/separation. Sulfamylon is contraindicated for use in patients with metabolic acidosis.[5] Other topical agents used in burn wound management include silver nitrate, which has broad antibacterial coverage and is applied as a solution on burn wounds or graft sites. Petroleum-based products such as neomycin and bacitracin are used on superficial burns or on areas where the skin is very thin (e.g., eyelids, scrotum).[38]

Acticoat dressing is another option to topical antimicrobial creams. It has been shown to be more effective than Silvadene and silver nitrate against gram-negative and gram-positive organisms. Acticoat is a three-ply gauze with an absorbent rayon and polyester core. The coating to Acticoat is non-adherent to the wound and is flexible. The child would need to undergo debridement prior to Acticoat placement. A bulky layer of wet gauze is wrapped around the Acticoat and then covered with dry gauze. Daily dressing changes include taking down the gauze dressings, inspecting the Acticoat for slippage from the wound bed, and reapplying wet gauze and dry gauze. Once adhered, the Acticoat is left in place until reepithelialization occurs. This process will decrease the risk of infection (from daily wound cleansing) and discomfort associated with dressing changes.[39]

AQUACEL Ag Hydrofiber is a moisture-retentive topical dressing used in the acute management of burns. It consists entirely of carboxymethylcellulose, which forms into a gel upon contact with burn exudate. This gel promotes a moist wound healing environment while still managing moderate amounts of burn exudate.[40] This hydrofiber with 1.2% ionic silver releases silver within the dressing for up to 2 weeks. It can be applied on an acute burn and left in place until healing occurs, thus decreasing pain and length of hospitalization.[41] Caruso et al. performed a randomized clinical study comparing AQUACEL Ag and silver sulfadiazine for the management of partial-thickness burns. Compared with silver sulfadiazine, AQUACEL Ag was associated with less pain and anxiety during dressing changes. Patients using the traditional silver sulfadiazine dressing had more flexibility and ease of movement during use in comparison with those using AQUACEL Ag. Overall, in this study the AQUACEL

Ag group demonstrated greater benefits with fewer dressing changes, less nursing time, and fewer pre-procedural opiate medications.[42] These benefits clearly support implementation of AQUACEL use in the pediatric setting where pain reduction and decreased length of hospitalization are overall patient care goals. Al-Ahdab and Al-Omawi reported use of AQUACEL Ag in a newborn with scald burns. They chose AQUACEL Ag due to the dressing being shown to be less painful as it required fewer dressing changes. The effectiveness of the dressing was noted by the rapid healing of the partial-thickness burns in their neonatal case study and absence of wound infection.[34]

Functional Dressings

Dressings should not excessively inhibit motion. The thumb, for example, should not be wrapped into the palm, nor should bandages restrict chest expansion. However, bandages can be used to help position the patient. For example, bulky bandages can be used in place of splints to support the fingers and wrists in infants and toddlers.

Additionally, applying the topical antimicrobial agent to the gauze and then applying the gauze to the wound (instead of applying the topical agent directly to the wound and then applying the gauze) will also help minimize pain during the dressing change. A non-adherent gauze such as Exu-Dry, Adaptic, or Xeroform will decrease the pain associated with dressing removal. A bulky bandage is used to secure the topical agent and non-adherent dressing in place. Tubular netting is then placed over the bulky bandage to secure it in place. The tubular netting can be cut/fabricated into many styles (e.g., sleeve, shirt, stocking) for the specific body part. Figure 17.9 shows a functional dressing for the hand, which allows the child more use of it for play or activities of daily living (ADLs).

Positioning with dressing application should be adhered to. Burns across joints or at the hands or feet require special attention with dressing application. Positioning is utilized to protect the burn wounds, decrease edema, and counteract

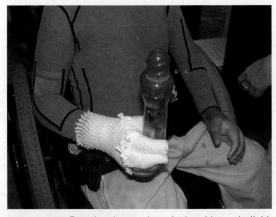

FIGURE 17.9 Functional wrapping of a hand burn. Individual finger dressings allow for easier movement and performance of activities of daily living.

wound and scar contraction by putting the tissue in an elongated position. For example, burns across the antecubital fossa should be wrapped and splinted into extension. Burns on the plantar/dorsal surface of the foot and calf should be wrapped and splinted into neutral dorsiflexion.[33]

Biologic Dressings

Advances in burn wound management surround the invention and improvements made in the area of biologic or synthetic dressings. Biobrane is a synthetic dressing that can be used on superficial partial-thickness burns, over autografts, on donor sites, and in the treatment of toxic epidermal necrolysis (TEN). It is a nylon fabric that is combined with a silicone film, where collagen is incorporated. The nylon fabric comes into contact with the burn wound and adheres until reepithelialization occurs. It is placed on the burn wounds in the operating room and secured with staples or sutures, and once adhered to the wound, no other dressing is necessary.[43]

Surgical Management

Once burn size and depth estimations have been made and the initial burn wound management has commenced, further wound management may include surgery.

Because a superficial partial-thickness burn will heal in approximately 2 weeks with normal skin, the goals of the surgeon in such cases are to keep the wound free of infection, to provide adequate nutrition and fluids, and to manage pain until the wound is healed. Depending on the size and location of the superficial partial-thickness burn, the age of the patient, and the ability of the parent, many of these burns can be treated on an outpatient basis and without surgery.

A deep partial-thickness burn can heal without surgical intervention if adequate medical treatment and wound management are provided. The progression of deep partial-thickness burns will usually take one of two pathways. The first includes the filmy eschar separating from the wound edges, allowing epithelial buds to resurface the wound. The other is following separation of eschar, the wound heals by granulation tissue. The presence of granulation tissue will increase the risk of hypertrophic scarring. This situation, along with large TBSA of deep partial-thickness burns, makes surgical intervention via grafting more probable. The surgeon may elect to graft the deep partial-thickness burn in a procedure called tangential excision and grafting.[5] Such excision and grafting can be done within the first week of the burn injury and is ideally performed 2 to 5 days after the burn injury (termed *early excision and grafting*). Early excision and grafting may also apply to other wounds, particularly full-thickness wounds, which may be excised to fascia. Tangential excision and grafting of deep partial-thickness wounds during the first week shortens the patient's hospital stay, lessens pain, decreases the incidence of infection, and improves cosmetic and functional outcome (by minimizing the amount of hypertrophic scar tissue development and scar contraction).[44]

There are drawbacks associated with early tangential excision and grafting of deep partial-thickness wounds, however, and not all patients are candidates for this procedure. Early excision and grafting of deep partial-thickness burns usually involves significant intraoperative blood loss that may require substantial transfusion; this may not be recommended for medically unstable patients or those with inhalation injury.[45] When a burn involves a significant percentage of TBSA, and particularly when the burn area consists of both deep partial-thickness and full-thickness burns with a limited number of donor sites for skin grafts, excision and grafting of deep partial-thickness burns is often delayed or such wounds are allowed to heal spontaneously.

Skin Graft and Donor Site

There are several different types of grafts, depending on the source of the skin. An autograft is skin that is surgically shaved from an unburned part of the patient's body (called the donor site) and placed on the burned area. Removal of the skin to be used for grafting is called harvesting. In the case where infection may be present, or due to a large TBSA, autografting may not be possible. In that case, alternative grafts can be used, including xenografts and allografts. A xenograft is skin harvested from a pig that can help protect and facilitate healing of partial-thickness burns as well as debriding exudative wounds. An allograft is a graft of skin from a cadaver, which has been harvested within 24 hours of death and preserved via cryopreservation (at a skin bank). These are often used in preparation for autografting to test the "receptivity" of the wound bed for an autograft.[46]

With an autograft, either a full thickness or partial thickness of skin can be harvested. If a full-thickness piece of skin from the unburned donor site was taken and placed on the burned area, the burn would heal, but a wound of similar dimensions to the burn would remain at the donor site. Full-thickness skin grafts (FTSGs) (0.025 to 0.030 inches thick) are used mostly in reconstructive surgery, over pressure points, or anywhere extra skin thickness is needed. More commonly, only a partial- or split-thickness (approximately 0.008-inch thick) portion of skin is taken (STSG). Some areas of the body are preferred donor sites because of the thickness, texture, or color of the skin; because they are areas that will heal well; and because they are in a region not usually visible. Common preferred donor sites include the lateral thighs and buttocks. However, when these areas are burned, or in an extensively burned individual, almost any skin on the body can be used. A split-thickness donor site is similar to a superficial partial-thickness burn, with healing occurring within 14 days via reepithelialization. After the patient has been anesthetized, the skin is shaved from the donor site with an electric knife—known as a dermatome—with settings to adjust the thickness of skin excised. The

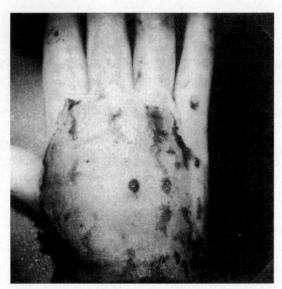

FIGURE 17.10 Example of a sheet graft to the dorsum of the hand.

procedure is called a sheet graft when the skin is placed "as is" on the excised burned area (also known as the recipient or graft site) (Fig. 17.10). Alternatively, the skin may be placed in a skin mesher before its application to the recipient site. The mesher cuts small slits in the graft, after which the graft may be stretched or expanded before placement on the recipient site. Such a graft is known as an expanded mesh graft (Fig. 17.11). The main purpose of meshing is to allow a skin graft to cover a larger area than could otherwise be covered using a sheet graft. The amount of graft expansion achieved is expressed as a ratio of the expanded to the unexpanded size. For example, an expanded mesh graft that covers one and a half times its original or unmeshed size would be referred to as a 1.5:1 mesh graft. One advantage of a mesh graft is that compared with a sheet graft, there is less likelihood that hematomas or serous fluid will collect under the graft, causing the graft to be non-adherent. A disadvantage of a mesh graft, particularly a large-ratio mesh graft, is scarring that occurs within the interstices or holes

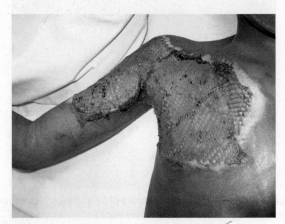

FIGURE 17.11 Meshed split-thickness skin graft.

and such scarring can hypertrophy and contract. The permanent meshed pattern of the graft may also be cosmetically unattractive.[47] Because sheet grafts provide a better cosmetic outcome with less contraction and hypertrophy, they are the graft of choice in burns involving less than 30% of TBSA that are not excessively colonized by bacteria and other microbes. Sheet grafts should also be used on the face, neck, and hands, and are often preferred for other functional areas of the body, such as the feet and the axillae. The surgeon may secure the graft with surgical staples, stitches, or Steri-strips. The graft usually requires 4 to 7 days to become adherent or to "take." The grafted area is protected during this period by bulky dressings. If the graft site is over a joint, the joint is usually immobilized with a splint during this initial period, and exercise of the joint is discontinued for that same period. Movement or shearing forces can result in graft loss. Infection, inadequate nutrition, a poor graft bed or inadequate debridement are other factors that can contribute to graft loss or less than optimal graft take.

Once healed, donor sites can be "re-harvested," up to three or four times in the case of a large TBSA burn. Harvesting of the skin over irregular surfaces can be achieved by injecting saline to contour such areas.[48]

Before the skin graft can be placed, the burned, necrotic skin, called *eschar*, must be removed. This is usually accomplished surgically, but enzymatic debrider may also be used on partial-thickness wounds. Surgical excision usually extends down to a level of viable tissue. Excision of eschar may occur immediately before placing the skin graft, or, depending on the depth and extent of the wound, it may be done earlier, in a separate operation. If an excised full-thickness wound is not grafted during the same procedure, granulation tissue will develop that will help prepare the site for grafting.

In the case of a burn involving a large percentage of TBSA, even when multiple donor sites are available, the surgeon may elect not to graft the entire burn at once because of the stress of surgery to the patient, particularly if the patient is already medically compromised or unstable. If the grafts do not take, not only is there still a large TBSA burn, but the donor sites are now additional wounds that must be healed, and the donor sites cannot be reused for about 10 days.

Cultured Autografts and Dermal Substitutes

Several advances in wound healing and surgical techniques during the past two decades have improved the outcome and increased survival of burn patients. Among these advances are two that increase survival in massively burned individuals who lack sufficient donor sites: cultured autografts and dermal substitutes.

In the 1980s, cultured epithelial autografts (CEAs) or keratinocytes were the newest advancement in wound closure of the severely burned individual. In the case of CEAs, a small piece of unburned skin measuring approximately 1 square inch is harvested from the patient and grown in a laboratory. Within several weeks or less, there is enough skin to cover an entire body, and this skin can be grafted onto the patient from whom the original sample was taken. However, there are drawbacks and problems with cultured autografted skin. Wound closure must be delayed until the skin is grown, and the rate of graft adherence varies from 15% to 80% depending on the occurrence of graft site infection.[49] Standard physical therapy regimens, in particular those involving ROM and mobilization, must be altered or their implementation delayed in many cases. Sood et al. in 2009 performed a retrospective study of pediatric patients with congenital nevi and burns who required CEA for wound coverage. They studied 29 children over 18 years old, with all participants surviving, and those with burns averaging over 50% TBSA. The final CEA "take" success rate was over 75%, with a 99-day mean length of hospitalization. Contractures were the major long-term complication in the majority of the children. The CEA proved to be a durable wound coverage option in large TBSA burns.[49]

Several dermal substitutes or dermal analogs are now available for us after decades of research. One such substitute, Integra (Integra LifeSciences Corp., Plainsboro, NJ), is an artificial dermis composed of two layers: a dermal replacement layer of bovine tendon collagen and a substitute epidermal layer of silicone.[33] Integra is placed on the excised wound. The porous dermal replacement layer serves as a matrix for the infiltration of elements from the wound bed that construct a neodermis. While the patient's own neodermis is being constructed, the bovine collagen dissolves. During the period of neodermis construction, about 2 weeks, the silicone epidermal layer acts to control moisture loss from the wound. After neodermis construction is complete, the surgeon removes the silicone layer and replaces it with very thin autografts from the patient. One major benefit of Integra is lack of scar formation associated with its use. Other benefits are

- its immediate availability for use,
- provision for immediate post-excisional wound coverage,
- early ambulation and rehabilitation,
- delayed autografting of the neodermis if necessary,
- more rapid healing and better cosmetic outcome of donor sites because of ultrathin autograft use, and
- ability to save certain donor sites for use on cosmetically sensitive areas.[50]

Some disadvantages of Integra are that it lacks hair follicles and sweat glands. However, sensory function returns at the same level and time course as with normal STSG autografting.[51] Integra is expensive, but may be justifiable if its use can decrease morbidity and mortality and improve outcome. Also, the high cost of the product may be offset by the lower costs associated as it can hasten wound closure and decrease the rehabilitation and future reconstructive needs of the patient.

Allografted skin (AlloDerm, LifeCell Corp., The Woodlands, TX), is another dermal replacement product. It is applied once the antigenic epidermis and antigenic cells from the dermis are removed. AlloDerm leaves a dermal matrix that will accept an ultrathin STSG. Less scarring and contraction result with AlloDerm and an ultrathin STSG than with an STSG alone, and the combination of ultrathin grafts with AlloDerm results in quicker healing and less scarring of donor sites.[33] The color of the combined AlloDerm and STSG closely resembles the surrounding skin. As is the case with Integra, the high cost of AlloDerm may be offset by the lower costs of decreased length of stay and fewer rehabilitation needs or future reconstructive surgeries.

▶ Physical therapy examination

The physical therapist plays a crucial role in the rehabilitation of the pediatric burn patient. The therapist's goals for the child who has been burned are

- to assist with burn wound management,
- to maintain or increase active and passive ROM,
- to manage soft tissue contours,
- to maintain and increase strength and endurance,
- to promote normal development and function,
- to inhibit loss of motion, deformity, hypertrophic scarring, and contractures.

The physical therapist is involved in the continuum of care for children with thermal injuries from the acute through the rehabilitative and reconstructive phases. The therapist is a member of the burn team and consults with other team members, including the patient and parents, when providing interventions and assisting with the plan of care.

Examination/Evaluation

Depending on the setting in which the physical therapist is working, the thermal injury will be in a different phase of healing (e.g., inflammation, proliferation, and maturation). You may be examining a new burn, one that has undergone excision and grafting, one that is healing following a graft, or one that has begun to demonstrate scarring months after the original injury.

History

Whether reviewing the patient's chart or conducting a detailed patient/parent interview, there are key pieces of information needed. These include the date of injury, the mechanism of injury, what the child was wearing, what was done immediately at the scene prior to emergency services arriving, and what medical or surgical interventions the child has had. The circumstances of the injury and the pattern of the burn will assist the team in ruling out child abuse. Knowing what the child was wearing may give a better idea of the appearance of the burn. For example, knowing whether a patient had clothing on that wasn't fire retardant or had a diaper on that spared the groin area will assist the therapist in a full evaluation. If there was clothing on, was it removed? Since there are still many home remedies for burns, it is important to ask the family members what first aid was provided at the scene. Was water poured on the area? Was any ointment or other substance applied to the burn? Many people still put ice, oils, ointments, or even butter on burns as these remedies have been passed down through generations; however, these can affect the healing process and influence the evaluation of the burn. A social and environmental history should be sought. What type of structure the child lives in, who lives in the home, in what grade is the child, and what mode of transportation the child uses are all questions to ask to assist with early discharge planning. If the child was burned in a house fire, is the home inhabitable, or does the family need assistance to secure safe housing prior to discharge? For the patient in the rehabilitation setting, return to and reintegration into the school setting need early planning to assist teachers and students in what to expect upon their return. Past medical history or developmental history that may influence the patient's recovery or physical therapy interventions is also important to document.

Review of Systems

CARDIOVASCULAR PULMONARY The circulatory changes following a thermal injury are called burn shock. Cardiac output is decreased due to fluid losses, vasodilation, and decreased circulating volume. Fluid resuscitation is key to regaining normal resting values of cardiac output.[16] Children with singed hair on the face or hairline, oral edema and blisters, hoarseness, and carbonaceous sputum have signs and symptoms of inhalation injury and need close monitoring of their respiratory status. They often require 100% oxygen or even intubation to protect their airway and provide adequate respiratory support.[16] The physical therapist in the acute care setting must be aware of normal vital signs, oxygen saturation, and the effects of interventions on these parameters. Severe thermal injuries will result in decreased pulmonary function, which can last several years. The initial obstructive respiratory phase often develops into a restrictive pattern as seen on pulmonary function tests.[52] Other factors that could influence pulmonary function include chest wall burns and the need for a tracheotomy. Suman et al.[52] reported increased pulmonary function in children who underwent exercise tolerance interventions, recommending it to be a component of a comprehensive outpatient intervention program for children following thermal injuries.

NEUROMUSCULAR Depending on the burn depth, circulatory compromise can result from edema formation. The patient is at risk for compartment syndrome (see Escharotomy), which can affect nerves and muscle viability.[16] The child is also at risk for peripheral nerve compression due to immobility and improper positioning (e.g., peroneal nerve compression with externally rotated lower extremities).

MUSCULOSKELETAL If the patient was involved in a motor vehicle accident with vehicle fire or jumped from a burning home, there is a fracture risk. The fractures may not be found initially if the patient is unresponsive and the initial trauma survey is concentrated on the thermal injury. With a deep hand burn, flexor or extensor tendons may be exposed, requiring careful attention to prevent tendon rupture. Heterotopic ossification is a complication that often occurs most often at the elbow in children following a thermal injury. Other joints affected due to immobility may be hip and shoulder, even if not directly affected by the thermal injury. In the acute phase, a ramification of heterotopic ossification is pain, while further into the child's recovery, function is limited. Surgical intervention is often required to improve ROM and ADLs such as feeding and self-care.[53]

INTEGUMENTARY As discussed previously, examination of the integumentary system needs to include estimation of burn depth and TBSA involved. The physical therapist can utilize a body diagram to make notations on the areas that are burned, as well as graft sites or scars that are present. The Lund and Browder chart should be utilized to determine TBSA. Identifying structures of the skin as well as tissue type, capillary refill, and mechanism of injury will aid in determining burn depth (see Burn Depth Estimation).

For a child following skin grafting, upon removal of the postoperative dressings, examination of graft adherence can be described in percentage of graft "take." For example, for an STSG that has completely adhered and with no signs of open wound, the graft has 100% take.

Scar-rating tools may be helpful in a more comprehensive examination/evaluation of burn scars. The Vancouver Scar Scale (VSS) is one such tool (Fig. 17.12). This visual examination tool rates the scar according to its pigmentation, vascularity, pliability, and height, assigning a score for each. The scores can then be compared over time.[54] In addition to such tools, the patient's perception of the scar should be taken into consideration.[55]

Examination of the non-burned skin is another component of the integumentary review. The acutely burned child may be immobile, due to medical instability, and careful inspection of non-burned skin must be done on at least a daily basis, as the immobile child is at risk for pressure ulcers. Contributing factors for pressure ulcers, in addition to immobility, are decreased nutrition, altered consciousness, and altered sensory perception in the case of compartment syndrome. Areas at risk for pressure ulcers include the occiput, sacrum, and heels. Splints are used to maintain joint position and preservation. Splints can also cause pressure ulcers due to improper fit or application and due to volume shifts from edema. Daily inspection of the skin and proper fit of splints is part of the acute care therapist's examination and subsequent interventions. The Braden Q scale is a skin risk assessment scale utilized in the pediatric population. It was adapted from the Braden scale, which was established for determining adults at risk for pressure sores. This scale is

often done by the bedside nurse, but can be implemented by any member of the health care team.[56]

Photography is another important component to the integumentary examination. In addition to the body diagrams, a photo may allow for further evaluation, once the burn has been covered by dressings. A photograph will also allow another clinician, who missed the dressing change, to view the wound. This approach avoids subjecting the child to an unnecessary dressing change. Advantages of digital photography (over 35-mm film) include image verification, immediate printing, and ease of collecting a series of photographs to document change. Photography can also be utilized as a communication tool between therapists and nurses in the case of specific dressing or splint application.[57]

Tests and Measures

PAIN The child's pain management should be a priority. Following an acute burn, children suffer pain not only from the original injury, but from daily procedures, including dressing changes and therapy. These procedures stimulate the nociceptive afferent fibers on a daily basis during their recovery.[35] Before physically examining the child (or during interventions), pain must be evaluated. Pain scales for children are readily available and valid measures. The Wong-Baker FACES scale is a self-reporting scale from which the child can pick from six different faces (no hurt to hurts as much as you can imagine) with a resultant score of 0 to 10.[58] For children older than age 7, a self-reporting numeric scale of 0 to 10 can be used. For unresponsive children or those unable to use the self-reporting scales, a behavioral scale should be used. The FLACC (Face, Legs, Activity, Cry, and Consolability) pain scale is a behavioral pain scale that has been validated for the evaluation of postoperative pain in children. FLACC is an acronym for five categories. Each category is scored 0 to 2, with a maximum score of 10. Analgesia should be considered for scores above 3, with narcotics utilized for scores above 7.[59] Documentation of the pain score is done daily by the therapist before, during, and after the interventions as well as periodically by nursing in the acute care setting.

SENSATION Sensory testing is part of examination for the acute burn. The patient's ability to detect touch or pain at the burn site indicates the depth of the burn. Insensate areas, which are not painful despite the burn, may indicate a full-thickness injury. As discussed earlier, edema in the acute phase of a burn formation may be rapid and extensive. Edema formation can be severe enough to compromise blood flow to the extremities and lead to compartment syndrome. Careful examination of skin color, temperature, and the presence of numbness/tingling are necessary.[16] Children with increased lower extremity or groin edema may assume a position of external rotation. This position can compress the peroneal nerve, causing numbness, tingling, or foot drop. For children in later stages of healing, or in the scar maturation phase, careful examination of sensation will aid in planning interventions. Children with foot burns, who

VANCOUVER GENERAL HOSPITAL
OCCUPATIONAL THERAPY DEPARTMENT

BURN SCAR ASSESSMENT
PATIENT NAME:

PIGMENTATION (M)
0   normal—color that closely resembles
    the color over the rest of one's body
1   hypopigmentation
2   hyperpigmentation

VASCULARITY (V)
0   normal—color that closely resembles
    the color over the rest of one's body
1   pink
2   red
3   purple

PLIABILITY (P)
0   normal
1   supple—flexible with minimal resistance
2   yielding—giving way to pressure
3   firm-inflexible, not easily moved,
    resistant to manual pressure
4   banding—rope-like tissue that
    blanches with extension of scar
5   contracture—permanent shortening of
    scar producing deformity or distortion

HEIGHT
0   normal—flat
1   < 2 mm
2   < 5 mm   Scale in mm
3   > 5 mm

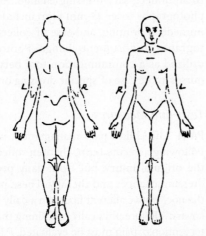

Date	Scar #	Pigmentation	Vascularity	Pliability	Height	Total	OT init

FIGURE 17.12 Vancouver Scar Assessment Scale.

lack normal sensation due to the depth of the burn or following a graft on the plantar surface, need to be instructed in safety concerns of going barefoot. Children and their parents must be aware of the dangers of walking barefoot and need to carefully inspect the skin for any cuts or infections.

RANGE OF MOTION On initial examination of the acute burn, careful attention should be given to examining ROM of all joints—affected and unaffected. If the patient can participate, active-assistive ROM is beneficial to give the child some form of control while also allowing you to get some idea of the ROM limits. Passive range of motion (PROM) can be performed with caution in the acute phase and especially in an unresponsive child. Aggressive PROM is

contraindicated over exposed tendons/joints owing to the risk of rupture. Care must also be taken at the shoulder to avoid joint or brachial plexus injury.

During the remodeling phase of healing, daily examination of ROM with the bandages removed is a necessity. Seeing the ROM without the dressings allows the therapist to view healing structures and to examine any scar tissue for blanching. Blanching tissue signifies the end of the ROM prior to tearing the skin.[33] Once blanching is noted, the clinician has a clear idea of what ROM to expect from the patient for the rest of the day during all therapies. Pushing the patient past the point of blanching can lead to a painful tearing of the skin that will create an unnecessary new open wound that needs to be dressed.

For patients well into the scar maturation phase, ROM determination of scarred joints needs to be done in multiple planes of movement to fully assess the ROM and scar blanching. For example, a child with a scar on the anterior shoulder may not show limitation in straight plane movements, but may be limited with overhead activities such as throwing a ball. Taking the shoulder and subsequent scars through multiplanar motions provides a more thorough examination.

MOBILITY/GAIT If the patient is allowed to mobilize, examine the level of independence with transfers in and out of bed and a chair, and with ambulating. With lower extremity burns, the child may have an antalgic gait, and may need an assistive device. Following grafts, the child may have pain/limitations at the donor sites, which are frequently on the upper legs, thus impeding mobility and gait. During the scar maturation phase, truncal and leg scars may inhibit normal walking or running patterns.

ACTIVITIES OF DAILY LIVING A thorough examination includes the child's ability to participate in ADLs. Depending on the child's age, the level of baseline participation will be different. For example, the toddler may be able to remove clothes/shoes, but will need assistance with donning those items. The child's ability to participate in ADLs may also include dressing changes in the acute phase, as well as scar management and donning compression garments during the scar maturation phase. The adolescent is expected to be independent with all ADLs.

▶ Interventions

Pain Management

Prior to any interventions for the child with a thermal injury, pain must be assessed. Use one of the self-reporting or behavioral pain scales described earlier to assess the child's pain level. There will be different types and causes of pain including those associated with the injury itself, wound care techniques, debridement, grafting, and therapies. Depending on the type and timing of interventions, pain assessment could determine a pharmacologic approach, nonpharmacologic approach, or a combination of the two.[60] Intervention strategies include premedicating the child prior to painful or anxiety-provoking procedures. Medications may include nonsteroidal anti-inflammatory agents, which reduce pain and modify the systemic inflammatory response. Opiates have been proven useful in alleviating burn pain. Benzodiazepines are effective for anxiety control. Ketamine, a dissociative anesthetic, is also widely used to provide comfort and has an amnesic effect so the child does not have memory of the painful procedure.[60]

Nonpharmacologic interventions include cognitive-behavioral therapy; relaxation training; hypnosis and guided imagery; biofeedback; distraction; and art, music, and play therapies.[60] In 2011, Miller et al. in Australia studied differences in pain experiences of children who used standard distraction techniques (TV, video games, stories, toys, and caregiver support) and those who used a multimodal distraction device (MMD). The MMD is a customized handheld device (console and content) that is interactive via movement, touch screen, and multisensory feedback. There are two components to the device, one for procedural preparation and one for distraction. The MMD group demonstrated a reduction in pain experiences during burn care procedures and decreased treatment length.[61]

If your institution has child life specialists, they should be included in either preparing the child for the procedure or aiding in distraction during the procedure. If you do not have access to a child life specialist or music therapist, you should be prepared, prior to providing interventions, with age-appropriate distraction activities. These may include bubbles, books, and magic wands for younger patients and portable radio/compact disc players, video games, or DVDs for older patients.

Wound Care

Acute Management

Depending on the institution at which you work, the mode of wound cleansing and dressing application will already be established. The physical therapist may play a primary role in wound care or an adjunctive role if nursing has the lead role in cleaning the wounds and applying dressings. Daily or twice-daily dressing changes may be ordered in the early stages of burn wound management.

Preparation for wound cleansing and dressing change includes premedicating the patient, coordinating staff who need to examine the patient, and preparing the room and supplies. The room temperature should be at least 86° F to minimize heat loss and lower the metabolic rate of the child.[16] Local wound care can occur in a whirlpool setting or more commonly with saline. Wounds should be gently cleansed to remove old topical agents and devitalized tissue and to decrease pain.[62] Wound beds should not be scrubbed to the point of bleeding, although bleeding may occur in the healing epithelium. Removal of intact blisters is controversial. Some believe that the area under the blister is sterile and can remain intact, unless it becomes very tense or erythematous. Others believe that remaining blisters may interfere with an ongoing examination process. Guidance from your trauma or plastic surgeon may dictate your institution's policies.

Once the wound is cleansed, timely application of the topical agents and dry dressings will aid in decreasing the child's pain when the wounds are left open to the air for prolonged periods.

Ideal burn dressings will serve multiple functions. They will be non-adherent to the healing wound; absorb exudates; provide a warm, moist environment for healing; protect the wounds from further damage; and allow for functional use of the affected area.[62] Functional wrapping of the affected areas is often best done by the physical therapist. The physical therapist can suggest positions for placement or positioning of extremities or affected joints and have the bandage applied so as to maximize function. Examples of this approach include wrapping the elbow into extension when a burn covers the antecubital fossa; individually wrapping fingers and toes; and positioning the ankle in neutral dorsiflexion to avoid a plantar flexion contracture, thereby inhibiting movement.

There are several layers to a good burn dressing. The contact layer is just that—it comes in contact with the burn and is low to non-adherent. The topical agent (most commonly Silvadene) should be applied onto the contact layer, not directly to the burn site due to pain concerns. Examples of commercially available contact layer dressings include Exu-Dry, Conformant, Xeroform, and Adaptic. The next layer is the intermediate absorbent layer and is usually dry gauze or absorptive pads (Exu-Dry). The outermost layer serves to hold the other two layers in place and includes rolls of gauze or tubular elastic netting. The netting can be made into garments, thus securing the bandages from slipping and exposing the burns. Tape should be avoided as it makes removal of the dressing more difficult and can also migrate onto good or burned tissue, thus creating pain and anxiety at dressing removal.[62] Ongoing wound/skin management includes moisturizing cream, sunscreen, and occasionally dressings for an open wound.

Splinting and Positioning

The purpose of splinting and positioning during the acute phase is to help control edema, provide support for edematous extremities, and inhibit wound contraction and loss of motion. Splinting children during this phase of care is often unnecessary, except in the case of older children and adolescents and those who are extensively burned. Care must also be taken to prevent pressure sores as these children are at high risk due to moisture and immobility. Pressure sores in the burn population can occur because of hypovolemia, decreased oxygenation, prolonged bed rest, or poorly fitting splints. Causes of pressure ulcers are attributed to shear, friction, and unrelieved pressure. The most common sites for pressure ulcers are the sacrum/coccyx and heels, with other areas at risk being the ankle, buttocks, and occipital area. The child who requires surgical intervention is also at risk during the operation if appropriate pressure-relieving devices are not used.[56]

For positioning in bed during the first few days of hospitalization, the child who is at bed rest must have appropriate devices in place. Heel and elbow protectors can be used as well as gel pillows for bony prominences. An interdisciplinary approach to proper positioning is key to tackling this problem. Appropriate positioning programs and devices are effective only when implemented correctly. Education and

communication between therapists and nurses will aid this process.

When using splints, the therapist must consider the skin integrity, edema formation, and proper fit of the device. As noted earlier, the zone of stasis lies immediately beneath the burn and has a compromised state of circulation; this area is sensitive to increased pressure. If splints or elastic bandages are applied too tightly, the zone of stasis could convert to a deeper burn. Care must also be taken when using devices on non-burned areas as they too could cause skin breakdown. Splints made to prevent contractures or protect structures during the early phase of wound healing must be monitored daily to ensure proper fit. They may need to be adjusted daily to accommodate for edema formation or changes in dressings. As edema increases, splints or elastic bandages holding the splints in place can cause increased compression, leading to a pressure sore. Meticulous skin inspection during dressing changes must occur during the edema formation stage and as the burn heals so as to ensure proper fit.[56]

Proper bed positioning must begin as soon as the child is admitted, either to an intensive care unit or regular unit. For patients at bed rest, care must be taken to avoid shear forces. The Agency for Healthcare Research and Quality has made recommendations to minimize shear, including avoiding elevating the head of the bed higher than 30 degrees for a prolonged time. The skin and fascia of the torso tend to remain static while the deep fascia and skeleton slide toward the bottom of the bed when the head is raised. The skin on the scapula and buttocks is then put on traction, causing a shearing force. With sufficient traction, blood supply is compromised and a pressure ulcer can develop. Transferring the patient in/out of bed to a stretcher should be performed via a lifting technique rather than sliding him or her across the support surfaces, again to further decrease the risk of shear.

Repositioning the patient in bed should occur at least every 1 to 2 hours, if the patient is medically stable. Keeping to the lower limits of this time frame will be helpful as different tissues have different tolerances to ischemia from pressure.[56]

There is an axiom that states that the position of comfort—flexion—is the position of contracture for burn patients. Patients are therefore splinted or positioned to counteract contracting forces. As mentioned previously, it is often not necessary to splint children during the acute care phase, although the therapist may elect to begin splinting and positioning children with severe burns or older children and adolescents later in this phase. The neck should be positioned in a neutral position or slight extension. Pillows under the head are prohibited because they promote cervical flexion. The shoulders should be positioned in approximately 90 degrees of abduction and in slight protraction. Elbows should be placed in extension and supination (Fig. 17.13). Wrist/hands should be positioned in slight wrist extension, slight metacarpophalangeal (MCP) joint flexion, proximal interphalangeal/distal interphalangeal extension, and thumb abduction as shown in Fig. 17.14. Hips are placed

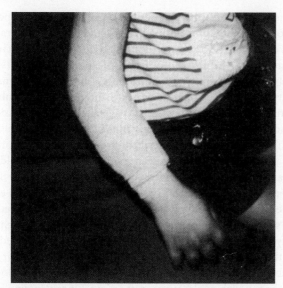

FIGURE 17.13 Elbow extension splint to prevent or correct elbow flexion contracture.

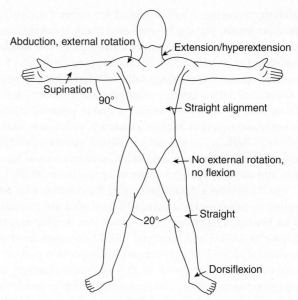

FIGURE 17.15 Positioning for contracture avoidance.

in neutral extension and slight abduction, neutral rotation. Knees are placed in full extension and ankles are in neutral dorsiflexion (no plantar flexion). Figure 17.15 shows recommended anti-contracture positioning. All of these anti-contracture positions can be attained either with towel rolls, splints, or other positioning devices that are commercially available.[33] Splints are fabricated over a uniform layer of dressings to ensure proper day-to-day fit and are monitored closely due to the edema issues discussed earlier.

Specialized splints can be fabricated for specific body parts. Airplane splints are made for axillary burns. Microstomias are special devices to assist in mouth/lip stretching. A multi-ring collar is a flexible neck orthosis that allows circumferential pressure to the neck to assist increasing ROM and is easier to fabricate than traditional thermoplastic splints.[63]

Casting

Casting may be used during both the acute and rehabilitation phases to maintain position in pediatric patients when

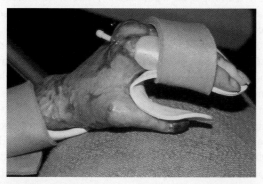

FIGURE 17.14 Example of a hand splint to prevent contractures.

a splinted position is difficult to sustain. For example, it may be preferable to immobilize the MCP joints in flexion while allowing active use of the distal joints. Serial casting is effective in correcting contractures in both pediatric and adult burn patients in whom other methods of regaining motion have failed, in noncompliant patients,[64] in patients whose splints easily slip or are removed, or in those for whom other methods, such as dynamic splinting, cannot be used. Once motion is regained through serial casting, it must be maintained through continued casting or splinting and ROM exercise. Depending on the particular patient and the phase of healing, casts made of either plaster or synthetic materials may be used. Soft Cast, a synthetic casting material, is particularly useful for children because it sets quickly. In addition, although the child cannot remove it, the therapist can simply unwrap it rather than using a cast saw, which might frighten the child or cause skin disruption due to vibration over fragile skin.

Range of Motion

Active ROM (AROM) exercises during the emergent phase help control edema and initiate early motion. Muscle contraction serves as a pumping mechanism to aid venous and lymphatic return.[65] As stated previously, ROM exercises should be performed during dressing changes when the bandages do not restrict motion, the therapist can see the limitations in motion resulting from edema, the wound can be viewed, and the patient has received pain medication.

Active ROM exercises should commence upon admission and continue throughout the rehabilitative and scar management phases. Active exercise will help decrease edema as well as preserve muscle, tendon, and joint function.[65] Activities that are fun will motivate the child to participate in active exercise. Such activities could include catching/throwing a ball overhead for upper extremity/shoulder burns, playing baseball (for trunk rotation), and riding a bike (for lower extremity burns). ADLs can also be implemented to gain active ROM. Stepping into/out of a bathtub requires increased hip/knee ROM; reaching up onto a counter or into a cabinet requires good shoulder ROM. Those patients with true weakness due to deconditioning or nerve damage may require assistance with active ROM exercises. Both active and active-assisted exercises provide sensory feedback, increase circulation, maintain muscle function, and allow for preserving fine and gross motor skills.[33]

PROM exercises are implemented for children who are unable to move on their own. Children who are critically ill or heavily sedated/medicated may not be able to participate in AROM exercises, and PROM exercises are then implemented. PROM exercises are an important part of a postburn therapy program as they maintain elasticity of joint structures, muscle, and tendons and help to minimize the formation of contractures.[65] Stretching exercises can be achieved either via traditional PROM by the therapist or by the patient using a self-stretch premise. Self-stretching can be achieved by using overhead pulleys for shoulder ROM or a towel stretch for ankle dorsiflexion. Stretching, no matter when it is done, should be slow, gentle, and sustained. Remember that blanching of tissue/scar is the sign of the appropriate stretch. PROM could be performed in the operating room if the child is undergoing a surgical procedure. For a child who is resistant to all stretching, active ROM, or positioning, the opportunity to examine ROM under anesthesia is invaluable. Caution must be taken, however, to protect joints from subluxation or dislocation during this exam.[33]

Massage

Massage of scar tissue and skin grafts helps maintain motion by freeing restrictive bands and increasing circulation.[66] Massage may also be helpful in decreasing itching. Initially, only gentle massage should be employed, because the newly healed tissue is often too fragile to tolerate much friction. Many children enjoy massage because it decreases itching, but other children find massage painful or will not sit still for such treatment. Although all patients should have scar tissue and skin grafts lubricated by lotions—preferably two to three times each day—the therapist may select particular areas of concern for massage and may also instruct the parent in massage of these areas. Massage should be done before specific ROM exercises, especially passive ROM exercises.

Ambulation

Once cleared by the physician, mobility should commence as soon as possible. For patients with donor sites on their legs, premedication may reduce pain during mobility. For those patients with lower extremity burns or grafts, elastic bandage compression is necessary to give vascular support prior to ambulating. Following a lower extremity graft, the child may be at bed rest for up to 5 to 7 days to permit graft adherence. The recent trend is to mobilize patients as early as possible to avoid joint stiffness and risks of immobility such as deep vein thrombosis and pulmonary embolism.[65] Once cleared to get up (usually after the first dressing change), gradual mobility activities may begin. Wrapping or use of an elastic cotton bandage (Tubigrip) should be applied to the lower extremities. To begin, the child is wrapped and then allowed to dangle the extremity for approximately 1 minute. The extremity is returned to an elevated position, the wrap taken off, and the graft inspected for signs of color change, bleeding, or breakdown. The child may progress with a dangling protocol, sitting at the edge of the bed for up to 15 minutes four times a day prior to ambulating. This approach should decrease the risk of blood pooling, which could cause graft failure. Once dangling has been successful, ambulation may begin, again with careful monitoring of color, discomfort, tingling, edema, bleeding, or breakdown.

Exercise

Sakurai et al. studied the benefits of exercise in children with burns. They found increased physical functioning, muscle mass, strength, and cardiovascular endurance.[67] Exercise that incorporates repetitive movement of extremities and increased core body temperature, thus increasing blood flow, may alter scar elasticity and increase ROM. Celis et al.[68] found that a supervised exercise program produced beneficial outcomes in children with thermal injuries. They reported a decreased number of scar releases needed for functional improvement in comparison with their control group.[68]

Children with an inhalation injury as well as thermal injury are at risk for decreased exercise tolerance due to decreased pulmonary function. Children may have an initial obstructive pattern of disease, which can last up to 2 years after the initial injury. This obstructive pattern then develops into a restrictive pattern for up to 8 years after burn. Suman et al.[52] examined the effects of an exercise program in severely burned children. The subjects did resistance and aerobic training 3 days per week. There were increases in pulmonary function and subsequent improved exercise tolerance due to the exercise program.[52]

Cucuzzo et al.[69] compared the efficacy and effects of an inpatient exercise program versus traditional outpatient therapy in burned children. The inpatient program included a general conditioning prescription for exercise. This program included moderate intensity, progressive resistance training with aerobic and general conditioning exercises for 1 hour three times per week. Strength training utilized free weights, and aerobic training included motorized treadmill, stationary bike, or independent walking. The results showed that severely burned children could participate safely in this type of supervised exercise program, as their study group showed gains in strength and functional outcomes.[69]

With the advent of more sophisticated computer software, video games have started to play a role in burn rehabilitation. In 2011, Yohannon et al.[70] looked at the adjunctive use of the Nintendo® Wii™ during sessions. Patients in this study received traditional PROM and exercises, and either designated Wii™ games or therapist-chosen interventions. Those in the Wii™ group showed less pain responses, decreased anxiety, and greater enjoyment.[70]

Scar Management

Following burn wound healing, or skin grafting, scar formation may occur. Skin and scar care progresses from the initial open wound phase into the scar maturation phase as the wounds heal. Once the wounds or grafts have healed, it is important to keep the skin well moisturized. Application of a moisturizer throughout the day will decrease the risk of skin cracks and decrease itching. Massaging in the lotion with enough pressure to create blanching may assist in releasing the scar tissue and increase ROM.[33] Avoid putting too much pressure too soon on the scars as blisters can form, thus requiring massage to be discontinued. Massage may help break up collagen fibers, which in turn will soften the scar.[71]

Compression has also been used to combat the formation of hypertrophic scarring. Early compression can begin once the wounds or grafts have healed. Compression can begin in the form of Ace wrapping, elastic cotton tubular stockings, or adhesive wraps (Figs. 17.16 and 17.17). Once edema has stabilized and the grafts or burns are completely healed, the child may be measured for a custom compression garment. Pressure garments have four main functions. They restore function, relieve symptoms, prevent scar recurrence,

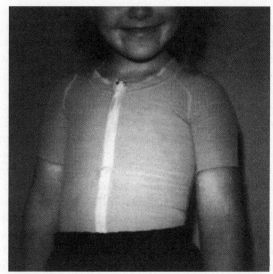

FIGURE 17.17 Child wearing the temporary compression vest from Figure 17.16.

and promote an aesthetic appearance. Pressure results in the reduction of intercollagen fibers, which helps to flatten the excessive collagen that is deposited during the proliferative phase of healing. Pressure levels for these garments should be 24 mm Hg or above and applied for a minimum of 12 months. Pressure garments are worn for 23 hours a day, allowing removal for bathing/skin care. Pressures over 24 mm Hg occlude vessels, which leads to hypoxia and fibroblast degeneration and altered collagen synthesis. This process then helps flatten the scar.[71] Early application of pressure is necessary for optimal outcomes. Pressure is applied as soon as reepithelialization has occurred and continues through the maturation phase. Children are issued two sets of garments due to the constant wear and the need for the garments to be washed. They will need to be refit periodically due to wear from usage, growth, or surgical interventions.[72] Several commercially available options are made for children, with a wider variety of colors and appliqués to try to increase patient use (Fig. 17.18).

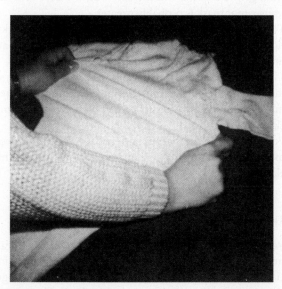

FIGURE 17.16 Example of a compression vest made out of tubular elastic netting.

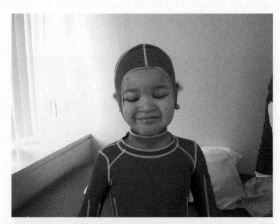

FIGURE 17.18 Example of custom compression mask and jacket.

To apply uniform pressure over convex or concave areas, foam, rubberized materials, or thermoplastic splinting material may be used as inserts under the garments. Areas often needing more custom pressure include finger web spaces, the palm, the interscapular area, and the central face.[33] Silicone linings and inserts have also been used as an adjunct to compression therapy. The mechanism of action by silicone is hydration and occlusion of the scar. Silicone elastomers (putty) were made to solve concavity problems, especially in web spaces. Benefits of using silicone sheets include comfort in application and little to no hindrance of movement. Disadvantages include frequent need to renew the sheets, loss of mobility when used over a joint, and excessive sweating.[73] Most manufacturers of compression garments offer some form of silicone lining that can be sewn directly into the garment over specified areas. Use of compression and silicone combined was studied in 2009 by Harte et al.[74] Their randomized controlled trial included patients using compression garments with silicone sheeting or compression garments alone for burn scar management. There were no statistically significant changes in the VSS scores between the groups, but both groups showed a reduction in the scores with use of both types of garments.[74]

Facial burns require special attention, given the importance of cosmetic appearance following a burn. Children with facial burns will have the social stigma of looking different and may have a long-term psychological impact of disfigurement. Compression therapy for the face can occur in three different ways. Custom compression garments are available for the face, but usually cover the entire face and head, thus "hiding" the deformities. Clear plastic masks allow the clinician to see the pressure applied to the scars directly under the mask; however, the child's face and scars are fully visible. A third option is a silicone mask held in place with a facial pressure garment.[75]

The transparent plastic face mask was introduced in 1979 by Rivers et al. as an alternative to the elastic face mask to control facial scarring (Fig. 17.19).[76] As its name implies, the transparent face mask is a piece of hard, transparent plastic in the form of a custom-fitting face mask secured to the face by means of straps. The mask is constructed by forming heated plastic over a modified positive mold of the patient's

face. In the past, the mold would need to be made in the operating room with the child anesthetized due to using plaster, which requires that the patient not move. New digital scanning technology has made that procedure obsolete. The Total Contact Scanner, by Total Contact Inc. (www. totalcontact.com), is a digital surface scanner, which allows for noncontact scanning. This system uses a low-power helium-neon laser projected from the moving scanner head to the patient's face. The scan is transmitted to a computer, which captures all the surface data. These data are then sent to the company, which produces a positive mold, over which a negative mold of the plastic/silicone face mask is made. The therapist can then adjust the fit of the mask by making the necessary changes to the positive mold and reheating the mask. The time and resources saved by not having the patient undergo anesthesia are quite beneficial.

The advantages of the transparent face mask versus the elastic face mask are as follows:

- The mask can be constructed and applied to the patient within 24 hours. (There is no waiting for the elastic garment to return from the manufacturer.)
- The therapist can see exactly where pressure is being adequately applied by observing blanching of the scar. The transparent mask can be adjusted accordingly by the therapist to increase or decrease pressure in specific areas.
- The patient's face is visible to other people and is not covered by a "mask."
- The transparent mask usually does not require the construction and exact placement of inserts.
- The transparent face mask may cause fewer problems with head growth and malocclusion than the elastic mask.

There are also several disadvantages of the transparent face mask, including the following:

- Although both types of mask must be replaced as the child grows and the mask wears out, the cost of a new transparent mask is probably greater.
- The plastic used to construct the transparent mask is rigid, permits little movement of the facial muscles, and often limits mandible motion.
- The transparent mask may not cover as many areas on the head as the elastic mask. (However, the transparent mask can be used with a chin strap or alternated with an elastic mask.)
- Perspiration is increased underneath the transparent mask, and plastic may be more uncomfortable than elastic.

Patient/Client-related Instructions

Throughout the continuum of care following a burn injury, the child and caregivers will need ongoing teaching. Initially, the parents may help with burn dressing changes, application of splints, and exercises. As the child returns to home and school, caregivers must assume all care, including

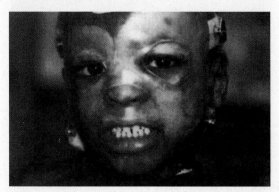

FIGURE 17.19 Transparent face mask for facial burn compression.

skin and graft care, scar management, night splints, day splints, compression garments, massage, and, in many cases, being parents to other siblings. When possible, practicing interventions in a controlled setting may help parents be more comfortable than carrying out the intervention on their own child. This can occur in a classroom-type setting where parents can practice on mannequins or each other, gain confidence, and then work with their own child. Children who are old enough to follow directions and a schedule are able to learn their self-care and often prefer to have control over parts of their care. A written home program for exercises, splint application, and compression garment wearing schedules will aid in the caregiver's carryover.

Outcomes

Children who suffer a burn injury, especially one of extensive TBSA, have cosmetic and functional impairments that may never be completely corrected. Psychosocial implications for children include acceptance by their family, peers, and schoolmates, with potentially disfiguring and disabling effects of their original injury. A study by Sheridan et al. in 2000[77] showed that massively burned children do not necessarily suffer from a poor quality of life. Even though they can't be returned to their pre-burn status, appearance, and function, their acute care team, support after discharge, and family support can produce satisfying long-term outcomes for children with massive burns.[77]

The child who sustains a burn injury undergoes long-term hospitalization, painful procedures and rehabilitation, and lifelong disfigurement. Landolt et al. in 2002 looked at predictors of quality of life in pediatric burn survivors. Their results demonstrated an almost normal outcome concerning health-related quality of life. The family environment was one of the main predictors of quality-of-life outcome. The overall quality of life and psychological adjustment were best predicted by greater family cohesion, higher expressiveness, and fewer conflicts within the family. Age at injury was the second most important variable to predicting quality of life. Children burned at a younger age had a better quality of life at follow-up. Younger children may more easily deal with their scars and integrate disfigurement into their developing body image. Older children may have more difficulties with the need for changing their body image. Their study noted that there was a quality-of-life scale pending from the ABA.[78]

The impact of a thermal injury on the family and siblings was reviewed by Mancuso et al. in 2003.[79] Sibling research has shown that relationships among themselves are among the most significant in preparing a child for adulthood. The studies revealed that siblings had fewer signs of internalizing problems and were less withdrawn and showed fewer depressive symptoms and fewer somatic problems than the control group. Compared with the control group, those siblings of children with moderate to severe injuries did have more difficulties with social competence. This finding corresponds with the severity of injury causing an increased duration of care, potentially more absence of parents, and more family attention to the injured sibling. The siblings appeared to do well at school, and the social competence piece may have been related to their ability to have friends at their home, in light of the disfigurement of their sibling. Even under stressful events, the well siblings are adjusting socially, emotionally, and behaviorally.[79]

Burn camp

Just as there are camps for children with various diseases or disabilities (e.g., diabetes camp, spina bifida camp, etc.), there are also about 40 burn camps in North America offering a variety of programs for children who had sustained burn injuries. Several camps are coordinated or staffed by therapists, and therapists are encouraged to attend the camp to help with programs or to assist campers. The purpose of most of the camps is to provide a safe, recreational environment in which children with burns can interact with one another, build self-esteem, learn new skills, and have fun.

SUMMARY

Physical therapists play a vital role on the interdisciplinary burn care team. They function in many different roles from acute burn wound management to positioning, splinting, ROM, and functional mobility, to scar management and return to home and school. Pediatric physical therapists in any setting across the continuum of care need to be prepared to provide interventions for these children as well as to be advocates for their psychosocial needs upon reentry into the community. Ongoing continuing education and mentorship will provide the best experience to gain clinical competence in the area of care for the child with thermal injuries.

CASE STUDIES

CASE STUDY 1 **Jade** Jade is a 6-year-old girl who was admitted to her local hospital following an accident at home. Jade was leaning over a candle in her mom's bedroom when her braids caught fire and set her shirt on fire. Her mom put out the flames with a blanket and removed her shirt immediately, calling 911 in the process. Jade received emergency care within minutes and was transported to the hospital. She was referred to physical therapy on postburn day 1.

Upon initial examination, she appeared to have superficial partial-thickness burns to her face and deep partial-thickness burns to her arm and chest, with some questionable areas of deeper burns at her right upper chest and arm (Fig. 17.4). She received local wound care and ongoing burn depth estimation as structures evolved. On postburn day 2, the areas at the upper right chest and upper right arm appeared to have a brown coloration and no capillary refill and did not cause her pain upon palpation. It was determined at that time that these areas were full-thickness injuries, and the plastic surgeon decided upon skin grafting. On postburn day 6, she underwent excision of the eschar and split-thickness grafting with her right thigh as the donor site (Fig. 17.11). She was immobilized in the operating room with an airplane splint to protect the graft from shearing as well as to maintain preoperative ROM.

On postoperative day 5, the dressings were taken down with 100% graft take (Fig. 17.20). She was allowed to mobilize on postoperative day 5, with pain limiting her right lower extremity ROM from the donor site. She required assistance with ambulating short distances. She remained in the airplane splint until postoperative day 7, when she began gentle active-assisted ROM exercises. She was discharged on postoperative day 8 to home, with follow-up therapy for ROM and scar management. She was also seen by occupational therapy for ROM, splinting, and ADLs as well as compression garments.

CASE STUDY 2 **Frankie** Frankie is a 3-year-old boy who was involved in a house fire, sustaining 60% TBSA burns to his face, trunk, upper extremities, and lower extremities. He developed severe compartment syndrome, sepsis, and respiratory complications in addition to his massive burns. He was treated at a local burn center. During his acute hospitalization, he developed decreased circulation to both feet and required bilateral below-knee amputations. He underwent local wound care and multiple grafting procedures to achieve wound closure. After a prolonged hospitalization, he was transferred to our rehabilitation hospital for further care.

Initially, he had multiple open wounds that required daily dressing changes as well as graft care. He had significant loss of ROM at both knees (stuck in extension) as well as limited ROM at

his upper extremities. He underwent serial casting of both knees into flexion, which was quite successful in achieving functional ROM. He required occupational therapy and physical therapy to regain the use of his hands, ADLs, bed mobility, and preparation for prosthetic training. He began prosthetic training but had a setback as he developed an open wound at the end of one stump and accentuated growth of his fibula faster than his tibia on the other stump. This precluded gait training for several months.

Once his open wound had healed, new liners and sockets were developed to relieve pressure on both areas, and he was cleared to begin standing. He began a standing program both static at the edge of a mat and in a mobile prone standing frame. He had stubbies, which he tolerated well, and began ambulation about 4 days after starting standing (Fig. 17.21). He progressed to platforms on his pylons and quickly to SACH feet. He is ambulating 200 feet with a rolling walker and supervision (Fig. 17.22). His lack of normal knee flexion is limiting his ability to transition as well as ascend and descend stairs. Owing to nerve damage to his left hand, he was unable to utilize Lofstrand crutches and worked toward independent ambulation without an assistive device. He continues to work on fine motor skills with occupational therapy (Fig. 17.23).

He has developed several sites of hypertrophic and keloid-type scarring at his face, neck, upper extremities, trunk, and lower extremities (Fig. 17.7). He is utilizing custom compression garments with a mask, jacket, and pants. His new prosthetic liners are actually custom fit and are providing excellent

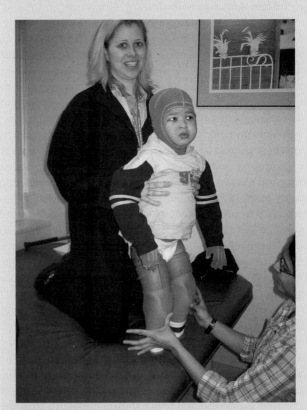

FIGURE 17.21 Patient attempting to stand, utilizing stubbies as prostheses.

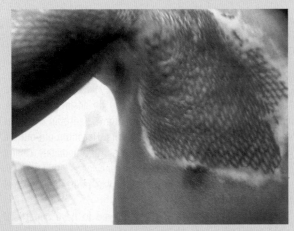

FIGURE 17.20 Healed meshed split-thickness skin graft (same patient from Figure 17.4)

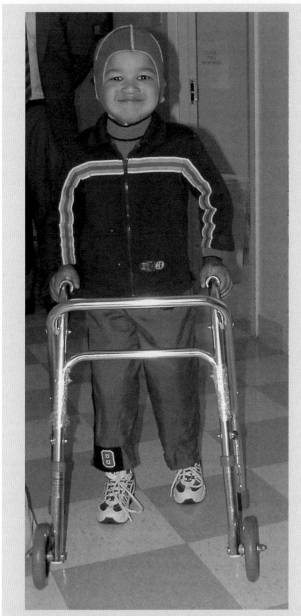

FIGURE 17.22 Patient progressed to pylons and SACH feet and was able to ambulate with supervision with a rolling walker.

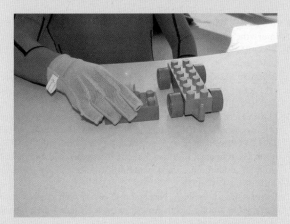

FIGURE 17.23 Patient using play to increase hand function.

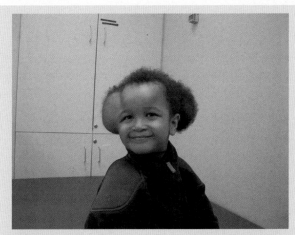

FIGURE 17.24 Patient with tissue expanders in his scalp.

compression for his lower extremities while being worn. While out of the prostheses, he has a custom compression garment that he tolerates well (Fig. 17.18). He has undergone injections of steroids at his keloid scar on his neck and had a Z-plasty done to release the neck scar. He participated in our day hospital rehabilitation program for 5 months and then transitioned to outpatient care. He required scar revision surgery for the back and side of his head/neck. For this, he underwent tissue expander placement (Fig. 17.24) at his scalp. This enabled the surgeon to have enough non–burn/scar tissue to cover the previous defect (Fig. 17.7). Once the tissue expanders were removed, the scarred tissue was excised and the nonscarred tissue moved into its place (Fig. 17.25).

He is now independently ambulating community distances with new prostheses and Impulse feet by Ohio Willow Wood (Fig. 17.26). This energy-storing foot has allowed him to achieve better heel strike and push-off during the gait cycle. He can now ascend and descend a full flight of stairs and practice bus steps with supervision. He will receive school-based physical therapy services as well as continue with outpatient services to address his ongoing scar management and prosthetic needs.

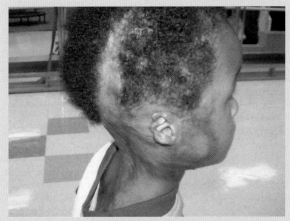

FIGURE 17.25 Patient status after tissue expander removal and corrective surgery.

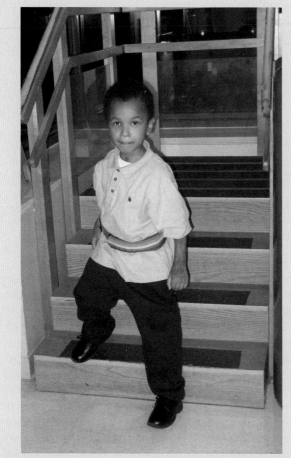

FIGURE 17.26 Patient ambulating independently with bilateral prostheses.

REFERENCES

1. National Center for Injury Prevention and Control. WISQARS: 2010 United States Unintentional Injuries. www.cdc.gov. Accessed October 2013.
2. National Center for Injury Prevention and Control. WISQARS: 2011 United States Overall Fire/Burn Nonfatal Injuries. www.cdc.gov. Accessed May 2013.
3. National Center for Injury Prevention and Control. WISQARS: 2007 United States 10 leading causes of nonfatal violence-related injury. www.cdc.gov. Accessed May 2013.
4. Safe Kids Worldwide. Burn and scalds safety. www.safekids.org. Accessed May 2013.
5. Johnson RM, Richard R. Partial thickness burns: identification and management. *Adv Skin Wound Care.* 2003;16(4):178–187.
6. The Burn Foundation. Safety facts on scald burns. www.burnfoundation.org/programs. Accessed October 2013.
7. Lorch M, Goldberg J, Wright J, et al. Epidemiology and disposition of burn injuries among infants presenting to a tertiary-care pediatric emergency department. *Pediatr Emerg Care.* 2011;27(11):1022–1026.
8. Shah A, Suresh S, Thomas R, et al. Epidemiology and profile of pediatric burns in a large referral center. *Clin Pediatr.* 2011;50(5):391–395.
9. Children's Bureau Express. *New child welfare outcomes, AFCARS reports.* https://cbexpress.acf.hhs.gov. Accessed October 2013.
10. Zenel J, Goldstein B. Child abuse in the pediatric intensive care unit. *Crit Care Med.* 2002;30(11)(suppl):S515–S523.
11. Gornor G. Medical evaluation for child physical abuse: what the PNP needs to know. *J Pediatr Health Care.* 2012;26(3):163–170.
12. Safe Kids Worldwide. Burn and scald prevention tips. www.safekids.org. Accessed September 2013.
13. Dowd MD, Keenan HT, Bratten SL. Epidemiology and prevention of childhood injuries. *Crit Care Med.* 2002;31(11)(suppl):S385–S392.
14. Consumer Product Safety Commission. Children's sleepwear regulations. www.cpsc.org. Accessed January 2005.
15. Lockhard RD, Hamilton GF, Fyfe FW. *Anatomy of the Human Body.* Philadelphia, PA: JB Lippincott; 1969.
16. Merz J, Schrand C, Mertens D, et al. Wound care of the pediatric burn patient. *AACN Clin Issues Adv Pract Acute Crit Care.* 2003;14(4):429–441.
17. Lund CC, Browder NC. The estimation of areas of burns. *Surg Gynecol Obstet.* 1944;79:352.
18. Chan Q, Barzi F, Cheney L, et al. Burn size estimation in children: still a problem. *Emerg Med Australas.* 2012;24:181–186.
19. American Burn Association. Burn center referral criteria. www.ameriburn.org. Accessed September 2013.
20. Sussman C, Bates-Jensen B. Wound healing physiology: acute and chronic. In: Sussman C, Bates-Jensen B, eds. *Wound Care: A Collaborative Practice Manual.* Philadelphia, PA: Wolters Kluwer/Lippincott Williams & Wilkins; 2007:26–33.
21. Ward RS. Management of scar. In: Sussman C, Bates-Jensen B, eds. *Wound Care: A Collaborative Practice Manual.* Philadelphia, PA: Wolters Kluwer/Lippincott Williams & Wilkins; 2007:309–318.
22. Hunt TK. *Fundamentals of Wound Management in Surgery—Wound Healing: Disorders of Repair.* South Plainfield, NJ: Chirurgecom; 1976.
23. Chan Q, Harvey J, Graf N, et al. The correlation between time to skin grafting and hypertrophic scarring following an acute contact burn in a porcine model. *J Burn Care Res.* 2012;33(2):e43–e48.
24. Diegelmann RF, Rothkop LC, Cohen LK. Measurement of collagen biosynthesis during wound healing. *J Surg Res.* 1975;19:239–243.
25. Barnes MK, Morton LF, Bennett RC, et al. Studies on collagen synthesis in the mature dermal scar in the guinea pig. *Biochem Soc Symp.* 1975;3:917–920.
26. American Burn Association. Guidelines for the operation of burn centers. www.ameriburn.org. Accessed October 2013.
27. Kim L, Martin H, Holland A. Medical management of paediatric burn injuries: best practice. *J Paediatr Child Health.* 2012;48:290–295.
28. Orgill D, Piccolo N. Escharotomy and decompressive therapies in burns. *J Burn Care Res.* 2009;30(5):759–768.
29. Blasier RD. Treatment of fractures complicated by burn or head injuries in children. *J Bone Joint Surg.* 1999;81(A7):1038–1043.
30. Barret JP, Herndon DN. Modulation of inflammatory and catabolic responses in severely burned children by early burn wound excision in the first 24 hours. *Arch Surg.* 2003;138(2):127–132.
31. Huckleberry Y. Nutritional support and the surgical patient. *Am J Health Syst Pharm.* 2004;61(7):671–684.
32. Tengvall O, Wickman M, Wengstrom Y. Memories of pain after burn injury-the patient's experience. *J Burn Care Res.* 2010;31(2):319–327.
33. Ward RS. Physical rehabilitation. In: Carrougher GJ, ed. *Burn Care and Therapy.* St. Louis, MO: Mosby; 1998:293–327.
34. Al-Ahdab M, Al-Omawi M. Deep partial scald burn in a neonate: a case report of the first documented domestic neonatal burn. *J Burn Care Res.* 2011;32(1): e1–e6.
35. Martin-Herz SP, Patterson DR, Honari S, et al. Pediatric pain control practices of North American burn centers. *J Burn Care Rehabil.* 2003;24(1):26–36.
36. Bayat A, Ramaiah R, Bhananker S. Analgesia and sedation for children undergoing burn wound care. *Expert Rev Neurother.* 2010;10(11):1747–1759.
37. Davison PG, Loiselle F, Nickerson D. Survey on current hydrotherapy use among North American burn centers. *J Burn Care Res.* 2010;31(3):393–399.

38. Patel P, Vasquez S, Granick M, et al. Topical antimicrobials in pediatric burn wound management. *J Craniofacial Surg.* 2008;19(4): 913–922.

39. Tredget EE, Shankowsky HA, Groeneveld A, et al. A matched-pair, randomized study evaluating the efficacy and safety of acticoat silver-coated dressing for the treatment of burn wounds. *J Burn Care Rehabil.* 1998;19(6):531–537.

40. AQUACEL Ag. The dual-purpose antimicrobial dressing: absorbency with the power of silver. www.convatec.com. Accessed October 2013.

41. Caruso DM, Foster KN, Hermans MH, et al. AQUACEL Ag in the management of partial-thickness burns: results of a clinical trial. *J Burn Care Rehabil.* 2004;25(1):89–97.

42. Caruso DM, Foster KN, Blome-Eberwein SA, et al. Randomized clinical study of hydrofiber dressing with silver or silver sulfadiazine in the management of partial-thickness burns. *J Burn Care Res.* 2006;27(3):298–309.

43. Barre JP, Dziewulski P, Ramzy PI, et al. Biobrane versus 1% silver sulfadiazine in second-degree pediatric burns. *Plast Reconstr Surg.* 2000;105:62–65.

44. Xiao-Wu W, Herndon DN, Spies M, et al. Effects of delayed wound excision and grafting in severely burned children. *Arch Surg.* 2002;137(9):1049–1054.

45. Sheridan FL. Burns. *Crit Care Med.* 2002;30(11S):S500–S514.

46. Carrougher GJ. Burn wound assessment and topical treatment. In: Carrougher GJ, ed. *Burn Care and Therapy.* St. Louis, MO: Mosby; 1998:133–165.

47. Parks DH, Wainwright DJ. The surgical management of burns. In: Carvajal HF, Parks DH, eds. *Burns in Children: Pediatric Burn Management.* Chicago, IL: Year Book Medical Publishers; 1988: 158, 166.

48. Mozingo DW. Surgical management. In: Carrougher GJ, ed. *Burn Care and Therapy.* St. Louis, MO: Mosby; 1998:233–248.

49. Sood R, Balledux J, Koumanis D, et al. Coverage of large pediatric wound with cultured epithelial autografts in congenital nevi and burns: results and technique. *J Burn Care Res.* 2009;30(4):576–583.

50. Integra LifeSciences Corp. Medical economics of integra artificial skin. www.integralife.com. Accessed October 2013.

51. Burk JF. Observations on the development and clinical use of artificial skin: an attempt to employ regeneration rather than scar formation in wound healing. *Jpn J Surg.* 1987;17:431–438.

52. Suman O, Mlcak RP, Herndon DN. Effect of exercise training on pulmonary function in children with thermal injury. *J Burn Care Rehabil.* 2002;23(4):288–293.

53. Gaur A, Sinclair M, Caruso E, et al. Heterotopic ossification around the elbow following burns in children: results after excision. *J Bone Joint Surg.* 2003;85-A(8):1538–1543.

54. Baryza MJ, Baryza GA. The Vancouver Scar Scale: an administration tool and its inter-rater reliability. *J Burn Care Rehabil.* 1995;16: 535–538.

55. Martin D, Umraw N, Gomez M, et al. Changes in subjective vs. objective burn scar assessment over time: does the patient agree with what we think. *J Burn Care Rehabil.* 2003;24(4):239–244.

56. Gordon M, Gottschlich, MM, Helvig EI, et al. Review of evidence-based practice for the prevention of pressure sores in burn patients. *J Burn Care Rehabil.* 2004;25(5):388–410.

57. Van LB, Sicotte KM, Lassiter RR, et al. Digital photography: enhancing communication between burn therapists and nurses. *J Burn Care Rehabil.* 2004;25(1):54–60.

58. Wong D, Baker C. Pain in children: comparison of assessment scales. *Pediatr Nurs.* 1988;14(1):9–17.

59. Merkel S, Voepel-Lewis T, Malviya S. Pain assessment in infants and young children: the FLACC scale: a behavioral tool to measure pain in young children. *Am J Nurs.* 2002;102(10):55–58.

60. Stoddard FJ, Sheridan RL, Saxe GN, et al. Treatment of pain in acutely burned children. *J Burn Care Rehabil.* 2002;23(2):135–156.

61. Miller K, Rodger S, Kipping B, et al. A novel technology approach to pain management in children with burns: a prospective randomized controlled trial. *Burns.* 2011;37:395–495.

62. Taylor K. The management of minor burns and scalds in children. *Nurs Stand.* 2001;16(11):45–52.

63. Hurlin FK, Doyle B, Paradis P, et al. Use of an improved Watusi collar to manage pediatric neck burn contractures. *J Burn Care Rehabil.* 2002;23(3):221–226.

64. Ridgway CL, Daugherty MB, Warden GD. Serial casting as a technique to correct burn scar contractures: a case report. *J Burn Care Rehabil.* 1991;12:67–72.

65. Whitehead C, Serghiou M. A 12-year comparison of common therapeutic interventions in the burn unit. *J Burn Care Res.* 2009; 30(2):281–288.

66. Cyriax JH. Clinical application of massage. In: Licht S, ed. *Massage, Manipulation, and Traction.* New Haven, CT: Elizabeth Licht Publisher; 1960.

67. Sakurai Y, Aarsland A, Herndon DN, et al. Stimulation of muscle protein synthesis by long-term insulin infusion in severely burned patients. *Ann Surg.* 1995;222:283–297.

68. Celis MM, Suman OE, Huang TT, et al. Effect of a supervised exercise and physiotherapy program on surgical interventions in children with thermal injury. *J Burn Care Rehabil.* 2003;24(1):57–61.

69. Cucuzzo NA, Ferrando A, Herndon DN. The effects of exercise programming vs. traditional outpatient therapy in the rehabilitation of severely burned children. *J Burn Care Rehabil.* 2001;22(3):214–220.

70. Yohannon S, Tufaro P, Hunter H, et al. The Utilization of Nintendo® Wii™ during burn rehabilitation: a pilot study. *J Burn Care Res.* 2012;33(1):36–45.

71. Edwards J. Scar management. *Nurs Stand.* 2003;17(52):39–42.

72. Williams F, Knap D, Wallen M. Comparison of the characteristics and features of pressure garments used in the management of burn scars. *Burns.* 1998;24:329–335.

73. Van den Kerckhove E, Stappaerts K, Boeckx W, et al. Silicones in the rehabilitation of burns: a review and overview. *Burns.* 2001;27(3):205–214.

74. Harte D, Gordon J, Shaw M, et al. The use of pressure and silicone in hypertrophic scar management in burns patients: a pilot randomized controlled trial. *J Burn Care Res.* 2009;30(4):632–642.

75. Serghiou MA, Holmes CL, McCauley RL. A survey of current rehabilitation trends for burn injuries to the head and neck. *J Burn Care Rehabil.* 2004;25(6):514–518.

76. Rivers EA, Strate RG, Solem LD. The transparent facemask. *Am J Occup Ther.* 1979;33:109–113.

77. Sheridan RL, Hinson MI, Liang MH, et al. Long-term outcome of children surviving massive burns. *JAMA.* 2000;283(1):69–73.

78. Landolt MA, Grubenmann S, Meuli M. Family impact greatest: predictors of quality of life and psychological adjustment in pediatric burn survivors. *J Trauma.* 2002;53(6):1146–1151.

79. Mancuso MG, Bishop S, Blakeney P, et al. Impact on the family: psychosocial adjustment of siblings of children who survive serious burns. *J Burn Care Rehabil.* 2003;24(2):110–118.

Children with Obesity and the Role of the Physical Therapist

Kathy Coultes

Children with Obesity

Scope of the Issue

Definitions

Role of Physical Therapists in Pediatric Obesity

Health Consequences of Obesity

How Obesity Treatment Fits Within the ICF
  Framework

Physical Therapy History and Examination
  of the Child with Obesity
  Systems Review
  Tests and Measures

Determining Functional Outcome Expectations
  for the Child with Obesity

Therapeutic Interventions to Address Obesity
  in the Pediatric Population

Summary

Children with obesity

Pediatric physical therapists can be found in a variety of practice settings. Whether practicing in early intervention, acute care, and educational or community settings, the epidemic of pediatric obesity can be appreciated. As this issue has become a health crisis, this chapter is dedicated to increasing the knowledge base of pediatric physical therapists in the definitions, prevalence, trends, and health impacts as well as suggesting clinical paths that might be taken to begin halting this epidemic. As obesity has formally been established as a diagnosis by the American Medical Association (AMA) in June 2013, the International Classification of Functioning, Health and Disability (ICF) framework as well as the American Physical Therapy Association Guide to Physical Therapy Practice 2 will be considered in the call to action for pediatric physical therapists to become primary service providers in health promotion and wellness.[1,2]

Scope of the issue

Despite the comprehensive efforts of health policymakers, industry, and media to bring to light the major health consequences related to obesity, research indicates that it remains an issue of epidemic proportion. The American College of Sports Medicine (ACSM) has defined obesity as "percent fat at which disease risk increases."[3] The Centers for Disease Control and Prevention (CDC) report that findings from the National Health and Nutrition Examination Survey (NHANES) 2009–2010 continue to suggest alarming statistics regarding obesity in the United States. Findings show that 35.7% of adults and 16.9% of children and adolescents in the United States were found to be obese. This indicates that there are more than 78 million U.S. adults and 12.5 million children considered obese. Further data suggest that one in three children and adolescents between the ages of 6 and 19 years are overweight or obese, with one in six within that age range found to be obese.[4] While this survey did suggest that the rapid increases seen in childhood obesity in the 1980s and 1990s have not continued, current estimates by the AMA have suggested that rates of childhood obesity have increased more than threefold in the last 30 years.[5] Table 18.1 shows the increase in childhood obesity as described by NHANES in selected years.[6]

Another area of concern for health care providers is the rise in the number of young children, between 3 and 5 years of age, who are now identified as overweight or obese. Estimates in 2007 to 2008 were that 21.2% of these young children were overweight or obese.[5,7] In addition to the prevalence information available regarding age variations in

TABLE

18.1   Prevalence of Obesity (≥95th Percentile) Among U.S. Children and Adolescents[6]

Age (in yr)[1]	NHANES 1963–1965 1966–1970[2]	NHANES 1971–1974	NHANES 1976–1980	NHANES 1988–1994	NHANES 1999–2000	NHANES 2001–2002	NHANES 2003–2004	NHANES 2005–2006	NHANES 2007–2008
Total	(3)	5.0	5.5	10.0	13.9	15.4	17.1	15.5	16.9
2–5	(3)	5.0	5.0	7.2	10.3	10.6	13.9	11.0	10.4
6–11	4.2	4.0	6.5	11.3	15.1	16.3	18.8	15.1	19.6
12–19	4.6	6.1	5.0	10.5	14.8	16.7	17.4	17.8	18.1

[1]Excludes pregnant women starting with 1971–1974. Pregnancy status not available for 1963–1965 and 1966–1970.

[2]Data for 1963–1965 are for children aged 6–11 yr; data for 1966–1970 are for adolescents aged 12–17, not 12–19 yr.

[3]Children aged 2–5 yr were not included in the surveys undertaken in the 1960s.

NOTE: Obesity defined as body mass index (BMI) greater than or equal to sex- and age-specific 95th percentile from the 2000 CDC Growth Charts.

obesity, it is important that health care providers recognize racial and ethnic disparities in obesity rates. Again, referring to the NHANES 2007–2008, obesity rates are highest among non-Hispanic Black girls and Hispanic boys. Furthermore, the highest rate of childhood obesity was found in American Indian/Native Alaskan children when compared with rates in White or Asian children.[8] This information can provide physical therapists with a profile of at-risk populations whose children are seen for developmental, orthopedic, or other diagnoses that may decrease the child's overall activity level. Table 18.2 further defines the disparity among racial and ethnic population data.

In the adult population, obesity rates were inversely associated with income and educational level in women, that is, increased body mass index (BMI) was found in those adults with less income and education. However, the relationship between income and obesity in children is less consistent, with some indication of the opposite relationship being true.[8] This finding led to the recommendation by the White House Task Force on Childhood Obesity in 2010 that "efforts to reeducate ethnic disparities in obesity must target factors other than income and education, such as environmental, social, and cultural factors."[8]

TABLE

18.2   Obesity Among Children and Adolescents in the United States by Gender, Age, and Ethnicity

Table 69 (page 1 of 2). Obesity among children and adolescents aged 2–19 years, by selected characteristics: United States, selected years 1963–1965 through 2007–2010

Updated data when available. Excel, PDF, more data years, and standard errors: http://www.cdc.gov/nchs/hus/contents2012.htm#069. (Data are based on physical examinations of a sample of the civilian noninstitutionalized population)

Age, Sex, Race and Hispanic Origin[1] and Percent of Poverty Level	1963–1965 1966–1970[2]	1971–1974	1976–1980[3]	1988–1994	1999–2002	2003–2006	2007–2010
2–5 years			Percent of population				
Both sexes[4]..........	---	---	---	7.2	10.3	12.5	11.1
Not Hispanic or Latino:							
White only..........	---	---	---	5.2	8.7	10.8	9.0
Black or African American only..........	---	---	---	7.7	8.8	14.9	15.0
Mexican..........	---	---	---	12.3	13.1	16.7	14.6
Boys..........	---	---	---	6.1	10.0	12.8	11.9
Not Hispanic or Latino:							
White only..........	---	---	---	*4.5	*8.2	11.1	8.8
Black or African American only..........	---	---	---	7.7	*8.0	13.3	15.7
Mexican..........	---	---	---	12.4	14.1	18.8	19.1
Girls..........	---	---	---	8.2	10.6	12.2	10.2
Not Hispanic or Latina:							
White only..........	---	---	---	5.9	*9.0	10.4	*9.2

Age, Sex, Race and Hispanic Origin[1], and Percent of Poverty Level	1963–1965 1966–1970[2]	1971–1974	1976–1980[3]	1988–1994	1999–2002	2003–2006	2007–2010
Black or African American only.........	---	---	---	7.6	9.6	16.6	*14.2
Mexican.........	---	---	---	12.3	*12.2	14.5	*9.9
Percent of poverty level:[5]							
Below 100%.........	---	---	---	9.7	10.9	14.3	13.2
100%–199%.........	---	---	---	7.2	*13.8	12.7	11.8
200%–399%.........	---	---	---	5.6	*7.6	11.9	13.9
400% or more.........	---	---	---	*	*	*10.0	*5.8
6–11 years							
Both sexes[4].........	4.2	4.0	6.5	11.3	15.9	17.0	18.8
Boys.........	4.0	*4.3	6.6	11.6	16.9	18.0	20.7
Not Hispanic or Latino:							
White only.........	---	---	6.1	10.7	14.0	15.5	18.6
Black or African American only.........	---	---	6.8	12.3	17.0	18.6	23.3
Mexican.........	---	---	13.3	17.5	26.5	27.5	24.3
Girls.........	4.5	*3.6	6.4	11.0	14.7	15.8	16.9
Not Hispanic or Latina:							
White only.........	---	---	5.2	*9.8	13.1	14.4	14.0
Black or African American only.........	---	---	11.2	17.0	22.8	24.0	24.5
Mexican.........	---	---	9.8	15.3	17.1	19.7	22.4
Percent of poverty level:[5]							
Below 100%.........	---	---	---	11.4	19.1	22.0	22.2
100%–199%.........	---	---	---	11.1	16.4	19.2	20.7
200%–399%.........	---	---	---	11.7	15.3	16.7	18.9
400% or more.........	---	---	---	*	12.9	9.2	*12.5
12–19 years							
Both sexes[4].........	4.6	6.1	5.0	10.5	16.0	17.6	18.2
Boys.........	4.5	6.1	4.8	11.3	16.7	18.2	19.4
Not Hispanic or Latino:							
White only.........	---	---	3.8	11.6	14.6	17.3	17.1
Black or African American only.........	---	---	6.1	10.7	18.8	18.4	21.2
Mexican.........	---	---	7.7	14.1	24.7	22.1	27.9
Girls.........	4.7	6.2	5.3	9.7	15.3	16.8	16.9
Not Hispanic or Latina:							
White only.........	---	---	4.6	8.9	12.6	14.5	14.6
Black or African American only.........	---	---	10.7	16.3	23.5	27.7	27.1
Mexican.........	---	---	8.8	*13.4	19.6	19.9	18.0
Percent of poverty level:[5]							
Below 100%.........	---	---	---	15.8	19.8	19.3	24.3
100%–199%.........	---	---	---	11.2	15.1	18.4	20.1
200%–399%.........	---	---	---	9.4	15.7	19.3	16.3
400% or more.........	---	---	---	*	13.9	12.6	14.0

Beyond racial, ethnic, and socioeconomic disparities, there exist regional disparities regarding obesity within the United States. The CDC released data from 2012 suggesting that the prevalence of adult obesity ranged by state from 20.5% in Colorado to 34.7% in Louisiana. While no state had a prevalence of obesity less than 20%, higher prevalence was found in the Midwest (29.5%) and the South (29.4%). The Northeast (25.3%) and the West (25.1%) were observed to have lower prevalence. See Figure 18.1 for the CDC Self-reported obesity map of the United States.

As a clearly identified national health crisis, obesity in both children and adults has taken a huge financial toll on the health care system. While specific health impairments will be addressed later in the chapter, it is important to point out here that obesity has been estimated to cause 112,000 deaths per year in the United States.[8] The White House Task Force on Childhood Obesity Report to

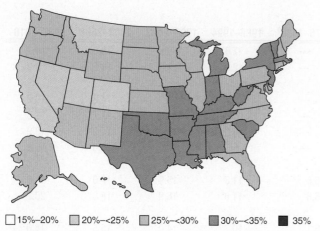

☐ 15%–20%　☐ 20%–<25%　☐ 25%–<30%　☐ 30%–<35%　■ 35%

FIGURE 18.1 CDC Self-reported obesity map of the United States. http://www.cdc.gov/obesity/images/brfss-self-reported-obesity-2012.gif (9)

the President in 2010 documents the financial burden to the health care system, with an estimated $1429 more in medical expenses incurred by adults with obesity as compared with normal-weight peers. Medical spending estimates attributed to obesity in adults topped $40 billion in 1998, with an increased estimate to $147 billion in 2008. Direct medical costs due to excess body weight were estimated at $3 billion per year for children. The report also found alarming statistics on how overweight and obese children are more likely to become obese adults. A study was revealed which suggested that obese 6- to 8-year-olds were approximately 10 times more likely to become obese adults than those with lower BMIs. Moreover, the association may be stronger for obese adolescents than for younger children.[8]

In 2000, the American Physical Therapy Association (APTA) House of Delegates adopted its official vision statement for the future of physical therapy entitled "Vision 2020." The following excerpt relates to how this obesity epidemic is within the scope of practice for physical therapists: "By 2020, physical therapy will be provided by physical therapists who are doctors of physical therapy, recognized by consumers and other health care professionals as the practitioners of choice to whom consumers have direct access for the diagnosis of, interventions for, and prevention of impairments, activity limitations, participation restrictions, and environmental barriers related to movement, function, and health." Of importance to the discussion of the role of physical therapists in the treatment of pediatric obesity is the commitment to both prevention and health promotion. The vision statement went on to say:

"Physical therapy, by 2020, will be provided by physical therapists who are doctors of physical therapy and who may be board-certified specialists. Consumers will have

direct access to physical therapists in all environments for patient/client management, prevention, and wellness services. Physical therapists will be practitioners of choice in patients'/clients' health networks and will hold all privileges of autonomous practice. Physical therapists may be assisted by physical therapist assistants who are educated and licensed to provide physical therapist directed and supervised components of interventions. Guided by integrity, life-long learning, and a commitment to comprehensive and accessible health programs for all people, physical therapists and physical therapist assistants will render evidence-based services throughout the continuum of care and improve quality of life for society. They will provide culturally sensitive care distinguished by trust, respect, and an appreciation for individual differences. While fully availing themselves of new technologies, as well as basic and clinical research, physical therapists will continue to provide direct patient/client care. They will maintain active responsibility for the growth of the physical therapy profession and the health of the people it serves."[10]

Physical therapists must advance their position to become the practitioners of choice to maximize the prevention of impairments, activity limitations, participation restrictions, and environmental barriers related to movement, function, and health of children with obesity and who are overweight. Furthermore, proponents have defined "integration of prevention and wellness strategies into the physical therapy intervention" as a critical role in the practice of physical therapy[1] (Guide to Physical Therapy Practice, APTA, 2001).

▶ Definitions

The classification of childhood obesity is distinct from that of adult obesity, as it is dependent not only upon height and weight, but also age and gender, owing to the variations in a maturing body. The BMI, typically utilized as the measure of adult obesity, is defined by the CDC as a number calculated from the measure of a person's height and weight. BMI expresses this relationship as a ratio of weight (in kilograms) divided by height (in meters) squared. The ratio is considered to be a reliable measure of body fat, as a relatively easy and inexpensive screening tool for weight categories that may be used as health indicators. Experts recommend BMI because it correlates strongly with body fat percentage and is associated weakly with height. It also identifies the most obese individuals correctly, with "acceptable accuracy at the upper end of the distribution."[11] For children and adolescents, BMI is calculated and compared with others of the same age to determine the percentile for age. It is advantageous to use this body mass index–for–age (BMI-for-age) value as the indicator for nutritional status in children because it provides a guideline based on weight and height while considering that interpretation depends on age, as normal body fat differs in boys and girls as they mature. As of April 2012, the CDC defined overweight children between the ages of 2 and 18 years as having a BMI at or above the 85th percentile and lower than the 95th percentile for children of the same age and sex. Childhood obesity was defined as a BMI at or above the 95th percentile for children of the same age and sex using the 2000 CDC growth chart.[12] See Figures 18.2 and 18.3 for males and females, respectively.

This more recent definition represents a departure from the original language used in describing overweight and obesity in children. The Expert Committee on Clinical Guidelines for Overweight in Adolescent Preventive Services had originally recommended in 1994 that the word "obese" be avoided in describing youth greater than or equal to the 95th percentile for BMI for age due to the inability of the measure to quantify the total body fat specifically. Instead, they had suggested the term *"at risk of overweight"* be used to describe those between the 85th and up to the 95th percentile in BMI for age. Those children at or above the 95th percentile were categorized as *overweight*. In an attempt to show the breadth and urgency of the issue of pediatric obesity, the Institute of Medicine elected in 2005 to depart from that recommendation and began to refer to those individuals between 2 and 18 years of age with a BMI for age greater than or equal to the 95th percentile for age as *"obese."* For those children 2 years of age and younger, it was recommended to continue to refrain from use of the term *obese* and utilize *overweight* to describe those children at or above the 95th percentile in BMI for age.[11]

To truly be practitioners of choice for wellness, physical therapists must learn to integrate prevention and wellness strategies into interventions. It is also necessary for physical therapists to have a working knowledge of the various aspects of health-related fitness and wellness terminology so as to increase the impact they might have working with the pediatric client with obesity. The ACSM clearly defines physical fitness as "a multidimensional concept" consisting of "a set of attributes that people possess or achieve that relates to the ability to perform physical activity, and is comprised of skill-related, health-related, and physiologic components."[3] Physical therapists are often involved in return to skill-related component of fitness, such as rehabilitation following a sports injury. Agility, balance, coordination, and speed are just a few of the functional skills often included in treatment. Health-related fitness measures include the ability of an individual to perform activities of daily life with stamina. It precludes the effects of inactivity, such as an overall state of deconditioning. This type of fitness may have the greatest impact in children with obesity, as they are not able to perform many activities enjoyed by same-aged peers. The physical therapist must understand that health-related fitness includes body composition, muscular strength and endurance,

cardiovascular endurance, as well as flexibility, and should be considered in designing long- and short-term goals. To attain a role in promoting fitness, health, and wellness for the pediatric population, physical therapists must understand other components of obesity and measurement. To review, *body composition* refers to the relative amount of fat versus fat-free body mass. A healthy body composition in youth is associated with improved cardiovascular profile later in life and a decreased morbidity. A balance of caloric intake and energy expenditure determines body composition. Recent studies have examined the question of whether calories are weighted differently, with the consumption of certain types of foods being better for burning calories and maintaining weight loss than others.[13] (See Display 18.1 for more information) *Waist circumference measurements* have also been used as a health indicator, along

---

DISPLAY 18.1 Nutrition Updates

While pediatric physical therapists are not experts in the area of nutrition, some basic information is valuable in being an integral part of an interdisciplinary team working together to combat childhood obesity.

Recent evidence alters the long-held theory of "energy in equals energy out."[13,16,17] While it is still an undeniable truth that calories taken in through food must be burned through physical activity and basal metabolic functioning to avoid being stored in the body, just how this occurs is being called into question. Robert Lustig, MD, has done significant research in this area and is now suggesting the theory that the quality of the calorie determines how much is burned and how much is stored. Breaking it down further, he describes four examples of calorie categories:

Fiber: Fiber delays absorption of calories; for example, eating 160 calories in almonds leads to the absorption of only 130. Recent evidence suggests that bacteria in the intestine use some of the calories, therefore delaying the absorption of the remaining calories into the bloodstream.

Protein: Due to the thermic effect of food, metabolizing proteins requires about twice the energy than with carbohydrates. This leads to proteins using more energy and therefore calorie burn in its processing. It is also stated that proteins reduce hunger better than carbohydrates by reducing hunger hormones.

Fat: Fats release nine calories per gram when burned. Some fats, such as trans fats, can cause plaque development in arteries and are considered "bad" fats. But other fats are considered "healthy" fats, such as Omega-3 fats, which are considered heart healthy.

Sugar: Consists of two chemicals—fructose and glucose. Every cell in the body uses glucose for energy, while fructose is metabolized in the liver as fat and not used for energy like glucose. Fructose is the key ingredient in soda, candy, and processed foods.

In keeping abreast of nutrition evidence and research, physical therapists may be able to dispel myths patients and their families may hold in developing a healthier diet.

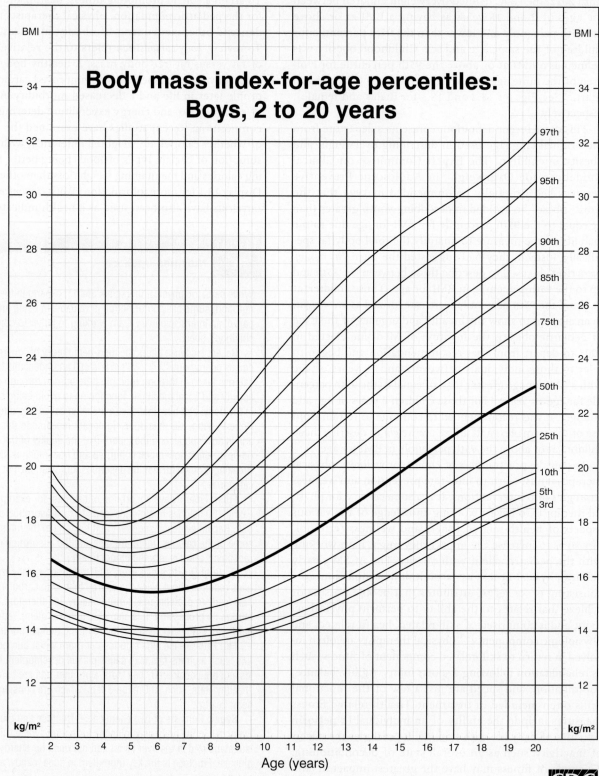

CDC Growth Charts: United States

Body mass index-for-age percentiles: Boys, 2 to 20 years

Published May 30, 2000.
SOURCE: Developed by the National Center for Health Statistics in collaboration with the National Center for Chronic Disease Prevention and Health Promotion (2000).

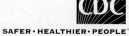

FIGURE 18.2 BMI-for-age for boys. http://www.cdc.gov/growthcharts/data/set1/chart15.pdf

CDC Growth Charts: United States

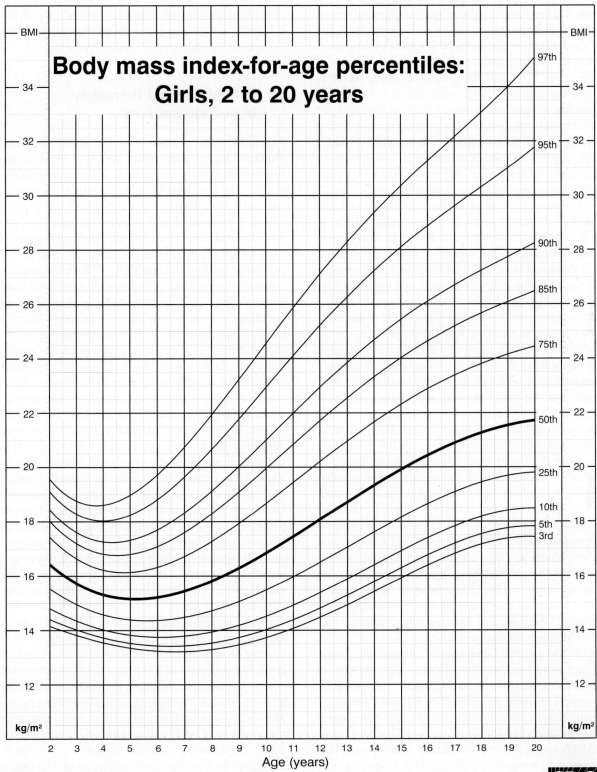

Body mass index-for-age percentiles:
Girls, 2 to 20 years

Published May 30, 2000.
SOURCE: Developed by the National Center for Health Statistics in collaboration with
the National Center for Chronic Disease Prevention and Health Promotion (2000).

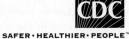

SAFER·HEALTHIER·PEOPLE™

FIGURE 18.3 BMI-for-age for girls. http://www.cdc.gov/growthcharts/data/set1/chart16.pdf

with BMI-for-age. Central adiposity, which is measured by circumferential measurement, is associated with hyperlipidemia, cardiovascular disease risk factors, and Type 2 diabetes. Studies have suggested that an increased measure of central adiposity at age 8 years could increase the risk of cardiovascular disease in adolescence by four times over that of children with smaller waist circumferential measurements.[14] *Muscular strength and endurance* are often measured using standardized youth fitness tests, such as those used in physical education curriculum. Examples of such tests might include curl-up or push-up tests, as well as more comprehensive tests such as the FITNESSGRAM.[15] Pediatric physical therapists routinely measure strength as part of the subtests of gross motor tests such as the Peabody Developmental Motor Scales–2nd edition or the Bruininks-Osertesky Test of Motor Proficiency 2nd edition, though these test items do use jumping, which requires the children to overcome body weight to complete the task (see Chapter 3). In "typical" scenarios such as this, physical therapists must use their judgment to determine whether the risk for injury of testing a young child who is obese balances the benefits of the standardized testing results. *Cardiorespiratory endurance* is the ability of the body to deliver oxygen to tissues at levels appropriate to the activity. Children who are physically active have more high density lipoproteins, lower triglycerides, reduced low density lipoproteins, lower BMI, improved insulin sensitivity, and lower systolic blood pressure when compared with sedentary children.[14] Flexibility is another aspect of fitness often tested in children to help determine their overall fitness level. The ACSM defines flexibility as the ability of a joint to move through the full range of motion. Many factors influence the flexibility of a joint, including extensibility of muscle, tendons, ligaments, and the joint capsule.[3] Education of the physical therapist routinely includes measurements of flexibility, such as use of a goniometer or tape measure. In the fitness arena, field tests include sit and reach tests and the v-sit and reach. Both tests measure flexibility across multiple joints, and therefore offer more information to a more general state of the flexibility of the individual than joint specific goniometric tests. Furthermore, the field tests have normative data to compare the children with their peers.[14]

The ACSM describes elements of physiologic fitness as distinct from health-related fitness components "in that it includes nonperformance components that relate to biological systems influenced by habitual activity."[3] Metabolic fitness, morphologic fitness, and bone integrity may be included in this category. The previously cited APTA vision statement includes health promotion and wellness as integral to practice. This arena of physiologic fitness growth is necessary for youth with obesity. Tests and measures in the physical therapy evaluation will help to identify goals to maximize all fitness measures in children with obesity, even if not directly related to the primary diagnosis for which physical therapy was sought.

Applying the multifactorial concepts of fitness within the treatment program for children with obesity and continuing to employ evidence-based research in the design of such programs will help enhance the role of physical therapists within the multidisciplinary team focused on decreasing the incidence of pediatric obesity.

Role of physical therapists in pediatric obesity

Physical therapists have been defined by the American Physical Therapy Association (APTA) as "health care practitioners who maintain, restore, and improve movement, activity, and health enabling individuals of all ages to have optimal functioning and quality of life" and who "are involved in promoting health, wellness, and fitness through risk factor identification and the implementation of services to reduce risk, slow the progression of or prevent functional decline and disability."[10] Within this definition, the role of a physical therapist within pediatric obesity is defined. The battle to combat the growing incidence of childhood obesity begins with the concepts of active living and healthy lifestyle. Considering the definition of "active living" as a way of life incorporating physical activity into daily routine, there is a unique opportunity to promote this healthy living as pediatric physical therapists, whether in the educational setting, or community, or in a medically based facility. Because physical therapists are experts in the musculoskeletal system and gross motor development, and are practitioners who assist in health promotion and prevention of impairment, their role is clear in the treatment of pediatric obesity. Because promoting the opportunity for independent movement and quality of life are key objectives of physical therapists in pediatric populations, their function within the care of children with obesity is multifactorial. Beyond interventions for specific physical impairments, a physical therapist should be part of the multidisciplinary team working with families in the education and prevention of comorbid impairments in virtually all professional settings. In 2008, the U.S. Department of Health and Human Services established the guidelines for physical activity to maximize healthy growth and development in children and adolescents. Sixty minutes of physical activity, or more, each day was recommended, including the components of aerobic training, muscle strengthening, and bone strengthening. The daily hour of physical activity should incorporate the concepts of health-related fitness. The guidelines further delineate aerobic recommendations to include at least moderate- to vigorous-level activity most days and vigorous level 3 days a week. Muscle- and bone-strengthening activities are also recommended at least 3 days a week.[18] These guidelines should be considered in developing a comprehensive home exercise program for all pediatric patients, especially those with increased weight status.

Physical activity refers to a movement of the body by the skeletal muscles that result in energy expenditure. To differentiate, *exercise* is physical activity that is planned, structured, and repetitive and has the purpose of improvement or maintenance of one or more components of physical fitness.[3,14] While physical therapists may be considered experts in therapeutic exercise as a key component of the rehabilitation, a research report in 2011 by Schlessman et al. suggests only one in three physical therapists "were thinking of or preparing to incorporate wellness promotion into practice and only 54% were incorporating wellness into practice."[19] The increased attention to health promotion and obesity prevention in postbaccalaureate physical therapy degree programs has strengthened the perception of physical therapists as leaders in this area of practice.[19]

The general public has not yet fully recognized the role of physical therapists as leaders in health promotion and wellness. Studies of parents of preschoolers indicate they did not recognize weight concerns in their children, nor did they know what action to take when presented with the issue. This finding suggests a lack of public knowledge and awareness of the role physical therapists play in pediatric health promotion and suggests a need for physical therapists to explore the opportunities available in this arena. As important participants on the early intervention team, physical therapists are charged with increasing the gross motor skill acquisition of the children and education of their families. As Nervik et al. suggested in a study in 2011, gross motor development in children aged 3 to 5 years may be impacted by higher BMIs.[7] The timing of development of fat tissue between the ages of 3 and 7 years makes this a critical time for obesity prevention and recognition. physical therapists can begin the education of both parents and early education professionals at preschool and day care centers about the importance of physical activity for this young population.[8,20] Barriers do exist in putting wellness promotion into practice, including a lack of resources, time, and funding as well as difficulty with keeping the families and children engaged in programs.[19] Physical therapists often interact with children and families in the course of rehabilitation for the comorbidities of obesity. This interaction offers a unique opportunity to begin promoting a healthy lifestyle choice and educating families in health-related fitness guidelines for children.

▶ Health consequences of obesity

The numbers of children who are overweight and obese have increased at an alarming rate as have the health consequences in this population, long and short term, being seen at hospitals and clinics throughout the country. The impact of obesity not only exists in the medical arena, but can also be seen throughout the educational system. It is well documented that associated with primary childhood obesity are increases in high blood pressure, Type 2 diabetes, respiratory disorders, sleep disorders, chronic low grade systemic inflammation, orthopedic musculoskeletal issues, and psychosocial impacts. As noted above, studies have suggested that children with obesity may have difficulty with developmental motor skill acquisition.[7] There is an increased risk for long-term consequences such as adult obesity, with over 50% of overweight adolescents now meeting the criteria for the metabolic syndrome (insulin resistance, hypertension, hyperlipidemia, and abdominal obesity), adverse socioeconomic impact, cardiovascular disease, and premature morbidity.[21] Current estimates are that up to one-third of the population of the United States will develop Type 2 diabetes during their lifetime. There is a twofold increase in the mortality risk as early as the fourth decade of life for those adolescents who are obese. This epidemic threatens to reverse the gains in life expectancy occurring through improvements in clinical treatments of hypertension, hyperlipidemia, and smoking cessation. Most drastically, data suggest that this generation of children will be the first not to outlive their parents.[8,21]

While many of the secondary impairments of pediatric obesity are beyond the scope of the physical therapy practice, orthopedic and musculoskeletal dysfunction are often evaluated and treated by physical therapists. Blount disease, slipped capital femoral epiphysis, spinal dysfunction, and fractures are just a few of the diagnoses that may be directly related to the child being overweight or obese. Treatment approaches for these various conditions are specifically addressed in Chapter 12. Research suggests that being overweight can impact the body's response to weight-bearing activities that are a part of regular physical activity. Gait dysfunction, including changes in velocity, cadence, energy usage, biomechanical changes leading to abnormal knee loading, and foot discomfort have also been linked to children who are overweight or obese.[22]

In addition to comorbidities related to obesity, pediatric physical therapists must also be aware of those children most frequently seen in therapy and the impact the primary dysfunction may have on their ability to be physically active. There is a paucity of research into the area of physical activity behavior among children with a disability. The positive effects of physical activity on overall health and well-being have been well documented; however, for people with a disability, an active lifestyle may be even more beneficial.[23] As individuals with childhood-onset physical disabilities such as cerebral palsy (CP), myelomeningocele (MMC), or brain injury are living longer, health care is shifting focus for this group toward health promotion and wellness to help prevent secondary conditions and improve quality of life into adulthood.[24] Buffart et al. found that overall health-related physical fitness was poor in youth with MMC. This is of particular concern when considering that life expectancy of persons with MMC has increased and lifestyle-related diseases such as cardiovascular disease and diabetes will be of increasing concern.[25]

Pan and Frey published a study outlining the paucity of information surrounding the physical activity level of children with autism spectrum disorders (ASD). They found that youth with ASD might have less opportunity for physical activity as a result of social and behavioral deficits as well as difficulty with peer interaction. Although the authors found no consistent pattern in physical activity of youth with ASD, findings suggested that increasing opportunities were needed to address extracurricular physical activity, particularly during adolescence.[26] These findings present another opportunity for PTs in the educational setting to provide assistance and adaptations to improve participation of the students with whom they work in physical activity opportunities. Children with CP may live the most sedentary lifestyles among those with pediatric disabilities.[27] In a study examining self-reported levels of activity in adolescents with CP, the authors found that physical activity participation was related to level of gross motor function and that physical activity decreased with increasing age. The inverse relationship between physical activity level and age is consistent with data on the physical activity of nondisabled peers. There was notable decrease in variation and intensity level of the physical activity among those with CP when contrasted with their same-aged peers.[28] A strategy of lifelong fitness and physical activity should help focus the treatment approach, home exercise programs, and discharge planning in physical therapy with a goal to maximize the potential of those patients with CP. Encouraging increased physical activity is important for health promotion and may help improve overall functional independence, social integration, and life satisfaction for all children, with and without childhood-onset physical disabilities.[24] A qualitative study examined personal and environmental barriers to physical activity in young adults with childhood-onset physical disabilities. As with the general population, perceived barriers to physical activity were related to attitude and motivation, particularly in conjunction with fatigue, injuries related to the condition, and lack of information and professional support.[24] This suggests yet another role physical therapists might have as health care providers who can promote physical activity in these pediatric patients. By helping alleviate barriers, educating clients and families about the recommendations for physical activity from the CDC, and helping determine the correct balance between activity and rest to reduce fatigue, physical therapists can begin to bridge the gap in activity levels for children with physical impairments. Studies have been reported documenting improved levels of physical activity for those with acquired short- and long-term physical disability. Future studies are warranted to determine the efficacy of rehabilitation professionals to provide counseling and advice on physical activity and whether such intervention would impact physical activity levels of youth with childhood-onset physical disabilities.[24] (See Display 18.2 for an example of increasing opportunities for physical activity for those with special needs.)

▶ How obesity treatment fits within the ICF framework

The World Health Organization's (WHO) ICF framework can serve as a guide to guide clinical pathways and critical thinking in the treatment of impairments related to pediatric obesity (Fig. 18.4).[29] In contrast to the Guide to Physical Therapist Practice 2, the ICF offers a model of health and functioning as opposed to a disability model. This classification system describes human functioning within the daily lives of individuals with a health condition. It is generally agreed that individuals with obesity experience disability in terms of their ability to participate in activities within both daily and community functioning. In a pediatric population, these activities could include mobility in and around an educational setting, recreational activities, or even their ability to progress with self-care activities. Intolerance for physical activity could impede social development and lead to further issues. Looking only at the presence of obesity, whether as a primary or secondary diagnosis, does not offer a clinician

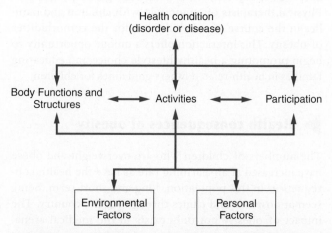

FIGURE 18.4 Visualization of the current understanding of interaction of various components of the International Classification of Functioning, Disability and Health (ICF).[30]

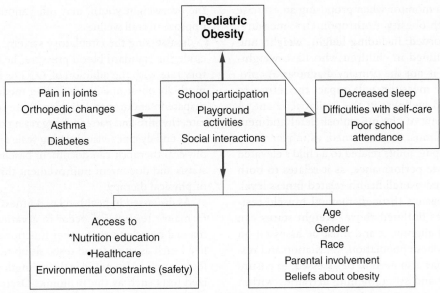

FIGURE 18.5 ICF as model for pediatric obesity effects on health and functioning of a pediatric patient.

enough information on how the child's participation in daily activities may be affected. The ICF can be used to assess the dynamic impact obesity can have on the function, activities, and participation looking at two distinct components. First are the impairments that might be present with the disability of obesity on the body structures and functioning and the impact this might have on performance and participation in activities. Second, the contextual component of obesity is examined in the psychosocial views of health and well-being and includes personal and environmental factors. This dynamic interaction between health conditions and environmental and personal factors moves away from the disablement models emphasizing the individual as being handicapped by the diagnosis (Fig. 18.5). The APTA has been clear in identifying the ICF as a means of using the language of function and health, understood by those both in and out of the health care arena, which might be utilized to enhance communication between health care provider and patient, policy makers, and payers. By using this language, communication within the health care community might be enhanced, leading to a clearer picture of the role physical therapists might play in the broader concept of rehabilitation of those children with obesity. Furthermore, conversations might be stimulated regarding interdisciplinary collaboration in research, resulting in overall improved clinical care.[29–31] Figure 18.6 suggests a model related to the ICF format.

Physical therapy history and examination of the child with obesity

In the case of pediatric obesity, it is very important to recognize the patient may *not* be seeking physical therapy for diagnosis and treatment of obesity; rather, obesity may exist as a comorbidity of a more specific physical impairment, such as back or knee pain. A comprehensive history and physical examination must include the patient's entire body structure and impairments responsible for functional limitations of the presenting diagnosis. Particular attention must be paid to risk factors, including ethnicity, cultural beliefs, family/caregiver resources, education, social interaction, activities, and support systems. General health status questions will lead to information regarding physical functioning, psychological functioning, level of physical fitness, and general health perception. Physical functioning should include perceived mobility difficulty or sleep patterns and related issues. Psychological functioning might include existing conditions such as depression, anxiety, memory, or social issues related to weight status. The family history is important as it might relate to the overall home environment and health-related fitness. Intake information about medications currently being used by the child for comorbidities may also offer vital information regarding weight status in the patient. Knowledge of the potential for weight gain as a side effect of some antipsychotic drugs used to treat attention-deficit hyperactivity disorder or autism; mood stabilizers, antidepressants, and oral steroids are also important medications to note.[32,33] In some cases, parents or educational staff may need education regarding these side effects that may be contributing to changes in weight status of a child.

Systems Review

Within a systems review, attention should be paid to cardiopulmonary-related measures, as indicated above in the discussion of health-related fitness measures. Blood pressure, resting heart rate, and respiratory rate are important factors to monitor when proposing an exercise plan for a child with obesity. Anthropometric measurements must be recorded, including height, weight, and BMI-for-age determined in children who have weight-related issues, even if not the primary diagnosis. As previously noted, these measures will impact the return to maximal health and wellness in the pediatric client. A comprehensive review of the musculoskeletal and neuromuscular systems must be performed, as impairments may occur in developing joints related to a child's elevated weight status. Muscle performance, as it relates to both primary diagnosis and overall health-related fitness level, is important to measure through manual muscle testing and other modes outlined above. Weight status can impact posture and alignment and must be assessed on evaluation. For the obese population, ventilation and respiration measures may also need to be assessed, to ensure safety with aerobic and strengthening activities within the treatment plan. As previously noted, gross motor skills and coordinated movements may also be impacted if a child is obese. The child and family's motivation for change and expectations for results must be measured as well to determine goal-attainment strategies.

Tests and Measures

While the physical therapist may use a variety of specific tests and measures in the evaluation of a pediatric client for a specific diagnosis, it is important to address those measures that quantify the effect weight status may have on overall prognosis and outcomes. As previously noted, there are a variety of tests to look specifically at both health- and skill-related fitness measures that may be useful in some patient populations. For other patients, the Guide to Physical Therapy Practice supplies a framework with which to specifically measure impairments in children with obesity. Aerobic capacity and endurance testing may necessitate standardized testing protocols such as arm, cycle, or wheelchair ergometer tests, step tests (such as the Harvard step test), or walk/run testing such as the 6-minute walk test. All of these measures offer standards with which to compare results.

Measuring anthropometric characteristics, including body composition and dimensions, has already been discussed. In the area of arousal, attention, and cognition, it may be beneficial to assess motivation and expectation level as well as overall quality-of-life ratings by using a self-assessment tool such as the *Child Health Questionnaire*.[34] This type of assessment may be necessary, because, as previously stated, severely obese children report lower health-related quality of life. In view of the fact that weight status can be associated with a stigma within the pediatric population, the child with obesity often displays lower self-esteem and reports feeling sad, lonely, and nervous more than typical-weight peers.[8] Although not always included in a physical therapy assessment, quality-of-life measures, particularly in

the overweight youth, may offer another outcome area to improve overall wellness.

In assessing the circulatory system, measures should include the standard blood pressure, heart rate, and respiratory rate with the addition of ECG or EKG if the patient is morbidly obese and needs further medical clearance to participate in endurance activities. Pulse oximetry, respiratory rate, rhythm, and pattern, Borg rating of perceived exertion scale, and dyspnea visual analog scale are means for which a physical therapist can document baseline cardiorespiratory status and document improvement throughout the course of physical therapy.

As discussed in health-related fitness testing, muscle performance testing can occur in a variety of ways. Beyond manual muscle testing, other functional tests might be utilized such as sit-to-stand tests, sit-up tests, or squat testing, for example. Also noted is the strength portion of standardized tests such as the Bruininks-Oseretsky Test of Motor Proficiency–2 subtest.

In the evaluation of the child with obesity, particular attention should be paid to posture and alignment to assess further risk factors related to weight status, such as increased genu valgus at the knees, or issues at the subtalar joint resulting in pain with activity. An assessment of self-care issues may also be necessary with the patient population in the highest weight percentile for children to help with problem solving for the family in the area of home management when the child cannot be safely lifted due to weight.

 Determining functional outcome expectations for the child with obesity

The physical therapist should focus interventions for children with obesity and increased weight status on decreasing the risk of cardiovascular, pulmonary, and musculoskeletal disorders. Therapeutic exercise, aerobic conditioning, functional training, education and training of patients and their families, and overall lifestyle modifications are all strategies used to attain the overarching goal of improved health status and well-being. Anticipated functional outcomes affecting participation aspects of activity could include the following:

- Improved ability to perform physical actions such as jumping activities is documented
- Awareness and use of community resources is improved
- Behaviors that foster healthy habits, wellness, and prevention strategies are acquired and documented through self-assessments
- Decision making is enhanced regarding patient health and use of health care resources by the patient and family both at home and in school
- Patient and family knowledge of personal and environmental factors associated with weight status and obesity is increased

- Performance levels in self-care, school, play, community, or leisure activities are improved by self-reported measures
- Attendance at school is improved

More outcomes related to body structure and function related to obesity might include the following:

- Increased muscle performance, strength, and joint range of motion
- Improved aerobic capacity and endurance
- Improved tolerance of positions and activities both at home, in school, and within the community
- Improved sense of well-being as documented through questionnaires or surveys
- Improved measures of skill-related fitness
- Decrease in risk factors

Other secondary outcomes that are broader in spectrum would include decreasing utilization and cost of health care services and optimizing use of physical therapy services. This utilization of physical therapy to include attention to weight status in pediatric patients who present with other primary impairments results in a more efficient use of health care dollars.

▶ Therapeutic interventions to address obesity in the pediatric population

Whether the child with obesity is receiving physical therapy in a medical setting or in the educational environment, particular attention must be paid to structuring therapeutic interventions in a safe and effective manner to meet goals. Increased monitoring of perceived level of exertion, respiratory rate, blood pressure, and heart rate may be indicated

in this population to maintain a safe working zone. Patient and family education is often necessary to properly monitor heart rate. Because of the variation in resting heart rate in children, target heart rate for children under 18 years is not as reliable a measure as in adults. Rating perceived exertion is a safe way to monitor exercise intensity.[35] There are options beyond the Borg for rating exertion in children. The Pictorial Children's Effort Rating Table (PCERT) and OMNI child scales are two other self-rating scales that offer a physical therapist the ability to grade exercise intensity.[36,37] In terms of health-related fitness, aerobic capacity

---

DISPLAY 18.3   Recommendations to Motivate Children and Families to Exercise.

Encourage	Discourage
Fitness education for family members	Comparing child with physically active Peers
Having fun with activities	
Begin with lower intensity exercises	Participation more important than winning
Include child/family in goal identification	Gradual progression of exercise program
Develop achievable goals that enhance quality of life	Maintain appropriate level of reinforcement
	Do not be demanding, exercise should be its own reward
Give positive reinforcement as appropriate	

Adapted from McWhorter JW, Wallmann HW, Alpert PT. The obese child: motivation as a tool for exercise. *J Pediatr Health Care*. 2003;17:11–17.

DISPLAY 18.4   Pennsylvania's Growth Screening Program

In response to the growing obesity epidemic, some states developed school health initiatives to begin to gain control over the issue. In 2003, PA Department of Health initiated the Nutrition and Physical Activity Plan to Prevent Obesity and Related Chronic Diseases. Parental awareness of the BMI-for-age measure as a tool to measure growth was set as one of the goals of the program. Over the course of three school years, the program was mandated for all students in the kindergarten through twelfth grade to have BMI for age documented with notifications being offered to parents should the measure fall outside the norms for age. The procedure set forth by the state includes annual screening of height and weight, with attention given to the average growth velocity as a measure of normal growth, and use of the CDC growth charts to determine BMI for age statistics for each student in the district. Interpretation of the findings fall into one of three categories:

Weight within acceptable range—Even when findings are within a normal range for testing, parent notification of results are recommended to decrease possibility of a student being singled out for being overweight.

Weight less that 5th percentile—includes both BMI for age <5th percentile and stature for age <5th percentile; recommendations include sending parent/guardian notification home in a timely manner with additional recommendation for follow up by primary care provider for nutritional concerns and information on community-based food supplementation programs.

Weight equal to or greater than 85th percentile—includes BMI for age greater than or equal to 85th percentile; recommendations include parental notification, encouraging healthy eating and regular physical activity, and recommendation for follow up with primary care provider for blood pressure, total cholesterol, family history, assess exogenous causes of overweight, and for Type 2 diabetes screening.

Furthermore, the PA Department of Health requests each school district to submit the data each school year. On the website, the Department of Health offer variety of handouts and resources accessible to both the districts and the families to increase knowledge base of healthy nutrition and living an active lifestyle.[39]

www.dsf.health.state.pa.us

18.5   Towards a Larger Wellness Community: A Physical Therapist Collaborates with a Community Elementary School in Securing a Federal Grant

Through the Carol M. White Physical Education Program (PEP), the US Department of Education provides grants "to LEAs and community-based organizations (CBOs) to initiate, expand, or enhance physical education programs, including after-school programs, for students in kindergarten through 12th grade. Grant recipients must implement programs that help students make progress toward meeting state standards."[40] In 2007, a physical therapist partnered with a community elementary school nurse and physical education department to procure a 2-year grant in the amount of 175,000 dollars. The physical therapist served as the project director and chief investigator for the grant, which opens up a new role in the wellness arena. The following is an excerpt from the grant report: "The purpose of *The Healthy Kids/Healthy Community Program* is to ensure students in a high risk population are healthier and therefore better able to learn and that the staff at Penrose Elementary will be properly trained and supported to promote a healthy school environment. This has been a collaborative effort between (school) and (health system) with other community partners, focusing on the needs of this underserved population, with particular attention to ensure specific needs are being met for those children already at risk for adult obesity. Specifically, three areas were identified as focal points for this project.

1. Students will receive nutrition education both as a classroom based curriculum and as a component of after-school wellness programs.
2. Children identified as overweight or at risk of overweight as per the established CDC guidelines of a BMI-for-age at or above the 85th percentile, will be eligible and encouraged to participate in after-school programming which will focus on teaching these children how to live an active, healthy lifestyle. For those children who have special needs, a separate program will focus on increasing their activity levels by adapting current PE/fitness programming or by establishing individualized fitness plans. Use of components of the Fitnessgram will be used to assess fitness changes as related to activity levels in random group of students.
3. Promote comprehensive increases in moderate to vigorous activity throughout the school day by increasing the number of playground activities available to all students, and

improving the organization of the recess yard. Fitnessgram measures as part of the PE program will be used to assess the overall fitness changes with increasing activity options at lunch recess. Furthermore, professional development of the staff, towards creating a healthy school environment will be available. As a final component in achieving an inclusive program, parents will be invited to participate in fitness nights to further their knowledge and experience of wellness.

Using a collaborative approach, exploring available resources from the (school district), an after-school program, nutrition education professionals, and utilizing and training the current staff on available low/no cost programs (such as professional student capital) has enabled (health system), a community-based health system with strong ties to the community, to assist (elementary school) to utilize its expertise in health and wellness to meet the current standards for Health, Safety and Physical Education. The overarching goal of the PEP program this year is to increase the activity levels of students in Kindergarten to 5th Grade to 150 minutes a week and those students in 6th through 8th Grade to 225 minutes a week.

Web resources for physical therapists, pediatric patients, and families as of October 2013:

Centers for Disease Control and Prevention (CDC), National Center for Chronic Disease Prevention and Health Promotion. BMI for children and teens growth charts. http://www.cdc.gov/growthcharts
Action for Healthy Kids. http://www.actionforhealthykids.org
American Dietetic Association. http://www.eatright.org
BMI-for-Age Calculator for Children. http://www.cdc.gov/healthyweight/assessing/bmi/
National Institutes of Health. National Heart, Lung, and Blood Institute. Obesity education initiative. http://www.nhlbi.nih.gov/about/oei/index.htm
President's Council on Fitness, Sports & Nutrition. http://www.fitness.gov
The President's Challenge. https://www.presidentschallenge.org
Shapedown: weight management for children and adolescents. http://www.shapedown.com
Shape Up America! Healthy weight for life. http://www.shapeup.org
Child and teen health and nutrition information. http://kidshealth.org/teen/index.jsp?tracking=T_Home
Portion distortion information. www.kidnetic.com

---

and endurance conditioning require specific attention. Interventions to improve cardiovascular endurance may include aquatics, walking or wheelchair propulsion programs, gait training on treadmills, cycle ergometers, as well as elliptical training activities.

In the area of flexibility, beyond the typical interventions such as manual and self-stretching, group activities such as yoga have become available to children both in the educational setting and in the community. Strength and endurance for more skill-related fitness is also to be considered in the interventions for children with obesity. Beyond active assisted, active, and resistive exercises, more comprehensive

exercise approaches have been used such as Pilates or Power Yoga.

Motivation is another key aspect of therapeutic intervention to be understood by the physical therapist working with a child with obesity. To encourage optimal effort in exercises and interventions, it is necessary to properly motivate these youth who may already have a negative view of physical activity. Display 18.3 offers guidelines for increasing participation in therapeutic exercise in children.[38]

There are various approaches taken by physical therapists who treat children with obesity. As with many patients, it is clear that interventions need to be individualized for each client. Furthermore, as obesity in children has become a health problem of epidemic proportions, it is also clear that an interdisciplinary approach provides a comprehensive means to achieving the goal of reducing the incidence of obesity in general. Health care providers, such as primary care physicians and physical therapists, must partner with the community through the educational team, and those with an "environmental" stake in the effort such as local and state governments and health insurers who are in a position to extend the reach of strategies to promote a healthy lifestyle. Display 18.4 describes part of a Commonwealth of Pennsylvania growth screening program related to body weight determination. Taking advantage of unique opportunities to be part of a larger wellness community may be available to physical therapists as primary interventionists in the treatment of pediatric obesity. Display 18.5 shows a recent report about a physical therapist-led project to partner with a local school district. The physical therapist is this chapter's author.

SUMMARY

As physical therapists strive to achieve the designation of health care professionals who are experts in health promotion and wellness, it is imperative that clinicians achieve a level of knowledge regarding assessment and intervention for pediatric patients who are obese. The role of a physical therapist within the larger interdisciplinary team allocated to begin the process of reversing the epidemic of childhood obesity continues to be defined. As experts in the area of gross motor development, and as part of a larger response to optimize function and enhance movement in children with obesity, physical therapists have an opportunity to upgrade the overall quality of life for these patients. There is an additional case to be made for physical therapists to be educators for families and the larger community in addressing pediatric health promotion and wellness.

REFERENCES

1. APTA. Guide to physical therapist practice. Second edition. *Phys Ther.* 2001;81(1):9–746.
2. AMA adopts new policies on second day of voting at annual meeting. Released June 18 2013. www.ama-assn.org/AMA/pub/news/news/2013/2013-06-18-new-AMA-policies-annual-meeting.page. Accessed September 2013.
3. American College of Sports Medicine. *ACSM's Guidelines for Exercise Testing and Exercise Prescription.* Baltimore, MD: Williams and Wilkins; 1995.
4. National Health and Nutrition Examination Survey, 2009–2010. www.cdc.gov/nchs/data/databriefs/DB82.htm. Accessed February 2013.
5. Ogden CL, Carroll MD, Kit BK, et al. Prevalence of obesity and trends in BMI among US children and adolescents, 1999–2010. *JAMA.* 2012;307(5):483–490.
6. Centers for Disease Control and Prevention. NCHS Health E-Stat. www.cdc.gov/NCHS/data/hestat/obesity_Child_07_08/obesity_child_07_08.htm. Accessed March 2013.
7. Nervik D, Martin K, Rundquist P, et al. The relationship between body mass index and gross motor development in children aged 3 to 5 years. *Pediatr Phys Ther.* 2011;23:144–148.
8. White House Task Force on Childhood Obesity Report to the President: Solving the Problem of Childhood Obesity Within a Generation. May 2010. www.letsmove.goc/sites/letsmove.gov/files/TaskForce_on_Childhood_Obesity_May2010_FullReport.pdf. Accessed March 2013.
9. Prevalence of self-reported obesity among U.S adults. BRFSS 2011 State Obesity Map. http://www.cdc.gov/obesity/data/adult.html. Accessed February 2013.
10. Vision 2020. American Physical Therapy Association. http://www.apta.org/vision2020/. Accessed March 2013.
11. Krebs NF, Himes JH, Jacobson D, et al. Assessment of child and adolescent overweight and obesity. *Pediatrics.* 2007;120(4):S193–S228.
12. Centers for Disease Control and Prevention. Overweight and Obesity. http://www.cdc.gov/obesity/childhood/basics.html. Accessed February 2013.
13. Ebbeling CB, Swain JF, Feldman HA, et al. Effects of dietary composition on energy expenditure during weight-loss maintenance. *JAMA.* 2012;307(24):2627–2634.
14. Ganley KJ, Paterno MV, Miles C, et al. Health related fitness in children and adolescents. *Pediatr Phys Ther.* 2011;23:208–220.
15. FITNESSGRAM. www.cooperinstiture.org/fitnessgram. Accessed May 2013.
16. Lustig RH. Still Believe "A Calorie is Just a Calorie?" Huffington Post Healthy Living. www.huffingtonpost.com/rober-lustig-md/sugar-toxic_b_2759564.html. Accessed October 2013.
17. Gelman L. 3 reasons a calorie is not a calorie. *Reader's Digest.* July 2013;26.
18. 2008 Physical Activity Guidelines for Americans. www.health.gov/paguidelines/pdf/paguide.pdf. Accessed July, 2013.
19. Schlessman AM, et al. The Role of physical therapists in pediatric health promotion and obesity prevention: comparison of attitudes. *Pediatr Phys Ther.* 2011;23:79–86.
20. Whitaker RC, Pepe MS, Wright JA, et al. Early adiposity rebound and the risk of adult obesity. *Pediatrics.* 1998;101(3) e5. http://pediatrics.aappublications.org/content/101/3/e5. Accessed October 2013.
21. Lynn CH, Miller JL. Bariatric surgery for obese adolescents: should surgery be used to treat the childhood obesity epidemic? *Pediatr Health.* 2009;3(1):33–40.
22. Pathare N, Haskvitz EM, Selleck M. Comparison of measures of physical performance among young children who are healthy weight, overweight, or obese. *Pediatr Phys Ther.* 2013;25:291–296.
23. Saebu M. Physical disability and physical activity: a review of the literature on correlates and associations. *Euro J Adapted Phys Activity.* 2010;3(2):37–55.
24. Buffart LM, Westendorp T, van den Berg-Emons RJ, et al. Perceived barriers and facilitators of physical activity in young adults with childhood-onset physical disabilities. *J Rehabil Med.* 2009;41:881–885.
25. Buffart LM, van den Berg-Emons RJ, van Wijlen-Hempel MS, et al. Health related physical fitness of adolescents and young adults with myelomeningocele. *Euro J Appl Physiol.* 2008;103:181–188.
26. Pan CY, Frey GC. Physical activity patterns in youth with autism spectrum disorders. *J Autism Dev Disord.* 2006;36:597–606.
27. Longmuir PE, Bar-Or O. Factors influencing the physical activity levels of youths with physical and sensory disabilities. *Adapted Physical Activity Q.* 2000;17:40–53.
28. Maher C, Williams MT, Olds T, et al. Physical and sedentary activity in adolescents with cerebral palsy. *Dev Med Child Neurol.* 2007;49(6):450–457.
29. Winstein C, et al. The Physical therapy clinical research network (PTClinResNef), methods, efficacy, and benefits of a rehabilitation research network. *Am J Phys Med Rehabil.* 2008;87:937–950.
30. World Health Organization. *International Classification of Functioning, Disability, and Health.* Geneva, Switzerland: World Health Organization; 2001.

31. Forhan M. An analysis of disability models and the application of the ICF to obesity. *Disabil Rehabil.* 2009;31(16):1382–1388.

32. American Academy of Child and Adolescent Psychiatry. Preventing and Managing Medication–Related Weight. www.aacap.org/AACAP/Families_and_Youth/Facts_for_Families/Facts_for_Families_Pages/Preventing_and_Mananging_Medication_Related_Weight_94.aspx. Accessed September 2013.

33. UCLA Department of Medicine. Drug-induced weight gain. www.med.ucla.edu/modules/wfsection/article.php?articleid=371. Accessed September 2013.

34. CHQ: Child Health Questionnaire TM. www.healthactchq.com/chq.php. Accessed October 2013.

35. National Council on Strength and Fitness. Heart rate guidelines for adults and children. National Council on Strength and Fitness. www.ncsf.org/enew/articles/articles-heartrateguidelines.aspx. Accessed September 2013.

36. Lagally KM. Using rating of perceived exertion in physical education. *J Phys Educ Recreation Dance.* 2013;84(5):35–39.

37. Roemmich JN, Barkley JE, Epstein LH, et al. Validity of PCERT and OMNI walk/run ratings of perceived exertion. *Med Science Sports Exercise.* 2006;38(5):1014–1019.

38. McWhorter JW, Wallmann HW, Alpert PT, et al. The obese child: motivation as a tool for exercise. *J Pediatr Health Care.* 2003;17:11–17.

39. Procedures for the growth screening program for Pennsylvania's school-aged population. www.portal.state.pa.us. Accessed October 2013.

40. Carol M. White physical education program. www2.ed.gov/programs/whitephysed/index.html. Accessed September 2013.

41. Overweight and Obesity. www.cdc.gov/obesity/data/adult.html. Accessed February 2013.

42. van den Berg-Emons, Saris WH, de Barbanson DC, et al. Daily physical activity of school children with spastic diplegia and of healthy control subjects. *J Pediatr.* 1995;127(4):578–584.

Cardiac Disorders

Heather Hanson

Introduction
Cardiac System Development
  Normal Fetal Circulation
  Changes Associated with Birth
  Normal Circulation After Birth
Congenital Heart Defects
  Acyanotic Congenital Heart Defects
  Cyanotic Heart Defects
Heart Transplantation
Physical Therapy Examination
  History
  Laboratory Values
  Vital Signs
  General Appearance
  Pain
  Equipment and Devices

  Integument
  Thorax and Respiratory Examination
  Musculoskeletal Examination
  Strength
  Functional Mobility
  Aerobic Capacity and Endurance
Physical Therapy Evaluation, Diagnosis, and Prognosis
  Coordination, Communication, and Documentation
Physical Therapy Intervention
  Patient- and Family-Related Instruction
  Procedural Interventions
Neurodevelopmental Outcomes of CHD
Summary
Case Study

 ## Introduction

Congenital heart disease (CHD) occurs in varying severities, ranging from mild to severe.[1] Moderate and severe CHD occurs in approximately 2.5 to 3 of every 1000 births, whereas mild CHD can occur up to 10 per 1000.[1] There are 25,000 babies born each year with a CHD, and more than 1,000,000 individuals have reached adulthood and are living in the United States with a functionally significant CHD.[2] The mortality rates in infants with CHD have declined dramatically as a result of medical and surgical advances for their care, with up to 85% of infants born with CHD surviving to adulthood.[2] As more children are surviving, more and more research is being done regarding many domains of neurodevelopmental outcomes in children with all types of CHD, including cognition, language skills, gross and fine motor skills, and quality of life.[3–11] Pediatric physical therapists are likely to encounter infants, children, and adolescents with a cardiac disorder in every setting in which they practice. A physical therapist may see a child with CHD in the acute care setting preoperatively and/or postoperatively, in rehabilitation settings, in schools and home care, or in the outpatient setting. When treating patients with CHD, physical therapists should be familiar with the basics of the congenital heart defect, how it affects the child's cardiovascular system during exercise, and the complications that are prevalent in this population. It is also important to note that CHD commonly accompanies other genetic disorders linked to developmental delays, for which they may see a physical therapist.[9]

Most congenital abnormalities of the heart can be detected between 8 and 12 weeks of gestation, and when the heart is no larger than a peanut, although some may not be diagnosed until further in gestation because of imaging technique and growth.[12,13] In most CHD, it is speculated that genetic factors play a role in the acquisition of the defect, but the patterns of inheritance are not always clear, and likely multifactorial.[9,14] There are several single gene mutations that have been identified in relation to genetic syndromes that include CHD (e.g. DiGeorge/22q11.2 microdeletion; CHARGE/CHD7 deletion/mutation).[9] There are numerous types of CHDs, each having its own incidence. Table 19.1 lists the more common of the congenital defects of the heart and their incidence in the general population.

To understand the various types of CHD, one needs to have a clear understanding of normal cardiac development, anatomy, and physiology. It is beyond the scope of this text

TABLE 19.1 Incidence per Live Births of Congenital Heart Lesions	
Ventricular septal defects	1/1000
Patent ductus arteriosus (excluding preterm neonates)	1/2000
Coarctation of the aorta	1/2500
Atrial septal defects	1/3000
Tetralogy of Fallot	1/3500
Transposition of the great arteries	1/3500
Pulmonary stenosis	1/4000
Aortic valve stenosis	1/4500
Hypoplastic left heart syndrome	1/5500
Total anomalous pulmonary venous return	1/15,000
Tricuspid atresia	1/15,500
Truncus arteriosus	1/16,000
Pulmonary atresia	1/16,500

Wernovsky G, Gruber P. Common congenital heart disease: presentation, management and outcomes. In: Taeusch H, Ballard R, Gleason C, eds. *Avery's Diseases of the Newborn. 8th ed*. Philadelphia, PA: Elsevier Saunders; 2004:827–872.

to review cardiopulmonary physiology in detail; there are numerous excellent cardiopulmonary texts to which you can refer.[15,16]

Cardiac system development

The heart begins to form with four main components: (1) primary cardiac tube, (2) secondary, anterior heart field, (3) tertiary field cells, and (4) cardiac neural crest cells.[12] These four components combine in a modular fashion to eventually develop into the basic four ventricles in the fetus. The primary cardiac tube forms the majority of the left ventricle, the secondary anterior field cells develop into the right ventricle and outflow tract, the tertiary field cells contribute to the atrial chambers and to portions of each ventricle. The cardiac neural crest cells contribute to the aortic arch and coronaries. The component cells balloon and divide to connect to form the heart. Initially, there is a single ventricle leading into a large single vessel called the truncus arteriosus, and eventually the components bend and loop around to form two ventricles that separate as the septum grows vertically, and the truncus arteriosus separates into the aorta and pulmonary artery. The aortic and pulmonary valves develop, and the pulmonary artery loops around to lie in front of the aorta and attaches to the right ventricle. The foramen ovale remains open to allow blood to pass between the two atria, and the ductus arteriosus (DA) allows a connection between the aorta and the pulmonary artery. The four-ventricle heart is complete by 8 weeks of gestation, at which point the atria come to lie near the embryo's head and the ventricle toward the feet.[12] By 12 weeks, the heart is positioned normally in the fetal chest and is approximately 8 mm in length.[12] Development is primarily complete between the 10th and 12th weeks of gestation; thus these first weeks are the critical period of cardiac development. Between 12 and 17 weeks, the heart doubles in size, and by 21 weeks' gestation triples in size.[12] During life in the womb, the right ventricle is dominant, with most of the fetal blood bypassing the lungs and reaching the left ventricle through the foramen ovale or the DA[17] (see Fig. 19.1).

Normal Fetal Circulation

The fetal heart does not depend on the lungs for respiration, owing to high pulmonary resistance.[17] Rather, the fetus uses the low-resistance circulatory pathway of the

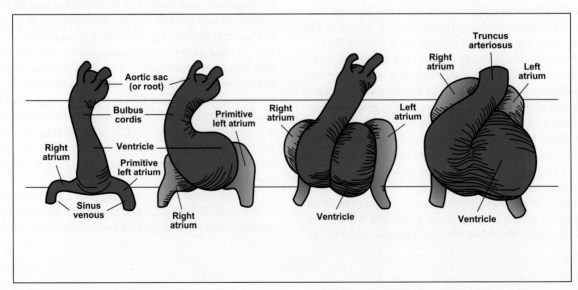

FIGURE 19.1 Cardiac system development in the fetus.

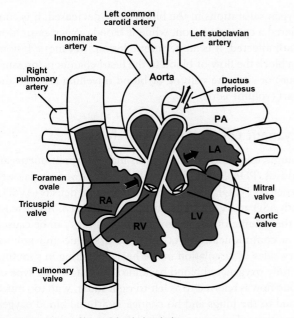

FIGURE 19.2 Normal fetal circulation.

placenta to obtain oxygen and to get rid of carbon dioxide (Fig. 19.2). In the fetus, the right and left ventricles exist in a parallel circuit. Blood travels through the umbilical vein through the ductus venosus to the fetal heart via the inferior vena cava to the right atrium, and through the foramen ovale to the left atrium. The superior vena cava leads to the right atrium, to the right ventricle, to the pulmonary artery, to the lungs or DA, bypassing the lungs, into the descending aorta to perfuse the bilateral lower extremities and body, then travels back to the placenta via

the umbilical arteries.[17] The blood travelling through the left ventricle to the aorta perfuses the brain and upper extremities.[17] All of the blood flowing through the various chambers of the heart, as well as the arteries and veins, are rich in oxygen. In the fetus, the vessels of the pulmonary circulation are vasoconstricted, leading to high pulmonary vascular resistance.[17] Any blood travelling to the lungs, all of which is oxygen rich, will be utilized to develop and nourish lung tissue.

Changes Associated with Birth

At birth, several changes occur within the circulatory system. Figure 19.3 shows normal cardiac anatomy before and after birth. As the first breath is taken, the lungs expand with air, and lung pressure falls; this allows blood to flow more easily into the lungs.[17] After reaching the lungs, the blood returns to the left atrium, which causes pressure to be higher on the left of the atrial septum than on the right. This pressure differential and the increase in oxygen levels causes the foramen ovale, DA, and ductus venosus to functionally close shortly after birth.[17] The foramen ovale closes anatomically by 9 to 30 months, the DA by 2 to 3 months, and the ductus venosus by 7 to 14 days of life.[17] The body now relies on the lungs for obtaining oxygen and expelling carbon dioxide, and maintains separation of oxygenated and deoxygenated blood.

Normal Circulation After Birth

The heart is now essentially two pumps working in unison to propel blood through the blood vessels to the body. The

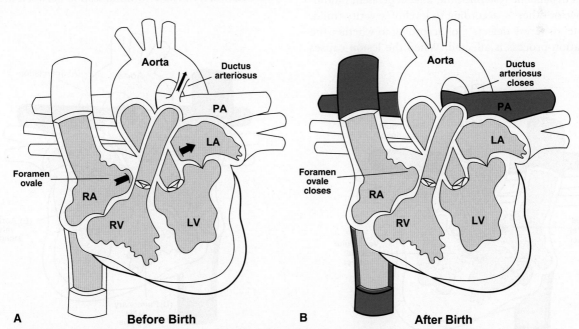

FIGURE 19.3 Normal cardiac structures **(A)** before and **(B)** after birth. (From Neill C, Clark EB, Clark C. *From Birth to Adolescence, from Doctor's Office to Playground. The Heart of a Child: What Families Need to Know about Heart Disorders in Children.* London, England: Johns Hopkins University Press; 1992)

right side of the heart receives deoxygenated blood from the body and pumps it through the pulmonary artery to the lungs. The left side receives oxygenated blood from the lungs and pumps it through the aorta to the body. Blood enters the right atrium via the inferior vena cava and superior vena cava and travels through the tricuspid valve to the right ventricle and then through the pulmonary valve. The pulmonary valve consists of three semilunar cusps and prevents blood from returning to the right ventricle from the lungs. The blood then travels through the pulmonary artery to the lung and back through four pulmonary veins, which enter the posterior wall of the left atrium with no valves at the openings. The left atrioventricular valve, or the mitral valve, sits between the left atrium and ventricle and allows oxygenated blood from the left atrium to pass into the left ventricle. The left ventricle pumps the blood through the aortic valve, which also has three semilunar cusps leading to the aorta. The aortic valve is similar to the pulmonary valve except that its cusps are thicker and placed slightly differently. The left ventricle has a greater amount of pressure than the right ventricle on account of higher systemic pressure of the body versus the lungs. Figure 19.3B demonstrates normal cardiac anatomy.

▶ Congenital heart defects

At any point in the development of the cardiac system, problems can arise leading to a CHD. It may be a persistent fetal pathway or a problem due to development of the heart. Congenital heart defects are traditionally classified by the direction of altered blood flow (left-to-right shunting, duct dependent systemic flow, duct dependent pulmonary flow, or other[14]), according to level of severity (mild, moderate, or severe defects[1]), or according to whether the oxygenation process is affected. When the lesion causes

oxygen saturations in the blood to be decreased, it is considered a cyanotic lesion, while if blood oxygen saturation is not affected, it is an acyanotic lesion. Acyanotic lesions can block the flow of blood to the heart chambers (pressure issue) or alter the volume of blood travelling through the heart (volume issue).

Acyanotic Congenital Heart Defects

Volume-related acyanotic lesions include patent ductus arteriosus (PDA), atrial septal defects (ASD), ventricular septal defects (VSD), and atrioventricular canal defects (AVSD). Both ASD and VSD are pictured in Figure 19.4. An increase in the volume of blood flowing to the lungs can be caused by a communication between the systemic and pulmonary sides of circulation in the heart, resulting in shunting of fully oxygenated blood back into the lungs. This type of blood flow is referred to as left-to-right shunt, with too much blood to the lungs and no change in arterial blood oxygen saturations. The symptoms for defects that lead to increased pulmonary blood flow include rapid breathing, even when asleep, as a consequence of congested lungs; delayed growth, as the extra calories are used by abnormal circulation and rapid breathing; sweating; heart failure; and severe difficulty in feeding.[14] Pressure-related acyanotic lesions include coarctation of the aorta, aortic stenosis, and pulmonary stenosis, and lead to increased pressure as blood leaves either ventricle. These lesions are demonstrated in Figure 19.5A–C.

Patent Ductus Arteriosus

PDA is associated with maternal rubella and prematurity. It occurs when the fetal communication between the aorta

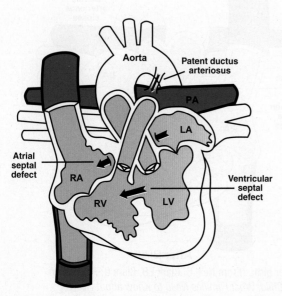

FIGURE 19.4 Atrial and ventricular septal defects and PDA.

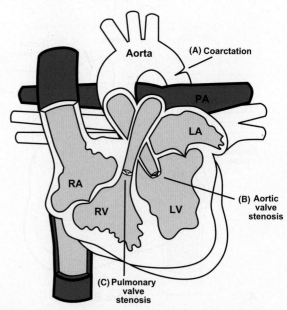

FIGURE 19.5 Several common congenital heart defects. **(A)** Coarctation of the aorta. **(B)** Pulmonary valve stenosis. **(C)** Aortic valve stenosis.

and the pulmonary artery (the DA described above) remains open after birth and allows blood flow between the two vessels. When the shunt does not close as it should, this is a PDA, and the pressure differential between the left and right sides of the heart causes too much blood to go to the lungs. The symptoms depend on the size of the opening and the degree of prematurity. A large opening can cause pulmonary congestion, congestive heart failure (CHF), and edema. Indomethacin may be given to decrease prostaglandin production to close the PDA in premature infants. In a full-term baby, surgery may be required if prostaglandins are unable to close the DA (see Fig. 19.4).

Atrial Septal Defects

An ASD is a hole in the wall separating the atria. This is most often caused by a patent foramen ovale, where the oval-shaped hole in the atrial wall that should close soon after birth does not close. Many ASDs will close spontaneously in the first few years of life. If it does not close, over many years, an ASD causes low pressure at the atrium and, consequently, results in gradual enlargement of the right atrium and ventricle. Symptoms include a heart murmur, an overactive right ventricle, and a large pulmonary artery. Surgery is usually performed if the ASD does not get closed by 2 to 3 years of age.[14] Surgery generally includes placing a Dacron patch or inserting a clamshell device via a catheter. Some surgeons will anticoagulate up to 6 months postoperatively to prevent clotting.

Ventricular Septal Defects

The ventricular septum consists of three distinct areas that fuse together to form the singular solid muscle wall of the ventricles. A VSD occurs when there is a failure of this fusion. With a VSD, some of the oxygen-rich blood in the left ventricle that should be pumped through the aorta is ejected directly to the right ventricle through a hole in the ventricular wall. Up to 50% of small VSDs close spontaneously and never become symptomatic.[14] With a large defect, excess blood goes to the lung and causes pulmonary congestion, which leads to shortness of breath. A large volume of blood returns from the lungs to the left heart, which, over time, becomes overburdened and enlarged. Heart failure may even occur causing a backup of fluid in the lungs and other body tissues. For individuals with a large VSD, the signs and symptoms include dyspnea, feeding difficulties, poor growth, profuse perspiration, recurrent pulmonary infections, cardiac failure in early infancy, respiratory distress, and growth failure. If a VSD becomes symptomatic, it will require surgery, which is similar to that with the ASD with a Dacron patch to close the defect in the ventricle wall.

Atrioventricular Septal Defects

A complete AVSD involves the portion of the heart where the atrial septum meets the ventricular septum as well as the mitral and tricuspid valves. The result is a large hole spanning the septum and the presence of one large valve on both sides. If the defect includes the entire septum, it is considered a complete common atrioventricular canal (CAVC). Blood flow shunts left to right because of the greater force generated by the left myocardium. Signs and symptoms include lung congestion, pulmonary hypertension, increased work of breathing, and feeding intolerance. AVSDs are associated with Down syndrome: 70% of patients with CAVC have Down syndrome.[14] This defect will require surgery in the first few months of life.

Coarctation of Aorta

In coarctation of the aorta, the aorta is pinched or narrowed after it leaves the heart. This defect increases pressure in the arteries closest to the heart, the head, and the arms, causing upper body hypertension, with reduced circulation and diminished pulses in the lower extremities. Coarctation in newborns is not evident until the DA closes and the obstruction of blood flow from the left ventricle results in heart failure and shock, requiring respiratory support and prostaglandin E_1 to reopen the ductus.[14] The problem occurs after DA closure because as the ductus closes, it shortens into a thin cord, and like a noose, this cord pinches off the aorta, making it narrower where the DA was located. The left ventricle then has to pump blood directly through the constriction, often resulting in left ventricular failure and symptoms including increased work of breathing, sweating, and wheezing. Symptoms in older children may include headache, leg cramps, and a pale appearance. Blood pressure differs from upper extremities (high) to lower extremities (low). Most children require surgery to remove the constriction and reconnect the aorta.[14] In 10% to 15% of children, re-coarctation occurs, requiring further intervention, often with balloon dilation via angioplasty.[14]

Aortic Stenosis

Aortic stenosis occurs when there is a fusion, thickening, or narrowing of the aortic valve. This valve defect leads to obstruction of flow from the left ventricle to the aorta, increasing the work of the left ventricle to pump to the body. Aortic stenosis is often identified at birth when an infant is critically ill with left ventricular failure and shock.[14] If found later, signs and symptoms may include fatigue, murmur, chest pain, fainting, or arrhythmia. Surgical intervention options include using balloon dilation via catheterization, performing valvuloplasty to separate fused leaflets of valve or artificial valve replacement.

Pulmonary Stenosis

Pulmonary stenosis occurs with a fused, thickened, or missing pulmonary valve or thickening of the area below or above the valve. This stenosis leads to pulmonary valve obstruction, causing increased work of the right ventricle to pump to the lungs. Signs and symptoms may include respiratory distress, fatigue, murmur, or chest pain. Just as with aortic stenosis, surgical intervention options include using balloon dilation via catheterization, performing valvuloplasty to separate fused leaflets of the valve, or using a homograft to replace the stenotic valve or artery.[14]

Cyanotic Heart Defects

A cyanotic heart defect causes a decrease in oxygen saturation, which causes the lips, toes, toenail beds, and fingernails to appear blue (*cyanosis* is Greek for blue). The resulting chronic arterial oxygen desaturation stimulates erythropoiesis, increased red blood cell formation, which results in polycythemia, an overabundance of red blood cells. This condition increases blood viscosity, which heightens the risk of cerebrovascular accidents and microvascular problems. The cyanotic heart defects include tetralogy of Fallot (TOF), double-outlet right ventricle (DORV), transposition of the great arteries (TGA), and hypoplastic left heart syndrome (HLHS) as shown in Figures 19.6–19.9.

Tetralogy of Fallot

TOF is the most common cyanotic congenital heart defect and has four components.[14] The first basic component is a large VSD with blood mixing freely between the ventricles. The second component is pulmonary stenosis, which causes a right ventricular outflow tract obstruction. The third component is an aorta positioned above the VSD (overriding aorta). Finally, hypertrophy of the right ventricle is caused by increased pressure due to the right ventricular outflow obstruction. Blood flow to the pulmonary artery is obstructed, so oxygen-poor blood finds it easier to enter the aorta than the pulmonary artery. The resulting

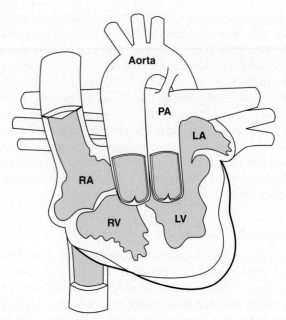

FIGURE 19.7 Transposition of the great arteries.

decreased oxygen levels in the arteries and tissues of the body cause cyanosis with symptoms of tiring easily, fainting, and shock.[14] Surgical correction to optimize outcomes is typically performed as early in a child's life as possible.[14] Figure 19.6 depicts TOF.

TGA and DORV

TGA (Fig. 19.7) occurs when the aortic artery arises from the right ventricle and the pulmonary artery from the left ventricle.[14] These errors cause deoxygenated blood to circulate around the body and the already oxygenated blood returns to the lungs. In DORV (Fig. 19.8), the aorta and the

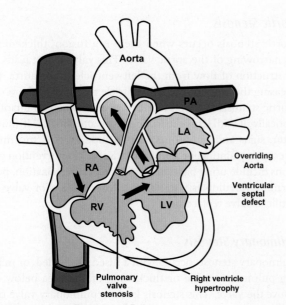

FIGURE 19.6 Tetralogy of Fallot.

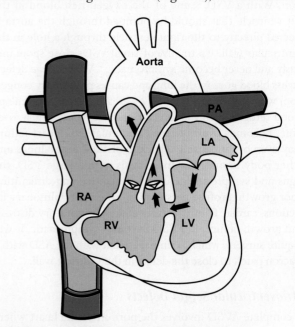

FIGURE 19.8 Double-outlet right ventricle.

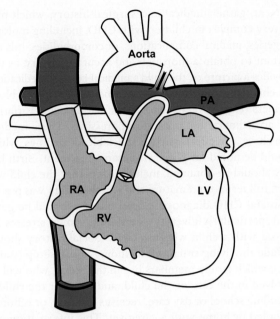

FIGURE 19.9 Hypoplastic left heart syndrome.

pulmonary artery arise from the right ventricle. The only outlet from the left ventricle is via a VSD, which shunts blood into the right ventricle and causes mixing of oxygenated and deoxygenated blood leaving the heart.[14] Signs and symptoms include cyanosis, poor feeding, poor weight gain, decreased appetite, and increased respiratory rate. One-third of children with TGA require urgent intervention within hours of birth to create an ASD to allow mixing of blood. All children with TGA eventually have an arterial switch operation to repair the defect a few days after birth.[14]

Hypoplastic Left Heart Syndrome

HLHS is the most serious of the congenital malformations with the poorest prognosis (Fig. 19.9). In HLHS, the left ventricle is underdeveloped or absent, and the mitral valve and/or aortic valve is atretic or too small. The presence of a PDA keeps the child alive by allowing flow from the left atrium back to the right heart. Signs and symptoms include cyanosis, poor feeding, poor weight gain, increased work of breathing, lethargy, and ultimately shock and multiorgan failure. Symptoms are usually minimal until the DA closes. Keeping the DA open with prostaglandin E_1 until surgery can be performed keeps the child alive. Children with HLHS typically undergo a three-stage repair.[18] In the first stage, the Blalock–Taussig shunt or Norwood procedure, a shunt is placed between innominate or aorta and pulmonary arteries to balance blood flow between heart and lungs. This typically occurs in the first few months of life. The second stage, the bidirectional Glenn procedure, occurs around 8 months of age. In this operation, the shunt is taken down, and the superior vena cava is connected to the pulmonary artery, allowing more venous blood to be oxygenated. The inferior vena cava still does not go to the lungs. The final stage,

or Fontan surgery, is typically done between 3 and 6 years of age.[18,19] The inferior vena cava is attached directly to the pulmonary artery, and an opening or fenestration is made to allow extra blood to go back to the right atrium. Following the Fontan completion, all venous blood goes to the lungs. This staged repair is a palliative surgery and may have late complications.[18,19] If the palliation fails, heart transplantation may be suggested as an option.[18]

▶ Heart transplantation

Heart transplantation may be recommended for children with less than 2 years of predicted survival due to heart failure, which may be associated with CHD, but may also be caused by cardiomyopathy. Congestive heart failure is a syndrome with many pathophysiologic and compensatory mechanisms in the body's attempt to maintain the normal ventricular ejection of blood from the heart to the vital organs. Right heart failure presents with hepatomegaly, peripheral edema, and cyanosis. Left heart failure presents with pulmonary edema and poor perfusion. The clinical presentations of CHF are listed in Table 19.2. Heart failure occurs in some children with CHD owing to the nature of their artificial circulatory systems. For example, the use of the right ventricle as the main systemic circulation ventricle may cause the right ventricle to fail, as it is not intended to pump against systemic pressures.[19]

Heart transplantation is generally considered for children with end-stage heart disease that is unresponsive to medical management or when conventional surgical intervention is not a realistic or viable option.[20,21] Transplantation is truly the exchanging of a set of undesirable lethal circumstances for another set of circumstances. Transplantation presents a lifelong risk of graft loss (acute and chronic rejection), graft coronary disease, nonspecific graft failure, death from infection, oncogenesis, and other organ failure.[21] Complex CHD and cardiomyopathy account for 90% of pediatric heart transplantations; however, two-thirds of *infant* heart transplants are due to CHD, while two-thirds of *adolescent*

TABLE 19.2 Clinical Presentation of CHF	
Onset of Rapid Breathing	**Change in Behavior**
Edema	Irritability
Fatigue	Excessive sweating
Poor feeding	Vomiting
Oliguria	Tachycardia
Pulmonary/systemic vein	Peripheral vasoconstriction
Engorgement	Wheezing
Tachypnea	Nasal flaring
Chest retractions	
Failure to thrive	

heart transplants are due to cardiomyopathy.[21,22] In 2009 (latest report), nearly 550 heart transplants were performed, with the distribution evenly spread between three age groups (infants, children aged 1 to 10, and adolescents).[22] In the first year of life, children with a single ventricle, such as HLHS and DORV, have the greatest risk of requiring transplantation.[21]

A heart transplant operation involves excising the original heart, inserting the donor heart, and then performing a re-anastomosis of atria and great arteries to the donor heart. The vagus nerve is removed, and the sympathetic cardiac nerves are severed. This means that a transplanted heart is denervated. Without the vagus nerve there is loss of sympathetic control of heart, which causes an altered heart rate response, higher resting heart rate, and lower heart rate increase with exercise.[20,23]

Survival data continue to improve each year as techniques and postoperative management is refined.[21] The overall 5-year survival rate for pediatric cardiac transplant is about 70%. The median survival (the age at which 50% of recipients are still alive) for children receiving transplants is 18.4 years in infancy, 16.4 years during childhood, and 12.0 years during adolescence.[22]

Heart transplantation has its own set of circumstances, of which the physical therapist must be aware. Physical therapists mainly need to be aware of the denervation of the heart posttransplantation. Immediately after heart transplantation, patients have a higher resting heart rate, lower exercise heart rate, and a lower heart rate recovery.[23] One longitudinal study showed that each year following transplant, patients' resting heart rate drops, and exercise heart rate and heart rate recovery increase, suggesting that pediatric heart transplant recipients may have the ability for long-term reinnervation.[23] For the physical therapist this means that warm ups and cooldowns are vital for exercise, which we will talk about in more detail later in the chapter.

▶ Physical therapy examination

History

A physical therapy examination should begin with a thorough history, including demographic information, medical/surgical history, family and social history, developmental history, and chief complaint. Demographics of the patient and family include age, date of birth, primary language, and race. It is important to recognize that families come from all over the world to centers that perform the delicate operations for children with CHD. The family should be an integral part of physical therapy intervention, so understanding the family structure, culture, and background will assist you in involving the family in all aspects of the care of their child.[24] A complete discussion of family-centered care is found in Chapter 1.

Next, gather medical and surgical history, which may be very complex in children with CHD, including multiple surgeries, medical complications, or comorbidities. It is important to obtain a thorough and accurate history, as this provides a picture of the child's medical course. Medications the child is taking should be documented, including blood thinners (e.g., Lovenox/enoxaparin, Coumadin/warfarin), anti-arrhythmics, and immunosuppressives. These medications have side effects such as quick bleeding times, which should be noted for physical therapy treatment. Birth history should be obtained, including whether the child was born full term or premature and whether there was pre- or postnatal CHD diagnosis. Social history should be gathered, particularly given the numerous family stresses involved with a child who has CHD. Social history should include the living situation, including house setup (stairs, etc.), which family members live in the home, who will be involved in the care of the child, and whether the child is attending school or day care, receives tutoring, or is homeschooled or home with a caregiver. This information can help determine who needs to be involved in care, as well as discharge recommendations or education/training needs. Family history is also important information to gather, including birth order, siblings or relatives with CHD, or other medical history. It may be important to discuss with the family that a child with a CHD is very different from, for example, an uncle who died from atherosclerosis.

Developmental history includes gathering information about developmental skill achievement and the age at which the child achieved various developmental milestones. Is the child or are siblings receiving early intervention services or have they ever received other therapies? A developmental history should also include questions regarding daily schedules, sleep patterns, prior level of function, and ability to perform activities of daily living (ADLs).

A final component of history gathering is the child and family's chief complaint. The chief complaints for infants with CHD are generally poor feeding, failure to thrive, or delayed milestones. Chief complaints for adolescents are often lethargy, fatigue, general malaise, and exercise intolerance. It is important to understand what the family believes is the main reason for a hospitalization, episode of outpatient therapy, or early intervention services. A thorough history of current signs and symptoms will assist the physical therapist in determining appropriate examination techniques.

Laboratory Values

Numerous laboratory values are important to the physical therapist. The most basic of these is a complete blood count (CBC). A CBC gives information about hemoglobin levels, white blood cells, and other basic functions. Along with a CBC, some children may have International normalized ratio (INR) or Anti-Xa levels that indicate how much the blood is thinned or thickened. A higher value indicates the blood is thinner and represents a higher risk of bleeding,

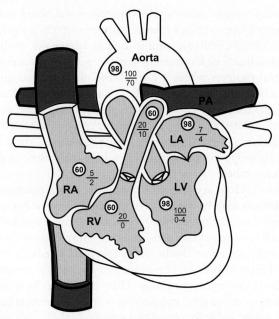

FIGURE 19.10 Cardiac catheterization values in a normal heart.

TABLE 19.3	Age-Appropriate Arterial Blood Gases		
	pH	PCO$_2$	PO$_2$
Preterm infant at 1–5 hr	7.29–7.37	39–56	52–67
Term infant at 5 hr	7.31–7.37	32–39	62–86
Preterm and term infant at 5 days	7.34–7.42	32–41	62–92
Children, adolescents, adults	7.35–7.45	35–45	80–100

acidosis. Hyperventilation causes a shift to the left with a decrease in CO$_2$ and an increase in pH, causing a respiratory alkalosis. A PaO$_2$ of 60 to 80 mm Hg corresponds with a SaO$_2$ of 90% to 95%, which is mild hypoxia. A PaO$_2$ of 40 to 60 mm Hg corresponds with a SaO$_2$ of 60% to 90%, or moderate hypoxia. A PaO$_2$ of less than 40 mm Hg corresponds with a SaO$_2$ of less than 60% and is considered severe hypoxia.

Vital Signs

Arterial blood gas determination often requires an invasive line and is not always indicated. Pulse oximeters may provide a proxy for saturations. Other vital signs to consider are heart rate, blood pressure, and respiratory rate. Consider these values for patients at rest, and observe how they change with position changes and activity to give an indication of the child's cardiovascular response to activity. The trends of the vital signs are very important. If possible, a resting cardiac rhythm strip should be examined for arrhythmia. A sinus tachycardia is commonly found in response to low cardiac output. Be aware of other conditions, such as transplantation, that may impact heart rate or rhythms as noted above. Be sure to monitor vital signs as you assess strength, functional mobility, and exercise tolerance.

General Appearance

During any physical examination of a child, always discuss with the parents the best way to approach the infant or toddler. For young children, begin with play when able. Let them explore the equipment you have with you, including stethoscopes or blood pressure cuffs. For adolescents, explain what your purpose is for being there, and explain to them and their caregiver what you will be doing. Utilize age and cognitively appropriate descriptions of the activities that you will be performing. This explanation should precede the actual examination. While introducing yourself and explaining your role, assess the child's state of consciousness. Some children with CHD will be very ill at initial examination. Some patients may be on musculoskeletal blockade, due to the inability of their cardiovascular system to tolerate any movement or excitement, while others may be more lightly sedated or fully engaged. The state of consciousness

while a lower number represents a greater risk of clotting. If the child has had a recent cardiac catheterization, the values from that procedure identify the central pressures and oxygen saturations. These values provide a baseline for how much mixing between oxygenated and deoxygenated blood occurs, and the degree to which central pressures are altered. As oxygen saturations decrease, there may be increasing complaints of fatigue, dizziness, lethargy, and general malaise. Figure 19.10 shows normal heart catheterization values for the various chambers of the heart. The values in the circles are the oxygen saturations, and the other values are the normal pressures for the various chambers and vessels of the heart.

A cardiac catheterization is an invasive examination where catheters are inserted into a vein in the groin and threaded into the heart under fluoroscopic guidance. The catheter enters the systemic venous and arterial systems to measure hemodynamic pressures and oxygen saturations. Radiographic material may be injected through the catheters to take cine radiographs of the heart and its structures. The right ventricle and pulmonary artery pressures are usually about one-fifth that of the left ventricle and aorta because of the high systemic pressure the left side of the heart must overcome to pump blood out of the aorta. The right heart is the deoxygenated side and generally has oxygen saturations in the 60s; the left side is the oxygenated side with the oxygen saturations in the high 90s (98% to 100%).

Age-Appropriate Arterial Blood Gas Values

Arterial blood is the most reliable way to assess O$_2$ transport (Table 19.3). Hypoventilation causes a shift to the right on the normal oxyhemoglobin dissociation curve with an increase in CO$_2$ and a decrease in pH, causing a respiratory will dictate the level to which the patient can cooperate with simple commands appropriate for age. Document the use or discontinuation of any supportive equipment or devices to give you an idea of the child's current or past health status, as well as to begin to consider needs for positioning and scar management. These devices and lines will vary by setting and acuity, and will be discussed in more detail later in the chapter. Assess the child for edema or ascites, which may result from retained fluid or abdominal fluid overload when the heart becomes unable to maintain adequate cardiac output. Note general coloring—anemia causes paleness, polycythemia causes plethora, and oxygen desaturation causes cyanosis. Assess the individual's body type as cachectic, obese, or appropriate for age.

Pain

Pain should be well documented with age-appropriate pain scales. For children who can verbalize and rate their own pain, a self-report of pain is preferred using a visual analog scale (VAS) or the Wong-Baker FACES scale.[25,26] An observational/behavioral pain scale may be used. These include the face, legs, activity, cry, consolability (FLACC) or the COMFORT scale, which have been validated for infants and young children,[27] in postoperative cardiac care,[28] and for critically ill children in intensive-care settings.[29,30]

A simple rating scale or VAS has a child rate their pain on a scale from 0 to 10 or to mark along a 10-cm line, with 0 being no pain and 10 the worst pain.[26] The Wong-Baker FACES is for children with a cognitive age of 3 to 7 years and uses a VAS from no hurt to hurts worst.[25] The FLACC assessment scale is a behavioral scale that has the rater observe five categories: face, legs, activity, cry, and consolability. Each category is scored from 0 to 2: A 0 is a relaxed and calm behavior, a 1 is an increase in pain behaviors noted, and a 2 is the most pain in each category. Therefore, a total score of 10 means the worst pain, and the range of scores is 0 to 10.[27] The COMFORT scale, another behavioral scale, has the observer examine and rate seven areas: alertness, calmness, respiratory response, cry, physical movement, muscle tone, and facial tension. Each area is rated 1 through 5, with 1 being the least pain and 5 the most pain, with the highest score being 35.[29] The management of pain is very important, as it impacts both movement and respiratory function. You will be better able to treat your patients if there is good pain control. This may mean requesting a directed time for pain medication and scheduling therapy around pain medications.

Equipment and Devices

Most children in the inpatient setting with CHD will have cardiorespiratory monitors and pulse oximetry continuously monitoring their vital signs. Many children will have a peripheral intravenous line, arterial line, or central line. An arterial line is placed directly into the artery and can be used to continuously monitor blood pressure and blood gases. A central line, such as a Broviac catheter or port, is inserted into central circulation and is used to administer medications or fluids, or for drawing blood. A peripherally inserted central catheter is also a central line that is placed more distally to the heart, generally in an arm. Postsurgically, patients may have chest tubes in place to help drain fluid. Some children may have supplemental oxygen delivered by oxygen masks, nasal cannulas, or oxygen hoods. Those requiring supplemental nutrition may have nasogastric or gastrotomy tubes.

As children require more support, other equipment or devices may be introduced, including pacer wires, mechanical ventilation, extracorporeal membrane oxygenation (ECMO), or ventricular assist devices (VAD). Pacer wires are centrally placed on the heart for emergent needs for electrical intervention for the heart and are usually removed within 7 days postoperatively. These lines must be treated with respect and care, and patients with pacer wires in place may not be stable for out-of-bed activity.

ECMO is similar to a heart–lung machine, supplying an artificial heart and lung outside the body. The machine adds oxygen into the blood and removes carbon dioxide, giving the patient's heart and lungs time to rest and heal. ECMO does not cure the disease; it just gives the child physiological support as he or she heals. Indications for ECMO include acute transplant rejection and respiratory failure. ECMO is generally used for short-term treatment and is considered a bridge to transplant or recovery.[31] In Figure 19.11, a child is receiving ECMO. During ECMO, a physical therapist will provide a positioning program to maintain midline orientation of the limbs, especially positioning of the lower extremities to prevent contractures. It is important not to kink the blood flow circuit; therefore, passive range of motion of some joints may be contraindicated. There are many sequelae of ECMO including stroke, necrosis of the extremities (especially distally), and thrombosis. It is important to be aware of these sequelae as a child is being removed from ECMO.

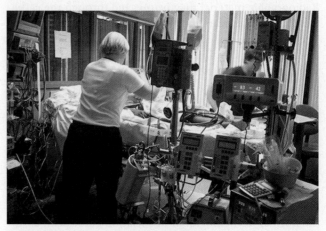

FIGURE 19.11 A child receiving ECMO.

A VAD is an external device that assists the right or left ventricle to pump blood. A left VAD will assist pumping to systemic circulation, while a right VAD will assist pumping to pulmonary circulation. Adults have been using VADs for many years and include internal device options. To date, only external VAD options are approved for use in children of all ages, although internal options for pediatric populations are under development.[31]

VADs can be utilized over a long period, often as a bridge to transplantation, and they allow for exercise conditioning and training while awaiting transplantation.[32] The VAD monitors heart rate, stroke volume, and cardiac output, but blood pressure and oxygen saturation are monitored manually. It is important to consider subjective reports of exertion, pain, and dyspnea.[32] The literature suggests patients should participate in early mobilization as soon as medically stable following VAD placement.[32] Exercise training should progress as tolerated while a VAD remains in place. A child with a left VAD can be seen ambulating in Figure 19.12. It may be helpful to have patients with a VAD use an athletic support or abdominal binder for upright activities.

Mechanical ventilation is utilized both pre- and postoperatively for children with CHD. Preoperatively, the ventilator is used to assist with breathing during respiratory distress. Postoperatively, it is used while returning to breathing independently. The ventilator may be connected to an endotracheal tube or tracheostomy tube. An endotracheal tube may be placed in the nose or mouth to assist with breathing. Figure 19.13 shows a postoperative patient with a nasotracheal tube. Airway suctioning to keep the child clear of secretions is of the utmost value when a child is intubated. Always be sure to clear the ventilator tubing of water prior

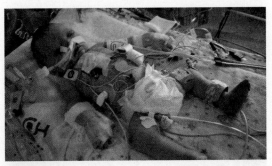

FIGURE 19.13 An infant postoperatively with a nasotracheal tube.

to listening to breath sounds because the water may distort the actual sounds. If physical therapists do not perform suctioning in your venue, make sure a person who is able to suction the child is aware of your interventions, should suctioning be necessary during your treatment. Without a clear airway it is unlikely that gross motor skills will be optimal. Providing midline orientation, especially to prevent a head preference, is very important. Some children will pull away from the ventilator and will have a head preference facing away from the ventilator, while some will hold still facing the ventilator, afraid to move and pull the tubing. Less invasive modes of ventilation may include continuous positive airway pressure (CPAP), bi-level positive airway pressure (BiPAP), nitric oxide ventilation, or oxygen via nasal cannula. Children may require these modes of ventilation continuously or intermittently while sleeping or with activity. It is important to communicate with the medical team to understand the reasons for noninvasive ventilation, as well as to monitor vital signs while working with children using these ventilator modes.

Integument

Examine the state of the integumentary system, beginning with the general appearance of the skin. Does it look glossy, turgid, loose, bruised, or broken down? Anticoagulation can lead to bruising and skin breakdown, and fluid retention can lead to glossy or turgid skin. Examine surgical sites and incisions, including clamshell, median sternotomy, thoracotomy, and small incisions for chest tubes, central lines, or other tubes. These sites may be sutured or stapled closed, but occasionally may be left open with a surgical dressing. Examine scar mobility in all directions. Document whether scars move well or are bound to the tissue underneath, as well as whether scars are painful. A typical chest of a child following heart surgery is seen in Figure 19.14.

Digital clubbing should be examined, and is a sign of prolonged hypoxia, where the tip of the distal phalanx becomes bulbous and the nail of the digit exits at an increased angle. Clubbing is common in patients with cyanotic CHD or chronic lung disease leading to hypoxia. An example of clubbing is presented in Figure 19.15. Examine capillary refill in

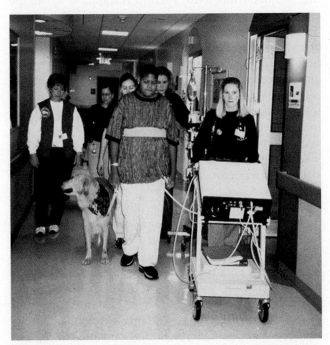

FIGURE 19.12 A child with a left ventricular assist device ambulating with a physical therapist.

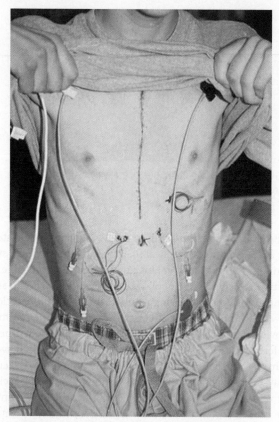

FIGURE 19.14 A child following transplantation with numerous lines and surgical incisions.

the extremities. Push down on the nail bed, which should blanch and rebound 1 to 2 seconds after pressure is relieved. Capillary refill ideally should be assessed by compression of the big toe. Children with CHD are at risk for wounds after their surgical procedures because of long operative times

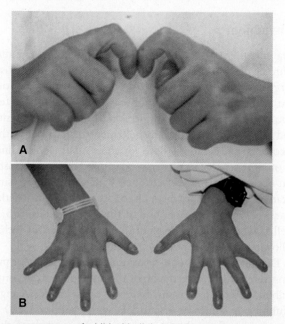

FIGURE 19.15 A child with digital clubbing and cyanosis in his extremities.

with positioning on hard surgical tables at awkward angles to access the necessary organs. Children should be examined after each surgical procedure to view their skin over bony prominences.

Edema should also be assessed. The most common method of assessing edema is to apply pressure with one or two fingers to the affected area for several seconds, then observe how deep the area depresses and how long it takes to return to normal. The result is graded on a 1+ to 4+ scale, where 1+ is the least and 4+ is the worst. Edema may also be assessed using circumferential measurements of the affected area. This method may be helpful to compare changes in the amount of edema over time. Peripheral and central edema may be evident with children with CHD. Peripheral edema is due to the inability of the heart to maintain adequate cardiac output. The autonomic nervous system is attempting to increase cardiac output by retaining fluid from the kidneys. This makes the heart work even harder, and the fluid accumulates in the periphery in the dependent extremities. Central edema or jugular venous distention results from fluid overload as the fluid is retained centrally because the heart's ability to pump is compromised and fluid backs up into the lungs and venous system. Adolescents with Fontan circulation are at risk for lymphatic dysfunction due to increased pulmonary lymphatic pressures, which can result in peripheral or central edema.[19]

Thorax and Respiratory Examination

Thoracic deformities should be examined, including the pectus excavatum, pectus carinatum, barrel chest, rib flaring, and mid-trunk folds. Pectus excavatum is where the chest caves inward, resulting in the tightening of the upper chest musculature. Pectus carinatum is where the chest bows outward, resulting in a deformity of the sternum. Both pectus excavatum and carinatum may be due to surgical procedures or due to altered chest pressures due to respiratory status.[33] Barrel chest deformities can be due to the overinflation of the lung tissue, rib flaring is due to an imbalance of the abdominal muscles with the diaphragm, and a mid-trunk fold is due to muscle imbalance of the chest wall to counteract the diaphragm. Examination of the rib angles and intercostal spaces for age appropriateness and mobility is important.[33–35]

To evaluate the thoracic cage of a child with CHD, the therapist must have knowledge of what an age-appropriate thoracic cage should look like. Newborns have narrow rib spaces, horizontal ribs, a triangular shape to the chest wall, minimal neck space, and chest separate from the abdomen.[35] Three- to six-month-old children will have a normal pectus, more rectangular shape, and horizontal ribs. They will be normal upper chest breathers with only anterior expansion possible. Six- to twelve-month-old children will have an even more pronounced rectangular shape, and lateral expansion will be added to their respiratory

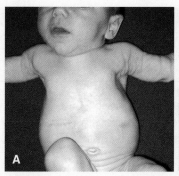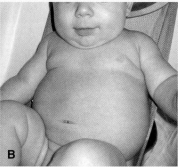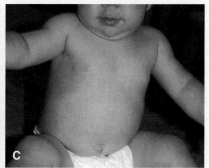

FIGURE 19.16 (A) A newborn and a normal chest wall shape. **(B)** A normal 3-month-old's chest wall shape. **(C)** An 8-month-old child with a normal chest wall.

repertoire, giving them rib space opening as well as increasing the length of the neck. This is a significant stage in the respiratory development of the thorax.[35] There will be a more barrel-shaped appearance of the chest. The rib cage is beginning to be pulled downward owing to a more upright posture and the more continuous effects of gravity on the thorax. This change provides the child a better length-tension relationship for the diaphragm and the intercostal muscles. In this stage, the diaphragm and all the accessory musculature patterns of breathing are available. This trend in the development of the thorax continues for several more years as the rib cage gradually rotates downward and the intercostal spaces widen.[35] Figure 19.16A–C shows a newborn, a 3-month-old, and an 8-month-old with normally configured chest walls. An infant with CHD may have respiratory compromise, which may alter typical muscular function of the chest and, if not addressed, may lead to chest wall deformities.

Examining thoracic cage mobility means ascertaining movement of the ribs. Can the child flex laterally? Do the ribs move with respiration? How is abdominal and upper chest movement? Muscular development should be symmetric without hypertrophy of accessory muscles of respiration. Chest wall movement can be examined by palpation and measurement. By placing your hands over the upper lobe of the lungs with the heel of the hand at the fourth rib, fingertips at the upper trapezii, and thumb at the sternal angle, you may examine symmetry, extent of movement, and general movement. Measure the thoracic circumference with a tape measure at three levels: axilla/3rd rib, xiphoid, and half way from xiphoid to umbilicus. Wrap a tape measure around the thorax until it overlaps, then measure the change in circumference during normal inhalation and exhalation. Adult data suggest that during quiet breathing, the chest wall should move approximately 2 to 3 mm at the upper chest, 3 to 4 mm at the lower chest, and 6 to 7 mm at the abdomen; during deep inhalation, it should move 19 to 18 mm at the upper chest, 16 to 20 mm at the lower chest, and 17 to 25 mm at the abdomen.[36] These values vary slightly by gender. No published data exist for pediatric values.

Children with CHD may present with respiratory issues as their primary complaint, given the integral relationship between the heart and lungs. Including respiratory examination as detailed in Chapter 20 will assist in your evaluation of the patient's status.

Musculoskeletal Examination

An examination of range of motion, postural alignment, and sensation is also necessary. Scoliosis, kyphosis, or a syndromic deviation of the musculoskeletal system may be present and can impact the child's posture, respiration, and pain before, during, or after surgery for CHD. Figure 19.17 shows common postural deviations in a child with CHD. Flexibility can be examined by functional range of motion, a sit-and-reach test, and lateral flexion measurements. Measure from the axilla to the base of the ribs and then the base of the ribs to the pelvis; there should be a 1:2 ratio. Nerve palsies and signs of thrombosis are also important to screen for as they can happen during prolonged positioning or with altered anticoagulation.

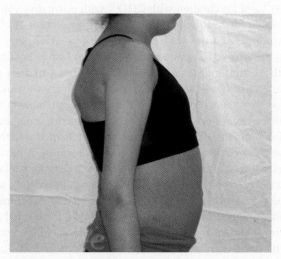

FIGURE 19.17 A child with common postural deviations associated with CHD.

Strength

Measurement of strength must consider children who are at risk for myopathy, osteopenia, and osteoporosis secondary to steroids preoperatively or following transplantation. Consider both manual muscle testing and dynamometry. Manual muscle testing may not offer an accurate measure of the child's strength, whereas dynamometry can provide an alternative, objective means to specifically assess strength. Be sure to teach breathing techniques while assessing strength to avoid Valsalva maneuver during exertion. Consider using an eight-repetition maximum to fatigue, rather than a one-repetition maximum so as to determine initial level of resistance.

Functional Mobility

Functional mobility examination includes bed mobility, transfers, balance, gait, and stairs, as well as developmentally appropriate activities. These activities can be evaluated on the first day postoperatively, and again as medical status improves, as well as in the outpatient and early intervention settings. Timing various functional activities, such as transfers, ambulation over a specified distance, or stair climbing, provides useful test–retest data by which to measure progress and may also motivate children to improve. Developmental motor skills should be assessed as able and standardized assessment tools provide an objective assessment of gross motor skills.

Aerobic Capacity and Endurance

Aerobic capacity can be assessed using formal exercise testing or timed walk tests. The 6-minute walk test is a self-paced walking test designed to measure the submaximal level of functional exercise, and is endorsed by the American Thoracic Society as the gold standard for assessment of functional exercise capacity.[37] It has been validated in children[38] and for children with CHD,[39] with normative values available for healthy children as young as 3 years old.[40,41] During a 6-minute walk test, the child is given specific and age-appropriate directions to walk as fast as possible, without running, for a total of six minutes. Children are instructed to walk at their own pace, but to try to walk as far as they can to cover the greatest distance possible in the allotted time. Rest breaks are allowed, but the time keeps going. Patients should be instructed to inform you if they have chest discomfort, dizziness, severe shortness of breath, unsteadiness, or blurred vision. Record the distance walked, rates of perceived exertion (RPE), dyspnea index (DI), and vital signs before, during, and after the testing. Six-minute walk distance correlates with oxygen uptake at maximal exercise (VO$_2$max),[38,39] which has been shown in children with CHD to be correlated with increased risk of heart failure, hospitalization, and death when below 50% of predicted values.[42–44] Thus, the 6-minute walk test can give the physical

TABLE 19.4 Dyspnea Index	Score
Breathlessness barely noticeable	1
Breathlessness moderately bothersome	2
Breathlessness severe, very uncomfortable	3
Most severe breathlessness ever experienced	4

therapist an idea of functional capacity compared with peers, prognostic information, and assist in goal setting.

While assessing aerobic capacity, observe shortness of breath and level of exertion. Breathlessness can be assessed using the DI (Table 19.4). Patients rate how breathless they feel with certain activities, and they respond with a number from a chart you show them. Breathlessness can also be examined by counting how many syllables they are able to speak per breath (8 to 10 syllables per breath is normal) or how long they can maintain a vowel sound without taking a breath (10 to 15 seconds is normal). These measures provide a baseline value to reexamine over time to determine whether ratings, syllables, or time change. Perceived exertion can be monitored using the Borg RPE scale (Table 19.5). Ask the patient, "How hard do you feel you are working?" This is meant to include overall work, breathing, muscle exertion, and fatigue. You want the patient to integrate information from the peripheral working muscles and joints, the cardiovascular and pulmonary systems, and the central nervous system. A rating of 6 is analogous to no work at all, while a rating of 20 is the hardest work ever done. A newer Borg scale from 0 to 10 points is also commonly used.

TABLE 19.5 Borg Rate of Perceived Exertion Scale	
6	
7	Very, very light
8	
9	Very light
10	
11	Fairly light
12	
13	Somewhat hard
14	
15	Hard
16	
17	Very hard
18	
19	Very, very hard
20	

Physical therapy evaluation, diagnosis, and prognosis

Following the physical therapy examination, the therapist must fit all the pieces together and integrate the findings to synthesize the individual's physical therapy diagnosis and prognosis. This process helps to determine the plan of care and the outcomes expected. The goals of a physical therapy plan of care are directly related to examination findings and may include improving the individual's endurance, strength, range of motion/flexibility, balance, functional mobility or gross motor skills, posture, respiratory/ventilatory status, scar and chest wall mobility, chest expansion, airway clearance, and providing patient and family education (Table 19.6). The plan of care should specify the anticipated frequency and duration of physical therapy intervention, as well as the areas to be addressed. Frequency and duration will vary according to individual needs, as well as the setting (e.g., acute care, outpatient, or community settings).

Coordination, Communication, and Documentation

Physical therapists should collaborate with other services, including cardiology, genetics, neurology, otolaryngology, orthopedics, social work, feeding team, occupational therapy, or speech therapy, and recommend consults as needed for specialists not involved. It is important to advocate for the child to gain the services he or she deserves. In the inpatient setting, participating in rounds with the medical team will allow collaboration. In the outpatient or community settings, establishing a relationship with the child's care team will help to determine important medical information or change in status. Several tertiary hospital centers have initiated team-based neurodevelopmental follow-up programs for children with CHD to enable collaboration and regular follow-up on issues across disciplines.

Physical therapy intervention

Patient- and Family-Related Instruction

Family and caregiver education should focus on the family unit as a whole, including the specific needs of the child. It is important to emphasize the difference between CHD and adult coronary artery disease. The child should be able to explore and play within boundaries based on his or her specific CHD, not based upon fear of participation as may happen in adults. Patient and family education should include discussion about sternal precautions, optimal positioning options for different ages, therapy outcomes and role of early intervention, importance of physical activity, and understanding self-limitation. Children and families should start to understand that exercise should be a lifelong habit. Health, wellness, and fitness programs including cardiac rehabilitation programs and YMCA programs are an important component of lifelong health habits. In addition, literature has shown that long-term cardiac outcomes, mortality, self-esteem, and emotional state are all improved with increasing exercise tolerance and motor skills.[42–46]

TABLE 19.6	Physical Therapy Goal Areas and Sample Goals

Endurance
Patient will have improved endurance as evidenced by increased 6-minute walk distance to at least 450 m to keep up with peers.

Strength
Patient will have improved strength by at least 5 lbs on dynamometry in bilateral gluteus maximus and quadriceps to climb stairs independently.

Respiratory/ventilatory status
Patient will have improved respiratory coordination during functional mobility as evidenced by ability to coordinate inhale and exhale with sit-to-stand transfer while maintaining saturation >90%.

Balance
Patient will have increased balance as evidenced by increased score on the Pediatric Balance Scale to 56/56 to maintain safe functional mobility without falls.

Functional mobility or gross motor skills
Patient will have improved gross motor skills to at least 37th percentile on standardized gross motor testing to age-appropriately interact with environment.

Posture
Patient will have improved posture with ability to maintain scapular retraction, chin tuck, and shoulders back for at least 5 minutes while sitting without verbal cues.

Range of motion/flexibility
Patient will have improved hip flexor flexibility with Thomas test to neutral to maintain upright posture for standing and walking.

Scar and chest wall mobility
Patient will have increased sternal scar mobility as evidenced by Vancouver Scar Scale score decrease by at least 3 points to allow full trunk rotation without pain.

Chest expansion
Patient will have improved chest wall expansion while seated as evidenced by increased circumferential excursion by at least 0.5 cm at diaphragm level to improve oxygenation.

Airway clearance
Patient will be independent with use of home airway clearance device with proper technique demonstrated on 3/3 trials without verbal cues.

Patient and family education
Patient's family will be independent with home positioning program as evidenced by 100% return demonstration without cues.

Procedural Interventions

Positioning

Providing and promoting varied positions will enable the physical therapist to begin to achieve goals related to preventing musculoskeletal abnormalities, improving pulmonary parameters, and promoting age-appropriate skills. Proper positioning can help provide midline orientation, prevent contractures, promote development, and improve pulmonary status. Positioning may include turning schedules, special devices or equipment, or recommendations for postures and positions. While a child is inpatient and has had a neuromuscular blockade or sedation, decreased mobility and in-dwelling lines and tubes, rotation schedules can reduce the possibility of skin pressure and breakdown. The therapist must coordinate changes in the infant's position with other nursing procedures to avoid unnecessary stimulation. Positioning devices such as Multi-Podus boots help control plantar flexion contractures, enhance hip rotation, and protect the heel. Molded foot and ankle orthoses, towel rolls, and gel pillows will help prevent secondary integument issues for children with CHD who are not mobile. Scar massage can help prevent binding down of scars after skin healing, enhance skin movement to reduce range-of-motion limitations, and limit deformities from surgical scars. Scar massage can begin 6 weeks after a sternal incision to allow time for bone healing of the sternum.

Positioning can also enhance oxygen transport and pulmonary function. Infants, even those with endotracheal tubes, have increased oxygenation while in prone versus other positions, especially supine.[47] A mismatch of ventilation and perfusion is a common cause of arterial hypoxemia. Small children have better ventilation to the uppermost lung. Larger children have better ventilation to the dependent lung, similar to the adult pattern. Specific body positioning can allow matching of ventilation and perfusion to a specific lobe of the lung.[48] Consider whether the lung has atelectasis versus hyperinflation. Utilize a chart like the one shown in Table 19.7 to place the child in different positions and see where the best ventilation–perfusion matching may be so as to raise SpO_2 and decrease heart rate, blood pressure, and respiratory rate. Prone positioning in infants with CHD can assist with maintaining hip extension range of motion, chest expansion, trunk and head strength, and attainment of gross motor skills.[49,50] Positioning should also play a role in the outpatient or early intervention plan of care to promote optimal lung function, developmental skills, and to allow engagement with the environment. These positions may include prone (as described above) and side lying to encourage reaching in a gravity-eliminated position. Other positioning should be specific to the child's needs.

Postural Education and Awareness

Most therapeutic exercises and activities can begin with postural training and education. This may mean using elastic wrap or other tools for tactile cues during upright posture to minimize thoracic kyphosis and rounded shoulders. Other techniques include exercises to improve postural control, strengthen postural muscles, and hands-on interventions for postural education.

Flexibility

Flexibility exercises should also begin early and, depending on the patient presentation, commonly include stretches for muscles, including pectoralis major, Achilles/gastrocnemius/soleus group, hip flexors, hamstrings, upper extremities, and chest expansion for thoracic cage mobility. Bolsters, balls, and towel rolls for thoracic cage stretching may assist in making stretching tolerable. Stretches may need to be held for long periods and may be completed as part of a home program while a child watches television or reads. All flexibility activities should consider sternal precautions that are present for 6 weeks postoperatively.

Breathing Exercises

Breathing activities should be incorporated into intervention to foster deep breathing, help maintain ventilation, assist with pain control, and promote coordinated breathing patterns. Breathing games such as blowing bubbles, air hockey, blowing a windmill, and sniffing stickers are an excellent start to improve the child's respiratory status. Diaphragmatic breathing training, inspiratory muscle trainers, incentive spirometers, and deep-breathing techniques can be utilized in children as young as 18 months. Finding a strategy that works with the developmental level of the child and one that the child finds "fun" is the goal. More extensive information about breathing exercises can be found in Chapter 20.

TABLE 19.7	Vital Sign Trends								
Breathing Patterns/Vital Sign Trends		RR		SpO$_2$%		HR		BP	
Position	Sequence	1 min	3 min	1 min	3 min	1 min	3 min	1 min	3 min
Supine									
Side lying									
Sitting/upright									
Prone									

BP, blood pressure; HR, heart rate; RR, respiratory rate.

Aerobic and Endurance Training

Aerobic exercise prescription should be individualized on the basis of the previous testing during the physical therapy examination. An exercise regimen should include principles of mode, frequency, duration, and intensity[51] and identified precautions. Mode may be a bicycle, treadmill, elliptical, upper body ergometer (UBE), or may be over-ground exercise such as walking. The frequency should be a minimum of three times a week and up to seven times a week. When a child is very ill, the duration may be as little as short bouts of 2 to 5 minutes, with rest breaks between bouts. Lower-intensity stretching may be tolerated during rest breaks. Duration should progress to 30 to 45 minutes as the child improves or transitions to the outpatient or early intervention setting. Intensity can be determined from a stress or functional exercise test performed prior to training. Generally, intensity should begin at 60% to 65% of the maximal level of work. Intensity can also be prescribed on the basis of RPE with the Borg scale, which should fall between 11 and 15 on the 20-point scale. Very deconditioned children may need to start with lower-intensity activities or alternate short-duration and higher-intensity activities with lower-intensity activities. During activity, the therapist should monitor the vital signs, including heart rate, blood pressure, RPE, DI, respiratory rate, and SpO_2. Some children may benefit from electrocardiogram (EKG) monitoring during aerobic activity. During training, the therapist can instruct some patients to take their own heart rate, respiratory rate, RPE, and DI. Identifying their own vital signs will foster the independence necessary to continue exercise independently once they are ready to move to autonomous activity. It is important to remember that following heart transplant, a patient does not have normal exercise response due to loss of the vagus nerve, and therefore requires warm-up to increase the heart rate in order to have an effect from the circulating catecholamines in the blood, followed by a cooldown.

Strength Training

Strength training is an important component of physical therapy for children of an appropriate age. Following cardiac surgery, children generally have sternal precautions in place for 6 to 8 weeks, which may include lifting precautions for greater than 10 pounds. With this caveat, strength training is a valuable tool in the treatment of children with CHD both pre- and postoperatively. Patients should always be taught proper breathing techniques with lifting to prevent a Valsalva maneuver and an unnecessary rise in blood pressure. Figure 19.18 shows a child participating in strength training.

Airway Clearance Techniques

These topics will be covered in detail in Chapter 20. Positioning, as discussed above, as well as postural drainage should be utilized immediately postoperatively. Mechanical airway clearance techniques such as percussion, vibration,

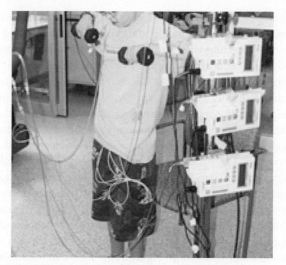

FIGURE 19.18 A child with a congenital heart defect participating in strength training.

shaking, and the high-frequency chest wall oscillation may require a short wait postoperatively, but other airway clearance techniques, such as Acapella or autogenic drainage, can be utilized as appropriate.

Functional Mobility

Transfer training, gait training, balance training, and stair climbing are functional tasks that should be included as necessary in physical therapy intervention. Transfer training should include ways to move that decrease discomfort and improve independence. This may mean teaching log rolling postoperatively while using deep-breathing techniques, or giving a child a "hug pillow" to hold over surgical sites. For small children this may mean teaching family members how to pick up and hold their child in such a way as to pose as little discomfort as possible. Gait training, balance training, and stair climbing should be initiated as soon as patients are able and medically stable. This may involve coordinating care with nursing staff, respiratory staff, or medical team members to allow safe completion. Once children are discharged to outpatient or early intervention programs, gait training, balance training, or stair training may need to continue to improve speed, stability, or technique.

Developmental Activity

Play is the means by which young children explore their world. A child with CHD who is awaiting surgery or is very ill and hospitalized has little exposure to physical exploration. Age-appropriate gross and fine motor play is very important for this population. Although there may be many tubes and wires to manage in the acute care setting, an infant should be exposed to all positions, including prone. Parent education and involvement of early intervention personnel in the home should also promote position changes, prone position, and progression of motor skills as tolerated. This effort may start with getting the infant accustomed to prone by starting with semi-prone positioning over a towel roll or prone on the shoulder of the caregiver. Prone positioning is the forerunner for many early developmental skills, including creeping, crawling, and upper extremity weight bearing and will assist in promoting infant development.[49,50] This position is important for children with poor feeding, reflux, and respiratory issues. Families should be encouraged to promote prone positioning during awake, alert, and calm periods during the day to help the infant gain head control and feel comfortable in prone. It is unusual for a child to have difficulty in prone after practice. Prone is seldom a contraindicated position, with the exception of a thoracic wound that is not closed or for the first 2 weeks following a sternal incision. Figure 19.19 shows an infant with a nasotracheal tube being placed in prone, and an infant following two cardiac surgeries working on prone skills in the home setting. Crawling should be encouraged in children with CHD as it improves upon all the muscle groups that are impacted by the surgical procedures done to correct or palliate CHD. Ambulatory children should be encouraged to ambulate postoperatively as soon as they are medically stable. Children receiving mechanical ventilation can ambulate with a team effort to maintain their ventilatory support and the safety of their airway. Children with chest tubes can also ambulate with little limitation, and ambulation may help to hasten chest tube removal. Higher-level motor skills may be delayed in children with CHD and should be promoted during therapy sessions.[3–6,10]

Home Programming

Recommendations should be made for home exercise programs, according to the patient's needs and age. Any of the above activities can be transitioned to home program activities as the patient is safe and stable to complete them without supervision. Parents should be encouraged to participate in sessions, and to assist with carryover of home activities.

▶ Neurodevelopmental outcomes of CHD

Children with CHD are at high risk for a myriad of neurodevelopmental challenges, the causes of which are multifactorial and not yet fully understood. Early developmental milestones, including cognition, language, and motor skills, are often delayed. One report found that 54% of infants with any type of single ventricle defect were receiving early intervention for any developmental domain by 6 months, 62% by 12 months, and 67% by 2 years, while 45% of infants with two ventricle defects were receiving developmental intervention by 6 months, 43% at 12 months, and 52% at 2 years.[6] Another study reported an overall rate of developmental delay of 25% for children following Fontan completion.[10] Uzark et al. demonstrated that 46% of children status post–heart transplantation present with language delay and 63% with visual motor deficits.[52] They also found a decrease in intelligence quotient (IQ), with the lowest IQs being in children with CHD as the primary reason for transplant.[52] Seventy-four percent of children with single ventricle defects and 29% of children with two ventricle defects scored below the 5th percentile on specific gross motor testing at 6 months.[6] Up to 50% of children with TGA present with decreased psychomotor skills at 1 year of age[3], up to 40% present with motor or gait abnormalities at 4 years of age,[5] and by 8 years of age, 54% present with gait abnormalities and 63% with motor abnormalities.[4]

While the factors causing neurodevelopmental challenges are not fully known, they likely involve an interaction of the preoperative, intraoperative, and postoperative events. Oxygenation levels following the first stage of single ventricle repair have been found to be associated with composite developmental score.[53] Whether a child undergoes circulatory arrest or low flow cardiopulmonary bypass during surgery may also impact outcomes, as children with TGA who underwent circulatory arrest have been shown to have up to 30% more delays at 1, 4, and 8 years of age.[3–5] In addition, several studies have found that length of stay following surgical intervention can impact neurodevelopmental

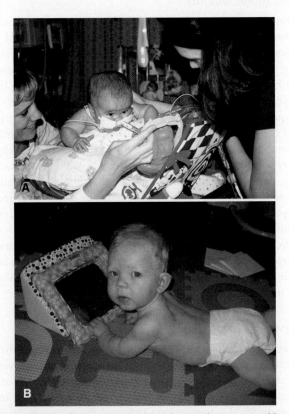

FIGURE 19.19 (A) An infant awaiting cardiac surgery with nasotracheal intubation working on prone skills in physical therapy with physical therapist and mother. **(B)** An infant with congenital heart defect following two surgeries working on prone skills in the home setting.

outcome, such that each increased day of length of stay was shown to lead to a 1.4-point decrease in full scale IQ and a 1.6-point decrease in math IQ.[54,55] Increased length of stay has been shown to be the greatest predictor of decreased motor skills at 1 year for children with HLHS.[7]

Concern regarding the neurodevelopmental implications in children with CHD has become a significant focus of cardiac management for these children. A recent scientific statement from the American Heart Association recommends regular surveillance for neurodevelopmental delays in children with CHD with referral for full evaluation and intervention when there is concern for delay.[9] While initial surveillance may often occur in the cardiology or pediatrician visits, physical therapists should be involved for evaluation and monitoring of motor skills in early intervention, outpatient, and hospital-based settings for children with CHD.

SUMMARY

Physical therapy is an integral component of the care of a child with CHD in the inpatient, outpatient, and community-based settings. Physical therapists are a vital component of the care of all children with cardiac disorders to improve posture, mobility, development, and ultimately ability to keep up with peers and participate and thrive in their family, school, and community environments.

CASE STUDIES

CASE STUDY 1

TODDLER WITH HLHS FOLLOWING TWO CARDIAC SURGERIES

History of Present Illness and Chief Complaint
Baby X is a 13-month-old male with HLHS who presents for developmental assessment in a multidisciplinary outpatient clinic setting. Baby X has a history of gross motor delay, and his parents are concerned that he does not put his feet down to stand.

Birth and Medical History
Baby X was diagnosed prenatally with HLHS and was born full term in the Special Delivery Unit at a children's hospital and transferred immediately to the Cardiac Intensive Care Unit for stabilization.

Surgical History
Baby X underwent a stage one repair with Blalock–Taussig shunt on day of life three (Fig. 19.20), which was complicated by left vocal cord paralysis and venous sinus thrombus. He had a bidirectional Glenn procedure at 4.5 months.

Current Medications
Lasix 0.8 mg 1/day; Lovenox 0.7 mg 1/day; Benefiber 1 tsp/day.

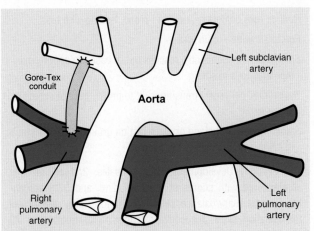

FIGURE 19.20 Modified Blalock–Taussig shunt.

Social History
Baby X's parents are very involved in his care, and his mother stays home with him. He has been receiving early intervention physical therapy weekly since 8 months of age.

Physical Therapy Examination
General appearance/Lines/Tubes: Baby X presents with mild cyanosis and no external supportive devices or lines.

State of consciousness: He is awake, alert, and oriented and interactive with parents in the exam room.

Pain: FLACC score of 0 out of 10.

Vital signs at rest: Heart rate = 130, SpO_2 = 87%, blood pressure in the right upper extremity = 92/59, respiratory rate = 30.

Integument/Skin integrity: Median sternotomy scar well healed with good scar mobility. Capillary refill: <3 seconds.

Thoracic Cage and Respiratory Examination
Baby X presents in no obvious distress, with a respiratory rate of 30 breaths/min. He uses primarily upper chest breathing, although he has some diaphragmatic excursion. When working hard, he demonstrates increased cyanosis and mild intercostal retractions. He clears his lungs using cough and sneeze independently. Baby X has a mild pectus carinatum with age-appropriate rib spacing and good chest wall mobility. He does not tolerate chest wall circumferential measurements due to age.

Musculoskeletal Examination
Baby X presents with full passive range of motion in bilateral upper and lower extremities, with mild hypotonia in bilateral lower extremities. Formal manual muscle test not performed due to age, but presents with decreased lower extremity strength evidenced by decreased standing skills detailed below. Functional skills are detailed under developmental assessment.

Developmental assessment
Supine: brings feet to mouth, reaches across midline, and tracks bilaterally.

Prone: pushes up onto palms, reaches with either upper extremity in prone, starting to move onto all fours.

Rolling: rolls bilaterally supine to prone, leading with hips.

Pull to sit: with + chin tuck.

Sitting: sits independently, reaches out of base of support, manipulates toys in sitting.

Transitions: per report transitions sit to prone, but not supine or prone to sit.

Standing: does not stand or place feet on ground, very resistant to lower extremity weight bearing.

The Peabody Developmental Motor Scales, 2nd edition was administered with scores at the 16th, 2nd, and 37th percentile for stationary/balance skills, locomotor skills, and object manipulation skills, respectively. Gross motor quotient is 79 (8th percentile).

Physical Therapy Evaluation and Diagnosis

Baby X is a 13-month-old male with HLHS s/p stage two repair. He presents to physical therapy with decreased leg strength and decreased weight bearing, impacting his standing and walking skills, leading to delayed gross motor skills. He presents with overall gross motor skills at the 8th percentile on the Peabody Developmental Motor Scales, 2nd edition, with performance at the 16th, 2nd, and 37th percentile for stationary/balance skills, locomotor skills, and object manipulation skills, respectively. This corresponds to the 7- to 12-month level. His delayed motor skills impact his ability to age-appropriately interact with his environment.

Plan of care

Early intervention physical therapy once per week, with a focus on standing skills. Parent education for standing skills and shoe wear.

Goals (for 12 weeks)

1. Baby X will stand at a support surface when placed for 5 minutes without loss of balance.
2. Baby X will pull to stand at support surface independently.
3. Baby X will cruise laterally for 5 feet each direction.
4. Baby X will take steps for 10 feet forward with one hand held.

Procedural interventions

Parent education: Role of shoe wear, ways to encourage standing and walking, continue scar massage.

Developmental skills: Play activities to encourage standing, transfers to standing, cruising and walking.

Strengthening: Via standing and walking repetition activities.

REFERENCES

1. Hoffman JI, Kaplan S. The incidence of congenital heart disease. *J Am Coll Cardiol.* 2002;39(12):1890–1900.
2. Green A. Outcomes of congenital heart disease: a review. *Pediatr Nurs.* 2004;30(4):280–284.
3. Bellinger DC, Jonas RA, Rappaport LA, et al. Developmental and neurologic status of children after heart surgery with hypothermic circulatory arrest or low-flow cardiopulmonary bypass. *N Engl J Med.* 1995;332(9):549–555.
4. Bellinger DC, Wypij D, duPlessis AJ, et al. Neurodevelopmental status at eight years in children with dextro-transposition of the great arteries: the Boston circulatory arrest trial. *J Thorac Cardiovasc Surg.* 2003;126(5):1385–1396.
5. Bellinger DC, Wypij D, Kuban KC, et al. Developmental and neurological status of children at 4 years of age after heart surgery with hypothermic circulatory arrest or low-flow cardiopulmonary bypass. *Circulation.* 1999;100(5):526–532.
6. Hoskoppal A, Roberts H, Kugler J, et al. Neurodevelopmental outcomes in infants after surgery for congenital heart disease: a comparison of single-ventricle vs. two-ventricle physiology. *Congenit Heart Dis.* 2010;5(2):90–95.
7. Knirsch W, Liamlahi R, Hug MI, et al. Mortality and neurodevelopmental outcome at 1 year of age comparing hybrid and Norwood procedures. *Eur J Cardiothorac Surg.* 2012;42(1):33–39.
8. Majnemer A, Limperopoulos C, Shevell M, et al. Long-term neuromotor outcome at school entry of infants with congenital heart defects requiring open-heart surgery. *J Pediatr.* 2006;148(1):72–77.
9. Marino BS, Lipkin PH, Newburger JW, et al. Neurodevelopmental outcomes in children with congenital heart disease: evaluation and management: a scientific statement from the American Heart Association. *Circulation.* 2012;126(9):1143–1172.
10. McCrindle BW, Williams RV, Mitchell PD, et al. Relationship of patient and medical characteristics to health status in children and adolescents after the Fontan procedure. *Circulation.* 2006;113(8):1123–1129.
11. Newburger JW, Sleeper LA, Bellinger DC, et al. Early developmental outcome in children with hypoplastic left heart syndrome and related anomalies: the single ventricle reconstruction trial. *Circulation.* 2012;125(17):2081–2091.
12. Cook AC, Yates RW, Anderson RH. Normal and abnormal fetal cardiac anatomy. *Prenat Diagn.* 2004;24(13):1032–1048.
13. Godfrey ME, Messing B, Cohen SM, et al. Functional assessment of the fetal heart: a review. *Ultrasound Obstet Gynecol.* 2012;39(2):131–144.
14. Wernovsky G, Gruber P. Common congenital heart disease: presentation, management and outcomes. In: Taeusch H, Ballard R, Gleason C, eds. *Avery's Diseases of the Newborn.* 8th ed. Philadelphia, PA: Elsevier Saunders;2004:827–872.
15. Frownfelter D, Dean E, eds. *Cardiovascular and Pulmonary Physical Therapy: Evidence and Practice.* 5th ed. St. Louis, MO: Elsevier Mosby; 2005.
16. Hillegass E, ed *Essentials of Cardiopulmonary Physical Therapy.* Philadelphia, PA: Saunders; 2011.
17. Blackburn S. Placental, fetal, and transitional circulation revisited. *J Perinat Neonatal Nurs.* 2006;20(4):290–294.
18. Feinstein JA, Benson DW, Dubin AM, et al. Hypoplastic left heart syndrome: current considerations and expectations. *J Am Coll Cardiol.* 2012;59(1)(suppl):S1–S42.
19. Fredenburg TB, Johnson TR, Cohen MD. The Fontan procedure: anatomy, complications, and manifestations of failure. *Radiographics.* 2011;31(2):453–463.
20. Mendeloff EN. The history of pediatric heart and lung transplantation. *Pediatr Transplant.* 2002;6(4):270–279.
21. Webber SA, McCurry K, Zeevi A. Heart and lung transplantation in children. *Lancet.* 2006;368(9529):53–69.
22. Kirk R, Edwards LB, Kucheryavaya AY, et al. The registry of the International Society for Heart and Lung Transplantation: fourteenth pediatric heart transplantation report—2011. *J Heart Lung Transplant.* 2011;30(10):1095–1103.
23. Singh TP, Gauvreau K, Rhodes J, et al. Longitudinal changes in heart rate recovery after maximal exercise in pediatric heart transplant recipients: evidence of autonomic re-innervation? *J Heart Lung Transplant.* 2007;26(12):1306–1312.
24. Kuhlthau KA, Bloom S, VanCleave J, et al. Evidence for family-centered care for children with special health care needs: a systematic review. *Acad Pediatr.* 2011;11(2):136–143.
25. Garra G, Singer AJ, Taira BR, et al. Validation of the Wong-Baker FACES Pain Rating Scale in pediatric emergency department patients. *Acad Emerg Med.* 2010;17(1):50–54.

26. Howard R, Carter B, Curry J, et al. Pain assessment. *Paediatr Anaesth.* 2008;18(suppl 1):14–18.

27. Merkel S, Voepel-Lewis T, Malviya S. Pain assessment in infants and young children: the FLACC scale. *Am J Nurs.* 2002;102(10):55–58.

28. Bai J, Hsu L, Tang Y, et al. Validation of the COMFORT Behavior scale and the FLACC scale for pain assessment in Chinese children after cardiac surgery. *Pain Manag Nurs.* 2012;13(1):18–26.

29. Johansson M, Kokinsky E. The COMFORT behavioural scale and the modified FLACC scale in paediatric intensive care. *Nurs Crit Care.* 2009;14(3):122–130.

30. Voepel-Lewis T, Zanotti J, Dammeyer JA, et al. Reliability and validity of the face, legs, activity, cry, consolability behavioral tool in assessing acute pain in critically ill patients. *Am J Crit Care.* 2010;19(1):55–61; quiz 62.

31. Potapov EV, Stiller B, Hetzer R. Ventricular assist devices in children: current achievements and future perspectives. *Pediatr Transplant.* 2007;11(3):241–255.

32. Corra U, Pistono M, Mezzani A, et al. Cardiovascular prevention and rehabilitation for patients with ventricular assist device from exercise therapy to long-term therapy. Part I: exercise therapy. *Monaldi Arch Chest Dis.* 2011;76(1):27–32.

33. Massery M. Musculoskeletal and neuromuscular interventions: a physical approach to cystic fibrosis. *J R Soc Med.* 2005;98(suppl 45):55–66.

34. Massery M. The Linda Crane Memorial Lecture: the patient puzzle: piecing it together. *Cardiopulm Phys Ther J.* 2009;20(2):19–27.

35. Massery M. Chest development as a component of normal motor development: Implications for pediatric physical therapists. *Pediatr Phys Ther.* 1991:3–8.

36. Ragnarsdottir M, Kristinsdottir EK. Breathing movements and breathing patterns among healthy men and women 20-69 years of age. Reference values. *Respiration.* 2006;73(1):48–54.

37. ATS statement: guidelines for the six-minute walk test. *Am J Respir Crit Care Med.* 2002;166(1):111–117.

38. Li AM, Yin J, Yu CC, et al. The six-minute walk test in healthy children: reliability and validity. *Eur Respir J.* 2005;25(6):1057–1060.

39. Moalla W, Gauthier R, Maingourd Y, et al. Six-minute walking test to assess exercise tolerance and cardiorespiratory responses during training program in children with congenital heart disease. *Int J Sports Med.* 2005;26(9):756–762.

40. Geiger R, Strasak A, Treml B, et al. Six-minute walk test in children and adolescents. *J Pediatr.* 2007;150(4):395–399, e391–e392.

41. Li AM, Yin J, Au JT, et al. Standard reference for the six-minute-walk test in healthy children aged 7 to 16 years. *Am J Respir Crit Care Med.* 2007;176(2):174–180.

42. Diller GP, Dimopoulos K, Okonko D, et al. Exercise intolerance in adult congenital heart disease: comparative severity, correlates, and prognostic implication. *Circulation.* 2005;112(6):828–835.

43. Fredriksen PM, Therrien J, Veldtman G, et al. Lung function and aerobic capacity in adult patients following modified Fontan procedure. *Heart.* 2001;85(3):295–299.

44. Inuzuka R, Diller GP, Borgia F, et al. Comprehensive use of cardiopulmonary exercise testing identifies adults with congenital heart disease at increased mortality risk in the medium term. *Circulation.* 2012;125(2):250–259.

45. Fredriksen PM, Kahrs N, Blaasvaer S, et al. Effect of physical training in children and adolescents with congenital heart disease. *Cardiol Young.* 2000;10(2):107–114.

46. Rhodes J, Curran TJ, Camil L, et al. Sustained effects of cardiac rehabilitation in children with serious congenital heart disease. *Pediatrics.* 2006;118(3):e586–e593.

47. Balachandran R, Nair SG, Sivadasan PC, et al. Prone ventilation in the management of infants with acute respiratory distress syndrome after complex cardiac surgery. *J Cardiothorac Vasc Anesth.* 2012;26(3):471–475.

48. Bhuyan U, Peters AM, Gordon I, et al. Effects of posture on the distribution of pulmonary ventilation and perfusion in children and adults. *Thorax.* 1989;44(6):480–484.

49. Kennedy E, Majnemer A, Farmer JP, et al. Motor development of infants with positional plagiocephaly. *Phys Occup Ther Pediatr.* 2009;29(3):222–235.

50. Kuo YL, Liao HF, Chen PC, et al. The influence of wakeful prone positioning on motor development during the early life. *J Dev Behav Pediatr.* 2008;29(5):367–376.

51. Medicine ACoS. *ACSM's Guidelines for Exercise Testing and Prescription.* 6th ed. Philadelphia, PA: Lippincott, Williams & Wilkins; 2000.

52. Uzark K, Spicer R, Beebe DW. Neurodevelopmental outcomes in pediatric heart transplant recipients. *J Heart Lung Transplant.* 2009;28(12):1306–1311.

53. Hoffman GM, Mussatto KA, Brosig CL, et al. Systemic venous oxygen saturation after the Norwood procedure and childhood neurodevelopmental outcome. *J Thorac Cardiovasc Surg.* 2005;130(4):1094–1100.

54. Mahle WT, Visconti KJ, Freier MC, et al. Relationship of surgical approach to neurodevelopmental outcomes in hypoplastic left heart syndrome. *Pediatrics.* 2006;117(1):e90–e97.

55. Newburger JW, Wypij D, Bellinger DC, et al. Length of stay after infant heart surgery is related to cognitive outcome at age 8 years. *J Pediatr.* 2003;143(1):67–73.

Pulmonary and Respiratory Conditions in Infants and Children

Jan Stephen Tecklin

Introduction

Growth and Development of the Lungs

Predisposition to Respiratory Failure

Physical Therapy Examination of Children with Respiratory Disorders
History
Review of Systems
Tests and Measures

Physical Therapy for Children with Pulmonary Disease and Respiratory Disorders
Airway Clearance
Breathing Exercises and Retraining
Physical Development

Atelectasis
Medical Information
Physical Therapy Examination
Physical Therapy Procedural Interventions

Respiratory Muscle Weakness
Medical Information
Physical Therapy Examination
Physical Therapy Interventions

Asthma
Medical Information
Medical Management
Physical Therapy Examination
Physical Therapy Interventions

Cystic Fibrosis
Medical Information
Medical Management
Physical Therapy Examination
Physical Therapy Management

Summary

Case Study

Introduction

Pulmonary diseases and respiratory disorders continue to be major causes of both mortality and morbidity for children in the United States and throughout the world. Respiratory viruses and bacteria continue to cause acute and sometimes fatal respiratory infections in infants and children. Vaccines against both bacterial and viral agents have decreased the incidence of certain acute respiratory infections and are commonly employed for children at risk for respiratory disease.

In the United States, up to 20% or more of children younger than 18 years of age have been reported to have a chronic respiratory problem such as asthma, wheezing, bronchial hyper-reactivity, cystic fibrosis (CF) and bronchopulmonary dysplasia.[1] Chronic lung disease in children has morbidity statistics that are staggering. An estimated 7.1 million children (9.5%) in the United States have been diagnosed with asthma,[2] which is responsible for missed days of school in almost 50% of those children diagnosed.[3] It is also important to note that childhood asthma is most prevalent among those of black and multiracial (non-Hispanic) ethnicity. In addition, respiratory illness is the most common reason for hospitalization in children with severe neurological impairment and is the most common cause of death in these children.[4,5] These statistics may seem surprising but not to health professionals who spend a great deal of time treating children with primary pulmonary diseases or respiratory problems secondary to other conditions.

This chapter provides background information to enable readers to understand more completely the fragility of the neonatal and pediatric respiratory system, the process of development of that system, and the need for aggressive treatment of disorders of the system. These introductory topics include growth and development of the respiratory tract, and predisposition to acute respiratory failure in children and infants. Physical therapy examination and intervention skills for infants and children with pulmonary disorders follow. Medical information and a discussion of physical therapy for four major respiratory problems of children—atelectasis, respiratory muscle weakness, asthma, and CF—are next presented, followed by questions about future research.

Growth and development of the lungs

A brief review of the major periods of lung development is useful in discussing the interrelationship between lung and airway growth and specific childhood diseases. A description of lung development also provides insight into some unique aspects of the growth, particularly in number, of pulmonary alveoli.

Four specific periods of lung growth have been confirmed and include the embryonic, pseudoglandular, canalicular, and saccular periods from post-conception weeks 0 to 6, 6 to 16, 16 to 24, and 24 to 40(term), respectively.[6] Because alveolar growth continues after birth, a 5th period, alveolar, is also noted. The earliest sign of lung development occurs during the *embryonic period*, from 0 to 6 weeks' gestation. Endodermal tissue of the primitive foregut expands into an anterior lung pouch when the embryo is 4 mm long. During this period, in which there is a separation of the trachea and esophagus, aberrations in development may lead to one of several configurations of tracheoesophageal fistulae—abnormal communication between the two structures. (Fig. 20.1) Four days later, the future trachea differentiates into right and left bronchial buds—the precursors of each lung. Mesenchymal cellular tissue surrounding the developing bronchial buds will later differentiate to become muscle, connective tissue, and cartilage within the bronchial walls. Also developing from the mesenchyme is vascular tissue that will soon connect the primitive pulmonary artery to the pulmonary veins. Noncellular tissue will provide the elastic and collagen fibers that support the lung structures.[7] Vascular development is congruent with bronchial buds and airway branching.[8]

The lung buds continue to grow and subdivide into smaller airways during the 5th to 16th week of gestation, termed the pseudoglandular period because the lung tissue looks similar to glandular cells. During this period, many of the early cells differentiate into specific types of airway cells. Tall bronchial epithelium lines the primitive airways, and there is a burst of growth between the 10th and 14th weeks. Mucus-secreting glands and supportive cartilage

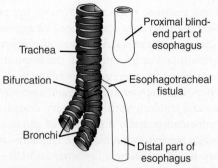

FIGURE 20.1 Tracheoesophageal fistula. (From Sadler TW. *Langman's Medical Embryology.* 9th ed. Baltimore, MD: Lippincott Williams & Wilkins; 2002.)

appear late in the pseudoglandular period and continue their growth through the canalicular period. Branching and subdivision produces 8 to 32 bronchial generations, with the greatest number of divisions occurring in those lung areas that are most distant from the hilum, or root of the lungs. The bronchial tree is complete from the glottis to the terminal bronchioles by the end of the pseudoglandular period, and the diaphragm is beginning to form. Similar development of the pulmonary vascular system occurs concurrently.[8]

The major events that mark the 16th to 26th week, the canalicular period, are thinning and flattening of the epithelium that will become the type I pneumocytes or alveolar cells. Type II cells also begin to appear at this time and are the lamellar cells that ultimately produce surfactant. In addition, a critical occurrence is the appearance of pulmonary capillaries. The capillaries, which protrude into the epithelium, provide close proximity of the blood supply to the airways. Thinning of the epithelium and capillary development provide the apparatus—the air–blood interface—for respiration. Gas exchange can take place by the end of the canalicular period.[8]

At approximately 26 weeks, the energy of the developing lung begins to form outpouchings of the terminal bronchioles called saccules. This "terminal sac" or "saccular" period continues until about birth when the alveolar period begins, at which time the saccules have begun to branch into many alveolar pockets or ducts. These ducts are in continued proximity to the tiny capillaries formed during the canalicular period. Once sufficient numbers of alveolar/capillary units are present, life may be sustained, provided that the biochemical substance surfactant is present within the alveoli.

Surfactant, as noted, is a phospholipid material secreted by Type II cells that line the pulmonary alveoli. Surfactant reduces surface tension within the alveolus, thus allowing inflation of the alveolus with smaller pressures and less work by the infant than would be needed to inflate a surfactant-deficient alveolus. Surfactant appears at its mature chemical level at approximately 34 weeks of gestation and indicates maturity of the lung by allowing the maintenance of continuous respiration.[9]

The postnatal period is characterized initially by an 18- to 24-month period of rapid growth of both surface area and volume of lung tissue for gas exchange through continued subdivision of the alveolar ducts to form alveolar sacs (i.e., the true alveoli). The current consensus is that alveolar number is largely completed by 6 months of age, although some development may continue through 24 months.[8] Of note is that the vasculature grows to an even greater degree than the air spaces in this earlier of the postnatal phases. In the second of the postnatal phases, there is more parallel growth in the alveoli and capillaries. From the 25 million alveoli present at birth, there is a 12-fold increase by 8 to 10 years, at which time the adult number of approximately 300 million is achieved. Destructive processes within the period of alveolar multiplication may limit the potential for achieving the adult number of pulmonary alveoli.[10]

Predisposition to respiratory failure

The following information is presented to describe more fully several mechanisms of acute respiratory failure and its rapid development in children and infants. Although acute respiratory failure is not a disease, it is often the final common pathway for many diseases that affect the developing respiratory system.

Several structural and metabolic factors in the pediatric population, although entirely normal, predispose them to acute respiratory failure. Respiratory failure can be defined as a condition in which impairment of gas exchange within the lungs poses an immediate threat to life. Downes and associates were among the first to state that clinical signs and arterial blood gas determinations should be used to monitor infants and children for the development of acute respiratory failure.[11] The arterial blood gas levels compatible with respiratory failure are 75 mmHg of carbon dioxide and 100 mmHg of oxygen when the patient is receiving an inspired oxygen concentration of 100%. Respiratory failure exists when either of these arterial levels is reached in the presence of any of the following clinical signs—decreased or absent inspiratory breaths sounds, severe inspiratory retractions with accessory muscle use, cyanosis with inspiration of 40% oxygen, depressed consciousness and response to pain, and poor skeletal muscle tone.

The most important general factor predisposing infants and children to acute respiratory failure is their high incidence of respiratory tract infections. During the first several years of life, when immunologic defenses are developing, the child is at risk for infections. This risk increases as the environment of the toddler expands, particularly with early enrollment in day care, preschool, and other similar exposures to various infectious agents transmitted by classmates, teachers, and other personnel. As the number of children in day care programs has increased in recent decades, the concurrent increase in the incidence of respiratory infections has been predictable. Indeed, recent research has focused on the economic impact of these infectious episodes and the economic benefits to developing and instituting infection control programs.[12]

Two major structural factors—airway size and poor mechanical advantage for the respiratory muscles—contribute to respiratory failure in a young child. According to calculations applied to the work of Effmann, the diameter of the tracheal lumen in children less than 1 year of age is smaller than the diameter of a lead pencil.[13] A large percentage of the young child's peripheral bronchioles are smaller than 1 mm in diameter. A small amount of mucus, bronchospasm, or edema can effectively not only occlude the peripheral airways but may also obstruct the larger, more proximal bronchi. With sufficient airway blockage, respiratory failure may quickly ensue.

Additional major structural issues that predispose infants and children to respiratory failure involve several items that cumulatively cause poor mechanical advantage to the respiratory bellows of the child's thorax:

1. Type I fatigue-resistant muscle fibers are not present in adult proportions in the diaphragm or other ventilatory muscles of the infant until 8 months of age.[14] This lack of fatigue-resistant fibers allows the infant's respiratory muscles to tire quickly, causing alveolar hypoventilation that may lead to respiratory failure.
2. There is a greater work of breathing cost that may reach 10% of basal metabolic rate when the preterm infant must use the diaphragm to distort its ribcage in times of stressful breathing. Should the infant have lung disease as well, the increased metabolic demands of the diaphragm may predispose preterm infants to fatigue and may contribute to respiratory failure.[15]
3. Poor development of the ability to cough either spontaneously or with direct laryngeal stimulation renders the infant's airways susceptible to obstruction by mucus.[16]
4. Horizontal alignment of the infant's rib cage and the round (rather than oval) configuration of the chest provide poor mechanical advantage to the intercostal and accessory muscles of respiration. These muscles lift the ribs and sternum to increase thoracic diameter and lung volume.
5. Increased chest wall compliance during infancy can result in sternal retractions associated with increased inspiratory effort during times of illness. The relative lack of stiffness in the infant thorax can simulate a flail chest. Intense inspiratory efforts may paradoxically decrease thoracic volume at a time when just the opposite response is necessary, and ventilation is further compromised with the potential for hypoventilation. Developmental changes in the chest wall during the second year of life result in chest wall compliance similar to that of adults.[17]
6. The baby's position may affect diaphragmatic excursion. The infant who is in a supine position works harder to ventilate because the abdominal viscera may impede the full descent of the diaphragm.

A third important issue for the physical therapist is respiratory metabolism. The high metabolic rate of the child causes increased consumption of oxygen, increased heat loss, and increased water loss secondary to a faster respiratory rate. The range of normal respiratory rates for children is shown in Table 20.1.

In addition to having muscle fibers that are susceptible to early fatigue, as noted above, the young child or infant has a relatively poor muscle fuel supply. Glycogen supply in the muscle tissue is small in the infant, and is depleted quickly when muscular activity is increased, which occurs during respiratory distress.[18]

The factors described above—general, structural, and metabolic factors—although developmentally and chronologically normal and appropriate, may combine to render the young

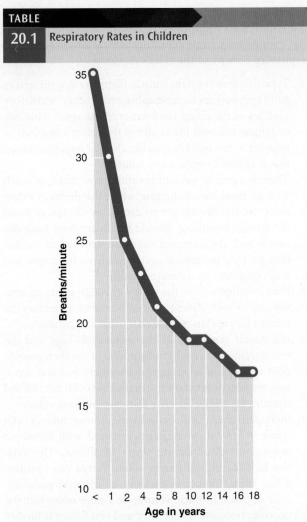

TABLE
20.1   Respiratory Rates in Children

Age in years

This graph shows normal respiratory rates in children, which are higher than normal rates in adults. Accordingly, bradypnea and tachypnea in a child are defined by the child's age.

respiratory tract fragile and prone to failure during periods of stress, which are commonly seen in respiratory diseases.

▶ Physical therapy examination of children with respiratory disorders

Careful examination of the infant or child with respiratory distress can offer useful information. The younger the patient, the more the therapist may need to rely on careful observation, because the infant or young child cannot participate actively in a chest assessment. An age-appropriate description of the activities that the therapist will be performing should precede the actual physical examination. The following organization of the examination is based upon the Guide to Physical Therapist Practice.[19]

History

A complete medical chart review should be the first aspects of the physical therapy assessment of a child. The review should provide information regarding the child's medical history—the clinical course of the child's current illness, including signs and symptoms and their precipitating factors; any previous treatment for the illness; and reasons for the referral for physical therapy. In addition to the information in the chart, physicians and nurses can often provide invaluable and immediate information regarding the child's current state. The chest radiographs and other forms of imaging are useful in identifying specific areas of the lung or thorax that may be affected by the illness. A complete radiographic interpretation is beyond the scope of physical therapy practice.

Living Environment

Does the home or other discharge destination provide the space and resources needed for respiratory items such as oxygen, ventilator, and suction device?

General Health Status

Has the infant or child displayed a normal developmental history? Have motor milestones been reached at appropriate times? Is there a history of ongoing or recurrent medical problems?

Medical/Surgical History

Have there been recent hospitalizations, illnesses, or surgical interventions of note? Does the patient or parent report comorbidities or past illnesses that may affect the current condition? Is there knowledge of genetic diseases within the family?

Current Condition/Chief Complaint

What is the recent concern leading to the request for physical therapy? Is this a recurrence of a previous problem? Is the child receiving physical therapy, including airway clearance (AC), at home? What are the patient/family expectations for this episode of care?

Functional Status/Activity Level

Has the child been functioning at an age-appropriate level? Chapter 3 presents numerous tests of development.

Medications

What medications is the child taking, and is there any potential impact on the physical therapy regimen? (Aerosol medications such as bronchodilators, mucolytics, and hypertonic saline often precede AC.)

Other Clinical Tests

Review all laboratory values, including pulmonary function tests, arterial blood gas values, and pulse oximetry, all imaging information, exercise tests, and any other potentially informative studies.

Review of Systems

The systems review is a brief and gross examination, a "quick check," used to gather additional information and to detect other health problems that should be considered in the diagnosis, prognosis, and plan of care.

Cardiovascular/Pulmonary Systems

This brief review of the child should include blood pressure determination, measurement of pulse and respiratory rate, and documentation of any gross indications of edema.

Integument

Are the color and integrity of the skin normal? Are any old or new scars apparent? Are current wounds healing properly?

Musculoskeletal System

Measure and record the patient's height and weight. Identify any obvious physical asymmetries. Assess gross muscle strength and range of motion to the degree possible, depending upon the age of the child and the ability to cooperate.

Neuromuscular System

Determine whether grossly coordinated and age-appropriate movement or movement patterns are seen.

Tests and Measures

Ventilation and Respiration/Gas Exchange

Of all the tests and measures administered to the child with pulmonary disease, none is more important than those assessing ventilation and respiration. Many signs and symptoms associated with ventilation and gas exchange have a direct bearing on the interventions that the therapist will choose. A traditional chest examination includes the four classic approaches of inspection, auscultation, palpation, and mediate percussion.

The physical therapist has several objectives related to the chest examination:

- Identify the pulmonary problems and symptoms noted
- Assess coexisting signs of pulmonary disease
- Determine the need for additional tests and measures such as exercise testing when appropriate
- Formulate a prognosis and a plan of care
- Identify treatment goals.

Inspection

The inspection phase of the chest examination documents clinical characteristics of the presenting symptoms, which may indicate what other components of the examination are necessary.

Inspection includes:

- Examining the child's general appearance
- Inspecting the head and neck
- Observing the chest
- Considering the child's breath, speech, cough, and sputum

GENERAL APPEARANCE First, the therapist should note the state of consciousness of the child and the level to which the child can cooperate with simple commands. Is the child's body habitus normal, obese, or cachectic. Are there obvious postural issues such as kyphosis, scoliosis, and forward bent or unusual postures. Children who are dyspneic often assume a forward bent position.

During the extremity examination, the therapist notes digital clubbing, painful swollen joints, tremor, and edema. Clubbing of the fingers or toes is associated with CF, as shown in Figure 20.2 A and B.[20] Painful swollen joints may indicate pseudohypertrophic pulmonary osteoarthropathy[21] rather than the osteoarthritis or rheumatoid arthritis more familiar to physical therapists. Bilateral pedal edema may indicate cor pulmonale or right heart failure in those with long-standing CF and chronic lung disease with hypoxemia.[22]

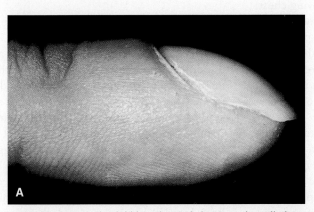
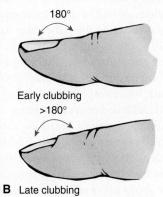

FIGURE 20.2 In clubbing, the angle between the nail plate and the proximal nail fold increases to 180 degrees or more. Clubbing of the fingers is seen in patients with cystic fibrosis and other respiratory and cardiovascular disease.

The therapist also notes all equipment and monitoring devices used in managing the patient and the impact of those devices on planned interventions. (e.g., mechanical ventilator, oxygen hood or mask, intravenous or arterial lines).

INSPECTION OF THE HEAD AND NECK The child's face often shows signs of respiratory distress and oxygen deficit. Of these signs, *flaring of the alae nasi* and *cyanosis* of the mucous membranes are commonly seen in those with acute respiratory distress. *Head bobbing* that coincides with the respiratory cycle may be the result of attempts to use the accessory muscles of inspiration by an infant who has inadequate strength to stabilize the head and neck. *Audible expiratory grunting* is thought to be an effort by the infant and young child to maintain airway patency and prevent airway collapse during expiration. Grunting is most commonly heard during lower respiratory tract disorders.

EXAMINATION OF THE UNMOVING CHEST In this portion of the physical examination, the shape and symmetry of the thorax are noted, as are any unusual characteristics of the skin, including rashes, scars, and incisions. The thorax of the infant is more rounded in configuration than the adult thorax, and the ribs attach to the vertebrae almost at 90 degrees, which makes further elevation almost impossible.[23] The anteroposterior diameter of the thorax in the infant is likely to be equal to its transverse diameter, whereas in the adult's thorax, there is usually a much greater transverse diameter. Among the more common abnormalities of the thorax are congenital defects, including pectus excavatum (or funnel chest) and pectus carinatum (or pigeon-breast); barrel-chest, usually associated with hyperinflation of the lungs, in which the anterior-to-posterior measurement of the thorax is greater than the lateral measurement; and the several thoracic deformities associated with scoliosis. Muscle development of the thorax should also be examined for symmetry and for the presence of hypertrophy of the accessory muscles of inspiration, which suggests chronic dyspnea.

EXAMINATION OF THE MOVING CHEST Respiratory rate is the first item assessed when examining the moving chest. Counting respirations should be done inconspicuously and is often done when counting the pulse rate. As previously noted, in Table 20.1, the younger the patient, the greater the normal resting respiratory rate. Tachypnea refers to an abnormally high respiratory rate and bradypnea refers to a low respiratory rate, while keeping in mind the normal variation in infant and childhood respiratory rates.

The pattern and regularity of breathing should also be evaluated, particularly in neonates and in children with neuromuscular disorders. Short periods of apnea are not particularly unusual and may be referred to as periodic breathing in neonates. True apnea exists when apneic periods exceed 20 seconds. Apnea can be associated with respiratory distress, sepsis, and central nervous system (CNS) hemorrhage.

In addition to the rate and regularity, the ratio of inspiration to expiration (I:E) should be determined. This I:E ratio is usually approximately 1:2. Infants and children with obstructive airway disease, such as asthma and bronchiolitis, may have a marked increase in expiratory time; as a result, their I:E ratio may become 1:4 or 1:5. Synchronous motion of the abdomen and thorax should be observed. On inspiration, both thoracic expansion and abdominal bulging should be noted. When this synchrony is lost, a "seesaw" motion of thoracic expansion with abdominal in-drawing occurs on inspiration, with the opposite movements being noted on expiration. The presence of chest wall retractions should be noted. Retractions, or in-drawing, may occur in suprasternal, substernal, subcostal, or intercostal areas. Retractions, seen more frequently in pediatric patients, occur as a result of the compliant thorax of the infant and young child and an increased respiratory effort. During respiratory distress, the muscles of either inspiration or expiration, or both, place sufficient pull on the as yet largely cartilaginous thorax to cause an in-drawing in several areas. When retractions are severe, they may reduce effective inspiration.

Audible sounds during breathing can be heard and may be notable. *Stridor*, a crowing sound during inspiration, suggests upper airway obstruction or possible laryngospasm. During expiration, one may also hear grunting sounds, particularly in infants with respiratory distress. Expiratory *grunting* may represent a physiological attempt to prevent premature airway collapse. *Gurgling* sounds heard during both ventilatory phases commonly indicate copious secretions in the larger airways.

EVALUATION OF COUGHING AND SNEEZING Infants probably use sneezing more than coughing as both a protective and a clearance mechanism for the airway. Older infants and children must be able to cough effectively to clear secretions or other debris from their airway. It is important to determine the ability to cough in a child with neuromuscular disease. With neuromuscular disease and associated abdominal muscle weakness the child may be at risk for secretion retention and aspiration of feedings, which may require some mechanical assistance for secretion removal, to be discussed later.

Auscultation

Auscultation—listening to the lungs with a stethoscope—is a useful method of assessment. The stethoscope used for auscultation of the infant and young child is a smaller version of that used for adults. The therapist should warm the stethoscope before using it, and, depending on the age of the child, the therapist may show how it is used by demonstrating on a child's doll or on a puppet. Because of the proximity to the thoracic surface of the child's airways, as well as the thin chest wall in the young child and infant, sounds are easily transmitted, and anatomic specificity may be reduced. A particular sound, therefore, although heard in one area of the thorax, may not correspond to the lung segment directly below the area in which the sound is heard. As a result, auscultation, particularly in the neonate or premature neonate, may not be as precise as in the older child or adult. Nonetheless, the therapist should attempt to ascertain the presence of normal and abnormal breath sounds throughout the lung fields. The therapist should also try to identify adventitious sounds, such as wheezes, crackles, rubs, and crunches.

Wheezes are musical sounds thought to be produced by airflow through narrowed airways. They may be inspiratory or expiratory and may be monophonic or polyphonic. Expiratory wheezes are probably more common and represent airways obstruction from bronchospasm or secretions.

Crackles (sometimes called *rales)* are non-musical sounds that may be heard during inspiration or expiration. They may represent previously deflated airways opening suddenly. Expiratory crackles often denote fluid in the larger airways.

Rubs are coarse, grating leathery sounds that often indicate inflammatory tissues rubbing against one another.

Crunches are crackling sounds often heard over the mediastinum when air has leaked into that area.

The audible sounds of stridor, and expiratory grunting were mentioned earlier. Because of the ease of transmission of sound through the infant's thorax, the therapist should attempt to correlate auscultatory findings with roentgenographic changes and other physical findings during the evaluation and treatment planning portion of the patient encounter.[24]

Palpation

Palpation of the thorax in the infant or child can help to identify the following circumstances:

- Position of the mediastinum via palpation of the trachea
- Palpation for rhonchal fremitus (the feeling of turbulent airflow around secretions) is also a useful means to localize secretion in the larger airways.
- Palpation for local areas of rib cage motion and the symmetry of that motion as the chest expands is also useful in older children.
- The activity of muscles of inspiration can be determined via their direct palpation

Palpation can also be employed to help identify and localize areas of chest pain in the child.

Mediate Percussion

This last of the four skills in a traditional respiratory examination enables the therapist to identify areas of abnormal lung density, and evaluate the extent of diaphragmatic motion. The technique requires tapping the finger of one hand against the nail of a finger placed firmly in a rib interspace. The actual sound or percussion note can denote air-filled versus non–air-filled lung tissue. The more hollow/resonant

the sound, the greater is the likelihood of air-filled lung. The more dull or flat the sound, the more likely the lung is poorly aerated in that specific area.

In addition, percussion can also identify diaphragmatic motion. The percussion note changes from resonant (air-filled) to dull (airless) at the base of the lungs, where the diaphragm is located. The therapist percusses the rib interspaces from lung apex to base. When dullness is encountered, the therapist has the patient exhale fully, causing the diaphragm to ascend. The therapist percusses to mark the highest level of ascent. Next, the patient inspires completely, and percussion tracks the descending diaphragm until the limit of descent is identified. Diaphragmatic excursion is the distance traveled between maximum ascent and maximum descent.

Aerobic Capacity and Endurance

Aerobic capacity and endurance are commonly defined by the term maximal oxygen uptake. This measurement is an indication of (1) the ability of the cardiovascular system to provide oxygen to working muscles and (2) the ability of those muscles to extract oxygen for energy generation. Such testing can provide much useful information about the patient such as the following:

- Identify the baseline ability
- Determine aerobic capacity during functional activities
- Predict the response to physiological demands during periods of increased or stressful activity
- Recognize limitations in the face of an increased workload.

Many modes of testing are used that range from observation of symptomatic responses during a standard exercise challenge to instrumented, technically sophisticated invasive aerobic testing in an exercise laboratory. Exercise testing in a laboratory typically involves progressive and incremental increases in exercise intensity while the patient is walking on a treadmill or riding a bicycle ergometer. Exercise testing sites should have the capacity for continuous electrocardiographic monitoring, periodic heart rate and blood pressure measurement, cutaneous oximetry and arterial blood gas determination, and expired gas analysis; they should also have an oxygen source. In addition, a cardiac defibrillator, other emergency equipment and supplies, and proper personnel for their use must be immediately available in case of cardiopulmonary emergency. Maximal and submaximal testing may be performed.

When a formal laboratory is not available or not practical, a 6- or 12-minute timed walking test,[25,26] a shuttle walking test,[27] or a step test[28] are simple and well-studied alternatives to be discussed later in the chapter.

Anthropometric Characteristics

Assessment of height and weight percentiles, body mass index, and peripheral edema are all important measures of anthropometric characteristics for children with pulmonary disorders. Height and weight along with body mass index values are important in determining physical growth, stature, and nutrition in the child. Nutritional status has a significant impact on lung function and, hence, on exercise capacity in children.[29] Monitoring of cor pulmonale—congestive right heart failure—is an important reason for measuring edema in the child with chronic lung disease, particularly those with CF and severe asthma. Cor pulmonale often results from long-standing arterial hypoxemia, hypercapnia, and respiratory acidosis, all of which add to right ventricle afterload, leading to right ventricular hypertrophy.[30] Right ventricular failure is associated peripheral edema, likely manifested as pedal and ankle edema. The physical therapist may use simple girth measurements, volumetric displacement, and figure-of-eight girth measurements to monitor the early development of peripheral edema and its progression.[31] In addition, sudden gross weight gain may indicate a rapid onset of cor pulmonale; therefore, periodic weight measurement is useful.

Arousal and Cognition

The child should be oriented to time and space and should be able to respond both to questions of a cognitive nature and to varied environmental stimuli given the limitations of developmental age. The therapist should determine the general state of consciousness and ability to respond to questions and requests.

Assistive and Adaptive Devices

Assistive and adaptive devices such as crutches, walkers, wheelchairs, splints, raised toilet seats, environmental control systems, and the like are not inherent needs for most children who have acute or chronic pulmonary problems. Some pulmonary-related devices that children might use include nebulizers, supplemental oxygen by nasal cannula or mask, mechanical ventilator, tracheotomy tube, and in some cases a port for provision of supplemental nutrition. A major exception to this pattern concerns children whose respiratory impairment is secondary to a musculoskeletal or neuromuscular disease for which such devices as walkers, wheelchairs, and others would be appropriate.

Environmental, Home, and Work (Job/School/Play) Barriers

Major environmental barriers of importance for the child with pulmonary disease involve the physical demands of attending school and playing in various environments. In addition, the therapist should inquire about the presence or absence within the home or school environment of dust, vapors, known or possible allergens or other inhalation hazards. These can be evaluated through interviews of the child and parent or caretaker regarding the home, school, and play environments.

Integumentary Integrity

The review of systems above will have been useful to the clinician in identifying any existing or potential skin impairments. Major findings are likely to involve pallor or cyanosis in individuals who are hypoxemic. Patients with CF are also likely to exhibit digital clubbing.[20]

Muscle Performance

Gross muscle performance should be documented in the review of systems. However, because increasing evidence indicates that peripheral muscle dysfunction exists independent of ventilation limitations in persons with CF, the physical therapist must be particularly careful to document and follow strength measures. Studies indicate that chronic lung disease results in muscle weakness, placing voluntary maximal strength measures at about 80% of similar persons without chronic lung disease. Mechanisms leading to this strength deficit have been identified as inactivity that leads to muscle deconditioning, malnutrition, and a myopathic process. Regardless of their cause, it is clear that peripheral muscle strength deficits lead to exercise limitation and intolerance.[32,33] More recently, a great deal of attention has focused on physical rehabilitation of patients in intensive care and the development of intensive care unit–acquired weakness.[34,35] Although this recent work refers to adult care, it is likely that children suffer from similar deficits following long periods of intensive care.

Muscle performance can be measured in many different ways, including manual muscle testing, dynamometry using handheld devices or more sophisticated technology-assisted systems, and functional muscle testing. Functional muscle testing often employs timed walking tests, a shuttle walking test, or a step test.[20–24] Although these several approaches examine more than discrete muscle function, they offer a more practical examination of muscle performance as it occurs during a child's daily activities.

Other Important Tests and Measures

Although this chapter deals with disorders of the pulmonary system, the therapist must consider all systems when assessing a child. A functional combination of several systems can be assessed by considering exertion and dyspnea.

EXERTION AND DYSPNEA Perceived exertion is quantified commonly with the revised 10-point Borg scale and dyspnea is quantified by using various dyspnea scales. These measures are described below. The Borg scale of perceived exertion was originally designed as a scale with a range of scores from 6 to 20. The scale was later revised to a 10-point scale ranging from 0 to 10, with 0 equating to no exertion at all and 10 identifying very strong exertion. The Borg scale correlates well with physiological measures of maximal oxygen uptake and others. However, recent work has questioned the strength of validity for the Borg scales.[36] There is some indication that the Borg scale has validity in the pediatric and adolescent population, though perhaps not as robust a scale as in adults.[37]

Quantification of dyspnea in children is a new endeavor with very little support in the literature. Prasad et al. described a 15-count dyspnea test in which the child simply inhaled deeply and counted aloud to 15. The authors stated:

> The 15-count score has been evaluated as an objective measure of breathlessness. It is easy to explain and perform, and can be used by any child capable of counting fluently to 15 in any language. It is best used in conjunction with a subjective score, and either the Borg scale or a visual analogue score is appropriate.[38]

A group of visual dyspnea scales for children was published by McGrath et al. in 2005. The descriptive drawings demonstrated and measured throat closing, chest tightness, and effort in a group of 79 children, including those with asthma, CF and lung disease. The authors stated that the measures appeared to measure the three constructs built into the visual aids.[39]

Neuromotor development and sensory integration testing is often necessary for a child who has experienced periodic or chronic episodes of hypoxemia that often occur with pulmonary disorders. Inadequate oxygenation for a period of time may cause minor or major CNS deficit, resulting in a developmental delay. (Normal development and tests of development are discussed in Chapters 2 and 3 of this text.)

Assessment of pain—both its source and perceived level—is an important part of the examination. Identification of painful areas of the thorax is often accomplished via palpation and questioning the child or parent. If a painful site is identified, it is appropriate for the clinician to use some pain scale or pain diary to determine the patient's level of pain, its attributes, and its effect on daily activity, as well as methods of reducing or modifying the painful stimulus. This issue of an age and developmentally appropriate rating scale for pain in children has been addressed in the past two decades. The Faces Pain Scale, developed by Bieri, was an early and significant attempt to use a scale that was suitable for children but suffered from having 7 faces on the scale and was difficult to correlate with the more commonly employed 5- or 10-point analogue pain scales.[40] More recently, Hicks and colleagues revised the scale by Bieri in a manner that made it more easily comparable with either a 5- or 10-point analogue pain scale. The revised Face Pain Scale was not significantly different from either of the analogue scales previously noted.[41] Figure 20.3 shows the Faces Pain Scale.

Postural abnormalities can result from *or* can cause respiratory disorders. Scoliosis with a primary curvature of greater than 60 degrees often results in thoracic restriction and a decrease in lung volumes, as will severe pectus

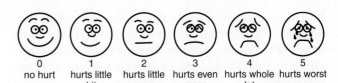

FIGURE 20.3 The Wong-Baker FACES Pain Rating Scale. (Reprinted with permission from Hockenberry MJ, Wilson D, Winklestein ML. *Wong's Essentials of Pediatric Nursing.* 7th ed. St. Louis, MO: Mosby; 2005:1259.)

excavatum.[42] Some chronic lung diseases, such as severe recurring asthma and CF, lead to hyperinflated, barreled chest with abducted and protracted scapulae. These possibilities must be considered in the assessment of the child with pulmonary disorders. Common orthopedic disorders, some of which have respiratory complications, are discussed in Chapter 13.

Finally, an assessment of the family's knowledge and ability to participate in the child's care is important when planning discharge from the hospital. Many pediatric pulmonary disorders are chronic, and will require continuing and effective care at home. The physical therapist is an important family educator and troubleshooter and must participate in formal and informal teaching.

▶ Physical therapy for children with pulmonary disease and respiratory disorders

Physical therapy for the infant or child with pulmonary disease or respiratory disorder can be categorized into three general areas that often overlap:

1. AC for removal of secretions, either by traditional postural drainage with percussion and vibration (PDPV) or more contemporary techniques that will be discussed at some length.
2. Breathing exercises and retraining.
3. Physical reconditioning including aerobic exercise, strength training, and other types of exercise for the thorax.

Of course, the degree to which these three areas are used and the specific interventions employed will depend not only on the disease process, but also on the age and level of ability and cooperation of the child. Neonates and infants will be treated almost exclusively with traditional AC procedures, including positioning to alter ventilation and perfusion. Simple breathing games and activities can be incorporated into the regimen as needed when the child becomes a toddler. As the child grows older, exercises for breathing retraining, physical reconditioning, and postural exercises become possible. Also, measures for AC that depend on breathing control, such as autogenic drainage, active cycle of breathing, and positive expiratory pressure devices become more applicable as the older child can coordinate the necessary breathing maneuvers. The next section of the chapter presents the more classic studies that helped to establish the efficacy of the numerous types of intervention.

Airway Clearance

Removal of secretions from the child's airway is the main goal of AC. Of all types of physical therapy treatment for patients with respiratory problems, AC in its many formats and approaches has been most extensively studied. Despite limited compelling evidence based upon controlled studies, AC is widely accepted and used universally. Perhaps the universal use of AC suggests that "lack of evidence does not mean lack of effectiveness." AC includes both traditional methods—positioning for gravity-assisted drainage of the airways, manual techniques for loosening secretions, and removal of secretions by coughing and suctioning of the airway. AC has also come to include active cycle of breathing techniques (ACBT), positive expiratory pressure (PEP) devices, oscillating PEP (Flutter® and Acapella®), high-frequency chest wall oscillation (HFWCO), and intrapulmonary percussive ventilation (IPV). Each of these techniques will be described below.

Postural Drainage with Percussion and Vibration
POSITIONING FOR GRAVITY-ASSISTED DRAINAGE Using a working knowledge of bronchopulmonary segment anatomy, the therapist can position the infant or child to drain areas of the lung in which secretions are found during the chest examination. The positions place the segment or lobe of lung to be drained uppermost, with the bronchus supplying that lung area in as close to an inverted position as possible. In adults and older children, specific positioning for segmental drainage often involves the use of treatment tables or tilting beds. In infants and young children, the therapist's lap and shoulder serve as the "treatment table." The infant or toddler can be held and comforted while in each of the drainage positions (Fig 20.4A and B). When the child reaches 3 or 4 years of age, the transition may be made from lap to treatment table, but many therapists and parents will continue to use the lap for children up to 4 or 5 years of age. The older child or teen can use an exercise table or pillows for proper positioning.

One point of caution must be raised regarding tipping infants into traditional head-down positions. In a series of well-designed studies over a period of 8 years, Button et al. clearly demonstrated that infants with CF had significant gastroesophageal reflux and resulting decreased long-term lung function associated with head-down positioning during PDPV.[43,44] With this clear evidence, the use of head-down positions for PDPV has become unpopular in CF centers around the world.

MANUAL TECHNIQUES OF PERCUSSION AND VIBRATIONS
The manual techniques of percussion and vibration are used to loosen or dislodge secretions from the bronchial wall, thus allowing easier removal when the child coughs, sneezes, or undergoes airway aspiration with a suction catheter. Although some obvious differences exist, the techniques used are quite similar to those performed on adults. One of the major differences is the amount of force used for either percussion or vibration. Common sense should dictate that minimal amounts of force should be used on the thorax of a premature infant who weighs 1 to 2 kg or less. Increased amounts of percussion and vibration force can be safely applied as the infant grows and as the bones and muscles of the thorax become stronger.

As with adults, the percussion and vibration should be applied to the area of thorax that corresponds to the lung and airways in which secretions are present. Another difference in the pediatric group is that a therapist's percussing or vibrating hand often covers the entire thorax of an infant or toddler. As a result, other implements have been suggested for percussion and vibration in the infant. Several items used for percussion are shown in Figure 20.5, and different hand configurations for percussion of the infant are shown in Figures. 20.6 A–E. Contraindications for chest percussion in the neonate commonly include a significant drop in transcutaneous (or arterial) oxygen level during percussion; rib fracture or other thoracic trauma; and hemoptysis.[45] There are also various conditions in which percussion for a child should be used carefully: poor condition of the infant's skin; coagulopathy; osteoporosis or rickets; cardiac arrhythmias; apnea and bradycardia; increased irritability during treatment; subcutaneous emphysema; and subependymal or intraventricular hemorrhage.[46] Vibration, which may be used in addition to or in place of percussion, is less vigorous than percussion. There are few true contraindications to vibration with the exception of hemoptysis and reduced oxygenation during treatment. Because vibration is usually done during the expiratory phase of breathing, and because the infant with respiratory disease often has a rate of 40 or more breaths per minute, it is difficult to coordinate manual vibration with the expiratory phase of breathing. Some persons use various battery-powered vibrators that can be held against the infant's thorax during expiration and then quickly removed during inspiration. The modifications and precautions for both percussion and vibration become fewer as the infant grows, and treatment begins to parallel more closely that used for an adult.

COUGHING AND SUCTIONING Infants and young children will seldom cough on request. Toddlers and school-aged children have the language skills to understand the request for coughing but will often choose not to cough. Imaginative means, including storytelling, coloring games, and nursery rhymes have been suggested to entice young children to cooperate.[47] In addition, the author has found

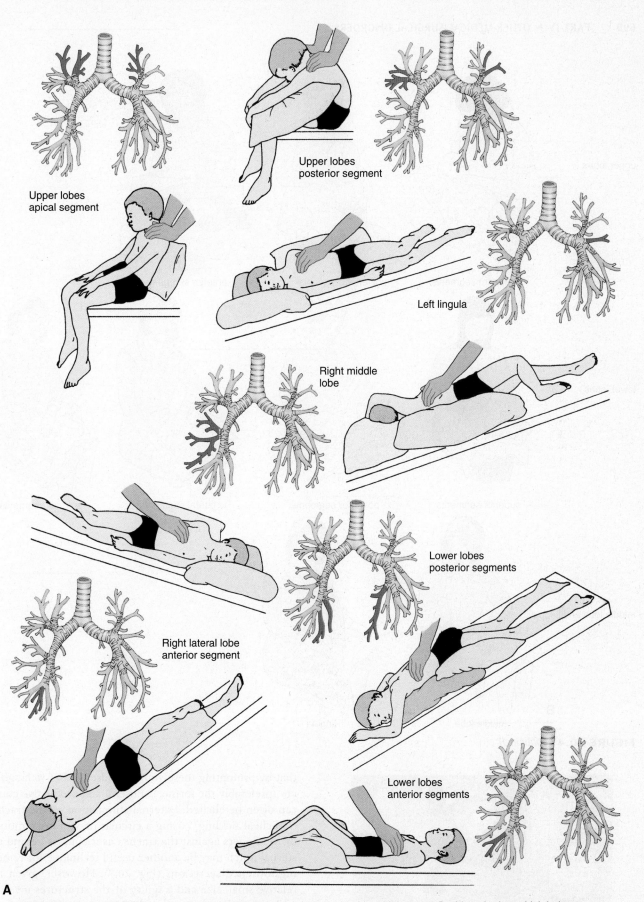

Upper lobes apical segment

Upper lobes posterior segment

Left lingula

Right middle lobe

Lower lobes posterior segments

Right lateral lobe anterior segment

Lower lobes anterior segments

A

FIGURE 20.4 **(A)** Positions for gravity-assisted postural drainage in older children. **(B)** Positions for bronchial drainage for major segments of all lobes in infants and toddlers. Note that head-down positions may be contraindicated in children with gastroesophageal reflux. This procedure is most readily performed with the infant in your lap, with your hand on the chest over the area to be cupped or vibrated. (From Pillitteri A. *Maternal and Child Nursing*. 4th ed. Philadelphia, PA: Lippincott, Williams & Wilkins; 2003.)

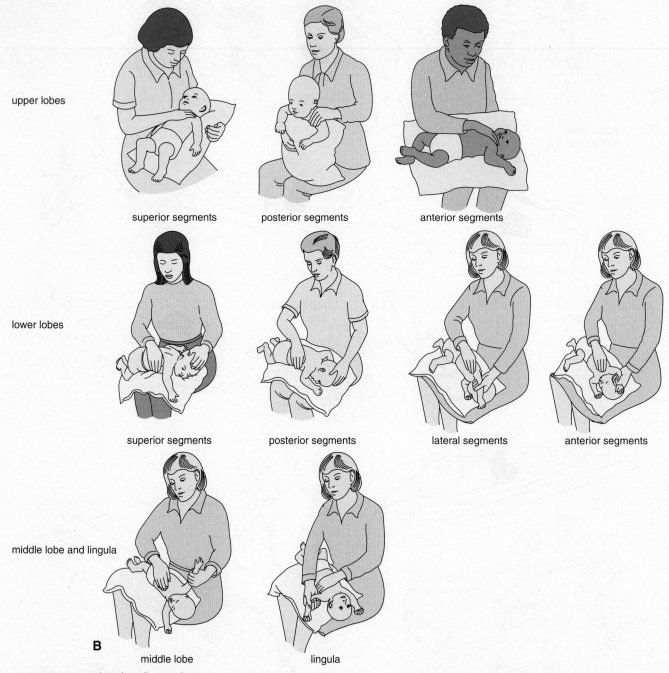

upper lobes

superior segments   posterior segments   anterior segments

lower lobes

superior segments   posterior segments   lateral segments   anterior segments

middle lobe and lingula

B

middle lobe   lingula

FIGURE 20.4 *(continued)*

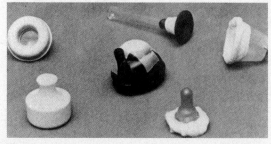

FIGURE 20.5 Commercially available and adaptable devices for percussion. (Reproduced by permission from Irwin S, Tecklin JS. *Cardiopulmonary Physical Therapy.* St. Louis, MO: CV Mosby; 1985.)

that by prompting these young children either to laugh or cry (preferably the former), a useful and productive cough can often be elicited. External stimulation of the trachea ("tracheal tickling") using a circular or vibratory motion of the fingers against the trachea as it courses behind the sternal notch may be another useful technique for removing loosened secretions (Fig. 20.7). However, given the relative small size and fragility of the structures involved with this technique, great care must be employed to avoid injury. Coughing is particularly difficult for the child who has undergone thoracic surgery. Splinting the incision with the hands or with a doll or stuffed animal pressed close to

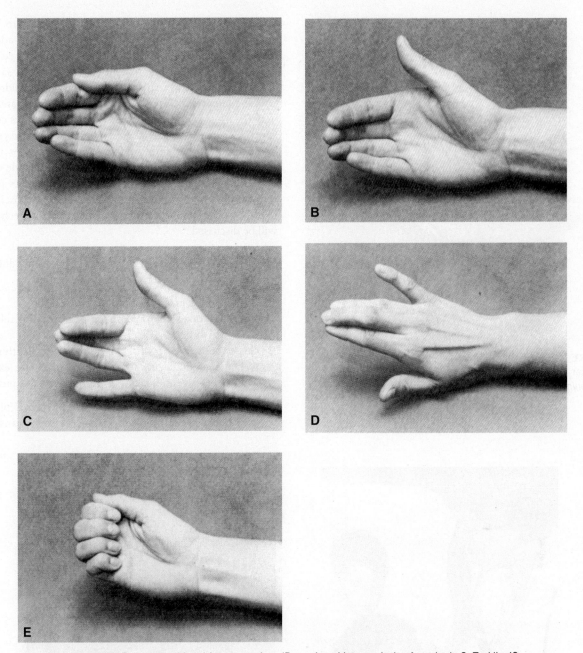

FIGURE 20.6 **(A)** Fully cupped hand for percussion. (Reproduced by permission from Irwin S, Tecklin JS. *Cardiopulmonary Physical Therapy.* St. Louis, MO: CV Mosby; 1985.) **(B)** Four fingers cupped for percussion. (Reproduced by permission from Irwin S, Tecklin JS. *Cardiopulmonary Physical Therapy.* St. Louis: CV Mosby; 1985.) **(C)** Three fingers cupped for percussion with the middle finger "tented" (anterior view). (Reproduced by permission from Irwin S, Tecklin JS. *Cardiopulmonary Physical Therapy.* St. Louis, MO: CV Mosby; 1985.) **(D)** Three fingers cupped for percussion with the middle finger "tented" (posterior view). (Reproduced by permission from Irwin S, Tecklin JS. *Cardiopulmonary Physical Therapy.* St. Louis: CV Mosby; 1985.) **(E)** Thenar and hypothenar surfaces for percussion. (Reproduced by permission from Irwin S, Tecklin JS. *Cardiopulmonary Physical Therapy.* St. Louis: CV Mosby; 1985.)

the child's chest promotes the development of an effective cough (Fig. 20.8).

Airway aspiration by suctioning is often needed, particularly in the neonate, to remove secretions. Suctioning must always be done carefully because it has significant risks, even when performed under the best circumstances. Despite the many protocols available, endotracheal suctioning is always

a potential hazard, particularly in the pediatric and neonatal populations.[48]

Contemporary Approaches to AC

During the past two or three decades several new approaches to AC were developed. The earlier of the new

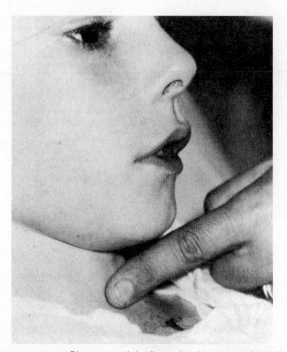

FIGURE 20.7 Placement of the finger for the tracheal "tickle" maneuver. (Reproduced by permission from Irwin S, Tecklin JS. *Cardiopulmonary Physical Therapy*. St. Louis, MO: CV Mosby; 1985.)

approaches included breathing maneuvers used to loosen and transport mucus as the common feature. In addition, the techniques were designed to eliminate the need for an individual other than the patient to perform necessary AC. These approaches were developed primarily for children and young adults with CF, although they are appropriate for all individuals with chronic lung disease that produces copious sputum. The 1990s saw the development of several new AC techniques that employed various modes of oscillation to either the chest wall or the airway. These include oscillatory PEP (Flutter® and Acapella®), intrapulmonary percussive ventilation, and high-frequency chest wall oscillation (The Vest® and SmartVest®). Each of these AC techniques will be discussed.

AUTOGENIC DRAINAGE This approach was introduced by Chevalier and described by Dab and Alexander:

1. The child sits in an upright or sitting position.
2. The child takes deep breaths at a "normal or relatively slow" rhythm.
3. Secretions move upward as a result of the breathing.
4. When secretions reach the trachea, they are expelled with either a gentle cough or slightly forced expiration.

The authors recommend that slightly forced expiration be used because of their belief that the high transmural

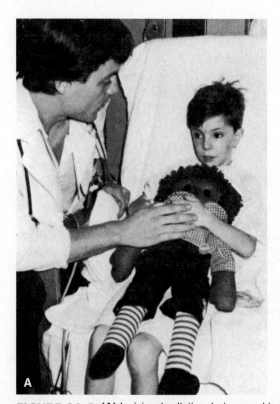

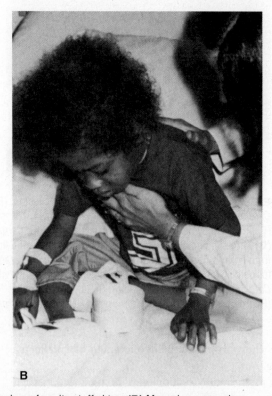

FIGURE 20.8 (A) Incisional splinting during coughing using a favorite stuffed toy. **(B)** Manual compression over the midsternum to facilitate expectoration of sputum. (Reproduced by permission from Irwin S, Tecklin JS. *Cardiopulmonary Physical Therapy*. St. Louis, MO: CV Mosby; 1985.)

pressures that develop during coughing effectively cause airway collapse, thereby rendering the coughing effort ineffective.[49,50]

Current use of autogenic drainage recommends tidal breathing at differing lung volumes rather than deep breathing. That is, the child will breathe at a normal volume but will begin this controlled breathing with most of the resting lung volume previously expelled. After several breaths at low lung volume, the child moves the tidal breathing to a midlung volume and then, following several additional breaths, to a higher lung volume. The movement of air through the smaller to the larger airways is thought to loosen secretions in the smaller more peripheral airways and move them proximally. The child should be taught to suppress active coughing until huff coughing (controlled coughing with an open glottis) can clear the secretions from the respiratory system. Although controlled research is minimal, at least two studies have shown autogenic drainage to be effective and equivalent to other accepted AC techniques.[46,51] In addition, evidence exists to support Autogenic Drainage (AD) as a well-accepted method of AC.[52] The author has worked with many patients in whom this technique has been successful in clearing the airways, particularly with copious thick secretions. A notion has circulated that autogenic drainage is a difficult technique to teach and learn. I believe that this is a highly overstated and essentially incorrect idea. Autogenic drainage is most commonly used for patients who are highly motivated and old enough to control their breathing well.

FORCED EXPIRATORY TECHNIQUE

The forced expiratory technique (FET) was developed in New Zealand, but was popularized in the late 1970s and into the 1980s by Pryor, Webber, Hodson, and Batten, all from Brompton Hospital in London.[53] As with autogenic drainage, the primary benefit derived from FET is that it can be performed without an assistant. Because the Brompton group has expressed great concern about what they believed to be misinterpretations of their original description, their description of FET is provided here in a direct quotation from the original article.

> The forced expiratory technique (FET) consists of one or two huffs (forced expirations), from mid-lung volume to low lung volume, followed by a period of relaxed, controlled diaphragmatic breathing. Bronchial secretions mobilized to the upper airways are then expectorated and the process is repeated until minimal bronchial clearance is obtained. The patient can reinforce the forced expiration by self compression of the chest wall using a brisk adduction movement of the upper arm.[54]

In a subsequent article that attempts to clarify the various components of FET, the authors place particular emphasis on huffing to low lung volumes in an effort to clear peripheral secretions. In addition, the phrase "from midlung volume" has been clarified to mean taking a medium-sized breath before initiating the huffing. The authors recommend that patients use FET while in gravity-assisted positions, and further suggest that pauses for breathing control and periods of relaxation are part of the overall technique.[48]

Owing to continuing differences in interpretation of the FET, it was reconstituted by the Brompton group into series of activities called ACBT. The ACBT employs a number of individual skills, including controlled breathing, FET, huff coughing, and thoracic expansion exercises. As was the case for the FET, there have been no attempts at controlled research for the ACBT by the individuals who developed the technique but some data exist to support ACBT.[44,45]

PEP BREATHING

PEP breathing was developed in Denmark in an attempt to maintain airway patency and employ channels of collateral ventilation to provide airflow distal to accumulated secretions. Airflow in the distal portions of the airway is presumed to dislodge and move secretions proximally toward larger airways. In addition, PEP provides expiratory resistance that appears to stabilize smaller airways, thereby preventing their early collapse during expiration and huff coughing. PEP is thought to be effective in both reducing air-trapping and enhancing secretion removal. The original technique relied upon breathing through an anesthesia face mask but more recent devices use mouthpieces.

When using PEP, the therapist attempts to have patients breathe with a level of expiratory pressure of approximately 15 cm H_2O. Devices to provide PEP usually offer varied resistance and have some type of indicator to identify when the 15 cm of pressure has been achieved. The child attempts to maintain that level of pressure throughout the expiratory phase of breathing for 10 to 15 breaths followed by ACBT with huff coughing to clear the secretions. Some recommend using PEP breathing while the child assumes each of the several bronchial drainage positions.[55] Figure 20.9 shows a commercially available PEP device. (Smith's Medical, St.Paul MN).

FLUTTER®

The Flutter is a small, handheld pipelike device that produces an oscillating resistance during expiration. The oscillations are created by a small ball within the device that is moved out of its seat during expiration but then rapidly moves back into its seat through the effects of gravity. The ball is then moved out of the seat again by the continuing force of the expiratory airflow. This repeated movement of the ball rapidly opens and occludes the orifice of the device that results in the rapid oscillations or vibrations transmitted into the airway. These rapid oscillations are thought to loosen the secretions for ease of removal. As with PEP breathing, airway collapse is reduced by the PEP generated by the device. Use

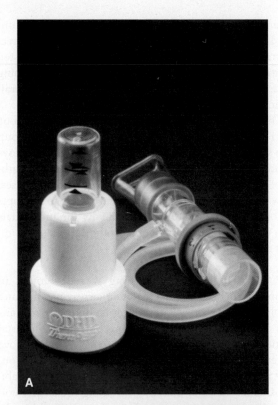

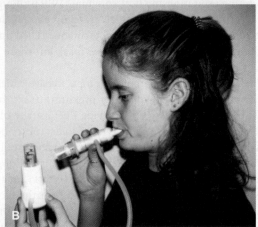

FIGURE 20.9 (A) An example of a positive expiratory pressure device (TheraPEP, DHD Healthcare, Canastota, NY). **(B)** TheraPEP device in use (compliments of A. Tecklin).

of the Flutter is followed by attempts to clear secretions by ACBT or huff coughing. Figure 20.10 A–E shows the Flutter device (Vario Raw SA; distributed by Scandipharm, Inc., Birmingham, AL). Research has shown Flutter to be an effective AC treatment when compared with PDPV for hospitalized patients with CF.[56]

ACAPELLA® This is another small handheld device capable of providing both PEP and oral oscillation. Unlike Flutter, Acapella generates oscillation by using a special valve. A benefit of the Acapella is that it is capable of providing

oscillation in any position, thereby being less technique-dependent than the Flutter. There are two versions of the device. I recommend the Acapella Choice® because that model can be disassembled for more complete disinfection and cleaning. Figure 20.11 shows the Acapella Choice (Smith Medical, St. Paul, MN).

HIGH-FREQUENCY CHEST WALL OSCILLATION (HFCWO)

HFCWO is a newer means of AC that employs an air pulse generator and a garment—a vest—that has inflatable bladders attached to the compressor by large, flexible tubing. The air pulse generator provides pulses at varying frequencies (5 to 20 Hertz) and at varying pressures into the inflatable bladders. The air pulses entering the bladder produce oscillations that are transmitted to the chest wall. King's work on dogs suggested that the bursts of air produced a shearing force on secretions within the airways and actually increased airflow into and out of the airways.[57] At least one researcher has referred to this air movement as a "staccato cough."[58] These rapidly recurring bursts of air, or staccato coughs, provide a shear force that cleaves the secretions from the walls of the airways. In addition to the shear forces, the air bursts reduce the viscosity of the secretions[59] and move the secretions upward where they can be coughed or suctioned out.[60] All lobes of the lungs are treated at the same time and the patient may sit upright throughout the entire treatment without having to assume the 10 to 12 different positions required for PDPV. Figure 20.12 is the MedPulse Smart Vest® (Electromed-USA, New Prague, MN).

Breathing Exercises and Retraining

Because many of the commonly used breathing exercises require voluntary participation by the child, the classic methods for teaching improved diaphragmatic descent, increased thoracic expansion, and pursed-lip breathing may not be useful in the infant or young child. Some therapists employ neurophysiologic techniques, such as applying a quick stretch to the thorax to facilitate contraction of the diaphragm and intercostal muscles, to increase inspiration for the baby or young child.

The toddler can participate in games that require deep breathing and control of breathing. Asking the child to breathe in time to music or to the beat of a metronome can present the skill of paced breathing. Blowing bubbles from a bubble wand or blowing a pinwheel will help emphasize increased control and prolonged expiration, which may be useful for the child with obstructive disease. Numerous types of incentive spirometers are also useful for enhancing deep inspiration after either medical or surgical diseases. Incentive spirometry has been studied extensively and is generally considered to be a useful adjunct to postoperative pulmonary care and a means of strengthening respiratory muscles. Improving ventilation

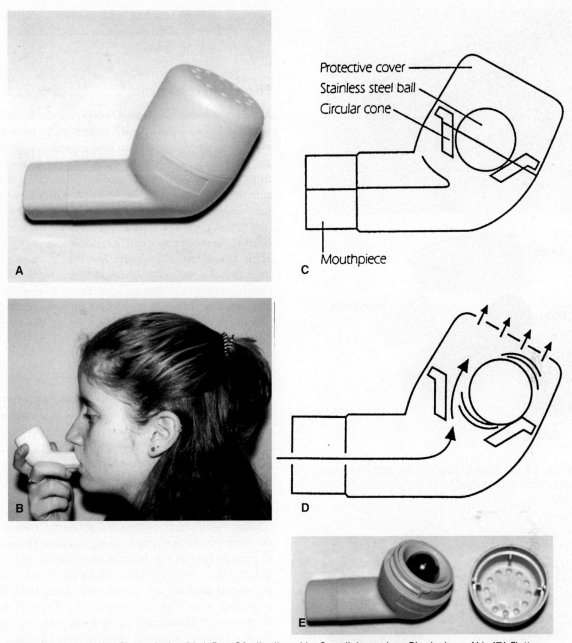

FIGURE 20.10 **(A)** Flutter device (VarioRaw SA, distributed by Scandipharm, Inc., Birmingham, AL). **(B)** Flutter device in use (compliments of A. Tecklin). **(C)** Cross section of Flutter device. **(D)** Cross section of Flutter device with representation of oscillating ball. **(E)** Flutter device with oscillating ball.

to the lower lobes by using diaphragmatic breathing and lateral costal expansion may help reduce postoperative pulmonary complications, but as with other breathing techniques, evidence for efficacy is lacking in both adult and pediatric care.

Participation in and cooperation with breathing exercises usually improves as the child grows older. When appropriate, the therapist may use manual contact to teach diaphragmatic breathing, lateral costal expansion, and segmental expansion. Depending on the findings from the assessment

of the moving chest, the therapist will choose one or more of these types of breathing exercises. The older child with severe, perennial asthma and the child or adolescent with advanced CF will often exhibit many of the same characteristics as adults with chronic obstructive pulmonary disease (COPD). Paced diaphragmatic breathing may be very useful for these children and young adults. Reduced energy expenditure of breathing is often considered a benefit of diaphragmatic breathing. Because exercise intolerance becomes a problem for children with asthma and CF, paced

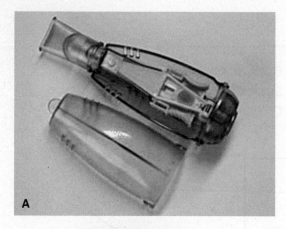

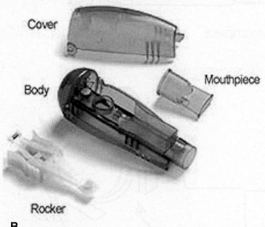

FIGURE 20.11 **(A)** Acapella Choice airway clearance device. **(B)** Acapella Choice disassembled for cleaning (Smith's Medical, Watford, UK).

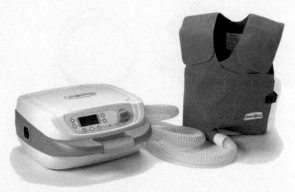

FIGURE 20.12 The MedPulse SmartVest Airway Clearance System (Electromed, New Prague, MN).

diaphragmatic breathing may improve the child's ability to walk, climb stairs, and perform other vigorous physical activities. Pursed-lip breathing may also be useful for breath control in the child with chronic lung disease. Relaxation exercise for the child with asthma is often suggested as a means of reducing breathlessness. Although there is little or no scientific evidence of any change in the pulmonary

function of these children with relaxation exercise, there is strong anecdotal evidence of a reduction in the anxiety associated with dyspnea.

Physical Development

Activities to improve physical function in the infant or child with a pulmonary disorder may begin in the neonatal nursery. When physiological conditions permit, physical therapy interventions should be done with the infant removed from the isolette or warming bed. The handling and tactile stimulation provided by the AC session may be helpful adjuncts to the sensorimotor development of the infant, who may spend great amounts of time in a supine position. Of course, this type of movement is not always possible, particularly for the critically ill baby. As the pulmonary condition improves, the infant should begin to receive, in addition to respiratory physical therapy, appropriate intervention to assess and, if necessary, to treat delays in motor development. Chapter 4, devoted to the high-risk infant, describes an approach to this type of child.

Physical Training

Children with asthma and CF and those with respiratory disease secondary to neuromuscular or musculoskeletal problems represent two distinct groups for whom physical training is important. A case example of each group follows in this chapter. Programs of physical training usually include exercises to improve strength and range of motion (ROM), posture, and cardiovascular endurance.

Strength training is helpful in both groups of children. Children with severe asthma and moderately advanced CF are often limited in strength owing to inactivity and chronic or periodic hypoxemia. In addition, evidence in the past decade has shown that children with CF have weakness in their peripheral muscles associated with diminished maximal workload, even without diminished pulmonary or nutritional status.[32] Darbee and Cerny advocated a strengthening program involving isotonic resistive exercise performed at a high number of repetitions rather than high levels of resistance. They also recommended that exercise should stress the shoulder girdle and thoracic musculature as a means of facilitating the respiratory pump.[61] Orenstein et al. demonstrated increased upper-body strength and physical work capacity over a one-year training program for children with CF.[62]

Decreased ROM is more commonly a problem for those with neuromuscular/musculoskeletal problems than for those with asthma and CF. Nonetheless, children with asthma and CF have been found to have reduced thoracic motion associated with chronic hyperinflation, and may be at risk for both loss of shoulder motion and development of kyphoscoliosis. Exercises for deep breathing, thoracic expansion, segmental expansion, and upper extremity function can help either prevent loss of motion or regain motion that has been lost.

Just as other skeletal muscles respond to training for both endurance and strength, the muscles of inspiration and expiration will respond similarly. Studies of children with chronic lung disease and groups with specific respiratory muscle weakness have shown that significant improvement in respiratory muscle function accompanies breathing activities aimed at either endurance or strength, or both. Inspiratory muscle endurance training and strengthening have resulted in improvement in numerous physiologic indices and have also shown functional and psychosocial benefits.[63,64] Expiratory muscle strengthening may benefit exercise tolerance and surely should enhance the force of expiratory maneuvers, including coughing.[65] These exercises are described later in this chapter.

The child with chronic lung disease will benefit from a program of cardiovascular training or conditioning. Because running precipitates exercise-induced bronchospasm in children with asthma, this group of young patients seems to respond much better to swimming programs.[66] Children and young adults with CF participate throughout the United States in organized walking or jogging groups. The popularity of these groups can be traced to Orenstein and colleagues, who first popularized jogging for children with CF and who then studied the benefits for those children.[67]

Regardless of the specific exercise or physical reconditioning program, and regardless of the pediatric pulmonary problem, there is a major role for the physical therapist in treating children with lung disease.

The next section of this chapter describes four common disorders of the respiratory tract in children and their physical therapy evaluation and treatment.

▶ Atelectasis

Atelectasis, or incomplete expansion of a lung or a portion thereof, was first described by Laennec in 1819.[68] Primary atelectasis occurs in the neonate as a result of pulmonary immaturity, and at any age as a result of inadequate respiratory effort. Secondary atelectasis occurs when gas in a lung segment is reabsorbed without subsequent refilling of that segment. Common causes of secondary atelectasis in children include external compression of lung tissue, obstruction of the bronchial or bronchiolar lumen, and respiratory compromise secondary to musculoskeletal or neuromuscular disorders.[69]

Primary atelectasis in small areas of the newborn lung is a common finding during the first few days of life. The sick neonate with poor respiratory effort and generalized weakness may not fully expand all areas of the lung for several weeks. Major areas of secondary atelectasis may be the result of abnormal thoracic content such as an enlarged heart or great vessels, congenital or acquired lung cysts, diaphragmatic hernia, and congenital lobar emphysema, each of which compresses lung tissue or the airways. Atelectasis seen by the physical therapist is caused frequently by airway obstruction secondary to accumulation of mucus or other debris, including meconium, amniotic content, foreign bodies, and aspirated gastrointestinal contents. Various AC techniques as part of pre-operative preparation followed by early post-operative mobility when possible can be an effective approach when treating atelectasis following surgery.[70]

Medical Information

Signs and symptoms of atelectasis depend on the degree of involvement of the lungs. Small areas may be asymptomatic, but common findings in larger areas of atelectasis include decreased chest wall excursion of the affected hemithorax, tachypnea, inspiratory retractions, and cyanosis if the atelectasis is large. The trachea, which can be palpated, will deviate toward the involved lung because of volume loss, and a dull percussion note, which indicates an airless lung, will be present. By auscultation, breath sounds will be reduced or absent. The radiograph will often demonstrate a sharply demarcated area of consolidation, although patchy areas of atelectasis are not uncommon in acute respiratory tract infection.

Medical management of obstructive atelectasis is directed toward removal of the obstructing material or condition. When atelectasis is associated with an acute infection, therapy to treat the infection will often eradicate the atelectasis. Good hydration may decrease the viscosity of the mucus, thereby aiding in its removal. A bronchodilator may widen the bronchus, thus allowing air past the obstruction to enhance AC techniques, including PDPV, PEP, various forms of oscillation—internal and chest wall and autogenic drainage. Finally, early patient mobilization while in bed is an important consideration.[66]

When an obstruction is caused by a neoplasm or other structure that occludes the airway or exerts pressure over the lung parenchyma, surgical removal of the item may be indicated. Endobronchial aspiration using a suction catheter may help remove airway debris, and repositioning of a poorly placed endotracheal tube may correct atelectasis. If none of these more conservative measures is successful, particularly in an acute scenario, bronchoscopy, using either a rigid or a flexible bronchoscope with administration of general or local anesthesia, is indicated to remove the intraluminal mucus or debris.[63]

Prognosis is usually good if the underlying disease process is not life-threatening and if the duration of the atelectasis has not been prolonged. Permanent damage to the bronchial architecture and lung parenchyma can occur with delayed or incomplete resolution of atelectasis and related postoperative pulmonary complication.

Physical Therapy Examination

A thorough review of the patient's chart is necessary to fully understand the pathophysiology of the condition and to identify the type and etiology of atelectasis (primary or secondary). The treatment for each type will include similar efforts to increase respiratory effort, but only secondary atelectasis requires AC.

Review of the radiographic findings will identify the location of the atelectasis. The therapist should use the roentgenogram as a clinical tool when treating a patient with atelectasis. Lateral and posteroanterior exposures provide a three-dimensional view of the lung fields to more accurately locate the area of atelectasis. Figure 20.13 A show two radiographs with different types of atelectasis. The patient's chest configuration and breathing pattern should be noted. A large atelectasis narrows the rib interspaces and decreases excursion of the involved hemithorax. The muscular pattern of respiration should be noted—diaphragmatic versus accessory—and the patient's respiratory rate should be determined. Palpation may indicate a shift of the trachea toward the atelectasis owing to volume loss in the involved lung as noted in Figure 20.13 A. The airless lung area has a dull percussion note that helps the therapist locate the atelectasis. Auscultatory findings will vary. The most frequent change is a diminution of breath sounds in the involved area. Complete obstruction of a large or main bronchus associated with the atelectasis may result in complete absence of breath sounds. With patchy or incomplete atelectasis, crackles may be heard for the first of several deep breaths; however, with subsequent deep breaths, the alveoli may open and the crackles may decrease.

Other considerations in evaluating the child include the following:

1. mobility—has the child been at bedrest for a long period of time?
2. pain—can the child take a deep breath and cough despite the level of pain?
3. cough—can the child cough, or is there insufficient strength or neurologic competence for an effective cough?

Physical Therapy Procedural Interventions

Several studies support physical therapy interventions for the ***prevention*** of postoperative atelectasis in adult and pediatric surgical patients. Therapeutic methods used in these studies included bronchial drainage, percussion, vibration, deep breathing[71-73] maximal inspiratory efforts,[74] and electrical stimulation of the thorax with direct current.[75] The success of each treatment regimen was unequivocal.

Finer and associates found a significant decrease in the incidence of postextubation atelectasis in infants who were treated with bronchial drainage, vibration, and oral suctioning when compared with a similar control group treated only with bronchial drainage.[76] A more recent Cochrane Review by Flenady and Gray found that AC techniques reduced postextubation atelectasis in a small group of infants who were being extubated.[77] A methodologically sound study by Wong compared traditional chest physical therapy techniques with a lung-squeezing approach. There was clear evidence of decreased non-resolution of atelectasis following lung-squeezing than with traditional treatment.[78] Atelectasis after extubation occurs commonly in infants, and is presumably caused by excessive bronchial secretions. These studies have not evaluated the treatment of atelectasis; however, they have evaluated its prevention, which is the best treatment.

Postoperative atelectasis is often a combination of primary and secondary atelectasis. Secretions are more abundant owing to irritation of the airway by the anesthetic gases and tube manipulations. With incisional pain, and with the generalized weakness that accompanies thoracic or abdominal surgery, the child has a less effective cough and the volume of inspirations is decreased. Deep breathing to achieve maximal inspiration will often be sufficient to resolve small areas of atelectasis. These efforts should be initiated early in the postoperative period—in the recovery room if possible—to

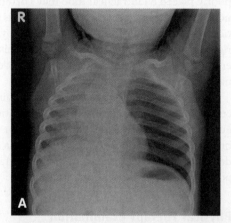
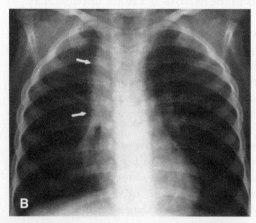

FIGURE 20.13 (A) The chest film shows tracheal deviation and mediastinal shift, and compression atelectasis of the right lung due to hyperinflation of the left lung, which compresses the lung on the right side. **(B)** Sublobar atelectasis. Asthmatic child with acute asthma attack. Note area of apparent consolidation in the right paratracheal region (*arrows*). This represents collapse of one portion of the right upper lobe.

prevent atelectasis. Coaching the child to breathe deeply, splinting the incision to reduce pain, and using propioceptive techniques to facilitate the inspiratory musculature can help the child increase the depth of respiration. Positioning the patient to drain the major lung fields and percussion/vibration followed by attempts to cough will aid in the prevention of pulmonary complications. Incentive spirometers, used as a breathing game, will stimulate deeper inhalations. Percussion and coughing become critical components of the treatment if the patient develops atelectasis despite preventive measures. Aggressive percussion of the chest over the atelectasis and splinted coughing will work to mechanically dislodge and clear the obstructing mucus. Should percussion prove too aggressive and result in increased pain, vibration of the chest is a good alternative intervention.[79] Endotracheal suctioning to remove accumulated mucus and to further stimulate coughing is often employed for postoperative atelectasis. Early mobilization of the patient after surgery and the resultant need for increased ventilation may help mobilize secretions by causing the patient to breathe deeply.

Children with medical chest conditions develop atelectasis as a result of retained secretions, and one of the many types of AC may be employed. These children without incisional pain can often tolerate liberal and more aggressive use of manual techniques. Bronchial drainage with localized percussion will often dislodge the obstructing secretions, and coughing will clear the airway. Other techniques such as ACBT, PEP, intra-airway oscillation and HFCWO are also likely to be effective in loosening the obstructing debris. Many physicians also suggest nebulized mucolytics and bronchodilators as well as bland aerosols to thin and moisten the secretions and to deliver a bronchodilator. The rationale for these procedures of inhalation is that thinned, moist secretions will drain more easily from a bronchus that is maximally dilated. Primary atelectasis caused by respiratory muscle weakness can be resolved by deep breathing and strengthening of the respiratory muscles and change in position to afford better aeration to the poorly ventilated lung areas.

▶ Respiratory muscle weakness

Respiratory muscle weakness in children, as in adults, may result from any disorder affecting any link in the chain of neuromuscular events that produce contraction of the respiratory muscles. Weakness or paresis of the respiratory muscles may be either mild and transient or severe and irreversible. The underlying pathologic process is the primary determinant of the duration and severity of the weakness. The physical therapist should develop a therapeutic regimen to treat the muscle weakness and to prevent or treat the resultant pulmonary symptoms within the limitations imposed by the disorder.

In the past two decades, a growing population of community-living ventilator-dependent children has arisen as a result of improved technology and care for chronic ventilatory failure.[80] A major improvement in the ability of families and caregivers to maintain these children at home has been due to the acceptance and *relative* ease of care through non-invasive ventilation and improved secretion control.[81,82] Many of these children require physical therapy for deficits and impairments associated with respiratory pump failure and for the delay in motor skill development caused by reliance on the mechanical ventilator be it invasive or non-invasive ventilation provided in a hospital, residential facility, or home.

Medical Information

Diffuse pathology of the CNS (e.g., viral encephalitis or barbiturate intoxication) may lead to respiratory failure by paralyzing portions of the respiratory muscle pump. Abnormal neural control mechanisms and reflexes may ablate or reduce the physiologic response to chemical and mechanical stimuli. These stimuli may occur within the lungs, the brain stem, the blood, and cerebrospinal fluid (CSF). Examples of childhood disorders that result in a reduced response to respiratory stimuli are familial dysautonomia, sleep apnea, and obesity-hypoventilation syndrome. Focal lesions may affect many nervous system sites such as the medullary centers that generate the inspiratory drive and may cause marked changes in ventilatory patterns.

Spinal cord lesions in the high cervical region may result in total ventilatory paralysis. Because the phrenic nerve, which innervates the diaphragm, leaves the spinal cord at the C3 to C5 level, a lesion at or above that level will likely affect many muscles of respiration. Injury to the high-thoracic or low-cervical cord often results in decreased lung volume and reduced chest wall compliance due to impairment of thoracic musculature. Coughing, which is critically important for removing debris from the airways, will be inadequate if the abdominal muscles are paralyzed. These factors may cause respiratory insufficiency that may progress to respiratory failure, which may be an early sign of neuromuscular disease.[83] Acute respiratory care and long-term rehabilitation are essential components of a treatment plan for the child with a spinal cord lesion or injury.

Diseases of the neuromuscular system are not uncommon in children, as was discussed in Chapter 9. Respiratory deficits can result from acute inflammatory polyneuritis (Guillain-Barré syndrome). Because recovery from Guillain-Barré syndrome is often complete, the respiratory weakness must be treated aggressively, and rehabilitation should include acute and long-term measures. The progressive loss of anterior horn cells seen in the spinal muscular atrophies may reduce respiratory muscle function, leading to paralysis and death secondary to respiratory failure. Degenerative diseases of the muscle (e.g., Duchenne myopathy) are characterized by progressive deterioration of pulmonary function later in the course of the disease. Adequate arterial oxygen and carbon dioxide values are maintained only through active efforts. Death is often the direct result of respiratory failure, which often follows the development of pneumonia. When these syndromes are fatal, it is usually attributable to respiratory failure.

The thoracic cage normally provides for adequate function of the respiratory musculature. Abnormalities of the thorax, such as idiopathic scoliosis, scoliosis secondary to neuromuscular disease, and other specific congenital abnormalities, may result in a loss of mechanical advantage of the respiratory muscles. In addition to specific abnormalities, chest wall compliance in individuals with chronic neuromuscular disease appears to decrease through the lifespan, which results in increased work of breathing.[84]

The examples just mentioned can cause respiratory muscle weakness or mechanical disadvantage, which may also lead to the requirement for long-term management by mechanical ventilation, as noted above. Mallory and Stilwell identify the physical therapist as a member of the typical team of caregivers for these technology-dependent children. In addition, of the seven rehabilitation goals they have identified for the ventilator-dependent child, six are directly related to physical therapy knowledge, skills, and scope of practice. These seven goals follow:

1. Increase in muscle strength
2. Increase in attention and cognition
3. Decrease in spasticity
4. Increase in chest wall movement
5. Accessory muscle breathing while upright
6. Diaphragmatic breathing
7. Assisted cough

All goals, with the possible exception of the second one, are direct benefits derived from physical therapy.[85]

Physical Therapy Examination

The physical therapy examination for a child with respiratory muscle weakness should follow the recommended sequence presented earlier.[23] Specific attention should be paid to breathing pattern, respiratory muscle strength, chest and shoulder mobility, and AC (see Case Study, H. E., and Table 14.2).

Determining breathing pattern is a major part of the examination. Minute ventilation—the product of the respiratory rate and the tidal volume—determines the arterial $PaCO_2$. The respiratory rate can be counted for 30 seconds or 1 minute, remembering that the child's normal respiratory rate at rest varies with age (a younger child will have a higher rate). Table 20.1 presents respiratory rates in children. Tidal volume can be easily measured with a mechanical or electronic handheld spirometer used at the bedside. Figure 20.14 shows a teenager using a handheld spirometer.

TABLE **20.2**	Recommendations for Varied Types of Exercise in Cystic Fibrosis

TABLE 1: General Exercise and Training Recommendations

	Patients with mild to moderate CF lung disease	Patients with severe CF lung disease
Recommended activities	Cycling, walking, hiking, aerobics, running, rowing, tennis, swimming, strength training, climbing, roller-skating, (trampolining)	Ergometric cycling, walking, strengthening exercise, gymnastics, and day-to-day activities
Method	Intermittent and steady-state	Intermittent
Frequency	3–5 times per week	5 times per week
Duration	30–45 minutes	20–30 minutes
Intensity	70%–85% HRmax; 60%–80% peak VO_2; LT; GET	60%–80% HRmax; 50%–70% peak VO_2; LT; GET
Oxygen supplementation	Indicated, if SaO_2 drops below 90% during exercise	Indicated, if SaO2 drops below 90% during exercise (cave: resting hypoxia)
Activities to avoid	Bungee-jumping, high diving, and scuba diving	Bungee-jumping, high diving, scuba diving, and hiking in high altitude
Potential risks associated with exercise, and training	Dehydration Hypoxemia Bronchoconstriction Pneumothorax Hypoglycaemia* Hemoptysis Oesophageal bleedings Cardiac arrhythmias Rupture of liver and spleen Spontaneous fractures**	

HRmax: maximum heart rate; peak Vo_2: peak oxygen consumption; LT; lactate threshold; GET: gas exchange threshold; SaO_2: oxygen saturation.

*Depending on the existence of an impaired glucose tolerance.

**Depending on the existence of untreated CF-related bone disease.

From Williams CA, Benden C, Stevens D, et al. Exercise training in children and adolescents with cystic fibrosis: theory into practice. *Int J Pediatr.* 2010;2010:670640.

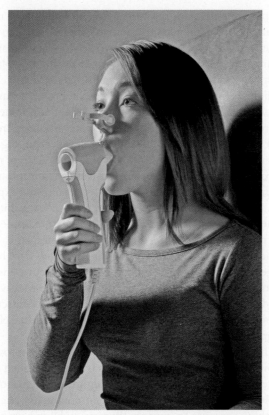

FIGURE 20.14 Use of a Spirometer to Evaluate Lung Function. Person being tested takes in a full breath, seals their lips over the mouthpiece of the spirometer, and then blows out as hard and as fast as possible for at least 6 seconds. Nose clips may be applied to ensure no air escapes through the nose. (Courtesy of Midmark Diagnostics, Versailles, Ohio.)

As with respiratory rate, tidal volume varies depending on the child's height. A taller child has a larger predicted tidal volume. The pattern and symmetry of muscular effort should be identified. Is the child using primarily the diaphragm, intercostal muscles, accessory muscles, or glossopharyngeal muscles? Is the muscular pattern similar for each hemithorax?

The therapist has several methods available for evaluating respiratory muscle strength. The measurement of maximal static inspiratory and expiratory pressures is simple and inexpensive, but requires the child's full cooperation. These pressures can be measured with appropriate pressure manometers, and measurements can be repeated as often as necessary. Reference values for maximal static respiratory pressures in children and adolescents were established by Domenech-Clar et al. In their conclusion, they state that both maximum inspiratory and expiratory pressures increase with age and are consistently higher in males.[86] Infants have also been studied. Airway pressures during crying have been an index of respiratory muscle function in infants for many years with differences in normal infants clearly distinguished from infants with neuromuscular disorders.[87,88]

Evaluation of chest wall mobility includes determining expansion of the chest wall in anteroposterior, transverse, and vertical directions during inspiration. Thoracic dimensions should be measured with a tape measure or chest calipers during inspiration and expiration to document chest motion. Active range of motion in the spine and the shoulder girdle should be examined, including glenohumeral, acromioclavicular, and sternoclavicular joints. Decreased motion at any one of these joints may result in reduced thoracic expansion.

Auscultation of the lungs of a child with respiratory weakness will serve several functions. Decreased breath sounds will help identify areas that are poorly ventilated. Lung areas with decreased or absent sounds may correlate with decreased chest motion or muscular effort. Breath sounds are the most reliable clinical tool for ensuring good ventilation. Breath sounds can help the therapist evaluate the need for AC. If crackles and wheezes are heard, AC and removal of secretions are probably necessary. Breath sounds may indicate the resolution or progression of pulmonary complications, such as pneumonia or atelectasis, and the therapist may choose to modify treatment accordingly.

The therapist should evaluate the child's cough. Integral components of a cough include several distinct phases. Stimulation or triggering of a cough is related to some irritant in the tracheobronchial system, which activates a deep inspiration. Normally, the increased inspiratory volume flows into small airways behind secretions or debris. Coordinated glottis closure is followed by sudden contraction of the expiratory muscles to markedly increase intrathoracic pressure, which can reach 300-mmHg pressure. The glottis opens, pressure is released, and secretions and other debris are sheared from the airway walls and moved proximally in the tracheobronchial tree. With neuromuscular dysfunction, the child may lack any or all cough-related function. Evaluation of inspiratory effort and volume, and abdominal muscle strength is important in assessing coughing and can be objectively done with maximal inspiratory and expiratory pressure measurements. The child must also coordinate the three components—inspiratory, glottis closure, and expiratory effort—into an effective, sputum-producing skill.[89]

Cough effectiveness can be determined by cough peak flow measurements. The child attempts to produce a cough after a maximal inspiration. The cough force is measured via a peak flow meter attached to the child by a mouthpiece or mask. Cough peak flows of less than 160 L/min during respiratory exacerbation are considered inadequate to protect against secretion retention and respiratory failure.[90]

Overall strength, mobility, and coordination, as well as the developmental level of the child, must be evaluated to plan a realistic rehabilitation program. A child who can actively locomote in some manner is less likely to suffer pulmonary complications and may improve pulmonary function as a by-product of the rehabilitative effort. An aggressive therapeutic regimen is necessary, both to provide

early mobility and to strengthen the respiratory musculature, thus improving ventilatory function.

Evaluation of oral motor function—swallowing and
feeding—is beyond the realm of physical therapy and often
requires an interdisciplinary effort by physicians, physical
therapists, occupational therapists, speech pathologists,
other therapists, and nurses. Swallowing should be evaluated for two reasons: eating is the best way for a child to
thrive nutritionally, and aspiration of feedings is a major
cause of respiratory problems in developmentally delayed
and neurologically impaired children.[91] It is clear that as
muscle weakness progresses, swallowing dysfunction and
aspiration of saliva and food can be problematic.[92]

Physical Therapy Interventions

Physical rehabilitation for the child with neurologic impairment should include an exercise program to improve
or maintain respiratory function. The exercises should
strengthen inspiratory and expiratory muscles, especially
the abdominal muscles that are necessary for effective
coughing. In addition, exercise, AC, and related techniques
are among the recommendations of the British Thoracic
Society guideline for respiratory management of children
with neuromuscular weakness.[93]

A traditional method of "strengthening" the diaphragm
by using abdominal weights has not withstood rigorous
scientific evaluation.[94] More physiologically appropriate
methods of improving inspiratory muscle strength and
endurance are currently used. Resistive breathing for improving inspiratory and expiratory strength will improve
maximal respiratory pressures. Endurance studies have similarly shown the benefit of repetitive inspiratory and expiratory exercise with increasing periods of time and increasing
resistive loads. Respiratory muscle training is a recognized
approach to reduce the progressive decline in respiratory
function in children with Duchenne myopathy and spinal
muscular atrophy (SMA). Studies have shown continuing
improvement over a period of up to 6 months of training,
with much of the improvement sustained at a point as long
as 6 months following the cessation of the formal exercise
regimen.[84,91] Training effects are dose-dependent but appear
most effective in children who have more slowly progressive
neuromuscular disease.[95] Despite numerous studies showing at least short-term benefit to respiratory muscle strength
and endurance, there is little evidence on the functional benefit of this exercise in the long term.

Active and resistive exercises for the neck will strengthen
the accessory muscles of inspiration (i.e., the sternocleidomastoid muscles and scalene muscles). Although accessory
muscle use increases the energy cost of breathing, the accessory muscles may provide increased inspiratory volume
to prevent respiratory insufficiency in the child with neuromuscular disease. Active and resistive exercises for strengthening of the abdomen, which may help develop a strong,
effective cough, are well known by physical therapists.

Improving the pattern of breathing of a child with neuromuscular disease may provide two benefits. First, an improved ratio of alveolar ventilation to dead space ventilation
occurs when a slower, deeper pattern of breathing replaces
a fast and shallow mode. The therapist may have the child
attempt a slower and deeper pattern of breathing using
various clinical cues, including counting, a metronome, or
a spirogram. Avoiding inefficient or counterproductive muscular effort is the second possible benefit of changing the
pattern of breathing. A child with respiratory distress may
appropriately use the accessory muscles to aid inspiration
and may use the abdominal muscles to enhance full expiration. This muscular pattern, however, can become habitual.
If the diaphragm provides adequate ventilation, unnecessary muscular effort is exerted if the child continues to use
the accessory muscles. Various training methods have been
suggested, including relaxation exercises and neurosensory
techniques, but no scientific data support these endeavors,
nor do they suggest that short-term changes in muscular
patterns during the therapeutic session have a residual effect
or replace the inefficient patterns.

Although the importance of maintaining or improving
mobility of the thorax in children has been identified and
related treatment plans have been outlined, no controlled
studies of the techniques have been conducted. Active
breathing exercises to improve thoracic mobility have been
suggested for localized areas or for the entire chest. Manual
stretching of the chest wall has been advocated, but has not
been tested. Active or passive exercise to improve shoulder
girdle mobility in children with paralysis may also improve
thoracic excursion. Clinical studies must be undertaken to
justify the time-consuming procedures used in the name of
respiratory exercises. This notion of little evidence has been
supported by a recent Cochrane Review[96] and an independent systematic review of breathing exercises.[97] The authors
of the Cochrane Review stated:

> The results of this systematic review cannot inform clinical
> practice as no suitable trials were identified for inclusion.
> Therefore, it is currently unknown whether these interven-
> tions offer any added value in this patient group or whether
> specific types of breathing exercise demonstrate superiority
> over others.[98]

AC is an important therapeutic regimen for hospital,
residential, and home treatment programs because many
children with respiratory weakness and general inactivity
accumulate secretions. If the parent suspects an increase
in secretions as a result of a respiratory tract infection, AC
techniques described above may prevent the development
of pneumonia or atelectasis. If the child cannot cough well
and if secretions are problematic, oral or nasal suctioning may be necessary to maintain a clear airway. Parents
should be trained in aspiration techniques and should
have proper suctioning equipment in the home. Two additional approaches may help evacuate secretions when
a child with neuromuscular weakness is unable to cough

effectively. Manually assisted cough is achieved by helping the child inhale to maximal capacity by performing an "air-stacking" maneuver, being insufflated via a bag and mask effort, or with a breath provided by a mechanical ventilator. The caregiver then performs an abdominal thrust or thoracic squeeze as the child relaxes the glottis. The sudden expulsive thrust or squeeze attempts to mimic a cough by promoting a higher expiratory flow than is possible by the weakened musculature. The second approach uses mechanical insufflation/exsufflation (MIE). This mechanical device, originally described during the polio epidemics of the early 1950s, can produce positive pressure that will insufflate the lungs followed by pressure reversal to an expiratory pressure that simulates a cough.[99] MIE has been shown useful in children with neuromuscular disease and impaired cough in numerous studies including children with DMD, and SMA.[100,101] Despite many articles and textbooks that describe detailed physical therapy programs for patients with neuromuscular weakness of the chest, there is a dearth of well-substantiated clinical research to support many of the suggested treatment procedures.

▶ Asthma

The following description of asthma is a direct quotation from An Official American Thoracic Society/European Respiratory Society Statement.[102]

> Asthma is a heterogeneous condition. Its natural history includes acute episodic deterioration (exacerbations) against a background of chronic persistent inflammation and/or structural changes that may be associated with persistent symptoms and reduced lung function. Trigger factor exposure combines with the underlying phenotype, the degree of hyperresponsive- ness and of airflow obstruction, and the severity of airway inflammation to cause wide variability in the manifestations of asthma in individual patients.

Medical Information

Asthma is among the most prevalent chronic childhood conditions in the United States affecting approximately 7 million children, which accounts for 9.6% of children. Asthma is more prevalent in non-Hispanic black children, with the percentage for this group at 16%.[103] There is enormous morbidity associated with the condition, including days lost from school, emergency room (ER) visits, hospitalizations, and health care costs. There are approximately 2 million yearly visits to the ER in the United States related to acute asthma among all ages.[104] Further, from 6% to 13% of those with asthma exacerbations require hospital admission.[13,14,105]

Asthma in children is characterized by several factors. Boys seem to predominate over girls by as much as a 2:1 ratio. Exercise-induced bronchoconstriction is common in most children with asthma, and may be a specific phenotype for some children, with a reported incidence of up to 90%.[106] Children with asthma are often allergic, with the inhaled or ingested allergen triggering a type 1 immunoglobin E (IgE)–mediated response. Symptoms may also be provoked by viral infections and by dry, cold air in some. Finally, the increasing mortality and continuing high morbidity associated with childhood asthma are attributable, in part, to an increasing incidence of asthma in the inner city populations.[104]

The physiologic changes responsible for the signs and symptoms of asthma are thought to be initiated when IgE in the sensitized child binds with receptor sites on mast cells. The IgE binding causes the release of histamine and tryptase from mast cells in the airways. Histamine provokes bronchoconstriction, vasodilation within the bronchial walls, and mucous secretion. Tryptase has similar effects but also generates bradykinin a very powerful bronchoconstrictor. The activated mast cells begin to manufacture numerous inflammatory mediators, including prostaglandins and leukotriene. These inflammatory mediators—histamine, prostaglandin D_2, leukotriene C_4, and others—stimulate a response that increases bronchial smooth muscle contraction, causes mucous secretions from the airways, and causes bronchial edema.[107] The result of these three processes is often an obstruction of the airways. As airway obstruction progresses, expiratory airflow decreases, lung volumes and airway resistance increase, airway conductance decreases, and ventilation/perfusion inequality leads to arterial hypoxemia. The various pathophysiologic aspects of asthma appear to have a major hereditary component. However, asthma seems to have a complex genetic model without any clear pattern of inheritance.

A fascinating aspect of asthma in children is the exercise-induced component. With strenuous exercise for a period of time, usually 5 to 10 minutes, a child can develop many manifestations of asthma (e.g., dyspnea, wheezing, and airway obstruction) that may reverse spontaneously or with treatment.[98] This exercise component is important to the physical therapist developing a conditioning program to increase exercise tolerance in the child with asthma. The response can be managed by having the child premedicate using appropriate oral or inhalation medications before the exercise session to counteract the likely asthmatic response.

Medical Management

Medical management of the child with asthma has two major phases—treatment of the acute attack and control of chronic asthma.

Treatment goals for the acute attack in the ER include reversal of hypoxemia, if present; reduction in airway obstruction; and treatment of airway inflammation. β2-agonists, which can be administered in several modes—including inhalation, subcutaneously, and intravenously—relax bronchial smooth muscle. Short-acting β2-agonists are the recommended first-line therapy for the acute asthma exacerbation. Albuterol sulfate is the most commonly used β2-agonist for acute asthma.[108] Anticholinergic medications, most commonly, ipratropium bromide, produce bronchodilation by blocking the effects of acetylcholine on the parasympathetic autonomic nervous system in the airways. The parasympathetic response includes bronchial smooth muscle constriction. β2-agonists are often used with anticholinergics in multiple doses for best effects.[109] Systemic corticosteroids in the ER are recommended for patients with moderate or severe asthma to help reduce the inflammatory changes within the airways. A study of almost 900 patients found a reduction in hospital admission rates when corticosteroids were given within 1 hour of ER presentation.[110] Supplemental oxygen is used to maintain an O_2 saturation of approximately 95%.

The long-term medical management for control of chronic asthma has several components: pharmacologic, environmental, and immunologic. The pharmacologic agents used may include β2 sympathomimetic agents delivered orally or by aerosol; oral preparations of theophylline; antiinflammatory agents including inhaled and oral corticosteroids; and cromolyn sodium delivered by inhalation. Two newer groups of medication for long-term treatment of asthma include leukotriene receptor antagonists (LTRA) and long-acting β2-agonists (LABA). LTRA reduce the ability of certain leukotrienes—inflammatory mediators—to produce bronchial constriction by interfering with their attachment to receptor sites. LABAs have been in use for almost two decades, but their safety and efficacy are still unsure. A recent Cochrane Review states: "The current systematic review seriously questions the benefit of LABAs in children, although it also demonstrates that they appear safe when combined with inhaled corticosteroids."[111]

Control of environmental factors plays a major role in asthma therapy. A dust-free environment is imperative for the child, and special air-filtration units may be required for the child's room. Several multifaceted, randomized controlled trials have shown that reducing multiple early allergen exposures with environmental controls is associated with a decreased risk of asthma.[112] Among the several major allergens noted for removal from the child's environment are dust mites, pets, cockroach, mouse, mold, tobacco smoke, endotoxin, and air pollution. If the youngster chooses to be active in athletics, care must be taken either to avoid levels of activity that may provoke bronchospasm or to use appropriate medication before engaging in asthmainducing levels of physical exertion.

Immunotherapy (allergy shots) is another method of long-term therapy for allergic asthma. Once allergens are identified by skin testing, extracts of these allergens are given in gradually increasing strengths via periodic subcutaneous injections. The rationale is that the child's immunologic system will respond to the small doses of allergen by producing circulating antibodies. Once sufficient levels of antibodies are developed, environmental exposure to the allergen will result in no symptoms of asthma because the acquired antibodies will alleviate the allergic response of the child. A recent review has established the efficacy of both subcutaneous immunotherapy and sublingual immunotherapy.[113]

Physical Therapy Examination

As with medical care, physical therapy examination and management of children with asthma is largely based on the clinical situation at the time (i.e., whether the child is in an acute, subacute, or chronic stage of the disease). The hospitalized child with status asthmaticus (intractable acute asthma) will not tolerate either AC or physical training. A notable exception for AC is when the patient is intubated and mechanically ventilated and control of airway secretions is part of care.

The physical therapist's examination of a child receiving mechanical ventilation should include lung auscultation to identify the location of bronchial secretions and to assess whether areas of the lungs are poorly ventilated. The pattern of ventilation and use of accessory muscles should be noted. Measurements of the thorax, including thoracic index, should be made during inspiration and expiration to determine chest mobility. Several or all of these evaluated items will be abnormal. The therapist must reevaluate these items with each treatment until the thoracic index, breath sounds, and pattern of breathing have improved.

A long-term rehabilitation plan for the child with asthma must also examine exercise tolerance, strength, and posture. Exercise tolerance may be evaluated by several well-studied and easily performed tests. These commonly include the six-minute walk test,[114] the step test,[115] and the 20-minute shuttle run test.[116] Quantitative strength measurement of major muscle groups can be made with equipment that is readily available in the physical therapy department. Posture can be evaluated using a grid system.

Physical Therapy Intervention

As noted above under Examination, there is little, if any, rationale for physical therapy for the child with status asthmaticus.[117] Status asthmaticus renders a child too dyspneic, anxious, scared, and physically unable to cooperate with the therapist for AC, breathing activity, posture and ROM evaluation, or any rehabilitative endeavors.

When the severe bronchospasm begins to reverse, accumulated secretions are often encountered in the previously narrowed airways. Aggressive AC is imperative during this subacute stage, but must be administered within tolerance. Secretions retained in the airways predispose the patient to atelectasis and bronchial infection. AC at this time is indicated within the limits of the youngster's tolerance and endurance. Secretion volume, color, consistency, and the child's vital signs including pulse oximetry before, during, and after treatment should be recorded.

In the long-term care of asthmatic children, intermittent AC treatments may be useful when secretions are present, but treatments are not used routinely as in other conditions, such as CF. Parents should use AC techniques at the first sign of a respiratory infection or increased mucous production and should know the drainage positions and manual techniques and the techniques of use of newer AC modalities in order to treat the child at home. One of the only reported controlled studies of the effects of AC via bronchial drainage and percussion in children with asthma involved 21 outpatients. These children, who had mild to moderate asthma, were divided into a treatment group and a control group. The mean FEV_1 for the treatment group increased by 10.5% 30 minutes after therapy. The control group had a slight decrease in mean FEV_1 during the same period. The difference in mean FEV_1 values was significant at the 0.05 level.[118]

In previous editions of this chapter, various traditional breathing exercises for children with asthma were discussed. They are omitted in this edition owing to a complete lack of supporting evidence for their efficacy.

Relaxation techniques have also been advocated to reduce the anxiety and physical stress associated with an episode of asthma. Many anecdotal and verbal reports lend support to the benefits of relaxation techniques in patients with asthma, but controlled studies are lacking. Two systematic reviews have been published—one regarding relaxation exercises for asthma and the second, more recent, review on psychological interventions for children with asthma. Huntley et al. found some evidence for muscular relaxation exercises improving lung function, but no other benefits were noted owing to poor methodology and inherent difficulties with this type of study.[119]

The second systematic review found some data to suggest relaxation therapy was beneficial, but in general, studies showed widely varied approaches and lack of sufficient data.[120]

Physical rehabilitation to improve aerobic endurance, work capacity, and strength are major goals in the long-term management of asthmatic children. Children with chronic asthma are often less physically active than their unaffected peers. Exercise-induced bronchospasm may restrict a child with asthma from participating in vigorous exercise, and the child may, therefore, be unable to respond to physical demands in daily life. Appropriate medication before vigorous exercise may attenuate the bronchospastic response, and the child can derive the enjoyment, social interaction, and physiological benefits of exercise.[121] A formal physical training program should be preceded by quantitative evaluation of the child's response to strenuous exercise. The initial evaluation determines the level of exercise needed to improve strength and endurance, and is a baseline against which the results of subsequent studies can be compared to determine improvement or deterioration. Among the more commonly used methods of physical training are free running, treadmill running, bicycle ergometry, and swimming.

There is conclusive evidence supporting physical training and exercise for individuals with asthma. Most significant is that physical training/activity does not exacerbate asthma symptoms or disease control.[122,123] Mancuso et al. recently demonstrated an improved quality of life following a one-year program of increased physical activity. Asthma Quality of Life Quotient improved during the year of activity from 5.0 to 5.9, a clinically important difference. Although not specifically for children, there were children 12 years old and above who participated in the program.[124] A Cochrane Review of physical exercise in asthma found that many modes of exercise—(running, walking, cycling, swimming, and others)—were well tolerated without detrimental effects on symptoms. Cardiopulmonary and aerobic fitness levels improved along with quality of life measures. However, as is also found in adults with COPD, physical training had no significant effect on resting lung function.[125]

In addition to traditional land-based exercise showing promise for improving physical status and quality of life in individuals with asthma, swimming as a training mode also has been shown to have beneficial effects for children with asthma. Sly and associates studied the effects of swimming by assigning children to either a treatment group or a control group. The treatment group participated in a swimming program for 2 hours three times a week for 13 weeks. Although no changes were recorded in pulmonary function or basic personality traits, a marked decrease in wheezing days was noted in the treatment group, as was also seen with land-based exercise studies cited above. The mean number of days of wheezing for the treatment group was 31.3 during the 13 weeks before the training program; this figure declined to 5.7 days of wheezing during the swimming program. A similar control group of asthmatic children had a mean of 10.1 and 13.2 days' wheezing, respectively, before and during the 3-week control period.[126]

Fitch and associates published the results of a 5-month swimming program in 46 asthmatic children compared with a control group of 10 non-asthmatic children. Outcome measures included asthma score (based on wheeze, cough, and sputum), physical work capacity at a heart rate of 170, drug score (based on the amount of medication), FEV_1 values, and response to an exercise challenge on a treadmill. A marked improvement in asthma score, drug score, and physical work capacity followed the training period. A concomitant improvement in posture was noted. No change was reported in FEV_1 or the severity of exercise-induced asthma. The authors concluded that swimming is an effective method of physical training in asthmatic children.[127]

More recent studies include a 2009 report by Wang and Hung, who followed 30 children with asthma randomly assigned to a swimming group or usual care during a 6-week period. There was a significant improvement in peak expiratory flow rate in the experimental group compared with the control group (330 L/min, 95% CI: 309–351 vs. 252 L/min, 95% CI: 235–269) after the swimming intervention. There was also a significant decrease in the severity of asthma in the experimental group compared with the control group. The authors suggested swimming may be an effective non-pharmacological intervention for the child or adolescent with asthma.[128] A 2011 study using a prospective longitudinal examination of data on 5738 children sought to find information on recreational swimming pool attendance and asthma and allergy at 7 and 10 years of age. The results showed that by 7 years of age, more than 50% of the children swam once a week or more. Children with high cumulative totals of swimming had a decreased likelihood of developing asthma at both 7 and 10 years of age and also showed a significant improvement in forced mid-expiratory flow of 0.2 standard deviations. As seen with land-based physical training, swimming provided clinical and physiological benefits to a large cohort of children as regards development of asthma.[129] A recent systematic review supported swimming as a safe and effective means of physical training for children with asthma. The authors stated that swimming is "well-tolerated in children and adolescents with stable asthma, and increases lung function (moderate strength evidence) and cardiopulmonary fitness (high strength evidence)."[130]

It is very clear that children with asthma will benefit from physical training using the more traditional modes of treadmill, bicycle, and running or jogging as well as swimming.

▶ Cystic fibrosis

Medical Information

CF is the most common life-limiting genetic disorder affecting primarily Caucasians. The disease is inherited in an autosomal recessive pattern. It is estimated to occur in 1 of every 3500 births in the United States, and has a carrier rate of approximately 1 in 29 persons. When two carriers have a child, there is a 25% chance that the child will have CF, a 50% chance that the child is a carrier of the gene, and a 25% chance that the child will be completely free from the CF gene. Accurate genetic testing is currently available when CF is suspected or when there is a high risk of inheritance due to family history of the disorder. CF is a generalized disorder of the exocrine glands, which, in its fully manifested state, produces elevated sweat electrolyte concentrations, pancreatic enzyme deficiency, and chronic inflammatory and suppurative pulmonary disease. The clinical presentation of CF varies, but usually includes combinations of productive cough, abnormally frequent and large stools, failure to thrive, recurrent pneumonias, rectal prolapse, nasal polyposis, and clubbing of the digits. Because of its variable presentation, CF is often misdiagnosed as asthma, allergy, celiac disease, and chronic diarrhea. The well-informed health professional should consider CF when any of these symptoms are encountered.

The gene for CF, the cystic fibrosis transmembrane conductance regulator (CFTR), was identified in 1989 on the long arm of chromosome 7.[131] Although one mutation is responsible for approximately 85% of all cases of CF - F508del - more than 1000 mutations of the CFTR gene are

recognized. The major hypothesis of CFTR dysfunction states that the absence of CFTR is responsible for a decrease in chloride and water secretion and transport by airway epithelial and submucosal cells, thereby resulting in thick and dehydrated mucus.[132] However, the diversity of organ system involvement in CF suggests that other mechanisms are also associated with the CFTR. Regardless of the specific mechanisms, it is agreed that all exocrine glands are impaired to some degree and the variable dysfunction results in a wide spectrum of symptoms and complications for CF.

The incidence in the United States has been mentioned. CF is much less common in the black population, occurring in 1 of about 17,000 births among African Americans. CF is considered uncommon in the Asian population. The course of the disease, like its presentation, is variable. Although severe lung and gastrointestinal disease can be fatal for children with CF, survival rates have improved steadily over the last several decades with an increasing percentage of individuals living beyond 40 years in developed countries.[133]

The pulmonary disease associated with CF causes the greatest mortality. Pulmonary involvement in CF begins with the production and retention of thick, viscous, poorly hydrated secretions within the airways. These secretions provide a medium in which bacterial pathogens flourish. The resultant infections produce inflammation, more secretions, additional obstruction, and a vicious cycle is begun. The earliest pathologic changes may be reversed with aggressive treatment. With continued reinfection, bronchiolitis and bronchitis progress to bronchiolectasis and bronchiectasis. The latter two processes, which are irreversible, destroy elements within the walls of the airways.

In addition to these destructive processes, hyperplasia of mucus-secreting glands and cells occurs within the lungs. Large quantities of thick, purulent mucus are produced, causing the airway obstruction that is common in CF. If the obstruction is partial, a ball-valve process may result in which airways that widen on inspiration allow air into the lungs. When those same airways narrow with expiration, the air becomes trapped, thereby producing hyperaeration of the lung distal to the obstruction. Complete airway obstruction results in absorption atelectasis distal to the obstruction. Small areas of hyperaeration and atelectasis often exist in adjacent areas, and present a honeycomb pattern on a chest roentgenogram. The rapidity of pulmonary progression and success of treatment play major roles in determining the survival of a child with CF.

Pulmonary complications often include massive hemoptysis, pneumothorax, lobar atelectasis, and pulmonary hypertension with cor pulmonale. These problems have been discussed at length by others.[134–137]

Medical Management

Management of CF is directed toward decreasing pulmonary infection and airway obstruction, replacing pancreatic enzymes to help reverse the nutritional deficiency, and providing appropriate psychosocial and emotional support to the child and family. Control of pulmonary infection is the major therapeutic objective. Sputum culture and sensitivity tests to identify pathogens and determine appropriate antimicrobial drugs enable the physician to plan a rational course of medications. The most common bacteria-causing infections in patients with CF vary with patient age. *Staphylococcus aureus, pseudomonas aeruginosa,* and *heamophilus influenzae* are the most frequently identified pathogens in the early years of life. H. influenzae infection decreases as the child ages. Antimicrobial agents are used aggressively and may be given orally, parenterally, and by inhalation. In the past two decades, the bacterium *Burkholderia cepacia* has become recognized as contributing to infection in people with CF. *B. cepacia* is largely antibiotic-resistant and may be transmitted in epidemic-like fashion. Some strains of *B. cepacia* are associated with a syndrome of rapid progression of lung disease, ending in death within several months. It must be noted, however, that not all *B. cepacia* infections react in this manner. The Cystic Fibrosis Foundation (CFF), in 2013, recommended isolating individuals with CF at CFF events to prevent or reduce the likelihood of cross-infection.[138]

Reduction of airway obstruction is the most time-consuming aspect of comprehensive treatment for CF. Reduction of sputum viscosity by aerosolized or oral medications is thought to enhance physical efforts to loosen and drain mucus from the airways. Physical therapy is a major part of the care and will be detailed later.

Replacement of pancreatic enzymes is essential for the 85% of patients with pancreatic dysfunction. Traditionally, the recommended diet for patients with CF has included high-protein, high-carbohydrate, and low-fat foods. With more effective pancreatic preparations, many children have liberalized their intake of fat. Despite apparent control of pancreatic insufficiency with enzymes, patients with CF may need up to 50% more calories than their age- and weight-matched peers. Continually underweight children, or those who experience weight loss with a progression of disease, may benefit from commercial dietary supplements. Supplements must be chosen carefully and added to the diet, and a nutritionist's counseling is necessary.

Psychosocial and emotional support for patients with CF and their families is the responsibility of all professionals who work with this population. Issues that must be confronted include chronic life-shortening illness, genetic disease, cost of drugs and care, time-consuming treatments, death of a child, denial, and guilt. Other issues emerge as patients reach adulthood: marriage, occupations, and dependence on others for treatment. A counselor or social worker plays a major role on the CF team. A large literature is available regarding psychosocial aspects of the patients with CF and their families.

Two newer approaches to pulmonary treatment include lung transplantation and gene therapy. Lung transplantation for those with end-stage disease has been successful. Unfortunately, there are major problems with transplantation, including an uncertain waiting time for donor organs and the development of obliterative bronchiolitis following transplantation. A study published in 2007 in the New England Journal of Medicine and a related editorial provide varied perspectives on this extraordinarily difficult treatment.[139,140] More recent work by Thabut et al. shows a significant survival benefit after lung transplant, with approximately 68% of patients surviving at 3 years following transplantation.[141] Lung transplantation for CF will continue to develop as a major treatment option for advanced lung disease in CF.

Gene therapy trials followed the identification of the CFTR in 1989. Researchers attempted to introduce normal versions of the CFTR into the airways, but successes were limited. One of the biggest issues in gene therapy has been finding a way to introduce the normal genes into the airways of patients. The most commonly tried approach was using a viral vector as a gene transfer agent to carry the genes into the lungs. To date, results have been limited owing to many different factors and lack of an effective gene transfer agent.

A nationwide network of centers is dedicated to the treatment of CF. These centers are sponsored by the CFF and can reach almost every population center in the United States. The CFF sponsors research projects, fellowships, conferences, fund raising, and other activities in its mandated task of providing the best care for children and adults with CF. (See CFF.org) As a result of the CFF Drug Development Pipeline, a medication developed by Vertex Pharmaceuticals was approved by the Food and Drug Administration for use in individuals with one specific mutation of the CFTR gene – G551D - which represents approximately 4% of the population with CF. The medication, called Kalydeco® (ivacaftor), helps improve the function of the specific CFTR in this group and improves pulmonary function values and reduces sweat chloride values.[142] This medication is considered a proof of concept breakthrough with work on Kalydeco and similar possible medications continuing.

Physical Therapy Examination

Physical therapy examination for the child with CF is similar to the process described early in this chapter based upon the Guide to Physical Therapist Practice.[23] Emphasis in CF must be placed on the bronchial secretions that cause the numerous pulmonary problems and complications.

Auscultation for secretions must be done with the expectation of finding many areas with sonorous wheezes, harsh breath sounds, and crackles (all abnormal breath sounds), which are associated with secretions. Of course, the findings will vary depending upon the degree of lung impairment in the child. The sounds may not change for several days in a patient with advanced disease, and auscultation on an intermittent, rather than daily, basis may be helpful.

A determination of the child's ability to cough and raise secretions is very important. An acutely ill child with

CF who cannot cough effectively risks further deterioration in airway function. The chest radiograph and other imaging are useful in identifying specific anatomical areas of lung disease and infection. Many believe that the three-dimensional view of the lungs afforded by posteroantero and lateral chest films provides specific information to help direct treatment.

Also, the child's physical capabilities, including strength and aerobic fitness, should be a focus of the examination. Children with CF participate in less physical activity than their healthy non-CF peers despite those with CF having good lung function.[143] Therefore, strength testing and cardiopulmonary exercise testing should be performed when appropriate to develop an exercise reconditioning program appropriate to the child's tolerance.

The most valid and accurate manner for formal exercise testing includes laboratory maximal exercise testing by treadmill for measurement of peak oxygen consumption (peak VO_2), which is considered the best index of cardiopulmonary function.[144] Orenstein developed a group of runners with CF in the late 1970s. He reported safe and beneficial results of a three-month cardiopulmonary fitness program, which heralded more and more importance ascribed to cardiopulmonary or aerobic "fitness" in the population with CF.[67] In addition to enhancing exercise, fitness, and quality of life, the concept of exercise capacity has been shown to have prognostic features for survival in CF.[145,146] Owing to limitations of time, space, and financial concerns related to laboratory exercise testing, several widely used "clinical tests" of exercise among physical therapists working with patients with CF have been popularized and included in exercise evaluation. The following are three commonly used clinical tests for exercise evaluation in CF.

1. The 6-minute walk test is well known by physical therapists. The patient is asked to walk as far as possible in a 6-minute period, with the distance walked being the primary outcome. Other values can be measured but should not interfere with the time or distance. The patient walks alone at a self-paced speed on a straight, flat course of no less than 30 meters with small traffic cones at each end of the course for a turnaround point. If the patient is receiving supplemental oxygen, it should be used.[147]

2. Subjects performing a step test are instructed to step up and down on a step at a height of 15 cm. The step frequency is kept constant at a pace controlled by a metronome. The duration of the test is 3 minutes, with the subject maintaining a rate of 30 steps per minute for 3 minutes by stopwatch. The child is encouraged to switch the leading leg during the 3-minute test period. If the test is aborted early, owing to muscle fatigue or dyspnea, the number of steps taken must be counted.[148]

3. The modified shuttle walking test may be performed in either 12-level or 15-level formats. Patients must move around two markers over a 10-meter course in cadence with "beeps" from a prerecorded tape. Work at each level—12 or 15—continues for 1 minute, and the speed of the cadence increases by 0.61 km/h each minute. There are a maximum of 15 levels. The test ends when subjects have completed the required work, state that they are unable to continue, or fail to achieve the course marker on two consecutive beeps. Selvaduri et al. validated the 10-meter modified shuttle walk test in children with CF.[149]

Evaluation of the child's posture, including mobility of the chest wall, should be determined for several reasons. Children with CF often have hyperinflated lungs, so the chest wall may appear barreled and fixed, very similar to adults with COPD. Figure 20.15 shows a young child with CF and thoracic changes due to advanced pulmonary disease. A noncompliant thorax increases the work of breathing. If chest wall changes occur, the child may have difficulty developing the necessary inspiratory and expiratory pressures and flow rates to cough effectively and to increase ventilation during physical stress. Thoracic index, thoracic girth, and rib motion should be determined during full inspiration and full expiration.

The barrel-shaped configuration of the hyperinflated thorax will likely increase the normal thoracic kyphosis. Scapular protraction also becomes evident. With the anatomic

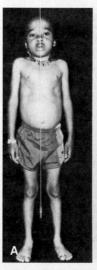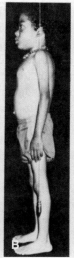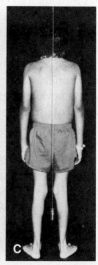

FIGURE 20.15 Postural abnormalities in a child with cystic fibrosis. **(A)** Anterior view. Notice that the shoulders are held high, especially on the right. This posture appears to offer better mechanical advantage to the accessory muscles for breathing. The lower ribs are flared, and the thorax appears barreled and elongated because of the hyperinflation of the lungs. A full postural evaluation might reveal other, less obvious abnormalities. **(B)** Lateral view. The thoracic kyphosis and barreled chest seen here are common findings in children with obstructive pulmonary disease and hyperinflation of the lungs. **(C)** Posterior view. The shoulders appear high, with a protraction of the scapulae. Notice the enlargement of the thorax in relation to the rest of this patient's body. Pronated feet are also noticeable. (Reproduced by permission from Irwin S, Tecklin JS. *Cardiopulmonary Physical Therapy*. St. Louis, MO: CV Mosby; 1985.)

changes in the upper thorax that accompany hyperaeration, range of motion of the shoulder girdle must be measured too. A comprehensive examination should include those postural items that may affect both function and cosmesis.

Physical Therapy Management

Physical therapy for infants and children with CF begins invariably with AC techniques taught to the parents of newly diagnosed children. This usually includes positioning for gravity drainage, and manual techniques of percussion and vibration, keeping in mind the concern previously noted regarding head-down drainage positions. As the child ages, other AC techniques can begin at age-appropriate times. Exercise for both aerobic fitness and strengthening will begin at differing times in a child's life, depending upon the specific progression of lung disease and activity levels of the individual.

Airway Clearance

A major role of physical therapy for the child with CF is in the aggressive use of AC—including bronchial drainage, chest percussion, vibration, and suctioning (if necessary) and the many newer and effective techniques developed and popularized in the last three decades. Treatment should be generalized as needed because mucus is produced in all areas of the lungs, but if the examination identifies specific lobes or segments with advanced disease or that appear to have increased production of mucus, emphasis for treatment should center on these segments. Early studies of conventional bronchial drainage, percussion, and vibration in CF during the 1960s and 1970s helped document their efficacy. Lorin and Denning, for instance, demonstrated that twice the amount of sputum per cough and per treatment was obtained when a combined treatment regimen of gravity drainage, percussion, and vibration was compared with cough alone.[150] Tecklin and Holsclaw found improvement in forced vital capacity and peak expiratory flow rate after bronchial drainage, percussion, and vibration in 26 children with CF.[151] Feldman and associates have demonstrated remarkable improvement in flow rates at low lung volumes 45 minutes after treatment in nine patients with CF.[152] In Feldman's study, the isovolume flow rate near 25% of forced vital capacity increased from baseline by 70% 45 minutes after treatment.[153] These changes in small airway flow rates are consistent with the results of Motoyama.[154]

Desmond and coworkers employed a crossover design to determine whether pulmonary function decreased over a 3-week period during which physical therapy was withheld. There was a statistically significant decrease in flow rates reflective of small airway function, forced expiratory flow (FEF 25% to 75%) and Vmax60 (total lung capacity [TLC]), each of which declined by 20% after 3 weeks of no therapy. These values returned to their prior levels shortly after resumption of physical therapy.[155]

Current AC Techniques

As individuals with CF have grown older to the point where the median age of survival approaches 40 years, the importance of independent treatment is now paramount. The contemporary techniques are used extensively throughout the world because they provide independence in self-care without the need for an assistant to provide the manual techniques.

AUTOGENIC DRAINAGE Autogenic drainage, described previously, improves pulmonary function and secretion removal when compared with several other AC techniques.[156–159] Autogenic drainage is most commonly used by teenagers and adults with CF owing to the need for good breathing control and personal motivation required. One of the drawbacks with autogenic drainage is that it requires individual training by the physical therapist, and some individuals have difficulty learning and performing the technique. Those who are able to participate report good acceptance and use of the procedure and independence in its use.

PEP MASK The PEP mask, described earlier in the chapter, may hold the greatest promise in terms of independent removal of excess secretions in children with CF and is used throughout the world. Two long-term studies of PEP breathing have been reported. McIlwaine et al., a long-time supporter of PEP, recently compared two groups of subjects with CF who were assigned randomly to a PEP group or a HFCWO group. At the end of 12 months, the PEP group had a lower frequency of pulmonary exacerbations, but there were no differences in lung function, health-related quality of life scores, or personal satisfaction with treatments.[160] Darbee et al. found notable improvements in pulmonary function following low-PEP or high-PEP treatment in individuals with CF. In addition to increased lung function, including oxygen saturation, those using PEP had increased sputum expectoration with high PEP. Darbee also discussed the physiologic rationale for PEP.[161]

FLUTTER AND ACAPELLA The Flutter® was developed to offer a measure of independence to young adults with CF and included an oscillatory aspect to PEP. Several studies of the Flutter found no difference between the device and other modalities of AC. It appears that the Flutter is well accepted by many patients and is equivalent to the effects on sputum clearance and pulmonary function of other types of AC.[162] A negative aspect of the Flutter is its dependence on gravity for proper use. The Acapella is a device with a specific valve that enables oscillation without regard to position, and for this reason may be easier to use than the Flutter. As with many AC devices, the Acapella provides AC effects similar to most other techniques.[163]

HIGH FREQUENCY CHEST WALL OSCILLATION HFCWO has gained acceptance throughout many CF centers in the United States and internationally largely because of its ease of application. Warwick and Hansen examined the efficacy of HFCC in a long-term but uncontrolled study of 16 subjects with CF. All but one of those subjects showed improvement in their respiratory impairment during the trial.[153] Subsequent evaluations of HFCWO demonstrated that the technique was at least as beneficial to subjects with CF as conventional physical therapy and PEP breathing both in short-term and in long-term studies.[164,165] The "vest," as HFCWO is called by patients, has provided a useful, independent means for both children and adults with CF to perform daily AC without an assistant to provide manual techniques. The only drawback to the vest is its high cost, but many insurance carriers will provide excellent levels of support for this device.

In summary, gravity-assisted bronchial drainage with manual techniques as the "gold standard" for children with CF is no longer the case as numerous other interventions have been determined to be equally efficacious. When working with children and adults with CF, the therapist must consider many alternatives for AC and secretion removal. Despite the publication and presentation of several hundred comparisons of the many AC techniques, I concur with the comments by Jennifer Pryor and Eleanor Main. Pryor stated in 1999:

> If objective differences are small, individual preferences and cultural influences may be significant in increasing adherence to treatment and in the selection of an appropriate regimen or regimens for an individual patient.[166]

Main, in 2013, reflected upon the lack of conclusive evidence regarding AC in CF despite numerous Cochrane Reviews and several unsuccessful recent attempts at long-term comparative studies:

> Strong patient preference, lack of blinding and the requirement for effortful and demanding participation over long intervals will continue to derail efforts to find the best ACT for CF, unless they are addressed in future clinical trials.[167]

Given the current evidence, this author believes that the choice of procedures should be based upon age, disease severity, caregiver availability, need for independence, and patient/family preference. The decision falls largely on the patient and family members who are ultimately responsible for this daily procedure.

MODIFICATIONS OF AC PROCEDURES Modifications of usual treatment procedures are often necessary for acutely ill children or for those with certain complications. There is little or no evidence to support one technique versus another. In a patient with major hemoptysis, chest percussion and vibration should be discontinued temporarily because the physical maneuvers may dislodge a blood clot and prolong the bleeding. AC techniques that employ breathing—PEP, autogenic drainage, Flutter and Acapella—may be useful in an attempt to remove accumulated blood from the airways.

Pneumothorax is a complication of CF and is commonly treated with an intrapleural chest tube with suction. Gravity drainage is appropriate, although percussion and vibration at the site of tube insertion are contraindicated. PEP and other breathing approaches to AC may enable continued treatment of excessive secretion. With advanced lung disease, the child may benefit from any of the techniques that they are able to use and find tolerable and acceptable.

Physical Exercise

There is little question about the benefits of exercise and physical conditioning for children with CF. More than 30 years ago, Cropp and associates showed that children with CF, excepting those with advanced lung disease, had a normal *cardiovascular* response to exercise. Children with advanced disease were likely to have arterial oxygen desaturation during exercise due to ventilator limitations.[168] Marcus and colleagues demonstrated that patients with advanced CF who exercised with an FIO_2 of 30% worked longer, had higher maximal oxygen consumption, and experienced less oxygen desaturation than while exercising at room air. This suggested that patients with advanced disease were also able to improve their exercise tolerance with supplemental oxygen during training.[169] Muscle fatigue as a limiting factor in physical exercise was identified by Moorcraft et al. on the basis of 78 of 104 subjects with CF who reported needing to stop exercise owing to muscular fatigue.[170]

Treadmill walking or running, cycle ergometer training, free running or walking, and strengthening exercises are useful methods of increasing cardiovascular fitness, endurance, and general muscular strength. See Table 20.2.[171]

The relevance of these findings is that physical training and reconditioning, in a formal or informal program, is safe and beneficial in all patients except those with severe lung disease. Even those with severe disease have been shown to benefit from an exercise program if supplemental oxygen is provided.

SUMMARY

This chapter has attempted to provide a summary of unique characteristics of lung disease in children, growth and development of the respiratory system, and the reasons why children and infants are predisposed to acute respiratory failure. Assessment of the child with pulmonary disease and treatments aimed at reducing the severity of pulmonary disease in infants and children have been reviewed. Four major respiratory disorders have been described, along with a discussion of appropriate physical therapy assessment and management. Published evidence for the physical therapy methods has been reviewed. Physical therapy for children with lung disease has been shown to be efficacious, depending on the treatment employed and the problems addressed.

CASE STUDY

H.E., a 14-year-old Caucasian boy with a history of Duchenne muscular dystrophy diagnosed at 4 years of age, was referred for pulmonary physical therapy evaluation. This case study will focus on the cardiovascular/pulmonary needs of this patient.

Examination

HISTORY

H.E. was a full-term infant who appeared to be developing normally until approximately 3 years of age, when his parents noted that he had difficulty rising easily from the floor and could not easily ascend stairs. Upon stating their concerns to the pediatrician, H.E. was sent for laboratory testing and a muscle biopsy. The testing indicated abnormally high serum creatinine kinase, and a muscle biopsy was performed. The resulting diagnosis of Duchenne muscular dystrophy was made. He was referred to a large children's hospital for follow-up and continuing care. As the years progressed, H.E.'s weakness became more pronounced, and he developed some of the classical physical characteristics including increasingly severe lumbar lordosis, several contractures including plantar flexion, and hip and knee flexion contractures. He was still ambulatory, although he and his mother reported that the distance was steadily decreasing and the speed was getting slower.

REVIEW OF SYSTEMS

Integument: There were no obvious or stated problems in this area.

Musculoskeletal: Numerous contractures in the lower extremities were obvious along with severe lumbar lordosis. Elbow contractures were also noted, although not as severe as those of the lower extremities. There was obvious weakness, particularly in the shoulders and hip musculature.

Neuromuscular: Ambulation, balance, and transfers were all significantly abnormal and limited. H.E. currently functions from a power wheelchair.

Cardiovascular/Pulmonary: Heart rate, respiratory rate, and blood pressure were all within normal limits.

Communication, affect, cognition, language, and learning style appeared unimpaired.

TESTS AND MEASUREMENTS

General Summary of Function: At the time of his referral, an examination of overall physical function revealed that H.E. could ambulate 25 feet in 20 seconds, roll from a prone to a supine position and back to a prone position, and had adequate sitting balance. He was unable to run, ascend or descend stairs, rise from the floor or from a chair, sit up from a supine position, or assume a posture on all fours. A modified manual muscle examination indicated strength that was graded from "poor" to "absent" for all isolated muscle groups, with the exception of wrist extensors, which were graded as "fair" to "good." H.E. could function from an electric wheelchair, and he could ambulate slowly using a walker with supervision.

Ventilation, Respiration/Gas Exchange: H.E.'s breathing pattern was examined and was found to be a diaphragmatic pattern with appropriate intercostal muscle use while at rest and during exertion; his accessory respiratory muscles became active during inspiration and expiration. His respiratory muscle strength was measured using maximum static inspiratory pressure (MSIP), inspiratory capacity (IC), and slow inspiratory vital capacity (IVC). The MSIP was 60% of predicted values; the IC was 45% of predicted values; and the IVC was 45% of predicted values. His maximal static expiratory pressure, a measure of expiratory muscle strength, was 35% of predicted values.

Chest wall expansion was determined with a tape measure and found to be approximately 2.5 cm at maximal inspiratory effort. Passive motion was adequate at the glenohumeral joints. Coughing was evaluated as being weak and questionably functional. As previously noted, his limited IC and reduced expiratory pressures were largely responsible for the impaired cough.

Evaluation, Diagnosis, and Prognosis

On the basis of the data gathered specific to his current pulmonary issues, H.E. would receive a classification at cardiovascular/pulmonary pattern 6E ventilatory pump dysfunction or failure. This would be a pattern specific to his respiratory muscle impairment for which he was referred. His prognosis would be 8 to 10 weeks of care with episodes of physical therapy two times per week for the first several weeks, and reduced to weekly thereafter.

Interventions

Coordination, communication, and documentation would focus upon interaction with the muscular dystrophy center at the children's hospital where H.E. is followed. Patient instruction would focus on instruction of H.E. and his parents and other caregivers regarding a home exercise program to improve his respiratory muscle strength, enhance his coughing, and provide for AC as needed. In addition, they would be trained in proper AC and assisted cough techniques, including various devices to support AC.

PROCEDURAL INTERVENTIONS

Therapeutic Exercise: Active cycle of breathing to enhance diaphragmatic excursion, maximal inspiration, and FET to aid in improving ventilation to the lower lobes, maintain/improve chest expansion, and aid in secretion removal.

Continuing with ongoing strength training and range-of-motion exercise with emphasis on thorax and shoulder girdle to maintain thoracic compliance.

Inspiratory muscle and expiratory muscle strengthening using simple handheld devices to maintain/increase respiratory muscle strength.

AC as needed using high-frequency chest wall oscillation with SmartVest or airway oscillation with either Acapella or Flutter device; should secretion removal become problematic, equipment for airway aspiration or insufflation–exsufflation recommended.

REFERENCES

1. Yeatts K, Davis KJ, Sotir M, et al. Who gets diagnosed with asthma? Frequent wheeze among adolescents with and without a diagnosis of asthma. *Pediatrics*. 2003;111(5, pt 1):1046–1054.

2. CDC. *National Health Interview Survey (NHIS) Data: 2011 Lifetime and Current Asthma*. Atlanta, GA: US Department of Health and Human Services, CDC; 2012. Available at: http://www.cdc.gov/asthma/nhis/2011/data.htm. Accessed January 24, 2013.

3. Barnett SBL, Nurmagambetov TA. Costs of asthma in the United States: 2002–2007. *J Allergy Clin Immunol*. 2011;127:145–152.

4. Mahon M, Kibirige MS. Patterns of admissions for children with special needs to the paediatric assessment unit. *Arch Dis Child*. 2004;89:165–169.

5. Westbom L, Bergstrand L, Wagner P, et al. Survival at 19 years of age in a total population of children and young people with cerebral palsy. *Dev Med Child Neurol*. 2011;53:808–14.

6. Boyden E. Development and growth of the airways. In: Hodson AW, ed. *Development of the Lung*. New York, NY: Marcel Dekker Inc; 1977:3–35.

7. Haddad GG, Fontan JJP. Development of the respiratory system. In: Berman RE, Kliegman RM, Jensen HB, eds. *Nelson's Textbook of Pediatrics*. 17th ed. Philadelphia, PA: Saunders; 2004:1357–1359.

8. Smith LJ, McKay KO, van Asperen PP, et al. Normal development of the lung and premature birth. *Peaditr Respir Rev*. 2010;11:135–142.

9. Avery ME. Hyaline membrane disease. *Am Rev Respir Dis*. 1975;111:657–688.

10. Polgar G, Weng TR. The functional development of the respiratory system. *Am Rev Respir Dis*. 1979;120:625–695.

11. Downes JJ, Fulgencio T, Raphaely RC. Acute respiratory failure in infants and children. *Pediatr Clin North Am*. 1972;19:423–445.

12. Ackerman SJ, Duff SB, Dennehy PH, et al. Economic impact of an infection control education program in a specialized preschool setting. *Pediatrics*. 2001;108(6):E102.

13. Effmann EL, Fram EK, Vock P, et al. Tracheal cross-sectional area in children: CT determination. *Radiology*. 1983;149(1):137–140.

14. Siren PMA, Siren MJ. Critical diaphragm failure in sudden infant death syndrome. *Ups J Med Sci*. 2011;116(2):115–123.

15. Guslits BG, Gaston SE, Bryan MH, et al. Diaphragmatic work of breathing in premature human infants. *J Appl Physiol*. 1987;62(4):1410–1415.

16. Leith DE. The development of cough. *Am Rev Respir Dis*. 1985;131(5):S39–S42.

17. Papastamelos C, Panitch HB, England SE, et al. Developmental changes in chest wall compliance in infancy and early childhood. *J Appl Physiol*. 1995;78:179–184.

18. Pagliara AS, Karl IE, Haymond M, et al. Hypoglycemia in infancy and childhood. *J Pediatr*. 1973;82:365–379.

19. American Physical Therapy Association. *Interactive Guide to Physical Therapist Practice*. 2003.

20. Nakamura CT, Ng GY, Paton JY, et al. Correlation between digital clubbing and pulmonary function in cystic fibrosis. *Pediatr Pulmonol*. 2002;33(5):332–338.

21. Nathanson I, Riddlesberger MM Jr. Pulmonary hypertrophic osteoarthropathy in cystic fibrosis. *Radiology*. 1980;135(3):649–651.

22. Boat TA. Cystic fibrosis. In: Berman RE, Kliegman RM, Jensen HB, eds. *Nelson's Textbook of Pediatrics*. 17th ed. Philadelphia, PA: Saunders; 2004:1447.

23. Gaultier C. Respiratory muscle function in infants. *Eur Respir J*. 1995;8:150–153.

24. Tecklin JS. The patient with airway clearance dysfunction. In: Irwin S, Tecklin JS, eds. *Cardiopulmonary Physical Therapy–A Guide for Practice*. Mosby, MO: St. Louis; 2004:290–292.

25. Li AM, Yin J, Yu CC, et al. The six-minute walk test in healthy children: reliability and validity. *Eur Respir J*. 2005;25(6):1057–1060.

26. Gulmans VA, van Veldhoven NH, de Meer K, et al. The six-minute walking test in children with cystic fibrosis: reliability and validity. *Pediatr Pulmonol*. 1996;22(2):85–89.

27. Tomkinson GR, Leger LA, Olds TS, et al. Sports Med. Secular trends in the performance of children and adolescents (1980-2000): an analysis of 55 studies of the 20m shuttle run test in 11 countries. *Sports Med*. 2003;33(4):285–300.

28. Holland AE, Rasekaba T, Wilson JW, et al. Desaturation during the 3-minute step test predicts impaired 12-month outcomes in adult patients with cystic fibrosis. *Respir Care*. 2011;56(8):1137–1142.

29. Steinkamp G, Wiedemann B. Relationship between nutritional status and lung function in cystic fibrosis: cross sectional and longitudinal analyses from the German CF quality assurance (CFQA) project. *Thorax*. 2002;57(7):596–601.

30. Palevsky HI, Fishman AP. Chronic cor pulmonale. Etiology and management. *JAMA*. 1990;263:2347.

31. Mawdsley RH, Hoy DK, Erwin MP: Criterion-related validity of the figure-of-eight method of measuring ankle edema, *J Orthop Sports Phys Ther*, 30:149, 2000.

32. de Meer K, Jeneson JA, V. A. Gulmans VA, et al. Efficiency of oxidative work performance of skeletal muscle in patients with cystic fibrosis. *Thorax*. 1995;50:980–983.

33. de Meer K, Gulmans VA, van Der Laag J. Peripheral muscle weakness and exercise capacity in children with cystic fibrosis. *Am J Respir Crit Care Med*. 1999;159(3):748–754.

34. Engel HJ, Tatebe S, Alonzo PB, et al. Physical therapist–established intensive care unit early mobilization program: quality improvement project for critical care at the University of California San Francisco Medical Center. *Phys Ther*. 2013;93:975–985.

35. Nordon-Craft A, Moss M, Quan D, et al. Physical rehabilitation of patients in the intensive care unit requiring extracorporeal membrane oxygenation: a small case series. *Phys Ther*. 2012;92:1494–1506.

36. Chen MJ, Fan X, Moe ST. Criterion-related validity of the Borg ratings of perceived exertion scale in healthy individuals: a meta-analysis. *J Sports Sci*. 2002;20(11):873–899.

37. Pfeiffer KA, Pivarnik JM, Womack CJ, et al. Reliability and validity of the Borg and OMNI rating of perceived exertion scales in adolescent girls. *Med Sci Sports Exerc*. 2002;34(12):2057–2061.

38. Prasad SA, Randall SD, Balfour-Lynn IM. Fifteen-count breathlessness score: an objective measure for children. *Pediatr Pulmonol*. 2000;30(1):56–62.

39. McGrath PJ, Pianosi PT, Unruh AM, et al. Dalhousie dyspnea scales: construct and content validity of pictorial scales for measuring dyspnea. *BMC Pediatr*. 2005;5:33.

40. Bieri D, Reeve R, Champion G, et al. The Faces Pain Scale for the self-assessment of the severity of pain experienced by children: development, initial validation and preliminary investigation for ratio scale properties. *Pain*. 1990;41:139–150.

41. Hicks CL, von Baeyer CL, Spafford PA, et al. The Faces Pain Scale-Revised: toward a common metric in pediatric pain measurement. *Pain*. 2001;93(2):173–183.

42. Koumbourlis AC, Stolar CJ. Lung growth and function in children and adolescents with idiopathic pectus excavatum. *Pediatr Pulmonol*. 2004;38(4):339–343.

43. Button BM, Heine RG, Catto-Smith AG, et al. Postural drainage in cystic fibrosis: is there a link with gastro-oesophageal reflux? *J Peadiatr Child Health*. 1998;34(4):330–334.

44. Button BM, Heine RG, Catto-Smith AG, et al. Chest physiotherapy in infants with cystic fibrosis: to tip or not? A five-year study. *Pediatr Pulmonol*. 2003;35(3):208–213.

45. Crane L. Physical therapy for the neonate with respiratory disease. In: Irwin S, Tecklin JS, eds. *Cardiopulmonary Physical Therapy*. 3rd ed. St. Louis, MO: CV Mosby; 1995.

46. Savci S, Ince DI, Arikan H. A comparison of autogenic drainage and the active cycle of breathing techniques in patients with chronic obstructive pulmonary diseases. *J Cardiopulm Rehabil*. 2000;20(1):37–43.

47. DeCesare J. Physical therapy for the child with respiratory dysfunction. In: Irwin S, Tecklin JS, eds. *Cardiopulmonary Physical Therapy*, 3rd ed. St. Louis: CV Mosby; 1995.

48. Morrow BM, Futter MJ, Argent AC. Endotracheal suctioning: from principles to practice. *Intensive Care Med.* 2004;30(6):1167–1174.

49. Dab I, Alexander F. Evaluation of a particular bronchial drainage procedure called autogenic drainage. In: Baran K, Van Bogaert K, eds. *Chest Physical Therapy in Cystic Fibrosis and Chronic Obstructive Pulmonary Disease.* Ghent, Belgium: European Press; 1977:185–187.

50. Dab I, Alexander F. The mechanism of autogenic drainage studied with flow volume curves. *Monogr Paediat.* 1979;10:50–53.

51. Miller S, Hall DO, Clayton CB, et al. Chest physiotherapy in cystic fibrosis: a comparative study of autogenic drainage and the active cycle of breathing techniques with postural drainage. *Thorax.* 1995;50(2):165–169.

52. Davidson AGF, Wong LTK, Pirie GE, et al. Long-term comparative trial of conventional percussion and drainage physiotherapy to autogenic drainage in in cystic fibrosis [abstract]. *Pediatr Pulmonol.* 1992;14(suppl 8).

53. Pryor JA, Webber BA, Hodson ME, et al. Evaluation of the forced expiratory technique as an adjunct to postural drainage in treatment of cystic fibrosis. *Br Med J.* 1979;2:417–418.

54. Partridge C, Pryor J, Webber B. Characteristics of the forced expiratory technique. *Physiotherapy.* 1989;75:193–194.

55. Hofmyer JL, Webber BA, Hodson ME. Evaluation of positive expiratory pressure as an adjunct to chest physiotherapy in the treatment of cystic fibrosis. *Thorax.* 1986;41:951–954.

56. Gondor M, Nixon PA, Mutich R, et al. Comparison of Flutter device and chest physical therapy in the treatment of cystic fibrosis pulmonary exacerbation. *Pediatr Pulmonol.* 1999;28(4):255–260.

57. King M, Zidulka A, Phillips DM, et al. Tracheal mucus clearance in high-frequency oscillation: effect of peak flow bias. *Eur Respir J.* 1990;3:6.

58. Warwick W. High frequency chest compression moves mucus by means of sustained staccato coughs. *Pediatr Pulmonol.* 1991;(suppl 6): 283, A219.

59. Tomkiewicz RP, Biviji A, King M. Effects of oscillating air flow on the rheological properties and clearability of mucous gel simulants. *Biorheology.* 1994;31(5):511–520.

60. King M, Phillips DM, Zidulka A, et al. Tracheal mucus clearance in high-frequency oscillation. II: Chest wall versus mouth oscillation. *Am Rev Respir Dis.* 1984;130(5):703–706.

61. Darbee J, Cerny F. Exercise testing and exercise conditioning for children with lung dysfunction. In: Irwin S, Tecklin JS, eds. *Cardiopulmonary Physical Therapy.* 3rd ed. St. Louis, MO: CV Mosby; 1990:570.

62. Orenstein DM, Hovell MF, Mulvihill M, et al. Strength vs aerobic training in children with cystic fibrosis: a randomized controlled trial. *Chest.* 2004;126(4):1204–1214.

63. Keens TG, Krastins IRB, Wannamaker EM, et al. Ventilatory muscle endurance training in normal subjects and patients with cystic fibrosis. *Am Rev Respir Dis.* 1977;116:853–860.

64. Enright S, Chatham K, Ionescu AA, et al. Inspiratory muscle training improves lung function and exercise capacity in adults with cystic fibrosis. *Chest.* 2004;126(2):405–411.

65. Weiner P, Magadle R, Beckerman M, et al. Comparison of specific expiratory, inspiratory, and combined muscle training programs in COPD. *Chest.* 2003;124(4):1357–1364.

66. Weisgerber MC, Guill M, Weisgerber JM, et al. Benefits of swimming in asthma: effect of a session of swimming lessons on symptoms and PFTs with review of the literature. *J Asthma.* 2003;40(5):453–464.

67. Orenstein D, Franklin BA, Doershuk CF, et al. Exercise conditioning and cardiopulmonary fitness in cystic fibrosis. *Chest.* 1981;80:392.

68. Laennec RTH; Forbes J, trans. *Diseases of the Chest.* 4th ed. London, UK: 1819.

69. Rosenfeld R. In: Behrman RE, Kliegman RM, Jensen HB, eds. *Nelson Textbook of Pediatrics.* 17th ed. Philadelphia, PA: Saunders, An Imprint of Elsevier; 2004:1459–1461.

70. Felcar JM, Guitti JCS, Marson AC, et al. Preoperative physiotherapy in prevention of pulmonary complications in pediatric cardiac surgery. *Rev Bras Cir Cardiovasc.* 2008;383–388.

71. Ferreyra G, Long Y, Ranieri VM. Respiratory complications after major surgery. *Curr Opin Crit Care.* 2009;15(4):342–348.

72. Thoren L. Postoperative pulmonary complications: observations on their prevention by means of physiotherapy. *Acta Chir Scand.* 1954;107:193–205.

73. Stein M, Cassara EL. Preoperative pulmonary evaluation and therapy for surgery patients. *JAMA.* 1970;211:787–790.

74. Bartlett RH, Gazzinga AB, Graghty JR. Respiratory maneuvers to prevent postoperative complications. *JAMA.* 1973;224:1017–1021.

75. Hymes AC, Yonehiro EG, Raab DE, et al. Electrical surface stimulation for treatment and prevention of ileus and atelectasis. *Surg Forum.* 1974;25:222–224.

76. Finer MN, Moriartey RR, Boyd J, et al. Postextubation atelectasis. A retrospective review and a prospective controlled study. *J Pediatr.* 1979;94:110–113.

77. Flenady VJ, Gray PH. Chest physiotherapy for preventing morbidity in babies being extubated from mechanical ventilation. *Cochrane Database Syst Rev.* 2002;(2):CD000283.

78. Wong I, Fok TF. Randomized comparison of two physiotherapy regimens for correcting atelectasis in ventilated pre-term neonates. *Hong Kong Physiother J.* 2003;21:43–50.

79. Chen YC, Wu LF, Mu PF, et al. Using chest vibration nursing intervention to improve expectoration of airway secretions and prevent lung collapse in ventilated ICU patients: a randomized controlled trial. *J Chin Med Assoc.* 2009;72(6):316–322.

80. Graham RJ, Fleegler EW, Robinson WM. Chronic ventilator need in the community: a 2005 pediatric census of Massachusetts. *Pediatrics.* 2007;119:e1280–e1287.

81. Kennedy JD, Martin AJ. Chronic respiratory failure and neuromuscular disease. *Pediatr Clin North Am.* 2009;56:261–273.

82. Wolfe LF, Joyce NC, McDonald CM, et al. Management of pulmonary complications in neuromuscular disease. *Phys Med Rehabil Clin N Am.* 2012;23(4):829–853.

83. Yang ML, Finkel RS. Overview of paediatric neuromuscular disorders and related pulmonary issues: diagnostic and therapeutic considerations. *Paediatr Respir Rev.* 2010;11(1):9–17.

84. Martin AJ, Stern L, Yeates J, et al. Respiratory muscle training in Duchenne muscular dystrophy. *Dev Med Child Neurol.* 1986;28: 314–318.

85. Mallory GB, Stillwell PC. The ventilator-dependent child: issues in diagnosis and management. *Arch Phys Med Rehabil.* 1991;72:43–55.

86. Domènech-Clar R, López-Andreu JA, Compte-Torrero L, et al. Maximal static respiratory pressures in children and adolescents. *Pediatr Pulmonol.* 2003;35(2):126–132.

87. Shardonofsky FR, Perez-Chada D, Carmuega E, et al. Airway pressures during crying in healthy infants. *Pediatr Pulmonol.* 1989;6:14–18.

88. Shardonofsky FR, Perez-Chada D, Milic-Emili J. Airway pressures during crying: an index of respiratory muscle strength in infants with neuromuscular disease. *Pediatr Pulmonol.* 1991;10:172–177.

89. Finder JD. Airway clearance modalities in neuromuscular disease. *Paediatr Respi Rev.* 2010;11:31–34.

90. Gauld LM, Boynton A. Relationship between peak cough flow and spirometry in Duchenne muscular dystrophy. *Pediatr Pulmonol.* 2005;39:457–460.

91. Wanke T, Toifl K, Formanek D, et al. Inspiratory muscle training in patients with Duchenne muscular dystrophy. *Chest.* 1994;105: 475–482.

92. Aloysius A, Born P, Kinali M, et al. Swallowing difficulties in Duchenne muscular dystrophy: indications for feeding assessment and outcome of videofluoroscopic swallow studies. *Eur J Paediatr Neurol.* 2008;12:239–245.

93. Hull J, Aniapravan R, Chan E, et al. British Thoracic Society guideline for respiratory management of children with neuromuscular weakness. *Thorax.* 2012;67(suppl 1):i1–i40. doi: 10.1136/thoraxjnl-2012-201964.

94. Merrick J, Axen K. Inspiratory muscle function following abdominal weight exercises in healthy subject. *Phys Ther.* 1981;61:651–656.

95. Winkler G, Zifko U, Nader A, et al. Dose-dependent effects of inspiratory muscle training in neuromuscular disorders. *Muscle Nerve.* 2000;23(8):1257–1260.

96. Barker NJ, Jones M, O'Connell NE, et al. Breathing exercises for dysfunctional breathing/hyperventilation syndrome in children. *Cochrane Database Syst Rev.* 2013;12:CD010376. doi: 10.1002/14651858.CD010376.pub2.

97. Cup EH, Pieterse AJ, ten Broek-Pastoor JM, et al. Exercise therapy and other types of physical therapy for patients with neuromuscular diseases: a systematic review. *Arch Phys Med Rehabil.* 2007;88: 1452–1464.

98. Crapo RO, Casaburi R, Coates AL, et al. Guidelines for methacholine and exercise challenge testing–1999. *Am J Respir Crit Care Med.* 2000;161(1):309–329.

99. Barach AL, Beck GL, Bickerman HA, et al. Physical methods simulating mechanisms of the human cough. *J Appl Physiol.* 1952;5:85–91.

100. Miske L, Hickey E, Kolb S, et al. Use of the mechanical in exsufflator in pediatric patients with neuromuscular disease and impaired cough. *Chest.* 2004;125:1406–1412.

101. Bach JR. Amyotrophic lateral sclerosis: prolongation of life by noninvasive respiratory aids. *Chest.* 2002;122:92–98.

102. Reddel HK, Taylor DR, Bateman ED, et al. Asthma control and exacerbations. *Am J Respir Crit Care Med.* 2009;180:59–99.

103. Adams PF, Kirzinger WK, Martinez ME. Summary health statistics for the U.S. population: National Health Interview Survey, 2011. National Center for Health Statistics. *Vital Health Stat.* 2012; 10(255).

104. Moorman JE, Rudd RA, Johnson CA. National surveillance for asthma–United States, 1980-2004. *MMWR Surveill Summ.* 2007;56:1–54.

105. Rowe BH, Bota G, Clark S. Comparison of Canadian versus American emergency department visits for acute asthma. *Can Respir J.* 2007;14:331–337.

106. Milgrom H, Taussig LM. Keeping children with exercise-induced asthma active. *Pediatrics.* 1999;104:e38.

107. Haslett C. Asthma: cellular and humoral mechanisms. In Seaton A, Leitch AG, Seaton D, eds. *Crofton and Douglas's Respiratory Diseases.* Wiley Publishers; 2008:916–917.

108. National Asthma Education and Prevention Program. *Expert panel report III: guidelines for the diagnosis and management of asthma.* Bethesda, MD: National Heart, Lung, and Blood Institute; 2007 (NIH publication no. 08-4051).

109. Craven D, Kercsmar CM, Myers TR, et al. Ipratropium bromide plus nebulized albuterol for the treatment of hospitalized children with acute asthma. *J Pediatr.* 2001;138(1):51–58.

110. Rowe BH, Spooner CH, Ducharme FM, et al. Early emergency department treat- ment of acute asthma with systemic corticosteroids. Cochrane Database Syst Rev 2001;1:CD002178.

111. Ni Chroinin M, Lasserson TJ, Greenstone I, et al. Addition of long-acting beta-agonists to inhaled corticosteroids for chronic asthma in children. *Cochrane Database Syst Rev.* 2009;3:CD007949.

112. Rao D, Phipatanakul W. Impact of environmental controls on childhood asthma. *Curr Allergy Asthma Rep.* 2011;11(5):414–420.

113. Kim JM, Lin SY, Suarez-Cuervo C, et al. Allergen-specific immunotherapy for pediatric asthma and rhinoconjunctivitis: a systematic review. *Pediatrics.* 2013;131(6):1155–1167.

114. Andrade LB, Silva DA, Salgado TL, et al. Comparison of six-minute walk test in children with moderate/severe asthma with reference values for healthy children. *J Pediatr (Rio J).* 2013; pii: S0021-7557(13)00209-X. doi: 10.1016/j.jped.2013.08.006. [Epub ahead of print].

115. Jinzhou Y, Fu Y, Zhang R, et al. The reliability and sensitivity of indices related to cardiovascular fitness evaluation. *Kinesiology.* 2008;40(2):139–146.

116. Liu L, Plowman S, Looney M. The reliability and validity of the 20-metre shuttle test in American students 12-15 years old. *Res Q Exerc Sport.* 1992;63:360–365.

117. Schechter MS. Airway clearance applications in infants and children. *Respir Care.* 2007;52(10):1382–1390; discussion 1390–1391.

118. Huber AL, Eggleston PA, Morgan J. Effect of chest physiotherapy on asthmatic children (abstract). *J Allergy Clin Immunol.* 1974;53:2.

119. Huntley A, White A, and Ernst E. Relaxation therapies for asthma: a systematic review. *Thorax.* 2002;57(2):127–131.

120. Yorke J, Fleming SL, Shuldham C. A systematic review of psychological interventions for children with asthma. *Pediatr Pulmonol.* 2007;42(2):114–124.

121. Bonini M, Di Mambro C, Calderon MA, et al. Beta2-agonists for exercise-induced asthma. *Cochrane Database Syst Rev.* 2013;10: CD003564.

122. Mendes F, Cukier A, Stelmach R, et al. Which asthmatic patients benefits most from aerobic training program? Paper presented at: European Respiratory Society Annual Congress; 2010; Barcelona.

123. Moreira A, Delgado L, Haahtela T, et al. Physical training does not increase allergic inflammation in asthmatic children. *Eur Respir J.* 2008;32(6):1570–1575.

124. Mancuso CA, Choi TN, Westermann H, et al. Improvement in asthma quality of life in patients enrolled in a prospective study to increase lifestyle physical activity. *J Asthma.* 2013;50(1):103–107.

125. Carson KV, Chandratilleke MG, Picot J, et al. Physical training for asthma. *Cochrane Database Systematic Rev.* 2013;9:CD001116.

126. Sly RM, Harper RT, Rosselot I. The effect of physical conditioning upon asthmatic children. *Ann Allerg.* 1972;30:86–94.

127. Fitch KD, Morton AR, Blanksby BA. Effects of swimming training on children with asthma. *Arch Disease Childhood.* 1976;51(3): 190–194.

128. Wang JS, Hung WP. The effects of a swimming intervention for children with asthma. *Respirology.* 2009;14(6):838–842.

129. Font-Ribera L, Villanueva CM, Nieuwenhuijsen MJ, et al. Swimming pool attendance, asthma, allergies, and lung function in the Avon Longitudinal Study of Parents and Children cohort. *Am J Respir Crit Care Med.* 2011;183(5):582–588.

130. Beggs S, Foong YC, Le HC, et al. Swimming training for asthma in children and adolescents aged 18 years and under. *Cochrane Airways Group Cochrane Database of Systematic Reviews.* 4, 2013.

131. Rommens JM, Iannuzzi MC, Kerem B, et al. Identification of the cystic fibrosis gene: chromosome walking and jumping. *Science.* 1989;245:1059–1065.

132. Pilewski JM, Frizzell RA. Role of CFTR in airway disease. *Physiol Rev.* 1999;79(1)(suppl):S215–S255.

133. Simonds NJ. Ageing in cystic fibrosis and long-term survival. *Paediatr Respir Rev.* 2013;14(supp 1):6.

134. Flume PA, Yankaskas JR, Ebeling M, et al. Massive hemoptysis in cystic fibrosis. *Chest.* 2005;128:729–738.

135. Flume PA, Strange C, Ye X, et al. Pneumothorax in cystic fibrosis. *Chest.* 2005;128:720–728.

136. Slattery DM, Waltz DA, Denham B, et al. Bronchoscopically administered human DNase for lobar atelectasis in cystic fibrosis. *Pediatr Pulmonol.* 2001;31:383–388.

137. Bright-Thomas RJ, Webb AK. The heart in cystic fibrosis. *J R Soc Med.* 2002;95(suppl 41):2–10.

138. Cystic Fibrosis Foundation. Infection Prevention and Control Policy. Bethesda, MD. http://www.cff.org/aboutCFFoundation/InfectionPreventionControlPolicy/Policy/. Accessed January 9, 2014.

139. Liou TG, Adler FR, Cox DR, et al. Transplantation and survival in children with cystic fibrosis. *N Engl J Med.* 2007;357:2143–2152.

140. Allen J, Visner G. Lung transplantation in cystic fibrosis—primum non nocere? *N Engl J Med.* 2007;357:2186–2188.

141. Thabut G, Christie JD, Mal H, et al. Survival benefit of lung transplant for cystic fibrosis since lung allocation score implementation. *Am J Respir Crit Care Med.* 2013;187(12):1335–1340.

142. Ramsey BW, Davies J, McElvaney NG, et al. A CFTR potentiator in patients with cystic fibrosis and the G551D mutation. *N Engl J Med.* 2011;365:1663–1672.

143. Nixon PA, Orenstein DM, Kelsey SF. Habitual physical activity in children and adolescents with cystic fibrosis. *Med Sci Sports Exerc.* 2001;33(1):30–35.

144. Radtke T, Stevens D, Benden C, et al. Clinical exercise testing in children and adolescents with cystic fibrosis. *Pediatr Phys Ther.* 2009;21(3):275–281.

145. Nixon PA, Orenstein DM, Kelsey SF, et al. The prognostic value of exercise testing in patients with cystic fibrosis. *N Engl J Med.* 1992;327:1785–1788.

146. Moorcroft AJ, Dodd ME, Webb AK. Exercise testing and prognosis in adult cystic fibrosis. *Thorax.* 1997;52:291–293.

147. ATS Statement: guidelines for the six-minute walk test. *Am J Respir Crit Care Med.* 2002;166:111–117.

148. Narang I, Pike S, Rosenthal M, et al. Three-minute step test to assess exercise capacity in children with cystic fibrosis with mild lung disease. *Pediatr Pulmonol.* 2003;35:108–113.

149. Selvadurai HC, Cooper PJ, Meyers N, et al. Validation of shuttle tests in children with cystic fibrosis. *Pediatr Pulmonol.* 2003;35(2):133–138.

150. Lorin MI, Denning CR. Evaluation of postural drainage by measurement of sputum volume and consistency. *Am J Phys Med.* 1971;50:215–219.

151. Tecklin JS, Holsclaw DS. Evaluation of bronchial drainage in patients with cystic fibrosis. *Phys Ther.* 1975;55:1081–1084.

152. Feldman J, Traver GA, Taussig LM. Maximal expiratory flows after postural drainage. *Am Rev Respir Dis.* 1979;119:239–245.

153. Warwick WJ, Hansen LG. The long-term effect of high frequency chest compression therapy on pulmonary complications of cystic fibrosis. *Pediatr Pulmonol.* 1991;11:265–271.

154. Motoyama EK. Lower airway obstruction. In: Mangos JA, Talamo RD, eds. *Fundamental Problems of Cystic Fibrosis and Related Diseases.* New York, NY: Intercontinental Medical Book Corp; 1973.

155. Desmond KF, Schwenk F, Thomas E, et al. Immediate and long-term effects of chest physiotherapy in patients with cystic fibrosis. *J Pediatr.* 1983;103:538–542.

156. McIlwaine PM, Davidson AGF. Cystic fibrosis, basic and clinical research. Comparison of expiratory pressure and autogenic drainage with conventional percussion and drainage therapy in the treatment of cystic fibrosis (abst.). In: *Proceedings of the 17th European Cystic Fibrosis Conference, Copenhagen, Denmark.* Amsterdam, Netherlands: Elsevier Science BV; 1991:54.

157. Pfleger A, Theissl B, Oberwalder B, et al. Self-administered chest physiotherapy in cystic fibrosis: a comparative study of high-pressure PEP and autogenic drainage. *Lung.* 1992;170:323–330.

158. Miller S, Hall D, Clayton CB, et al. Chest physiotherapy in cystic fibrosis: a comparative study of autogenic drainage and active cycle of breathing technique (formerly called FET). *Pediatr Pulmonol.* 1993;(suppl 9):267.

159. Butler-Simon N, McCool P, Giles D, et al. Efficacy and desirability of autogenic drainage vs. conventional postural drainage and percussion. *Pediatr Pulmonol.* 1995;(suppl 253):(abst 265)

160. McIlwaine MP[1], Alarie N[2], Davidson GF, et al. Long-term multicentre randomized controlled study of high frequency chest wall oscillation versus positive expiratory pressure mask in cystic fibrosis. *Thorax.* 2013;68(8):746–751.

161. Darbee JC, Ohtake PJ, Grant BJ, et al. Physiologic evidence for the efficacy of positive expiratory pressure as an airway clearance technique in patients with cystic fibrosis. *Phys Ther.* 2004;84(6):524–537.

162. Gondor M, Nixon PA, Rebovich PF, et al. A comparison of the Flutter device and chest physical therapy in the treatment of cystic fibrosis pulmonary exacerbation. *Pediatr Pulmonol.* 1999;28:255–260.

163. West K, Wallen M, Follett J. Acapella vs. PEP mask therapy: a randomised trial in children with cystic fibrosis during respiratory exacerbation. *Physiother Theory Pract.* 2010;26(3):143–149.

164. Arens R, Gozal D, Omlin KJ, et al. Comparison of high frequency chest compression and conventional chest physiotherapy in hospitalized patients with cystic fibrosis. *Am J Respir Crit Care Med.* 1994;150(4):1154–1157.

165. Tecklin JS, Clayton R, Scanlin T. High frequency chest wall oscillation vs. traditional chest physical therapy in cystic fibrosis—A large one-year, controlled study. Paper presented at: 14th Annual North American Cystic Fibrosis Conference; Nov 11, 2000; Baltimore, MD. Nov. 11, 2.

166. Pryor JA. Physiotherapy for airway clearance in adults. *Eur Respir J.* 1999;14:1418–1424.

167. Main E. What is the best airway clearance technique in cystic fibrosis? *Pediatr Respir Rev.* 2013;14(suppl 1):10–12.

168. Cropp GJA, Pullano TP, Cerny FJ, et al. Adaptation to exercise in cystic fibrosis. *CF Club Abstr.* 1979;20:32.

169. Marcus CL, Bader D, Stabile MW, et al. Supplemental oxygen and exercise performance in patients with cystic fibrosis with severe pulmonary disease. *Chest.* 1992;101:52–57.

170. Moorcraft AJ, Dodd ME, Howarth C, et al. Muscular fatigue, ventilation, and perception of limitation at peak exercise in adults with cystic fibrosis. *Pediatr Pulmonol.* 1996;(suppl 13):306(abst 349).

171. Williams CA, Benden C, Stevens D, et al. Exercise training in children and adolescents with cystic fibrosis: theory into practice. *Int J Pediatr.* 2010;2010:670640.

Physical Therapy in the Educational Environment

Karen Yundt Lunnen and Rita F. Geddes

Introduction
Historical Background
Service Provision for Children Aged 3 to 21 (Part B)
Educational Team
Referral
Assessment/Evaluation
Eligibility for Related Services under IDEA
Eligibility Under Rehabilitation Act
Individualized Education Program
Service Provision for Infants/Toddlers (Part C)
Evaluation Under Part C
Infant Family Service Plan
Program Development/Intervention under Parts B and C
Meaningful Collaboration with Parents
IEP/IFSP Goals and Objectives

Inclusive Education
Models of Service Delivery
Role of the Physical Therapist Assistant
Assistive Technology
Transition Planning
Re-evaluation
Documentation
Extended School Year
Reimbursement for Services
Role of the Physical Therapist in Program-related Areas
Points to Ponder
Summary

▶ Introduction

Services for children with disabilities in the educational setting are guided by comprehensive federal legislation, the Individuals with Disabilities Education Improvement Act (IDEA).[1] In the legislation, physical therapy is considered a related service and may be required to enable a child with a disability to benefit from special education. The educational environment is a rewarding one and challenges physical therapists to use the best of their professional abilities within a unique context.

▶ Historical background

Physical therapists have been practicing in the educational environment in the United States since the 1930s. During those early years, children with physical disabilities were usually segregated in special orthopedic schools or in separate classrooms within the school building. Typically, children with intellectual impairment or more severe disabilities did not have access to public education.

Often, physical therapists were employed as "special teachers, with the same privileges and responsibilities."[2] They met the same educational requirements as teachers and had, in addition, "a course in physical therapy from an approved school."[2] Physical therapists practicing in educational environments were already addressing the benefits of including children with disabilities in activities with "normal" children. Ruth De Young (1932) describes an orthopedic school housed under the same roof as the high school allowing a "complete curriculum for little cripples."[3] Hutchinson (1944) comments that "it is easier for the crippled child to grow normally when he is in association with regular school children."[4] Yet, for approximately 30 more years, segregation for those with physical handicaps and exclusion for those with intellectual disabilities and/or severe physical disabilities was the prevailing norm.

In the 1960s and 1970s, parents and other advocates became active in the so-called normalization movement and found support from President John F. Kennedy's administration. Several landmark decisions in the Supreme Court in the early 1970s paved the way for subsequent legislation guaranteeing the rights of those with disabilities. It is essential that physical therapists understand this legislation at both federal and state levels, because it has directed the provision of special education for children and defined the role of the physical therapist in the educational environment.

The first significant civil rights legislation for individuals with disabilities was PL 93-112, the Rehabilitation Act of

1973.[5] Section 504 of the Rehabilitation Act states that "no otherwise qualified disabled individual would be excluded from the participation in, be denied the benefits of, or be subjected to discrimination under any program or activity receiving federal financial assistance."[5] Section 504 paved the way for subsequent legislation impacting the provision of special education for children with disabilities in the public schools.

In 1975, the U.S. Congress passed the Education for All Handicapped Children Act (PL 94-142),[6] which was the template for dramatic changes in the responsibility of public schools to educate children with disabilities. PL 94-142 provided for a "free appropriate public education" for all children with disabilities from the age of 6 to 21 years (or from 5 years if that was the age in a particular state when children normally began their participation in public school).[6] Special education and related services provided in accordance with an individualized education program were emphasized to address each child's unique needs. Related services encompassed a broad range of support services, including physical therapy.

Further provisions of PL 94-142 described a number of important new concepts for the public education of children with disabilities that remain part of the current legislation.

1. *Zero reject:* No child is excluded from receiving a free appropriate public education regardless of the type or severity of his or her disability.
2. *Least restrictive environment:* School systems are required to ensure that "[t]o the maximum extent appropriate, children with disabilities are educated with children who are non-disabled; and that special classes, separate schooling or other removal of children with disabilities from regular classes occurs only when the nature or severity of the disability is such that education in the regular classroom with the use of supplementary aids and services cannot be achieved satisfactorily."[6]
3. *Parent participation:* Parents or primary caregivers are essential members of the team approach to evaluation, planning, and intervention and are assured various rights.
4. *Nondiscriminatory evaluation:* Evaluation of a child is free from racial or cultural bias, no one test is used as the sole criterion for placement decisions, and the test is administered in the child's native language.
5. *Individualized Education Program (IEP):* Every child receiving special education must receive an individualized education program. This is a comprehensive individualized plan developed by a multidisciplinary team in cooperation with the parents that outlines the special education and related-service needs of the child.

The government built into PL 94-142 the requirement that it be periodically reviewed, revised, and reauthorized. Over the past several decades, several amendments have been made to PL 94-142, and other legislation has been introduced that has impacted services for children with disabilities (Table 21-1).

The impact of the legislation on the delivery of services in the educational environment for children with a wide range of disabilities has been dramatic. The reader is urged to explore further the interesting progression of federal mandates over time. However, the remainder of this chapter will focus on IDEA and the framework it provides for the education of children with special needs. The full text of the IDEA legislation and related resources are available on the following Web site: http://idea.ed.gov/.

IDEA impacts the education of almost 7 million American children with disabilities. The assumption underlying IDEA is that, on average, the cost of educating children with disabilities is twice the average cost of educating other children. Congress determined that the federal government would pay up to 40% of this additional cost, but with the exception of a 1-year increase in 2009 from the American Recovery and Reinvestment Act, the actual federal allocation has always been less than half the amount promised (16.5% in 2012), resulting in a significant burden for the states.[17] In 2002, a large number of professional organizations, including the National Education Association, formed the IDEA Funding Coalition and developed a proposal for full funding by the federal government that could be phased in over a predetermined time period.[18] These organizations are still advocating increased federal support.

The overall purpose of IDEA is to "ensure that all children with disabilities have available to them a free appropriate public education that emphasizes special education and related services designed to meet their unique needs and prepare them for further education, employment, and independent living."[1] The purpose has changed little since PL 94-142, but what is notable is the inclusion of *all* children and the emphasis on planning for a child's lifetime.

IDEA has four major sections: (A) General Provisions, (B) Assistance for All Children with Disabilities, (C) Infants and Toddlers with Disabilities, and (D) National Activities to Improve Education of Children with Disabilities (including personnel development).[1]

In substantiating the reauthorization of IDEA, Congress noted the overall success of the federal legislation to assure access to free appropriate public education and to improve educational outcomes for children with disabilities. Cited as impediments to the success of the legislation were low expectations and "insufficient focus on applying replicable research on proven methods of teaching and learning for children with disabilities."[1]

The overall tenets supported by IDEA include:[1]

- having high expectations for children and "ensuring their access to the general education curriculum, to the maximum extent possible";[1]
- strengthening the role and responsibility of parents;
- providing appropriate special education and related services;
- supporting the development and use of assistive technology to maximize accessibility;
- supporting high-quality, intensive preservice preparation and professional development for all personnel who work with children with disabilities;

TABLE 21.1	Legislation Impacting Provision of Services for Children with Disabilities in Educational Environments	

Year Enacted	Title of Legislation	Impact
1986	PL 99-457 Education of the Handicapped Act Amendments[7]	Expanded the provisions of PL 94-142 to include infants and toddlers (Birth to 3 years) and preschool children (3–5 years).
1988	PL 100-360 Medicare Catastrophic Coverage Act [8]	Allowed Medicaid funds to pay for needed services identified in the formal education plan. The intent of this act was to improve access to therapy for children by allowing federal resources other than education to pay for some related services.
1988	PL 100-407 Technology-Related Assistance for Individuals with Disabilities Act (Tech Act)[9]	Mandated that states address policies, practices, and structures to promote access to appropriate assistive technology (AT). Public schools were obligated to provide needed AT services and/or devices.
1990	PL 101-336, The Americans with Disabilities Act (ADA)[10]	Extended comprehensive civil rights protection to individuals with disabilities. The law's major impact on public education was the provision that all public buildings must be accessible.
1991	PL 102-119 Individuals with Disabilities Education Act Amendments of 1991 (IDEA)[11]	Supported most of the provisions of PL 94-142 and PL 99-457 with amendments that expanded or modified the provisions of the law in other areas.
1997	PL 105-17 Individuals with Disabilities Education Act Amendments of 1997[12]	Reauthorization of IDEA Supported most of the provisions of earlier legislation and expanded or modified other provisions.
1998	PL 105-394 Assistive Technology Act of 1998[13]	Reauthorization of PL 100-407 (Tech Act)
2001	PL 107-110 No Child Left Behind Act of 2001[14]	Addressed the quality of education for all children; included annual testing and mandate for adequate progress.
2004	PL 108-446 Individuals with Disabilities Education Improvement Act of 2004[1]	Reauthorization of PL 102-119
2004	HR 4278 Assistive Technology Act of 2004 (Putting technology into the hands of Individuals with disabilities)[15]	Reauthorization of PL 105-394
2009	American Recovery and Reinvestment Act[16]	Appropriated significant new funding (although for 1 year) to state and local educational agencies to implement statewide systems of coordinated, comprehensive, multidisciplinary programs for children with disabilities.

- recognizing the increasing number of racial and ethnic minorities and the need for equitable treatment and for increased participation of minorities in the teaching profession; and
- emphasizing the importance of effective transition services to promote independence and success in employment or further education after leaving public education.

▶ Service provision for children aged 3 to 21 (Part B)

Part B of IDEA addresses the provision of services for children aged 3 to 21 years and includes a set of operational definitions that are important to understand.[1] A few key definitions are included below:

Educational Team

IDEA stipulates that assessment, planning, and service delivery must be provided by a "multidisciplinary team of qualified professionals and the parent of the child."[1] More specifically, the IEP team must include the parent(s), a regular education teacher, a special education teacher, a representative of the local educational agency (LEA), and "at the discretion of the parent or LEA, other individuals who have knowledge or special expertise regarding the child, including related services personnel as appropriate."[1]

The federal legislation labels teams as "multidisciplinary," although the description of membership, roles, and responsibilities is closer to what most would define as a transdisciplinary or collaborative team model. In the transdisciplinary model, team members jointly assess the child; parents are full and active participants; a primary service provider is

Child with a disability	a child ". . . with mental retardation, hearing impairments (including deafness), speech or language impairments, visual impairments (including blindness), serious emotional disturbance, orthopedic impairments, autism, traumatic brain injury, other health impairments, or specific learning disabilities . . . who, by reason thereof, needs special education and related services."[1]
Child with a disability for a child aged 3 through 9 (or any subset of that age range)	". . . may, at the discretion of the State and the local educational agency, include a child experiencing developmental delays, as defined by the State and as measured by appropriate diagnostic instruments and procedures, in 1 or more of the following areas: physical development, cognitive development; communication development; social or emotional development; or adaptive development . . . who, by reason thereof, needs special education and related services."[1]
Related services	". . . transportation, and such developmental, corrective, and other supportive services (including speech-language pathology and audiology services, interpreting services, psychological services, physical and occupational therapy, recreation, including therapeutic recreation, social work services, school nurse services designed to enable a child with a disability to receive a free appropriate public education as described in the IEP of the child, counseling services, including rehabilitation counseling, orientation and mobility services, and medical services, except that such medical services shall be for diagnostic and evaluation purposes only) as may be required to assist a child with a disability to benefit from special education, and includes the early identification and assessment of disabling conditions in children."[1]
Special education	". . . specifically designed instruction, at no cost to parents, to meet the unique needs of a child with disability."[1]
Supplementary aids and services	". . . aids, services and other supports that are provided in regular education classes or other education-related settings to enable children with disabilities to be educated with non-disabled children to the maximum extent appropriate. . . ."[1]

assigned to implement the plan with the family; information, knowledge, and skills are continuously shared among team members; and there is a commitment to teach, learn, and work together across disciplinary boundaries to implement a unified service plan.[19] The collaborative model is a combination of a transdisciplinary team functioning in an integrated service delivery model.[20,21] Palisano conceptualized a collaborative model of service delivery as a framework for evidence-based decision making.[22]

When the Education for All Handicapped Children's Act was passed in 1976, there was suddenly a legal mandate for physical therapy services in the public schools. Therapists to provide those services were in high demand and short supply. The section on pediatrics was created, at least in part, to define the competencies required to practice in the educational environment and to establish a process for specialty certification in pediatric physical therapy.[23]

The qualifications of personnel working with children who have disabilities received increased emphasis in the 2004 reauthorization of IDEA and is a matter of increasing concern to various agencies and associations. An American Physical Therapy Association (APTA) task force initially established competencies for physical therapists in early intervention that were published in 1991 and updated by Effgen and Chiarello in 2006.[24] Effgen and Chiarello have also published updated competencies for physical therapists working in schools (ages 5 to 21).[25] The authors used a four-step process to define the following nine major competency areas for physical therapists practicing in educational environments:

1. Context of therapy practice in education settings
2. Wellness and prevention
3. Team collaboration
4. Examination and evaluation
5. Planning
6. Intervention
7. Documentation
8. Administration
9. Research

Specific skills and competencies are outlined for each of the nine competency areas that conform to the *Guide to Physical Therapist Practice*[26] as well as the International Classification of Functioning, Disability and Health (ICF) model.[27] Clinicians desiring to practice in the educational setting, or students preparing for a clinical rotation in a school setting, can utilize this information to prepare for an interview, improve baseline knowledge of educational services, assess professional development needs, and prioritize a professional development plan.

The Association for Persons with Severe Handicaps (TASH), an international association of people with disabilities that broadly advocates inclusion, developed a *Resolution on Preparation of Related Services Personnel for Work in Educational Settings*.[28] The TASH resolution is aimed at the preparation of related-service providers at the university level and addresses both entry-level and advanced competencies in a comprehensive manner. In all of the competency areas of this resolution, emphasis is placed on maximizing participation and meaningful involvement at school and in the community for children with disabilities.

Referral

Referral for evaluation to determine whether a child is a child with a disability (as defined by the law) can be made by a parent, a state agency, or LEA. Referral for a related service, including physical therapy, can be initiated by anyone on the child's team, but an IEP must be developed for the student before initiation of a related service. Physical therapists may screen a child as a preliminary step and help direct the process of subsequent referral in that way. The referral process can be cumbersome, especially for a child who is not already receiving special education services. Results of survey research by Goodrich et al.[29] indicated that developing a specific form, providing training on an education-based decision-making process, and implementing a classroom-based support service significantly increased the number of appropriate referrals for physical and occupational therapy over a 5-year period. If a student is determined ineligible for special education, a physical therapist may (at the discretion of the LEA) offer limited consultation to the classroom teacher, physical education teacher, or parent.

If the state practice act for physical therapy requires physician referral for a client to access physical therapy, then it is necessary to obtain that medical referral in addition to the procedural steps outlined by legislative guidelines. In states with direct access, a physician referral is not necessary unless dictated by a third-party payer (e.g., Medicaid). A physician referral is recommended for students with complex medical needs to formalize a process for needed communication with the referring physician. Children with disabilities are frequently served by a variety of professionals and social agencies. Communication with others involved in providing care for the child outside of the educational environment is crucial regardless of the decision about medical referral.

Assessment/Evaluation

IDEA requires a "full and individualized initial evaluation" to determine whether the child has a disability and, if so, whether the disability limits in some way the student's ability to benefit from special education or participate optimally in the educational environment.[1] An evaluation requires parental consent and must be completed within 60 calendar days after receiving consent. IDEA requires the use of a variety of assessment tools and strategies to gather functional, developmental, and academic information. Progressively more importance has been given in the federal legislation to using assessment instruments that are nondiscriminatory, administered in the language and form most likely to yield accurate information, by appropriately trained personnel, according to the purpose for which reliability and validity were established, and in accordance with instructions specific to the instrument.

A physical therapy evaluation may be part of the initial evaluation to determine eligibility for special education/related services or may be a recommendation of the team after eligibility has been established. A physical therapy evaluation should include traditional elements as suggested by the *Guide to Physical Therapist Practice*[26] or other models. At least one standardized measure, either norm-referenced or criterion-referenced, is recommended. Summaries of assessment instruments available to use with children who have developmental delays are available in Chapter 3 of this textbook and in other published materials.[29] Instruments in common use in the educational environment are:

1. *Bruininks-Oseretsky Test of Motor Proficiency, 2nd Edition*[30]—a standardized, norm-referenced test for children from 4 to 21 years of age who range from those who are developing normally to those who have moderate motor skill deficits. The complete battery includes eight subtests: (1) fine motor precision, (2) fine motor integration, (3) manual dexterity, (4) bilateral coordination, (5) balance, (6) running speed and agility, (7) upper limb coordination, and (8) strength. Together the items provide a comprehensive index of motor proficiency plus separate measures of both gross and fine motor skills. A test kit contains all items necessary for administration. The complete battery requires approximately 45 to 60 minutes to administer. A short form includes a subset of items from the complete battery and can be used as a screening tool. Clinical validity studies have been conducted on children with high-functioning autism, developmental coordination disorder, and mild to moderate intellectual impairment.

2. *Children's Assessment of Participation and Enjoyment (CAPE) and Preferences for Activities of Children (PAC)*[31]—a student-rated questionnaire that looks at five dimensions of participation: (1) recreational, (2) physical, (3) social, (4) skill-based, and (5) self-improvement. The CAPE documents the child's daily participation, and the PAC explores the child's preferences for activities. Both are intended for use with students 6 to 21 years of age. The CAPE takes approximately 30 to 45 minutes to administer and the PAC approximately 15 to 20 minutes.

3. *Gross Motor Function Measure (GMFM)*[32]—a criterion-based observational measure designed and validated for use by pediatric physical therapists as an evaluative measure for assessing change over time in gross motor function of children with cerebral palsy. The GMFM has been validated for use with children and adolescents with traumatic brain injury[33] and found to be reliable when administered to children with osteogenesis imperfecta.[34] It may be appropriate for other populations as well. The GMFM was designed for children whose motor skills are at or below those of a 5-year-old child without motor disability. Motor function is assessed in five dimensions: (1) lying and rolling, (2) sitting, (3) crawling and kneeling, (4) standing, and (5) walking, running, and jumping. Performance with or without assistive device(s) can be assessed and compared. The option to delineate goal areas from among the five dimensions increases the test's sensitivity to change in a particular individual. The GMFM-88 contains 88 items, while a more recent, shorter version, the GMFM-66, contains only 66 items (taken from the original 88) and can be scored electronically.

4. *Mobility Opportunities Via Education (MOVE)*[35]—a full curriculum developed specifically for children with severe/profound disabilities over the age of 7 who have not developed the physical skills necessary to sit independently, bear weight on their feet, or take reciprocal steps.

The curriculum is designed as a comprehensive, interdisciplinary approach to teach students basic, functional motor skills needed for adult life in home and community environments. The Top-Down Motor Milestone Test, part of the MOVE curriculum, is an interview-based assessment tool that rates a child's performance in 16 categories of basic motor function.

5. *School Function Assessment*[36]—a criterion-referenced standardized survey instrument that utilizes the responses of one or more individuals familiar with the child's function in the educational environment as the basis for scoring. Items cover a comprehensive array of functional behaviors categorized in five areas: (1) participation, (2) task supports, (3) activity performance, (4) physical tasks, and (5) cognitive/behavioral tasks. The content is specifically relevant for children with physical or sensory impairments and can reveal patterns of strength and weakness. Individual items on the test are worded in behavioral, measurable terms that allow them to be easily converted to IEP goals. Completing the whole assessment can be time-consuming (approximately 2 hours), but this is strongly recommended as a baseline. Individual sections can also be administered separately.

6. *School Outcomes Measure*[37]—a minimum data set, comparable to the Functional Independence Measure for Children (WeeFIM)[38] but specific to the educational environment, that can be used to measure population-based outcomes data (demographic and functional ability information) of primary and secondary students (ages 3 to 21 years) receiving school-based occupational or physical therapy. The authors have published information on the content validity and inter-rater reliability and are continuing to determine psychometric properties of the measure.[39]

7. *Test of Gross Motor Development 2*[40]—a norm-referenced measure of gross motor skills in children aged 3 through 10 years who are significantly behind their peers in gross motor skill development. Results produce standard scores, percentile scores, and age equivalents. Detailed descriptions/illustrations and the availability of a test kit standardize administration. The test can be administered in about 20 minutes.

In addition to the standardized, norm-referenced or criterion-referenced component, the evaluation should include an ecological component, or assessment of the student's ability to participate in and benefit from the educational environment and activities. An ecological assessment is an approach that focuses on the activities necessary for a student to function in various environments and the skills required to perform the specified activities. Examples of ecological assessment may include reporting on the level of assistance, time, prompts, and/or adaptations needed for the student to:

access transportation on the school bus;
enter and exit the bathroom, including toileting;

eat/navigate in a cafeteria setting; and
negotiate hallways, doors, and stairs.

As part of the ecological assessment, the physical therapist may have to complete a task analysis of activities that the student performs routinely at school to identify the specific areas of need that must be addressed in order to improve the student's level of independence.[41] Ecological assessment may also provide baseline information from which goals can be set and measured (e.g., walking speed in elementary school hallways of a student with a disability compared with walking speed of nondisabled peers).[42]

It is especially important in an educational environment that the physical therapist interpret the results of testing for other team members. Depending on their background, team members may have varying levels of understanding about concepts and terms common to a physical therapist. Documentation of the testing must also be written in language that can be understood by nonmedical personnel.[1]

Eligibility for Related Services under IDEA

Determining who is eligible for related services in the educational environment is often a challenging process. Decisions about educational relevance are made by the team, not any one service provider. It is important to remember that related services support the educational process and not the medical well-being of the child, and that related services are provided to help a child benefit from special education. Under the provisions of IDEA, if a child does not need special education, he or she is not eligible to receive related services. Eligibility determination can vary significantly from state to state, so the physical therapist in an educational setting should be familiar with the eligibility standards set by the state in which he/she practices.

Faced with financial constraints, shortages of physical therapy personnel, and legal accountability, many states struggle to improve the objectivity of the process for determining eligibility without losing the mandate for individualized program plans. As a result, several states are developing clinical reasoning tools to assist IEP teams with determining educational needs for related services. A current example is the Considerations for Educationally Relevant Therapy (CERT) for Occupational Therapy and Physical Therapy.[43] Tools such as the CERT are designed to be used by physical or occupational therapists in collaboration with the IEP team to help guide the decision as to whether physical or occupational therapy services are relevant and necessary as well as to guide decisions regarding the intensity and frequency of services. Additional tools that are not specific to the school environment are also available to assist physical therapists with clinical reasoning. The Hypothesis-Oriented Pediatric Focused Algorithm (HOP-FA), for example, provides a framework or step-by-step guide with respect to clinical reasoning using the ICF model.[44] While it does not yield the same end information as the CERT, it does assist the therapist with identifying and prioritizing areas of need and the development of interventions to address those needs. Such tools are especially valuable to therapists who are new to pediatrics.

Eligibility under Rehabilitation Act

The Rehabilitation Act[5] is a federal statute designed to assure that individuals with disabilities are provided equal opportunities. Provisions of the Rehabilitation Act are generally broader than those in IDEA, and it is often used as a justification for expanding a student's eligibility for related services within the educational environment and/or the scope of intervention. It ensures that students with disabilities receive an appropriate education even if special education is not required, and it is an important source of support and funding for children who do not qualify for services under other legislative acts. Students who receive services under the provisions of the Rehabilitation Act will have a 504 Plan rather than an IEP.

Individualized Education Program

If the team identifies the student as being eligible for special education services, then the process advances to IEP development. An IEP must be developed within 30 calendar days of the determination of eligibility. In developing the IEP, the law emphasizes the importance of considering the strengths of the child, the concerns of the parents for enhancing the education of their child, the results of the initial (or most recent) evaluation, and the academic, developmental, and functional needs of the child. The written program must include the following:[1]

1. Statement of the child's present levels of academic achievement and functional performance, including how the child's disability affects the child's involvement and progress in the general education curriculum (or for preschool children, the child's participation in age-appropriate activities).
2. Statement of measurable annual goals, including academic and functional goals designed to enable the child

to make progress in the general education curriculum and meet each of the child's other educational needs that result from the child's disability.
3. Description of the child's progress toward meeting the annual goals.
4. Statement of the special education and related services and supplementary aids and services (based on peer-reviewed research to the extent practical) to be provided. Explanation of the extent, if any, to which the child will not participate with nondisabled children in the regular class and in other activities.
5. Statement of accommodations that are necessary to measure the academic achievement and functional performance of the child on state- and district-wide assessments. Accommodations and modifications are typically included in the Supplementary Aids and Services portion of the IEP.
6. Projected date for the beginning of the services and modifications described and the anticipated frequency, location, and duration of those services and modifications.
7. Beginning not later than the first IEP to be in effect when the child is 14, and updated annually, appropriate measurable postsecondary goals based upon age-appropriate transition assessments related to training, education, employment, and, where appropriate, independent living skills; and the transition services needed to assist the child in reaching those goals.

On the United States Department of Education Web site is a sample form that outlines the IEP content required by IDEA (http://www.ed.gov/policy/speced/guid/idea/modelform-iep.doc).[45] Physical therapists are typically responsible for the following IEP input:

1. A statement of the child's present levels of functional performance (including a statement of progress toward the prior year's annual goal if appropriate).
2. Development of (a) child-centered, measurable annual goal(s) if indicated (Refer Table 21-3).
3. Recommendations for service levels, including frequency, duration, and location.
4. Recommendations for supplementary aids and services, examples of which are given in Table 21-2.

TABLE 21.2	Examples of Recommendations for Supplementary Aids				
Adaptation	**Location**	**Frequency**	**Beginning Date**	**Duration**
Allow James to leave class 3 minutes early to avoid crowded hallways.	All classes	Daily for hallway mobility	05/01/2014	04/30/2015
Use an adapted chair to compensate for decreased postural stability.	Classroom	Daily for desktop activities	03/20/2015	03/19/2016
Modify distance and/or time allotted to complete tasks in PE class (e.g., run 40 feet instead of 100 feet).	Gym	Weekly in PE class	05/17/2016	05/16/2017

An IEP must be reviewed at least annually and revised as appropriate.[1] IDEA provides the option to develop "a comprehensive multi-year IEP, not to exceed 3 years, that is designed to coincide with the natural transition points for the child."[1] These transitions include the transition from preschool to elementary, elementary to middle, middle to secondary, and secondary to postsecondary.

A number of procedural safeguards are stipulated, and states must establish mechanisms for due process, mediation, and appeal. States are required to establish quantifiable indicators in specified priority areas and to report data on outcomes. A continuing area of federal focus is evidence that education is occurring in the least restrictive environment and that no discriminatory activity is occurring in relation to minorities.

Service provision for infants/toddlers (Part C)

Part C of IDEA describes infants and toddlers with disabilities and the services provided for them. IDEA recognizes that significant brain development occurs in the first 3 years of life and that early intervention is important to enhance development, reduce educational costs to society, and maximize the ability of individuals with disability to live independently.

The basic tenets of IDEA are the same for this age group as for older children, but there are important differences. Since the providers of early intervention services were much more diverse, the federal government allowed more discretion at the state level in Part C. Every state must use the federal assistance "to develop and implement a statewide, comprehensive, coordinated, multidisciplinary, interagency system . . ." coordinated by an Interagency Coordinating Council.[1] The council must meet at least quarterly, and its composition must include parents (not less than 20% of the members), public or private providers of early intervention services (not less than 20% of the members), and at least one representative from the state legislature, the state Medicaid program, and the state welfare agencies responsible for foster care, children's mental health, and homeless children.

IDEA mandates that states must develop specific policies and procedures for children under 3 years who have experienced substantiated physical, emotional, or sexual abuse or neglect or who have been affected by the abuse of illegal substances or withdrawal symptoms as a result of prenatal drug exposure. APTA has published a monograph, *Guidelines for Recognizing and Providing Care for Victims of Child Abuse*, and incorporated it into their Learning Center with the option of earning continuing education credit with purchase.[46] It is an important resource.

The services identified for early intervention are expansive and include physical therapy; occupational therapy; speech therapy; assistive technology devices and services; psychological services; family training and counseling; diagnostic medical services; special instruction; social work; vision; hearing; and related transportation. As for older children, an important stipulation is that services should be provided in a natural environment, which for infants and toddlers is typically in the home or in day-care centers.

Important definitions in Part C include the following[1]:

At-risk infant or toddler	". . . an individual under 3 years of age who would be at risk of experiencing a substantial developmental delay if early intervention services were not provided to the individual."
Infant or toddler with a disability	". . . an individual under 3 years of age who needs early intervention services because the individual is experiencing developmental delays, as measured by appropriate diagnostic instruments and procedures, in 1 or more areas of cognitive development, physical development, communication development, social or emotional development, and adaptive development . . ." or "has a diagnosed physical or mental condition that has a high probability of resulting in developmental delay; and . . . may also include, at State's discretion, at risk infants . . ."
Developmental delay	Defined by each state

Evaluation under Part C

The same federal mandates and guidelines for evaluation apply under Part C. For this younger population, however, physical therapists may use other assessment instruments described in Chapter 3, including:

1. *Bayley Scales of Infant and Toddler Development, Third Edition (Bayley III)*[47]—a standardized, norm-referenced test that measures a child's competency in five major developmental domains that correspond with those stipulated in IDEA: (1) cognitive, (2) language, (3) motor,

(4) social-emotional, and (5) adaptive behavior. Physical therapists would typically complete the Motor Scale.

2. *Peabody Developmental Motor Scales 2*[48]—a standardized, norm-referenced test of motor skills in children from birth to 5 years of age. Six subtests assess motor skills in the following areas: reflexes, stationary, locomotion, object manipulation, grasping, and visual motor integration. A motor activities program with instructional objectives, reasons for teaching the skill, examples of related skills as they occur in the natural environment, and suggested instructional strategies supplements the assessment.

3. *Pediatric Evaluation of Disability Inventory*[49]—a functional assessment instrument for the evaluation of children with disabilities from age 6 months to 7 years. On the basis of an interview with a primary caregiver, the inventory measures functional status and change in three domains: self-care, mobility, and social function. Scoring is done to indicate functional skill level, the amount of caregiver assistance required, and modifications or adaptive equipment used.

Infant Family Service Plan

The Infant Family Service Plan (IFSP) is the equivalent of the IEP for older children. The IFSP must be developed by a multidisciplinary team that includes the parents and must include a description of appropriate transition services (e.g., transition from Part C to Part B at 3 years of age). The IFSP must be evaluated once a year but should be reviewed with the family at 6-month intervals or more often when appropriate. Timeliness of assessment, IFSP development, and beginning of services is crucial. The IFSP must include at a minimum the following elements:[1]

1. Statement of the infant's or toddler's present levels of physical development (vision, hearing, motor, and health), cognitive development (thinking, reasoning, learning), communication development (responding, understanding, using language), social or emotional development (feelings, playing, interacting), and adaptive development (bathing, feeding, dressing, etc.) based on objective criteria.
2. Statement of family's resources, priorities, and concerns related to enhancing the development of the family's infant or toddler with a disability.
3. Statement of the measurable results or outcomes expected to be achieved for the infant or toddler and family, the criteria, procedures, and timelines used to determine the degree to which progress toward achieving the results or outcomes is being made, and whether modifications or revisions of the result or outcomes or services are necessary.
4. Statement of specific early intervention services based on peer-reviewed research necessary to meet the unique needs including frequency, intensity, and method of delivering services.
5. Statement of natural environments in which early intervention services will appropriately be provided.
6. Projected dates for initiation of services and the anticipated length, duration, and frequency of the services.
7. Identification of the service coordinator from the profession most immediately relevant to the needs of infant or toddler and family.
8. Steps to be taken to support the transition of the toddler with a disability to preschool or other appropriate services (which must include a formal plan and team conference 3 to 9 months prior to anticipated transition).
9. Provision for parental consent.

 ## Program development/intervention under Parts B and C

Meaningful Collaboration with Parents

Parents' involvement in the planning process facilitates focus on meaningful functional goals for the child and family and consideration of the child's unique needs within a broader context. Physical therapists share with other professionals the responsibility of ensuring that parents are aware of their rights and encouraged to be active participants in program planning for their children. Adherence to the principles of family-centered care requires that every effort is made to customize communication to the unique needs of each family partner. Parents and their children may feel overwhelmed by the planning process and may need guidance to facilitate their meaningful involvement in planning. Several instruments are available that lend structure and guidance to the process: (1) McGill Action Planning System (MAPS),[50] (2) Choosing Options and Accommodations for Children (COACH),[51] (3) Canadian Occupational Performance Measure,[52] (4) Planning Alternative Tomorrows with Hope (PATH),[53] and (5) Transition Planning Inventory-2.[54]

IEP/IFSP Goals and Objectives

IDEA requires "measurable annual goals" as part of the IEP and a statement of the "measurable results or outcomes expected to be achieved" for the infant or toddler and family as part of the IFSP.[1] Short-term objectives are not required by current federal legislation, although state regulations may vary. Ideally, IEP/IFSP goals are developed by the team in a collaborative process and not by specific disciplines in isolation. Writing meaningful goals is an important framework for the delivery of services but can be challenging. Well-developed goals and objectives should be[55]:

1. Educationally relevant and linked with state standards.
2. Functional (i.e., will increase a student's ability to interact with people and objects within the daily environment and would have to be performed by someone else if the student could not).
3. Stated as behaviors the student will demonstrate (i.e., not what will be done with or to the student or what the student may think or feel).
4. Measurable, including performance criteria, conditions, frequency of data collection, and time frame for achievement. *Note:* A skill is measurable if it can be seen and/or heard, can be directly counted (frequency, duration, or distance measures), and lends itself to determination of performance criteria. The conditions for performance should be clearly stated.
5. Practical (i.e., work on the skill can be integrated into daily routines).
6. Linked to assessment that is valid and reliable, when possible.

7. Generalizable (i.e., the identified skill represents a general concept as opposed to a particular task, allows for individual adaptations and modifications for a variety of disabling conditions, and can be generalized across settings, materials, and people).

Dole et al.[56] utilized the Delphi technique to establish consensus among a sample of expert occupational therapy and physical therapy practitioners on characteristics necessary for IEP objectives to be educationally relevant, measurable, and appropriate in content (Table 21-3). Characteristics with 90% or greater agreement include the following:

1. Measurability—IEP objectives should:
   a. Use an identified method for measuring achievement
   b. Describe an observable behavior or functional skill
   c. Utilize valid and acceptable measurement strategies/tools
   d. Specify the level or amount of assistance of cuing needed
2. Education Relevance—IEP objectives should:
   (e) Enhance school function or the child's ability in school
   (f) Be easily understood by all those involved
3. Overall Content—IEP objectives should:
   (g) Be well-defined, specific, clear, and without jargon
   (h) Relate to a functional or educational skill
   (i) Be realistic and achievable within the time frame
   (j) Relate to the long-term goals
   (k) Be child-focused

Inclusive Education

IDEA requires that states develop policies and procedures to ensure, to the maximum extent appropriate, that children with disabilities, including children in public or private institutions or other care facilities, are educated with children who are not disabled, and special classes, separate schooling, or other removal of children with disabilities from the regular educational environment occurs only when the nature or severity of the disability of a child is such that education in regular classes with the use of supplementary aids and services cannot be achieved satisfactorily. The terminology used in Part B is "least restrictive environment" and in Part C is "natural environment."[1] The IEP or IFSP must identify the least restrictive or natural environment where services will be provided or justify why services might be provided in a more isolated environment.

Establishing the necessary support so that every student with a disability is able to participate to the maximum extent possible in the general education environment is beneficial to students with and without disabilities. It presents unique challenges, however, to all service providers. The most appropriate placement might be any of the following: (1) a regular classroom with an aide, (2) a primary placement in a classroom for children with special needs but inclusion for music, mealtimes, and other activities as appropriate, (3) an alternative school with specialized services and processes for children with similar diagnoses (e.g., autism), or (4) home-based services (e.g., a medically fragile child).

Models of Service Delivery

Various authors use different terminology to describe models of physical therapy service in the educational setting, but categories commonly referred to are (1) direct, (2) indirect (monitoring), and (3) consultation.[57] Although these are described separately below, they often occur together as complementary components of a comprehensive intervention plan for an individual student.

- *Direct service* involves hands-on intervention directly from a physical therapist or physical therapist assistant. Direct service can be offered in an isolated manner (e.g., in a separate physical therapy treatment area) or integrated (provided within the context of normal routines/activities in

TABLE 21.3	**Components of an IEP Goal and Examples**				
Condition	**Student**	**Activity**	**Criteria**	**Responsible Parties**	**Baseline & Standard**
Describe when and where the activity will take place	[Name]	Describe the desired activity and the level of prompting-assistance	Indicate the performance level for achievement.	Who will collect and report on the data?	Current level of performance of the task
When transitioning between activities in the classroom,	Tiffany	will stand from her classroom chair given only verbal prompts	in at least 3 out of 5 daily trials per week across 4 consecutive weekly data collections.	Personal Care Assistant, Teacher, Physical Therapist	Minimal physical assistance(State Academic Standard #)
When walking in line from his classroom to the cafeteria,	Joey	will maintain his walking speed to keep pace with peers with a maximum of one direct verbal prompt	in at least 3 out of 4 trials across 4 consecutive weekly data collections.	Teacher, Personal Care Assistant, Physical Therapist	4 physical prompts(State Academic Standard #)

least restrictive or natural environments). The mandates in IDEA for service in inclusive environments make it preferable for direct physical therapy to be integrated. The needs of individual children, however, may be better served in an isolated area via a "pull-out" model of service delivery. This might be true for a child who is easily distracted or in a classroom where the therapy might be distracting for other children. The need for special equipment or safety concerns may be other factors. Scheduling can be one of the limitations of the pull-out direct service model, because if a child is receiving physical therapy, he or she is not participating in the normal academic curriculum.

- *Indirect service (monitoring)* involves establishing a management program for a student, instructing others to carry it out, and monitoring the process to ensure positive outcomes. The indirect model requires physical therapists to teach others and "sell" their "product" (i.e., the functional importance of the recommended intervention). A study by Otto and Effgen,[58] although limited in scope, suggests that inactive, stability behaviors occur naturally at high rates and are easily integrated into a classroom routine, but that movement activities like walking, creeping, or transferring require more direct assistance before they will be integrated and practiced.
- *Consultation* involves an exchange of information with a defined purpose and can be an effective preliminary step in determining the appropriateness of a referral or collaborating on resolution of a problem. Bundy describes consultation as "extraordinarily powerful" and recommends it as the primary form of service delivery for most students.[59]

Decision making about the delivery of physical therapy services is a complex process, guided by numerous considerations. Kaminker et al.[60] conducted a nationwide survey of pediatric physical therapists to explore their recommendations for the models, contexts, frequency, and intensity of service delivery and the factors that influenced their decision making. Therapists were asked to make clinical decisions on the basis of four clinical cases that varied by age, cognitive ability, and condition. Respondents had a strong preference for direct services, especially for the younger children, and for services delivered in a combination of natural (integrated) and isolated settings. Factors that strongly impacted their decision making were the students' functional levels and the students' goals. Factors with minimal impact included administrative influence and budgetary constraints. A follow-up study by some of the same authors investigated the impact of geographic region on decision making, and results indicated considerable variability in recommendations across regions.[61]

In a survey of pediatric physical therapists practicing in early intervention, Sekerak et al.[62] found that in typical practice therapists selected an in-class model more often than an out-of-class model, but that physical therapists are less likely to select an in-class model than occupational therapists, speech and language pathologists, or special educators.

A more recent study by Nolan et al.[63] surveyed pediatric occupational therapists and physical therapists and results indicated that 55.3% of children received the majority of services in isolated settings and 24.7% received the majority of services in integrated settings, with the remainder equally blended between the two models.

Kingsley and Mailloux[64] conducted a review of literature to determine the effectiveness of different service delivery models for occupational therapists providing early intervention services and found little consensus. Parents were most positive about family-centered and routine-based approaches. A systematic review of existing research indicated that service delivery factors do not appear to have a significant effect on speech and language outcomes in young children.[65] More evidence is needed to guide best-practice recommendations.

Role of the Physical Therapist Assistant

The section on pediatrics addressed the role of the physical therapist assistant in the provision of pediatric physical therapy in a formal position statement that was approved by the APTA Board Review Committee in April 1997.[66] The statement supports the qualifications of physical therapist assistants to assist in the provision of pediatric physical therapy services with the exception of services for children who are physiologically unstable. The level of supervision required for physical therapist assistants varies significantly from state to state, so it is imperative that physical therapist and physical therapist assistants are familiar with the supervision requirements outlined in their state's Practice Act. For example, the Pennsylvania Practice Act states, "When care is provided to an individual [by a physical therapist assistant] in a preschool, primary school, secondary school or other similar educational setting, a licensed physical therapist shall make an onsite visit and examine the patient at least every four patient visits or every 30 days, whichever occurs first."[67] The New Jersey Practice Act, however, states, "The licensed physical therapist supervisor shall be in the same building or, where physical therapy is rendered in several contiguous buildings, in one of the contiguous buildings, while the licensed physical therapist assistant is rendering care."[68]

Assistive Technology

Appropriate assistive technology for individuals with disabilities empowers those individuals to have greater control over their lives and to participate more fully in their home, school, and work environments and in their communities. As defined in IDEA, an assistive technology device is ". . . any item, piece of equipment, or product system, whether acquired commercially off the shelf, modified, or customized, that is used to increase, maintain, or improve functional capabilities of a child with a disability."[1] Assistive technology devices include such items as communication devices, adaptive equipment (e.g., standers, wheelchairs), environmental control devices, adapted computers, and specialized software.[1] The Assistive Technology Act ("Tech Act"), originally enacted in 1988, was most recently reauthorized in 2004 and will likely be revised to coincide with the next reauthorization of IDEA.[15]

An assistive technology service is ". . . any service that directly assists a child with a disability in the selection, acquisition, or use of an assistive technology device."[1] Services include evaluation of the child's needs; acquisition of device (e.g., purchase or lease); selection, design, fit, adaptation, application, maintenance/repair; coordinating other services/interventions; training or technical assistance for child/family; and service providers or employers.

Physical therapists are often involved with other team members in the selection and use of assistive technology, and it is a crucial role. Thousands of items are available from a variety of vendors, and the cost is typically high. It is imperative that decisions about assistive technology consider the individual needs of a child and family; the environment in which the equipment is to be used; sources of funding; training for caregivers; safety; evidence to support its use; and the potential for the technology to be used by other children. Therapists should be aware of assistive technology resources in the state, which might include specialists to assist with evaluation and selection of appropriate devices or centers that will loan equipment on a trial basis.

A physical therapist will need to be knowledgeable about many types of assistive technology, but supported standing is a particularly important and somewhat controversial area. Supported standing programs are often recommended for students in the educational environment, but evidence to support effective dosing has been lacking. On the basis of a systematic review of 687 studies and their clinical judgment, Paleg et al.[69] in 2013 made the following clinical recommendations: standing programs 5 days per week positively affect bone mineral density (60 to 90 minutes per day); hip stability (60 minutes per day in 30 to 60 degrees of total bilateral hip abduction); range of motion of hip, knee, and ankle (45 to 60 minutes per day); and spasticity (30 to 40 minutes per day).

Transition Planning

IDEA identifies two critical transition periods for children with disabilities and mandates effective results-oriented planning by the IEP or IFSP team. The identified periods are the transition from early intervention services covered under Part C to the preschool programs covered under Part B and the transition from school to community living. Transition typically results in new personnel working with the child and family, a new environment, and a new lead agency with new policies and processes. It can be very stressful for both children and families. The transition to community living can be especially challenging for students with severe/profound disabilities because of the lack of resources.[70]

The goal of transition planning should be to ensure continuity of service, minimize disruption to the student and family, and promote optimum service delivery. For transition from early intervention (Part C) to public school, STEPS (Sequenced Transition to Education in the Public Schools) is a helpful model for facilitating interagency collaboration at both state and local levels.[71] Components of the STEPS model include creation of a responsive administrative structure, active involvement of families, preparation of the child, and training for staff so that they can effectively facilitate the process. A Web site, Florida's Transition Project for Infants, Young Children and Their Families, provides valuable resources.[72]

Physical therapists can and should play an active role in transition planning. A study by Myers and Effgen[73] provided some preliminary data on physical therapists' participation in early childhood transitions. In their survey of pediatric physical therapists, they found varying levels of participation across settings, but the majority of respondents (54.8%) believed they were not participating fully in the transition process. Perceived barriers included a lack of time and lack of administrative support for their involvement. Only 16.6% of the respondents had received training on transition.

Re-evaluation

General guidelines for re-evaluation of a child with a disability are not more frequently than once a year and at least every 3 years unless the parent and LEA agree to a different schedule. Physical therapists must use their clinical judgment to determine an appropriate schedule for re-evaluation. This will vary depending on the nature of the child's problems, the goals established, and whether a physical therapist assistant is involved in-service delivery.

Terminating physical therapy services for children in school settings can be challenging because multiple factors must be considered and the physical therapist must remain focused on the overall purpose of related services under IDEA, to allow the child to benefit from special education. Effgen[74] found that therapists generally based their decision to terminate physical therapy services on the child's attainment of functional goals without influence from school administrators. Many of the assessment and clinical reasoning tools described earlier can help guide decisions in regard to discontinuation of school-based physical therapy services.

Documentation

Although requirements for documentation are not stipulated in IDEA, and practice acts and Medicaid requirements vary substantially from state to state, therapists are encouraged to document every contact, especially if a physical therapist assistant is involved in the provision of care or Medicaid or other third-party payment is involved. Using an electronic format and/or flowcharts may streamline the process. Documentation should contain a minimum of the activities/interventions in which the student participated during the session, the student response to the interventions, and the length of time for the session. It is essential that the school-based therapist become familiar with the documentation guidelines of their state's practice act as well as Medicaid guidelines.

Extended School Year

The IEP team can consider the necessity of related services outside of the regular school year if it is determined that a child served under Part B will experience substantial regression or loss of functional abilities if services are suspended (typically over the summer months) or if the child failed to make adequate progress toward his/her annual IEP goals.

Reimbursement for Services

The mandate of IDEA is to provide free and appropriate education to qualified individuals with disabilities, but the cost can be staggering to LEAs. PL 100-360 was enacted in 1988 to allow states to utilize Medicaid funds to supplement the cost of providing related services for eligible children. Rules and regulations about Medicaid eligibility and allocation of funds vary significantly from state to state but are frequently restricted to direct service, which can limit the ability of providers to select a delivery mode that is most appropriate and is the most efficient use of resources. Private insurance may also be billed if parents give informed consent to do so, but it is important that they are aware of the specifics of their policy so that they do not negatively impact long-term coverage (e.g., a policy that has lifetime caps on therapy services).

▶ Role of the physical therapist in program-related areas

The majority of the functions and roles assumed by physical therapists in the public school setting that have been described so far have been student-related. Physical therapists can also make significant contributions to program-related needs. Physical therapists may assist others in the educational setting to:

- identify architectural barriers and plan for accessibility modifications;
- establish guidelines and child-specific modifications for the transport of children with disabilities on school-owned vehicles (e.g., buses);
- promote acceptance of students with disabilities by both educational personnel and students;
- plan recreational areas for accessibility;
- contribute to the development of safety procedures for emergency evacuation of students with disabilities;
- collaborate with physical educators to develop "mutually supportive and effective motor programs";
- participate with others in various prevention activities, including screening programs (e.g., musculoskeletal for athletes, scoliosis, and developmental); prevention and treatment of sports-related injuries; prevention of neck and back pain secondary to backpack use[75]; physical

activity and fitness promotion[76]; and/or educational programs for coaches, parents, and students; and
- suggest general environmental modifications to promote independence.

Frequently, physical therapists are the liaison between the educational and medical communities. They may provide background information about various conditions, interpret medical reports, facilitate communication between educational and medical personnel, and assist with access to resources in the medical community.

Physical therapists may also be expected to provide educational personnel with information about physical therapy and topics related to intervention with children who have physical disabilities. Hardy and Roberts[77] recommend conducting a survey of educators' interests and needs to structure in-service education programs that are meaningful. Topics of interest identified from the authors' survey of special educators included specific student disabilities, classroom adaptations, referral guidelines, physical therapist roles and responsibilities, and the difference between an occupational therapist and a physical therapist. A helpful resource is an article by Dole, *Collaborating Successfully with Your School's Physical Therapist*, that was published by the Council for Exceptional Children.[78] Physical therapists frequently provide training for support personnel; all trainings should be documented, and both the trainer and the trainee should sign an outline of the training to verify that the training has been completed.

Management functions are important in the educational environment to ensure that decisions affecting job descriptions, delivery of care, supervision, and so on are compatible with best-practice models. It is not possible, as it was in the 1930s, for physical therapists to have the same job description and qualifications as teachers. Shortages are common, and therapists must understand and communicate to school administrators recruitment and retention strategies for physical therapists that are often very different than those for educational personnel. In a survey, by Keppler and Effgen,[79] of physical therapists practicing in educational settings, the areas of job dissatisfaction most frequently mentioned were lack of continuing education opportunities, insufficient peer contact, lack of an identified place to work, lack of time allotted for administrative tasks and meetings, and too much travel.

A variety of other management tasks are essential as a framework for best practice, and time should be negotiated to ensure that they can be given adequate attention. Efficient systems should be in place for documentation, record keeping, and billing, and these components should be reviewed on a regular schedule. Job descriptions should be comprehensive, state essential functions, and may form the basis for annual performance evaluations of individual physical therapists. Many states are also in the process of developing standardized performance assessments for all educational personnel, including physical therapists.[80]

North Carolina Dept. of Public Instruction, Exceptional Children Division; Physical Therapist Performance Appraisal

A physical therapist should have his/her clinical performance evaluated by another physical therapist, which may require special, formalized arrangements. Both the job descriptions and the performance evaluations should be reviewed annually.

A plan for program evaluation, quality assurance, and peer review should be in place and reviewed regularly (at least annually). Agreement should be reached on reasonable caseloads and guidelines for determining eligibility for physical therapy as a related service. Lines of communication and authority should also be clearly established.

Many references are now available to guide the physical therapist in the educational environment, including guidelines published at the state level. APTA's Section on Pediatrics and the special interest group on School-based Physical Therapy within the section provide valuable resources on a variety of topics that can be accessed on their Web page (www.pediatricapta.org). Table 21-4 lists some of the more applicable resources.

TABLE 21.4	Selected Resources for School-based Physical Therapists

APTA RESOURCES:

FACT SHEETS from APTA Section on Pediatrics:
- Clinical Reasoning in Pediatric Physical Therapist Practice
- FAQs on Response to Intervention for School-Based Physical Therapists
- List of Pediatric Assessment Tools Categorized by ICF Model
- Team-based Service Delivery Approaches in Pediatric Practice
- The Role of School-based Physical Therapy: Successful Participation for Every Student
- What Providers of Pediatric Physical Therapy Services Should Know About Medicaid
- Intervention for Youth Who Are in Transition from School to Adult Life
- Assistive Technology and the Individualized Education Program
- Assistive Technology Resources
- Natural Environments in Early Intervention Services

http://www.pediatricapta.org/members/member-fact-sheets.cfm

APTA Section on Pediatrics: *List of Assessment Tools Used in Pediatric Physical Therapy* (updated November 2011)
http://www.pediatricapta.org/members/pdfs/PedsAssessmentScreeningTools.pdf

APTA Section on Pediatrics School-Based Special Interest Group:
National organization working to provide opportunities for school-based physical therapists to confer, meet, and promote high standards of practice. Sponsors an annual meeting/conference.
www.pediatricapta.org

APTA Section on Pediatrics School-Based Special Interest Group Brochure: *Providing Services Under IDEA 2004* (2010)
www.pediatricapta.org

McEwen I, *Providing Physical Therapy Services under Parts B and C of the Individuals with Disabilities Education Act (IDEA)*–2009
APTA Section on Pediatrics
www.pediatricapta.org

APTA Pediatric Listserv: on-going email discussion forum for current issues in pediatric physical therapy:
http://www.pediatricapta.org/members/listserve.cfm

Pediatric Physical Therapy: Quarterly peer-reviewed publication
http://journals.lww.com/pedpt/pages/default.aspx

RELATED ORGANIZATIONS/ASSOCIATIONS:

US Department of Education: *Building the Legacy–IDEA 2004*–provides resources for IDEA and its implementation.
http://idea.ed.gov

National Education Association–A professional employee organization committed to advancing public education.
http://www.nea.org/

IDEA Partnership-reflects the collaborative work of more than 50 organizations, technical assistance providers, and organizations and agencies at state and local levels.
http://ideapartnership.org/

The National Early Childhood Technical Assistance Center–funded through the Office of Special Education Programs this website provides resources to promote evidence based practices to improve child outcomes.
www.nectac.org

National Early Childhood Transition Center promotes successful transitions from early childhood to school-age services.
www.igdi.uky.edu/nectc

TASH: Equity, Opportunity and Inclusion for People with Severe Disabilities TASH is an international organization that advocates for human rights and inclusion for people with severe disabilities.
http://tash.org/

CanChild: Center for Childhood Disability Research–a research and educational center focused on improving the lives of children with disabilities.
www.canchild.ca

▶ Points to ponder

The educational environment presents on going challenges for the team of professionals who serve children with disabilities. Policies and procedures vary from state to state and even within districts. Therapists struggle on a daily basis to make the "right" decisions that most appropriately address the needs of individual students within the context of federal regulations. Below are examples of some of the kinds of questions that therapists must address.

- Do we have evidence to support many of the common recommendations in the school setting? For example:
  - manual stretching to increase range of motion or prevent contractures
  - supported standing in various types of adaptive equipment
- Do we have reliable, valid assessment tools and evidence-based intervention options for children with severe/profound disabilities?
- For many children with severe/profound disabilities, acquiring basic motor skills (e.g., head control) may be a primary focus of an educational plan. Do these children warrant more attention from physical therapists or less?
- Do we have evidence to support our prognosis for potential functional gains that can appropriately guide decisions related to frequency and duration of intervention?
- Can life skills like riding a bicycle be justified within an educational program plan?
- Should a school-based physical therapist increase services for a child on his/her caseload who receives surgical intervention?

▶ SUMMARY

The educational environment is a challenging and rewarding environment for the physical therapist. To be effective in the public school setting in the United States, a physical therapist must have an understanding of the federal legislation that has shaped the delivery of special education for children from infancy to young adulthood. Most significant was PL 94-142, passed in 1975, which mandated physical therapy as a related service and created a variety of conceptually new ways of thinking about the educational needs of children with disabilities. Local, state, and federal rules and regulations must be understood and adhered to.

Physical therapists must be willing and able to participate actively as part of a collaborative team and to consider parents an integral part of that team. They must acknowledge that their intervention is limited to the educational needs of the child. They must utilize models of service delivery that most effectively address the individualized needs of each child. Practice in the educational environment requires the knowledge, skills, and abilities of a specialist in pediatric physical therapy, but with the grounding to always be able and willing to

interpret physical therapy intervention so that it is understood and appreciated by nonmedical personnel. The rewards include the benefits of functioning as part of a team, following a child long-term, and having the opportunity to observe the child in his or her daily functions within the school environment.

Below are examples of translating evidence into practice in the school-based setting.

CASE STUDIES

CASE STUDY 1   A 13-year-old student named Elizabeth has spastic cerebral palsy and multiple disabilities, including moderate to severe cognitive impairments and severely limited motor abilities. Her age-equivalent performance of motor skills is less than 12 months. While attending Elizabeth's IEP meeting, her parents asked for physical therapy for 30-minute range of motion/stretching sessions three times per week to prevent dislocation of her hips.

- What factors should the IEP team consider when discussing the parents' request?

The primary factor to be determined in consideration of the request is whether or not limitations in Elizabeth's hip stability impact her performance at school or her ability to participate in her educational program. Therefore, the IEP team should examine Elizabeth's goals and performance at school in an effort to examine the educational impact of Elizabeth's hip stability deficits. If Elizabeth's limitations are relatively minor, do not affect her ability to access her curriculum, have not progressed significantly, and do not predispose her to significant complications that could potentially impact her education, then the IEP team would likely conclude that addressing these issues would not be educationally relevant. If, however, the limitations are more severe and interfere with Elizabeth's school performance (e.g., inability to assist with transfers), then the maintenance of hip integrity may be deemed educationally relevant. In this case, the team would then progress through the IEP process and determine how the maintenance of hip stability can best be met in Elizabeth's school environment.

- Is there evidence in the literature to support or refute this requested service?

Evidence to support these intervention strategies is improving, and therapists must increasingly use the evidence to support their school-based interventions. In Elizabeth's case, evidence is best for the use of a supported standing program in order to address her parents' concerns. A supported standing program consisting of at least 60 minutes per day in 30 degrees of abduction is recommended.[69] Continued research is needed if we are to advocate appropriately for children and make effective recommendations to educational personnel.

- What is the role of the physical therapist in the implementation of a supported standing program?

The physical therapist may be involved with the selection of standing equipment, staff training for transfers and use of the stander, developing a compliance monitoring system (e.g., chart to track time in stander and level of assistance needed), and for monitoring and updating the parameters of the standing program on the basis of student response. Issues to consider with the delegation and implementation of this program are the severity of the hip involvement and other risk factors that might include osteopenia or osteoporosis and behavioral concerns. Once the support staff has been trained and the training has been documented, the physical therapist should not need to be present when the student is using the supported standing device.

CASE STUDY 2 A 12-year-old student named Rasheen has normal cognitive function and a midthoracic spinal cord injury (since 4 years of age). He is independent with mobility using a manual wheelchair throughout the school environment: the classroom, hallways, playground, cafeteria, special classes, and curbs. Rasheen is transported to/from school on a lift bus. Rasheen has a stander that he uses on a daily basis at school and he transfers into/out of the stander independently. Rasheen participates in physical education class with minimal adaptations. Given his diagnosis and prognosis, Rasheen is not a candidate for functional independent ambulation.

- Would Rasheen likely qualify for physical therapy services?

Since Rasheen's disability does not affect his independence and performance in the educational environment, the IEP team may not recommend physical therapy as a related service. Rasheen may receive services under a 504 Plan.

- What would likely be the primary focus of physical therapy intervention for Rasheen under the 504 Plan agreement?

The focus of the services under the Section 504 agreement would likely be to address emergency evacuations, assistance with and access to catheterization, use of the stander, and adaptations for physical education class.

- What model of service delivery would be utilized?

Rasheen would likely be monitored by the physical therapist to ensure that his stander and wheelchair are properly fitted, he continues to participate to the maximum extent possible in his physical education class, to address any questions or concerns of the PE teacher, and to ensure that Rasheen complies with emergency evacuation procedures.

- Do you expect that Rasheen would receive additional physical therapy services on an outpatient basis (i.e., outside the educational environment)? If so, what would be the primary focus of Rasheen's outpatient services?

Outpatient services for Rasheen might be recommended to intensify intervention when working on a particular functional skill or following a medical intervention. For example, Rasheen might benefit from a neuromuscular electrical stimulation program established and monitored on an outpatient basis to maintain leg strength. The outpatient physical therapist might also assume a more active role in developing and monitoring a comprehensive home program for prevention of contractures that would involve adaptive equipment for the home environment and night splinting[81]. Regardless of the circumstances, Rasheen's parents, physician, and therapists should all work collaboratively to comprehensively address his needs.

- How might the focus of Rasheen's services change as he progresses through middle school and high school?

As Rasheen approaches middle school and high school, planning for the school-to-adulthood transition will play a larger role in his educational programming. Exploring Rasheen's vocational interests and linking them to his physical abilities will become increasingly important. Investigating potential living arrangements, identifying community agencies, and examining recreational options should be addressed via transition planning.

REFERENCES

1. Individuals with Disabilities Education Improvement Act of 2004, 20 USC § 1401 (2004).
2. Pratt RE. Physical therapy in schools for crippled children. *Phys Ther Rev.* 1950;30(6):233.
3. DeYoung R. Child cripples get full course at Morton High. *Physiother Rev.* 1932;12:24.
4. Hutchinson E. The physical therapist looks at the school child. *Physiother Rev.* 1944;24:6–9.
5. Section 504 of the Rehabilitation Act, 29 USC § 701 (1973).
6. Education for All Handicapped Children Act, 20 USC § 1400 (1975).
7. Education of the Handicapped Act Amendments of 1986, 20 USC § 1401 (1986).
8. Medicare Catastrophic Coverage Act, 42 USC § 1305 (1988).
9. Technology-Related Assistance for Individuals with Disabilities Act, 29 USC § 2201 (1988).
10. Americans with Disabilities Act, 42 USC § 12101 et seq. (1990).
11. Individuals with Disabilities Education Act Amendments of 1991, 20 USC § 1401 (1991).
12. Individuals with Disabilities Education Act Amendments of 1997, 20 USC § 1401 (1997).
13. Assistive Technology Act of 1998, 29 USC § 3001 (1998).
14. No Child Left Behind Act of 2001, 20 USC § 6301 (2001).
15. Assistive Technology Act of 2004, 29 USC § 3001 (2004).
16. American Recovery and Reinvestment Act. http://www2.ed.gov/policy/gen/leg/recovery/factsheet/idea.html.
17. National Education Association. http://www.nea.org/assets/docs/IDEA_Full_Funding_Chart_FY1981-2012.pdf. Accessed October 10, 2013.
18. IDEA funding coalition offers proposal: plan would make funding mandatory; 2002. http://www.nea.org/home/18750.htm. Accessed October 10, 2013.
19. Ogletree BT, Bull J, Drew R, et al. Team-based service delivery for students with disabilities: practice options and guidelines for success. *Interv Sch Clin.* 2001;36(3):138–145.
20. Thousand JS, Villa RA. Collaborative teaming: a powerful tool in school restructuring. In: Villa RA, Thousand JS, eds, *Restructuring for Caring and Effective Education: Piecing the Puzzle.* Baltimore, MD: Paul H. Brookes Publishing; 2000:254–292.

21. Hunt P, Soto G, Maire J, et al. Collaborative teaming to support students at risk and students with severe disabilities in general education classrooms. *Council Except Child*. 2003;69:315–332.

22. Palisano RJ. A collaborative model of service delivery for children with movement disorders: a framework for evidence-based decision making. *Phys Ther*. 2006;86:1295–1305.

23. DeHaven GE. Is selective hearing an occupational hazard in physical therapy? *Phys Ther*. 1974;54:1301–1305.

24. Chiarello L, Effgen SK. Updated competencies for physical therapists working in early intervention. *Pediatr Phys Ther*. 2006;18:148–158.

25. Effgen SK, Chiarello L. Updated competencies for physical therapists working in the schools. *Pediatr Phys Ther*. 2007;19:266–274.

26. American Physical Therapy Association. Guide to physical therapist practice. Second Edition. *Phys Ther*. 2001;81(1):9–746.

27. International classification of functioning, disability and health (ICF). World Health Organization web site. http://www.who.int/classifications/icf/en/. Accessed October 31, 2013.

28. TASH. Preparation of related services personnel for work in educational settings. http://tash.org/advocacy-issues/inclusive-education/. Accessed October 5, 2013.

29. Goodrich B, Hawkins J, Burridge A, et al. Facilitating appropriate referrals for related service in schools. *J Occup Ther*. 2012;5(3/4): 221–239.

30. Bruininks RH, Bruininks, D. *Bruininks-Oseretsky Test of Motor Proficiency*. 2nd ed. Minneapolis, MN: Pearson Assessments; 2005.

31. King G, Law M, King S, et al. *Children's Assessment of Participation and Enjoyment (CAPE) and Preferences for Activities of Children (PAC)*. San Antonio, TX: Pearson Assessment; 2004

32. Russell DJ, Rosenbaum PL, Avery LM, et al. *Gross Motor Function Measure (GMFM-66 and GMFM-88) User's Manual*. High Holborn, UK: Mac Keith Press; 2002.

33. Stein S, Weissenmayer H, Korinthenberg R, et al. Validation of Gross Motor Function Measure for use in children and adolescents with traumatic brain injury. *Pediatrics*. 2007;120:e880–e886.

34. Ruck-Gibis J, Plotkin H, Hanley J, et al. Reliability of the Gross Motor Function Measure for children with osteogenesis imperfecta. *Pediatr Phys Ther*. 2001;13:10–17.

35. Blanton KF. *M.O.V.E.: Mobility Opportunities Via Education*. Bakersfield, CA: MOVE International; 1991.

36. Coster W, Deeney T, Haltiwanger J, et al. *School Function Assessment*. San Antonio, TX: Pearson Assessments; 1998

37. Department of Rehabilitation Science. *School Outcomes Measure: Administrative Guide*. http://www.ah.ouhsc.edu/somresearch/adminGuide.pdf. University of Oklahoma Health Sciences Center, PO Box 26901, Oklahoma City, OK, 73190–1090; 2013.

38. Granger CV, Hamilton BB, Kayto R. Guide for the use of the Functional Independence Measure for Children (WeeFIM) of the Uniform Data Set for Medical Rehabilitation. Buffalo, NY: Research Foundation, State University of New York; 1989. Available at: http://www.udsmr.org/Documents/WeeFIM/WeeFIM_II_System.pdf. Accessed October 9, 2013.

39. McEwen IR, Arnold SH, Hansen LH, et al. Inter-rater reliability and content validity of a minimal data set to measure outcomes of students receiving school-based occupational therapy and physical therapy. *Phys Occup Ther Pediatr*. 2003;23(2):77–95.

40. Dale Ulrich. *Test of Gross Motor Development 2*. San Antonio, TX: Pearson Assessments; 2000

41. Kaplan SL, O'Connell MD. Task analyses identify coat-donning delays in preschoolers in special education. *Pediatr Phys Ther*. 2011;23:62–69.

42. David KS, Sullivan M. Expectations for walking speeds: standards for student in elementary schools. *Pediatr Phys Ther*. 2005;17:120–127.

43. Considerations for Educationally Relevant Therapy for Occupational Therapy and Physical Therapy (CERT). http://www.fldoe.org/ese/CERT/cert-script.pdf. Accessed October 12, 2013.

44. Kenyon L. The Hypothesis-Oriented Pediatric Focused Algorithm: a framework for clinical reasoning in pediatric physical therapist practice. *Phys Ther*. 2013;93:413–420.

45. Office of Special Education Programs, Office of Special Education and Rehabilitative Services, U.S. Department of Education (2006). Model Form: Part B: Individualized Education Program. http://www.ed.gov/policy/speced/guid/idea/modelform-iep.doc.

46. Potter SL. *Guidelines for Recognizing and Providing Care for Victims of Child Abuse*. Alexandria, VA: American Physical Therapy Association; 2005

47. Bayley N. *Bayley Scales of Infant and Toddler Development*. 3rd ed. San Antonio, TX: Pearson Assessments; 2005.

48. Folio MR, Fewell RR. *Peabody Developmental Motor Scales*. 2nd ed. San Antonio, TX: Pearson Assessments; 2000.

49. Haley SM, Coster WJ, Ludlow LH, et al. *Pediatric Evaluation of Disability Inventory*. San Antonio, TX: Pearson Assessments; 1992.

50. Vandercick T, Your J, Forest M. The McGill Action Planning System (MAPS): a strategy for building the vision. *J Assoc Persons Severe Handicaps*. 1989;14:205–215.

51. Giangreco MG, Cloninger, CJ, Iverson VS. *Choosing Outcomes and Accommodations for Children (COACH): A guide to educational planning for students with disabilities*. 2nd ed. Baltimore, MD: Paul H. Brookes Publishing; 1998.

52. Law M, Baptiste S, Carswell A, et al. *Canadian Occupational Performance Measure*. 4th ed. Ottawa, Ontario, Canada: Canadian Association of Occupational Therapists Publications ACE; 2005.

53. Pearpoint J, O'Brien J, Forest M. *PATH: Planning Alternative Tomorrows with Hope*. Toronto, Canada: Inclusion Press; 1992.

54. Patton JR, Clark GM. *Transition Planning Inventory*. 2nd ed. Austin, TX: Pro-Ed, Inc.; 2006.

55. McCormick L. Assessment and planning: the IFSP and IEP. In Noonan MJ, McCormick L, eds. *Young children with disabilities in natural environments: Methods and procedures*. Baltimore, MD: Paul H. Brookes; 2006:47–76.

56. Dole R, Arvidson K, Byrne E, et al. Consensus among experts in pediatric occupational and physical therapy on elements of individualized education programs. *Pediatr Phys Ther*. 2003;15:159–166.

57. McEwen I. *Providing Physical therapy Under Parts B and C of the Individuals with Disabilities Education Act (IDEA)*. 2nd ed. Alexandria, VA: Section on Pediatrics, American Physical Therapy Association; 2009.

58. Otto DS, Effgen SK. Occurrence of gross motor behaviors in integrated and segregated preschool classrooms. *Pediatr Phys Ther*. 2000;12:164–172.

59. Bundy AC. Assessment and intervention in school-based practice: answering questions and minimizing discrepancies. *Phys Occup Ther Pediatr*. 1995;15(2):69–87.

60. Kaminker MK, Chiarello LA, O'Neill ME, et al. Decision making for physical therapy service delivery in schools: a nationwide survey of pediatric physical therapists. *Phys Ther*. 2004;84:919–933.

61. Kaminker MK, Chiarello LA, Chiarini Smith JA. Decision making for physical therapy service delivery in schools: a nationwide analysis by geographic region. *Pediatr Phys Ther*. 2006;18:204–213.

62. Sekerak DM, Kirkpatrick DB, Nelson KC, et al. Physical therapy in preschool classrooms: successful integration of therapy into classroom routines. *Pediatr Phys Ther*. 2003;15(2):93–104.

63. Nolan KW, Mannato L, Wilding GE. Integrated models of pediatric physical and occupational therapy: regional practice and related outcomes. *Pediatr Phys Ther*. 2004;16:121–128.

64. Kingsley K, Mailloux Z. Evidence for effectiveness of different service delivery models in early intervention services. *Am J Occup Ther*. 2013;67:431–436.

65. Cirrin FM, Schooling TL, Nelson NW, et al. Evidence-based systematic review: effects of different service delivery models on communication outcomes for elementary school-age children. *Lang Speech Hear Serv Sch*. 2010;41:233–264.

66. Section on Pediatrics. Utilization of Physical Therapist Assistants in the Provision of Pediatric Physical Therapy. Approved by the APTA Board Review Committee, April 1997.

67. Regulations of the State Board of Physical Therapy, 49 PA Code § 40.173 (c) 2.

68. New Jersey Physical Therapy Practice Act, N.J.S.A. 45 § 39A - 7.2.

69. Paleg GS, Smith BA, Glickman LB. Systematic review and evidence-based clinical recommendations for dosing of pediatric supported standing programs. *Pediatr Phys Ther*. 2013;25:232–247.

70. Certo N, Luecking R, Murphy S, et al. Seamless transition and long-term support for individuals with severe intellectual disabilities. *Res Pract Pers Severe Disabil*. 2008;33(3):85–95.

71. Rous B, Hemmeter ML, Schuster J. Sequenced transition to education in public schools: A systems approach to transition planning. *Topics Early Childhood Spec Educ*. 1994;10.

72. (http://www.floridatransitionproject.ucf.edu/history.html).

73. Myers CT, Effgen SK. Physical therapists' participation in early childhood transitions. *Pediatr Phys Ther*. 2006;18:182–189.

74. Effgen SK. Factors affecting the termination of physical therapy services for children in school settings. *Pediatr Phys Ther*. 2000;12:121–126.

75. Mehta TB, Thorpe DE, Freburger JK. Development of a survey to assess backpack use and neck and back pain in seventh and eighth graders. *Pediatr Phys Ther*. 2002;14:171–184.

76. Racette SB, Cade WT, Beckmann LR. School-based physical activity and fitness promotion. *Phys Ther*. 2010;90(9):1214–1218.

77. Hardy DD, Roberts PL. The educational needs assessment on physical therapy for special educators: enhancing in-service programming and physical therapy services in public schools. *Pediatr Phys Ther*. 1989;1:109–114.

78. Dole RL. Collaborating successfully with your school's physical therapist. *Teach Exceptional Child*. 2004;36(5):28–35.

79. Effgen SK, Keppler S. Survey of physical therapy practice in educational settings. *Pediaatr Phys Ther*. 1994;6:15–21.

80. School-based Physical Therapist Development Team. *NC School-Based Physical Therapist Evaluation Process*. Raleigh, NC: NC Department of Public Instruction; June 2013.

81. Stuberg W, DeJong S. (February 4, 2006). Contracture management of children with neuromuscular disabilities. Paper Presented at: *Combined Sections Meeting*,. American Physical Therapy Association, San Diego, IL; February 4, 2006.

Page numbers in italics *denote figures; those followed by a t denote tables; those followed by a b denote display boxes.*

A

Abasia, 19t, 51
Abnormal extraocular movements, Chiari II malformation and, 250b
Abnormal tone, 312
Acapella device, 694, 696, 709
Acceleration–deceleration injuries, 303–304
Acceptability, of screening test, 70
Access technologies, 455–457
Accessory navicular, 530
Achilles tendon reflex, 594
ACL injuries, 519–520
Acquired Brain Injury-Challenge Assessment (ABI-CA), 314
Acromioclavicular (AC) joint separations, 512
Active cycle of breathing technique (ACBT), 693, 694
Active range of motion (AROM), 227
Activities of daily living (ADLs), 425
    arthritis and, 571
    assessment of, 553–554b, *562*
    burns and, 629
    equipment for, 454–455
    instrumental, 337–338
    muscular dystrophy and, 364
    spinal cord injury and, 337–338, 340, 348
Activity Scales for Kids (ASK), 96, 552
Acute disseminated encephalomyelitis (ADEM), 330
Acute lymphoblastic leukemia (ALL), 590, 597, 603–605, *605*
Acute myeloid leukemia (AML), 590
Acute patella dislocations, 522–523
Acute transverse myelitis (ATM), 330, 334
Acyanotic congenital heart defects, 660–662
Adaptive Behavior and Social-Emotional Scales, 84
Adaptive skills, assessment of, 204–205
Adductor angle, *156*
Adelaide Pediatric Coma Scale, 307t
ADLs (*see* Activities of daily living)
Aerobic capacity, 685 (*see also* Conditioning)
Affect, brain trauma and, 311
Age
    adjusted, 21, 21b, 123
    blood gas values and, 665, 665t
    brain trauma and, 308–309
    burns and, 611
    calculation of, 18, 21, 21b, 123
    chronologic, 123
    coma scale and, 306, 307t
    corrected, 123
    gestational, 21b, 123
    motor milestones and, 18, 19t
    and obesity, 642–643t
Age-equivalent score, 71
Ages and Stages Questionnaire (ASQ), 72, 73, 411
Agitated patients, 318–319
Airway clearance, 673, 688–694, *689–692, 694–696*
    for asthma, 704–705
    for cystic fibrosis, 709–710

Alberta Infant Motor Scale (AIMS), 73, 75–77, *76,* 145t, 314, 411t, *412*
Alcohol (*see* Fetal alcohol syndrome)
Alcohol-related birth defects (ARBD), 19
Alcohol-related neurodevelopmental disorder (ARND), 19
Allergen immunotherapy (AIT), 704
Allergy, latex, 286–287, 287b
    and spinal cord injury, 331b
AlloDerm, 625–626
Allografts, 624
Alpha-fetoprotein (AFP), 251
Als, Heidelise, 116, 122, 122t, 145t
Alternative technology, 424
Ambulation, 599t, 600 (*see also* Walking)
    aids, 219–220
    burns and, 632, *636–638*
    motor development and, 55–57, *55–58,* 57t, 64t
    muscular dystrophy and, *354, 355,* 356t, 362
    spina bifida and, 272–285, *273–275, 277,* 278t, *279, 281*
    spinal cord injury and, 338–340, *339,* 339b, 347
American Academy of Orthopedic Surgeons (AAOS), 95
American Academy of Pediatrics (APA), 104, 450, 563b
    "Black to Sleep" program, 476
    Committee on Child Health Financing, 434
    Committee on Sports Medicine of, 394
American College of Rheumatology (ACR), 563b, 541, 542t
American Physical Therapy Association (APTA), 434, 720, 724, 730
    Board Review Committee, 727
    Vision 2020, 644
American Recovery and Reinvestment Act, 719t
American Spinal Injury Association (ASIA), 333–334
    ASIA Impairment Scale, 334b
    clinical syndromes, 334b
    International Standards for Neurologic Classification of Spinal Cord Injury (ISNCSCI), 333–334
Americans with Disabilities Act (ADA), 3, 343, 719t
Amnesia, 312
    posttraumatic, 306, 307
Amputation, 470, 471, 596, 596t
Androids, 457
Anemia, 597
Angular alignment, 466–468
Ankle
    arthritis of, 556, 557t
    deformities of, 228–230
    enthesitis of, *545*
    fractures, 527–528
    impingement, 528
    injuries, 526–528, *527,* 527t
    sprains, 526–527
Ankle–foot orthoses (AFO), 201
    articulating, 231–234
    after brain trauma, 321
    dynamic, 232–233t, 235
    ground-reaction, 203, 229, 231, 233t, 234

hinged, 203
    for knee flexion contracture, 228
    molded, 202, 203, 229, 231, 232–233t
    for muscular dystrophy, 362
    posterior leaf spring, 234
    solid, 203, 229
    solid molded, 231, 232–233t
    for spina bifida, 277–280, *279, 281*
    for spinal cord injury, 335t
Ankylosing spondylitis, 542t, 544, 548
Anorexia, from medications, 546b
Anterior cord syndrome, 334b
Anterior cruciate ligament (ACL) tears, 504, 505
Anterior inferior iliac spine (AIIS), pelvic apophysitis in, 514
Anterior superior iliac spine (ASIS), 561
    pelvic apophysitis in, 514
Anterior talofibular ligament (ATFL), 526, 528
Antinuclear antibodies (ANAs), 542
Aorta, coarctation of, 658t, 660, 661
Aortic valve stenosis, 658t, 660, 661
Apgar scores, 123, 125, 125t, 140, 153, 190b
Apley compression or distraction, 522
Apnea, 684
    Chiari II malformation and, 250b
Apophysitis, 524, 532
Applied Behavioral Analysis (ABA), for autism spectrum disorder, 414–415
Appropriate for gestational age (AGA), 123
Appropriateness, of screening test, 70
AQUACEL Ag Hydrofiber, 622–623
Aquatic therapy, 214, 564b
    for autism spectrum disorder, 417
Arm(s)
    congenital deficiency of, 468–475, *469, 471*
    muscular dystrophy and, *354,* 356t
Armrests, 438
Arnold–Chiari malformation (*see* Chiari II malformation)
Arousal level, brain trauma and, 311
Arthritis, 542t, 543, 548–550, 559 (*see also* Juvenile idiopathic arthritis)
    and activities of daily living, 571
    of ankle, 556, 557t
    and caregiver education, 572–573
    and conditioning, 559–560, 559b, 566b, 569
    of elbow, 557t
    and endurance training, 568–569
    enthesitis-related, 543t, 544, 551, 561
    ethnicity and, 545
    exercises for, 562, 566, 566b
    of foot, 556, 557t
    and functional abilities, 571–572
    of hand, *543,* 555, 557t
    of hip, 557t
    and home management, 572–573, 577
    juvenile idiopathic, 541–578
    juvenile rheumatoid, 541, 542t
    of knee, *547,* 557t
    rheumatoid, 543
    of shoulder, 556, 557t
    of spinal cord, 557t
    of wrist, 557t

Arthritis Foundation (AF), 586
Arthrodesis, 223t, 565
Arthrogryposis multiplex congenita (AMC), 480–482, *481*
Arthroplasty, 565–566
Articular severity score (ASS), 559
Articulating ankle–foot orthoses, 231–234, 232–233t
ASIA Impairment Scale, 334b
Asperger syndrome, 403–404, 404t
Asphyxia, perinatal, 153–154, 154t, 157, 190b
Assessment
  of adaptive skills, 204–205
  of ADLs, 553–554b, *562*
  of educational needs, 721–722
  equipment, 427–432
  of fine motor skills, 204–205
  of functional abilities, 72, 87–93
  of gait, 199–204
  hearing, 386
  of intellectual disabilities, 382, 382t
  of language skills, 205
  methods of, 69–70
  of motor function, 74–82
  of movement, 195–196
  musculoskeletal, 197–199
  outcome measures, 93–96
  of posture, 196
  of preterm infants, 121–123, 122t, 140–146, 144–145t
  of self-care skills, 204–205
  speech, 205
  terms for, 71–72
  visual, 385
Assessment of Preterm Infant Behavior (APIB), 145t
Assistive technology, 423–424, 727–728
Assistive Technology Acts, 719t, 728
ASSIST™ software, 82
Association for Persons with Severe Handicaps (TASH), 720
Astasia, 19t, 51
Asthma, 703–706
  assessment of, 703
  definition of, 703
  incidence of, 679, 703
  interventions for, 704–706
  management of, 696, 703–704
Astrocytoma, 590t
Asymmetric tonic neck reflex (ATNR), 24, 25t, 37–38
  embryogenesis and, 117
  inhibition of, 38–40, *39*, 61
  persistence of, 43
Ataxia, 193, 210b
  brain trauma and, 312
  Chiari II malformation with, 250b
  Friedreich, 383t
Ataxic gait, 204
Atelectasis, 697–699
Athetosis, 193, 206b, 209b, 384t
Athetotic gait, 204
Atkinson, Heather, 329–348
ATNR (*see* Asymmetric tonic neck reflex)
Atrial septal defects (ASD), 658t, 660, *660*
Atrioventricular septal defect (AVSD), 660, 661
Attention
  autism spectrum disorder and, 406
  brain trauma and, 311
  deficit disorder, 147
Aubert, Emilie, 17–65, 423–457
Auditory impairment, autism spectrum disorder and, 406–407

Auditory system, 121
Augmentative technology, 424
Auscultation, 684–685
Autism, 86
Autism Diagnostic Interview–Revised (ADI-R), 405
Autism Observation Schedule (ADOS), 405
Autism Observation Schedule for Infants (AOSI), 411, 411t
Autism spectrum disorders (ASDs), 403–419
  case study, 417–419
  classification of, 403–404, 404t
  definition of, 403
  diagnosis of, 405–406
  etiology of, 404–405
  examination of, 409–413, 411t
  impairments, 406–409, 407t
  incidence of, 404
  interventions for, 414–417
  neuropathology of, 405
  obesity and, 650
  physical therapy for, 413t
  prevalence of, 404t
  prognosis of, 405–406
  risk factors of, 404–405
  team approach to, 414
Autogenic drainage, 692–693, 709
Autografts, 624, 625–626
Autonomic dysreflexia, 331b
Ayres, A. Jean, 212

B
"Back-to-Sleep" program, 143, 476
Backrest, 437–438
Baclofen
  intrathecal pump, 222
  for pain, 336
  for spasticity, 221, 336
Balance, 58–60, *59*, *60*, 64t, 266
  CNS tumor and, 600
  loss, brain trauma and, 313
Balance Error Scoring System (BESS), 534
Ballismus, 193
Barlow test, *479*
Barrel chest, 668
Bathing, 454
Battelle Developmental Inventory–Second Edition (BDI-2), 69, 86
Bayley Infant Neurodevelopmental Screener (BINS), 73–74
Bayley Scales of Infant and Toddler Development–Third Edition (Bayley-III), 71, 82, 84–86, 85b, 162, 724
Bayley Scales of Infant Development (BSID), 20, 77, 411
  Movement Assessment of Infants versus, 194
Bayley Scales of Infant Development II (BSID II), 73, 74, 80
Beaman, Jason, 187–241
Becker muscular dystrophy (BMD), 351, 353, 355
Behavior(ism), 20, 21
  brain trauma and, 311
Behavior Observation Inventory, 84
Beighton Scale for Joint Mobility, 486, 486t
Beighton–Horan ligament laxity scale, 503, 504b
Benign joint hypermobility syndrome (BJHS), 485, 487
Bertoti, Dolores B., 379–399
Bethlem myopathy, 369
Bhat, Anjana, 403–419
Bicycles, 450
  helmets, 324
  injuries, 302

Bimanual Fine Motor Function Classification System (BFMFCS), 191
Birth
  cardiovascular changes associated with, 659, *659*
  normal cardiac circulation after, 659–660, *659*
  weight, 104, 123, *124*
Blalock-Taussig shunt, 663, 675, *675*
Blindness (*see* Visual impairment)
Blood gas values, 665, 665t
Blount disease, 490–491, *490*
Bobath approach (*see* Neurodevelopmental treatment)
Bobath, B., 211
Bobath, K., 211
Body composition, 645
Body mass index (BMI), 642, 644
  and slipped capital femoral epiphysis, 518
Bonding, 18t, 114
Bone (*see also* Osteoporosis)
  composition, skeletally immature athlete, 501–503
  density, spinal cord injury and, 343
  marrow
    aspiration of, 593
    transplant of, 596–597
  tumors of, *591–592*, 593, 594t, 601t
Bony abnormalities, foot, 530
Borg Rate of Perceived Exertion scale, 670t, 673, 686–687
Boston brace, 495, *496*
Both, Amy, 301–325
Botulinum toxin A (BTX-A) injection, 214
  for equinus deformity, 229
  for gastrocnemius stretching, 201
  for knee flexion contracture, 227
  and phenol, 222
  for spasticity, 221–222, 336
Bowel continence/incontinence, spina bifida and, 253b
Boxer's fracture, 513
BPD (*see* Bronchopulmonary dysplasia)
Brace(s) (*see also* Orthosis)
  Boston, 495, *496*
  for spina bifida, 268, *270*, *272–275*, 279, *281*
  after spinal cord injury, 338–340, *338*, *339*
Brachial plexus injury, 123, 162
Brachycephaly, 392
Braden Q scale, 627
Brain (*see also* Hydrocephalus; Traumatic brain injury)
  abnormalities, congenital muscular dystrophy and, 368
  embryogenesis of, *115*
  herniation of, 305
  intracranial hemorrhage of, 128–129, 304–305, 383t
  intraventricular hemorrhage of, 127, 134–136, *135*, 135t, 190
  tumors of, 590, 590t, 594t, 595, 601t
Brainstem auditory-evoked response audiometry (BAER), 410
Brainstem auditory-evoked potentials (BAEP), 250
Brazelton, T. Berry, 104, 116, 122, 144t
Breath sounds, 685, 707
Bridgman, Laura, 380
Broader autism phenotype (BAP), 404t
Bronchial aspiration, Chiari II malformation and, 250b
Bronchopulmonary dysplasia (BPD), 146–147, 679
Broviac catheter, 595, 666
Brown–Séquard syndrome, 334b
Bruininks-Oseretsky Test of Motor Proficiency (BOTMP), 71, 81, 411, 411t
  brain trauma and, 314

Bruininks-Oseretsky Test of Motor Proficiency, Second Edition (BOT-2), 81–82, *81, 83,* 648, 652
  arthritis and, 555
  educational needs and, 721
Bruininks Pediatric Clinical Test of Sensory Integration for Balance and the Postural Stress Test, 309
Bruininks, Robert H., 81
Bubela, D., 403–419
Burkholderia cepacia, 707
Burkitt lymphoma, 591
Burn camp, 635
Burn centers, 618
Burn team, 618–619
Burns, 611–638
  assessment of, 614–616, *616,* 626–629, *628*
  case studies of, *635–638*
  classification of, 614–617, *615*
  depth, 614–615
  dressing, 622
  epidemiology of, 611–612
  etiology of, 612–613
  interventions for, 629–635, *631, 633–634*
  minor, 617
  moderate, 617
  nutritional concerns with, 620
  outcomes, 635
  pain management for, 620–621, 621t, 627, 629
  pathophysiology of, 617
  prevention of, 613
  scarring from, 617–618, 627, *633–634*
  size, 615–616
  surgery for, 623–625
  systems review, 619–620
  wound care for, 621–623, *623,* 629–630

C

Cadence, 56, 57t
Calcaneofibular ligament (CFL), 526
Calpain-3, 366
Campbell, S. K., 145t
Canadian Occupational Performance Measure, 725
Cancer, 589–607
  assessment of, 597–601
  case studies of, 603–607, *605*
  chemotherapy for, 594–595, 594t, 600, 603
  diagnosis of, 601–603, 601t
  exercise program for, 593–594, 593t, 603–606
  incidence of, 589
  interventions for, 601–603, 602t
  radiation therapy for, 595, 595t
  staging of, 593–594
  surgery for, 595–596, 596t
  types of, 589–593, 590t
Canes, 220, 450
Car safety belts, 324, 330, 344
Car seats, 344
Carbohydrate disorders, 383t
Cardiomyopathy, *357*
Cardiopulmonary fitness, Down syndrome and, 395
Cardiorespiratory endurance, 648
Cardiovascular system, 657–676
  burns and, 619, 626
  development of, 658–660, *658–660*
Caregiver Assistance Scales, 88, 89
Caregiver education (*see also* Home management)
  arthritis and, 572–573
  burns and, 634–635
  cancer and, 602
  cultural background and, 4–6, 12–13, 430–431

family dynamics and, 3–4
  heart disease and, 671
  literacy issues with, 8
  muscular dystrophy and, 360
  NICU and, 141–142
  spinal cord injury and, 341
Carol M. White Physical Education Program, 654b
Cascade DAFO, Inc., 236
Cast(s)
  bivalved inhibitive, *316*
  for burns, 631
  Petrie, *488*
  after spinal bifida surgery, 282–285, *283, 284*
CAT$_{CHAQ-38}$, 554, 555b
Catheterization, 595, *665,* 666
Cauda equina syndrome, 334b
CDH (*see* Congenital diaphragmatic hernia)
Center-Based Delivery, 2b
Centers for Disease Control and Prevention (CDC), growth charts, 646, *647*
Central cord syndrome, 334b
Central line placement, 595
Central nervous system (CNS) (*see also* Brain)
  embryogenesis of, *115*
  tumors of, 590, 590t, 601t
Central pattern generators (CPGs), 20–21, 213
Cerebral edema, 305
Cerebral palsy (CP), 187–241
  assessment of, 78, 194–199, 194–195b
  botulinum toxin A for, 221–222, 228
  case studies of, 12, 237–241
  classification of, 191–194, 191b
  definition of, 187–188
  diagnosis of, 189–191
  equipment issues with, 215–220
  etiology of, 188–189
  gait in, 199–204
  home management of, 236
  incidence of, 188
  interventions for, 206–215, 221–222
  IVH and, 135
  lower extremity orthoses, 230–236
  neuromuscular blocks, 221–222
  obesity and, 649, 650
  oral medications, 221
  orthoses for, 232–233t
  perinatal causes of, 189b
  postneonatally acquired, 189b
  prenatal causes of, 188b
  prognosis of, 189–191
  risks for, 189–190b
  school-based therapy for, 236–237
  surgery for, 222
CF (*see* Cystic fibrosis)
Chairs, *435,* 437–439, *439, 441, 442*
Charcot–Marie–Tooth (CMT) disease, 352, 373–374, *373*
CHDs (*see* Congenital heart defects)
Chemotherapy, 594–595, 594t, 600, 603, 605
Chiari II malformation, 249–250, 250b, 261, 288, *289*
Child abuse, 189b, 302
  burns and, 612–613, *613*
  of intellectual disabilities, 383t
  spinal cord injuries from, 330
Child-Centered Services, 2b
Child Health Questionnaire (CHQ), 95, 96, 652
Childhood disintegrative disorder (CDD), 405
Childhood Health Assessment Questionnaire (CHAQ), 552, 552t, 554, 555b
Children's Assessment of Participation and Enjoyment (CAPE), 410, 721
Children's Medical Ventures, *141, 142, 143*

Children's Orientation and Amnesia Test (COAT), 307
Chlamydia trachomatis, 146
Choosing Options and Accommodations for Children (COACH), 725
Choreoathetosis, 193, 384t
Chorioamnionitis, 139, 146
Christopher and Dana Reeve Foundation, NeuroRecovery Network, 340
Chromosomal abnormalities
  collagen VI and, 369
  cystic fibrosis and, 706
  dystrophin and, 351, *352, 353*
  intellectual disabilities with, 383t
  myotonia and, 365
  sarcoglycan and, 366t
  SMN protein and, 370
  Down syndrome and, 391
Chronic exertional compartment syndrome (CECS), 525–526
Chronic lung disease of infancy (CLDI), 146–147
Chronic obstructive pulmonary disease (COPD), 695
Cigarette smoke, 18t, 137, 151
Circulation, spinal cord injury and, 342
Circulatory system, burns and, 619–620
Cisplatin, 594t
Clavicle fractures, 512
Clinton, Bill, 11
Clonidine
  for pain, 336
  for spasticity, 336
Clubbing, digital, *668,* 683
Clubfoot deformity, 477–478 (*see also* Talipes equinovarus)
CMV (*see* Cytomegalovirus)
Cobblestone lissencephaly, 368
Cognitive function
  brain trauma and, 310–312
  intellectual disabilities and, 389–390
  pulmonary and respiratory disorders and, 686
Cognitive impairments, autism spectrum disorder and, 406
Cognitive skills, equipment selection and, 429
Collagen, *352,* 369, 617, 618
Colles fracture, 60
Coma, 302
  assessment of, 307t
  depth of, 307
  duration of, 306
  scales, 306, 307t
  stimulation program for, 317–318, 317b, 318b
COMFORT scale, 666
Committee on Children with Disabilities of the American Academy of Pediatrics, 69
Communication systems, 455–456
Community programs, 215
Compartment syndrome, 525–526
Competent feeder, 116
Complete blood count (CBC), 664
Computed tomography (CT) scan
  for accessory navicular, 530
  for pelvic avulsion fractures, 515
  for tarsal coalition, 530
  for traumatic hip dislocation, 518
  for traumatic shoulder dislocation, 512
Concurrent validity, 71
Concussion, 304, 383t
Conditioning (*see also* Endurance, training)
  arthritis and, 559–560, 559b, 566b, 569
  cardiac disorders and, 670
Confused patients, 319–321
Congenital diaphragmatic hernia (CDH), 127–129

Congenital heart defects (CHDs), 149, 157, 392, 657, 660–663
  assessment of, 664–670, 665, 665t
  case study of, 675–676, 675
  equipment for, 666, 667
  incidence of, 657, 658t
  interventions for, 671–674
  neurodevelopmental outcomes of, 674–675
  types of, 660, 662–663
Congenital limb deficiencies, 468–475, 469–475
Congenital muscular dystrophy, 368–369
Congenital muscular torticollis (CMT) (see Torticollis)
Congenital myopathy, 367–368
Congestive heart failure (CHF)
  clinical presentation of, 663t
  cor pulmonale and, 686
  muscular dystrophy and, 357
  transplant for, 663–664
Connective tissue diseases, 541
Considerations for Educationally Relevant Therapy (CERT), 722, 723
Constraint-induced movement therapy (CIMT), modified, 212–213
Content-Balanced CAT, 89
Content validity, 71
Continuous positive airway pressure (CPAP), 125t, 126
Contracture management, 315–316
Contusion, 304, 383t
Conus medullaris syndrome, 334b
Coping strategies, 113–114 (see also Stress management)
Cor pulmonale, 686
Corner chair, 439, 439
Corticosteroids
  for arthritis, 550
  for muscular dystrophy, 356, 362
  nutritional concerns with, 546b
Cost, of screening test, 70
Coultes, Kathy, 641–655
Coup injuries, 533
CP (see Cerebral palsy)
Crackles, 685, 707
Craniopharyngioma, 590
Creatine monohydrate, for muscular dystrophy, 357
Cri-du-chat syndrome, 384t
Criterion-related validity, 71
Crouch gait, 202–203
Crutches, 220
  for spina bifida, 273, 275t, 282
Culturally and Linguistically Appropriate Services (CLAS) standards, 9b
Culture (see Multiculturalism)
Cultured epithelial autografts (CEAs), 625
Cushing's syndrome, 550
Cyanotic heart defects, 662–663
Cyclosporine, 597
Cystic fibrosis (CF), 679, 683, 706–710
  assessment of, 706–710
  exercise for, 700t
  gene for, 706
  interventions for, 709–710
  management of, 696–697, 706–707
  postural drainage for, 688–691, 689–690
Cytomegalovirus (CMV)
  BPD and, 146
  and cerebral palsy, 188b
  intellectual disabilities and, 384t

D

Dactylitis, 544, 545
Dance classes, 215
Dance Dance Revolution, 417
Dantrium (see Dantrolene)

Dantrolene (Dantrium), for spasticity, 316
Dantrolene sodium, for spasticity, 221, 336
Dargassies, Suzanne Saint-Anne, 116
De Lange syndrome, 384t
Death and dying, 7, 114
Debridement, 621, 625
Deflazacort, for muscular dystrophy, 357
Dejerine–Sottas (DS) disease, 373
Dermatomyositis, 541
Development
  cardiac system, 658–659
  of central nervous system, 115
  fine motor, 60–64, 60–64, 64t
  motor, 17–65
  pulmonary system, 680–681
  tests of, 69–97
Developmental care, 110–112
Developmental Coordination Disorders Questionnaire (DCDQ), 410
Developmental delay
  myotonic dystrophy with, 365
  risks for, 104, 724b
  Down syndrome and, 393–394
Developmental dysplasia of hip (DDH), 478–480
  assessment of, 478–480, 479
  classification of, 479t
  management of, 480, 480
Developmental quotient (DQ), 71, 86
Dexamethasone, 594t
Diabetes mellitus
  gestational, 123
  obesity and, 649
  steroid use and, 550
  type 2, 649
Diagnostic and Statistical Manual of Mental Disorders, 4th ed. (DSM-IV-TR), 383
Diagnostic and Statistical Manual of Mental Disorders, 5th ed., 381
Diazepam (Valium), for spasticity, 316, 336
Dickens, Charles, 380
Diffuse axonal injury (DAI), 305
DiGeorge syndrome, 657
Digital clubbing, 668, 683
DiLenno, Michael, 463–496
Diplegic gait, 202–203, 206b
Disability index, 552
Discharge planning, spinal cord injury and, 341 (see also Home management)
Disease-modifying antirheumatic drugs (DMARDs), 549
Distal forearm fractures, 513
Distal interphalangeal (DIP) joint of finger, 514
DMD (see Duchenne muscular dystrophy)
Documentation, 728–729
Dolichocephaly, 117, 144
Double-outlet right ventricle (DORV), 662–663, 662
Down syndrome, 379–399
  assessment of, 382–387, 382t, 384t
  case study, 397–399
  complications with, 391–392, 590
  definition of, 391
  history of, 391
  incidence of, 381, 391
  interventions for, 390–396, 392–395
  neuropathology for, 391–392
  pathophysiology of, 391
Doxorubicin, 594t
Dubowitz, V., 144t
Duchenne muscular dystrophy (DMD), 351–375, 699
  ambulation with, 354, 355, 356t, 362
  assessment of, 359–360
  case studies of, 374–375, 711
  clinical presentation of, 353–356

  complications with, 356–357
  diagnosis of, 352–353, 353
  functional abilities with, 354, 355, 355, 356t, 359
  interventions for, 359–365
  pathophysiology of, 353
  progression of, 353–356
  proteins implicated in, 352
  pulmonary problems with, 711
  school issues with, 358
  treatment for, 357–358
Dynamic ankle–foot-orthoses (DAFO), 232–233t, 235
Dynamic Orthotic Cranioplasty (DOC) band, 477
Dynamic systems theory, 20, 106–108, 107
Dynamometry, 465, 466, 670
Dysautonomia, 306
Dyskinesia, 193, 428
Dyspnea, 686–687 (see also Pulmonary and respiratory disorders)
  index, 670, 670t
Dysreflexia, autonomic, 342
Dystonia, 193
Dystrophinopathy, 352, 352

E

ECMO (see Extracorporeal membrane oxygenation)
Education, 380 (see also Caregiver education; School issues)
  inclusive, 726
  legislation on, 718, 719t
  sex, 3, 343
  supportive, 382–383, 390, 394
Education for All Handicapped Children Act, 104, 718, 720
Educational team, 719–720
Ege's test, 522
Ehlers–Danlos syndrome (EDS), 485–487, 486t
Elbow
  arthritis of, 557t
  injuries, 510–511
Electromyography (EMG), 256, 438–439
  for Duchenne muscular dystrophy, 353
  for limb-girdle muscular dystrophy, 366
  for spinal muscular atrophy, 370
Embryogenesis, 114–116, 115
Enablement models, 109
Encephalopathy
  hypoxic–ishemic, 153, 154t, 189b
  metabolic, 189b
Endocrine disorders, 306
Endurance, 685
  autism spectrum disorder and, 408–409
  cardiorespiratory, 648
  muscular, 648
  training (see also Conditioning)
    arthritis and, 568–569
    heart disease and, 670, 673
Enthesitis, 545, 548
Enthesitis-related arthritis (ERA), 543t, 544, 551, 561
Environmental controls, 456–457
Environmental influences, on brain trauma, 309
Ependymoma, 590t
Epilepsy, myoclonic, 383t (see also Seizures)
Equilibrium reaction, 59b
Equinus deformity, 228–230
Equinus gait, 202
Equipment, 423–457
  activities of daily living, 454–455
  assessment for, 427–432
  for cerebral palsy, 215–220

classification of, 423–424
fabricating, 434–436, *435*
for family environment, 430–432
for heart defects, 666–667, *666, 667*
for home care, 430–432
for joint hypermobility syndromes, 487
manufacture of, *435, 436*
for NICU, 125–129, 125–126t, *127, 128*
playground, 324
for positioning, 215–217
precautions with, 425–427
for pulmonary and respiratory
    disorders, 685
purchasing, 432–434
renting or borrowing, 434
role of, 424–425
for school environment, 430–432
seating, 215–217
selection of, 432–436
for side-lying, *316, 442*
for spina bifida, 267–268
for standing, 439–442, *440*
universal design, 457
Escharotomy, 620, *620,* 626
Etanercept, 550
Ethnicity
    arthritis and, 545
    asthma and, 703
    child abuse and, 612
    cystic fibrosis and, 706
    and obesity, 642–643t
    spina bifida and, 248
Ethyl alcohol, for spasticity, 221
European League Against Rheumatism
    (EULAR), 541, 542t
Ewing's sarcoma, 591–592
Executive functioning (EF), 312, 405
    autism spectrum disorder and, 406
Exercise-induced compartment
    syndrome, 525
Exercises (*see also* Range of motion, exercises)
    for arthritis, 562, 566, 566b
    blood counts and, 593t
    for burns, 632–633
    for cerebral palsy, 208–211
    for cystic fibrosis, 696, 700t
    distinguished from physical activity, 649
    heart defects and, 672–673, *673*
    for leukemia, 593t, 603–606
    for muscular dystrophy, 361
    for spina bifida, 257–258, *258,* 280
    for spinal cord injury, 337
    stretching, 567
Exertion, 686–687
Extended school year, 729
Extracorporeal membrane oxygenation (ECMO),
    125t, 127, 128–129, *128*
    for CDH, 149
    for heart defects, 666, *666*
    for PPHN, 157
Extradural hematoma, 304
Eye(s) (*see also* Vision)
    congenital muscular dystrophy and, 368
    infections of, 550
    retinoblastoma of, 592
    sunset sign of, 254, 259t

F
Fabricating equipment, 434–436
Face mask, *634*
Faces Pain Scale, 560b, 599t, 627, 666, 687
Failure to thrive, 18t, 612, 664
Falls, 302, 330
Family Bill of Rights, 11

Family-centered care, 1–13 (*see also* Caregiver
    education)
    barriers to, 2–3
    benefits of, 10–11
    case studies of, 11–13
    cultural factors in, 4–10
    interventions for, 7–10
    legal issues with, 2, 720, 725
Family environment, equipment needs and,
    430–432
Family Resource Center on Disabilities, 341
FAS (*see* Fetal alcohol syndrome)
Fasciotomy, 620
Fatiman, Anne, 6
Feeding, 454–455
    poor, Chiari II malformation and, 250b
Female athlete
    special considerations for, 536
    triad, 536–537, 537t
Femoral acetabular impingement (FAI) tears,
    517–518
Femoral stress fracture, 516
Femur (*see also* Hip)
    anteversion of, 198, 224–225
    focal deficiency of, 468, 470, *470*
Fencer's posture (*see* Asymmetric tonic neck
    reflex)
Ferguson, P., 3
Fetal alcohol spectrum disorder (FASD), 158–159
Fetal alcohol syndrome (FAS), 19, 158t (*see also*
    Substance abuse)
    intellectual disabilities and, 384t
Fetal surgery, 151–152, 251
Fine Motor Quotient (FMQ), 79
Fine motor skills
    assessment of, 204–205
    development of, 60–64, *60–64,* 64t
Finger fractures, 513–514
Finnegan scale, 159
FITNESSGRAM, 648
FLACC pain scale, 599t, 627, 666
Flat foot deformity (*see* Planovalgus deformity)
Flexibility, 648
    assessment, 503
Flexor digitorum profundus (FDP), 514
Flickinger, Jean M., 351–375
Floortime play, for autism spectrum disorder, 416
Fluid resuscitation, 619, 626
Flutter device, 693–694, *695,* 709
Folic acid, 247–248
Folk remedies, 6, 11–13
Foot (*see also* Talipes equinovarus)
    amputation of, 471, *472*
    arthritis of, 556, 557t
    assessment of, 199, 466, 467, 481
    deformities of, 228–230, 276–277, 276b
    drop, 600
    enthesitis of, *545*
    injuries, 528–531
    orthoses, 235–236
    Down syndrome and, 394
Foot-progression angle (FPA), 466, 467, 482
Forced expiratory technique (FET), 693
Forefoot fractures, 530–531
Forward-bend test, 495, *495*
Fracture(s), 613
    brain injury and, 313–314
    Colles, 60
    pelvic, 313–314
    Salter–Harris classification of, 502, *502,* 502b,
        513, 527, 528
    skull, 304
Fragile X syndrome, 384t, 405–406
French angles, 155, *156*
Friedreich ataxia, 383t

Fukutin-related protein (FKRP), 367
Functional abilities
    arthritis and, 571–572
    assessment of, 72, 87–93, 598–600, 599t
    after brain trauma, 309
    with muscular dystrophy, 354, 355, *355,*
        356t, 359
    neonatal, *107*
    after spinal cord injury, 334, 335t
Functional electrical stimulation (FES), 214, 230,
    340, 342
Functional Independence Measure for Children
    (WeeFIM), 89–91, 90b, 722
    brain trauma and, 314
    spinal cord injury and, 335
Functional outcomes, 205, 206b
Functional skills, equipment selection and,
    429–430
Functioning, defined, 423

G
Gait
    arthritis and, 561
    ataxic, 204
    athetotic, 204
    autism spectrum disorder and, 408
    after brain trauma, *319–323*
    after burns, 629
    in cerebral palsy, 199–204
    deviations, causes of, 200, 201t
    diplegic, 202–203, 206b
    hemiplegic, 200–202
    motor development and, 55–57, *55–57*
    in muscular dystrophy, 354
    observational analysis, 200
    parameters of, 57t
    prosthetic legs and, 473
    quadriplegic, 203–204
    robotic training, 213–214
    Down syndrome and, 393
    three-dimensional analysis of, 282
    trainers, 219, *220,* 450
Ganglioneuroblastoma, 591
Ganglioneuroma, 591
Gastrocnemius stretching, BTX-A injection
    for, 201
Gastroesophageal reflux (GER), 131–132
    Chiari II malformation with, 250b
    cystic fibrosis and, 688
    positioning for, 143
Gastrointestinal system disorders, muscular
    dystrophy and, 356
Gastroschisis (GS), 150–151
Geddes, Rita F., 717–732
Gender, and obesity, 642–643t
General Movements Assessment (GMA), 145t
Generalized ligamentous laxity, 503
Genetics (*see* Chromosomal abnormalities)
Germinal matrix–intraventricular hemorrhage
    (GM-IVH), 134–136, *135,* 135t, 190
Gesell, Arnold, 19
Gestural-assisted strategies, 456
Gestural strategies, 456
Glanzman, Allan M., 351–375
Glasgow Coma Scale (GCS), 306, 307t, 315
Glenohumeral internal rotation deficit
    (GIRD), 507
Glioblastoma multiforme, 590t
Glioma, 590t, 595, 599
Glucocorticoids, 550 (*see also* Corticosteroids)
GMFCS–E&R, 78, 78t
GMFM-66, 77, 78, 79, 721
GMFM-88, 77, 78, 79, 721
Goniometry, 197, 555, 599t

Gore, Al, 11
Gower's sign, 354, *354*
Graft-versus-host disease (GVHD), 131, 597
Grasp, 25, 25t, 45, 60–63, *60–64*, 64t
Grasp plantar, *54*
Greenberg, Elliot M., 501–537
Greenberg, Eric T., 501–537
Grieving, 7, 113–114
Gross Motor Ability Estimator (GMAE), 77, 79
Gross Motor Function Classification System for Cerebral Palsy (GMFCS), 78, 191, 191b, 199, 207, 221–223, 225
Gross Motor Function Measure (GMFM), 77–79, 207, 314, 335, 721
Gross Motor Performance Measure (GMPM), 77
Gross Motor Quotient (GMQ), 79
Ground-reaction ankle–foot orthoses (GRAFOs), 203, 229, 231, 233t
Ground-reaction orthoses, 234
Growth
  abnormalities, spinal cord injury and, 342–343
  arthritis and, 561
  charts, *124*
Guggenbuhl, Johann Jacob, 380
Guillain-Barré syndrome (GBS), 330, 699
Gunshot wounds, 302
Gymnast wrist, 513

H

Hamstring lengthening, 227–228
Hand(s)
  arthritis of, *543*, 555, 557t
  digital clubbing of, *668*, 683
  prosthetic, 473, *474*
  skin graft for, *624*
Hand grasp reflex, 45, 60–61, *61*, 64t
Handling, for spina bifida, 258–259
Hanson, Heather, 657–676
Harness, Pavlik, 480, *480*
Harrington rods, 496
Harris Infant Neuromotor Test (HINT), 72–73, 73t
Head trauma (*see* Traumatic brain injury (TBI))
Healing, 596, 596t
  burn, 620–622, *623*, 629–630
Health Assessment Questionnaire, 553–554b
Health consequences, of obesity, 649–650
Healthy Kids/Healthy Community Program, The, 654b
Heamophilus influenzae, 707
Hearing, 121
  impairment of, 386
  loss, brain trauma and, 313
Heart disease (*see also* Congenital heart defects (CHDs))
  intellectual disabilities and, 384t, 392
  muscular dystrophy and, 357, 358
  transplant for, 357, 663–664, 667, 668
Helmets, 324, 477
Hemiplegic gait, 200–202
Hereditary motor and sensory neuropathy (HMSN) (*see* Charcot–Marie–Tooth disease)
Hernia, diaphragmatic, 127–129, 149
Herniation syndromes, 305
Heterotopic ossification (HO), 313, 333b
Hickman catheter, 595
Hierarchical theory, 20, 21
High-frequency chest wall oscillation (HFCWO), 694, 696, 709
High-frequency ventilation (HFV), 125t, 126, 127, 129
High lumbar paralysis, 271
  orthotics for, 271–276
Higher education, spinal cord injury and, 343
Hip (*see also* Femur; Pelvis)

adductor contracture without subluxation, 226
arthritis of, 557t
arthroplasty of, 565
assessment of, 198
dislocation of, 225–226, 277, 479t
dysplasia of, 478–480, *479*, 479t
femoral anteversion, 224–225
muscular dystrophy and, *354*, 356t
pain, differential diagnoses of, 514, 514t
rotation of, 466, *467*, 482
subluxation of, 225–226, 342, 394, 479t
Hip-knee-ankle-foot orthosis (HKAFO)
  for osteogenesis imperfecta, 485
  for spina bifida, 273, *275*, 275t, 286
  for spinal cord injury, 335t, *339*, 340, 347
  for tibia vara, 491
Hip spica cast, 282–285, *283*, *284*
Hippotherapy, 214–215
  for autism spectrum disorder, 417
History-taking process, for sports injuries, 503
HIV disease, 10
Hodgkin disease, 590–591, 594t
Home management (*see also* Caregiver education)
  arthritis and, 572–573, 577
  burns and, 635
  cerebral palsy and, 236
  equipment needs and, 430–432
  Infant Family Service Plan and, 725
  spina bifida and, 257, 263–264, *263*, *264*, 289
Hook of hamate fractures, 513
Horseback riding, 215
Hospitalized children, movement in, 452
Household ambulator, seating for, 216–217
Howe, Samuel Gridley, 380
Human leukocyte antigen (HLA) B27, 543t, 544
Hurler syndrome, 384t
Hydrocephalus, 261
  case study of, 294
  from head injury, 305
  intellectual disabilities and, 384t
  IQ and, 288, 293, 383t
  management of, 254–255, *254*
  PVL and, 136
  spina bifida and, 249–250
Hydromyelia, 285, 286
Hydrotherapy, 621–622
Hyperactivity, 302
Hyperbilirubinemia, 130–131, *131*
Hyperinsulinism, 123
Hyperreflexia, 342
Hypertonia, 207–208b, 428
Hypopituitarism, 306
Hypoplastic left heart syndrome (HLHS), 658t, 663, *663*, 677
Hypothermia, 131
Hypothesis-Oriented Pediatric Focused Algorithm (HOP-FA), 722
Hypotonia, 208b
  Chiari II malformation with, 250b
  intellectual disabilities and, 384t, 393
Hypoxic–ischemic encephalopathy (HIE), 153, 154t, 189b, 305

I

ICF (*see* International Classification of Functioning, Disability, and Health)
Idiopathic toe-walking versus mild diplegic gait, 203
Ifosfamide, 594t
IFSP (*see* Infant Family Service Plan)
Ilizarov procedure, 491, *491*
Imitation, autism spectrum disorder and, 408
Impaired endurance, brain trauma and, 313
Impression injuries, 304
Individualized education program, 2

Individualized Educational Plan (IEP), 431, 572, 723–724
  components of, 726t
  goals and objectives, 725–726
Individualized Family Service Plan, 2, 416
Individuals with Disabilities Education Act (IDEA), 162, 323, 431, 433, 572, 717–732, 719t
  Part C, 82, 86
Infant and Toddler Sensory Profile, 410
Infant Family Service Plan (IFSP), 725
  goals and objectives, 725–726
Infants without physical impairments, 453–454
Infections, brain trauma and, 306
Inflammation, 617
Inflammatory bowel disease (IBD), 544
Instrumental activities of daily living (IADLs), 337–338
Integumentary system, assessment of, 667–668
Intellectual disabilities, 379–399 (*see also* Down syndrome)
  adults with, 396
  assessment of, 382–387, 382t, 384t
  case study, 397–399
  cerebral palsy and, 194
  classification of, 381–383, 383t
  definition of, 381
  diagnosis of, 381–382
  etiology of, 383, 383t
  incidence of, 381
  interventions for, 390–396
  pathophysiology of, 383
Intelligence quotient (IQ)
  heart disease and, 674, 675
  intellectual disabilities and, 382, 382t, 388
  muscular dystrophy and, 357, 358
  spina bifida and, 288, 293
Interleukin-6, 330, 334
International Classification of Functioning, Disability, and Health (ICF), 109, 468, 541, 552t, 598
International League of Associates for Rheumatology (ILAR), 541, 542–543t, 544
International Society for Prosthetics and Orthotics (ISPO), 468
Interobserver reliability, 71
Interpreters, language, 8, 13
Intra-articular injuries, 521–523
Intracranial hemorrhage (ICH)
  ECMO and, 128–129
  intellectual disabilities and, 383t
  from trauma, 304–305
Intracranial pressure (ICP), 305, 324
Intradural hematoma, 304–305
Intrathecal baclofen pump, 222
Intrauterine growth restriction (IUGR), 123
Intraventricular hemorrhage (IVH), 127, 134–136, *135*, 135t, 190
iPads, 457
Iritis, 550
Ischial tuberosity, pelvic apophysitis in, 514
Iselin's disease, 529
Isokinetic dynamometry, 332
Isolette, 125t, 140
Itard, Jean Marc, 380
IVH (*see* Intraventricular hemorrhage)

J

Jaundice, 130, 189b
Javits, Jacob, 381
JIA (*see* Juvenile idiopathic arthritis)
Job training, spinal cord injury and, 343
Joint Commission on the Accreditation of Health Care Organization (JCAHO), 2, 119
Joint hypermobility syndromes, 485–487, 486t

adaptive equipment for, 487
examination of, 486
functional training for, 487
management of, 486
orthoses for, 487
self-care for, 487
therapeutic exercise for, 486–487
Jump knee gait, 203
Juvenile ankylosing spondylitis (JAS), 542t, 548
Juvenile Arthritis (JA) Alliance, 563b
Juvenile Arthritis Functional Assessment Scale
(JAFAS), 552, 554
Juvenile Arthritis Quality of Life Questionnaire
(JAQQ), 552t, 555
Juvenile idiopathic arthritis (JIA), 541–578
assessment of, 551–561, 552t, 556, 557t,
574–575
case study of, 573–578
classification of, 541–545, 542t
etiology of, 545, 547
incidence of, 545
interventions for, 562–573, 562, 566b, 567, 568,
570, 576–577
management of, 548–550
nutritional concerns with, 546b
outcomes of, 550–551
pain with, 560–561, 560b
pathogenesis of, 545, 547
pathology of, 547–548
postoperative physical therapy for, 565–566
prevalence of, 545
prognosis with, 550–551
resources for, 572, 586
school issues with, 562, 572
surgery for, 565–566
Juvenile rheumatoid arthritis (JRA), 541, 542t

K

Kalisperis, Faithe, 187–241
Kangaroo care, 120, 142
Karate, 215
Kaufman Assessment Battery for Children, 382
Kaufman Brief Intelligence Test (KBIT), 410
Keloids, 617–618, 618
Keratinocytes, 625
Kleinman, A., 6
Klepper, Susan E., 541–578
Klinefelter syndrome, 383t, 590
Knee
arthritis of, 547, 557t
arthroplasty of, 566
assessment of, 198
enthesitis of, 545
extension test of, 465
flexion contracture, 227–228
injuries, 519–524
stiff knee gait due to rectus femoris
dysfunction, 228
Knee-ankle-foot orthosis (KAFO)
for spina bifida, 277, 282
for spinal cord injury, 335t
for spinal muscular atrophy, 371, 372
Knee Society Score (KSS), 566
Korner, A. F., 144t
KT-1000™ arthrometer, 520
Kugelberg–Welander disease, 369, 373
Kyphoscoliosis, 252, (see also Scoliosis)

L

Labral tears, 517–518
Labyrinthine reflex, 38, 58, 59
Laennec, RTH, 697
Landa, R., 403–419

Language skills
assessment of, 205
after brain injury, 312
communication systems and, 455–456
interpreters and, 8, 13
Large for gestational age (LGA), 123
Late term infants, physical therapy assessment
and intervention for, 159–160
Lateral collateral ligament (LCL)
injuries, 521
Lateral condyle fractures, 512
Latex allergy, 286–287, 287b
and spinal cord injury, 331b
Lead intoxication, 383t
Learning impairments, intellectual disabilities
and, 384–385
Left ventricular assistive devices (LVAD), 667
Leg(s)
alignment of, 466–468, 467
congenital deficiency of, 469–472
length discrepancy between, 199, 491–493,
493, 544, 571, 596
muscular dystrophy and, 354, 356t
osteogenesis imperfecta of, 483
osteosarcoma of, 591–592, 597
prosthetic, 472, 473–475, 475
Legg–Calvé–Perthes disease (LCPD), 468,
487–489, 488, 519
Lemon sign, 251
Lesch–Nyhan syndrome, 383t, 384t
Lester, B. M., 145t
Leukemia, 589–590, 601, 601t
bone marrow transplant for, 596–597
case study of, 603–605, 605
chemotherapy for, 594t, 603
stem cells for, 596–597
Leukocoria, 592
Licata, Ann Marie, 397–399
Lidocaine
for pain, 336
for spasticity, 336
Ligament laxity, 547
Ligament Sprain Grading Scale, 521b
Ligamentous injuries, 519–521
Limb deficiencies, 468–475, 469–472, 474–475
Limb-girdle muscular dystrophy (LGMD), 351,
365–367, 366t
Limb lengthening, 471–472
Limb-sparing procedures, 591–592, 596t, 597,
605–607
Limited-community ambulator, seating for,
216–217
Lipomeningocele, 249
Lisfranc (midfoot) injury, 529–530
Lissencephaly, 188
Literacy skills, 8
Little league elbow, 510
Little league shoulder, 508–509, 509t
Locomotion (see also Walking)
bipedal, 55–57, 55–57
in prone position, 35–36, 35–36
Locomotor training, 340
Longitudinal radial deficiency, 471
Low lumbar paralysis, 276–280
Lower extremity
alignment, 466
orthoses, 230–236
Lower leg
injuries, 524–526
tibial torsion in, 228
Lumbar puncture, 593
Lund and Browder chart, 615, 616, 627
Lung transplant, 707
Lunnen, Karen Yundt, 713–732
Lymphoma, 590–591, 594t, 601t

M

Maddocks Questions, 534
Mafenide acetate, 622
Magnetic resonance angiography (MRA)
for traumatic shoulder dislocation, 512
Magnetic resonance imaging (MRI)
for acute patella dislocations, 523
for femoral stress fracture, 516
for meniscus injury, 522
for muscle strains, 518
for osteochondral fractures, 523
for osteochondritis dissecans, 522
for pelvic avulsion fractures, 515
for spondylolysis, 532
for traumatic hip dislocation, 518
for traumatic shoulder dislocation, 512
Malaria, 189b
Malerba, Kirsten H., 69–97
Malnutrition, spina bifida and, 253b
Mann, Horace, 380
Manual muscle testing (MMT), 465, 466, 503–504
Marchese, Victoria Gocha, 589–607
Marginal ambulator, seating for, 216
Mask, face, 634
Massage, of burns, 632
Maturational theory, 20
McGill Action Planning System (MAPS), 725
McGraw, Myrtle, 19, 26
McMurray test, 521, 522
Meaningfulness, 389
Meconium aspiration syndrome (MAS), 156–157
Medial collateral ligament (MCL) injuries, 520–521
Medial epicondyle apophysitis, 510
Medial epicondyle avulsion fracture, 510
Medial patellofemoral ligament (MPFL)
reconstruction, 523
Medial tibial stress syndrome (MTSS), 524–525
Medicare Catastrophic Coverage Act, 719t
Medulloblastoma, 590t
Megalocephaly, 189
Memory impairment, 307, 311–312, 389
Menelaus, Malcolm, 268
Meningitis, 189b
Meningomyelocele (see Spina bifida)
Meniscus injury, 521–522
Merosin, 369
Metabolic bone disease of prematurity, 139–140
Metabolic disorders, 188b, 383t
Metatarsus adductus (MTA), 477–478
Methotrexate (MTX)
for arthritis, 549–550
for cancer, 594, 594t
nutritional concerns with, 546b
for transplant rejection, 597
Microcephaly, 189
Micrognathia, 548
Migliore, Suzanne F., 611–638
Mild traumatic brain injury (mTBI), 533
Miller-Skomorucha, Kathleen, 187–241
Minimal clinically important difference
(MCID), 555
Mobility Opportunities Via Education (MOVE),
721–722
Modified Ashworth Scale (MAS), 191, 192t, 332b
Modified Checklist for Autism in Toddlers
(MCHAT), 411
Modified constraint-induced movement therapy
(mCIMT), 212–213
Modified Florida Apraxia Battery, 411t, 412
Molded ankle–foot orthoses (MAFOs), 202, 203,
229, 231, 232–233t
Monteggia fracture, 513
Moro reflex, 441
Morphine (see Narcotics)
Morphogenesis, 468

Motor development, 17–65
    balance in, 58–60, *59, 60,* 64t
    extrinsic factors of, 18t
    fine, 60–64, *60–64,* 64t
    grasp in, 25, 25t, 45, 60–63, *60–64,* 64t
    of neonates, 25–26, 25t
    of preterm infants, 21, 21b, 25t
    prone progression in, 19t, 26–36, *26–36*
    rolling progression in, 19t, 41–43, *42, 43*
    sequences of, 21–66, 22t, *23–25,* 25t, 57t, 64t
    sitting progression in, 19t, 43–49, *44–50*
    spina bifida and, 261–263
    stair climbing in, 18t, 19t, 57–58, *57, 58*
    standing progression in, 49–57, *51–57,* 57t
    supine progression in, 18t, 19t, *37–43*
    theories of, 19–21
    variability in, 17–19, 18t, 19t
Motor function tests, 74–82
Motor impairments, autism spectrum disorder
    and, 407–409, 407t
Motor neuropathy, 352
Motor quotient (MQ), 71
Motor vehicle accidents (MVAs)
    brain trauma from, 302, 324
    spinal cord injuries from, 330
MOVE (Mobility Opportunities Via Education),
    721–722
Movement Assessment Battery for Children
    (MABC), 410, 411t
Movement Assessment in Infants (MAI), 194
Movement disorders, 191
    case study of, 237–238
Mullen Scales of Early Learning (MSEL), 411, 411t
Multi-Podus boots, 672
Multiculturalism, 4–10, 11–13, 430–431
Multidirectional instability (MDI)
    of shoulder, 511
Multimodal distraction device (MMD), 629
Multiple congenital contracture (MCC),
    480–482, *481*
Multiple sclerosis (MS), 330
Muscle control, equipment selection and, 428
Muscle-eye-brain disease, 368
Muscle imbalances, 332b
Muscle performance exercise, 567–569
Muscle strains, 518
Muscle strength
    autism spectrum disorder and, 408
    equipment selection and, 428
Muscle tone, equipment selection and, 428
Muscle transfers, 335–336
Muscular dystrophy, 351 (*see also* Duchenne
    muscular dystrophy)
    Becker, 351, 353, 355, 358
    congenital, 368–369
    Duchenne, 351–375
    limb-girdle, 351, 365–367, 366t
    spinal, 369–373, *370, 372*
Muscular endurance, 648
Muscular properties, skeletally immature
    athlete, 503
Muscular strength, 648
Musculoskeletal development, 463–464
Musculoskeletal examination, 464–468
Musculoskeletal problems, Down syndrome and,
    394–395
Musculoskeletal system, burns and, 620
Music therapy, for autism spectrum disorder, 417
MVAs (*see* Motor vehicle accidents)
Myelocele, 249
Myelomeningocele (MMC), obesity and, 649
    (*see also* Spina bifida)
Myelopathy, compressive, 330
Myoclonic epilepsy, 383t

Myopathy, 351, 352
    Bethlem, 369
    central core, 368
    congenital, 367–368
    nemaline, 367, 368
Myotonic dystrophy (MTD), 365, 383t

N

Narcotics (*see also* Substance abuse)
    for burns, 621
    during pregnancy, 383t
National Association for Retarded Citizens
    (NARC), 380, 381
National Parent Network on Disabilities, 341
National Spinal Cord Injury Association (NSCIA),
    329, 341
Naturalistic play observation, for autism
    spectrum disorder, 409–410
Near-drowning event, 189b
Necrotizing enterocolitis (NEC), 132–134, *134*
Negative predictive value, 72
Neglect, burns and, 612–613
Neonatal abstinence syndrome (NAS), 159
Neonatal Behavioral Assessment Scale (NBAS),
    104, 144t
Neonatal care, levels of, 105t
Neonatal follow-up services, 162–163
Neonatal intensive care unit (NICU), 103–104
    equipment for, 125–129, 125–126t, *127, 128*
    family-centered care in, 113–114
    language of, 123–125, *124*
    lighting in, 121, 140
    noise levels in, 121, *141*
    pain management in, 118–120, 119t
    physical therapists, role of, 104–106
    surgical patients in, 152–153
    theoretical frameworks for, 106–114, *107,*
        110–112, 112t
    therapists roles and competencies in, 106
    training for, 106, 106t
Neonates
    behavioral development of, *110, 112,* 122t
    competencies of, 115–116
    as medical specialty, 103–104
    musculoskeletal development of, 116–117
    neurological development of, 117–121
    pain management for, 118–120, 119t
    preterm infant versus, 17, 21, 21b, 25t
Nephroblastoma (*see* Wilms tumor)
Neural tube closure defects, 383t
Neural tube defects, 247–249 (*see also specific types,*
    e.g., Spina bifida)
Neuro-assisted strategies, 456
Neurobehavioral Assessment of the Preterm
    Infant (NAPI), 144t
Neuroblastic tumors, 591
Neuroblastoma, 591, 594t, 595
Neurochemical events, brain trauma and, 305
Neurodevelopmental treatment (NDT), 208, 211
Neurofibromatosis, 383t, 590
Neurofibromatosis type 1 (NF1), 82
Neurologic Assessment of Preterm and Full-
    Term Infants (NAPFI), 144t
Neuromotor impairments, intellectual disabilities
    and, 383–384
Neuromuscular blocks, for spasticity, 221–222
Neuromuscular electrical stimulation (NMES),
    214, 230
    for ligamentous injuries, 520
Neuromuscular scoliosis, cerebral palsy and, 223
Neuromyelitis optica (NMO), 330
Neuronal group selection theory (NGST),
    108–109, 211

Neuropathic pain, 336
Neurophysiologic testing, for sports-related
    concussion, 534–535
NeuroRecovery Network (NRN), 340
Newborn Individualized Developmental Care
    and Assessment Program (NIDCAP),
    108–112, *111*
Newton, M., 2b
NICU (*see* Neonatal intensive care unit)
NICU Network Neurobehavioral Scale (NNNS),
    145t, 159
Nitric oxide, inhaled, 125t, 127, 147
9-Minute Walk–Run Test (9MRW), 559
No Child Left Behind Act, 719t
Nociceptive pain, 336
Noise levels, in NICU, 121
Non-Hodgkin lymphoma (NHL), 590–591, 594t
Nonambulator, seating for, 216
Nonsteroidal anti-inflammatory drugs
    (NSAIDs), 549
Normal fetal circulation, 658–659, *659*
Normalization, 380–381
Nutrition updates, 645b
Nutritional concerns
    with arthritis, 546b
    with burns, 620
    with corticosteroids, 546b
    with spina bifida, 253b
    with spinal cord injury, 331b
    with traumatic brain injury, 303b
Nystagmus, 250b

O

Ober test, 359
Obesity, 641–655 (*see also* Overweight)
    defined, 641, 644–648
    functional outcome expectations,
        determining, 652–653
    health consequences of, 649–650
    muscular dystrophy and, 363
    pediatric obesity, physical therapists role in,
        648–649
    physical therapy history and examination,
        651–652
    prevalence of, 642t
    scope of, 641–644
    spina bifida and, 253b, 289
    steroid use and, 550
    therapeutic interventions for, 653–655
    treatment for, within ICF framework,
        650–651, *650, 651*
OCD (*see* Osteochondritis dissecans)
Olfactory development, 120
OMNI child scales, 653
Omphalocele, 150
Oncology, 589–607 (*see also* Cancer)
Open reduction internal fixation (ORIF), 513, 515, 531
Opioids (*see* Narcotics)
Orientation level, brain trauma and, 311
Orthopedic interventions, for cerebral palsy,
    222–230, 224t
Orthosis (*see also specific types, e.g.,* Ankle–foot
    orthoses)
    A-frame, *270, 272,* 275t
    ankle–foot (*see* Ankle–foot orthoses)
    Boston, 495, 496
    after brain trauma, 321
    for cerebral palsy, 230–236, 232–233t
    dial-lock, 568
    floor-reaction, 234
    foot, 235–236
    lower extremity, 230–236
    Orlau, 272

Scottish-Rite, 488
for spina bifida, 268–282, *270, 272–275, 279, 281*
after spinal cord injury, *339*
supramalleolar, 235
Ortolani maneuver, *479*
Osgood–Schlatter disease (OSD), 524
Ossification, heterotopic, 313, 333b
Osteochondral fractures, 522–523
Osteochondritis dissecans (OCD), 502, 511
knee, 522
Osteogenesis imperfecta (OI), 468, 483–485, *483*
classification of, 483, 483t, 484t
Osteopenia, 139
Osteoporosis, *547*, 550, 594t
Osteosarcoma, 591, *591–592*, 594, 594t, 605–607
Osteotomy, 223t
for arthritis, 565
for limb shortening, 492
tibial, 228
Ostomy, *134*
Ottawa ankle rules, 527, 527t, 530b
Oucher Scale, 560b
Overuse injuries
foot, 528–529
knee, 523–524
Overweight, 645 (*see also* Obesity)
spinal cord injury and, 342

P

Pain
assessment of, 119t, 560b, 560–561, *560*
cancer, 598, 601t
neonatal, 118–120
neuropathic, *336*
nociceptive, *336*
types of, 599–600
Pain management
for arthritis, 549, 563–564
for burns, 620–621, 621t, 627, 629
for muscular dystrophy, 360, 364–365
nonpharmacologic, 621t
for pulmonary and respiratory disorders, 686–687
for spinal cord injury, 336
Palsy, facial, 250b
Panner's disease, 511
Parapodium, 272, 275, 450
Parent Training and Information Center, 586
Parents (*see also* Caregiver education)
bonding difficulties of, 18t, 113
cultural background of, 4–6, 11–13, 431
family dynamics and, 3–4, 113, 309
Parents' Evaluation of Developmental Status (PEDS), 72
Partial body weight–supported treadmill training (PBWSTT), 213, 214
Passive range of motion (PROM), 201, 225, 227, 228
Patellar tendinopathy, 524
Patellofemoral dysfunction, 504
Patellofemoral pain syndrome (PFPS), 523
Patent ductus arteriosus (PDA), *130*, 660–661, *660*
cerebral palsy and, 190b
incidence of, 658t
ventilator for, 127
Pavlik harness, 480, *480*
Pavlov, Ivan, 20
Peabody Developmental Motor Scales (PDMS), 676, 724
Peabody Developmental Motor Scales–Second Edition (PDMS-2), 9, 71, 79–81, *80*, 411t, 555, 648

Pectus carinatum, 668
Pectus excavatum, 668
Pediatric Coma Scales (PCS), 306, 307, 307t
Pediatric Evaluation of Disability Inventory (PEDI), 87–89, 87b, 191, 314, 412, 419, 725
brain trauma and, 309
Mobility Functional Skills scale, 309
spinal cord injury and, 335
Pediatric Evaluation of Disability Inventory—Computer Adaptive Test (PEDI-CAT), 89
Pediatric Orthopedic Society of North America (POSNA), 95
Pediatric Outcomes Data Collection Instrument (PODCI), 552
Pediatric Pain Questionnaire (PPQ), 560
Pediatric Powered Wheelchair Screening Test (PPWST), 216
Pediatric Quality-of-Life Inventory™ (Peds-QL), 93–95, *94*, 552t, 599t, 600
Rheumatology Module 3.0, 555
Pediatric Rancho Scale, 307–308, 309b
Pediatric throwing athlete, injuries in, 508–510
Pelvic apophysitis, 514–515, 514t
Pelvic avulsion fractures, 515
Pelvis (*see also* Hip)
assessment of, 198
fracture of, 313–314
osteotomy of, 225–226, *225*
Penn Spasm Frequency Scale, 332
Pennsylvania, growth screening program, 653b, 655
Percentile score, 71
Percussion, for airway clearance, 685, 688, 691
Percutaneous lengthening, 223t
Peripheral stem cell transplantation (PSCT), 596–597
Periventricular hemorrhagic infarction (PHI), 135
Periventricular intraventricular hemorrhage (PIVH), 190
Periventricular leukomalacia (PVL), 136–137, *137*, 153, 383t
cerebral palsy and, 190
chorioamnionitis with, 139
IVH with, 135
ventilator for, 127
Persistent pulmonary hypertension of the newborn (PPHN), 127, 128, 157–158
Pervasive developmental disorders–not otherwise specified (PDD-NOS), 403, 404t, 405
Pes calcaneus, 276b
Petrie cast, 488
Phantom limb pain, 596
Phenol, for spasticity, 222, 336
Phenylketonuria, 383t
Phototherapy, 131, *131*
Physical activity
defined, 649
distinguished from exercise, 649
Physical examination
for sports injuries, 503–506
Physical fitness, 645
Physical therapists
defined, 648
role in pediatric obesity, 648–649
role in program-related areas, 729–730
school-based, resources for, 730t
Physical therapy assistant, role of, 727
Physiologic fitness, elements of, 648
Physiologic flexion, 19t, 24–28, 25t, *28*, *37*, *38*
Piaget, Jean, 19
theory of intellectual development, 388–389

Pictorial Children's Effort Rating Table (PCERT), 653
Picture Exchange Communication System (PECS), for autism spectrum disorder, 416
Piper, M., 145t
Plagiocephaly, 117, 475, 476, 477
Planning Alternative Tomorrows with Hope (PATH), 725
Planovalgus deformity, 230
Planovalgus gait, 202
Plantar fasciitis, 529, 571
Playground equipment, 324
Playing, 455
Plica syndrome, 524
Plus disease, 138
Pneumonitis, 157
Pneumothorax, 190b, 710
Poker Chip Tool, 560, 560b
Polycythemia, 123, 662
Popliteal angle, 25t, *156*
Porencephaly, 383t
Positioning
for airway clearance, 688–691, *689–690*
for brain injury, 316, *316*, *317*
for burns, 630–631
equipment for, 216–217
with heart defects, 672
of preterm infants, 142–144, *142–143*
for spina bifida, 258–259
Positive expiratory pressure (PEP) breathing, 693, *694*, 696, 709
Positive predictive value, 72
POSNA instrument (*see* Pediatric Outcomes Data Collection Instrument)
Postconcussion syndrome, 535–536
Posterior cruciate ligament (PCL) injuries, 521
Posterior element overuse syndrome, 532
Posterior leaf spring (PLS) orthoses, 234
Posterior talofibular ligament (PFL), 526
Posthemorrhagic ventricular dilation (PVD), 135–136
Postoperative physical therapy, for spina bifida, 257
Posttraumatic amnesia (PTA)
assessment, orientation and, 307
duration of, 307
Postural control loss, brain trauma and, 313
Postural drainage with percussion and vibration (PDPV), 688–691, *689–690*
Postural screen, musculoskeletal examination during, 464–465
Posture
arthritis and, 561
assessment of, 196
motor development and, 25t
static versus dynamic, 26
PPHN (persistent pulmonary hypertension of the newborn), 127, 128, 157–158
Prader–Willi syndrome, 383t, 384t
Praxis, autism spectrum disorder and, 408
Predictive validity, 71
Predictive value
negative, 72
positive, 72
Prednisone, 597
for muscular dystrophy, 357
Preferences for Activities of Children (PAC), 721
Pregnancy
cerebral palsy risks and, 188b, 189b
diabetes and, 123
drug use during, 383t
psychological tasks of, 113
Premature infant pain profile (PIPP), 119t, 120
Pretchl, H. F., 145t

Preterm infants
    assessment of, 121–123, 122t, 140–146, 144–145t
    BPD with, 146–147
    complications with, 129–140, *130, 131, 134, 135, 135t, 137, 138*
    full-term versus, 17, 21b, 22, 25t
    growth chart for, *124*
    metabolic bone disease of, 133
    positioning of, 142–144, *142–143*
    retinopathy of, 137–139, *138*
    stability of, *112*, 112t
    surgery for, 149–152, *152*
Prevent injury Enhance Performance (PEP), 520
Prewheelchair device, 443, *443*
PRICE (protection, rest, ice, compression, and elevation) principle, 518, 527, 527t, 531
PRINTO criteria, 559
Progressive muscular dystrophy (*see* Duchenne muscular dystrophy)
Prone progression, 19t, 26–36, *26–36*
Prone standers, 440–441, *440*
Prostaglandins, 130, 663, 703
Prosthesis, 596
    hand, 473, *474*
    leg, *472*, 473–475, *475*
    for limb-sparing surgery, *591–592, 596, 597*
Protective reactions, 59, *60*
Proximal femoral focal deficiency (PFFD), 468, 470, *470, 471–473, 471*
Pseudohypertrophic muscular dystrophy (*see* Duchenne muscular dystrophy)
Pseudomonas aeruginosa, 707
Psoriasis, 544
Puberty
    precocious, 306
    slipped capital femoral epiphysis and, 489
Pulmonary and respiratory disorders, 146–147, 679–711 (*see also* Respiratory distress syndrome)
    assessment of, 682–687
    heart disease with, 668–669, 670t
    interventions for, 687–697, 689–692, 694–696
    muscular dystrophy and, 356, 358–359, 364
    school issues with, 686
    vital signs and, 672t
Pulmonary system, burns and, 619
Pulmonary valve stenosis, 658t, 660, 661–662
Purchasing equipment, 432–434
PVL (*see* Periventricular leukomalacia)

Q

Quadriplegic gait, 203–204, 238–240
Quadruped posture, *23, 33–34, 58*
Quality improvement studies, 10
Quality of life questionnaires, 551, 552–555, 552t, 599t
Quality of My Life (QOML) Questionnaire, 555
Questions as selection guidelines, using, 70–71

R

Radiation therapy, 595, 595t, 600
Rales (*see* Crackles)
Rancho Los Amigos Levels of Cognitive Function Scale (Rancho Scale), 307, 308b, 315
Range of motion (ROM), 465, 503
    active, 227
    burns and, 618, 631–632
    cancer patients and, 598, 599t
    equipment selection and, 428
    exercises (*see also* Exercises)
        for arthritis, 567
        for spina bifida, 257–258, *258,* 280

goniometer for, 197
    knee, 520, 522
    loss, brain trauma and, 313
    muscular dystrophy and, 355
    passive, 201, 225, 227, 228
    shoulder, 507, 510
    spina bifida and, 256–257
    after spinal cord injury, 331–333
RAP Journal for teens with JIA, 586
Rapid eye movements, *110,* 122t
Rate of perceived exertion (RPE) scale, 670t, 673, 686–687
Rating Scale, 560b
Raw scores, 71
RDS (*see* Respiratory distress syndrome)
Re-evaluation, of child, 728
Recession, 223t
Reciprocating gait orthosis (RGO), 450
    for spina bifida, 273, *273–274,* 277, 286
    for spinal cord injury, 335t, 338–340, *339,* 347
Recreation and leisure activities, 290–291, 291b
    for autism spectrum disorder, 417
    and traumatic brain injury, 302–303
Rectus femoris dysfunction, stiff knee gait due to, 228
Recurvatum gait, 203
Referral for evaluation, 720–721
Reflex(es), 428–429 (*see also specific types, e.g.,* Asymmetric tonic neck reflex)
    Achilles tendon, 594
    developmental, 21–22, *23,* 25t
    encephalopathy and, 154t
    hand grasp, 45, 60–61, *61,* 64t
    labyrinthine, 38, 58, *59*
    Moro, 441
    newborn, 114
    plantar grasp, *54*
    primitive, 114, 117, *316*
    red, 592
Reflex hierarchy model, 2b
Reflex sympathetic dystrophy (RSD), 336
Rehabilitation Act, 717–718, 723
Reimbursement, for services, 729
Reiter's syndrome, 544
Relationship development intervention (RDI), for autism spectrum disorder, 416
Reliability
    defined, 71
    interobserver, 71
    of screening test, 70
    test–retest, 71
Renal disease, spinal cord injury and, 342–343
Renal failure, 619
Renting or borrowing equipment, 434
Respiratory distress syndrome (RDS), 126, 129–130 (*see also* Pulmonary and respiratory disorders)
Respiratory failure, 681–682
Respiratory muscle weakness, 699–703
Respiratory rates, 682t
Responsive teaching (RT), for autism spectrum disorder, 416
Retinal detachment, 368
Retinoblastoma, 592
Retinopathy of prematurity (ROP), 137–139, *138*
Rett syndrome, 383t, 384t, 405
Reye syndrome, 383t
Rhabdomyosarcoma, 592, 594t
Rheumatoid arthritis (RA), 543 (*see also* Arthritis)
Rheumatoid factor (RF), 542t, 550
Rheumatology transition checklist, 585
Rib flaring, 668
Rifton Equipment, Inc., 219
Rifton Pacer, 219, *219*
Robotic-assisted locomotion training (RALT), 213–214

Robotic gait training, 213–214
Robotic technologies, 417
Rolling progression, 19t, 41–43, *42, 43*
Rooting reflex, 25t
ROP (*see* Retinopathy of prematurity)
Rotational deformities, 482
Rotational injury, 304
Rotational profile, 466
Rotationplasty, 471, *472,* 596t
Rubella, and cerebral palsy, 188b
Rubs, 685
Rule of Nines, 615
Running, 57, 64t (*see also* Ambulation)

S

Sacral-level paralysis, 280–282
SAFE KIDS Campaign, 613
Salter–Harris classification of fractures, 502, *502, 502b,* 513, 527, 528
Sarcoglycanopathy, 352, 365, 366t
Sarcoma, *591–592,* 594t
Sarnat clinical stages, 153, 154t
Scaphoid fractures, 513
Scapular dysfunction, 507
Scarf sign, 25t, *156*
Scarring
    assessment of, *627, 628*
    from burns, 617–618, *618, 633–634*
    from child abuse, 613
    contraction, 617–618
    hypertrophy, 617–618
Schizencephaly, 188
Schober test, 561, *561*
School-based therapy, for cerebral palsy, 236–237
School Functional Assessment (SFA), 91–93, *92,* 412, 419, 555, 722
School issues, 717–732 (*see also* Education)
    adaptive equipment and, 430–432
    arthritis and, 562, 572
    brain trauma and, 323, 325
    case studies of, 731–732
    checklist for, 583–584
    muscular dystrophy and, 358
    pulmonary and respiratory disorders and, 686
    spinal cord injury and, 341, 348
School Outcomes Measure, 722
School systems, play therapy in, 416–417
Schreiner, Mary B., 379–399
Scobey, Kristin, 589–607
Scleroderma, 541
Scoliosis (*see also* Kyphoscoliosis)
    Down syndrome and, 394
    idiopathic, 494–496, *494, 495*
    muscular dystrophy and, 356, 361
    pulmonary and respiratory disorders with, 700
    spina bifida and, 252, 286
    after spinal cord injury, 332, 342
    surgery for, 496
    torticollis and, 477
Scooter board, 283, 348, 443, *443*
Scooter, motorized, 445, 572
Scottish-Rite orthosis, 488, *488*
Screening tests, 72–74 (*see also* Test(s))
    for scoliosis, 495, *495*
Seat belts, 324, 330, 344
Seat insert, *436*
Seat to backrest angle, 438
Seating equipment, 215–217
    household ambulatory, 216–217
    limited-community ambulatory, 216–217
    marginal ambulatory, 216
    nonambulator, 216

Second impact syndrome (SIS), 535
Secondhand smoke, 18t
Seizures, 154–155
    cerebral palsy and, 189b, 190b
    Chiari II malformation and, 250b
    head trauma and, 306
    intellectual disabilities and, 383t, 384t
Selective dorsal rhizotomy (SDR), 222
Self-care skills, assessment of, 204–205
Sensation, equipment selection and, 429
Sensitivity, 72
Sensorimotor skills, equipment selection
    and, 429
Sensory integration (SI), 212
    for autism spectrum disorder, 415–416
    disorder, 212
Sensory Integration and Praxis Test (SIPT),
    410, 412
Sensory modulation disorders, autism spectrum
    disorder and, 406
Sensory-perceptual impairments, autism
    spectrum disorder and, 406
Sensory responses, evolution of, 117–121
Sequin, Edouard, 380, 391
Service delivery, models of, 726–727
Sever's disease, 528
Sex education, 3
    spinal cord injury and, 343
Shaken baby syndrome, 189b (see also Child
    abuse)
Shelf procedure, 223t
Sherrington reflex model, 115
Shin splints, 524–526
Shoe inserts, 236
Short Sensory Profile, 410
Shoulder(s)
    arthritis of, 556, 557t
    assessment of, 197–198
    muscular dystrophy and, 354, 356t
    skin graft for, 624
    TV, 29
Shunt, ventriculoperitoneal, 254, 254,
    259t, 294
Sickle cell disease, 597
Side-lying, 428
    equipment for, 316, 442
    of preterm infants, 142, 143
SIDS (sudden infant death syndrome), 143, 476
Sign language, 456
Silfverskiold test, 229, 229
Silver sulfadiazine, 622
Simplicity, of screening test, 70
Sinding–Larsen–Johansson disease (SLJ), 524
Single-event multilevel surgery (SEMLS), 223
Single photon emission computed tomography
    (SPECT)
    for spondylolysis, 532
Sitting
    equipment for, 436–439
    progression, 19t, 43–49, 44–50
6-Minute walk test (6MWT), 559–560
Skeletally immature athlete, anatomic and
    physiologic differences of, 501–503
Skin
    assessment of, 599t, 600
    functions of, 613–614
    grafts, for burns, 624–625
    heart disease and, 667
    integrity, spinal cord injury and, 343
    spinal cord injury and, 331
    structures of, 613–614, 614
Skinner, B. F., 20
Skull abnormalities, 117, 143
Skull fracture, 304

Sleeping
    muscular dystrophy and, 364
    neonates and, 122, 122t
    positions for, 18t
Slipped capital femoral epiphysis (SCFE),
    489–490, 489, 518–519
Small Beginnings, Inc., 142
Small for gestational age (SGA), 123
Snapping hip syndrome, 515–516
Social skills, 3
Social/emotional skills, equipment selection
    and, 429
Sodium channel blockers, for pain, 336
Soft tissue releases (STRs), 565
Spasticity, 191–192, 200
    brain trauma and, 312
    functional outcomes for, 206b
    intellectual disabilities and, 384t
    medications for, 221–222, 316, 336
    after spinal cord injury, 332, 336
    surgery for, 222
Spearing, Elena M., 1–13, 329–348
Special Olympics, 214, 650b
Specificity, 72
Speech assessment, 205
Speedy-CAT, 89
Spina bifida, 247–295, 289
    ambulation with, 272–285, 273–275, 275t, 277,
        278t, 279, 281
    case study of, 294–295
    definitions of, 249
    embryology of, 249
    equipment for, 267–268, 449
    etiology of, 247–248
    incidence of, 247–248
    management of, 252–255, 253b, 254, 260–264,
        260b, 263, 264
    muscle testing for, 255b, 255–256, 255
    nutritional concerns with, 253b
    orthoses for, 268–282, 270, 272–275, 279, 281
    physical therapy for, 264–268, 265b, 266
    prenatal testing and diagnosis for, 250–251
    preoperative assessment of, 252–254
    prevention of, 247–248
    prognosis with, 248
    sensory assessment of, 259–260
    surgery for, 252–255, 252, 254, 277
    younger adults with, 292–293
Spina bifida occulta, 249
Spinal cord
    arthritis of, 557t
    assessment of, 197, 561, 561
    cerebral palsy and, 223, 225
    embryogenesis of, 115
    stimulators, 336–337
    tethered, 285–286, 286b
    tumors of, 595
Spinal cord injury, 329–348
    adolescents with, 337, 343
    ambulation after, 339b, 339, 347
    assessment of, 333, 334b
    brain trauma with, 333b, 348
    caregiver education for, 341
    case studies of, 345–348, 348
    discharge planning, 341
    exercises for, 337
    functional expectations after, 334, 335t, 339b
    illness prevention and wellness, 342
    incidence of, 329
    nutritional concerns with, 331b
    outcomes with, 343–344
    pain management for, 336
    patient history for, 330–331
    prevention of, 344, 344b

    research on, 344
    school issues with, 341, 348
    spasticity with, 336
    surgery for, 336
    systems review for, 331–333
    traumatic, 330
    wheelchairs for, 338, 338
Spinal cord injury without radiographic
    abnormality (SCIWORA), 330
Spinal muscular atrophy (SMA), 352, 369–373,
    370, 372
    genetics, 370
    pathophysiology of, 370
    type I, 370–371
    type II, 371–372
    type III, 373
Spine injuries, 531–533
Spirometers, 694
Splints
    for arthrogryposis, 481
    after brain trauma, 321
    for burns, 625, 630–631, 631
    congenital radial deficiency and, 471
    incisional, 690–691, 692
    muscular dystrophy and, 360
    night, 234
    resting, 564
    shin, 524–526
Split-thickness skin graft (STSG), 626, 627
Spondyloarthropathy, 544
Spondylolisthesis, 532, 532b
Spondylolysis, 531–532
Sports injuries, 501–537
    ankle injuries, 526–528
    brain trauma from, 302–303
    elbow injuries, 510–511, 512–513
    female athlete, 536–537
    foot injuries, 528–531
    forearm injuries, 513–514
    hand injuries, 513–514
    hip injuries, 514–519
    history-taking process, 503
    knee injuries, 519–524
    lower leg injuries, 524–526
    pediatric throwing athlete, 508–510
    pelvis injuries, 514–519
    physical examination for, 503–506
    shoulder injuries, 511–512
    spine injuries, 330, 531–533
    thigh injuries, 514–519
    upper extremity functional testing for, 506–514
    wrist injuries, 513–514
Sports-related concussion
    activity progression following, 535b
    assessment of, 534–535
    diagnosis of, 534–535
    management of, 535
    pathophysiology of, 533
    return to play, 535
    risk factors of, 534
    signs and symptoms of, 533–534, 534t
    special considerations for, 535–536
Sportsmetrics™, 520
Spranger's classification, 468
Staheli's rotational profile, 466, 467
Stair climbing, 18t, 19t, 57–58, 57, 58, 64t
Standard error of measurement (SEM), 71
Standard scores, 71
Standardized Assessment of Concussion (SAC), 534
Standers, 217–219
    prone, 440–441
    selection, guide to, 218t
    with sit-to-stand option, 441–442
    supine, 441

Standing
developmental progression of, 49–57, *51–57*, 57t
equipment for, 439–442, *440–441*
muscular dystrophy and, *354*, 356t
prosthetic legs and, 473–474
spina bifida and, *267*
Standing tables, 442
Stanford–Binet Intelligence Scale, 382 (*see also* Intelligence quotient)
Stanford–Binet Intelligence Test (SBIT), 410
Staphylococcus aureus, 707
Status asthmaticus, 704
Stem cells
for leukemia, 597
for spinal cord regeneration, 344
for transplants, 597
Sequenced Transition to Education in the Public Schools (STEPS), 728
Steroids (*see* Corticosteroids)
Stiff knee gait, 203
due to rectus femoris dysfunction, 228
Stimulus–response theory, 20, 22
Stingers, 532–533
Storage disorders, 189b
Strabismus, 592
Strength loss, brain trauma and, 312–313
Strength training, 465–466
arthritis and, 567–569
cerebral palsy and, 238
heart disease and, 670, 673
muscular dystrophy and, 361–362
Stress management, 3–4, 113
brain trauma and, 309
dyspnea and, 696
spina bifida and, 257
Stretching exercises, 567
Stride length, 56–57, 57t, 198, 200, 203, 220, 231, 234, 235
Stride width, 200
Stridor, 684
Chiari II malformation and, 250b
Strollers, 435, 451–452, *452*
Substance abuse, 19 (*see also* Narcotics)
intellectual disabilities and, 383t
pregnancy and, 383t
withdrawal symptoms and, 159
Sucking reflex, 25t
Sudden infant death syndrome (SIDS), 143, 476
Sulfamylon (*see* Mafenide acetate)
Sulfasalazine, 550
Sunset sign, 254, 259t
Superior labrum anterior-to-posterior (SLAP) lesions, 509–510
Supine progression, 18t, 19t, *37–43*, 142
Supine standers, 441, *441*
Supracondylar elbow fractures, 512
Supracondylar osteotomy, 565
Supramalleolar orthosis (SMO), 235
Surface electromyography, 332
Surfactant, 129, 146, 156, 680
Swallowing difficulty, Chiari II malformation and, 250b
Swimming, 215
Synactive theory, 109–110, *110*
Synchronized intermittent mandatory ventilation (SIMV), 127
Synovectomy, 565
Synovium, *547*
Syphilis, 5
Systemic lupus erythematosus (SLE), 541
Systems review, 651–652
for spinal cord injury, 331–333
Systems theory (*see* Dynamic systems theory)

T
Tablet computers, 457
Tactile system, 118–120, 386–387
Taking Responsibility for Adolescent/Adult Care (TRAC), 586
Talipes equinovarus, 277, 478
spina bifida and, 276–277
Taping, therapeutic, 277
Tappit-Emas, Elena, 247–295
Tarsal coalition, 530
Taste, sense of, 120–121
TBI (*see* Traumatic brain injury)
Technology-Related Assistance for Individuals with Disabilities Act, 719t
Tecklin, Jan Stephen, 679–711
Temporomandibular joint (TMJ), 543, 548, 557t
Tendoachilles lengthening (TAL), 229
Tendon
lengthening, 223t
release, 223t
transfer, 223t
Tendonitis, 529
Tenotomy, 223t
for hamstring lengthening, 227
Teratoma, 152
Term infants, physical therapy assessment and intervention for, 159–160
Test(s)
criterion-referenced, 71
developmental, 69–97
purposes of, 69, 70
reporting of, 96, 96b
screening, 72–74
selection guidelines, 70
standardized, 71
validity of, 71
Test of Gross Motor Development, 722
Test of Infant Motor Performance (TIMP), 73, 74–75, 145t
Test of Visual-Motor Skills, Revised (TVMS-R), 82
Test–retest reliability, 71
Tetralogy of Fallot (TOF), 658t, 662, *662*
Thelen, Esther, 49
Therapeutic handling, 212
Thessaly test, 522
Thigh–foot angle, 466, *467*
Thomas test, 198, 359
Thoracic deformities, 668–669, 684
Thoracic-level paralysis, 270–271
orthotics for, 271–276
Thoracic movement, assessment of, 197
Thoracolumbar sacral orthosis (TLSO), 346–348, 495, *496*, 532
Three-dimensional gait analysis, 282
Threshold electrical stimulation (TES), 214
Thyroid disease, 189b, 595t
Tibia vara, 490–491, *490*
Tibial stress fracture, 525
Tibial torsion, 198–199, 228
Tibialis anterior strengthening, 201
Tillaux fractures, 528
Tilting reaction, 58–59, *59*
Tizanidine, for spasticity, 221
Tobacco smoke, 18t
Toddlers without physical impairments, 453–454
Toileting, 454
"Tommy John" surgery, 511
Tongue fasciculations, Chiari II malformation and, 250b
Tonsillectomy, 10
Torticollis, 144, 475–476, *475*
head and neck features of, 475t
orthoses for, *475*, 476–477
surgery for, 477

Total Contact Scanner, 634
Total hip arthroplasty (THA), 565
Total joint arthroplasty (TJA), 565
Total knee arthroplasty (TKA), 566
Total Motor Quotient (TMQ), 79
Total parenteral nutrition (TPN), 190b
Total rotational motion (TRM), 507
Toxic epidermal necrolysis (TEN), 623
Toxoplasmosis, and cerebral palsy, 188b
Tracheal esophageal fistula (TEF), 151, *152*
Tracheal tickle maneuver, 690, *692*
Tracheoesophageal fistula, 680
Transdisciplinary model, 719
Transfer of learning, 389–390
Transfusions
cerebral palsy and, 190b
complications from, 131
twin-to-twin, 152
Transition planning, 728
Transition Planning Inventory-2, 725
Transition to home, 160–162
Translational injury, 304
Transmalleolar axis, 466, *467*
Transplantation
bone marrow, 596–597
heart, 357, 663–664, 667, 668
lung, 707
peripheral stem cell, 596–597
Transporting children with disabilities, 450–451
Transposition of the great arteries (TGA), 662–663, *662*
Trauma (*see specific types, e.g.,* Sports injuries)
Traumatic brain injury (TBI) (*see also* Brain)
assessment of, 309–314, 310b, 311b
case study of, 324–325
causes of, 302–303
classification of, 301–302, 302t
definition of, 301–302
diagnosis of, 314–315
environmental influences on, 309
evaluation of, 314
functional abilities and, 309
incidence of, 302
management of, 315–323, *316–317, 319–323*
mechanisms of, 303–304
mild, 533
nutritional concerns with, 303b
outcomes for, 306–309, 307t, 308b, 309b
patient history for, 309–310, 310b
plan of care, 315
predictors of, 306–309
prevention of, 323–324
prognosis of, 314–315
school issues with, 323, 325
spinal cord trauma with, 333b, 348
types of, 304–305
Traumatic hip dislocation, 518
Traumatic injuries, 529–530
Traumatic shoulder dislocation, 511–512
Treadmill training, 213–214
Treatment and Education of Autistic and related Communication-handicapped Children (TEACCH), for autism spectrum disorder, 414, 416
Tricuspid atresia, 658t
Tricycles, 450
Triplane fractures, 528
Trisomy 13, 150
Trisomy 15, 150
Trisomy 16, 150
Trisomy 18, 150
Trisomy 21, 150 (*see also* Down syndrome)

Truncus arteriosus, 658t
Tubular orthosis for torticollis (TOT), 477
Tumbling, 215
Turf toe, 531
Turner syndrome, 383t
Tuskegee Syphilis Research Experiment, 5
Twin-to-twin transfusion syndrome
    (TTTS), 152

U

Ulnar collateral ligament (UCL) injury, 510–511
Umbilical lines, 126t, 142
Uniform Data System for Medical Rehabilitation
    (UDS), 89
Universal design, 457
Upper extremity weakness, Chiari II
    malformation and, 250b
Urinary tract infection (UTI), 293
Urologic care, spina bifida and, 260b, 289, 293,
    342–343
U.S. Collaborative Perinatal Project, 188
Uveitis, 550

V

Valgus stress test, for medial collateral ligament
    injuries, 521
Validity, 71
    concurrent, 71
    content, 71
    criterion-related, 71
    predictive, 71
    of screening test, 70
Valium (see Diazepam)
Valproic acid, 248
Vancouver Scar Scale (VSS), 627, 628
Varus deformity, 230

VAS$_{CHAQ-38}$, 554, 555b
Vegetative state, 318
Ventilators, 125–129, 125t, 127, 128
    for BPD, 146–147
    for heart disease, 667
    for muscular dystrophy, 363
    respiratory muscle weakness from, 699
    strollers with, 451, 453
Ventricular septal defects (VSD), 658t, 660, 661
Ventriculoperitoneal shunt, 254, 254, 259t, 294, 595
Versaw-Barnes, Diane, 103–166
Vestibular system, 120, 386, 387
Vincristine, 594, 594t, 600
Vineland Adaptive Behavior Scale (VABS), 382, 412
Vision
    assessment of, 385
    development of, 121
    impairment of, 313
Visual analog scale, 332
Visual impairment, autism spectrum disorder
    and, 406–407
Visual system, 121
Visuospatial skills, brain injury and, 313
Vital signs, 672t
Vocal cord paralysis, Chiari II malformation and, 250b
Volpe, J. J., 135

W

"W" sitting, 262
Wagner procedure, 492
Waist circumference measurements, 645, 648
Walkers, 219–220, 450, 453, 454
Walker–Warburg syndrome, 369
Walking, 64t (see also Ambulation)
    assessment of, 199–204
    "bear," 36, 36
Wartenberg pendulum test, 332

Wechsler Intelligence Scale for children (WISC),
    382, 410
WeeFIM (see Functional Independence Measure
    for Children)
Werdnig–Hoffmann disease, 370–371
Wheelchair, 443–450, 443, 447
    for arthritis, 572
    for muscular dystrophy, 362–363
    ordering of, 444b
    positioning in, 316, 317
    for spina bifida, 275, 289–290, 290, 449
    for spinal cord injury, 338, 338
    standing devices, integrated, 442
Wheezes, 685, 701, 705, 707
Whole body vibration (WBV) systems, 485
Wii boards, 417
Williams syndrome, 384t
Wilms tumor, 592–593, 594t
Withdrawal syndromes, 159 (see also Substance
    abuse)
Wood, Audrey, 103–166
World Health Organization (WHO)
    cancer grading of, 593
    ICF of, 109, 468, 541, 552t, 598
Wound healing, 596, 596t
    dressings for, 622, 623, 629–630
    hydrotherapy for, 621–622
    topical agents for, 622–623
Wrist, arthritis of, 557t

X

Xenografts, 624

Y

Yoga, 215, 342
    for autism spectrum disorder, 417